# Lecture Notes in Computer Science 7724

Commenced Publication in 1973
Founding and Former Series Editors:
Gerhard Goos, Juris Hartmanis, and Jan van Leeuwen

## Editorial Board

David Hutchison
*Lancaster University, UK*

Takeo Kanade
*Carnegie Mellon University, Pittsburgh, PA, USA*

Josef Kittler
*University of Surrey, Guildford, UK*

Jon M. Kleinberg
*Cornell University, Ithaca, NY, USA*

Alfred Kobsa
*University of California, Irvine, CA, USA*

Friedemann Mattern
*ETH Zurich, Switzerland*

John C. Mitchell
*Stanford University, CA, USA*

Moni Naor
*Weizmann Institute of Science, Rehovot, Israel*

Oscar Nierstrasz
*University of Bern, Switzerland*

C. Pandu Rangan
*Indian Institute of Technology, Madras, India*

Bernhard Steffen
*TU Dortmund University, Germany*

Madhu Sudan
*Microsoft Research, Cambridge, MA, USA*

Demetri Terzopoulos
*University of California, Los Angeles, CA, USA*

Doug Tygar
*University of California, Berkeley, CA, USA*

Gerhard Weikum
*Max Planck Institute for Informatics, Saarbruecken, Germany*

Lecture Notes in Computer Science 7924

Kyoung Mu Lee   Yasuyuki Matsushita
James M. Rehg   Zhanyi Hu (Eds.)

# Computer Vision – ACCV 2012

11th Asian Conference on Computer Vision
Daejeon, Korea, November 5-9, 2012
Revised Selected Papers, Part I

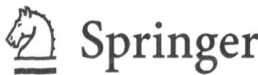 Springer

Volume Editors

Kyoung Mu Lee
Seoul National University
Department of Electrical and Computer Engineering
1 Gwanak-ro, Gwanak-gu, 151-744 Seoul, Korea
E-mail: kyoungmu@snu.ac.kr

Yasuyuki Matsushita
Microsoft Research Asia
No. 5, Danling st., Haidian District, 100080 Beijing, P.R. China
E-mail: yasumat@microsoft.com

James M. Rehg
Georgia Institute of Technology
School of Interactive Computing
801 Atlantic Drive, CCB 315, Atlanta, GA 30332, USA
E-mail: rehg@gatech.edu

Zhanyi Hu
Chinese Academy of Sciences
Institute of Automation
National Laboratory of Pattern Recognition
Zhong Quan Cun East Road 95, Haidian District, 100190 Beijing, P.R. China
E-mail: huzy@nlpr.ia.ac.cn

ISSN 0302-9743                e-ISSN 1611-3349
ISBN 978-3-642-37330-5      e-ISBN 978-3-642-37331-2
DOI 10.1007/978-3-642-37331-2
Springer Heidelberg Dordrecht London New York

Library of Congress Control Number: 2013934230

CR Subject Classification (1998): I.4.1-10, I.5.1-4, I.2.10, I.2.6, I.3.5, H.3.4, H.2.8, F.2.2

LNCS Sublibrary: SL 6 – Image Processing, Computer Vision, Pattern Recognition, and Graphics

© Springer-Verlag Berlin Heidelberg 2013
This work is subject to copyright. All rights are reserved, whether the whole or part of the material is concerned, specifically the rights of translation, reprinting, re-use of illustrations, recitation, broadcasting, reproduction on microfilms or in any other way, and storage in data banks. Duplication of this publication or parts thereof is permitted only under the provisions of the German Copyright Law of September 9, 1965, in ist current version, and permission for use must always be obtained from Springer. Violations are liable to prosecution under the German Copyright Law.
The use of general descriptive names, registered names, trademarks, etc. in this publication does not imply, even in the absence of a specific statement, that such names are exempt from the relevant protective laws and regulations and therefore free for general use.

*Typesetting:* Camera-ready by author, data conversion by Scientific Publishing Services, Chennai, India

Printed on acid-free paper

Springer is part of Springer Science+Business Media (www.springer.com)

# Preface

The 11th Asian Conference on Computer Vision (ACCV 2012) took place in South Korea in the city of Daejeon, a well-known center of research and high-tech industry. Following the tradition of previous meetings, ACCV 2012 had a number of events co-located with the main conference, including nine workshops, two tutorial sessions, 12 on-site demos featuring a wide range of advanced vision technology, and a special competition on RGB-D camera applications. In addition, there were three keynote speakers: Tomaso Poggio (Invariant Recognition in the Visual Cortex), Du Sik Park (The Color and Image Processing Technology for CE Device: Current and Future), and Andrew Fitzgibbon (3D Vision in a Changing World).

The ACCV Steering Committee, consisting of Katsushi Ikeuchi, Yasushi Yagi, and Tieniu Tan, provided guidance throughout the organizational process and we are grateful for their support. We were fortunate to be able to work closely with the General Chairs, In So Kweon, Chilwoo Lee, and Akihiro Sugimoto, who arranged the financing and logistics. Thanks to their efforts we were able to secure the Daejeon Convention Center as an excellent venue for our meeting. Special thanks go to our Publication Chairs In Kyu Park and Tae-Wuk Bae, for handling the daunting task of assembling the conference proceedings and meeting the publication deadlines.

Additional support for ACCV 2012 was provided by our 13 sponsors, who contributed at four levels: Platinum (Daejeon Metropolitan City, Daejeon International Marketing Enterprise, Daejeon Convention Center, Korea Tourism Organization, DigiCar Center, Mobile Device Interface Research Center, and Seoul National University), Gold (Samsung AIT and Puloon Technology), Silver (Mando Corporation, Qualcomm, and 4D View Solutions), and Bronze (NVIDIA Corporation).

In order to support an on-line review process, we utilized Microsoft's CMT system, with special thanks to Yasuyuki Matsushita for managing the CMT process. Continuing the trend of increasing submissions to ACCV, we received 869 submissions by the deadline of July 1, 2012. This represents an 18% increase in submissions over 2010. We received submissions from 43 countries, with Asia (63%), Europe (23%), and North America (12%) making up the bulk of the submissions by region. Submitted papers that did not conform to the submission criteria regarding author anonymity, formatting, and length, were desk rejected and removed from consideration.

The four Program Co-chairs assembled a group of 33 leading vision researchers to serve as Area Chairs (ACs) and conduct the review process. These Chairs managed a group of 479 reviewers, who provided expert assessment of the submitted papers. Each paper received a minimum of three reviews, as well as a consolidation report from the responsible AC, which detailed the outcome of the decision process. Review decisions were finalized at the AC meeting, which was held at Seoul National University during September 17–18, 2012. Special thanks to Kyoung Mu Lee for handling the arrangements for this meeting. ACs were organized into triples, so that papers with varying review scores could be discussed by multiple ACs. The triples in turn were organized into four panels, which finalized all of the paper decisions. The AC panels were instructed to use their best judgement in determining which papers to accept. While review scores were an input to the decision process, these scores alone did not determine the outcome. The Program Chairs strictly followed the recommendations of the panels with regard to acceptance. We asked for clarification where it was needed, and requested detailed and clear consolidation reports. Each consolidation report was checked by at least one Program Chair.

We wish to acknowledge the invaluable help of a number of people in making this conference possible. The logistical talents of the Organizing Committee made it possible to conduct a well-run meeting with a diverse set of activities. We extend our thanks to everyone who was involved in the submission and review process: the ACs, reviewers, and authors. Without your dedication and hard work there would be no meeting. We look forward to the continuing evolution of ACCV as one of the top conferences in the field.

November 2012

Kyoung Mu Lee
Yasuyuki Matsushita
James M. Rehg
Zhanyi Hu

# Organization

## Steering Committee

Katsushi Ikeuchi      The University of Tokyo, Japan
Yasushi Yagi      Osaka University, Japan
Tieniu Tan      The National Laboratory of Pattern
     Recognition, China

## General Chairs

In So Kweon      KAIST, Korea
Chilwoo Lee      Chonnam National University, Korea
Akihiro Sugimoto      National Institute of Informatics, Japan

## Program Chairs

Kyoung Mu Lee      Seoul National University, Korea
Yasuyuki Matsushita      Microsoft Research Asia, China
Jim Rehg      Georgia Institute of Technology, USA
Zhanyi Hu      Chinese Academy of Science, China

## Workshop Chairs

Jongil Park      Hanyang University, Korea
Junmo Kim      KAIST, Korea
Hideo Saito      Keio University, Japan
Yanxi Liu      The Pennsylvania State University, USA
Ming-Hsuan Yang      University of California at Merced, USA

## Finance Chair

Kiryong Kwon      Bukyung National University, Korea

## Publication Chairs

In Kyu Park      Inha University, Korea
Tae-Wuk Bae      Stanford University, USA

## Publicity Chairs

Chang-Su Kim                Korea University, Korea
Burkhard Wunsche            University of Auckland, New Zealand
Takeshi Oishi               The University of Tokyo, Japan
Robert Fisher               University of Edinburgh, UK

## Web Chair

Kanghyun Jo                 University of Ulsan, Korea

## Demo Chairs

Il dong Yun                 Hankuk University of Foreign Studies, Korea
Yongduek Seo                Sogang University, Korea
Hajime Nagahara             Kyushu University, Japan
Tat Jen Cham                Nanyang Technological University, Singapore

## Tutorial Chairs

Chang Dong Yoo              KAIST, Korea
Yoshinori Kuno              Saitama University, Japan
Michael S. Brown            National University of Singapore, Singapore

## Local Chairs

Kuk-Jin Yoon                GIST, Korea
Jongwoo Lim                 Hanyang University, Korea
Ju Yong Chang               ETRI, Korea

## Special Session Chair

Yu-Wing Tai                 KAIST, Korea

## Industrial Chair

Chang Yeong Kim             Samsung Advanced Institute of Technology,
                            Korea

## Area Chairs

Serge Belongie             University of California, San Diego, USA
Michael Brown              National University of Singapore, Singapore
Nam Ik Cho                 Seoul National University, Korea
Robert Collins             The Pennsylvania State University, USA

| | |
|---|---|
| Larry Davis | University of Maryland, USA |
| Kristen Grauman | University of Texas at Austin, USA |
| Abhinav Gupta | Carnegie Mellon University, USA |
| Bohyung Han | POSTECH, Korea |
| Richard Hartley | Australian National University, Australia |
| Jiaya Jia | Chinese University of Hong Kong, Hong Kong |
| Neel Joshi | Microsoft Research, USA |
| Koichi Kise | Osaka Prefecture University, Japan |
| Nikos Komodakis | University of Crete, Greece |
| Sang Wook Lee | Sogang University, Korea |
| Ales Leonardis | University of Ljubljana, Slovenia |
| Vincent Lepetit | EPFL, Switzerland |
| Yasuhiro Mukaigawa | Osaka University, Japan |
| Nikos Paragios | Ecole Centrale de Paris, France |
| Shmuel Peleg | The Hebrew University of Jerusalem, Israel |
| Hideo Saito | Keio University, Japan |
| Imari Sato | National Institute of Informatics, Japan |
| Shin'ichi Satoh | National Institute of Informatics, Japan |
| Shiguang Shan | Chinese Academy of Sciences, China |
| Jianbo Shi | University of Pennsylvania, USA |
| Cristian Sminchisescu | Universität Bonn, Germany |
| Chi-Keung Tang | HKUST, Hong Kong |
| Marshall Tappen | University of Central Florida, USA |
| Fernando de la Torre | Carnegie Mellon University, USA |
| Kenneth K.-Y.Wong | Hong Kong University, Hong Kong |
| Jianxin Wu | Nanyang Technological University, Singapore |
| Shuicheng Yan | National University of Singapore, Singapore |
| Ming-Hsuan Yang | University of California, Merced, USA |
| Ruigang Yang | University of Kentucky, USA |

## Program Committee Members

| | |
|---|---|
| Austin D. Abrams | Atsuhiko Banno |
| Catherine Achard | Yufang Bao |
| Emre Akbas | Adrian Barbu |
| Karteek Alahari | Nick Barnes |
| Mitsuru Ambai | John Barron |
| Bjoern Andres | Abdessamad Ben Hamza |
| Gaston R. Araguas | Chiraz BenAbdelkader |
| Nafiz Arica | Moshe Ben-Ezra |
| Yasuo Ariki | AndrewTeoh Beng-Jin |
| Chetan Arora | Achraf Ben-Hamadou |
| Abdullah Arslan | Benjamin Berkels |
| Xiang Bai | Horst Bischof |
| Vineeth Balasubramanian | Prabir Biswas |

Soma Biswas
Matthew Blaschko
Konstantinos Blekas
Adrian Bors
Michael Boshra
Nizar Bouguila
Edmond Boyer
Steve Branson
Michael M. Bronstein
Andres Bruhn
Asad A. Butt
Ricardo S. Cabral
David W. Cai
Jinhai Cai
Francesco Camastra
Xiaochun Cao
Xun Cao
Barbara Caputo
Joao Carreira
Yaron Caspi
Umberto Castellani
Turgay Celik
Kap Luk Chan
Kwok-Ping Chan
Sharat Chandran
Hong Chang
Vincent Charvillat
Rama Chellappa
Bing-Yu Chen
Chu-Song Chen
Haifeng Chen
Hwann-Tzong Chen
Jie Chen
Jiun-Hung Chen
Ling Chen
Qiang Chen
Terrence Chen
Tsuhan Chen
Xiangyu Chen
Xiaowu Chen
Hong Cheng
MingMing Cheng
Shyi-Chyi Cheng
Yuan Cheng
Liang-Tien Chia

Shao-Yi Chien
Tat-Jun Chin
Minsu Cho
Wen-Sheng Chu
Yung-Yu Chuang
Albert CS Chung
Pan Chunhong
Arridhana Ciptadi
Javier Civera
Carlo Colombo
Jason Corso
Marco Cristani
Beleznai Csaba
Jinshi Cui
Jeremiah D. Deng
Qieyun Dai
Kostas Daniilidis
Petros Daras
Francois de Sorbier
Fatih Demirci
Joachim Denzler
Anthony Dick
Santosh Divvala
Csaba Domokos
Qiulei Dong
Test Dong
Michael Donoser
Gianfranco Doretto
Bruce Draper
Fuqing Duan
Zoran Duric
Ulrich Eckhardt
Michael Eckmann
Wolfgang Einhauser
Hazim Ekenel
Francisco Escolano
Jialue Fan
Wen-Pinn Fang
Micha Feigin
Jianjiang Feng
Jiashi Feng
Francesc J. Ferri
Pierre Fite Georgel
Katerina Fragkiadaki
Juan Francisco Giro Martín

Chi-Wing Fu
Chiou-Shann Fuh
Hironobu Fujiyoshi
Giorgio Fumera
Ryo Furukawa
Juergen Gall
Li Gang
Jun Hong Gao
Yongsheng Gao
Weina Ge
Andreas Geiger
Arkadiusz Gertych
Bernard Ghanem
Guy Godin
Roland Goecke
Bastian Goldluecke
Yunchao Gong
Bogdan T. Goras
Stephen Gould
Hayit Greenspan
Irene Gu
Josechu Guerrero
Richard Guest
Guodong Guo
Yanwen Guo
Yaniv Gur
Vu Hai
Lin Hai-Ting
Kiana Hajebi
Peter Hall
Onur Hamsici
Hu Han
Mei Han
Tony Han
Allan Hanbury
Zhou Hao
Kenji Hara
Tatsuya Harada
Osman Hassab Elgawi
Jean-Bernard Hayet
Junfeng He
Ran He
Joon Hee Han
Shinsaku Hiura
Jeffrey Ho

Yo-Sung Ho
Christopher Hollitt
Hyunki Hong
Ki Sang Hong
Kazuhiro Hotta
Seiji Hotta
Edward Hsiao
Winston Hsu
Gang Hua
Chunsheng Hua
Chun-Rong Huang
Dong Huang
Fay Huang
Jonathan Huang
Kaiqi Huang
Peter Huang
Xinyu Huang
Benoit Huet
Yi-Ping Hung
Mohamed Hussein
Cong Phuoc Huynh
Sung Ju Hwang
Naoyuki Ichimura
Ichiro Ide
Yoshihisa Ijiri
Sei Ikeda
Nazli Ikizler-Cinbis
Atsushi Imiya
Kohei Inoue
Catalin Ionescu
Rui Ishiyama
Yoshio Iwai
Nathan Jacobs
Arpit Jain
Yangqing Jia
Yunde Jia
Shuqiang Jiang
Xiaoyi Jiang
Yu-Gang Jiang
Nianjuan Jiang
Yushi Jing
Kang-Hyun Jo
Matjaz Jogan
Manjunath V. Joshi
Frederic Jurie

Shingo Kagami
Zdenek Kalal
Amit Kale
George Kamberov
Kenichi Kanatani
Atul Kanaujia
Henry Kang
Sing Bing Kang
Mohan Kankanhalli
Abou-Moustafa Karim
Zoltan Kato
Harish Katti
Rei Kawakami
Hiroshi Kawasaki
Mark Keck
Sang Keun Lee
Saad-Masood Khan
Aditya Khosla
Hansung Kim
Kyungnam Kim
Sungwoong Kim
TaeHoon Kim
Tae-Kyun Kim
Benjamin Kimia
Ron Kimmel
Yasuyo Kita
Itaru Kitahara
Kris Kitani
Reinhard Klette
Georges Koepfler
Mario Koeppen
Kevin Koeser
Effrosyni Kokiopoulou
Iasonas Kokkinos
Alexander Kolesnikov
Sotiris B. Kotsiantis
Junghyun Kown
Norbert Kruger
Arjan Kuijper
Kashino Kunio
Yoshinori Kuno
Cheng-Hao Kuo
Suha Kwak
Bogdan Kwolek
Junseok Kwon

Ľubor Ladický
Alexander Ladikos
Shang-Hong Lai
Antony Lam
Zhiqiang Lao
Longin Jan Latecki
Francois Lauze
Duy-Dinh Le
Chan-Su Lee
Guee Sang Lee
Jae-Ho Lee
Seungyong Lee
Taehee Lee
Christian Leistner
Bocchi Leonardo
Marius Leordeanu
Matt Leotta
Wee-Kheng Leow
Bruno Lepri
Frederic Lerasle
Thomas Leung
Annan Li
Fuxin Li
Hongdong Li
Jia Li
Li-Jia Li
Rui Li
Yongmin Li
Yufeng Li
Chia-Kai Liang
Shu Liao
T. Warren Liao
Wen-Nung Lie
Jenn-Jier J. Lien
Jongwoo Lim
Joo-Hwee Lim
Joseph J. Lim
Ser-Nam Lim
Hai Ting Lin
Huei-Yung Lin
Weiyao Lin
Wen-Chieh(Steve) Lin
Zhouchen Lin
Haibin Ling
Baoyuan Liu

Cheng-Lin Liu
Hairong Liu
Jingchen Liu
Ligang Liu
Miaomiao Liu
Qingzhong Liu
Si Liu
Tianming Liu
Tyng-Luh Liu
Xiaobai Liu
Xiaoming Liu
Marco Loog
Huchuan Lu
Juwei Lu
Le Lu
Tong Lu
Ludovic Macaire
Anant Madabhushi
Subhransu Maji
Atsuto Maki
Yasushi Makihara
Koji Makita
Yoshitsugu Manabe
Rok Mandeljc
Al Mansur
Gian-Luca Marcialis
Tim Marks
Stephen Marsland
Jean Martinet
Aleix Martinez
Syed Zain Masood
Takeshi Masuda
Thomas Mauthner
Stephen J. Maybank
Kenton McHenry
Stephen McNeill
Gerard Medioni
Ramin Mehran
Domingo Mery
David Michael
Gregor Miller
Washington Mio
Ikuhisa Mitsugami
Anurag Mittal
Daisuke Miyazaki

Yoshihiko Mochizuki
Pascal Monasse
Vlad I. Morariu
Greg Mori
Bryan Morse
Yadong Mu
Jayanta Mukhopadhyay
Henning Müller
Hajime Nagahara
Shin-ichi Nakajima
Atsushi Nakazawa
Woonhyun Nam
Loris Nanni
Ram Nevatia
Shawn Newsam
Tian-Tsong Ng
Jifeng Ning
Masashi Nishiyama
Mark Nixon
Shohei Nobuhara
Vincent Nozick
Tom O'Donnell
Chi-Min Oh
Takeshi Oishi
Takahiro Okabe
Takayuki Okatani
Gustavo Olague
Maks Ovsjanikov
Yuji Oyamada
Paul Sakrapee Paisitkriangkrai
Kalman Palagyi
Gang Pan
Hailang Pan
Sharath Pankanti
In Kyu Park
Jong-Il Park
Ioannis Patras
Vladimir Pavlovic
Helio Pedrini
Pieter Peers
Yigang Peng
David W. Penman
Amitha Perera
Alessandro Perina
Janez Pers

Wong Ya Ping
Robert Pless
Thomas Pock
Dipti Prasad Mukherjee
Andrea Prati
Yael Pritch
Oriol Pujol Pujol
Amal Punchihewa
Zhen Qian
Xueyin Qin
Bogdan Raducanu
Luis Rafael Canali
Visvanathan Ramesh
Ananth Ranganathan
Nalini Ratha
Nilanjan Ray
EdelGarcia Reyes
Christian Riess
Tammy Riklin Raviv
Tron Roberto
Antonio Robles-Kelly
Mikel Rodriguez
Bodo Rosenhahn
Guy Rosman
Arun Ross
Peter Roth
Amit Roy Chowdhury
Xiang Ruan
Raif Rustamov
Fereshteh Sadeghi
Satoshi Saga
Ryusuke Sagawa
Fumihiko Sakaue
Mathieu Salzmann
Jorge A. Sanchez
Nong Sang
Angel Sappa
Michel Sarkis
Jun Sato
Tomokazu Sato
Walter Scheirer
Bernt Schiele
Frank Schmidt
Dirk Schnieders
William Schwartz

Stan Sclaroff
McCloskey Scott
Shuji Senda
Vinay Sharma
Chunhua Shen
Li Shen
Shuhan Shen
Qinfeng J. Shi
Hakjoon Shim
Nobutaka Shimada
Ikuko Shimizu
Ilan Shimshoni
Koichi Shinoda
Takaaki Shiratori
Abhinav Shrivastava
Leonid Sigal
Terence Sim
Sudipta Sinha
Danijel Skocaj
Eric Sommerlade
Jeany Son
Andy Song
Li Song
Zheng Song
Aristeidis Sotiras
Richard Souvenir
Jacopo Staiano
Chris Stauffer
Gideon Stein
Evgeny Strekalovskiy
Yu Su
Ramanathan Subramanian
Yusuke Sugano
Yasushi Sumi
Fengmei Sun
Jian Sun
Ju Sun
Min Sun
Weidong Sun
Xiaolu Sun
Yajie Sun
Jinli Suo
Rahul Swaminathan
Yu-Wing Tai
Taketomi Takafumi

Jun Takamatsu
Hugues Talbot
Toru Tamaki
Robby Tan
Tieniu Tan
Xiaoyang Tan
Masayuki Tanaka
Jinhui Tang
Jinshan Tang
Ming Tang
Rinichiro Taniguchi
João Manuel R. S. Tavares
Mutsuhiro Terauchi
Taipeng Tian
Joseph Tighe
Yu Ting
Reichl Tobias
Eno Toeppe
Matt Toews
Shoji Tominaga
Akihiko Torii
Bill Triggs
Werner Trobin
Ngo Thanh Trung
Yanghai Tsin
Pavan Turaga
Matt Turek
Matthew Turk
Seiichi Uchida
Hideaki Uchiyama
Toshio Ueshiba
Norimichi Ukita
Roberto Valenti
Michel F. Valstar
Pascal Vasseur
Changhu Wang
Chen Wang
Cheng Wang
Hanzi Wang
Hongcheng Wang
Liang Wang
Lu Wang
Min Wang
Ruiping Wang
Shiaokai Wang

Song Wang
Xianwang Wang
Xiaogang Wang
Yang Wang
Yu-Chiang Frank Wang
Yunhong Wang
Chaohui Wang
Li-Yi Wei
Yichen Wei
Chee Sun Won
Young W. Woo
John Wright
Tai Pang Wu
Xiaomeng Wu
Yi Wu
Peter Wurtz
Jianxiong Xiao
Jing Xiao
Yang Xiao
Xuehan Xiong
Changsheng Xu
Dong Xu
Li Xu
Ning Xu
Yong Xu
Jianru Xue
Yasushi Yagi
Osamu Yamaguchi
Pingkun Yan
Keiji Yanai
Fei Yang
Hao Yang
Herbert Yang
Jie Yang
Meng Yang
Ming Yang
Peng Yang
Yongliang Yang
Bangpeng Yao
Jong Chul Ye
Sai Kit Yeung
Alper Yilmaz
Zhaozheng Yin
Xianghua Ying
Kuk-Jin Yoon

Lap Fai Yu
Tianli Yu
Baozong Yuan
Junsong Yuan
Lu Yuan
Xenophon Zabulis
John Zelek
Gang Zeng
Zheng-Jun Zha

Cha Zhang
Changshui Zhang
Guofeng Zhang
Hong Hui Zhang
Hongbin Zhang
Hui Zhang
Lei Zhang
Li Zhang

Liqing Zhang
Xiaoqin Zhang
Yu Zhang
Xiao-Wei Zhao
Lu Zheng
Weishi Zheng
Wenming Zheng
Zhonglong Zheng
Baojiang Zhong
Feng Zhou
Zhi-Hua Zhou
Cai-Zhi Zhu
Feng Zhu
Jiejie Zhu
Zhigang Zhu
Ning Zhu
Danping Zou

# External Reviewers

Farnaz Abtahi
Yasuhiro Akagi
Rushil Anirudh
Hirooki Aoki
Indriyati Atmosukarto
Qinxun Bai
Somdutta Banerjee
Yosuke Bando
Loris Bazzani
J. Bermudez
Fatih Cakir
Kevin Cannons
Che-Han Chang
Ding-Jie Chen
Hsin-Yi Chen
James Chen
Xida Chen
Hong Cheng
Shinko Cheng
Hung-Kuo Chu
Ahmed Sheikh Deeb
Idit Diamant
Liana Diesendruck

Xiaoyu Ding
Yuanyuan Ding
Carl Doersch
Keisuke Doman
Ralf Dragon
Marco Fornoni
David Fouhey
Nathan Frey
Hua Gao
Jizhou Gao
Yuli Gao
Haokun Geng
Fabian Gigengack
Arjan Gijsberts
Hitoshi Habe
Ralf Haeusler
Hossein Hajimirsadeghi
Patrick Harding
Kun He
Ariane Herbulot
Simon Hermann
Jacob Hinkle
Shang-Hong Lai

Tzu-Wei Huang
Tomoya Ishikawa
Hiroyuki Iwama
Yoshihiro Kanamori
Swarna Kamlam
Phil Kang
Wai L. Khoo
Kazuaki Kondo
Hiroshi Koyasu
Ilja Kuzborskij
Po-Lun Lai
Tian Lan
Ken-Yi Lee
Tung-Ying Lee
Daniel Leung
Yi Li
Yang Liu
Shugao Ma
Rouzbeh Maani
Rok Mandeljc
Samuele Martelli
Lucas Marti
Alhayat Ali Mekonnen
Chhaya Methani
Ikuhisa Mitsugami
Oliver Müller
T. Nathan Mundhenk
Daigo Muramatsu
Amit Padhy
Samunda Parera
Liliana Lo Presti
Ajita Rattani
Mahdi Rezaei
Samuel Rivera
Mike Roberts

Guy Rosman
Mohammad Rouhani
Muhammad Rushdi
Christian Schmaltz
Nataliya Shapovalova
Bin Shen
Farzad Siyahjani
Marcos Slomp
Tomokazu Takahashi
Danhang Tang
Hao Tang
Junli Tao
Tatiana Tommasi
Arash Vahdat
Jinjun Wang
Jun Wang
Junqiu Wang
Qing Wang
Tsaipei Wang
Yu-Shuen Wang
ZhengXiang Wang
Donglai Wei
Jie Wei
Chenyu Wu
Herb Yang
Yi Yang
Thibault Yohan
Jianming Zhang
Tianzhu Zhang
Wei Zhang
Ji Zhao
Bineng Zhong
Shengqi Zhu
Gali Zimmerman

## ACCV 2012 Best Paper Award Committee

Sing Bing Kang        MicroSoft Research, USA
Ian Reid              University of Oxford, UK
Long Quan             HKUST, Hong Kong

## ACCV 2012 Best Paper (The Saburo Tsuji Award)

Detecting Partially Occluded Objects with an Implicit Shape Model Random
Field
Paul Wohlhart, Michael Donoser, Peter Roth, and Horst Bischof

## ACCV 2012 Best Student Paper
## (The Sang Uk Lee Award)

Discriminative Dictionary Learning with Pairwise Constraints
Huimin Guo, Zhuolin Jiang, and Larry Davis

## ACCV 2012 Best Application Paper
## (The Songde Ma Award)

Large-Scale Bundle Adjustment by Parameter Vector Partition
Shanmin Pang, Jianrue Xue, Le Wang, and Nanning Zheng

## ACCV 2012 Best Paper Honorable Mention

Rapid Uncertainty Computation with Gaussian Processes and Histogram
Intersection Kernels
Alexander Freytag, Erik Rodner, Paul Bodesheim, and Joachim Denzler

## ACCV 2012 Best Student Paper Honorable Mention

Robust Visual Tracking Using Dynamic Classifier Selection with Sparse
Representation of Label Noise
Yuefeng Chen and Qing Wang

## ACCV 2012 Best Application Paper Honorable Mention

Efficient Learning of Linear Predictors Using Dimensionality Reduction
Stefan Holzer, Slobodan Ilic, David Tan, and Nassir Navab

## ACCV 2012 Best Reviewers

| | |
|---|---|
| Mitsuru Ambai | Steve Maybank |
| Steve Branson | Paul Sakrapee Paisitkriangkrai |
| Joao Carreira | Arun Ross |
| Wen-sheng Chu | Walter Scheirer |
| Hu Han | Yu-Wing Tai |
| Gang Hua | Toru Tamaki |
| Ichiro Ide | Bill Triggs |
| Yu-Gang Jiang | Liang Wang |
| Mohan Kankanhalli | Ruiping Wang |
| Junseok Kwon | Jianxiong Xiao |
| Longin Jan Latecki | Li Xu |
| Marius Leordeanu | Bangpeng Yao |
| Fuxin Li | Sai-Kit Yeung |
| Jongwoo Lim | Guofeng Zhang |
| Cheng-Lin Liu | Lei Zhang |

## ACCV 2012 Sponsors

| | |
|---|---|
| Platinum | Daejeon Metropolitan City |
| | Daejeon International Marketing Enterprise |
| | Daejeon Convention Center |
| | Korea Tourism Organization |
| | DigiCar Center, KAIST |
| | Mobile Device Interface Research Center, Chonnam National University |
| | Seoul National University |
| Gold | Samsung Advanced Institute of Technology |
| | Puloon Technology |
| Silver | Mando Corporation |
| | Qualcomm |
| | 4D View Solutions |
| Bronze | NVIDIA Corporation |

# Table of Contents – Part I

## Oral Session 1: Object Detection and Learning

## Poster Session 1: Object Detection, Learning and Matching

## Oral Session 2: Object Recognition I

## Poster Session 2: Feature, Representation, and Recognition

## Oral Session 3: Segmentation and Grouping

## Poster Session 3: Segmentation, Grouping, and Classification

# Table of Contents – Part II

## Oral Session 4: Image Representation

## Poster Session 4: Image/Video Retrieval and Medical Image Analysis

## Oral Session 5: Object Recognition II

## Poster Session 5: Face/Gesture Analysis and Recognition

# Table of Contents – Part III

## Oral Session 6: Optical Flow and Tracking

## Poster Session 6: Motion, Tracking, and Computational Photography

## Oral Session 7: Video Analysis and Action Recognition

## Poster Session 7: Video Analysis and Action Recognition

# Table of Contents – Part IV

# Oral Session 9: Applications of Computer Vision

# Poster Session 9: Low-level Vision and Applications of Computer Vision

# Beyond Dataset Bias: Multi-task Unaligned Shared Knowledge Transfer

Tatiana Tommasi[1,2], Novi Quadrianto[3],
Barbara Caputo[1], and Christoph H. Lampert[4]

[1]Idiap Research Institute, Martigny, CH
[2] École Polytechnique Fédérale de Lausanne, CH
[3] University of Cambridge, UK
[4] IST Austria (Institute of Science and Technology Austria), Klosterneuburg, AT

**Abstract.** Many visual datasets are traditionally used to analyze the performance of different learning techniques. The evaluation is usually done within each dataset, therefore it is questionable if such results are a reliable indicator of true generalization ability. We propose here an algorithm to exploit the existing data resources when learning on a new multiclass problem. Our main idea is to identify an image representation that decomposes orthogonally into two subspaces: a part specific to each dataset, and a part generic to, and therefore shared between, all the considered source sets. This allows us to use the generic representation as un-biased reference knowledge for a novel classification task. By casting the method in the multi-view setting, we also make it possible to use different features for different databases. We call the algorithm MUST, Multitask Unaligned Shared knowledge Transfer. Through extensive experiments on five public datasets, we show that MUST consistently improves the cross-datasets generalization performance.

## 1 Introduction

The long standing ambition of the visual recognition community has been to enable artificial visual systems to recognize not only specific instances of a category, such as *my car*, but *cars* in general. Many visual databases (e.g. Caltech 101 [1], PASCAL VOC [2], Animals with Attributes [3], ImageNet [4]) have been created to support such quest. However, recent studies [5,6] have questioned if the results obtained so far are a reliable indicator of real generalization abilities. Indeed, it seems that high performance on a data collection often does not reflect on the ability to classify correctly the same classes, imaged in another dataset.

One of the main reasons behind this problem is the data selection bias [5]: images contained in two databases under the same category label can represent instead different related subcategories, e.g. in ImageNet the class "car" has a strong preference for race cars. Conversely (category label bias [5]), it might happen that different labels are used for the same type of object, e.g. the class "dog" in PASCAL presents images of "collie" and "dalmatian" breed dogs that correspond instead to two separate classes in Animals with Attributes.

K.M. Lee et al. (Eds.): ACCV 2012, Part I, LNCS 7724, pp. 1–15, 2013.
© Springer-Verlag Berlin Heidelberg 2013

When looking at the disappointing cross-dataset generalization results reported in [5] keeping in mind the biases described above, one could formulate an hypothesis: a classifier trained on a specific dataset learns, for each object class, a model containing some generic knowledge about the semantic categorical problem, and some specific knowledge about the bias contained into that dataset. For example for the object category "car", a classifier trained on ImageNet would learn a racing car model. Still, the specific ability to classify correctly race cars implies having some knowledge about the general category car.

Issues arise even when focusing only on common classes across multiple existing datasets, as their label name is not sufficient to select and align them. It is necessary to inspect visually their content or use a pre-defined hierarchical ontology (like Wordnet [7]). Moreover, analyzing one class at a time implies the definition of binary problems where the negative class is obtained by sampling from the remaining set of classes, specific to each database. Thus, the definition of *what an object is not* is intrinsically biased (negative bias [5]).

Here we propose a method to overcome these issues. We exploit existing visual datasets preserving their multiclass structure and relying on the fact that they are many: each of them presents specific characteristics, but all together they cover different nuances of the real world. As the data are not uniformly distributed [8], it often happens that some classes overlap across the datasets, giving us the possibility to learn on them decoupling explicitly the generic and specific knowledge. The common information can then be used on any new multiclass problem. Along this line our main contributions are (1) we generalize the dataset bias problem presented in [5] to multiclass and to heterogeneous features: often the biases are induced by a specific research focus which turns in some features being more appropriate for some databases; (2) we introduce our Multi-task Unaligned Shared knowledge Transfer (MUST) algorithm that learns jointly shared and private knowledge from multiple datasets, and then transfers the common information when training on a new dataset. By casting the problem within the multi-view learning setting, we are able to use, for each database, features previously proposed, pre-computed and publicly available for download; (3) we propose for the first time a leave-one-dataset-out experimental setup over five existing datasets that can be considered a valid test bed for any cross-dataset generalization method.

In the rest of the paper we define our learning problem, and review related work (Section 2). We then describe the model (Section 3) and its extension to the multi-view setting (Section 4). Experiments are presented in Section 5. We conclude the paper with an overall discussion.

## 2    Problem Statement and Related Work

We formalize here the problem of learning a classifier on a target set when many source sets are available, in the hypothesis of a distribution mismatch between the target and the sources, and across the sources.

Let's indicate with $X \in \mathcal{X}$ the data and with $Y \in \mathcal{Y}$ the corresponding labels, where $\mathcal{X}$ and $\mathcal{Y}$ specify respectively the feature and the label space. We call

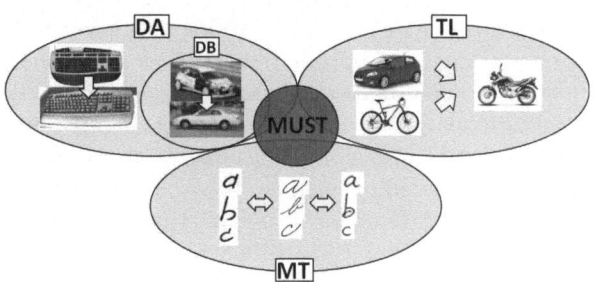

**Fig. 1.** Examples of existing approaches to the distribution mismatch problem. **DA:** adapt from Amazon keyboards to images of keyboards acquired in a specific office. **DB**: the difference between ImageNet cars and Caltech 101 cars is shown by the bad results obtained when learning on the first and testing on the second. **TL**: extract information from a car and a bicycle and use it when learning motorbikes from few examples. **MT**: learn to classify letters from the handwriting of many subjects. Our MUST algorithm partially overlap with all the described methods, filling in the empty space among them.

*domain* $D = \{\mathcal{X}, P(X)\}$ the couple of feature space and marginal distribution on the data, while a *task* $T = \{\mathcal{Y}, P(Y|X)\}$ is the couple of label space and prediction function written in probabilistic terms. Depending on (a) what gives rise to the distribution mismatch in terms of domain and task relations, and (b) if the learning process is symmetric or asymmetric over the multiple data sets, it is possible to consider different solutions to specific subparts of the general problem. We describe them below, giving corresponding examples in Figure 1.

**Domain Adaptation (DA)** aims at solving the learning problem on a target domain $D^t$ exploiting information from a source domain $D^s$, when both the domains and the corresponding tasks $T^s, T^t$ are not the same. In particular, the tasks have identical label sets $\mathcal{Y}^s = \mathcal{Y}^t$ but with slightly different conditional distributions $P^s(Y|X) \sim P^t(Y|X)$. The domains are different in terms of marginal data distribution $P^s(X) \neq P^t(X)$, and/or in feature spaces $\mathcal{X}^s \neq \mathcal{X}^t$.

DA is well studied in machine learning [9,10], speech and language processing [11,12] and more recently in computer vision, both in the semi-supervised [13] and unsupervised settings [14,15]. In case of multiple sources either the information extracted is averaged over all of them [14], or specific methods are proposed to select the best source [15]. The particular problem of domain shift across common classes in different datasets has been identified with the name of Dataset Bias (DB) [5].

**Transfer Learning (TL)** focuses on the possibility to pass useful knowledge from a source task to a target task with different label sets $\mathcal{Y}_s \neq \mathcal{Y}_t$, when the corresponding domains are not the same but the marginal distributions of data are related $P^s(X) \sim P^t(X)$. TL has been widely studied in the binary setting across couples of categories [16] and recently has been extended to multiclass problems [17]. One of the main issues here is how to evaluate the task relatedness before transferring, on the basis of only few available labeled samples in the target and eventually multiple sources.

**Multi-Task Learning (MT)** aims at learning jointly over $N$ available sets, leading to a symmetric share of information. This is particularly useful when each task has few data. The multi-task framework supposes that all the sets share the same feature space $\mathcal{X}^i = \mathcal{X}^j$ but present slightly different domains $P^i(X) \sim P^j(X)$ for $i, j \in \{1, \ldots, N\}$. Traditionally, one either assume that the set of labels for all the tasks are the same ($\mathcal{Y}^s = \mathcal{Y}^t$) or that it is possible to access to an oracle mapping function $\mathcal{Y}^s \mapsto \mathcal{Y}^t$ that aligns the classes. Many techniques for MT have been published in machine learning [18,19] with some applications in computer vision [20,21]. Most of the works suppose multiple binary tasks and only few attempts has been done in the multiclass case without label correspondences [22,23].

Our MUST algorithm fits in the general setting of all these approaches, while covering issues orthogonal across all of them. We are interested in multiple sources and a single target with domain shift and partially overlapping label sets: $\mathcal{Y}^i \cap \mathcal{Y}^j \neq \emptyset$ for all $(i, j) \in \{1, \ldots, N\}$. The difference in the domains can be caused by both $P^i(X) \neq P^j(X)$ and $\mathcal{X}^i \neq \mathcal{X}^j$. The aim is to extract general information from all the sources (in multi-task fashion) and to use it when learning on a new target with a general advantage both on the known categories (as in domain adaptation) and on new ones (as in transfer learning). With respect to classical multi-task learning, we break the symmetry adding a transfer part to a target problem. At the same time, we overcome the transfer learning problem of evaluating the task relatedness leveraging on the possibility to extract a common useful knowledge from multiple sources. Finally, we go beyond domain adaptation which does not cover the case of completely new classes in the target task. Moreover, considering multiple sources (with eventually different features) we show that the hypothesis of relying on a flat average knowledge is not helpful in the case of tasks with partially overlapping label sets.

We pursue our goal by defining a method that allows us to exploit existing visual resources with a *minimal effort*: (1) we do not need to know explicitly which classes are present in each task and therefore, no manual alignment is necessary, (2) we do not need to keep the source data when learning on the target, (3) we leverage over multiple sources regardless to their feature space. MUST is inspired by recent research on finding shared and private projections [24,25] for problems where multiple modalities or multiple views of the same data are available. This notion was also exploited in the context of Multi-Task learning in [23].

Recently the dataset bias problem has been explored in [26]. The proposed approach is based on the combination of a specific and a common discriminative model across several tasks, following the same idea of the original multi-task SVM [18]. The novelty is in the fact that the common model, apart from sharing information, is constrained to perform well on any task on its own. By using SVM, this strategy results intrinsically limited to binary problems: any SVM multiclass solution considers one model for each class and this would ask for class alignment.

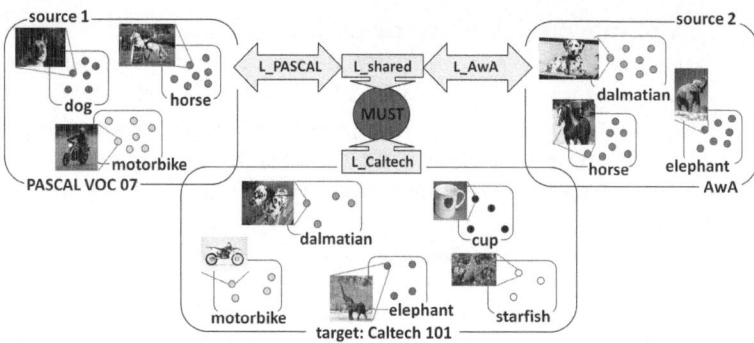

**Fig. 2.** Schematic representation of the MUST algorithm: shared and private information are extracted from two existing datasets. The shared knowledge is then transferred to solve a new multiclass problem on a different dataset. Notice that no explicit alignment is requested between "dalmatian" and "dog" classes.

## 3   The Model

Starting from multiple visual object datasets, our goal is to learn a projection function that maps the data points into one shared and several private latent spaces with an *orthogonality* constraint between them. We can then transfer the knowledge encoded in the shared space to a new dataset and use the available training samples to learn only the remaining private orthogonal part (see Figure 2). The new problem will benefit from this approach only if the shared space captures non-dataset-specific information which we will call *common sense*.

More formally, we are given $N$ sets of $m_n$ observed data points, $\mathcal{D}_n = \{(x_1^n, y_1^n), \dots, (x_{m_n}^n, y_{m_n}^n)\} \subset \mathcal{X}^n \times \mathcal{Y}^n$ for $n = 1, \dots, N$. Here we use $\mathcal{X}^n$ and $\mathcal{Y}^n$ to denote the input space and output space of the $n$-th dataset. For the purpose of explaining the key idea, we assume that the same representation is used for all the datasets, $\mathcal{X}^n = \mathbb{R}^d$ for all $n$. We further require some overlap in the output spaces, i.e. $\mathcal{Y}^i \cap \mathcal{Y}^j \neq \emptyset$ for all $(i, j) \in \{1, \dots, N\}$. The existence of such partial superposition in the label sets allows to introduce the notion of common sense as generic knowledge among the tasks. It is important to underline that we want an approach which does not require explicit label correspondences among datasets, and we are interested in models that do not build those correspondences as an intermediate learning step. We seek functions

$$g_n : \mathbb{R}^d \to \mathbb{R}^D \quad \text{for} \quad n = 1, \dots, N, \tag{1}$$

which project the original space into a novel one with potentially much smaller dimension $D \ll d$. We assume a *linear* parametrization of the functions and an *additive* model for the shared-private spaces. Thus, the projection functions admit the following form $g_n(x_i^n) := (L_n + L_s)\phi(x_i^n)$ for $H$ basis functions[1]

---

[1] We use $\phi(x_i)$ to indicate the possibility of non-linear mapping applied on the original feature vector $x_i$. The full method might be kernelized by building on [27].

$\{\phi_h(x_i)\}_{h=1}^H$, a private projection matrix for the $n$-th dataset $L_n \in \mathbb{R}^{D \times H}$, and a shared projection matrix $L_s \in \mathbb{R}^{D \times H}$. We learn those projection matrices based on the *folk-wisdom* principle [28,27,29] of pulling objects or data samples together if they are of the same type (keeping your friends close), and pushing them apart if they are not (keeping your enemies far away). This principle is formalized by the regularized risk functional described in the following Section.

## 3.1   Regularized Risk Functional

We want to learn a transformation over the data by minimizing a function which penalizes large distances between samples of the same class, and small distances between samples with non-matching class labels. We assume that for each sample, it is possible to identify a set of genuine neighbors or friends. The notation $i \sim j$ is used to indicate that $x_i$ and $x_j$ are friends as belonging to the same class, and the notation $i \nsim l$ describes that $x_i$ and $x_l$ are enemies as associated to different class labels. Our optimization problem has the following form:

$$\min_{\substack{L_s \\ L_1,\dots,N}} \underbrace{\sum_{n=1}^N \sum_{i \sim j} d_n^2(x_i^n, x_j^n) + \sum_{\substack{i \sim j \\ i \nsim l}} \max(0, 1 + d_n^2(x_i^n, x_j^n) - d_n^2(x_i^n, x_l^n))}_{\text{Loss}(\cdot)}$$

$$+ \eta \Omega(L_n) + \gamma \Omega(L_s) \qquad (2)$$

$$\text{subject to } L_s^\top L_n = 0 \quad \text{for all } n = 1, \dots, N,$$

where $d_n^2(x_i^n, x_j^n) := \left\| (L_n + L_s)(\phi(x_i^n) - \phi(x_j^n)) \right\|_{\ell_2}^2$ is the squared distance in the projected space. In (2), $\text{Loss}(\cdot)$ is the loss function, $\Omega(\cdot)$ is a regularizer on the projection matrices, and the trade-off variables $\eta$ and $\lambda$ control the relative influence of loss and regularization terms. For $\Omega(\cdot)$, one typically chooses the $\ell_2$ norm, or the $\ell_1$ norm if one wants to induce sparsity in the projection matrices. The loss function consists of two terms: the first requires small distances among friend samples, while the second asks that the distance between each sample and its enemies is a unit greater than the corresponding distance to the friends. Finally, the constraints ensure that the inferred shared space is orthogonal to each of the private spaces.

Given a new dataset of $m_t$ observed data points $\mathcal{D}_t = \{(x_1^t, y_1^t), \dots, (x_{m_t}^t, y_{m_t}^t)\} \subset \mathbb{R}^d \times \mathcal{Y}^t$ with $\mathcal{Y}^t \cap (\bigcup_{n=1,\dots,N} \mathcal{Y}^n) \neq \emptyset$ we want to learn its specific representation while enforcing it to be orthogonal to the common sense obtained from the previous $N$ datasets. This corresponds to finding a private projection matrix $L_t$ *given* the shared projection matrix $L_s$, and can be expressed with the following optimization problem:

$$\min_{L_t} \sum_{i \sim j} d_t^2(x_i^t, x_j^t) + \sum_{\substack{i \sim j \\ i \nsim l}} \max(0, 1 + d_t^2(x_i^t, x_j^t) - d_t^2(x_i^t, x_l^t)) + \eta \Omega(L_t) \qquad (3)$$

$$\text{subject to } L_s^\top L_t = 0,$$

---
**Algorithm 1.** MUST

---
**Input** $N$ source datasets $\mathcal{D}_n = \{(x_1^n, y_1^n), \ldots, (x_{m_n}^n, y_{m_n}^n)\} \subset \mathbb{R}^d \times \mathcal{Y}^n$
**Input** a target dataset $\mathcal{D}_t = \{(x_1^t, y_1^t), \ldots, (x_{m_t}^t, y_{m_t}^t)\} \subset \mathbb{R}^d \times \mathcal{Y}^t$
Solve optimization problem in (2) for shared $L_s$ and private $L_{1,\ldots,N}$
Transfer the common sense as captured by $L_s$ to a new dataset $\mathcal{D}_t$
Given $L_s$, solve optimization problems in (3) for private $L_t$
**Output** $L_t$

---

where $d_t^2(x_i^t, x_j^t) := \left\| (L_t + L_s)(\phi(x_i^t) - \phi(x_j^t)) \right\|_{\ell_2}^2$. Intuitively, whenever the common sense knowledge given by $L_s$ is sufficient to enforce the folk-wisdom principle, there is no penalty incurred in (3). The learning capacity of the private projection matrix $L_t$ can thus be focused on those hard cases specific to this new dataset. In the following Section, we go on describing the methods to optimize problems (2) and (3).

### 3.2 Optimization

The optimization problem (2) (and (3) likewise) is non-convex with respect to the projection matrices $L_s, L_1, \ldots, L_N$, thus it is hard to optimize. However, [27] and more recently [23] presented two ideas to turn the problem in (2) – excluding the orthogonality constraints – into a convex optimization problem, namely, a semi-definite programming. The first idea is to replace the second term of the loss function, with a soft margin constraint. This is achieved by introducing a non-negative slack variable for every pair of friends and enemies $\xi_{ijl}$ such that $d_n^2(x_i^n, x_l^n) - d_n^2(x_i^n, x_j^n) \geq 1 - \xi_{ijl}$. This will essentially allow the distance between samples and their enemies to be less than a unit greater than the distance with their friends. To avoid this behavior for occurring often, there is a budget on the slack variables $\sum_{\substack{i \sim j \\ i \not\sim l}} \xi_{ijl}$ that needs to be minimized. The second intuition is to substitute the optimization over the projection matrix $L$ with the optimization over the corresponding metric $M := L^\top L$, therefore imposing a semi-definite constraint on $M \succeq 0$.

Weinberger and Saul [27] described a convex solver based on alternating sub-gradient descent methods for the re-formulated problem. Recently, Kleiner, Rahimi, and Jordan [30] devised an approach to solve SDPs by repeatedly solving randomly generated optimization problems over two-dimensional subcones of the PSD cone. This approach produces only approximate solutions due to randomization, but it scales to number of samples orders of magnitude larger than have previously been possible. Here, we show that the same solvers can still be used for our constrained problem as the linearity and additive model assumptions allow us to write

$$d_n^2(x_i^n, x_j^n) = \left\| (L_n + L_s)(\phi(x_i^n) - \phi(x_j^n)) \right\|_{\ell_2}^2 \tag{4}$$

$$= \left\| L_n(\phi(x_i^n) - \phi(x_j^n)) \right\|_{\ell_2}^2 + \left\| L_s(\phi(x_i^n) - \phi(x_j^n)) \right\|_{\ell_2}^2, \tag{5}$$

and its analogous for $d_t^2(x_i^t, x_j^t)$. The last equality follows directly from our orthogonality assumptions. Note that $\left\| L_s(\phi(x_i^t) - \phi(x_j^t)) \right\|_{\ell_2}^2$ is fixed for each set of neighbors and thus can be pre-computed. In this paper, we use the solver presented in [27]. The full method MUST is summarized in Algorithm 1.

## 4   Multi-view on Multiple Datasets

We now consider the case where each of the given $N$ datasets lies in its own feature space, that is $\mathcal{X}^n = \mathbb{R}^{d_n}$ for $n = 1, \ldots, N$. This setting easily appears since most of the visual datasets are released together with their own pre-extracted features. For this multi-view problem, we seek additional projection functions $f_n : \mathbb{R}^{d_n} \to \mathbb{R}^d$ that map all inputs from different databases to an intermediate $\mathbb{R}^d$ space in addition to finding the shared and private metrics. We assume a linear parametrization for the multi-view functions $f_n := W_n x_i^n$ where $W_n \in \mathbb{R}^{d \times d_n}$ is the multi-view projection matrix for the $n$-th dataset. Our multi-view distance function with the orthogonality constraint between shared and private spaces made explicit is now:

$$\hat{d}_n^2(x_i^n, x_j^n) = (W_n(\phi(x_i^n) - \phi(x_j^n)))^\top (L_n^\top L_n + L_s^\top L_s)(W_n(\phi(x_i^n) - \phi(x_j^n))) \quad (6)$$
$$= \text{trace}(M_s W_n v_{ij}^n v_{ij}^{n,\top} W_n^\top) + \text{trace}(M_n W_n v_{ij}^n v_{ij}^{n,\top} W_n^\top)$$
$$\text{with } M_s \succeq 0 \text{ and } M_n \succeq 0,$$

where $v_{ij}^n = (\phi(x_i^n) - \phi(x_j^n))$. We use the above distance function as a drop-in replacement to the objective function in (2). Thus the optimization problem will be over the multi-view projection matrices $W_n$s and over the metrics $M_s$, $M_n$s. Similarly to the single-view case, given a new dataset, we will solve the optimization problem in (3), but now an additional projection matrix $f_t : \mathbb{R}^{d_t} \to \mathbb{R}^d$ that bring the new datasets to the same intermediate space of the old training datasets has also to be found.

*Optimization.* The optimization problem in (2) with the modified distance function $\hat{d}_n^2(x_i^n, x_j^n)$ is convex with respect to the metrics given all the multi-view projection matrices $W_n$s and is non-convex with respect to the multi-view projection matrices given the shared and private metrics $M_s$ and $M_n$. We pursue an alternating approach: fix all the multi-view projection matrices and solve the shared and private metrics $M_s$ and $M_n$ with [27]; subsequently, fix the metrics and optimize all the multi-view projection matrices $W_n$s with fast sub-gradient descent algorithm. In this paper, we use nonsmooth BFGS [31]. This procedure is repeated until a certain number of alternating steps is reached. The Multi-View (MUST-MV) version of our method is summarized in Algorithm 2.

---

**Algorithm 2.** MUST-MV

---

**Input** $N$ source datasets $\mathcal{D}_n = \{(x_1^n, y_1^n), \ldots, (x_{m_n}^n, y_{m_n}^n)\} \subset \mathbb{R}^{d_n} \times \mathcal{Y}^n$
**Input** a target dataset $\mathcal{D}_t = \{(x_1^t, y_1^t), \ldots, (x_{m_t}^t, y_{m_t}^t)\} \subset \mathbb{R}^{d_t} \times \mathcal{Y}^t$
**Input** number of alternations $A$
Initialize $W_n^{d_n} = W_n^{\text{PCA}} \ \forall \ n = 1, \ldots, N$
**for** $a = 1$ **to** $A$ **do**
    Solve optimization problem in (2) for shared $L_s$ and private $L_{1,\ldots,N}$
    Solve optimization problem in (2) for multi-view projections $W_n$
**end for**
Initialize $W_t^{d_t} = W_t^{\text{PCA}}$
Transfer the common sense as captured by $L_s$ to a new dataset $\mathcal{D}_t$
**for** $a = 1$ **to** $A$ **do**
    Given $L_s$, solve optimization problem in (3) for private $L_t$
    Solve optimization problem in (3) for multi-view projection $W_t$
**end for**
**Output** $L_t, W_t^{d_t} \in \mathbb{R}^{d_t \times d}$

---

# 5 Experiments

We present here two groups of experiments designed to study how MUST[2] performs on *cross-database* generalization problems both in the case with all sets
having the same feature representation (single-view setting, Section 5.1) and
when each of the datasets lies in its own feature space (multi-view setting, Section 5.2). To this purpose, we selected five visual object databases which are
actively used in present computer vision research and have some partial overlapping in the label space: Caltech 101 [1] with 101 class labels, PASCAL VOC07
[2] with 20 class labels, MSRCORID [32] with 20 class labels, Animals with
Attributes (AwA) [3] with 50 class labels, and CIFAR 100 [33] with 100 class
labels. We applied a one-dataset-out strategy, extracting the general knowledge
from four datasets and giving the chance to each database in turn to be used as
a new problem.

## 5.1 Single-View Setting

For the single view experiments we extracted Gist features [34] from the images
converted to grayscale and ran metric learning on the sources with 15 genuine
neighbors, both considering the multi-task approach (using [23]) and keeping
the task separated (using [27]). We fixed the maximum number of enemies to
a very high value ($10^6$), letting the algorithm almost free to find all the active
neighbors belonging to a different class. A first set of experiments was run on
a subset of the listed datasets described in Figure 3(top, left): each dataset has
a partial class overlapping with the others and two completely new categories.
Here for each source database we have randomly chosen 90/30/30 samples per

---

[2] The code for MUST containing all the scripts used for the experiments is available
online http://www.idiap.ch/~ttommasi/source_code_ACCV12.html

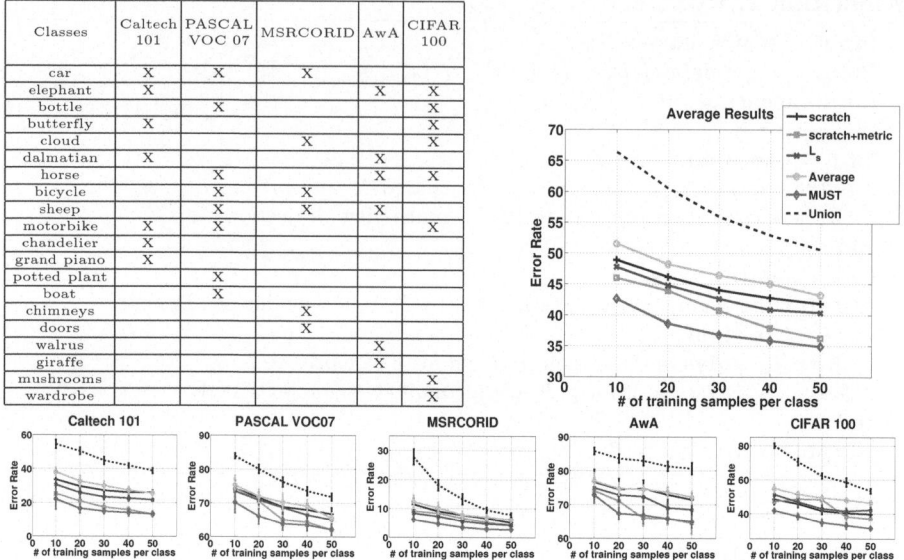

| Classes | Caltech 101 | PASCAL VOC 07 | MSRCORID | AwA | CIFAR 100 |
|---|---|---|---|---|---|
| car | X | X | X | | |
| elephant | X | | | X | X |
| bottle | | X | | | X |
| butterfly | X | | | | X |
| cloud | | | X | | X |
| dalmatian | X | | | X | |
| horse | | X | | X | X |
| bicycle | | X | X | | |
| sheep | | X | X | X | |
| motorbike | X | X | | | X |
| chandelier | X | | | | |
| grand piano | X | | | | |
| potted plant | | X | | | |
| boat | | X | | | |
| chimneys | | | X | | |
| doors | | | X | | |
| walrus | | | | X | |
| giraffe | | | | X | |
| mushrooms | | | | | X |
| wardrobe | | | | | X |

**Fig. 3.** Visual object classification across different datasets using the same feature. Top: (left) the table describing the experimental setup, (right) plot of the average results on five datasets. Bottom: separate results on each target dataset. Results over 10 repetitions for all methods except Union with 5 repetitions due to high computational demand.

class for training, validation and test. For the new target database we fixed a test set of 50 samples and considered an increasing number of available training samples $n = \{10, 20, 30, 40, 50\}$. Only for Caltech 101 we reduced the described sets respectively to 30/10/10 and we used 10 samples as test set, due to the smaller number of available data per class.

The performance of MUST is compared with four baselines, two corresponding to learning from scratch and two exploiting the shared knowledge with naïve transfer approaches:

**Scratch:** we used the Identity as projection matrix (Euclidean metric);

**Scratch+Metric:** we learn a metric from the available new training data; **$L_s$:** the shared projection matrix $L_s$ learned on multiple datasets is applied on the new one;

**Average:** projection matrices $L_n$ learned separately on each database; their average is applied on the new dataset.

We can in principle combine all the samples from the visual datasets. It is already known [5] that this simple solution is not helpful against the dataset bias problem, moreover, apart from suffering for an explosion in the number of data, it requires an explicit class alignment procedure. However, as a reference to the results that could be obtained in this setting, we ran metric learning [27] on the

**Table 1.** Error rate results obtained on the single-view experiments considering the whole datasets

| target | scratch+metric (%) | $L_s$(%) | Average (%) | MUST (%) |
|---|---|---|---|---|
| Caltech 101 | $65.69 \pm 0.99$ | $70.66 \pm 1.87$ | $75.35 \pm 1.56$ | $62.55 \pm 1.08$ |
| Pascal VOC07 | $84.94 \pm 3.14$ | $84.50 \pm 2.15$ | $85.38 \pm 3.42$ | $80.66 \pm 2.12$ |
| MSRCORID | $45.80 \pm 4.26$ | $51.79 \pm 2.73$ | $52.59 \pm 2.93$ | $40.24 \pm 3.11$ |
| AwA | $94.02 \pm 1.20$ | $93.98 \pm 0.84$ | $94.24 \pm 1.11$ | $92.32 \pm 1.18$ |
| CIFAR 100 | $90.91 \pm 0.97$ | $87.84 \pm 1.06$ | $92.76 \pm 0.80$ | $87.48 \pm 0.78$ |
| overall | 76.27 | 77.75 | 80.06 | 72.65 |

**Union** of all the training samples. All the final classification are performed using $k$-Nearest Neighbor with $k = 15$ ($k = 8$ only for 10 available training samples).

From the results in Figure 3 we can state that averaging over all the sources does not directly provide a good solution for the target problem. On the other hand, when only few training samples are available (10-20), by learning on them we get just slightly better performance w.r.t. using directly the general knowledge in $L_s$. However, when the number of samples increases, $L_s$ is no more enough by itself to solve the learning problem on the new task. Finally, inferring the specific private knowledge on the new dataset and combining it with the shared common sense with our MUST algorithm *always* improves the average classification performance. By looking closely at the results on each new dataset, MUST mostly improves but *never degrades* the performance in comparison to not utilizing the available sources (scratch+metric in the plot).

We also performed a second set of experiments considering all the available classes in each dataset. We defined ten splits randomly extracting 20/10 train/test samples from each class of the target task dataset, 15 genuine neighbors and 100 enemies. Since the test set changes at each run, the standard deviations are only barely indicative. We evaluated the difference between MUST and scratch+metric separately for all the splits: the sign test [35] on the obtained output confirms that MUST significantly outperforms scratch+metric with $p \leq 0.05$. There is only one exception for AwA, the animals are highly confused among each other and in this case it is probably necessary to increase the number of enemies in the method to reach significant results.

## 5.2 Multi-view Setting

In the multi-view setting we considered different features for each dataset. We used bag of words SIFT features[3] for Caltech 101, Hue color histogram[4] for PASCAL VOC07, the already calculated Gist for MSRCORID and PHOG features[5] for AwA. Finally we calculated PHOG for CIFAR but using different parameters with respect to the features used for AwA. We ran the experiments on the same data subset described above (Figure 3(top, left)): we applied PCA separately on the multiple tasks to project all of them in the same dimensional

---

[3] From http://www.vision.ee.ethz.ch/~pgehler/projects/iccv09/

[4] DenseHueV3H1 from http://lear.inrialpes.fr/people/guillaumin/data.php

[5] From http://attributes.kyb.tuebingen.mpg.de/

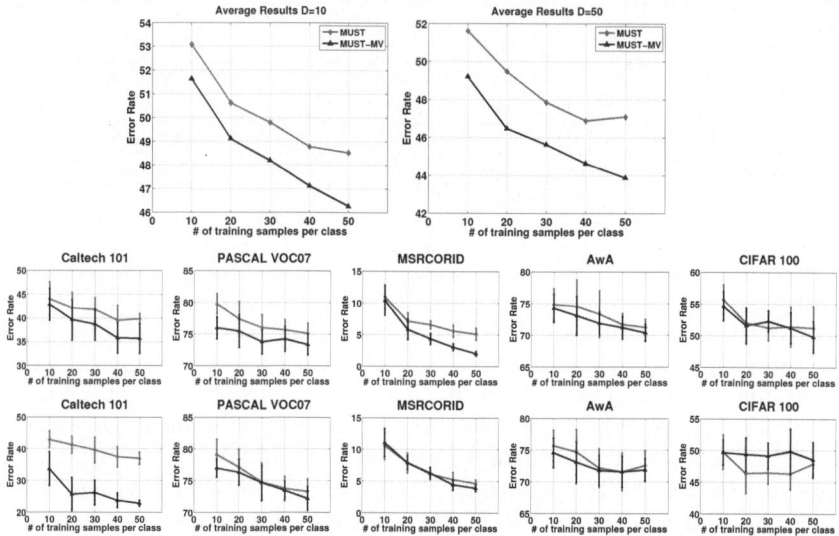

**Fig. 4.** Top: average error rate results on the five datasets considering the projection of all the different features to a space of dimension D=10,50 (left,right). Middle: separate results on each target datasets over 10 repetitions for D=10. Bottom: separate results on each target datasets over 10 repetitions for D=50. All the reported error rates for MUST-MV correspond to the best results obtained over the multiple iterations of the alternating optimization process.

space with $D = \{10, 50\}$ before running the metric learning process to define the shared knowledge. On the novel dataset, we can again use PCA and proceed with MUST to learn the specific metric, or we can activate the optimization for the projection matrix $W$. We consider the first approach as a reference baseline and compare with MUST-MV.

The number of genuine neighbors and enemies for these experiments are fixed to 3 to infer the general and specific knowledge on each task and to 5 for learning the multi-view projections. These choices are done on the basis of two considerations. First, we want a good balance between computational cost and accuracy performance. Further, we aim to put a little more emphasis on retaining dataset-specific characteristics before inferring the shared knowledge in successive iterations. The last point lead us also to observe that for the multi-view problem, it is beneficial to have a dataset specific constant in (2) and (3) when enforcing the large difference between friends and enemies. Thus we substituted the value 1 in the second term of the loss function with the median of the squared pairwise distances in each dataset own feature space.

The results reported in Figure 4 show that on average MUST-MV is more suitable for the multi-view problem than the original MUST. Looking at the single target results, the advantage given by learning the projection matrix $W_t$ is more evident the smaller is the dimension $D$. We also notice that MUST-MV performs always better (or at least equal) than MUST with one only exception when CIFAR 100 is used as target task with $D = 50$. We believe that in this particular case the combination of general and specific knowledge should be better weighted giving more importance to the common sense. This explanation is corroborated by the single-view CIFAR 100 results (Figure 3, bottom right) that show an initial abnormal increasing behavior for the scratch+metric baseline when the number of available training samples grows, while exploiting the common knowledge together with the specific one we get the best results.

## 6  Discussion and Conclusion

We presented here our MUST algorithm that decomposes multiple datasets into two orthogonal subspaces: one is specific to each dataset and the other is shared between all of them. Then the common information is transferred to help on a new task. On average, MUST *always* demonstrates cross-dataset generalization, assessed via a one-dataset-out strategy. We stress that the aim of our work was not to achieve the next state of the art accuracy on any of the considered databases, but rather to show that, in spite of the bias afflicting each of them, they do all carry a useful knowledge which is learnable and exploitable, significantly improving the generalization ability of a learning system.

By relying on metric learning and using a formulation similar to [27], MUST benefits of a max-margin framework analogous to that of SVM, but overcomes the class alignment limit of the SVM multiclass models. Moreover, the general and specific metrics produced by MUST can be used afterwords by any approach that requires distance computation among samples, including kernel methods.

Besides showing encouraging results, we have clearly only touched the surface of possibilities to be explored.

**Acknowledgements.** This work was supported by the PASCAL 2 Network of Excellence (TT) and by the Newton International Fellowship (NQ).

## References

1. Fei-Fei, L., Fergus, R., Perona, P.: Learning generative visual models from few training examples: An incremental bayesian approach tested on 101 object categories. Comput. Vis. Image Underst. 106, 59–70 (2007)
2. Everingham, M., Van Gool, L., Williams, C.K.I., Winn, J., Zisserman, A.: The PASCAL Visual Object Classes Challenge 2007 (VOC 2007) Results (2007), http://www.pascal-network.org/challenges/VOC/
3. Lampert, C.H., Nickisch, H., Harmeling, S.: Learning to detect unseen object classes by between class attribute transfer. In: CVPR (2009)
4. Deng, J., Dong, W., Socher, R., Li, L.J., Li, K., Fei-Fei, L.: ImageNet: A Large-Scale Hierarchical Image Database. In: CVPR (2009)
5. Torralba, A., Efros, A.A.: Unbiased look at dataset bias. In: CVPR (2011)
6. Perronnin, F., Sánchez, J., Liu, Y.: Large-scale image categorization with explicit data embedding. In: CVPR (2010)

7. Stark, M.M., Riesenfeld, R.F.: Wordnet: An electronic lexical database. In: Eurographics Workshop on Rendering. MIT Press (1998)
8. Salakhutdinov, R., Torralba, A., Tenenbaum, J.: Learning to Share Visual Appearance for Multiclass Object Detection. In: CVPR (2011)
9. Blitzer, J., Crammer, K., Kulesza, A., Pereira, O., Wortman, J.: Learning bounds for domain adaptation. In: NIPS (2008)
10. Ben-david, S., Blitzer, J., Crammer, K., Sokolova, P.M.: Analysis of representations for domain adaptation. In: NIPS (2007)
11. Blitzer, J., McDonald, R., Pereira, F.: Domain adaptation with structural correspondence learning. In: EMNLP (2006)
12. Daumé III, H.: Frustratingly easy domain adaptation. In: ACL (2007)
13. Saenko, K., Kulis, B., Fritz, M., Darrell, T.: Adapting Visual Category Models to New Domains. In: Daniilidis, K., Maragos, P., Paragios, N. (eds.) ECCV 2010, Part IV. LNCS, vol. 6314, pp. 213–226. Springer, Heidelberg (2010)
14. Gopalan, R., Li, R., Chellappa, R.: Domain adaptation for object recognition: An unsupervised approach. In: ICCV (2011)
15. Gong, B., Shi, Y., Sha, F., Grauman, K.: Geodesic flow kernel for unsupervised domain adaptation. In: CVPR (2012)
16. Pan, S.J., Yang, Q.: A survey on transfer learning. IEEE Transactions on Knowledge and Data Engineering 22, 1345–1359 (2010)
17. Jie, L., Tommasi, T., Caputo, B.: Multiclass transfer learning from unconstrained priors. In: ICCV (2011)
18. Evgeniou, T., Pontil, M.: Regularized multi–task learning. In: KDD (2004)
19. Kang, Z., Grauman, K., Sha, F.: Learning with whom to share in multi-task feature learning. In: ICML (2011)
20. Wang, X., Zhang, C., Zhang, Z.: Boosted multi-task learning for face verification with applications to web image and video search. In: CVPR (2009)
21. Vezhnevets, A., Buhmann, J.M.: Towards weakly supervised semantic segmentation by means of multiple instance and multitask learning. In: CVPR (2010)
22. Quadrianto, N., Smola, A.J., Caetano, T.S., Vishwanathan, S.V.N., Petterson, J.: Multitask learning without label correspondences. In: NIPS (2010)
23. Parameswaran, S., Weinberger, K.: Large margin multi-task metric learning. In: NIPS (2010)
24. Leen, G.: Context assisted information extraction. PhD thesis, University of the West of Scotland (2008)
25. Jia, Y., Salzmann, M., Darrell, T.: Factorized latent spaces with structured sparsity. In: NIPS (2010)
26. Khosla, A., Zhou, T., Malisiewicz, T., Efros, A.A., Torralba, A.: Undoing the Damage of Dataset Bias. In: Fitzgibbon, A., Lazebnik, S., Perona, P., Sato, Y., Schmid, C. (eds.) ECCV 2012, Part I. LNCS, vol. 7572, pp. 158–171. Springer, Heidelberg (2012)
27. Weinberger, K., Saul, L.: Distance metric learning for large margin nearest neighbor classification. Journal of Machine Learning Research 10, 207–244 (2009)
28. Goldberger, J., Roweis, S.T., Hinton, G.E., Salakhutdinov, R.: Neighbourhood components analysis. In: NIPS (2004)
29. Quadrianto, N., Lampert, C.H.: Learning multi-view neighborhood preserving projections. In: ICML (2011)
30. Kleiner, A., Rahimi, A., Jordan, M.I.: Random conic pursuit for semidefinite programming. In: NIPS (2010)
31. Lewis, A.S., Overton, M.L.: Nonsmooth optimization via quasi-newton methods. Math. Programming (to appear)

32. Microsoft Research Cambridge Object Recognition Image Database (2005),
    http://research.microsoft.com/en-us/downloads/
33. Krizhevsky, A.: Learning multiple layers of features from tiny images. Technical
    Report MSc thesis, University of Toronto, USA (2007)
34. Oliva, A., Torralba, A.: Modeling the shape of the scene: A holistic representation
    of the spatial envelope. IJCV 42, 145–175 (2001)
35. Gibbons, J.: Nonparametric Statistical Inference. Marcel Dekker, New York (1985)

# Cross-Database Transfer Learning via Learnable and Discriminant Error-Correcting Output Codes

Feng-Ju Chang[1], Yen-Yu Lin[1], and Ming-Fang Weng[2]

[1] Research Center for Information Technology Innovation, Academia Sinica, Taiwan
[2] Institute of Information Science, Academia Sinica, Taiwan
{fengju,yylin}@citi.sinica.edu.tw, mfueng@iis.sinica.edu.tw

**Abstract.** We present a transfer learning approach that transfers knowledge across two multi-class, unconstrained domains (source and target), and accomplishes object recognition with few training samples in the target domain. Unlike most of previous work, we make no assumption about the relatedness of these two domains. Namely, data of the two domains can be from different databases and of distinct categories. To overcome the domain variations, we propose to learn a set of commonly-shared and discriminant attributes in form of *error-correcting output codes*. Upon each of attributes, the unrelated, multi-class recognition tasks of the two domains are transformed into correlative, binary-class ones. The extra source knowledge can alleviate the high risk of overfitting caused by the lack of training data in the target domain. Our approach is evaluated on several benchmark datasets, and leads to about 40% relative improvement in accuracy when only one training sample is available.

## 1 Introduction

Object recognition is one of the most fundamental problems in vision research. Despite its importance, most of existing recognition techniques are still hindered by two main challenges: the large intra-class variation and the large number of categories to be identified. Recent research efforts, e.g., [2,3], on *multiple kernel learning* [4,5] overcome these difficulties via employing various powerful descriptors. However, these approaches rely on a large set of training samples to investigate data variations, such that the optimal kernel combination can be determined. In general, the cost of data labeling is quite expensive.

To reduce the labeling effort, *transfer learning* [6] has been demonstrated to be a promising technique for object recognition with few training samples. It delivers useful knowledge in the *source* to improve the *target* model learning. However, most transfer learning algorithms [7,8,9] handle merely the knowledge delivery *from either multiple classes or a single class in the source to a single class in the target*, and assume high correlation between the source and target domains. These two restrictions might reduce their applicability to object recognition, where diverse classes and multi-class classification are involved.

The proposed approach transfers knowledge *from muliple classes to multiple classes*, given two multi-class recognition tasks (one in the source domain and

K.M. Lee et al. (Eds.): ACCV 2012, Part I, LNCS 7724, pp. 16–30, 2013.
© Springer-Verlag Berlin Heidelberg 2013

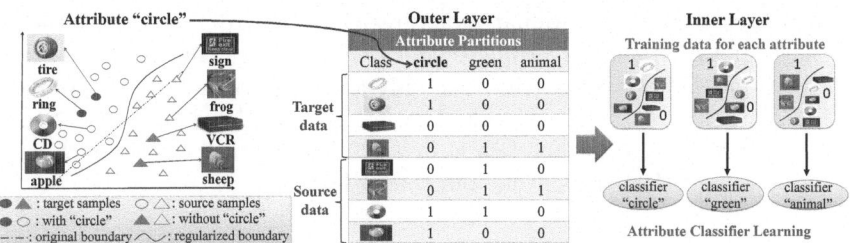

**Fig. 1.** The proposed two-layer boosting framework for transfer learning. While outer layer discovers attribute partitions, inner layer deals with classifier learning.

the other in the target domain). We leverage the extra source knowledge to learn a more robust multi-class classifier rather than a set of binary classifiers in the target domain. However, no assumptions about the relatedness between the two domains - data of the two domains can be from either the same or different databases, and their respective object categories may partially overlap or don't overlap at all - makes direct knowledge sharing infeasible.

Therefore, we propose to transfer knowledge through a sequence of the automatically learned *attributes*. Figure. 1 illustrates our idea. By associating with attribute circle, the *unrelated, multi-class* recognition tasks of the two domains become *correlative, binary-class* (i.e., with or without circle) ones. It follows that the extra source knowledge can be transferred to regularize the target classifier learning, which alleviates *overfitting* caused by the scarceness of target training data, and leads to a better classifier with the low generalization error.

To carry out our idea, we present a *two-layer (the outer and inner layers) boosting framework* that automatically derives a sequence of *discriminant* attributes, *commonly shared* by both the source and target domains, to facilitate knowledge transfer. Specifically, the outer layer implements a multi-task variant of *AdaBoost.OC* [10], which sequentially discovers a set of *attribute partitions* in form of *error-correcting output codes*. Each attribute divides all classes into two subsets - presence (1) or absence (0) of the attribute. With each attribute, the training data for learning the *attribute classifier* are of binary labels.

The inner layer exploits the training data from the outer layer to learn attribute classifiers by the principle of classifier sharing, which has been demonstrated to be effective in [11,12] for learning related tasks via sharing the weak learners in boosting. Namely, after associating the source and target data with each attribute partition, the learning of attribute classifiers in both two domains are cast into a joint optimizaiton problem.

Based on the two-layer boosting framework, our approach has the following three contributions. First, with the outer layer, the attribute partitions are complementary to each other due to the iterative minimization of the *pseudoloss* [10]. Second, with the inner layer, the robust and discriminant attribute classifiers can be learned in the target domain. Third, our formulation not only carries out knowledge transfer, but also supports multiple kernel learning for feature fusion, since attributes are high-level concepts and each of them might be captured by a distinct combination of low-level features.

The proposed method is evaluated on three benchmark datasets. Both the performances of *within-database transfer* and *cross-database transfer* demonstrate the effectiveness of our approach, when only few training samples are available. Section 2 shows several related work. The AdaBoost.OC is described in Section 3, and the details of our approach is presented in Section 4. Section 5 and 6 respectively show the experiments and conclusions.

## 2   Related Work

The task of object recognition is typically formulated as a multi-class classification problem. Much research effort has been devoted to the design of more discriminant features, e.g., [13,14], so as to minimize the intra-class variation while maximize the inter-class discrepancy simultaneously. On the other hand, many variants of multiple kernel learning algorithms, e.g., [1,2,3], are proposed to integrate various features in a unified fashion, and lead to higher recognition accuracy. However, most of these approaches require training on a sufficient number of data to build stable classifiers.

The early investigation into learning with few examples to recognize objects is pioneered by Fei-Fei et al. [8]. They suggest to extract visual knowledge from a set of previously learned object classes to represent a novel one. Intermediate features [15,16] such as attributes bridging low-level image features and high-level concepts have been shown potential for establishing a discriminant model with few, even zero new datum. In general, these attributes require tedious and expensive human efforts on labeling. Recently, Qi et al. [17] introduce a cross-category transfer learning algorithm, and explicitly transfer knowledge via label correlation between categories. Although improvement is demonstrated, their method depends on a large number of human-driven multi-label data.

The exploration of auxiliary data drawn from a different distribution for the target data has received a rapidly growing interest for visual object categorization [18,19]. The methods exploiting knowledge of either labeled or unlabeled data can be generally divided into several categories [6]: transfer by *model parameters* [20], by *data instances* [21], and by *feature representation* [22]. However, most of these approaches handle only transfer learning *from multiple classes to a single class*, in which knowledge from multiple sources is transferred to improve a single object category in the target. Thus it results in sub-optimal effectiveness on solving multi-class recognition problems.

Another notable category of work is to leverage auxiliary data to build a number of classifiers, and new feature representations of target data are yielded by applying these classifiers to themselves, e.g., *classemes* [23]. Along this line of thoughts, knowledge embedded within source domain can be revealed and then transferred to target domain for further use [24,25]. However, exploring good and proper features among such a rich set to address the target task still relies on a large number of training data in practice. In contrast, our method transfers knowledge by common attribute discovery instead of feature augmentation, and hence allows to account for such an ill-posed situation.

**Algorithm 1.** *AdaBoost.OC*

---

**Input:** Dataset $D = \{(\mathbf{x}_n \in \mathcal{X}, y_n \in \mathcal{Y})\}_{n=1}^N$ of $C$ classes, iteration $U$.

**Output:** Classifier $F(\mathbf{x}) = \arg\max_{c \in \mathcal{Y}} \sum_{t=1}^U \alpha_t [\![f_t(\mathbf{x}) = B_t(c)]\!]$.

**Initialize:** $\tilde{w}_{n,c} = [\![y_n \neq c]\!]/(N(C-1))$, for $1 \leq n \leq N$ and $1 \leq c \leq C$

**for** $t \leftarrow 1, 2, \ldots, U$ **do**

  1. Learn a class partition function $B_t : \mathcal{Y} \to \{-1, 1\}$.

  2. Compute data weights $\{w_n\}_{n=1}^N$ by

$$w_n = \frac{\sum_{c=1}^C \tilde{w}_{n,c} [\![B_t(y_n) \neq B_t(c)]\!]}{\sum_{j=1}^N \sum_{c=1}^C \tilde{w}_{j,c} [\![B_t(y_j) \neq B_t(c)]\!]}.$$

  3. Select weak learner $f_t : \mathcal{X} \to \{-1, 1\}$ by

$$f_t = \arg\min_f \sum_{n=1}^N w_n [\![f(\mathbf{x}_n) \neq B_t(y_n)]\!].$$

  4. Compute coefficient $\alpha_t = \frac{1}{2} \ln \frac{1-\epsilon}{\epsilon}$, where

$$\epsilon = \frac{1}{2} \sum_{n=1}^N \sum_{c \in \mathcal{Y}} \tilde{w}_{n,c}([\![B_t(y_n) \neq f_t(\mathbf{x}_n)]\!] + [\![B_t(c) = f_t(\mathbf{x}_n)]\!]).$$

  5. Update and normalize data weights $\{\tilde{w}_{n,c}\}_{n=1,c=1}^{N,C}$ by

$$\tilde{w}_{n,c} = \tilde{w}_{n,c} \cdot \exp\left(\alpha_t([\![B_t(y_n) \neq f_t(\mathbf{x}_n)]\!] + [\![B_t(c) = f_t(\mathbf{x}_n)]\!])\right)/Z.$$

---

## 3    AdaBoost.OC for Multi-class Classification

We introduce AdaBoost.OC [10] in this section, since some of its key elements are used in the establishment of the proposed approach. AdaBoost.OC is a multi-class boosting algorithm, which integrates *error-correcting output codes (ECOC)* [26] into the procedure of boosting, and solves a multi-class classification problem by reducing it to a set of binary ones. With dataset $D = \{(\mathbf{x}_n \in \mathcal{X}, y_n \in \mathcal{Y})\}_{n=1}^N$ of $C$ classes where $\mathcal{Y} = \{1, ..., C\}$, the steps of AdaBoost.OC are given in Algorithm 1.

AdaBoost.OC links the successive boosting iterations by keeping an array of weights $\{\tilde{w}_{n,c}\}_{c=1}^C$ for each $\mathbf{x}_n$. Except for $\{\tilde{w}_{n,y_n}\}_{n=1}^N$, weights $\{\tilde{w}_{n,c}\}_{n=1,c=1}^{N,C}$ are uniformly distributed in initialization. At iteration $t$, an *output code or partition function* $B_t$ is first built to divide the set of class labels into two subsets, i.e., $B_t : \mathcal{Y} \to \{-1, 1\}$. As suggested in [10], the optimal $B_t$ is obtained by maximizing

$$J(B_t) = \sum_{c,c' \in \mathcal{Y}} [\![B_t(c) \neq B_t(c')]\!] w(c, c'), \text{ where } w(c, c') = \sum_{n=1}^N \tilde{w}_{n,c} [\![c' = y_n]\!] \quad (1)$$

and $[\![\cdot]\!]$ denotes the indicator function. As $w(c, c')$ measures the *difficulty* of separating data of class $c$ and $c'$, maximizing $J(B_t)$ in Eq.(1) tends to assign two classes that currently mix together to opposite subsets. It follows that more emphases on separating these difficult classes will be given at this iteration.

Since partition function $B_t$ converts the multi-class learning problem to the binary one, the data weights, weak hypothesis, and its ensemble coefficient are respectively computed in step $2 \sim 4$ of Algorithm 1. Iteration $t$ is then completed by updating the data weights. Refer to [10] for the details of AdaBoost.OC.

# 4   Multi-class Transfer Learning

We carry out multi-class transfer learning by generalizing AdaBoost.OC to jointly deal with two multi-class learning tasks (one from source and the other from target). At each iteration, we discover a discriminant attribute that is commonly shared by the two domains via redesigning the partition function. By this attribute, the two learning problems become two *related, binary* (with or without this attribute) ones. It follows that knowledge transfer from source to target can be accomplished via the concept of classifier sharing. We summarize the proposed approach in Algorithm 2. In the following, we first give the problem definition. Then the two key components of our approach, including (i) *sharing the partition functions* for domain correlation and (ii) *jointly learning domain-dependent classifiers* for knowledge transfer, are respectively described.

## 4.1   Problem Definition

Given a *source domain* dataset $D_S = \{(\mathbf{x}_n^S \in \mathcal{X}, y_n^S \in \mathcal{Y}_S = \{1, ..., C_S\})\}_{n=1}^{N_S}$ of $C_S$ classes and a *target domain* dataset $D_T = \{(\mathbf{x}_n^T \in \mathcal{X}, y_n^T \in \mathcal{Y}_T = \{C_S + 1, ..., C_S + C_T\})\}_{n=1}^{N_T}$ of $C_T$ classes, our goal is to learn a classifier that recognize target data with low generalization error. This goal is achieved by considering not only information extracted from $D_T$ but also knowledge transferred from $D_S$. In the setting, the data space $\mathcal{X}$ in the source and target domains is the same. No assumption about the correlation between $D_S$ and $D_T$ is required.

To deal with complex visual recognition tasks, we consider using multiple descriptors to more precisely characterize the data, i.e., $\mathbf{x}_n = \{\mathbf{x}_{n,m} \in \mathcal{X}_m\}_{m=1}^M$. To handle the unfavorable diversity of representation among $\{\mathcal{X}_m\}$, we represent data under each descriptor by a *kernel matrix*. It allows that these features can be combined in the domain of kernel matrices. For each descriptor $m$, the corresponding kernel matrix $K_m$ and kernel function $k_m$ can be constructed by

$$K_m(n, n') = k_m(\mathbf{x}_n, \mathbf{x}_{n'}) = \exp\left(-\gamma_m d_m^2(\mathbf{x}_{n,m}, \mathbf{x}_{n',m})\right), \tag{2}$$

where $d_m$ is the associated distance function, and $\gamma_m$ is a positive constant. We empirically set $1/\gamma_m$ as the average of the pairwise distances. The resulting kernels $\{K_m\}_{m=1}^M$ will serve as the information bottleneck for data access.

## 4.2   On Sharing Partition Functions for Domain Correlation

At this stage, we aim to correlate two multi-class learning tasks to facilitate knowledge transfer. As mentioned before, this is fulfilled by deriving a class partition function at each iteration of AdaBoost.OC. Two criteria are considered: 1) As in AdaBoost.OC, the partition function should be discriminant for both domains; 2) As in transfer learning, a pair of similar classes (in the view of their data distributions) in the opposite domains should be partitioned into the same side. We propose an effective method to learn the discriminant, commonly-shared partition function, detailed in the following three steps.

**Algorithm 2.** *Multi-class Transfer Learning*

---

**Input:** source data $\{(\mathbf{x}_n^S \in \mathcal{X}, y_n^S \in \mathcal{Y}_S)\}_{n=1}^{N_S}$ of $C_S$ classes,
    target data $\{(\mathbf{x}_n^T \in \mathcal{X}, y_n^T \in \mathcal{Y}_T)\}_{n=1}^{N_T}$ of $C_T$ classes, iterations $U$
**Output:** target domain classifier $F(\mathbf{x}) = \arg\max_{c \in \mathcal{Y}_T} \sum_{t=1}^{U} \alpha_t^T [\![ f_t^T(\mathbf{x}) = B_t(c) ]\!]$
**Initialize:** $\tilde{w}_{n,c}^S = [\![ y_n^S \neq c ]\!]/(N_S(C_S - 1))$, for $1 \leq n \leq N_S$ and $c \in \mathcal{Y}_S$
    $\tilde{w}_{n,c}^T = [\![ y_n^T \neq c ]\!]/(N_T(C_T - 1))$, for $1 \leq n \leq N_T$ and $c \in \mathcal{Y}_T$.
**for** $t \leftarrow 1, 2, \ldots, U$ **do**
  1. Construct the class partition function $B_t$ via (6).
  2. Compute data weights $\{w_n^\ell\}_{n=1, \ell \in \{S,T\}}^{N_\ell}$ by
$$w_n^\ell = \frac{\sum_{c \in \mathcal{Y}_\ell} \tilde{w}_{n,c}^\ell [\![ B_t(y_n^\ell) \neq B_t(c) ]\!]}{\sum_{j=1}^{N_\ell} \sum_{c \in \mathcal{Y}_\ell} \tilde{w}_{j,c}^\ell [\![ B_t(y_j^\ell) \neq B_t(c) ]\!]}.$$
  3. Get a pair of weak classifiers $f_t^S$ and $f_t^T$ via Algorithm 3.
  4. Compute coefficient $\alpha_t^\ell = \frac{1}{2} \ln \frac{1 - \epsilon_\ell}{\epsilon_\ell}$, for $\ell \in \{S, T\}$, where
$$\epsilon_\ell = \frac{1}{2} \sum_{n=1}^{N_\ell} \sum_{c \in \mathcal{Y}_\ell} \tilde{w}_{n,c}^\ell ([\![ B_t(y_n^\ell) \neq f_t^\ell(\mathbf{x}_n^\ell) ]\!] + [\![ B_t(c) = f_t^\ell(\mathbf{x}_n^\ell) ]\!]).$$
  5. Update and normalize data weights $\{\tilde{w}_{n,c}^\ell\}_{n=1, c \in \mathcal{Y}_\ell, \ell \in \{S,T\}}^{N_\ell}$ by
$$\tilde{w}_{n,c}^\ell = \tilde{w}_{n,c}^\ell \exp\left(\alpha_t^\ell([\![ B_t(y_n^\ell) \neq f_t^\ell(\mathbf{x}_n^\ell) ]\!] + [\![ B_t(c) = f_t^\ell(\mathbf{x}_n^\ell) ]\!])\right)/Z_\ell.$$

---

**1. Construct *Intra-domain Graph* $G$:** The vertices of $G$ are over data classes of both domains. Its edge weights are defined in $W \in \mathbb{R}^{(C_S + C_T) \times (C_S + C_T)}$ by

$$W(c, c') = \begin{cases} w^S(c, c'), & \text{if } c \in \mathcal{Y}_S \wedge c' \in \mathcal{Y}_S, \\ w^T(c, c'), & \text{if } c \in \mathcal{Y}_T \wedge c' \in \mathcal{Y}_T, \\ 0, & \text{otherwise}, \end{cases} \tag{3}$$

where $w^S(c, c')$ is the same as $w(c, c')$ in Eq.(1) except only source data are considered. Similarly, $w^T(c, c')$ is computed for target data.

**2. Construct *Inter-domain Graph* $G'$:** Similar to $G$, the edges of graph $G'$ are recorded in $W' \in \mathbb{R}^{(C_S + C_T) \times (C_S + C_T)}$, defined by

$$W'(c, c') = \begin{cases} s(c, c'), & \text{if } c \in \mathcal{Y}_T \wedge c' \in \mathcal{Y}_S, \\ s(c', c), & \text{if } c' \in \mathcal{Y}_T \wedge c \in \mathcal{Y}_S, \\ 0, & \text{otherwise}, \end{cases} \tag{4}$$

where $s : \mathcal{Y}_T \times \mathcal{Y}_S \to \mathbb{R}$ measures the similarity between two classes of opposite domains. To account for the imbalance in data numbers, $s$ is defined by

$$s(c, c') = \sum_{\{\mathbf{x}_n^T | y_n^T = c\}} w_n^T \max_{\{\mathbf{x}_{n'}^S | y_{n'}^S = c'\}} k(\mathbf{x}_n^T, \mathbf{x}_{n'}^S), \tag{5}$$

where $w_n^T$ is the weight of $\mathbf{x}_n^T$ in AdaBoost.OC and $k$ is the kernel function. Note that $s$ is *asymmetrically* defined for classes in the source and target domains.

By Eq.(5), it measures how well source class $c'$ *covers* target class $c$. For multiple kernels, we simply adopt the average of the inter-domain graphs of all kernels.

**3. Establish Partition Function $B$:** The shared partition function $B : \mathcal{Y}_S \cup \mathcal{Y}_T \rightarrow \{-1, 1\}$ is built as follows

$$B(c) = \begin{cases} +1, & \text{if } \mathbf{b}^*(c) \geq \theta, \\ -1, & \text{otherwise,} \end{cases} \tag{6}$$

where $\theta$ is a threshold and $\mathbf{b}^*(c)$ is the $c$th element of $\mathbf{b}^* \in \mathbb{R}^{C_S + C_T}$, which is the generalized eigenvector corresponding to the largest eigenvalue of

$$L\mathbf{b} = \lambda L' \mathbf{b}. \tag{7}$$

$L = \text{diag}(W \cdot \mathbf{1}) - W$ and $L' = \text{diag}(W' \cdot \mathbf{1}) - W'$ in Eq.(7) are the *graph Laplacian* of $G$ and $G'$ respectively.

To gain insight into the learned partition function $B$ in Eq.(6), we consider the following optimization problem

$$B^* = \arg\max_B J_{dis}(B)/J_{shr}(B), \text{ where} \tag{8}$$

$$J_{dis}(B) = \sum_{c,c' \in \mathcal{Y}_S} [\![B(c) \neq B(c')]\!] w^S(c, c') + \sum_{c,c' \in \mathcal{Y}_T} [\![B(c) \neq B(c')]\!] w^T(c, c'), \tag{9}$$

$$J_{shr}(B) = \sum_{c \in \mathcal{Y}_T} \sum_{c' \in \mathcal{Y}_S} [\![B(c) \neq B(c')]\!] s(c, c'). \tag{10}$$

To optimize Eq.(8), maximizing $J_{dis}(B)$ and minimizing $J_{shr}(B)$ are required simultaneously. While the former makes the learned $B$ *discriminant* for both domains (cf. Eq.(1) and Eq.(9)), the latter connects the two domains by partitioning similar classes of opposite domains into the same side. Thus the yielded $B$ is commonly *shared* by two domains. Maximizing $J_{dis}(B)$ itself is a NP complete problem [10]. We instead adopt the continuous relaxation to solve Eq.(8). That is, an auxiliary variable $\mathbf{b} \in \mathbb{R}^{(C_S + C_T)}$ is adding, and terms $[\![B(c) \neq B(c')]\!]$ in Eq.(9) and Eq.(10) are replaced with $||\mathbf{b}(c) - \mathbf{b}(c')||^2$. It follows that the resulting optimization problem can be optimally solved via Eq.(7). The proof is omitted here for the sake of space. After $\mathbf{b}^*$ in Eq.(7) is obtained, the value of threshold $\theta$ in Eq.(6) can be determined by maximizing the objective function Eq.(8).

### 4.3   On Jointly Learning Classifiers for Knowledge Transfer

Once the partition function $B$ is solved, datasets $D_S$ and $D_T$ at the current iteration of boosting become *weighted, binary,* and *related,* i.e., $\{w_n^S, \mathbf{x}_n^S, B(y_n^S)\}_{n=1}^{N_S}$ and $\{w_n^T, \mathbf{x}_n^T, B(y_n^T)\}_{n=1}^{N_T}$. To learn an accurate target domain classifier, we use the principle of classifier sharing [11,12]. This way, not only information obtained in the target domain but also knowledge borrowed from the source domain can be considered. Apart from knowledge transfer, two additional requirements arise

---

**Algorithm 3.** *Dual-domain Boosting*

---

**Input:** weighted source data $\{(w_n^S, \mathbf{x}_n^S, y_n^S \in \pm 1)\}_{n=1}^{N_S}$,
        weighted target data $\{(w_n^T, \mathbf{x}_n^T, y_n^T \in \pm 1)\}_{n=1}^{N_T}$, iteration $V$.
**Output:** source classifier $f^S$ and target classifier $f^T$, where
$$f^{\ell}(\mathbf{x}) = \text{sign} \sum_{t=1}^{V} \beta_t^{\ell} h_t(\mathbf{x}) \text{ for } \ell \in \{S, T\}.$$
**for** $t \leftarrow 1, 2, \ldots, V$ **do**
   1. Select the optimal dyadic hypercut $h_t$ by
$$h_t = \arg\min_h \sum_{\ell \in \{S,T\}} \sum_{n=1}^{N_{\ell}} w_n^{\ell} [\![h_t(\mathbf{x}_n^{\ell}) \neq y_n^{\ell}]\!].$$
   2. Compute coefficient $\beta_t^{\ell} = \max\left(0, \frac{1}{2} \ln \frac{1-\epsilon_{\ell}}{\epsilon_{\ell}}\right)$, for $\ell \in \{S, T\}$ where
$$\epsilon_{\ell} = \sum_{n=1}^{N_{\ell}} w_n^{\ell} [\![h_t(\mathbf{x}_n^{\ell}) \neq y_n^{\ell}]\!].$$
   3. Update and normalize data weights $\{w_n^{\ell}\}_{n=1, \ell \in \{S,T\}}^{N_{\ell}}$ by
$$w_n^{\ell} = w_n^{\ell} \exp\left(-y_n^{\ell} \beta_t^{\ell} h_t(\mathbf{x}_n^{\ell})\right)/Z_{\ell}.$$

---

at this stage: 1) The learning process can deal with weighted data; 2) Multiple kernels should be considered jointly. We fulfill these requirements by introducing a boosting-based approach, whose two main elements are given below.

**The Design of Weak Learners.** To learn a boosted classifier with multiple kernels, we adopt the method proposed in [12]. The discriminant power of each kernel is first converted into a set of weak learners, called *dyadic hypercuts* [27]. It turns out that multiple kernel learning is achieved by boosting over the pool of dyadic hypercuts yielded from all the kernels.

A dyadic hypercut $h$ is composed of three elements: a positive sample $\mathbf{x}_p$ (i.e., $y_p = 1$), a negative sample $\mathbf{x}_n$ (i.e., $y_n = -1$), and a kernel function $k_m$. Note that $\mathbf{x}_p$ and $\mathbf{x}_n$ can be from the source or target domains. The yielded model is

$$h(\mathbf{x}) = \text{sign}(k_m(\mathbf{x}_p, \mathbf{x}) - k_m(\mathbf{x}_n, \mathbf{x}) - b), \tag{11}$$

where $b$ is a threshold, whose value is determined by error minimization in boosting. The size of the weak learner pool is $|\mathcal{H}| = N^+ \times N^- \times M$, where $N^+$ ($N^-$) is the number of positive (negative) data, and $M$ is the number of kernels.

**Dual-Domain Boosting for Knowledge Transfer.** To transfer knowledge from the source domain to the target domain, we follow the strategy of classifier sharing in [12] where the relatedness between tasks are modeled by the shared weak learners while the difference between tasks are reflected by their respective ensemble coefficients. That is, the binary classifiers $f^S$ and $f^T$ in the two domains are respectively given by

$$f^{\ell}(\mathbf{x}) = \sum_{t=1}^{V} \beta_t^{\ell} h_t(\mathbf{x}), \text{ for } \ell \in \{S, T\}, \tag{12}$$

where $\{h_t\}$ are the shared weak learners and $\{\beta_t^\ell\}$ are the respective coefficients.

Algorithm 3 provides a systematic way of learning $f^S$ and $f^T$ simultaneously. It can be proved that the dyadic hypercut $h_t$ picked in the step 1 will directly minimize the total *exponential loss* of the two domains, while the the ensemble coefficients defined in step 2 are respectively determined to minimize the exponential loss of the corresponding domains. Hence our approach comes with theoretical support of AdaBoost. It turns out that the high risk of overfitting resulting from insufficient samples in the target domain could considerably alleviated, since knowledge from the correlated source domain can smoothly regularize and benefit the process of learning $f^T$ via joint weak learner selection. Further, the intrinsic differences between the two domains can be properly addressed through their respective ensemble coefficients whose values are determined by considering data in individual domains. It hence relieves the unfavorable effect of *negative transfer*, which typically occurs if the underlying differences between the source and target domains are not properly modeled in knowledge transfer.

## 5 Experimental Results

The proposed method is evaluated in this section. We describe in turn the adopted datasets, features and kernels, baseline approaches, and the within-database and cross-database transfer learning settings along with their results.

### 5.1 Datasets

To evaluate the performance of the proposed method, we conduct experiments on three publicly available datasets, Caltech256 [28], SUN09 [29], and MSRC [30]. Although each of these datasets has its own emphasis [31], they are popular benchmarks of object recognition due to their broad coverage of object characteristics and divergent appearances of objects within a single category.

### 5.2 Features and Kernels

Generally speaking, there is no universal feature that can be effectively used to recognize diverse object categories. Hence, we select four representative features to capture various characteristics of images, including:

**GIST:** We apply the *gist* descriptor [14] to the resized images with an $128 \times 128$ pixel prior. Each dimension of the resulted vectors is normalized to have a standard normal distribution, i.e., zero-mean and unit-variance.

**BoW-SIFT:** We uniformly sample interesting points in an image and describe them by the SIFT descriptor [13]. With a dictionary of $1,000$ visual words, each image is represented as a histogram using this dictionary.

**Color Histogram:** We use a 166-bin color histogram extracted from the HSV color space to represent an image, where the hue, saturation, and intensity channels are divided into 18, 3, and 3 bins, respectively, and there are four additional scales of intensity for describing gray images.

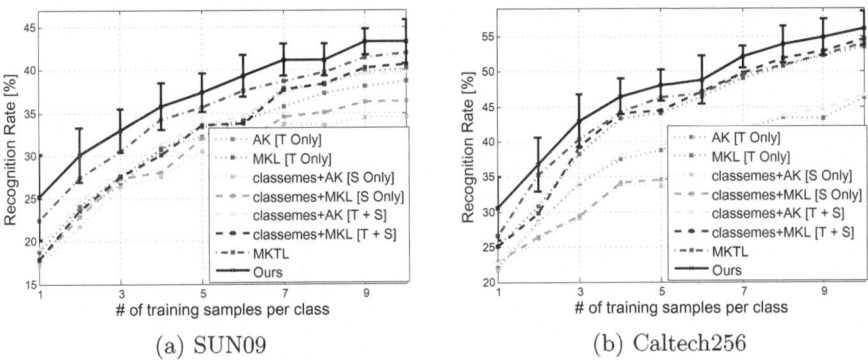

(a) SUN09                              (b) Caltech256

**Fig. 2.** Within-database transfer learning in (a) SUN09 and (b) Caltech256 datasets. Recognition rates of all the baselines and our approach are plotted.

**Texton:** We consider 99 filters from three filter banks to generate the vocabularies of texture prototypes [32]. Hence, an image can be represented by a histogram that records its probability distribution over all the generated textons.

For each feature, we construct its RBF kernel with the Euclidean distance.

### 5.3  Baselines

For comparison, we establish the following baselines:

**Target Only:** Neither auxiliary data nor prior knowledge are involved in the baselines of this category. Since kernel machines working with multiple kernels are the most powerful methodologies for object recognition, we adopt two multi-kernel extensions of SVMs, including the *average kernel* (AK) suggested in [3] and the ensemble kernel learned by the *multiple kernel learning* (MKL) software [5]. The two baselines are respectively denoted as *AK [T Only]* and *MKL [T Only]*.

**Source Only:** We implement the *classemes* [23], a set of powerful features designed for transfer learning, to deliver knowledge from source to target. To this end, an SVM-based classifier with probabilistic outputs is learned for each source object class. The classemes are the probabilistic estimates obtained by applying these classifiers to the target data. While the procedure is performed for each of the adopted features, four new kernels based on classemes are constructed. Baselines *classemes+AK [S Only]* and *classemes+MKL [S Only]* are then respectively established by coupling AK and MKL to the four new kernels.

**Target + Source:** To fuse the information of both the two domains, we jointly consider the kernels yielded by visual features and classemes. Similarly, baselines *classemes+AK [T+S]* and *classemes+MKL [T+S]* are established. Besides, our approach is compared with *multi kernel transfer learning* (MKTL) [25], which is one of the best transfer learning algorithms and supports heterogeneous transfer from different kinds of priors.

**Table 1.** The relative improvement in accuracy (%) and $p$ value w.r.t AK [T Only]

| Dataset | SUN09 | | | | | Caltech256 | | | | |
|---|---|---|---|---|---|---|---|---|---|---|
| No. of samples per class | 1 | 3 | 5 | 10 | $p$ | 1 | 3 | 5 | 10 | $p$ |
| AK [T Only] | — | — | — | — | — | — | — | — | — | — |
| MKL [T Only] | 5.39 | 3.91 | 3.60 | 3.56 | 0.97 | 14.00 | 7.70 | 13.73 | 15.40 | 0.11 |
| classemes+AK [S Only] | -3.03 | -0.90 | -5.34 | -10.78 | 0.31 | -1.64 | -14.39 | -12.91 | -18.81 | 0.03 |
| classemes+MKL [S Only] | 0.56 | 2.71 | -0.62 | -6.24 | 0.68 | 4.36 | -13.45 | -1.08 | -14.11 | 0.11 |
| classemes+AK [T + S] | 8.20 | 6.32 | 4.10 | 2.58 | 0.97 | 2.91 | 0.71 | 1.50 | 0.69 | 0.97 |
| classemes+MKL [T + S] | 0.79 | 3.53 | 4.10 | 4.80 | 0.97 | 14.09 | 15.45 | 14.82 | 17.73 | 0.03 |
| MKTL [25] | 19.78 | 5.94 | 7.39 | 2.73 | 0.68 | 15.00 | 10.00 | 8.00 | 11.17 | 0.03 |
| Ours | **41.80** | **23.83** | **16.09** | **11.76** | **0.11** | **38.82** | **26.38** | **24.01** | **20.88** | **0.006** |

## 5.4 Within-Database Transfer Learning

We first carry out within-database transfer learning on SUN09 and Caltech256 datasets. (MSRC dataset consists of only 22 categories, so it won't be adopted in the experiments of within-database transfer.) For each dataset, 10 target categories and 20 source categories are randomly selected. We extract 1 to 10 samples as well as 50 samples of each target class for training and testing respectively. The number of samples in each source class is set as 50. All experiments are repeated ten times to reduce the effect of sampling. As for boosting iterations, we set $U$ and $V$ in Algorithm 2 and 3 as 300 and 25 respectively.

In Fig. 2, the average recognition rates of our approach and other baseline methods are plotted. Note that only the standard deviations of our approach are shown for the sake of clearness. The consistent trend of curves indicates that our approach outperforms the other baselines. Although baselines with only source priors, e.g., classemes+AK [S only], don't work well, incorporating the source knowledge indeed helps in constructing more accurate classifiers, e.g., classemes+AK [T+S]. Besides, baselines with MKL work better than baselines with AK in most of the cases. This is because SimpleMKL [5] effectively selects the optimal kernel combination to emphasize discriminant features for the given data. With regard to MKTL, it works better than all other baselines.

The relative improvement of recognition rates with respect to AK [T Only] is reported in Table 1, in which entries for 1, 3, 5, 10 samples per class are computed via $(A-B)/B \times 100\%$ where $A$ is the recognition rate of each method and $B$ is the recognition rate of AK [T Only]. Besides, the widely-used Kolmogorov-Smirnov test (KS test), a type of significance test, is also applied to the recognition rates of 1 to 10 samples per class (quantified by $p$ value); the lower the $p$ value is, the better the relative performance is. We observe that the less the training samples, the more helpful the source information is. The quantitative results validate that our method is indeed effective for object recognition with few training examples.

It is worthy of noting that, the effect of *higher start* [18] in our approach is quite significant in the cases where one training sample per class is available. The relative performance w.r.t AK [T Only] is about 42% in SUN09 or 39% in Caltech256. Moreover, this improvement is consistent even in the cases of 10 training samples per class. It reveals the merit in the aspect of *higher asymptote* [18].

## 5.5    Cross-Database Transfer Learning

We evaluate if the proposed approach works for cross-database transfer. The experimental setting is the same as the one described in section 5.4, except for data of the source domain and the target domain are from different databases. With Caltech256, MSRC, and SUN09, totally we have six combinations.

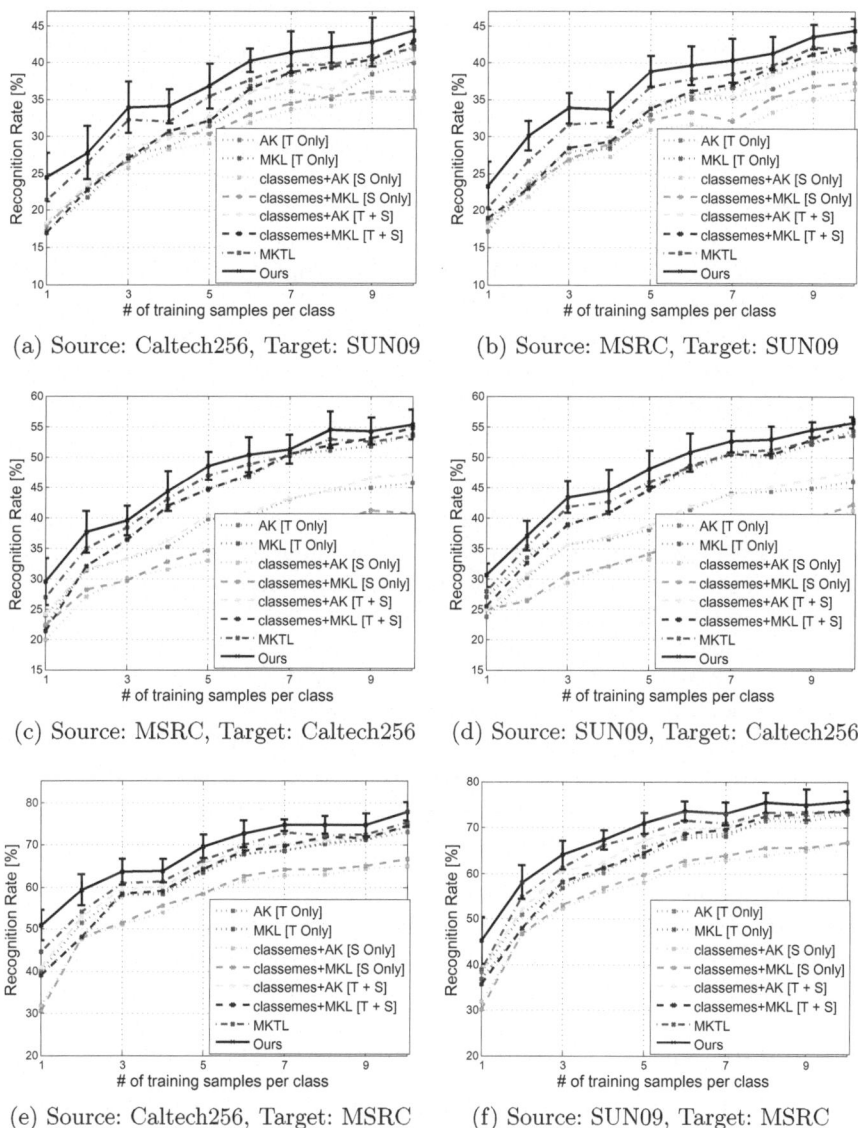

(a) Source: Caltech256, Target: SUN09    (b) Source: MSRC, Target: SUN09

(c) Source: MSRC, Target: Caltech256    (d) Source: SUN09, Target: Caltech256

(e) Source: Caltech256, Target: MSRC    (f) Source: SUN09, Target: MSRC

**Fig. 3.** Transfer learning across Caltech256, MSRC and SUN09 datasets. Recognition rates are plotted as a function of the number of training samples per class.

The recognition rates of our approach and all baselines are shown in Fig. 3. In the six settings of cross-database of transfer learning, our approach consistently achieves the best results. Besides, the effects of higher-start as well as higher-asymptote still remain in most cases. This validates that the proposed approach can explore commonly shared knowledge across databases, and use it to alleviate the difficulty caused by learning with few training examples.

In Fig. 3, it is observed that the performance gains of our approach with respect to baselines working on just target data, e.g., MKL [T Only], vary from case to case. We consider that it may result from the different degrees of similarity between the source and the target domains. As indicated in [31], each image in Caltech256 is usually pictured indoors, and always contains a single object. The images in MSRC, on the other hand, often contain the entire scene and are captured outdoors. For SUN09, objects may be photographed indoors or outdoors but are more similar to these in MSRC. Above observations explain why transferring knowledge between Caltech256 and MSRC is more difficult than between SUN09 and MSRC. Thus, the performance gains of our approach are relatively limited in cases of Fig. 3(c) and (e), but become significant in Fig. 3(b) and (f). To summarize, the proposed approach can effectively transfer useful knowledge from the source domain, and leads to significant improvements of performances in both the cases of within-database and cross-database transfer. This manifests its robustness and generality.

## 6     Conclusions

The proposed approach transfers knowledge from multiple classes to multiple classes by a two-layer boosting architecture. The outer layer discovers commonly shared attribute partitions, which cast two unrelated, multi-class learning problems into a series of binary, related ones. The inner layer explores useful source knowledge to learn discriminant and robust attribute classifiers in the target domain. Our approach is comprehensively evaluated with three benchmark datasets of object recognition. The significant improvements on recognition rates consolidate the usefulness of our approach. Moreover, the flexibility of our approach in cross-category and cross-database knowledge transfer makes it quite suitable to deal with increasingly complex recognition tasks, such as recognizing new categories or handling new datasets with few manually labeled data.

**Acknowledgement.** This study is conducted under the "III Innovative and Prospective Technologies Project" of the Institute for Information Industry which is subsidized by the Ministry of Economy Affairs of the Republic of China. It is also supported in part by grant NSC 101-2221-E-001-018.

## References

1. Lin, Y.Y., Liu, T.L., Fuh, C.S.: Multiple kernel learning for dimensionality reduction. TPAMI (2011)
2. Varma, M., Ray, D.: Learning the discriminative power-invariance trade-off. In: ICCV (2007)

3. Gehler, P., Nowozin, S.: On feature combination for multiclass object classification. In: ICCV (2009)
4. Bach, F.R., Lanckriet, G.R.G., Jordan, M.I.: Multiple kernel learning, conic duality, and the SMO algorithm. In: ICML (2004)
5. Rakotomamonjy, A., Bach, F.R., Canu, S., Grandvalet, Y.: SimpleMKL. JMLR (2008)
6. Pan, S.J., Yang, Q.: A survey on transfer learning. TKDE (2010)
7. Dai, W., Yang, Q., Xue, G.R., Yu, Y.: Boosting for transfer learning. In: ICML (2007)
8. Fei-Fei, L., Fergus, R., Perona, P.: One-shot learning of object categories. TPAMI (2006)
9. Yao, Y., Doretto, G.: Boosting for transfer learning with multiple sources. In: CVPR (2010)
10. Schapire, R.: Using output codes to boost multiclass learning problems. In: ICML (1997)
11. Torralba, A., Murphy, K., Freeman, W.: Sharing visual features for multiclass and multiview object detection. TPAMI (2007)
12. Lin, Y.Y., Tsai, J.F., Liu, T.L.: Efficient discriminative local learning for object recognition. In: ICCV (2009)
13. Lowe, D.: Distinctive image features from scale-invariant keypoints. IJCV (2004)
14. Oliva, A., Torralba, A.: Modeling the shape of the scene: A holistic representation of the spatial envelope. IJCV (2001)
15. Farhadi, A., Endres, I., Hoiem, D., Forsyth, D.: Describing objects by their attributes. In: CVPR (2009)
16. Lampert, C.H., Nickisch, H., Harmeling, S.: Learning to detect unseen object classes by betweenclass attribute transfer. In: CVPR (2009)
17. Qi, G.J., Aggarwal, C., Rui, Y., Tian, Q., Chang, S., Huang, T.: Towards cross-category knowledge propagation for learning visual concepts. In: CVPR (2011)
18. Tommasi, T., Orabona, F., Caputo, B.: Safety in numbers: Learning categories from few examples with multi model knowledge transfer. In: CVPR (2010)
19. Kulis, B., Saenko, K., Darrell, T.: What you saw is not what you get: Domain adaptation using asymmetric kernel transforms. In: CVPR (2011)
20. Duan, L., Tsang, I., Xu, D., Maybank, S.: Domain transfer SVM for video concept detection. In: CVPR (2009)
21. Bickel, S., Bruckner, M., Scheffer, T.: Discriminative learning for differing training and test distributions. In: ICML (2007)
22. Bart, E., Ullman, S.: Cross-generalization: Learning novel classes from a single example by feature replacement. In: CVPR, pp. 672–679 (2005)
23. Torresani, L., Szummer, M., Fitzgibbon, A.: Efficient Object Category Recognition Using Classemes. In: Daniilidis, K., Maragos, P., Paragios, N. (eds.) ECCV 2010, Part I. LNCS, vol. 6311, pp. 776–789. Springer, Heidelberg (2010)
24. Daume III, H.: Frustratingly easy domain adaptation. In: ACL (2007)
25. Jie, L., Tommasi, T., Caputo, B.: Multiclass transfer learning from unconstrained priors. In: ICCV (2011)
26. Dietterich, T., Bakiri, G.: Solving multiclass learning problems via error-correcting output codes. JAIR (1995)
27. Moghaddam, B., Shakhnarovich, G.: Boosted dyadic kernel discriminants. In: NIPS (2002)
28. Griffin, G., Holub, A., Perona, P.: Caltech-256 object category dataset. Technical report, California Institute of Technology (2007)

29. Xiao, J., Hays, J., Ehinger, K., Oliva, A., Torralba, A.: SUN database: Large-scale scene recognition from abbey to zoo. In: CVPR (2010)
30. Winn, J., Criminisi, A., Minka, T.: Object categorization by learned universal visual dictionary. In: ICCV (2005)
31. Torralba, A., Efros, A.A.: Unbiased look at dataset bias. In: CVPR (2011)
32. Varma, M., Zisserman, A.: A statistical approach to texture classification from single images. IJCV (2005)

# Human Reidentification
# with Transferred Metric Learning

Wei Li, Rui Zhao, and Xiaogang Wang

Electronic Engineering Department, The Chinese University of Hong Kong

**Abstract.** Human reidentification is to match persons observed in non-overlapping camera views with visual features for inter-camera tracking. The ambiguity increases with the number of candidates to be distinguished. Simple temporal reasoning can simplify the problem by pruning the candidate set to be matched. Existing approaches adopt a fixed metric for matching all the subjects. Our approach is motivated by the insight that different visual metrics should be optimally learned for different candidate sets. We tackle this problem under a transfer learning framework. Given a large training set, the training samples are selected and reweighted according to their visual similarities with the query sample and its candidate set. A weighted maximum margin metric is online learned and transferred from a generic metric to a candidate-set-specific metric. The whole online reweighting and learning process takes less than two seconds per candidate set. Experiments on the VIPeR dataset and our dataset show that the proposed transferred metric learning significantly outperforms directly matching visual features or using a single generic metric learned from the whole training set.

## 1 Introduction

Human reidentification has drawn great interest in video surveillance recently [1–4]. It is to match humans observed in non-overlapping camera views based on their visual features and is very important for inter-camera tracking. Human reidentification is a challenging problem, since the same person observed in different camera views undergoes significant changes of resolutions, lightings, poses and viewpoints. Because humans captured by surveillance cameras, especially in far-field video surveillance, are often in small sizes and a lot of their visual details such as facial components are indistinguishable in images, some of them look similar in appearance. The ambiguity increases with the number of persons to be distinguished. Many visual features of characterizing color [5, 6], shape [7, 8] and texture [9–11] of objects have been proposed. In order to overcome the large visual changes across camera views, learning approaches were typically adopted. They learned either the transformations of visual features between camera views [12–15] or visual distance metrics [16–18, 2, 19, 4] from a training set.

In inter-camera tracking, given a query sample observed in a camera view, simple temporal reasoning can be made by roughly estimating the transition time across cameras. Such reasoning can simplify the matching problem by pruning

K.M. Lee et al. (Eds.): ACCV 2012, Part I, LNCS 7724, pp. 31–44, 2013.
© Springer-Verlag Berlin Heidelberg 2013

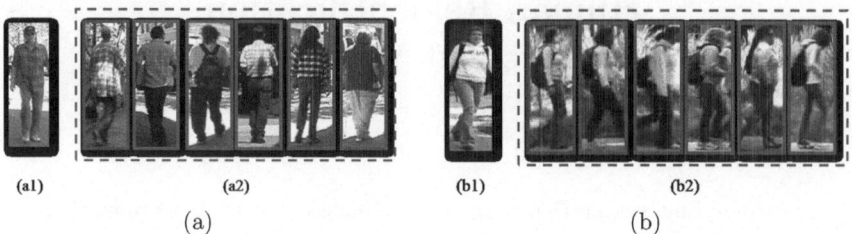

     (a1)              (a2)                 (b1)           (b2)

               (a)                                 (b)

**Fig. 1.** Examples of query samples and their corresponding candidate sets in human reidentification. (a1) and (b1) are query samples observed in a camera view. (a2) and (b2) are persons in the corresponding candidate sets observed in another camera view after pruning with temporal reasoning. The red windows indicate the truly matched persons. The persons in candidate set (a2) can be well distinguished with color histograms but some of them have similar texture. The persons in candidate set (b2) have similar color histograms. Therefore, distinguishing them has to rely more on other type of features.

the candidate set observed in another camera view. Existing approaches always use the same set of visual features and a fixed distance metric to match any query samples with any candidates, which is not an optimal solution. Since the goal is to distinguish a small number of persons in a particular candidate set, a candidate-set-specific visual metric is preferred. As an example shown in Figure 1, the persons in the first candidate set can be well distinguished with color histograms, while those in the second candidate set are similar in color and other features such as shape and texture could be more effective on them. Unfortunately, each person in the candidate set only has one sample observed in one camera view since the correspondences of samples across camera views are unknown during online tracking, while metric learning requires pairs of samples observed in different camera views with correspondence information. Therefore, directly applying existing metric learning algorithms to obtain a candidate-set-specific metric is infeasible. We tackle this problem under a transfer learning framework. As shown in Figure 2, for each sample in the candidate set, its nearest neighbors in the training set are found by directly matching their visual features. When the training set is large, the found nearest neighbors are likely to be visually similar to the sample in the candidate set and their corresponding training samples in another camera view are known with the ground truth labels. Therefore, the candidate-set-specific metric can be indirectly learned from the selected training pairs. These training pairs are weighted according to their visual similarities to the samples in the candidate set and the query sample. For each candidate set, a metric which maximizes the margin between the correctly matched pairs and wrongly matched pairs is learned [20]. In order to avoid overfitting, the candidate-set-specific metric is regularized by a generic metric learned from the whole training set. To the best of our knowledge, this is the first time for transfer learning to be applied to human reidentification. Experiments on the VIPeR database [21] and our dataset show that it significantly outperforms the approach of directly matching visual features or using a generic distance metric. The weighting and transfer learning process takes less than two seconds per candidate set. It can be applied to both online and offline human reidentification.

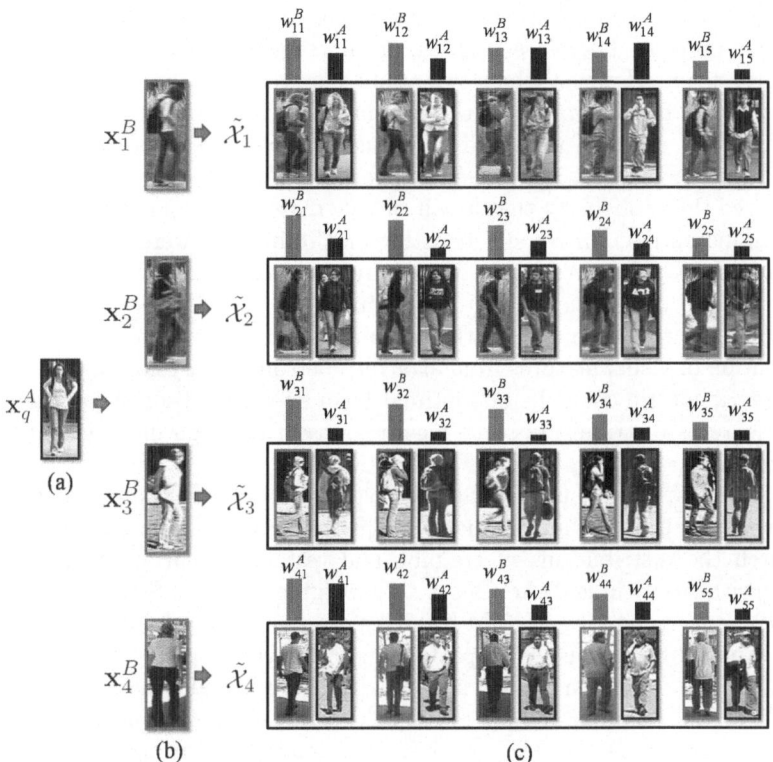

**Fig. 2.** (a) A query sample observed in camera view A. (b) Samples of four candidate persons observed in camera B based on temporal reasoning. (c) The nearest neighbors of each candidate in (b) found from a large training set by directly matching the visual features observed in camera B. Each person in the training set has a pair of samples observed in both cameras A and B according to manually labeled ground truth. Therefore the paired samples of the found nearest neighbors can be used to train the candidate-set-specific metric. Blue windows indicate samples observed in camera A and green windows indicate samples observed in camera B. $w_{ij}^A$ and $w_{ij}^B$ are the weights assigned to training samples according to their visual similarities with the candidates and the query sample respectively. See details in Section 3.2.

## 2    Related Work

Many approaches have been proposed to learn the distance metrics to match the visual features of image regions observed in different camera views. Schwartz and Davis [2] proposed an approach of projecting high dimensional features to a low dimensional discriminant latent space by Partial Least Squares reduction.

It weighted features according to their discriminative power to best distinguish the observations of one object with those of others in the training set in a one-against-all scheme. Lin and Davis [18] learned a different pairwise dissimilarity profile which best distinguished a pair of persons. It was assumed that a feature may be crucial to discriminate two very similar objects but not be effective for other objects. Therefore it is easier to train discriminative features in a pairwise scheme. However, these two approaches required that all the persons to be reidentified have examples in the training set. They can not re-identify a new person. Zheng *et al.* [4] proposed a *Probabilistic Relative Distance Comparison* model. It formulated object reidentification as a distance learning problem and maximized the probability that a pair of true match has a smaller distance than a wrong match pair. In [16, 19] boosting and RankSVM were used to select an optimal subset of features for matching objects across camera views. They could be generalized to persons outside the training set. They targeted on learning a generic metric to distinguish all the persons, which is very challenging since the distribution of visual features from arbitrary persons is very complex. Moreover, any generic metric could be suboptimal for a specific subset of persons whose visual features distribute in some local regions of the high dimensional feature space.

Transfer learning assumes that the distribution of the training data differs from the test data. It automatically adjusts the weights of training samples to match the distributions of training and test data. Various transfer learning algorithms, such as TrAdaBoost [22], weighted margin SVM [23], localized SVM [24] and cross-domain SVM [24] were proposed. Transfer learning has been widely applied to various vision problems such as object recognition [25], object detection [26], image and video retrieval [27], and visual concept classification [28, 24, 29, 30]. In cross-domain SVM [24], each training sample is weighted according to its closeness to the test data. It is related to our approach. However, different than [24], a distance metric instead of a hyperplane is learned in our case. Besides reweighting training samples, our adaptive metric is also regularized by a generic metric. Query-specific distance metric learning [31] optimally distinguishes query person with anyone else in the dataset, while ours optimally distinguish query person with others **ONLY** in the candidate set. So ours is both query-specific and candidate-set-specific which is the most important novelty of this paper.

## 3   Our Method

### 3.1   Visual Features

We employ five types of low-level visual features including dense color histograms, dense SIFT [32], HOG [7], Gabor [24] and LBP [10]. They characterize the color distributions, shape and texture of objects. Image regions are normalized to $160 \times 60$. For dense color histograms and dense SIFT, a uniform $20 \times 12$ grid is placed on the image region, and color histograms in the RGB color space and SIFT descriptors are densely computed on the grid. For each type of features, PCA is applied to retain 90% energy and then each feature vector is normalized to zero mean and unit variance. Different types of features are concatenated to form a single feature vector.

## 3.2   Searching and Weighting Training Samples

Our approach includes two key steps: searching and weighting nearest training samples for each candidate; and learning an adaptive metric for each candidate set. Let $\mathbf{x}_q^A$ be the visual feature vector of a query sample observed in camera A, and $\mathcal{X}_c^B = \{\mathbf{x}_1^B, \ldots, \mathbf{x}_N^B\}$ be a set of candidates observed in camera view B after pruning with temporal reasoning. For each candidate $\mathbf{x}_i^B$, a set of samples $\tilde{\mathcal{X}}_i^B = \{\tilde{\mathbf{x}}_{i_1}^B, \ldots, \tilde{\mathbf{x}}_{i_{K_i}}^B\}$ close to $\mathbf{x}_i^B$ is selected from the training set $\mathcal{S}$. A straightforward way is to set $\tilde{\mathcal{X}}_i^B$ as the $K$ nearest neighbors of $\mathbf{x}_i^B$ in $\mathcal{S}$ (denoted with $\mathcal{N}_K(\mathbf{x}_i^B)$) by comparing the visual features. However, this approach is not quite stable, since some $\mathbf{x}_i^B$ may be dissimilar with any samples in $\mathcal{S}$. In that case, none of the training samples should be selected and we should rely on the generic metric. We recompute the similarity between $\mathbf{x}_i^B$ and a sample $\tilde{\mathbf{x}}_j^B$ in $\mathcal{S}$ as following,

$$s(\mathbf{x}_i^B, \tilde{\mathbf{x}}_j^B) = \frac{|\mathcal{N}_K(\mathbf{x}_i^B) \cap \mathcal{N}_K(\tilde{\mathbf{x}}_j^B)|}{|\mathcal{N}_K(\mathbf{x}_i^B) \cup \mathcal{N}_K(\tilde{\mathbf{x}}_j^B)|}. \tag{1}$$

The intuition is that if $\mathbf{x}_i^B$ and $\tilde{\mathbf{x}}_j^B$ are visually similar, they should share more nearest neighbors in the training set[1]. $\tilde{\mathcal{X}}_i^B$ is selected by choosing $\tilde{\mathbf{x}}_j^B$ with $s(\mathbf{x}_i^B, \tilde{\mathbf{x}}_j^B) > s_0$, where $s_0$ is a threshold. $\mathcal{N}_K(\cdot)$ characterizes the geometric structures of the training set. It is more reliable than directly thresholding the visual distance $\|\mathbf{x}_i^B - \tilde{\mathbf{x}}_j^B\|_2^2$, whose value is difficult to be interpreted and whose threshold is hard to be decided. The nearest neighbors of training samples can be pre-computed offline and a reverse mapping maintains the neighbors of each sample. After $\mathcal{N}_K(\mathbf{x}_i^B)$ is online efficiently computed with Approximate Nearest Neighbor Search [33], $s(\mathbf{x}_i^B, \tilde{\mathbf{x}}_j^B)$ can be computed with a complexity of $O(K)$ using the reverse mapping. Once $\tilde{\mathcal{X}}_i^B$ is chosen, the corresponding training pairs $\tilde{\mathcal{X}}_i = \{(\tilde{\mathbf{x}}_{i_1}^A, \tilde{\mathbf{x}}_{i_1}^B), \ldots, (\tilde{\mathbf{x}}_{i_{K_i}}^A, \tilde{\mathbf{x}}_{i_{K_i}}^B)\}$ are obtained since the correspondences of training samples are known. In practice, one training sample $\tilde{\mathbf{x}}_j^B$ may correspond to multiple training samples in camera view A and more training pairs are obtained. In order to simplify the description, we assume that $\tilde{\mathbf{x}}_j^B$ only has one corresponding sample in another camera view without affecting the generalization of the proposed algorithm.

Each training pair $(\tilde{\mathbf{x}}_{i_j}^A, \tilde{\mathbf{x}}_{i_j}^B)$ is assigned with a weight $w_{ij}$ according to its visual similarities with the candidate sample $\mathbf{x}_i^B$ and the query sample $\mathbf{x}_q^A$. A training pair with a larger weight will have larger contribution for learning the adaptive metric. $w_{ij}$ is defined as following,

$$w_{ij} = w_{ij}^B \cdot w_{ij}^A, \tag{2}$$

---

[1] In our implementation $K = 10$.

$$w_{ij}^B = exp\left(-\frac{\|\mathbf{x}_i^B - \tilde{\mathbf{x}}_{ij}^B\|_2^2}{2\sigma_i^2}\right),$$ (3)

$$w_{ij}^A = exp\left(-\frac{\|\mathbf{x}_q^A - \tilde{\mathbf{x}}_{ij}^A\|_2^2}{2\sigma_0^2}\right),$$ (4)

where $\sigma_i^2 = \text{median}(\{\|\mathbf{x}_i^B - \tilde{\mathbf{x}}_{ij}^B\|_2^2\}_{\tilde{\mathbf{x}}_{ij}^B \in \tilde{\mathcal{X}}_i^B})$ and $\sigma_0^2 = \text{median}(\{\|\tilde{\mathbf{x}}_i^A - \tilde{\mathbf{x}}_j^A\|_2^2\}_{\tilde{\mathbf{x}}_i^A, \tilde{\mathbf{x}}_j^A \in \mathcal{S}})$. $w_{ij}^B$ is straightforward, since the selected training samples are supposed to be visually similar to the candidates. $w_{ij}^A$ has two purposes. (1) Even though some selected samples are similar with the candidate in camera B, their samples observed in camera A may be dissimilar with the query sample, because of pose variations. It is not useful to learn the adaptive metric from such training pairs, since their inter-camera variations are different than that of the query person. The learned adaptive metric is supposed to depress the inter-camera variation of the query person. (2) If the selected training samples are similar to $\mathbf{x}_q$ in camera A, their corresponding candidate persons are easy to be confused with the query person. Therefore, we should give more weights to their training samples to well distinguish them in transfer learning. Some examples are shown in Figure 2. $\{w_{2j}^A\}$ of the samples in $\tilde{\mathcal{X}}_2$ are low because their observations in A have very different colors than the query sample and the second candidate can be easily distinguished from the query person. $\{w_{3j}^A\}$ of the samples in $\tilde{\mathcal{X}}_3$ are also low because their pose variations are different than that of the query person. The inter-camera variation of the query person is not well captured by the training samples in $\tilde{\mathcal{X}}_3$. Both $\{w_{1j}^A\}$ and $\{w_{4j}^A\}$ have large weights because the first and the fourth candidates are similar to the query person and therefore a metric needs to be specially trained to extract their subtle differences. Also the inter-camera variations existing in $\tilde{\mathcal{X}}_1$ and $\tilde{\mathcal{X}}_4$ well match with that of the query person.

### 3.3 Learning Adaptive Metrics by Maximizing Weighted Margins

Given a positive semidefinite (PSD) matrix $M$, the distance between two samples $\mathbf{x}_i^A$ and $\mathbf{x}_j^B$ observed in two different camera views is computed as

$$d(\mathbf{x}_i^A, \mathbf{x}_j^B) = (\mathbf{x}_i^A - \mathbf{x}_j^B)^t M(\mathbf{x}_i^A - \mathbf{x}_j^B).$$ (5)

We first learn a generic metric $M_0$ from the whole training set $\mathcal{S}$. Given a query sample $\mathbf{x}_q$, its candidate set $\mathcal{X}_c^B$ and the selected training pairs $\{\tilde{\mathcal{X}}_i\}_{i=1}^N$, an adaptive metric $M$ is learned with a regularization added by $M_0$. It minimizes the following objective function with constraints,

$$\min \quad \|M - M_0\|_F^2 + C\sum w_{ij} \cdot w_{i'j'} \cdot \xi_{iji'j'},$$ (6)

$$s.t. \quad (\tilde{\mathbf{x}}_{i_j}^A - \tilde{\mathbf{x}}_{i'_{j'}}^B)^t M(\tilde{\mathbf{x}}_{i_j}^A - \tilde{\mathbf{x}}_{i'_{j'}}^B) - (\tilde{\mathbf{x}}_{i_j}^A - \tilde{\mathbf{x}}_{i_j}^B)^t M(\tilde{\mathbf{x}}_{i_j}^A - \tilde{\mathbf{x}}_{i_j}^B)$$

$$\geq 1 - \xi_{iji'j'} \quad \forall i, j, i', j', i \neq i'$$ (7)

$$M \succeq 0, \xi_{iji'j'} \geq 0$$ (8)

---

**Algorithm 1:** Learning an adaptive metric for each candidate set by optimizing (6-8) with the cutting plane method.

---

1  $\mathcal{W} = \emptyset$;
2  $M = M_0$;
3  $\xi_{iji'j'} = 0$;
4  **begin**
5     **repeat**
6        $(\hat{i}, \hat{j}, \hat{i}', \hat{j}') = \arg\max_{(i,j,i',j')} w_{ij} \cdot w_{i'j'}(1 - \psi_{iji'j'}(M))$;
7        **if** $1 - \psi_{\hat{i}\hat{j}\hat{i}'\hat{j}'}(M) > \xi_{\hat{i}\hat{j}\hat{i}'\hat{j}'} + \epsilon$ **then**
8           $\mathcal{W} = \mathcal{W} \cup \{(\hat{i}, \hat{j}, \hat{i}', \hat{j}')\}$;
9           Solve the following QP problem using ADMM;
10          $(M, \{\xi_{iji'j'}\}) = \arg\min \|M - M_0\|_F^2 + C\sum_{iji'j'} w_{ij} \cdot w_{i'j'} \cdot \xi_{iji'j'}$
11          $s.t. \; \forall (i,j,i',j') \in \mathcal{W}$
12          $(\tilde{\mathbf{x}}_{i_j}^A - \tilde{\mathbf{x}}_{i'_{j'}}^B)^t M(\tilde{\mathbf{x}}_{i_j}^A - \tilde{\mathbf{x}}_{i'_{j'}}^B) - (\tilde{\mathbf{x}}_{i_j}^A - \tilde{\mathbf{x}}_{i_j}^B)^t M(\tilde{\mathbf{x}}_{i_j}^A - \tilde{\mathbf{x}}_{i_j}^B) \geq 1 - \xi_{iji'j'}$
13          $M \succeq 0, \xi_{iji'j'} \geq 0$
14    **until** $\mathcal{W}$ *does not change*;

---

The distance between two metrics is define as

$$\|M - M_0\|_F^2 = \sum_{ij}(M[i,j] - M_0[i,j])^2 = \mathbf{tr}((M - M_0)(M - M_0)^t). \quad (9)$$

$(\tilde{\mathbf{x}}_{i_j}^A - \tilde{\mathbf{x}}_{i_j}^B)^t M(\tilde{\mathbf{x}}_{i_j}^A - \tilde{\mathbf{x}}_{i_j}^B)$ is the distance between two samples of the same person $(i,j)$ observed in different camera views under the metric $M$. It is supposed to be smaller than any $(\tilde{\mathbf{x}}_{i_j}^A - \tilde{\mathbf{x}}_{i'_{j'}}^B)^t M(\tilde{\mathbf{x}}_{i_j}^A - \tilde{\mathbf{x}}_{i'_{j'}}^B)$, which is the distance between the samples of $(i,j)$ and a different person $(i',j')$, with a margin. The slack penalties are weighted with $w_{ij}$ and $w_{i'j'}$. Here we require that $i \neq i'$. If $i = i'$, the two selected training persons $(i,j)$ and $(i,j')$ are actually related to the same candidate and we do not have to distinguish them.

Our objective function (6) is convex with liner constraints,

$$\psi_{iji'j'}(M) = (\tilde{\mathbf{x}}_{i_j}^A - \tilde{\mathbf{x}}_{i'_{j'}}^B)^t M(\tilde{\mathbf{x}}_{i_j}^A - \tilde{\mathbf{x}}_{i'_{j'}}^B) - (\tilde{\mathbf{x}}_{i_j}^A - \tilde{\mathbf{x}}_{i_j}^B)^t M(\tilde{\mathbf{x}}_{i_j}^A - \tilde{\mathbf{x}}_{i_j}^B)$$
$$= \mathbf{tr}(M(\tilde{\mathbf{x}}_{i_j}^A - \tilde{\mathbf{x}}_{i'_{j'}}^B)(\tilde{\mathbf{x}}_{i_j}^A - \tilde{\mathbf{x}}_{i'_{j'}}^B)^t) - \mathbf{tr}(M(\tilde{\mathbf{x}}_{i_j}^A - \tilde{\mathbf{x}}_{i_j}^B)(\tilde{\mathbf{x}}_{i_j}^A - \tilde{\mathbf{x}}_{i_j}^B)^t)$$
$$\geq 1 - \xi_{iji'j'}. \quad (10)$$

It can be solved by Semidefinite Programming (SDP). We did not choose the subgradient method [34], which has been used by many metric learning approaches [35], to solve this optimization problem, because it simultaneously considers all the constraints and the computational cost is high. Instead, we adopt the cutting plane method [36] and our learning steps are summarized in Algorithm (1). Since $M$ is initialized with $M_0$ which is a reasonably good starting point, only a small portion of samples violate the constraints of (7) during the optimization process.

At each of the iterative steps, we choose samples with the largest violation of the constraint of margin,

$$(\hat{i}, \hat{j}, \hat{i}', \hat{j}') = \arg\max_{(i,j,i',j')} w_{ij} \cdot w_{i'j'}(1 - \psi_{iji'j'}(M)), \qquad (11)$$

and add them to a working set $\mathcal{W}^2$. Then $M$ and $\{\xi_{iji'ji}\}$ are optimized only considering the constraints added by the samples in $\mathcal{W}$. The objective function (6) is quadratic in $M$ and linear in $\xi_{iji'j'}$, and can be solved using Quadratic Programming (QP). We implement the QP solver using the Alternating Direction Method of Multipliers (ADMM) [37][3] which was proven to have a fast convergence rate. Our optimization procedure is inspired by structural SVM [20] where the cutting plane method was also used and it converged fast. The convergence of our algorithm is guaranteed, since $\mathcal{W}$ cannot increase forever. The convergence rate of our algorithm is controlled by $\epsilon$ and a global optimal with $\epsilon$ violation of margin is obtained. Asymptotically, with $\epsilon \to 0$, the global optimal can be obtained. According to the suggestions of [20], we choose $\epsilon = 0.001$. The parameter $C$ is chosen as $1/\text{mean}(\{\|\tilde{\mathbf{x}}_i - \tilde{\mathbf{x}}_j\|_2^2\}_{\tilde{\mathbf{x}}_i, \tilde{\mathbf{x}}_j \in \mathcal{S}})$ referring to the recommendation of SVMLight[4].

From (2-4) and (6-8) it is observed that if a query sample and its candidate set are dissimilar with any samples in the training set, few training samples are selected and their weights are small. In that case, there are few constraints and the adaptive metric $M$ is very close to generic metric $M_0$. **Learning the generic metric.** $M_0$ is learned by minimizing the following objective function,

$$\min \quad \|M_0\|_F^2 + C \sum_{i,j} \xi_{ij},$$

$$s.t. \quad (\tilde{\mathbf{x}}_i^A - \tilde{\mathbf{x}}_j^B)^t M_0 (\tilde{\mathbf{x}}_i^A - \tilde{\mathbf{x}}_j^B) - (\tilde{\mathbf{x}}_i^A - \tilde{\mathbf{x}}_i^B)^t M_0 (\tilde{\mathbf{x}}_i^A - \tilde{\mathbf{x}}_i^B) \geq 1 - \xi_{ij}, \forall i, j, i \neq j$$

$$M_0 \succeq 0, \xi_{iji'j'} \geq 0 \qquad (12)$$

All the samples in the whole training set are included. $(\tilde{\mathbf{x}}_i^A, \tilde{\mathbf{x}}_i^B)$ are the training samples of the same person observed in different camera views, and $(\tilde{\mathbf{x}}_i^A, \tilde{\mathbf{x}}_j^B)$ are the training samples of different persons. Once $M_0$ is learned, it is normalized by $M_0 = \frac{M_0}{\text{tr}(M_0)}$.

## 4   Experimental Results

### 4.1   Dataset Description

Experiments are conducted on the VIPeR dataset [21] and the *Campus*[5] dataset built by us. The VIPeR dataset is a widely used benchmark for evaluating human

---

[2] $\mathcal{W}$ is initialized as empty and no samples are removed from $\mathcal{W}$ during the optimization procedure.

[3] In ADMM, after each gradient step, the updated $M$ is projected back onto the feasible set of PSD matrices by spectral decomposition.

[4] http://svmlight.joachims.org/

[5] http://www.ee.cuhk.edu.hk/~xgwang/CUHK_identification.html

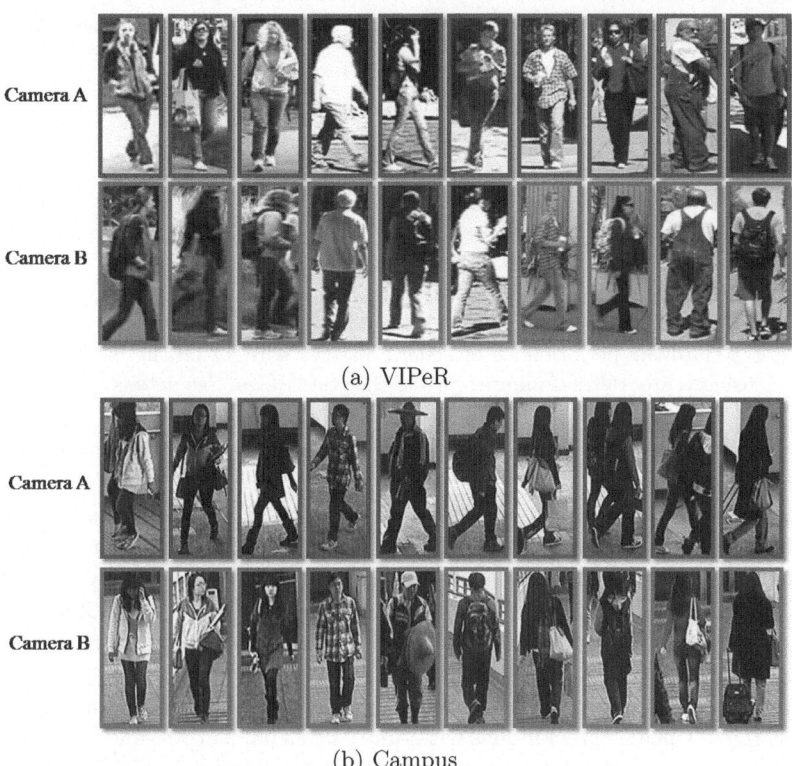

(a) VIPeR

(b) Campus

**Fig. 3.** Examples of images from the VIPeR dataset and the Campus dataset

reidentification algorithms. It includes 632 persons captured in two camera views. Each person has one image per camera view. The Campus dataset has 971 persons and each person also has two images captured in two disjoint camera views. Some examples of images from the two datasets are shown in Figure 3. Large inter-camera variations are observed in both datasets, which makes human reidentification challenging. The VIPeR dataset is even more challenging because even in the same camera view, persons appear in different poses and viewpoints, and lighting and background also change. It is difficult to learn a single generic metric to depress many kinds of inter-camera variations. In the Campus dataset, camera B mainly includes images of the frontal view and the back view, and camera A has more variations of viewpoints and poses.

## 4.2   Generic Metric Learning

We first test our generic metric learning algorithm, i.e., learning $M_0$ by minimizing (12), and compare it with other metric learning algorithms and the state-of-the-art human reidentification algorithms. The accumulative recognition accuracies on the VIPeR and Campus datasets are shown in Figure 4. For each of them, 50% persons are randomly selected for training and the remaining ones are used

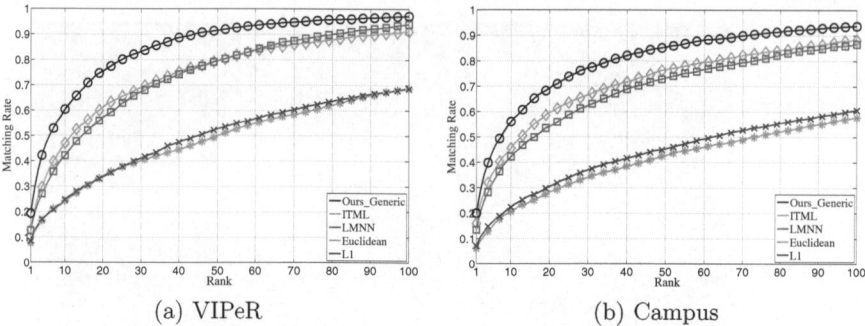

(a) VIPeR                          (b) Campus

**Fig. 4.** Evaluate the performance of generic metric learning on the whole gallery set without using temporal reasoning to prune the candidates. See details in Section 4.2.

for testing. The random partition is repeated for ten times and the average accuracies are computed. It is assumed that temporal reasoning is not used and each query sample matches the object from the whole gallery set. This is the scenario all the existing human reidentification algorithms assumed. We compare with two state-of-the-art metric learning algorithms, Large Margin Nearest Neighbor Classification (LMNN) [35] and Information-Theoretic Metric Learning (ITML) [38], as well as directly matching visual features with Euclidean distance (Euclidean) and $L_1$ distance ($L_1$). Our learned generic metric (Ours_Generic) has a better performance. Its rank-one accuracy is 19.3% on the VIPeR dataset. Some other state-of-the-art human reidentification techniques with different visual features and learning algorithms were also evaluated on the VIPeR dataset and published in literature with the same gallery size and in the same way of randomly partitioning the dataset [4]. The highest rank one accuracy reported so far is 15.66% [4]. Since their implementations are not available, we do not have their results on the Campus dataset. Compared to PRDC in [4], our methods enjoy a global optimal solution. Compared with ITML, our generic metric learning method employs a relative distance comparison rather than a hard global threshold between negative and positive pairs. For LMNN, as the distance is measured cross domain, the initial neighborhood selection will probability have no samples from the same identity selected which will bias the whole optimization procedure. Our generic metric learning algorithm for human reidentification is at least comparable with the state-of-the-art. However, this is **not** the main contribution of our framework. We focus on transferred metric learning.

### 4.3   Transferred Metric Learning

In this experiment, it is assumed that temporal reasoning can prune candidates and therefore for each query image the size of the candidate set could be much smaller than the gallery size. We have tried different sizes ($N$) of candidate sets from 5 to 50. The partitioning of training/test subsets is in the same way as Section 4.2. We design our experiment to simulate the real world scenario by random sampling the query-candidate configuration based on the assumption

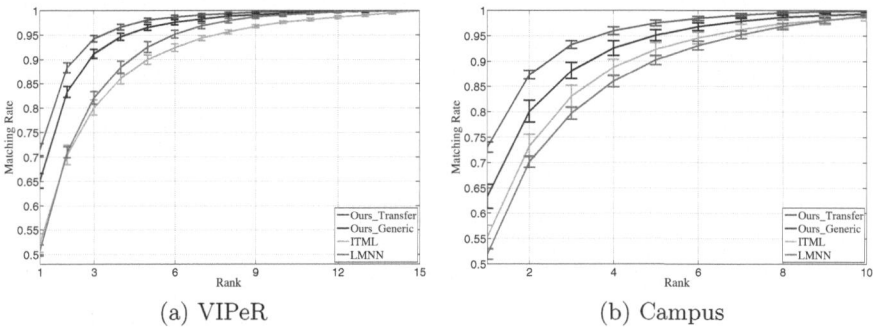

(a) VIPeR                                    (b) Campus

**Fig. 5.** Average accumulative recognition accuracies and their standard deviations on the candidate sets. The size of the candidate sets is fixed as 15. The bars indicate standard deviations.

that appearance is independent of the temporal reasoning. In order to validate our approach with a wide variety of configurations, for each query sample in the test set, we randomly select $N-1$ samples observed in the other camera view from the test set and also select the truly matched sample to form its candidate set. The same experimental design was also adopted in [3]. Human reidentification is to recognize the right person from the $N$ candidates. For each query image, this process is repeated for 50 times given a fixed training/test data partition. The partition of training/test data is repeated for 10 times. When the size of candidate sets is fixed as 15, the average accumulative recognition accuracies and their standard deviations on the two datasets are shown in Figure 5. Our transferred metric learning (Ours_Transferred) clearly outperforms our generic metric learning as well as other generic metric learning algorithms such as ITML and LMNN. The rank-one accuracy has been improved by 6.32% and 9.71% on the VIPeR dataset and the Campus dataset respectively. With an unoptimized matlab implementation and on a Core 8 2.27GHz CPU, it takes less than two seconds to train an adaptive metric for a candidate set of size 15. Figure 6 plots the average rank-one accuracies and their standard deviations when the size $(N)$ of the candidate sets varies from 5 to 50. When $N$ is small, the generic metric performs well and the improvement of the transferred metric learning is relatively small. When $N$ is too large $(> 50)$, the distributions of samples in the candidate set is complicated and close to the global distribution of the whole training set. In this case, the idea of adapting the metric to a local region of the training set is not feasible any more and most training samples are selected as the neighbors of the candidate set. Therefore, the learned adaptive metric is similar to the generic metric and the improvement becomes little. Compared with figure 4(b) in [3], the settings are same to ours and our approach outperforms the result test using the manually designed feature in VIPeR benchmark dataset with all candidate set size reported in their paper. The size of the training set is an important factor affecting the effectiveness of transfer learning. When the training set is large, it is more likely for the candidates to find similar training samples. Figure 7 plots the average rank-one accuracies when the size of the training set changes.

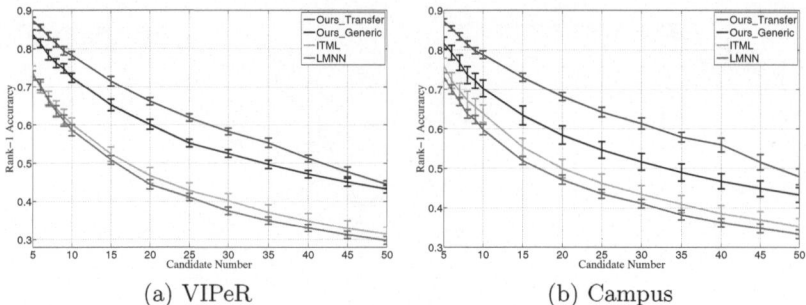

**Fig. 6.** Average rank-one accuracies when size of candidate sets varies from 5 to 50.

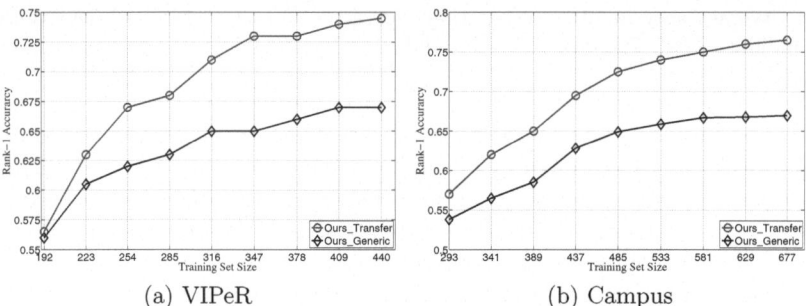

**Fig. 7.** Average rank-one accuracies when the size of the training set changes

When the training set gets large, the difference between the transferred metric learning and generic metric learning becomes large.

## 5   Conclusions and Discussions

In this paper, we solve the human reidentification problem from a new angle. Instead of trying to learn a generic metric to distinguish all the persons and to depress all types of inter-camera variations, we learn an adaptive metric for a specific candidate set under the framework of transfer learning. Given a query sample and its candidate set, the samples in the training set are selected and reweighted. An adaptive metric is learned by maximizing weighted margin of the selected training samples and being regularized by a generic metric. Experiments on the widely used VIPeR dataset and our Campus dataset shows that transferred metric learning is more effective than generic metric learning on human reidentification.

In this paper, we assume that the samples are from two fixed camera views. But the proposed approach also has good potentials to be generalized to the case when training and testing sets have multiple camera views or even the case when training and testing data are taken with different cameras. In the VIPeR dataset, persons captured by the same camera show a large diversity on poses, viewpoints, lightings and background. It is close to the general case of more camera views. In our approach, the training samples are selected and weighted by matching the visual features with the test samples. Therefore, the selected training samples should well match the query sample and candidate samples in pose, viewpoint and lighting even though they may be taken by different cameras. In the future work, we will build a new dataset with diversified camera views and will further improve our approach to make it work in more general camera settings.

**Acknowledgment.** This work is supported by the General Research Fund sponsored by the Research Grants Council of Hong Kong (project No. CUHK417110 and CUHK417011) and National Natural Science Foundation of China (project No. 61005057).

# References

1. Gheissari, N., Sebastian, T.B., Rittscher, J., Hartley, R.: Person reidentification using spatiotemporal appearance. In: CVPR (2006)
2. Schwartz, W., Davis, L.: Learning discriminative appearance-based models using partial least sqaures. In: Proc. XXII SIBGRAPI (2009)
3. Farenzena, M., Bazzani, L., Perina, A., Murino, V., Cristani, M.: Person re-identification by symmetry-driven accumulation of local features. In: CVPR (2010)
4. Zheng, W., Gong, S., Xiang, T.: Person re-identification by probabilistic relative distance comparison. In: CVPR (2011)
5. Park, U., Jain, A., Kitahara, I., Kogure, K., Hagita, N.: Vise: Visual search engine using multiple networked cameras. In: ICPR (2006)
6. van de Weijer, J., Schmid, C.: Coloring Local Feature Extraction. In: Leonardis, A., Bischof, H., Pinz, A. (eds.) ECCV 2006, Part II. LNCS, vol. 3952, pp. 334–348. Springer, Heidelberg (2006)
7. Dalal, N., Triggs, B.: Histograms of oriented gradients for human detection. In: CVPR (2005)
8. Wang, X., Doretto, G., Sebastian, T., Rittscher, J., Tu, P.: Shape and appearance context modeling. In: ICCV (2007)
9. Daugman, J.G.: Uncertainty relation for resolution in space, spatial frequency, and orientation optimized by two-dimensional visual cortical filters. Journal of the Optical Society of America A 2, 1160–1169 (1985)
10. Ojala, T., Pietikäinen, M., Mäenpää, T.: Multiresolution gray-scale and rotation invariant texture classification with local binary patterns. IEEE Trans. on PAMI, 971–987 (2002)
11. Torralba, A., Murphy, K., Freeman, W., Rubin, M.: Context-based vision system for place and object recognition. In: ICCV (2003)
12. Porikli, F.: Inter-camera color calibration by correlation model function. In: ICIP (2003)
13. Javed, O., Shafique, K., Shah, M.: Appearance modeling for tracking in multiple non-overlapping cameras. In: CVPR (2005)
14. Gilbert, A., Bowden, R.: Tracking Objects Across Cameras by Incrementally Learning Inter-camera Colour Calibration and Patterns of Activity. In: Leonardis, A., Bischof, H., Pinz, A. (eds.) ECCV 2006, Part II. LNCS, vol. 3952, pp. 125–136. Springer, Heidelberg (2006)
15. Prosser, B., Gong, S., Xiang, T.: Multi-camera matching using bi-directional cumulative brightness transfer function. In: BMVC (2008)
16. Gray, D., Tao, H.: Viewpoint Invariant Pedestrian Recognition with an Ensemble of Localized Features. In: Forsyth, D., Torr, P., Zisserman, A. (eds.) ECCV 2008, Part I. LNCS, vol. 5302, pp. 262–275. Springer, Heidelberg (2008)

17. Shan, Y., Sawhney, H.S., Kumar, R.: Unsupervised Learning of Discriminative Edge Measures for Vehicle Matching between Nonoverlapping Cameras. IEEE Transactions on Pattern Analysis and Machine Intelligence 30, 700–711 (2008)
18. Lin, Z., Davis, L.S.: Learning Pairwise Dissimilarity Profiles for Appearance Recognition in Visual Surveillance. In: Bebis, G., Boyle, R., Parvin, B., Koracin, D., Remagnino, P., Porikli, F., Peters, J., Klosowski, J., Arns, L., Chun, Y.K., Rhyne, T.-M., Monroe, L. (eds.) ISVC 2008, Part I. LNCS, vol. 5358, pp. 23–34. Springer, Heidelberg (2008)
19. Prosser, B., Zheng, W., Gong, S., Xiang, T., Mary, Q.: Person re-identification by support vector ranking. In: BMVC (2010)
20. Tsochantaridis, I., Joachims, T., Hofmann, T., Altun, Y.: Large margin methods for structured and interdependent output variables. Journal of Machine Learning Research 6, 1453–1484 (2005)
21. Gray, D., Brennan, S., Tao, H.: Evaluating appearance models for recognition, reacquisition and tracking (2007)
22. Dai, W., Yang, Q., Xue, G., Yu, Y.: Boosting for transfer learning. In: Proc. of ICML (2007)
23. Wu, X., Srihari, R.: Incorporating prior knowledge with weighted margin support vector machines. In: Proc. of SIGKDD (2004)
24. Jiang, W., Zavesky, E., Chang, S., Loui, A.: Cross-domain learning methods for high-level visual concept classification. In: ICIP (2008)
25. Saenko, K., Kulis, B., Fritz, M., Darrell, T.: Adapting Visual Category Models to New Domains. In: Daniilidis, K., Maragos, P., Paragios, N. (eds.) ECCV 2010, Part IV. LNCS, vol. 6314, pp. 213–226. Springer, Heidelberg (2010)
26. Yao, Y., Doretto, G.: Boosting for transfer learning with multiple sources. In: CVPR (2010)
27. Qi, G., Aggarwal, C., Huang, T.: Towards semantic knowledge propagation from text corpus to web images. In: Proc. of WWW (2011)
28. Yang, J., Yan, R., Hauptmann, A.G.: Cross-domain video concept detection using adaptive svms. In: Proc. of ACM Multimedia (2007)
29. Duan, L., Tsang, I.W., Xu, D., Maybank, S.J.: Domain transfer svm for video concept detection. In: CVPR (2009)
30. Qi, G., Aggarwal, C., Rui, Y., Tian, Q., Chang, S., Huang, T.: Towards cross-category knowledge propagation for learning visual concepts. In: CVPR (2011)
31. Zhan, D.C., Li, M., Li, Y.F., Zhou, Z.H.: Learning instance specific distances using metric propagation. In: Proc. of ICML, p. 154 (2009)
32. Sande, K., Gevers, T., Snoek, C.G.M.: Evaluating color descriptors for object and scene recognition. IEEE Trans. on PAMI 32, 1582–1596 (2010)
33. Liu, T., Moore, A.W., Gray, A.G., Yang, K.: An investigation of practical approximate nearest neighbor algorithms. In: Proc. of NIPS (2004)
34. Fletcher, R.: Semi-definite matrix constraints in optimization. SIAM J. Control Optim. 23, 493–513 (1985)
35. Weinberger, K.Q., Saul, L.K.: Distance metric learning for large margin distance metric learning for large margin. Journal of Machine Learning Research 10, 207–244 (2009)
36. Luenberger, D.G., Ye, Y.: Linear and Nonlinear Programming. Springer (2008)
37. Boyd, S., Parikh, N., Chu, E., Peleato, B., Eckstein, J.: Distributed optimization and statistical learning via the alternating direction method of multipliers. Foundations and Trends in Machine Learning 3, 1–122 (2011)
38. Davis, J.V., Kulis, B., Jain, P., Sra, S., Dhillon, I.S.: Information-theoretic metric learning. In: Proc. of ICML (2007)

# Tell Me What You Like and I'll Tell You What You Are: Discriminating Visual Preferences on Flickr Data

Pietro Lovato[1], Alessandro Perina[2], Nicu Sebe[3], Omar Zandonà[1],
Alessio Montagnini[1], Manuele Bicego[1], and Marco Cristani[1,4]

[1] University of Verona, Italy
[2] Microsoft Research, Redmond, WA
[3] University of Trento, Italy
[4] Istituto Italiano di Tecnologia (IIT), Genova, Italy

**Abstract.** The John Ruskin's 19th century adage suggests that personal taste is not merely an absolute set of aesthetic principles valid for everyone: actually, it is a process of interpretation which have also roots in one's life experiences. This aspect represents nowadays a major problem for inferring automatically the quality of a picture. In this paper, instead of trying to solve this age-old problem, we consider an intriguing, orthogonal direction, aimed at discovering how different are the personal tastes. Given a set of preferred images of a user, obtained from Flickr, we extract a pool of low- and high-level features; LASSO regression is then exploited to learn the most discriminative ones, considering a group of 200 random Flickr users. Such aspects can be easily recovered, allowing to understand what is the "what we like" which distinguish us from the others. We then perform multi-class classification, where a test sample is a set of preferred pictures of an unknown user, and the classes are all the users. The results are surprising: given only 1 image as test, we can match the user preferences definitely more than the chance, and with 20 images we reach an nAUC of 91%, considering the cumulative matching characteristic curve. Extensive experiments promote our approach, suggesting new intriguing perspectives in the study of computational aesthetics.

## 1 Introduction

People often get enjoyment from observing images and express preferences for some pictures over others. Surprisingly, there is as of yet no scientifically comprehensive theory that explains what psychologically defines such preferences [1]. However, certain guidelines which suggest principles of general gratification have been produced: for example, there has been an effort to infer the common aspects determining preference by checking whether average image preference for a group of observers can be reliably predicted from various factors in a test set [2]. Some of these guidelines have roots in the cognitive sciences: facial attractiveness of symmetric faces is one of the most known example [3]. For real-world scenes, there is high agreement in observer's preference ratings: factors such as

K.M. Lee et al. (Eds.): ACCV 2012, Part I, LNCS 7724, pp. 45–56, 2013.
© Springer-Verlag Berlin Heidelberg 2013

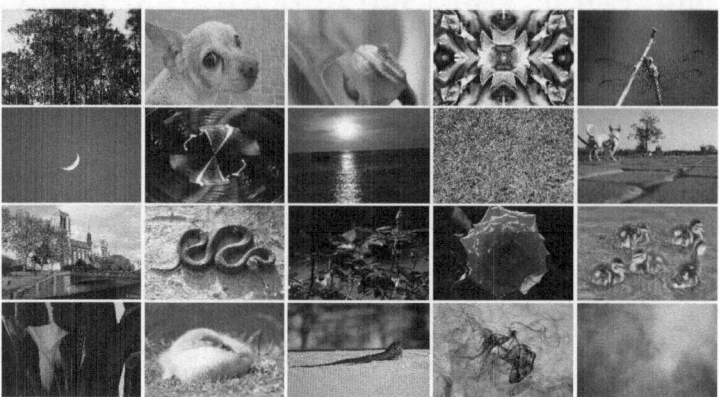

**Fig. 1.** Example of favourite images taken at random from a Flickr user

naturalness, complexity, coherence, legibility, vista, mystery and refuge seem to produce shared agreement [4], most probably due to the survival utility of a particular environment or viewpoint. Other guidelines are rules-of-thumbs (e.g., "rule of thirds","visual weight balance", etc. [5]) and all of them are modeled in a computational sense by the field of Computational Media Aesthetics (CMA) [6]. Many CMA applications have been developed: from aesthetic photo ranking [7,8] and preference-aware view recommendation systems [9], to picture quality analysis [10,11].

Nevertheless, these technologies ignore the potential role that factors internal to the observer may have on preference, summarized by the old adage "beauty is in the eye of the beholder". Recent studies have shown that preference formation is a result of the interplay between subjective novelty, e.g. how new a visual stimulus seems to an observer, and how well the observer is able to extract the sense of a stimulus and to relate it to previous knowledge, defined as interpretability [12]. Unfortunately, so far no automatic mechanism has been capable to subsume such experiences, limiting the effectiveness of the CMA applications to the sole manipulation of widely-shared preferences. Therefore, in this paper we do *not* propose a strategy for assessing the quality of an image; instead, we consider a brand-new orthogonal direction, learning the "personal aesthetics traits" of people, i.e. those visual preferences that distinguish people from each other. In particular, we take a crowdsearch approach [13] and we focus on Flickr[1], a popular website where every user can select his/her preferred photos, by tagging them as "favorites". This creates, for every user, a set of favorite photos, which is often very heterogeneous and whose modeling/recognition goes beyond standard computer vision tasks such as object/scene recognition (see fig. 1 for an example).

In this paper, we analyze the "favorites set" of 200 users to infer about their *personal* aesthetics traits. To this aim, we characterize each image with different

---

[1] http://www.flickr.com/

features, ranging from low-level color/edge statistics up to more high-level and semantic descriptors such as object detectors and overall scene statistics. LASSO regression is then exploited to learn the most discriminative aesthetic attributes, i.e., the aspects that an user likes that distinguish her/him from the rest of the community: such aspects can be easily recovered and visualized.

In the experiments, we show that personal tastes act like a blueprint for a user, allowing to recognize him with high accuracy; in particular, given just one image of an unknown user (the test samples), you can guess her/his identity more than the chance, and this probability dramatically raises as you consider a higher number of images.

Summarizing, the contributions of this paper are two:

1. A novel research direction: instead of studying which are the commonly liked visual aspects of an image (which is what computational aesthetics does), we explore the opposite direction, i.e., what are those aspects that allow to distinguish different users.
2. An inference method based on LASSO regression applied to heterogeneous visual features, which allows to obtain good recognition scores, and is highly interpretable, giving a clear idea of the aesthetic traits that distinguish an user from the other.

## 2 The Proposed Approach

Our approach is composed by two steps: feature extraction and feature weighting. In the next sections we will thoroughly detail each one of them.

### 2.1 Feature Extraction

In this step, the aim is to extract as much information as possible from an image. The idea is that we are not interested in extracting the classic aesthetic qualities of an image, but the aspects that make an image good for particular users; being this last goal slightly different, many factors and dimensions of analysis can be taken into consideration, each one considered for the purpose of describing different aspects of an image. Therefore, we wanted to span our selection from simple and standard image descriptors up to complex and state-of-the art ones.

In the following, we explain the cues we focus on, being aware that the list is neither exhaustive nor the best possible one; actually, our aim is to investigate how they should be properly treated for the task-at-hand.

1. **Color.** We calculated the average intensity of each channel (in the original RGB space).

2. **Edges.** We focused on the presence or absence of edges, as well as their predominant direction. Does a user have a tendency to like images with trees (lots of vertical edges)? Or maybe he is more fascinated by a sunset on the ocean or by a flat landscape, where horizontal edges are in abundance.

We extracted horizontal and vertical edges using the Prewitt filter, whereas the total edges have been computed with the Canny edge detector. We considered the number of horizontal, vertical and total point of edges. To avoid the dependence from the possible different sizes of images, the number of edge's pixels has been normalized by the total image area.

3. **Textures.** The repeated structures, or texture, in an image may be another important aspect; to extract this information we employed MTEX toolbox [14,15]. One of its major function is the suitability in analyzing very sharp texture symmetries. Among the many indices that MTEX computes, we retained the one called "texture index", that summarizes in one value all the information of the model fitted by the algorithm onto the image.

    In addition to that, we calculate the entropy of the image, a statistical measure to characterize the homogeneousness of an image.

4. **Regions.** As shown in the recent work of [16,17], objects and scene semantics are very important to understand the subjective judgement of a picture. Following this, we performed image segmentation collecting some low-order statistics.

    We employed the mean shift segmentation algorithm [18], and in particular the EDISON implementation [19][2]. After segmenting an image we extracted i) the number of segments – measuring the regions "density" which characterizes each image – and ii) the average extension of the regions. All the values have been normalized w.r.t. the total image area.

5. **Objects.** Once again motivated by [16,17], we employed the Deformable Part Models [20,21] system to detect objects. The algorithm works by detecting and localizing a specific object (for example a plane, a cat, a chair or a person), through the use of a model learned from a set of training examples. The system can detect different objects; in our approach we used as features the number of times every detectable object is present in the image (for a complete list of all detectable objects see [20]); we also retained the average area (the algorithm gives also the bounding box of the detected objects), to guess if objects are more towards the background or the foreground.

6. **Faces.** As a particular class of objects – which detection has been largely studied in the field of biometrics – we extracted the number and sizes of the faces present in the image. We employed the standard Viola-Jones face detection algorithm [22] implemented in the OpenCV libraries[3].

7. **Scenes.** Finally, we focused on describing the semantic of the whole scene, rather than the semantic of the single objects which appears in it. A very

---

[2] The code is freely available on:
   http://coewww.rutgers.edu/riul/research/code/EDISON/index.html
[3] http://opencv.willowgarage.com/wiki/

powerful scene descriptor is the GIST [23], which, roughly speaking, measures the responses of different Gabor filters. Such filters are built to describe the category of the scene in terms of openness, ruggedness, roughness and expansion[4].

The concatenation of all these descriptors, a vector $\mathbf{x}_m$ of 62 elements, represents the proposed signature for the image $m$. Since the value ranges are very heterogeneous, each feature/dimension is normalized across the images to have zero mean and unit standard deviation. More details are given in the experimental section.

It is worth noting that for the sake of reproducibility, every parameter of the different off-the-shelf computer vision libraries have been left as the default setting.

## 2.2   Feature Weighting

The main claim of this paper is that the discriminative aesthetical aspects of each user can be represented by a subset of all the features considered, opportunely weighted.

Given a pool of training images for $N$ users, we perform a sparse regression analysis using Lasso [24]. Lasso is a general form of regularization in a regression problem. In the simple linear regression problem every training image, described by the proposed feature vector and denoted with $\mathbf{x}_m$, is associated with a target variable $y_m$ (in our case, it can be the discrete label representing the user who posted it). Then, we can express the target variable as a linear combination of the image features:

$$y_m = \mathbf{w}^T \mathbf{x}_m \tag{1}$$

The standard least square estimate calculates the weight vector $\mathbf{w}$ by minimizing the error function

$$E(\mathbf{w}) = \sum_{m=1}^{M} \left( y_m - \mathbf{w}^T \mathbf{x}_m \right)^2 \tag{2}$$

where in our case $M$ correspond to the total number of images we have in the training set. The regularizer in the Lasso estimate is simply expressed as a threshold on the L1-norm of the weight $\mathbf{w}$:

$$\sum_j |w_j| \leq t \tag{3}$$

This term acts as a constraint that has to be taken into account when minimizing the error function.

By doing so, it has been proved that (depending on the parameter $t$), many of the coefficients $w_j$ become exactly zero [24]. Since each component $w_j$ of

---

[4] code is publicly available on
http://people.csail.mit.edu/torralba/code/spatialenvelope/

the weight vector weigh a different feature, it is possible to understand which features are the most important for a given user, and which ones are neglected.

In our particular scenario, where the aim is to capture the facets of the visual aesthetics of a user which discriminate him from other people, we performed Lasso regression for each user separately, considering all training images coming from that user to have positive label. In other words, we have to solve $N$ regression problems, each one returning a weight vector "user-specific" $\mathbf{w}^{(n)}$, $n = 1, \ldots, N$.

This way, by looking at the values in $\mathbf{w}^{(n)}$, we have that only the most important image features that characterize the preferences of the $n$-th user are retained.

# 3   Experiments

## 3.1   Data Collection

To test our approach, we consider a real dataset of 40.000 images, composed by 200 users chosen at random from the Flickr website. For each user, we retained the first 200 favourites[5].

## 3.2   Testing Protocol and Preliminary Evaluation

After computing all the images' signature, we randomly split the favorite images of each user into a training set and a testing set (here we used a 50%/50% splitting). Then, since the value ranges are very heterogeneous, each feature / dimension is normalized across all training images to have zero mean and unit standard deviation. The testing set is normalized with the constants calculated on the training set.

Then, as explained in the previous section, one Lasso regression is learned on the training set of each user, crossvalidating the parameter $t$. After estimating $\mathbf{w}^{(n)}$ for the $n$-th user, we calculated the regression scores $\beta_m^{(n)}$ for each testing image $m$ by simply applying the product described by eq. 1:

$$\beta_m^{(n)} = \mathbf{w}^{(n)T} \mathbf{x}_m \tag{4}$$

As a preliminary evaluation, we used these regression scores $\beta$ of the testing set to calculate a ROC curve for each user; basically, we are building a one-vs-all classifier that highlights the peculiar characteristics that distinguish a specific person. It turns out that Lasso is able to capture the differences between users, obtaining an average AUC of 69.4% with a standard deviation of 8%. Motivated by this promising result, we investigated in detail the issues discussed in the two next sections.

---

[5] The dataset is available upon request at
http://profs.sci.univr.it/~{}cristanm/projects/perpre.html

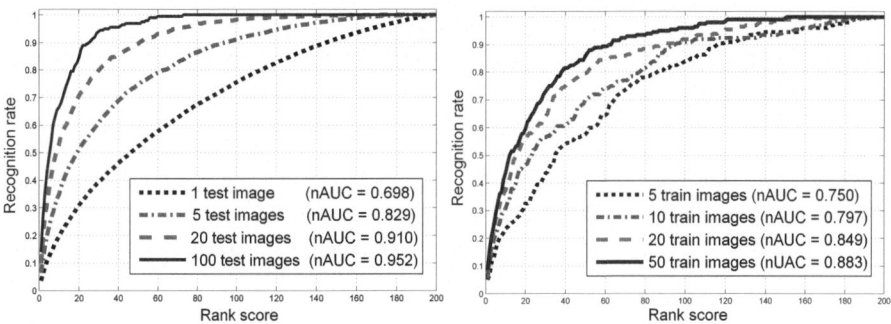

**Fig. 2.** CMC curves for our dataset. On the left: For each curve, we varied the number of testing images to be considered as a single "set". On the right: For each curve, we varied the number of images used to train Lasso.

### 3.3   Matching the Personal Aesthetics

In this section, we want to answer this question: how many images are needed to guess the personal aesthetics preferences of a person? Re-formulating the question, we want to prove if we are able to guess the user who tagged an image or a set of images. This task is intrinsically much more difficult than the previous one: instead of testing one user vs all the others, we are trying to predict which one tagged an image as favorite, on the basis of the "subjective" peculiar traits the image contains.

Intuitively, a single image does not contain every facet of the visual aesthetics sense of a person; the idea is to consider a *set* of testing images, and guess if the set contains enough information to catch the preferences of the user, allowing to identify him among all the others.

To do so, we exploit the fact that given a testing image $\mathbf{x}_m$ (or a set of images $\{\mathbf{x}_s\}_{s=1}^{S}$), we can evaluate – for each user $n$ – its corresponding lasso estimate $\beta_m^{(n)}$ (or, in the set case, the mean of the estimates of each image $\frac{1}{S}\sum_s \beta_s^{(n)}$). This value can be used as a score to rank the different users. Hopefully, the user with highest score is the one who originally faved the photo (or group of photos).

To show the results, we build a CMC curve [25], a common performance measure in the field of re-identification [26]: given a test set of images coming from a single user and the membership score discussed, the curve tells the rate at which the correct user is found within the first $k$ matches, with all possible $k$ spanned on the x-axis. Figure 2 shows various CMC curves for our dataset.

On the left, we reported four different CMCs, trying to vary the parameter $S$, which tells how many images are aggregated to form a single test object.

From the figure it is evident that performing the task of identifying correctly a user with a single image (black dotted line) is very difficult. However, as soon as the number of testing images grouped together increase a little, a consistent improvement can be noted. This is in line with our hypothesis: we are aggregating information from heterogeneous images, each one characterizing only a small portion of the user subjective tastes.

On the right, we assessed the importance of the training set size by keeping the test parameter $S$ fixed to 20. As expected, by lowering the number of training elements, it is more difficult to learn the users' preferences and their aesthetic sense uniqueness. For both figures, the normalized Area Under the Curve (nAUC) has been reported in the legend.

As a final comment, it is also worth noting that, even if at CMC rank 1 we achieve in the worst case a 3.9% rate of correct identification, this is higher that the probability we have to recognize the user by mere chance (which amounts to 0.5%).

## 3.4   Feature Analysis

This section is aimed at providing a qualitative evaluation of the proposed approach, showing that the regression score $\beta_m^{(n)}$ provides a valid measure of the preferences of an user, while the weight coefficients in the vector $\mathbf{w}^{(n)}$ provides an interpretable description for his visual aesthetic sense. First of all, we performed the following experiment: given a user, we considered all testing images $m$ we have, and we sorted them according to their regression score $\beta_m^{(n)}$ . The higher the score, the higher the probability that the user may have actually faved the image. Figure 3 briefly sketches the results; each column correspond to a Flickr user and the first 10 rows (before the white space) are favorite photos chosen from the training set of the user: we computed regression scores on the training set, and in the figure the top 10 are shown. The next images are the 10 testing images (coming from all users) with highest regression score; we highlighted with a blue box the ones that actually belong to the favorites of the user in hand.

The first column reveals some interesting information: although the highest test image for the user is not on his favorites set, it can have some visual appeals reflected on some of the images on his training set (see for example the lines on the spider web, or the red sunsets). It seems that a sort of "internal coherence" starts to show up.

We then looked into the weight coefficients for some users after learning the sparse regression model. For 3 random users, we reported the vector $\mathbf{w}$ in figure 4, on the right of their training and predicted preferred images. For visualization purposes, we labeled the 5 most prominent features (i.e. the ones with highest weight value): actually, the discriminative preferences of a user are determined by some features that have to be present in the pictures (high positive weight in the figure). As an example, by looking at the last bar-plot, it seems that faces, and some peculiarity in the textures are very important to the user; this is verified in his favorites, that contain faces, and gray-level images with a similar textural pattern.

As a final test, we have calculated the mean of the absolute values of the regression scores of all the subjects (Fig.5) This will show in general which are the most discriminative features for all the considered users. Interestingly, it seems that the low level features like color, texture, regions play a primary role compared to high-level cues like the scene or the objects.

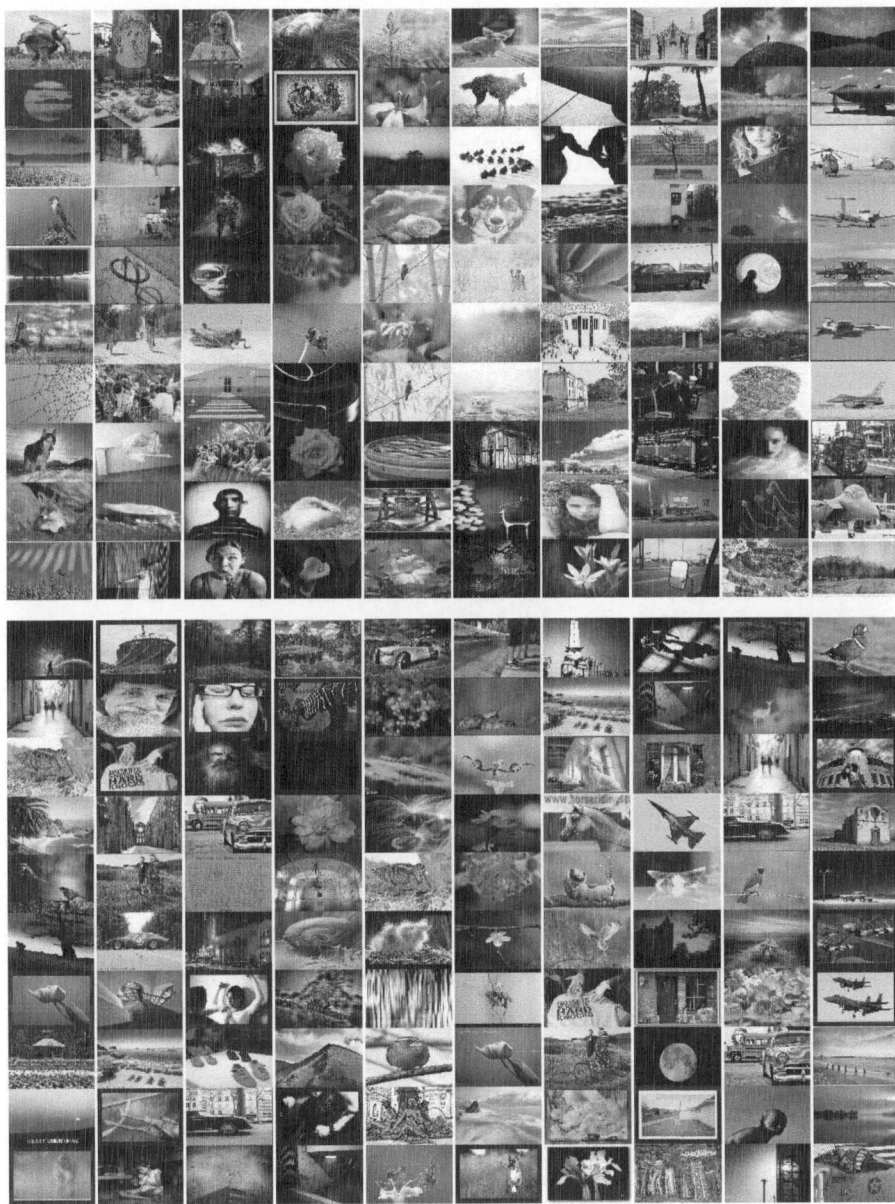

**Fig. 3.** Training and recognized testing images for different users. Each column is a user, and the first 10 images comes from his training set. In the half-bottom part, we show the first 10 testing images for that user, ranked on the basis of their regression score (the first being the one with highest score). In blue, correct matches are highlighted. A "coherence" between training and testing images can be seen.

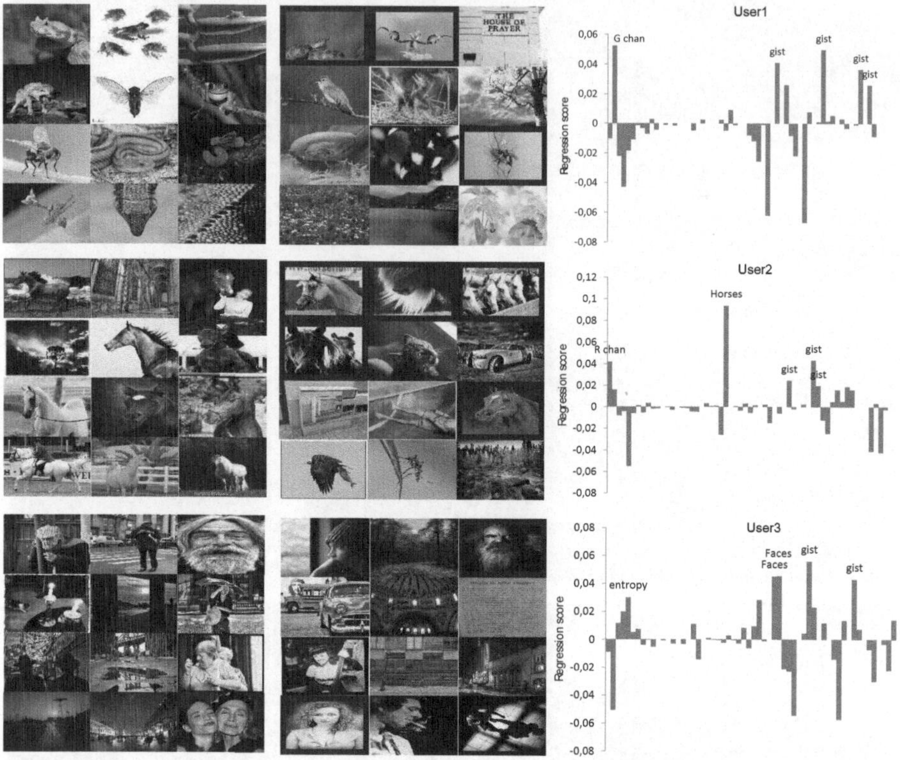

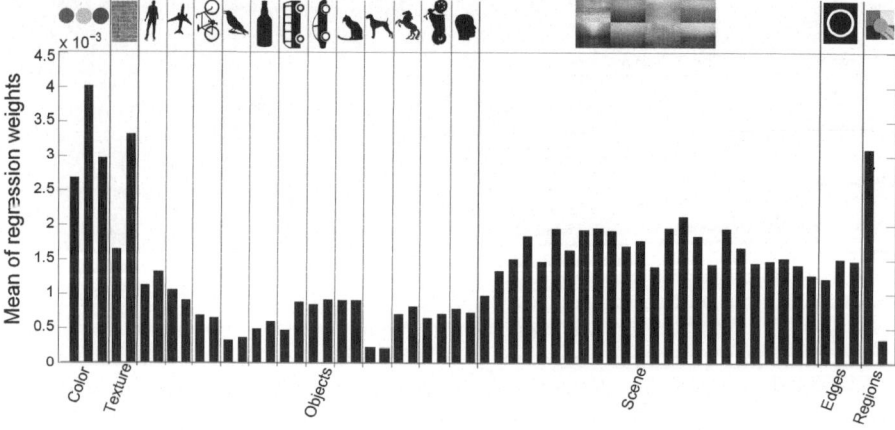

**Fig. 4.** Most prominent features for 3 users taken from the dataset. In the first two blocks of figures, training and testing elements are shown, in the same fashion of figure 3. On the right, for each user, a bar plot of each feature's importance is shown. The height of each bar represents the value of the corresponding weight.

**Fig. 5.** Mean of the absolute values of the regression weights over all users in the dataset

# 4    Conclusions

This paper proposed an innovative way to deal with image aesthetics: instead of focusing on the design of common rules of likeliness, we proceeded in an orthogonal direction, modeling the aesthetics differences which characterize many users. This is possible by crowdsearching huge Internet databases as the Flickr repository: we considered 200 users, 40.000 different images. The results may be summarized as follows: different users have different preferences, and these preferences can be employed to identifying the users with high precision; this precision depends on how many images you take into account, but with even an image, you can match the user preferences with an accuracy higher than the chance. This opens up to a set of interesting applications: given a set of images on a publication, you can infer who are the users that most probably will like them all; this could be a novel kind of recommender system, which subsume the aesthetic statistics of a set of images, matching with the personal preferences of each one of us. More intriguing, what if we consider a huge number of users? Imagine to have millions of users, and to apply our framework: the idea is that the classical image aesthetics could be found by checking the features that are not discriminative (i.e., they are liked by everyone), while discriminative aspects could be seen as outlier aspects that make our preferences so unique. These two perspectives are actually under study, with promising preliminary results.

# References

1. Leder, H., Belke, B., Oeberst, A., Augustin, D.: A model of aesthetic appreciation and aesthetic judgments. British Journal of Psychology 95, 489–508 (2004)
2. Martindale, C., Moore, K., Borkum, J.: Aesthetic preference: Anomalous findings for berlyne's psychobiological theory. American Journal of Psychology 103, 53–80 (1990)
3. Bronstad, P., Russell, R.: Beauty is in the "we" of the beholder: greater agreement on facial attractiveness among close relations. Perception 36, 1674–1681 (2007)
4. Kaplan, R., Kaplan, S.: The Experience of Nature: A Psychological Perspective. Cambridge University Press (1989)
5. Bhattacharya, S., Sukthankar, R., Shah, M.: A framework for photo-quality assessment and enhancement based on visual aesthetics. In: Proceedings of the International Conference on Multimedia, MM 2010, pp. 271–280. ACM, New York (2010)
6. Adams, B.: Where does computational media aesthetics fit? IEEE Multimedia 10, 18–27 (2003)
7. Yeh, C.H., Ho, Y.C., Barsky, B.A., Ouhyoung, M.: Personalized photograph ranking and selection system. In: Proceedings of the International Conference on Multimedia, MM 2010, pp. 211–220. ACM, New York (2010)
8. Datta, R., Joshi, D., Li, J., Wang, J.Z.: Studying Aesthetics in Photographic Images Using a Computational Approach. In: Leonardis, A., Bischof, H., Pinz, A. (eds.) ECCV 2006, Part III. LNCS, vol. 3953, pp. 288–301. Springer, Heidelberg (2006)
9. Su, H.H., Chen, T.W., Kao, C.C., Hsu, W.H., Chien, S.Y.: Preference-aware view recommendation system for scenic photos based on bag-of-aesthetics-preserving features. IEEE Transactions on Multimedia 14, 833–843 (2012)

10. Ke, Y., Tang, X., Jing, F.: The design of high-level features for photo quality assessment. In: CVPR 2006, pp. 419–426. IEEE Computer Society, Washington, DC (2006)
11. Luo, Y., Tang, X.: Photo and Video Quality Evaluation: Focusing on the Subject. In: Forsyth, D., Torr, P., Zisserman, A. (eds.) ECCV 2008, Part III. LNCS, vol. 5304, pp. 386–399. Springer, Heidelberg (2008)
12. Biederman, I., Vessel, E.: Perceptual pleasure and the brain. American Scientist 94, 1–8 (2006)
13. Bozzon, A., Brambilla, M., Ceri, S.: Answering search queries with crowdsearcher. In: WWW, pp. 1009–1018 (2012)
14. Hielscher, R., Schaeben, H.: A novel pole figure inversion method: specification of the *mtex* algorithm. Journal of Applied Crystallography 41, 1024–1037 (2008)
15. Bachmann, F., Hielscher, R., Schaeben, H.: Texture analysis with mtex–free and open source software toolbox. Solid State Phenomena 160, 63–68 (2010)
16. Isola, P., Jianxiong, X., Torralba, A., Oliva, A.: What makes an image memorable? In: 2011 IEEE Conference on Computer Vision and Pattern Recognition, CVPR, pp. 145–152 (2011)
17. Curran, W., Moore, T., Kulesza, T., Wong, W., Todorovic, S., Stumpf, S., White, R., Burnett, M.M.: Towards recognizing "cool": can end users help computer vision recognize subjective attributes of objects in images? In: ACM International Conference on Intelligent User Interfaces, pp. 285–288 (2012)
18. Comaniciu, D., Meer, P.: Mean shift: a robust approach toward feature space analysis. IEEE Transactions on Pattern Analysis and Machine Intelligence 24, 603–619 (2002)
19. Georgescu, C.: Synergism in low level vision. In: International Conference on Pattern Recognition, pp. 150–155 (2002)
20. Felzenszwalb, P.F., Girshick, R.B., McAllester, D.: Discriminatively trained deformable part models, release 4 (2010),
    http://www.cs.brown.edu/~pff/latent-release4/
21. Felzenszwalb, P., Girshick, R., McAllester, D., Ramanan, D.: Object detection with discriminatively trained part-based models. IEEE Transactions on Pattern Analysis and Machine Intelligence 32, 1627–1645 (2010)
22. Viola, P., Jones, M.: Rapid object detection using a boosted cascade of simple features. In: Proceedings of the IEEE Conference on Computer Vision and Pattern Recognition, pp. 511–518 (2001)
23. Oliva, A., Torralba, A.: Modeling the shape of the scene: A holistic representation of the spatial envelope. Int. J. Comput. Vision 42, 145–175 (2001)
24. Tibshirani, R.: Regression shrinkage and selection via the lasso. Journal of the Royal Statistical Society, Series B 58, 267–288 (1994)
25. Moon, H., Phillips, P.: Computational and performance aspects of pca-based face-recognition algorithms. Perception 30, 303–321 (2001)
26. Cheng, D., Cristani, M., Stoppa, M., Bazzani, L., Murino, V.: Custom pictorial structures for re-identification. In: Proceedings of British Machine Vision Conference (2011)

# Local Context Priors
# for Object Proposal Generation

Marko Ristin[1], Juergen Gall[2], and Luc Van Gool[1,3]

[1] ETH Zurich
[2] MPI for Intelligent Systems
[3] KU Leuven

**Abstract.** State-of-the-art methods for object detection are mostly based on an expensive exhaustive search over the image at different scales. In order to reduce the computational time, one can perform a selective search to obtain a small subset of relevant object hypotheses that need to be evaluated by the detector. For that purpose, we employ a regression to predict possible object scales and locations by exploiting the local context of an image. Furthermore, we show how a priori information, if available, can be integrated to improve the prediction. The experimental results on three datasets including the Caltech pedestrian and PASCAL VOC dataset show that our method achieves the detection performance of an exhaustive search approach with much less computational load. Since we model the prior distribution over the proposals locally, it generalizes well and can be successfully applied across datasets.

## 1  Introduction

Object detection is a well studied field in computer vision. While most works have focused on improving the accuracy [1], the computational burden of detectors is another important issue that needs to be solved. Object detectors commonly process the image at different scales, where only a small region of the image is processed for evaluating a single object hypothesis. In the extreme case, all possible rectangular regions, termed windows, are checked for whether they contain an instance of the object class. Although not all windows are classified in practice, a dense sampling of the windows with a small stride is necessary to obtain a high detection accuracy [2]. Since these sliding window approaches are very expensive, several strategies have been proposed for reducing the processing time. Among them, cascading [3, 4] is the most popular approach. It makes use of the fact that some parts of the image can be easily discarded with simple features and classifiers, such that a full processing of these image parts can be avoided. Cascading is specific for a classifier and can significantly reduce the computation time at a small expense of accuracy. When object detection is formulated as an optimization problem, where one searches for instances with the highest detection score in the full image, branch-and-bound techniques can be used to search the space of windows more efficiently [5].

K.M. Lee et al. (Eds.): ACCV 2012, Part I, LNCS 7724, pp. 57–70, 2013.
© Springer-Verlag Berlin Heidelberg 2013

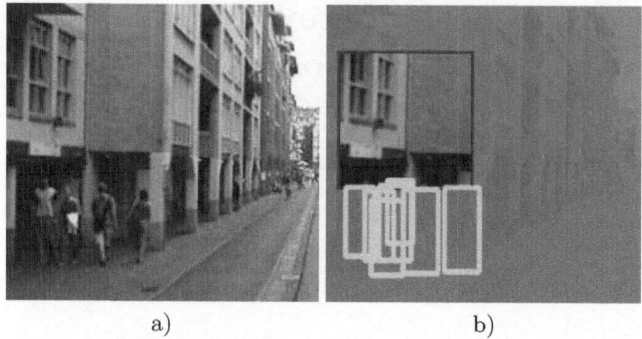

a)                                           b)

**Fig. 1.** When presented with an image a), our algorithm sees patches which might not contain any pedestrians, but whose visual appearance suggests that there could be some pedestrians walking on the sidewalk below

A different concept is followed by approaches that generate window proposals. While sliding window can be regarded as sampling uniformly from the set of windows, one can also learn a distribution over the set of windows that gives a higher probability to parts of the image where objects are expected and a lower probability to parts where objects are not expected. The advantage of the sampling methods is that highly probable candidates are processed first, such that the number of samples can be easily adapted to the available computational resources.

Previous work on proposal generation [6–10] has focused on disregarding windows that do not contain the object. For instance, sky or a building facade are ignored for detecting pedestrians. We propose to randomly sample very few, but large image patches and extract information about the image context from each one of them based on appearance. These nuggets of information are later combined to estimate a probabilistic prior distribution over object location in the image. For instance, instead of ignoring a facade of a building, it is a good indicator for pedestrians and their scales on the sidewalk below (see Fig. 1).

In order to model local probabilistic priors from image context, we learn a regression from large local image patches to its closest annotated object from training data. During testing, we combine the local probabilities from several patches to obtain a distribution over the space of windows. In our experiments, we show that on the challenging Caltech benchmark [11] as little as 0.2% of the windows need to be evaluated to achieve the same performance as processing all windows. Although local priors do not assume that the recording settings for training and testing data are the same, as we will show in a cross-dataset experiment, they can be combined with global priors if such global information is available.

## 2    Related Work

The exhaustive search methods based either on the sliding window approach [2] or on part-based models [4, 12, 13] are well-established approaches for detecting objects and proved to be the state-of-the-art according to recent Pascal VOC challenges [1]. The number of windows examined in an exhaustive search, however, grows at least linearly with the number of image pixels. Since the image needs to be upscaled for detecting small objects, the time for inspecting all windows can exceed the runtime requirements of real-world applications already for images as small as $320 \times 240$ pixels even on modern computers.

As there are usually far fewer windows containing an object of interest than the windows without it, methods were developed based on a cascade of classifiers [3, 14–17]. High-confident negatives are rejected in early stages of the cascade and more computational time is spent on windows that are more difficult to classify. The approach was improved by studying various combinations of features and attained state-of-the-art speed performance at a reasonable accuracy rate for pedestrian detection [18].

While conventional cascade classifiers still have to inspect the whole set of windows, the *Efficient Subwindow Search* (ESS) [5] and its cascaded variant [19] employ a branch-and-bound scheme to inspect only relevant regions. It approximates the response of the original classifier over a region by analytically derived bounding functions. For object detection, the image is first split into large regions and the search then continues recursively in the region ranked highest. The recursion stops when the window with the highest score is found. Since the performance of ESS depends on the tightness of the bounding functions, it has been also proposed to estimate the bounding functions [20].

Other methods focus on an efficient selective search for candidate windows which then serve as input for a classifier. In [7], it was proposed to estimate a likelihood function over the windows based on the response of some classifiers. The method refines the likelihood step-wise using Monte Carlo sampling to specifically draw samples from regions where target objects are more likely. Each refinement stage employs a more accurate and computationally more intensive classifier. This method basically combines coarse-to-fine search with cascading. The work in [6] employed a two-stage procedure. In the first stage, separate classifiers are applied, one for each aspect ratio/scale. The windows are then ranked by a pre-trained ranking classifier. In [21] and based on [22], the authors learn to predict candidate windows from discriminative visual words. A different bottom-up procedure was proposed in [23]: the image is first segmented by an unsupervised technique into locally coherent regions that are later reshaped and combined by the algorithm into rectangles, some of which are discarded as unlikely to contain an object. The approach of [9] begins with over-segmenting the image, proceeds with gradually joining similar regions to construct a hierarchical segmentation and then generates candidate windows based on such a pyramid of segmentations. In [10], a naïve Bayes model is trained to distinguish windows with high "objectness", defined as the probability of a window containing an object of all classes of interest, from windows containing background based on multiple cues. Given a testing image, windows on a regular grid are scored based on saliency. Candidate windows are then sampled from a distribution given by the saliency scores and the trained model. In [8], an initial set of about $10^5$ windows is generated based on super-pixel segmentation of the image and a global prior distribution estimated from the training images. The features measuring "objectness" are extracted for the windows and based on these features the final set of 100 or 1000 windows is selected. The approach of [24] estimates surface orientation and camera viewpoint to predict the scales and positions of the objects in order to improve the accuracy of object detectors. Since making these estimations in a general setting is still a very difficult problem, the method is not applicable for general, time-critical applications.

In contrast to previous approaches for proposal generation that focus on disregarding local image parts that are unlikely to contain an object, we propose a complementary approach where local image parts predict the occurrence of the closest object as shown in Fig. 1. While our approach uses image context to reduce the search space to promising windows, there are various methods that employ scene context or inter-object relations to boost the detection accuracy [25–29]. This is, however, not the focus of the paper.

## 3   Local Context Priors

Due to the high variation of objects with respect to image position, size, and aspect ratio, the number of image regions, termed windows, that need to be classified in order to detect an object, easily exceeds 1 million for a single image. In particular, detecting pedestrians on a wide range of scales as in the Caltech benchmark [11] is very expensive. In this work, we investigate a method to reduce the number of windows to be evaluated in order to get the same results as commonly used detectors like [2] that process all windows.

The sliding window principle can be formulated as sampling from the set of all windows $\mathcal{W}$, where a window is denoted by $W = (x, y, w, h)$ with $(x, y)$ being the center of the window, $w$ the width, and $h$ the height of the window. The sampling is performed according to a distribution $p(W|I)$, which depends on the image $I$. Each window is then classified according to a probability $p(c|W, I)$ or a scoring function that gives high values to windows that are tight bounds around an instance of the object class $c$. Although not all detectors are probabilistic, we use the probabilistic formulation:

$$p(c|W, I)p(W|I). \tag{1}$$

For sliding window detectors, $p(W|I)$ is a uniform distribution over $\mathcal{W}$. We aim to learn a distribution $p(W|I)$ that gives a higher probability to image regions where instances of the object class $c$ can be expected from the context. In our case, the probability is not modeled globally over the full space but locally over local image patches $\mathcal{P}(y)$ located at $y$ as illustrated in Fig. 1. In this way, we do not have to process the full image first and can thus compute very efficiently local priors over $\mathcal{W}$ from local image information. Another advantage is that the sampled patches do not need to include the objects of interest. Instead, the context gives information where relevant objects could be. For instance, the building in Fig. 1 gives information that the closest pedestrians are expected below the building. In order to handle $N$ local priors, we combine them by

$$p(W|I) = \frac{1}{N} \sum_i p(W|\mathcal{P}(\boldsymbol{y}_i)), \tag{2}$$

where   $\boldsymbol{y}_i = (x_i, y_i)$   and   $p(W|\mathcal{P}(\boldsymbol{y}_i)) = p((x - x_i, y - y_i, w, h)|\mathcal{P}(\boldsymbol{y}_i))$.   (3)

The right hand side of (3) models the relative location of a window with respect to the patch location $\boldsymbol{y}_i$. In this way, the probability becomes invariant to global translations. The context is also not learned explicitly, but implicitly and directly from the image data. Hence, the approach does not require any expensive computation and the prior (2) can be computed within 10ms as we will show in the experiments.

For learning the local priors, we use regression forests [30] that have been previously applied to a variety of regression problems in computer vision [31–34]. In the sequel, we outline the learning procedure of the priors and its application for object detection.

## 3.1   Training

For learning a local prior $p(W|\mathcal{P})$ given an image patch $\mathcal{P}$, we have to collect some training pairs $(\mathcal{P}_i, W_i)$. To this end, we randomly sample fixed-size patches $\mathcal{P}_i$ from images that contain at least one annotated object. For each patch, we then search for the closest annotated bounding box $(x, y, w, h)$, with $(x, y)$ being the center of the bounding box, to the patch center $\boldsymbol{y}_i$ and use the relative position as window:

$$W_i = (x - x_i, y - y_i, w, h). \tag{4}$$

In some cases, the closest bounding box does not correspond to the closest expected occurrence of an object. For instance, a building on the left hand side of a street might be associated with a pedestrian on the right hand side of the street since the training image captured only a scene where a pedestrian appeared on the right hand side. In order to enforce locality and reduce noise since not all plausible locations and scales of the objects are annotated, we only take patches that have at least some overlap with an annotated bounding box; see Fig. 1.

Having collected the training pairs $(\mathcal{P}_i, W_i)$, we learn a regression forest as in [30]. For each tree in the forest, we select a random subset of our training data and train each tree recursively. To this end, we generate at each node a set of binary tests. Each test $t$ is defined by a random feature and a random threshold and splits the training data arriving at the current node. We evaluate the splitting quality of each test $t$ using the information gain:

$$IG_t = H(A) - \sum_{k=\{0,1\}} \frac{|A_k(t)|}{|A|} H(A_k(t)) \tag{5}$$

where $H$ denotes the entropy, $A$ the samples arriving at the node and $A_k(t)$ the split sets of $A$ obtained by test $t$. For efficiency, we use a Gaussian approximation of the distribution over $\mathcal{W}$ as in [31, 33]:

$$H(A) = 2\left(1 + \log\left(2\pi\right)\right) + \frac{1}{2}\log\left(\left|\Sigma^W\right|\right), \tag{6}$$

where $\Sigma^W$ is the covariance matrix of the windows $W$ in the set $A$.

Once the optimal split which maximizes the information gain is found, the parameters of the test function are stored at the node and the construction of the tree continues recursively on the two subsets given by the split. As soon as the number of samples arriving at the node is below a threshold or the maximal depth is reached, a leaf node is created. At each leaf, we store the mean $\overline{W}$ and covariance matrix $\Sigma^W$ of the windows $W$ ending in the leaf during training.

## 3.2 Testing

For testing, we randomly sample a set of patches $\mathcal{P}(\boldsymbol{y}_i)$ from the image as illustrated in Fig. 2. Each patch is then passed through the random forest consisting of $L$ trees, ending in a leaf $l$ for each tree. Based on the normal distributions $p(W|l) = \mathcal{N}(W; \overline{W}_l, \Sigma_l^W)$ stored at the leaves, we compute the average of the leaves as in [30] and obtain the normal distribution given the patch $\mathcal{P}(\boldsymbol{y}_i)$:

$$p(W|\mathcal{P}(\boldsymbol{y}_i)) = \mathcal{N}(W; \overline{W}, \Sigma^W), \tag{7}$$

$$\overline{W} = \frac{1}{L}\sum_l (\overline{x}_l + x_i, \overline{y}_l + y_i, \overline{w}_l, \overline{h}_l), \tag{8}$$

$$\Sigma^W = \frac{1}{L^2}\sum_l \Sigma_l^W. \tag{9}$$

Since the regression forest models only the relative location of the windows, we have to add the patch center $\boldsymbol{y}_i = (x_i, y_i)$ to the mean in (8). To obtain a full distribution over the set of windows $\mathcal{W}$, we combine the local priors of the sampled patches $\mathcal{P}(\boldsymbol{y}_i)$ by a sum of Gaussians (2).

In order to use the local priors for object detection, we generate $N$ samples from the distribution and run an object detector on the image regions of the sampled windows. Note that the local priors are specific to an object category, but not to any detector. For each sampled patch $\mathcal{P}(\boldsymbol{y}_i)$, we sample $\rho$ windows from the corresponding normal distribution (7). Keeping the overall number of windows $N$ fixed, the number of sampled patches $\mathcal{P}(\boldsymbol{y}_i)$ is then given by $\frac{N}{\rho}$. The parameter $\rho$ is basically a trade-off between sampling locally based on (7) and exploring the full image by sampling more patches; see Fig. 2.

While (2) weights the Gaussians uniformly, we have also investigated to weight the Gaussians based on the variance. To this end, we weight each Gaussian $p(W|\mathcal{P}(\boldsymbol{y}_i))$ by $w_i \propto \frac{1}{\log(|\Sigma^W|)}$, where $\sum_i w_i = 1$. This is motivated by the observation that leaves with high variance are less confident about the location of the closest objects than leaves with low variance. Therefore, the weighting focuses the local sampling on the patches that are more confident. In our experiments, we observed that the weighting of the Gaussians improves the results slightly for small sample sizes, but the difference to (2) becomes negligible for larger sample sizes.

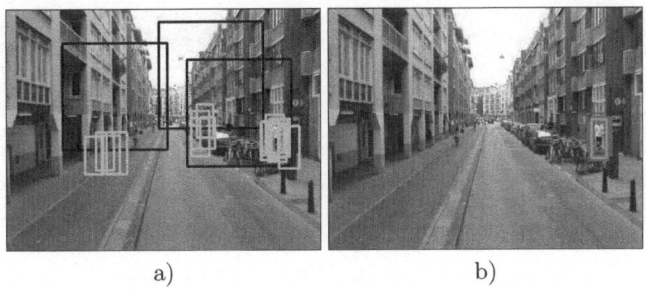

a)                                                    b)

**Fig. 2.** Example illustrating the local prior method. a) Exploration patches (blue) are generated uniformly at random and suggested windows (cyan) are sampled from the estimated distributions. b) Hits (ground truth is painted green, hits are painted purple).

# 4    Experimental Results

We focus our evaluation on three challenging datasets. The Caltech pedestrian detection benchmark [11] contains real-world sequences captured with a camera mounted on a car. The publicly available dataset consists of about 1M frames in $640 \times 480$ pixel resolution, split over a training and a testing set. A few example images are shown in Fig. 3. We followed the evaluation protocol of [11] and used the settings "reasonable" and "overall". The corresponding sets will be referred to as $caltech_{reasonable}$ and $caltech_{overall}$. For the parameter evaluation, we did not use all the frames, but subsets (every 300th frame; 402 frames in total). We denote them $caltech^{300}_{reasonable}$ and $caltech^{300}_{overall}$. The second dataset for pedestrian detection is taken from [35]. It was recorded from a mobile platform in an urban environment and contains 290 annotated images. We rescaled the images from the resolution $384 \times 288$ to $640 \times 480$ pixels. We will refer to this dataset as *amsterdam* and use it only for testing. We also evaluated our method on PASCAL VOC 2007 and 2006 [1] to further examine the performance on other object categories and non-urban environments. In the following figures, the mean value and standard deviation are reported over five runs.

## 4.1    Caltech

We chose patch size to be large relative to the image and fix $\mathcal{P}$ to $256 \times 256$ pixels. As image features, we use histograms of gradients [2] (*HOG*) or generalized Haar features [36] which can be efficiently implemented using integral images [37]. We will refer to these features as *Haar* features. As a pre-processing step before feature extraction, patches are down-sampled to the dimension of $128 \times 128$ pixels.

The regression forests have been trained with 5 trees, where each tree was trained on a random subset of 450 images containing at least one pedestrian. From these images, 50,000 patches $\mathcal{P}$ were extracted for training. For the training of a single node, 30,000 random tests were assessed. The minimal number of patches arriving at a leaf was set to 10 and the maximum tree depth was set to 20.

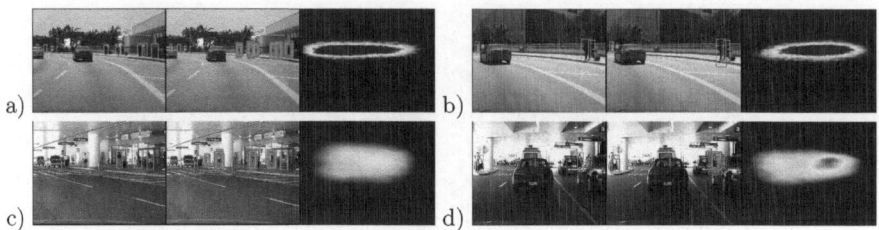

**Fig. 3.** Results on images from Caltech pedestrian benchmark [11] obtained by our method with $\rho = 20$, Haar features, and 5,000 sampled windows. Each image triple consists of: 1) ground truth (green), 2) suggested windows hitting the ground truth (purple), 3) density over the centers of the windows. a) The sidewalk area is correctly detected. b) 5,000 samples are not enough to obtain good hits for the pedestrians. c) Pedestrians are correctly recognized in an indoor setting. d) The method correctly detects that pedestrians are less likely to appear in the middle of the street. Best viewed in color.

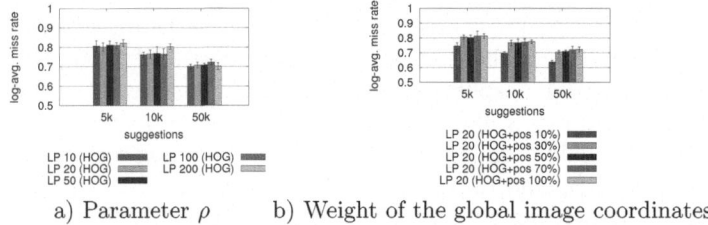

a) Parameter $\rho$    b) Weight of the global image coordinates

**Fig. 4. a)** Log-average miss rate with respect to parameter $\rho$. **b)** Log-average miss rate with respect to the weight of the global image coordinates (pos.). Parameter $\rho$ was fixed to $\rho = 20$. Both experiments were evaluated on $caltech_{reasonable}^{300}$ with HOG features and in conjunction with HOG classifier.

Fig. 3 shows a few example results from $caltech_{overall}$. Given an image, the method computes the distribution consisting of a sum of Gaussians over the windows $W = (x, y, w, h)$. The figure visualizes only the distribution over $(x, y)$. The distributions change depending on the image. While the distributions in Fig. 3a) and b) focus on the sidewalk which is nearly horizontal in these images, the distributions in c) and d) cover a larger area of the image. Since the sampled windows are limited to 5,000 in this example, some of the pedestrians are missed in b) although the estimated distribution is reasonable.

For quantitative evaluation, we classified the proposed windows using a SVM classifier and histogram of gradients features as in [2]. In our experiments, we used the OpenCV implementation of [2]. We will refer to it as *classifier HOG*. Although our method can generate continuous values for the windows, we limited the results to the set of windows generated by the sliding window approach in order to provide a fair comparison. We used a multiplicative scale stride of 1.05 and positional stride of 4 pixels. For the "reasonable" setting, the image scale range was $[0.5, 2.5]$ and for the "overall" setting, it spanned $[0.5, 5.2]$.

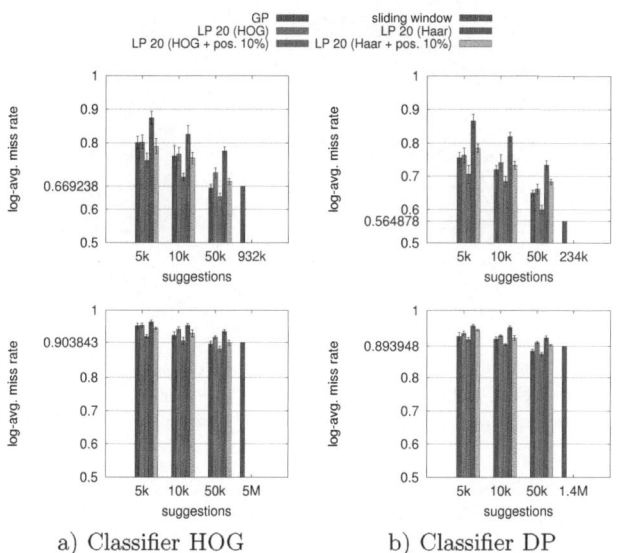

a) Classifier HOG            b) Classifier DP

**Fig. 5.** Comparison between HOG classifier and Deformable parts classifier (DP) performed on $caltech^{300}_{reasonable}$ (upper row) and $caltech^{300}_{overall}$ (bottom row). The global prior (GP) and sliding window serve as base line. The classifier HOG (a) is outperformed by the classifier DP (b).

In Fig. 4a), we show the performance with respect to the parameters $\rho$ and the number of sampled windows $N$ from the prior distribution. As measure, we use the log-average miss rate as in [18]. As one can see, the miss rate decreases with an increasing number of sampled windows. The impact of $\rho$ can be said to be negligible up to a certain level. For the rest of the experiments, we used $\rho = 20$ as parameter for the local priors ($LP$ 20).

To evaluate the impact of the patch size, we varied the patch size for LP 20 HOG with 10k windows on $caltech_{reasonable}$. The log-avg. miss rates were: 0.79 (32×32), 0.75 (64×64), 0.74 (128×128), 0.74 (256×256), 0.72 (384×384). This shows that the impact of the particular size is rather small as long as the patches are reasonably large. The patch size of 256×256 is used for the rest of the experiments.

In Fig. 5a) and 6, we compare our method with the sliding window approach on the Caltech dataset using classifier HOG. While the sliding window approach processes about 1 million windows in "reasonable" setting, LP 20 with HOG features requires only 10,000 - 50,000 windows to achieve a comparable performance. This corresponds to 1.1%-5.4% of all windows. In the "overall" setting (Fig. 6b), the computational advantage of our method becomes even more pronounced as the search space grows larger with the increasing number of scales: sliding window processes 5 million windows, while our method needs to inspect only 0.2%-1.0% thereof for a comparable performance. Since also detecting small objects is of utter importance for many real-world application like driver assistance systems [11], the "overall" setting is highly relevant.

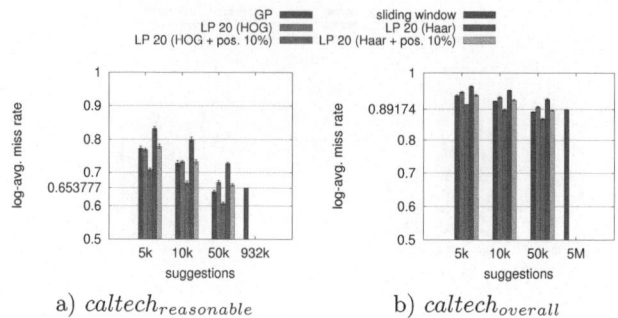

**Fig. 6.** Performance comparison evaluated on a) *caltech_reasonable* and b) *caltech_overall* using the classifier HOG. The local context priors were trained on corresponding *caltech_reasonable* and *caltech_overall* datasets.

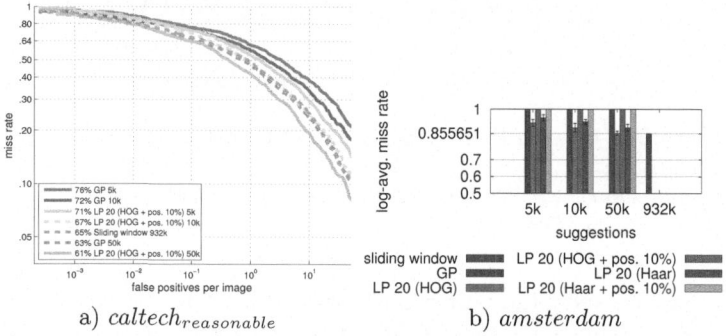

a) *caltech_reasonable*                          b) *amsterdam*

**Fig. 7. a)** Comparison of miss rate / false positive per image curves evaluated on *caltech_reasonable* with classifier HOG in a single run (log-avg. miss rate is indicated in the legend). The global prior (GP) and sliding window are used as base lines. The number of suggestions is indicated as suffix. The best performance is achieved by local priors combined with global image coordinates. **b)** Evaluation on *amsterdam* in "reasonable" setting with local priors trained on *caltech_reasonable*. Methods relying on global features fail, while the ones based only on local features successfully adapt.

We compared HOG features with Haar features for learning the local priors. While the Haar features perform worse than the HOG features, the Haar features are 9 times faster to compute.

The local priors were also compared to a global prior (GP). It has been shown that spatial Gaussian priors are the most important cue for modeling visual attention [38]. Hence, we model the global prior as Gaussian over the set of windows given in absolute spatial coordinates and estimated from the training annotations. Since in Caltech dataset the camera was mounted on a car, sampling from the global prior already improves the sliding window approach. Therefore, we combined the global and local priors by adding the absolute $(x, y)$ coordinates of the sampled training patch centers as additional features for learning the regression forests, where the impact of the local image features (HOG) and the global image coordinates (pos.) were weighted. The results for different settings are shown in Fig. 4b). Learning only with image coordinates corresponds to learning a global prior, which performs worse than HOG combined with patch position. Fig. 5 and Fig. 6 show that the global information improves the local prior for this dataset and performs as good or better than the global prior. The miss rate / false positive per image curves computed for a single evaluation run are shown in Fig. 7a).

In order to show that the learned priors are not specific to a detector, we employed a state-of-the-art classifier [4] (referred here as *classifier DP*). The evaluation with the classifier DP is presented in Fig. 5b). When Fig. 5a) and Fig. 5b) are compared, it becomes evident that the classifier DP has a lower miss rate than the classifier HOG, which agrees with the results presented in the literature [11]. The performance of our method changes accordingly.

We report here the average runtime of our method in conjunction with the classifier HOG. Sliding window approach took 18s to inspect 932k windows in "reasonable" setting, and 84s in "overall" setting (single-threaded; Intel Core i7-2600K CPU with 4 GB RAM). For benchmark, we used our method to sample 5k windows and run a classifier over them. The generation of windows ($\rho = 20$) with HOG features took 90ms and with Haar features 10ms, respectively. Adding location coordinates to the features did not affect the average runtime. Overall, our approach requires 0.8s for the "reasonable" and 1.3s for the "overall" setting, which corresponds to a runtime reduction by a factor of 23 and 65, respectively. Since the local priors are computed in few milliseconds, they can be used to speed up faster detectors like [18] or to use slower, but more accurate detectors.

Finally, we evaluated on *caltech*$_{reasonable}$ the benefit of a regression compared to a classification that just discards parts of the image. To this end, a random forest with HOG features was trained to discriminate patches containing objects with the same settings as before. During test time, we ranked patches on a dense grid and thoroughly explored the best ones by sliding window. The inspection stopped at 50k inspected windows. The classification with log-avg. miss rate 0.78 for 256×256 and 128×128 patch size performs worse than the regression LP 20 HOG (Fig. 6). When we ranked the patches based on the classification, but sampled windows with LP 20 HOG, the performance did not differ significantly for a patch size 256×256. For 128×128, however, the performance improved for 5k windows: 0.71 (5k), 0.70 (10k), 0.66 (50k). This shows that the combination of ranking or discarding image parts with predicting the scale and location of objects using a regression is worth to be explored more in detail in the future.

### 4.2   Amsterdam

To evaluate the generalizability of the local prior, we have performed a cross-dataset experiment. To this end, the local prior was trained on *caltech*$_{reasonable}$ and applied to *amsterdam*. The evaluation protocol and the parameters are the same as for the Caltech dataset. The results are presented in Fig. 7b). Due to variability in camera position, the global prior (GP) completely fails, while the local priors LP 20 without global features still perform well, thus indicating that the local prior does not overfit to the dataset bias in contrast to the global prior.

**Table 1. a)** Comparison of performance on PASCAL VOC 2007 by average precision (AP). Our method outperforms [20] and [10] and matches [9] at lower runtime cost. **b)** Comparison of performance on PASCAL VOC 2006 in terms of area under overlap-recall curves (AUC). We generally outperform [19] and in some categories come close to state-of-the-art [6]. Our method, however, is at least by a factor of 57 faster.

| a) VOC 2007, AP | Bird | Dog | Plant | Boat | Sheep | Cat | Chair | Table | Cow | Bottle | Aeroplane | Sofa | TV/Mon. | Person | Train | Motorbike | Bus | Horse | Car | Bicycle | Mean |
|---|---|---|---|---|---|---|---|---|---|---|---|---|---|---|---|---|---|---|---|---|---|
| LP 20 Haar 1k | 10.1 | 11.3 | 10.0 | 11.4 | 15.6 | 20.3 | 14.3 | 24.7 | 16.9 | 11.5 | 29.7 | 30.2 | 27.3 | 29.6 | 41.1 | 39.6 | 43.3 | 52.9 | 39.7 | 39.7 | 26.0 |
| LP 20 Haar 3k | 10.4 | 9.8 | 10.4 | 11.8 | 16.2 | 20.1 | 17.0 | 26.2 | 17.8 | 15.7 | 30.8 | 32.7 | 33.8 | 33.5 | 42.7 | 41.5 | 44.7 | 54.4 | 43.1 | 46.0 | 28.0 |
| [4] | 9.9 | 11.1 | 12.5 | 15.0 | 17.8 | 19.3 | 22.6 | 23.2 | 24.2 | 25.4 | 28.9 | 34.3 | 41.8 | 42.3 | 44.9 | 47.9 | 50.4 | 56.8 | 58.1 | 58.8 | 32.3 |
| [9] | 10.3 | 12.4 | 9.9 | 12.5 | 18.8 | 19.1 | 17.9 | 23.6 | 22.9 | 14.5 | 31.6 | 33.2 | 41.3 | 29.1 | 39.7 | 44.8 | 44.8 | 50.9 | 50.1 | 52.7 | 29.0 |
| [20] | 0.2 | 13.2 | 1.7 | 0.6 | 13.0 | 17.6 | 3.3 | 12.2 | 10.8 | 9.1 | 17.3 | 15.3 | 18.4 | 14.2 | 22.5 | 27.9 | 27.6 | 36.8 | 29.3 | 22.4 | 15.7 |
| [10] (2k windows) | - | - | - | - | - | - | - | - | - | - | - | - | - | - | - | - | - | - | - | - | 22.4 |

| b) VOC 2006, AUC | Bicycle | Bus | Car | Cat | Cow | Dog | Horse | Motorbike | Person | Sheep | Mean |
|---|---|---|---|---|---|---|---|---|---|---|---|
| LP 20 Haar 1k | 68.5 | 64.6 | 52.9 | 74.9 | 59.1 | 71.7 | 67.7 | 67.1 | 51.7 | 51.5 | 63.0 |
| LP 20 Haar 3k | 73.2 | 69.1 | 58.4 | 78.6 | 64.0 | 75.8 | 72.3 | 71.7 | 57.7 | 56.4 | 67.7 |
| [6] | 70.7 | 70.6 | 66.6 | 73.2 | 69.9 | 71.1 | 71.1 | 72.8 | 65.5 | 67.9 | 69.9 |
| [19] | 62.4 | 58.8 | 49.6 | 76.7 | 52.5 | 71.8 | 63.7 | 63.4 | 41.7 | 44.2 | 58.5 |

## 4.3   PASCAL VOC

In order to demonstrate that the approach also generalizes to other categories than pedestrians in urban environments, we have evaluated the approach on PASCAL VOC 2007 dataset [1].The evaluation protocol "comp3" was followed. The local priors were trained individually for each class on the "trainval" sets and applied to the respective "test" sets. Patch size was set to $128 \times 128$. Prior to feature extraction, patches were down-sampled once. Classifier DP [4] was used for the classification. In contrast to the pedestrian datasets, the performance of the Haar features is slightly better than the HOG features. While the HOG features capture shape better than Haar features, which is very important in urban environments, the Haar features also capture color information, which is a useful cue for the general categories. We therefore report results only for Haar features. Table 1a) shows the comparison with [4] as baseline, a related method for window proposal [9] and a branch-and-rank approach [20]. Except for one category, we outperform [20] in terms of average precision (AP), while we match the performance of [9] in many categories, but at significantly lower runtime cost. Our approach requires $7 \pm 2$ms for proposal generation whereas [9] takes at least 8s for the segmentation.

Due to the subsampling of window space, our approach misses some objects (see Table 1a)), but also removes some false positives. Since [4] is not perfect, subsampling can therefore even increase the AP. As the number of sampled windows increases, the AP converges to the baseline.

We evaluated our method with the same parameter settings on PASCAL VOC 2006 [1] to compare its sampling performance with two other selective search methods [6] and [19]. As in [6, 19], we use the area under overlap-recall curves as measure. Both reference methods proposed 1,000 windows. The results are presented in Table 1b). We outperform [19] on all but two categories and get close to the state-of-the-art [6] on some categories. While [6] and [19] require at least 400ms on average, our method is by more than a factor of 57 faster and requires only 7ms.

## 5 Conclusion

In this work, we presented a novel method for generating window proposals based on the local context. It sparsely examines the image and incorporates the knowledge extracted from a patch even if it does not contain an object of interest. While the approach generalizes well and can be successfully applied across datasets and for various categories, it can also be adapted to make use of global a priori knowledge. The experiments show that it achieves the detection performance of a computationally expensive exhaustive search in a fraction of the time. The approach also achieves competitive results compared to state-of-the-art approaches for proposal generation, but at significantly lower runtime cost. In further work, we would like to test the performance of our method with different features and other classifiers as well as to combine it with complementary methods for reducing the runtime, like cascading.

**Acknowledgement.** This work was partially supported by the EU projects FP7-ICT-24314 Interactive Urban Robot (IURO) and FP7-ICT-248873 Robotic ADaptation to Humans Adapting to Robots (RADHAR).

## References

1. Everingham, M., Van Gool, L., Williams, C., Winn, J., Zisserman, A.: The pascal visual object classes (VOC) challenge. IJCV 88, 303–338 (2010)
2. Dalal, N., Triggs, B.: Histograms of oriented gradients for human detection. In: CVPR (2005)
3. Viola, P., Jones, M.: Robust real-time face detection. IJCV 57, 137–154 (2004)
4. Felzenszwalb, P., Girshick, R., McAllester, D., Ramanan, D.: Object detection with discriminatively trained part based models. TPAMI 32 (2010)
5. Lampert, C., Blaschko, M., Hofmann, T.: Efficient Subwindow Search: A Branch and Bound Framework for Object Localization. TPAMI 31, 2129–2142 (2009)
6. Zhang, Z., Warrell, J., Torr, P.: Proposal generation for object detection using cascaded ranking SVMs. In: CVPR (2011)
7. Gualdi, G., Prati, A., Cucchiara, R.: Multi-stage Sampling with Boosting Cascades for Pedestrian Detection in Images and Videos. In: Daniilidis, K., Maragos, P., Paragios, N. (eds.) ECCV 2010, Part VI. LNCS, vol. 6316, pp. 196–209. Springer, Heidelberg (2010)
8. Rahtu, E., Kannala, J., Blaschko, M.: Learning a category independent object detection cascade. In: ICCV (2011)
9. van de Sande, K., Uijlings, J., Gevers, T., Smeulders, A.: Segmentation as selective search for object recognition. In: ICCV (2011)
10. Alexe, B., Thomas, D., Ferrari, V.: What is an object? In: CVPR (2010)
11. Dollár, P., Wojek, C., Schiele, B., Perona, P.: Pedestrian detection: An evaluation of the state of the art. TPAMI (2011)
12. Zhu, L., Chen, Y., Yuille, A., Freeman, W.: Latent hierarchical structural learning for object detection. In: CVPR (2010)
13. Pedersoli, M., Vedaldi, A.: Gonzàlez: A coarse-to-fine approach for fast deformable object detection. In: CVPR (2011)

14. Romdhani, S., Torr, P., Schölkopf, B., Blake, A.: Computationally efficient face detection. In: ICCV (2001)
15. Brubaker, S.C., Mullin, M.D., Rehg, J.M.: Towards Optimal Training of Cascaded Detectors. In: Leonardis, A., Bischof, H., Pinz, A. (eds.) ECCV 2006. LNCS, vol. 3951, pp. 325–337. Springer, Heidelberg (2006)
16. Zhang, W., Zelinsky, G., Samaras, D.: Real-time accurate object detection using multiple resolutions. In: ICCV (2007)
17. Felzenszwalb, P., Girshick, R., McAllester, D.: Cascade object detection with deformable part models. In: CVPR (2010)
18. Dollár, P., Tu, Z., Perona, P., Belongie, S.: Integral Channel Features. In: BMVC (2009)
19. Lampert, C.: An efficient divide-and-conquer cascade for nonlinear object detection. In: CVPR (2010)
20. Lehmann, A., Gehler, P., Van Gool, L.: Branch & rank: Non-linear object detection. In: BMVC (2011)
21. Vedaldi, A., Gulshan, V., Varma, M., Zisserman, A.: Multiple kernels for object detection. In: ICCV (2009)
22. Chum, O., Zisserman, A.: An exemplar model for learning object classes. In: CVPR (2007)
23. Russakovsky, O., Ng, A.: A steiner tree approach to efficient object detection. In: CVPR (2010)
24. Hoiem, D., Efros, A., Hebert, M.: Putting objects in perspective. IJCV 80 (2008)
25. Torralba, A., Murphy, K., Freeman, W.: Using the forest to see the trees: exploiting context for visual object detection and localization. Commun. ACM 53, 107–114 (2010)
26. Desai, C., Ramanan, D., Fowlkes, C.: Discriminative models for multi-class object layout. In: ICCV (2009)
27. Divvala, S., Hoiem, D., Hays, J., Efros, A., Hebert, M.: An empirical study of context in object detection. In: CVPR (2009)
28. Sadeghi, M., Farhadi, A.: Recognition using visual phrases. In: CVPR (2011)
29. Li, C., Parikh, D., Chen, T.: Extracting adaptive contextual cues from unlabeled regions. In: ICCV (2011)
30. Breiman, L.: Random forests. Machine Learning 45, 5–32 (2001)
31. Criminisi, A., Shotton, J., Robertson, D., Konukoglu, E.: Regression Forests for Efficient Anatomy Detection and Localization in CT Studies. In: Menze, B., Langs, G., Tu, Z., Criminisi, A. (eds.) MICCAI 2010. LNCS, vol. 6533, pp. 106–117. Springer, Heidelberg (2011)
32. Gall, J., Yao, A., Razavi, N., Van Gool, L., Lempitsky, V.S.: Hough forests for object detection, tracking, and action recognition. TPAMI 33, 2188–2202 (2011)
33. Fanelli, G., Gall, J., Van Gool, L.: Real time head pose estimation with random regression forests. In: CVPR (2011)
34. Girshick, R., Shotton, J., Kohli, P., Criminisi, A., Fitzgibbon, A.: Efficient regression of general-activity human poses from depth images. In: ICCV (2011)
35. Leibe, B., Cornelis, N., Cornelis, K., Van Gool, L.: Dynamic 3d scene analysis from a moving vehicle. In: CVPR (2007)
36. Dollár, P., Tu, Z., Tao, H., Belongie, S.: Feature mining for image classification. In: CVPR (2007)
37. Crow, F.: Summed-area tables for texture mapping. SIGGRAPH Comput. Graph. 18, 207–212 (1984)
38. Judd, T., Ehinger, K., Durand, F., Torralba, A.: Learning to predict where humans look. In: ICCV (2009)

# Arbitrary-Shape Object Localization
# Using Adaptive Image Grids

Chunluan Zhou and Junsong Yuan

School of EEE, Nanyang Technology University, Singapore

**Abstract.** Sliding-window based search is a widely used technique for object localization. However, for objects of non-rectangle shapes, noises in windows may mislead the localization, causing unsatisfactory results. In this paper, we propose an efficient bottom-up approach for detecting arbitrary-shape objects using image grids as basic components. First, a test image is partitioned into $n \times n$ grids and the object is localized by finding a set of connected grids which maximize the classifier's response. Then, graph cut segmentation is used to improve the object boundary by utilizing local image context. Instead of using bounding boxes, the proposed approach searches connected regions of any shapes. With the graph cut refinement, our approach can start with coarse image grids and is robust to noises. To make image grids better cover the object of arbitrary shape, we also propose a fast adaptive grid partition method which takes image content into account and can be efficiently implemented by dynamic programming. The use of adaptive partition further improves the localization accuracy of our approach. Experiments on PASCAL VOC 2007 and VOC 2008 datasets demonstrate the effectiveness of our approach.

## 1 Introduction

Given an image containing one or more objects of interest, object localization is to determine the position and scope of each object in the image. Object localization plays an important role in object detection systems [6,8,10,24], which need to determine whether there is any object of interest present in an image, and if any, where it is. Since the object of interest may only occupy a small region, it is usually difficult to judge its presence by the whole image. Generally, object detection first performs localization to obtain several candidates by assuming that the object is present, followed by a recognition step to verify each candidate. In such a case, localization accuracy is of fundamental importance to the subsequent recognition.

Sliding window search is widely used for object localization [1,8,11,12]. This localization approach searches all possible windows in an image, evaluating a score for each window, and then selects the windows with the highest scores as candidates for further verification. Since the object size is unknown in advance, for an $m \times n$ image, there are $O(m^2n^2)$ possible windows to be checked, leading to a high computational cost. Another drawback of this approach is that it

K.M. Lee et al. (Eds.): ACCV 2012, Part I, LNCS 7724, pp. 71–84, 2013.
© Springer-Verlag Berlin Heidelberg 2013

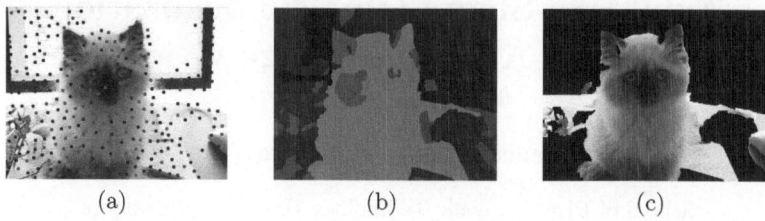

(a)          (b)          (c)

**Fig. 1.** A failed example of ERS. (a) Original image with positive-contribution features (red dots) and negative-contribution features (blue dots). (b) Super-pixel score map. Light regions and dark regions respectively denote positively scored and negatively scored super-pixels. (c) Optimal connected region. Some positively scored background super-pixels are included, while a few object super-pixels are lost due to their negative scores.

approximates the object shape as a rectangle. For non-rectangle objects, noises in the windows may misguide the localization [27].

To solve the above problems of sliding window search, efficient region search (ERS) [25] was recently proposed for localizing arbitrary-shape objects. This approach first segments a test image into super-pixels and each super-pixel is assigned a score by summing the contributions of its features. The object region is localized by selecting a set of connected super-pixels with the highest total score. The selection of super-pixels is converted to a graph search problem which is efficiently solved by a branch-and-cut algorithm. However, this approach largely depends on the quality of generated supper-pixels. If some super-pixels cover both object and background areas, part of the object region will be lost or part of the background region will be included in the localization result. The presence of noisy super-pixels, i.e. positive-score background super-pixels and negative-score object super-pixels, may also cause unsatisfactory results. Figure 1 shows a failed example of this approach. To exclude background super-pixels, the authors proposed to introduce contours into ERS (ERS-C). However, ERS-C depends on the robustness of contour evaluation, which makes it difficult to guarantee the performance.

To address the limitations of ERS, we propose an efficient bottom-up approach using image grids. An overview of our approach is shown in Fig. 2. A test image is uniformly partitioned into $n \times n$ grids and the branch-and-cut search is applied to these grids, instead of super-pixels, to obtain an optimal connected region (Fig. 2(a-c)). Then, the obtained region is enlarged and graph cut segmentation is applied to the enlarged region for refinement, i.e. retrieving lost object pixels and excluding background pixels (Fig. 2(d-f)). The introduce of graph cut refinement in our approach has two advantages. First, this refinement step makes it possible to use coarse basic components, e.g. image grids, which can be easily obtained. This is important to speed up the localization process as it is usually time-consuming to obtain high-quality super-pixels, like the segmentation method [2] used in ERS. Second, it makes our approach more robust to noises. To improve the localization accuracy, we also propose an efficient adaptive grid

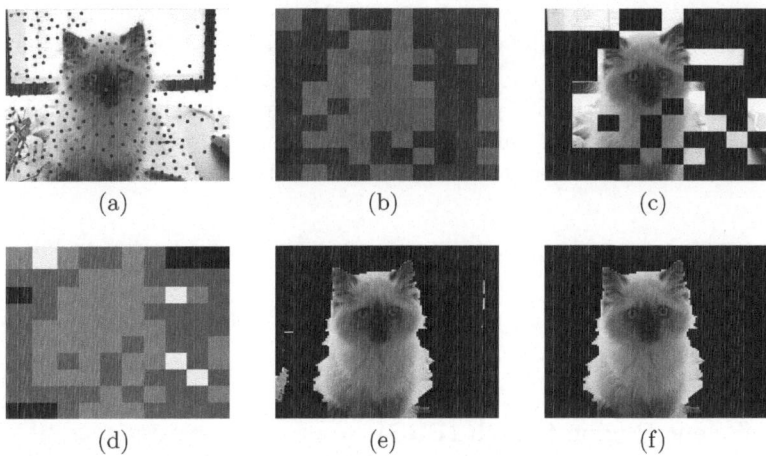

(a)  (b)  (c)

(d)  (e)  (f)

**Fig. 2.** Overview of our approach. (a) Original image with local features. (b) Grid score map. (c) Optimal connected region. (d) Initial background and foreground seeds for graph cut segmentation. Blue grids are newly added and selected as background seeds. Red grids are positive-score grids in the optimal region and selected as foreground seeds. Yellow grids are negative-score grids included by grid search to form the optimal region. The yellow grids may belong to either foreground or background and are left unlabeled initially. Graph cut segmentation relabels all the pixels in the image except the black area. (e) Result of graph cut segmentation. (f) Final object region.

partition method which takes image content into account. We demonstrate the effectiveness of our approach on PASCAL VOC 2007 and VOC 2008 datasets.

## 2 Related Work

Several approaches have been proposed for localizing arbitrary-shaped objects. In [26], extensions are made to efficient subwindow search [16] for localizing non-rectangle regions, $k$-composite boxes and $k$-side polygons, respectively. However, the parameter $k$ needs to be pre-determined, and to make the search efficient, its value cannot be too large, thereby limiting the shapes of objects the approach can detect. Voting approaches [17,18,21] are suitable for localizing objects of various shapes, but they may fail when the objects to be localized differ largely in shape and viewpoint from those used for training. Free-shape subwindow search [27] locates the object by connecting edge segments to form a closed region with its boundary and inner features maximizing the localization objective function. The approaches proposed in [13,23,25] use super-pixels as basic components and localize the object region by selecting a subset of super-pixels. Different from [13,23,25,27], our approach starts with coarse image grids, which are also used for object search [14,15] recently.

There are many object localization/detection approaches using segmentation for further processing [7,13,17,19,20,22,28]. In [17,20,22], more accurate segmentation is inferred from each localized object candidate and then used to verify the localized candidate. Several approaches [7,13,28] use segmentation to exclude background pixels from the localized object region and retrieve lost object pixels, as we do in this paper. With the observation that animals like cats and dogs have homogenous color and texture, segmentation is used to detect the rest parts of the body after the head is detected [19].

## 3   Grid-Based Object Localization

In this section, we first describe efficient region search [25], and then introduce our image-grid based object localization approach.

### 3.1   Efficient Region Search (ERS)

First, bag-of-visual-words representation and linear SVM are used to train a classifier. A set of features (e.g. SURF [3]) are collected from training images and quantized into a codebook of $K$ visual words. Using the codebook, an image region $R$ containing features $d_i$, $i = 1, ..., M$, is represented by a $K$-bin histogram $h(R)$. The classification function $f$ is learned by linear SVM:

$$f(R) = \sum_{j=1}^{N} \alpha_j \langle h(R), h(R_j) \rangle + \beta \tag{1}$$

where $N$ is the number of training examples, $R_j$ is the $j$-th training example, and $\alpha_j$ and $\beta$ are the weights and the bias respectively.

Let $h_k(R_j)$ be the count of the $k$-th bin of the histogram $h(R_j)$ and the expression of $f(R)$ is rewritten as

$$f(R) = \sum_{k=1}^{K} h_k(R) \sum_{j=1}^{N} \alpha_j h_k(R_j) + \beta = \sum_{i=1}^{M} c_{w_i} + \beta \tag{2}$$

where $c_k = \sum_{j=1}^{N} \alpha_j h_k(R_j)$ represents the contribution of the $k$-th visual word and $w_i$ is the index of the visual word associated with $d_i$. Therefore, the score of region $R$ is the sum of the contributions of its features plus the bias $\beta$.

Given a test image, the goal is to localize an optimal region that maximizes the learned classification function $f$. The image is first segmented into several super-pixels and each super-pixel is assigned a score according to the features extracted from the super-pixel by Eq. (2). And then object region is obtained by identifying a set of connected super-pixels with the highest total score. By viewing each super-pixel as a graph node with the weight its score and adding edges between adjacent super-pixels, the localization problem is converted to the following maximum-weight subgraph search (MWCS) problem:

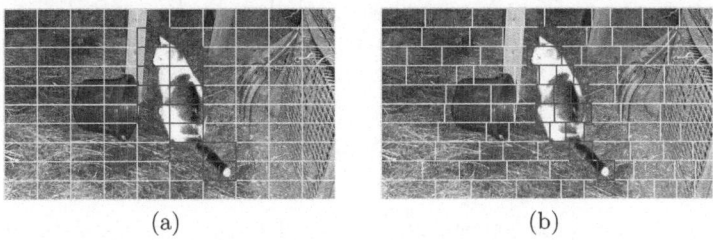

(a) (b)

**Fig. 3.** An example of uniform partition (a) and adaptive partition (b)

**MWSC Problem.** Given an undirected, vertex-weighted graph $G = (V, E)$ with weights $w : V \to \mathbb{R}$, find a connected subgraph $T = (V_T, E_T)$ which maximizes the score $W(T) = \sum_{v \in V_T} w(v)$.

With both positive and negative node weights, the MWCS problem is NP-complete, but in practice it can be efficiently solved by a branch-and-cut algorithm. See [25] for details.

### 3.2 Region Search Using Image Grids

For ERS, the quality of generated super-pixels has a considerable impact on the final localization result. The authors of ERS adopted a sematic segmentation method to obtain high-quality super-pixels but sacrificed computational efficiency. To speed up the component initialization, we start with a coarse grid partition. First, a test image is uniformly partitioned into $n \times n$ grids and each grid is assigned a score as described in section 3.1. By regarding grids as nodes and adding edges between each grid and its neighboring grids, we construct an undirected vertex-weighted graph. Then, the object region is localized by applying the branch-and-cut algorithm to the constructed graph. Figure 2(a-c) shows the search process. We refer to this process as grid search.

With uniform partition, some grids may be located at the object boundary, thus affecting the score evaluation of these grids. To make image grids better cover the object region, we propose an adaptive grid partition method: first, the image is evenly divided into $n$ bands in the horizontal direction; then, each band is vertically divided into $n$ grids satisfying the following two requirements:

1. The color distribution in each grid are as concentrated as possible;
2. The color difference between each two adjacent grids is as large as possible.

The first requirement forces grids to move off the object boundary and the second one prevents a region of homogeneous colors from being broken into many grids. Figure 3 shows an example of uniform partition and adaptive partition.

Now, we describe how to partition a band, denoted by $B$, of width $w$ into $n$ grids. A partition of the band into $n$ grids is represented by $P = \{p_i\}_{i=1}^{n+1}$, where $p_i$ is the position of the $i$-th vertical line and satisfies (1) $p_1 = 1$, (2) $p_{n+1} = w + 1$, and (3) $p_i < p_{i+1}$ for $1 < i \le n$. We denote a sub-band starting from position $s$ to position $t$ ($s$ and $t$ are included) by $B_{s,t}$ with $1 \leq s \leq t \leq w$. So, the $i$-th grid of the partition is the sub-band $B_{p_i,p_{i+1}-1}$, i.e. $g_i = B_{p_i,p_{i+1}-1}$. We obtain an optimal partition by minimizing the following cost function:

$$E(P) = \sum_{i=1}^{n} C(g_i) + \gamma \sum_{i=1}^{n-1} D(g_i, g_{i+1}) \tag{3}$$

where $C(g_i)$ is the color concentration of $g_i$, $D(g_i, g_{i+1})$ is the color difference between $g_i$ and $g_{i+1}$, and $\gamma$ is a parameter.

To calculate $C(g_i)$, we divide the RGB color space into $M = 16 \times 16 \times 16$ bins and compute for $g_i$ a color histogram $h(g_i)$ with $h_j(g_i)$ the count of the $j$-th bin. By normalizing $h(g_i)$ to sum to 1, we define the color concentration of $g_i$ using information entropy:

$$C(g_i) = \sum_{j=1}^{M} -h_j(g_i) log(h_j(g_i)) \tag{4}$$

With this definition, the more concentrated the colors of pixels in $g_i$ are, the smaller the value of $C(g_i)$ is. Typically, when the grid contains only one type of color, $C(g_i) = 0$.

We represent the color of a grid by the average color of the pixels in the grid. Some other representations are also applicable, e.g. color histogram. The color difference between $g_i$ and $g_{i+1}$ is defined as

$$D(g_i, g_{i+1}) = \exp\left(-\frac{\| c_{g_i} - c_{g_{i+1}} \|^2}{2\sigma^2}\right) \tag{5}$$

where $c_{g_i} \in \mathbb{R}^3$ is the color of $g_i$ and $\sigma = 32$ is used in our experiments.

Let $S(i,t)$ be the cost of the optimal partition of the sub-band $B_{1,t}$ into $i$ grids and $T(i,s,t)$ be the minimum cost of partitioning $B_{1,t}$ into $i$ grids with the last grid $g_i = B_{s,t}$. With these two definitions, minimizing the cost function in Eq. (3) is equivalent to compute $S(n,w) = \min_{p_n} T(n, p_n, w)$. By fixing $p_n$ and enumerating the $(n-1)$-th grid, $g_{n-1} = B_{p_{n-1},p_n-1}$, we have

$$T(n, p_n, w) = \min_{p_{n-1}} T(n-1, p_{n-1}, p_n - 1) + C(g_n) + \gamma D(g_{n-1}, g_n) \tag{6}$$

Generally, $T(i,s,t)$ has the following recursive solution:

$$T(i,s,t) = \begin{cases} C(g_1) & i = 1 \\ \min_r T(i-1, r, s-1) + C(g_i) + \gamma D(g_{i-1}, g_i) & i > 1 \end{cases} \tag{7}$$

where $r$, $s$ and $t$ determine the last two grids: $g_{i-1} = B_{r,s-1}$ and $g_i = B_{s,t}$. For the special case $i = 1$, the partition consists of only one grid, i.e. $g_1 = B_{1,t}$, so the partition cost is the color concentration of $g_1$.

According to Eq. (7), we design a dynamic programming algorithm for partitioning a band into $n$ grids (see Alg. 1). With $C(g_i)$ and $D(g_{i-1}, g_i)$ precomputed, this algorithm runs in $O(nw^3)$ time. As there are $n$ bands to be

---

**Algorithm 1.** Adaptive partition for one band

---

**Require:** a band $B$, band width $w$ and partition parameters $n$ and $\gamma$;
**Ensure:** the optimal partition $P^* = \{p_1^*, p_2^*, ..., p_{n+1}^*\}$;
1: $T(i, s, t) \leftarrow \infty, \forall i, s, t$;
2: **for all** $t \in [1, w]$ **do**
3:     $g_1 \leftarrow B_{1,t}$, $T(1, 1, t) \leftarrow C(g_1)$;
4: **end for**
5: **for** $i \leftarrow 2$ to $n$ **do**
6:     **for all** $t \le w$ **do**
7:        **for all** $s < t$ **do**
8:           $g_i \leftarrow B_{s,t}$;
9:           **for all** $r < s$ **do**
10:             $g_{i-1} \leftarrow B_{r,s-1}$, $c \leftarrow T(i - 1, r, s - 1) + C(g_i) + \gamma D(g_{i-1}, g_i)$;
11:             **if** $c < T(i, s, t)$ **then**
12:                $T(i, s, t) \leftarrow c$;
13:             **end if**
14:           **end for**
15:        **end for**
16:     **end for**
17: **end for**
18: $p_1^* \leftarrow 1$, $p_{n+1}^* \leftarrow w + 1$;
19: **for** $i \leftarrow n$ to $2$ **do**
20:     $p_i^* \leftarrow \arg\min_{p_i} T(i, p_i, p_{i+1}^*)$;
21: **end for**

---

partitioned, the total running time for adaptive partition is $O(n^2 w^3)$. To make adaptive partition robust to cluttered images, we restrict the width of each grid to the range $[\frac{1}{2} w_G, \frac{3}{2} w_G]$, where $w_G = \frac{w}{n}$ is the width of a grid obtained by uniform partition. With this restriction, the time needed to partition one band is reduced to $O(n \cdot w \cdot \frac{w}{n} \cdot \frac{w}{n}) = O(\frac{w^3}{n})$ with the total partition time $O(w^3)$. For a high-resolution image (e.g. $1280 \times 1024$ pixels), we first scale it down (e.g. to $320 \times 256$ pixels) and then perform the partition on the low-resolution image. Therefore, our adaptive partition is fast in practice.

### 3.3 Refinement with Graph Cut Segmentation

Due to noisy local features, a background grid may be assigned a positive score and included in the localized region. Similarly, some object grids possibly have negative scores and may therefore be excluded. We need to exclude the background pixels from the result region and retrieve the lost object pixels. To achieve this, we first enlarge the localized region to exploit local image context: the grids adjacent to the localized region are added to form a larger region (Fig. 2(d)). Then, graph cut segmentation [4] is applied to the enlarged region to refine the object boundary.

Graph cut segmentation divides the enlarged region into two parts, foreground (the object region) and background. Let $X$ be the set of pixels in the enlarged region and $Y$ be the set of adjacent pixel pairs. The goal is to seek a labeling $L = \{l_1, ..., l_x, ..., l_{|X|}\}$ such that $l_x = 1$ if pixel $x$ belongs to the foreground; otherwise, $l_x = 0$. The labeling $L$ is obtained by minimizing the following cost function:

$$E(X) = \sum_{x \in X} U(x) + \lambda \sum_{(x,y) \in Y} V(x,y) \cdot \delta(l_x, l_y) \qquad (8)$$

where

$$\delta(l_x, l_y) = \begin{cases} 0 & \text{if } l_x = l_y \\ 1 & \text{otherwise} \end{cases} \qquad (9)$$

Here $U(x)$ is the cost of assigning pixel $x$ to the foreground or the background, $V(x,y)$ is the cost incurred when two adjacent pixels $x$ and $y$ have different labels and $\lambda$ is a parameter. In this paper, we will focus on how to define $U(x)$ and $V(x,y)$. We refer readers to [4] for a fast solution to the minimization of Eq. (8).

To calculate $U(x)$, we select the positive-score grids in the localized region as foreground seeds and the newly added grids as background seeds (Fig. 2(d)). By dividing the RGB color space into $16 \times 16 \times 16$ bins, a foreground color histogram $h^{fg}$ and a background color histogram $h^{bg}$ are computed according to the foreground seeds and the background seeds, respectively, and each histogram is normalized with a summation of 1. With these two histograms, we estimate $p(x|l_x = 1) = h^{fg}_{b_x}$ and $p(x|l_x = 0) = h^{bg}_{b_x}$, where $b_x$ is the bin index of pixel $x$ in the histogram. By assuming $P(l_x = 1) = P(l_x = 0) = \frac{1}{2}$, we have the following two distributions

$$p(l_x = 1|x) = \frac{p(x|l_x = 1)P(l_x = 1)}{P(x)} = \frac{h^{fg}_{b_x}}{h^{fg}_{b_x} + h^{bg}_{b_x}} \qquad (10)$$

$$p(l_x = 0|x) = \frac{p(x|l_x = 0)P(l_x = 0)}{P(x)} = \frac{h^{bg}_{b_x}}{h^{fg}_{b_x} + h^{bg}_{b_x}} \qquad (11)$$

Using Eq. (10) and Eq. (11), we define $U(x)$ as

$$U(x) = -log(p(l_x|x)) \qquad (12)$$

As a result, the more likely a pixel $x$ belongs to the foreground(background), the less the cost is incurred if $l_x$ is set to 1(0).

We define $V(x,y)$ as

$$V(x,y) = \exp\left(-\frac{\| c_x - c_y \|^2}{2\sigma^2}\right) \qquad (13)$$

where $c_x$ is the color of pixel x, and as in Eq. (5), $\sigma$ is set to 32. If two adjacent pixels of similar colors are labelled differently, the value of $V(x,y)$ is large. Therefore, $V(x,y)$ imposes a smoothness constraint on the segmentation result.

To speed up the segmentation process, we scale the original test image to a lower resolution of $120 \times 120$ pixels. Graph cut segmentation is run on the smaller image to get the foreground which is then scaled up to the original size. After the graph cut segmentation, the obtained foreground may consist of several isolated regions (Fig. 2(e)). We select the region which maximizes the learned classification function as the final result (Fig. 2(f)).

### 3.4  Partition Parameter Selection

A coarse grid partition ($n$ is small) cannot cover the object region precisely, while a fine grid partition ($n$ is large) may make the grids too small to be sensitive to noisy features. In addition, a large $n$ causes a high computational cost for grid search. Therefore, the value of $n$ should not be too small or too large. Furthermore, since the objects to be localized can be of any sizes and at any positions, a single fixed partition may not work well for all cases. Without the prior knowledge of the object size and position, we apply to a test image several partitions which cover different scales, e.g. $9 \times 9$, $11 \times 11$ and $13 \times 13$. From these partitions, the optimal one is selected: first, for each partition, grid search and graph cut refinement are performed to get an object region; then, from these regions the one with the highest score is selected as the final result.

## 4  Experiments

To demonstrate the effectiveness of the proposed approach, we conduct object localization on PASCAL VOC 2007 and VOC 2008 datasets.

### 4.1  Experiment on VOC 2007 Dataset

We take cat and dog in the PASCAL VOC 2007 localization dataset as test categories. In this dataset, cats and dogs change in pose and viewpoint, and take on various shapes in images, so they are suitable for testing arbitrary-shape object localization. We compare our approach (GS-GC), i.e. grid search (GS) followed by graph cut (GC) refinement, with two state-of-the-art methods: efficient subwindow search (ESS) [16] and efficient region search (ERS) [25]. The former produces bounding-box localization results, and as ours, the latter produces object regions of any shapes.

The image set of each category consists of three parts: training set, validation set and testing set. We use the training set and the validation set for training and the testing set for evaluation. For local features, we extract SURF [3] from each image.[1] A codebook of 2000 visual words is generated for each category by collecting 500,000 features and quantizing them by $k$-means. As positive examples, we use the segmented training examples provided by the authors of [25]. We randomly sample some rectangular patches from image regions that are labelled as background or negative classes. The parameter $C$ for training linear SVM is selected by cross-validation. The parameter $\lambda$ for graph cut segmentation

---

[1] We keep all the features, while in [25] only features at Canny edge points are used.

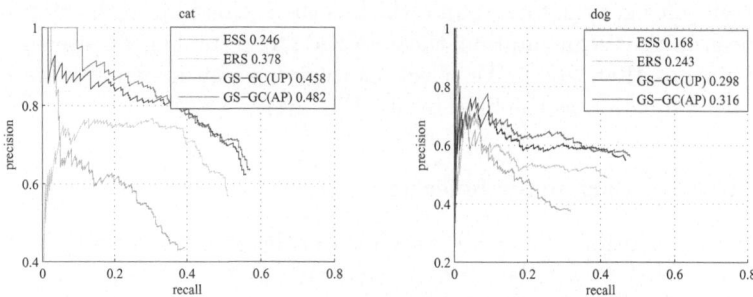

**Fig. 4.** Localization accuracy at bounding-box level

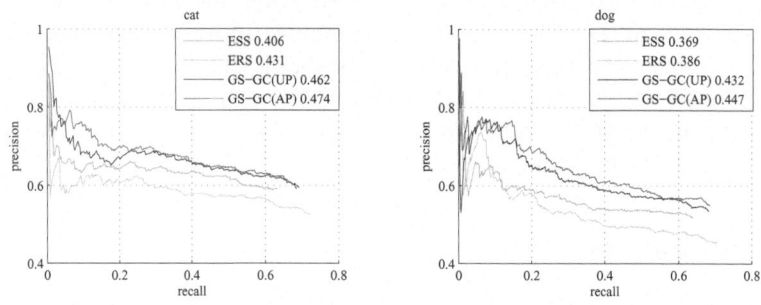

**Fig. 5.** Localization accuracy at pixel level

and the parameter $\gamma$ for adaptive partition are tuned so that our approach performs best on the validation set. For ESS, we use the authors' published code. The super-pixels used in ERS are kindly provided by the authors. To make a direct comparison, the same features and SVM models are used for ESS, ERS and our approach. Following [25], we apply each method to localize the optimal region in each test image and the confidence of the localized region is evaluated by a $\chi^2$-kernel SVM learned from the same training examples.

For evaluation, we use two types of precision-recall curves at bounding-box and pixel levels, respectively. At bounding-box level, a localized region is considered positive if the intersection area of the ground-truth bounding box and the bounding box that tightly surrounds the region divided by their union area

**Table 1.** Bounding-box level average precision of our approach using a single partition

| Category | cat | | | | | | | dog | | | | | | |
|---|---|---|---|---|---|---|---|---|---|---|---|---|---|---|
| n | 8 | 9 | 10 | 11 | 12 | 13 | 14 | 8 | 9 | 10 | 11 | 12 | 13 | 14 |
| GS(UP) | 32.6 | 31.2 | 29.1 | 30.0 | 28.6 | 29.4 | 29.1 | 19.5 | 20.7 | 18.9 | 19.5 | 20.2 | 18.8 | 18.3 |
| GS-GC(UP) | 41.8 | 41.8 | 37.9 | 41.9 | 38.4 | **45.3** | 39.8 | 27.4 | 27.3 | 28.7 | 31.7 | **31.0** | 29.6 | **30.1** |
| GS(AP) | 33.6 | 30.4 | 29.6 | 30.1 | 29.5 | 30.4 | 28.9 | 21.0 | 20.1 | 21.2 | 19.4 | 20.1 | 18.2 | 18.3 |
| GS-GC(AP) | **42.9** | **45.0** | **41.3** | **44.6** | **44.0** | 42.3 | **42.7** | **28.6** | **29.2** | **30.9** | **35.3** | 29.9 | **30.8** | **30.1** |

**Table 2.** Pixel level average precision of our approach using a single partition

| Category | cat | | | | | | | dog | | | | | | |
|---|---|---|---|---|---|---|---|---|---|---|---|---|---|---|
| n | 8 | 9 | 10 | 11 | 12 | 13 | 14 | 8 | 9 | 10 | 11 | 12 | 13 | 14 |
| GS(UP) | 32.6 | 31.3 | 30.5 | 30.5 | 28.7 | 28.0 | 28.7 | 28.6 | 28.0 | 26.8 | 26.5 | 26.5 | 25.3 | 24.6 |
| GS-GC(UP) | 43.3 | 44.0 | **44.4** | 44.8 | 44.4 | 45.9 | 44.4 | 41.7 | 41.8 | **42.3** | 43.1 | **43.1** | **43.1** | 42.7 |
| GS(AP) | 33.3 | 32.0 | 30.5 | 30.7 | 29.7 | 28.9 | 28.2 | 29.4 | 28.8 | 27.7 | 27.3 | 26.8 | 25.5 | 25.1 |
| GS-GC(AP) | **45.8** | **45.1** | 44.4 | **45.7** | **45.6** | **47.6** | **45.4** | **42.7** | **42.4** | 41.1 | **44.7** | 42.8 | 42.9 | **43.0** |

**Table 3.** Average runtime of grid search using single partitions

| Method | GS(UP) | | | | | | | GS(AP) | | | | | | |
|---|---|---|---|---|---|---|---|---|---|---|---|---|---|---|
| n | 8 | 9 | 10 | 11 | 12 | 13 | 14 | 8 | 9 | 10 | 11 | 12 | 13 | 14 |
| Average time (s) | 0.13 | 0.18 | 0.28 | 0.55 | 1.12 | 2.52 | 4.90 | 0.16 | 0.22 | 0.33 | 0.56 | 0.94 | 1.76 | 4.96 |

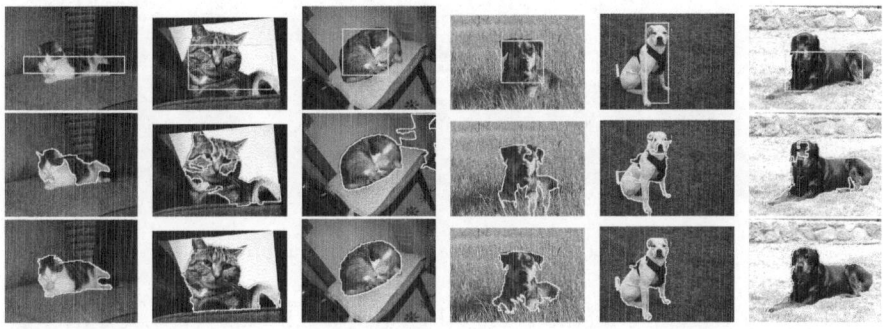

**Fig. 6.** Localization examples of different approaches. Results of EES, ERS and our approach are given in Row 1, Row 2 and Row 3 respectively.

is greater than 0.5. At pixel level, a pixel in the localized region is considered positive if it belongs to the true object region. Figures 4 and 5 show the results of ESS, ERS and our approach. For the two implementations of our approach, one with uniform partition (UP) and the other with adaptive partition (AP), we apply to each test image there different grid partitions, $9 \times 9$, $11 \times 11$ and $13 \times 13$. Both ERS and our approach outperform ESS, which indicates the advantage of arbitrary-shape region search over rectangle region search. Compared with ERS, our two implementations yield better localization accuracy with GS-GC(AP) performing best. Tables 1 and 2 give the results of our approach using a single grid partition with $8 \leq n \leq 14$. Due to the coarse initialization of image grids, GS(UP) and GS(AP) perform worse than ERS, but for all different $n$'s, GS-GC(UP) and GS-GC(AP) outperform ERS at both bounding-box and pixel levels, showing the effectiveness of the graph cut refinement. The advantage of using adaptive partition can be seen from Tabs. 1 and 2 that GS-GC(AP) improves the localization accuracy over GS-GC(UP) for most partitions. In addition, the use of multiple partitions further improves the performance, because it reduces the risk of single-partition failure and makes our approach more stable. Figure 6 shows some localization examples of ESS, ERS and our approach.

**Table 4.** Overlap accuracy on 20 categories of VOC 2008 dataset

| Category | aerop. | bicyc. | bird | boat | bottle | bus | car | cat | chair | cow |
|----------|--------|--------|------|------|--------|-----|-----|-----|-------|-----|
| ERS | 0.324 | 0.109 | 0.268 | **0.262** | 0.121 | 0.405 | 0.244 | 0.389 | 0.120 | 0.324 |
| GS-GC(UP) | **0.380** | 0.154 | 0.286 | 0.218 | 0.148 | 0.459 | 0.264 | 0.435 | **0.148** | 0.332 |
| GS-GC(AP) | 0.361 | **0.158** | **0.295** | 0.236 | **0.152** | **0.483** | **0.273** | **0.448** | 0.140 | **0.343** |
| Category | dinin. | dog | horse | motor. | person | potte. | sheep | sofa | train | tvmon. |
| ERS | 0.300 | 0.288 | **0.280** | 0.337 | 0.257 | 0.119 | 0.394 | 0.224 | 0.453 | 0.259 |
| GS-GC(UP) | **0.319** | 0.320 | 0.278 | **0.412** | 0.284 | 0.134 | 0.394 | 0.206 | **0.459** | 0.263 |
| GS-GC(AP) | 0.312 | **0.330** | 0.278 | 0.397 | **0.290** | **0.143** | **0.409** | **0.234** | 0.452 | **0.267** |

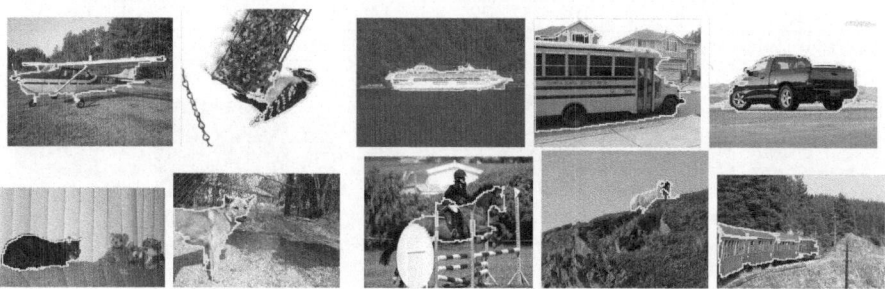

**Fig. 7.** Localization examples of our approach

We run all the three methods on a PC with a 3.2 GHz CPU. On average, the optimal region search takes about $0.06s$ for ESS and $0.26s$ for ERS (the time for segmentation is not counted). The average runtime of GS using a single partitions is listed in Tab. 3. When $n <= 11$, the runtime of GS and that of ERS are similar, as in one test image the number of super-pixels (about 100) is close to that of image grids ranging from 64 to 121. The runtime of GS gets longer as $n$ increases and we restrict $n < 15$. For graph cut segmentation, we use an efficient implementation of a min-cut/max-flow algorithm [5]. The average time to run graph cut segmentation on a test image is about $0.12s$.

## 4.2   Experiment on VOC 2008 Dataset

We further compare our approach with ERS on 20 object categories in the VOC 2008 segmentation dataset. Following the experimental setting in [25], we split the *trainval* set of each category into three parts and report the 3-fold cross-validation accuracy using the PASCAL segmentation criterion [9], overlap accuracy, defined by $\frac{TP}{TP+FP+FN}$, where $TP$, $FP$ and $FN$ are total true positives, false positives and false negatives, respectively. For each test image, $9 \times 9$, $11 \times 11$ and $13 \times 13$ grid partitions are used. We set $\lambda = 1.0$ and $\gamma = 3.0$ for all the 20 categories. Table 4 shows the results of 20 object categories. GS-GC(UP) and GS-GC(AP) outperform ERS on 16 and 17 categories respectively and improve the mean overlap accuracy on 20 categories: 0.274 for ERS, 0.295 for GS-GC(UP) and 0.3 for GS-GC(AP). Moreover, GS-GC(AP) improves the overlap accuracy over GS-GS(UP) on 14 categories. Some localization examples of our approach are given in Fig. 7.

## 5 Conclusions

We present an efficient bottom-up approach for arbitrary-shape object localization. Based on coarse image grids, the object region in an image is localized by searching an optimal connected region composed of image grids using the branch-and-cut algorithm, followed by graph cut segmentation for refinement. We also propose an efficient adaptive grid partition method which helps further improve the localization accuracy of our approach. We demonstrate the advantage of our approach on PASCAL VOC 2007 and VOC 2008 datasets.

**Acknowledgement.** This work was supported in part by the Nanyang Assistant Professorship (SUG M58040015) to Dr. Junsong Yuan. We thank Gangqiang Zhao for the help to proofread the paper.

## References

1. Agarwal, S., Roth, D.: Learning a Sparse Representation for Object Detection. In: Heyden, A., Sparr, G., Nielsen, M., Johansen, P. (eds.) ECCV 2002, Part IV. LNCS, vol. 2353, pp. 113–127. Springer, Heidelberg (2002)
2. Arbelaez, P., Maire, M., Fowlkes, C., Malik, J.: From Contours to Regions: An Empirical Evaluation. In: IEEE Conference on Computer Vision and Pattern Recognition, pp. 2294–2301 (2009)
3. Bay, H., Ess, A., Tuytelaars, T., Van Gool, L.: Speeded-Up Robust Features (SURF). Computer Vision and Image Understanding 110, 346–359 (2008)
4. Boykov, Y., Jolly, M.P.: Interactive graph cuts for optimal boundary & region segmentation of objects in N-D images. In: IEEE International Conference on Computer Vision, pp. 105–112 (2001)
5. Boykov, Y., Kolmogorov, V.: An Experimental Comparison of Min-Cut/Max-Flow Algorithms for Energy Minimization in Vision. IEEE Transaction on Pattern Analysis and Machine Intelligence 26, 1124–1137 (2004)
6. Chum, O., Zisserman, A.: An exemplar model for learning object classes. In: IEEE Conference on Computer Vision and Pattern Recognition, pp. 1–8 (2007)
7. Dai, Q., Hoiem, D.: Learning to localize Detected Objects. In: IEEE Conference on Computer Vision and Pattern Recognition, pp. 3322–3329 (2012)
8. Dalal, N., Triggs, B.: Histograms of oriented gradients for human detection. In: IEEE Conference on Computer Vision and Pattern Recognition, pp. 886–893 (2005)
9. Everingham, M., Van Gool, L., Williams, C.K.I., Winn, J., Zisserman, A.: The PASCAL Visual Object Classes Challenge 2008 Results (2008),
http://www.pascal-network.org/challenges/VOC/voc2008/workshop/index.html
10. Felzenszwalb, P.F., Girshick, R.B., McAllester, D., Ramanan, D.: Object Detection with Discriminatively Trained Part-Based Models. IEEE Transaction on Pattern Analysis and Machine Intelligence 32, 1627–1645 (2010)

11. Ferrari, V., Fevrier, L., Jurie, F., Schmid, C.: Groups of adjacent contour segments for object detection. IEEE Transaction on Pattern Analysis and Machine Intelligence 14, 36–51 (2008)
12. Fritz, M., Schiele, B.: Decomposition, discovery and detection of visual categories using topic models. In: IEEE Conference on Computer Vision and Pattern Recognition, pp. 1–8 (2008)
13. Fulkerson, B., Vedaldi, A., Soatto, S.: Class Segmentation and Object Localization with Superpixel Neighborhoods. In: IEEE Conference on Computer Vision and Pattern Recognition, pp. 670–677 (2009)
14. Jiang, Y., Meng, J., Yuan, J.: Grid-based Local Feature Bundling for Efficient Object Search. In: IEEE International Conference and Image Processing, pp. 113–116 (2011)
15. Jiang, Y., Meng, J., Yuan, J.: Randomized Visual Phrases for Object Search. In: IEEE Conference on Computer Vision and Pattern Recognition, pp. 3100–3107 (2012)
16. Lampert, C.H., Blaschko, M.B., Hofmann, T.: Efficient Subwindow Search: A Branch and Bound Framework for Object Localization. IEEE Transaction on Pattern Analysis and Machine Intelligence 31, 2129–2142 (2009)
17. Leibe, B., Leonardis, A., Schiele, B.: Robust object detection with interleaved categorization and segmentation. International Journal of Computer Vision 77, 259–289 (2008)
18. Opelt, A., Pinz, A., Zisserman, A.: A Boundary-Fragment-Model for Object Detection. In: Leonardis, A., Bischof, H., Pinz, A. (eds.) ECCV 2006, Part II. LNCS, vol. 3952, pp. 575–588. Springer, Heidelberg (2006)
19. Parkhi, O.M., Vedaldi, A., Jawahar, C.V., Zisserman, A.: The truth about cats and dogs. In: IEEE International Conference on Computer Vision, pp. 6–13 (2011)
20. Ramanan, D.: Using segmentation to verify object hypotheses. In: IEEE Conference on Computer Vision and Pattern Recognition, pp. 18–23 (2007)
21. Razavi, N., Gall, J., Van Gool, L.: Scalable Multi-class Object Detection. In: IEEE Conference on Computer Vision and Pattern Recognition, pp. 1505–1512 (2011)
22. Rihan, J., Kohli, P., Torr, P.H.S.: OBJCUT for Face Detection. In: Kalra, P.K., Peleg, S. (eds.) ICVGIP 2006. LNCS, vol. 4338, pp. 576–584. Springer, Heidelberg (2006)
23. Russakovsky, O., Ng, A.Y.: A Steiner tree approach to efficient object detection. In: IEEE Conference on Computer Vision and Pattern Recognition, pp. 1070–1077 (2010)
24. Vedaldi, A., Gulshan, V., Varma, M., Zisserman, A.: Multiple Kernels for Object Detection. In: IEEE International Conference on Computer Vision, pp. 606–613 (2009)
25. Vijayanarasimhan, S., Grauman, K.: Efficient Region Search for Object Detection. In: IEEE Conference on Computer Vision and Pattern Recognition, pp. 1401–1408 (2011)
26. Yeh, T., Lee, J.J., Darrell, T.: Fast Concurrent Object Localization and Recognition. In: IEEE Conference on Computer Vision and Pattern Recognition, pp. 280–287 (2009)
27. Zhang, Z., Cao, Y., Salvi, D., Oliver, K., Waggoner, J., Wang, S.: Free-Shape Subwindow Search for Object Localization. In: IEEE Conference on Computer Vision and Pattern Recognition, pp. 1086–1093 (2010)
28. Zhao, L., Davis, L.S.: Closely coupled object detection and segmentation. In: IEEE International Conference on Computer Vision, pp. 454–461 (2005)

# Disambiguation in Unknown Object Detection by Integrating Image and Speech Recognition Confidences

Yuko Ozasa[1], Yasuo Ariki[1], Mikio Nakano[2], and Naoto Iwahashi[3]

[1] Graduate School of System Informatics, Kobe University, 1–1, Rokkodaicho, Nada-ku, Kobe, Hyogo, 657–8501, Japan
y_ozasa@stu.kobe-u.ac.jp, ariki@kobe-u.ac.jp
[2] Honda Research Institute Japan Co., Ltd., 8–1 Honcho, Wako-shi, Saitama 351–0188, Japan
nakano@jp.honda-ri.com
[3] National Institute of Information and Communications Technology, Keihanna Research Laboratories, 3–5 Hikaridai, Seika-cho, Soraku-gun, Kyoto 619–0289, Japan naoto.iwahashi@nict.go.jp

**Abstract.** This paper presents a new method to detect unknown objects and their unknown names in object manipulation through man-robot dialog. In the method, the detection is carried out by using the information of object images and user's speech in an integrated way. Originality of the method is to use logistic regression for the discrimination between unknown and known objects. The accuracy of the unknown object detection was 97% in the case when there were about fifty known objects.

## 1 Introduction

The image features and names of the objects are associated when humans memorize the objects. The object name is represented as speech features spoken in the respective language. Therefore, image features and speech are memorized at the same time.

In the object recognition by computers, there is an ambiguity that the object is recognized as the different object with the similar image or speech features when recognized using the image or speech features separately. Since the image and speech features exist associatively, if they are used simultaneously, the ambiguity of object recognition will be dissolved and the recognition accuracy can be improved.

In a task where a robot brings a requested object to a human, the speech feature spoken by the human and image feature of the objects the robot watches can be utilized simultaneously. The most powerful method to integrate the features is the logistic regression method using feature confidences. If the integrated confidence measures are higher than a certain threshold, the robot can bring the object correctly. Otherwise, the robot does not know the object, namely, it is unknown object to the robot.

K.M. Lee et al. (Eds.): ACCV 2012, Part I, LNCS 7724, pp. 85–96, 2013.
© Springer-Verlag Berlin Heidelberg 2013

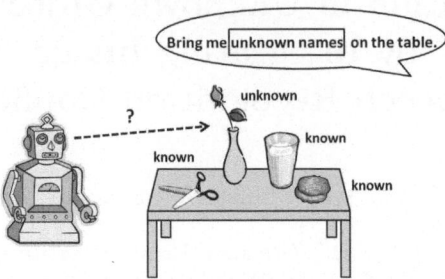

**Fig. 1.** Autonomous detection of unknown objects and their names by a robot

It is difficult to teach household robots every object in home environments. Therefore, robots need to learn unknown objects as well as recognize known objects. Few researchers have previously addressed such systems [1–3].

The most effective method is that robots can learn unknown objects in natural communication with humans using speech and physical actions in a home environment. Specifically, robots learn unknown objects during object manipulations requested by spoken dialogs[4, 5]. The learning is interactive and unsupervised learning. Most of the previously proposed methods are non-interactive and supervised learning [4–6].

In this paper, we propose an object recognition method using integrated confidence measure of image and speech, and the unknown object detection method by the extension of the object recognition method for the first step of the unknown object learning. The task which we set up has several objects on a table, and the user tells the robot "bring me ⟨object name⟩. " as shown in Fig.1, whether the robot knows the objects or not in the home environment. Under the assumption that the spoken object name is the name of an object on the table, the image feature of the objects on the table and human speech are integrated. Then, the robot brings the object indicated, no matter whether the objects are known or not. The proposed methods are more efficient than methods using image or speech features separately and the efficiency is shown by the experiments in this paper.

## 2   Proposed System

The proposed system diagram is shown in Fig.2. It is composed of two parts, estimating confidence and detecting unknown objects and their names. The proposed method for unknown object detection uses both image and speech information in an integrated way. The confidence of the recognition results for input speeches and images are estimated. Then, the confidences are integrated via logistic regression and are detected by thresholding the integrated confidence.

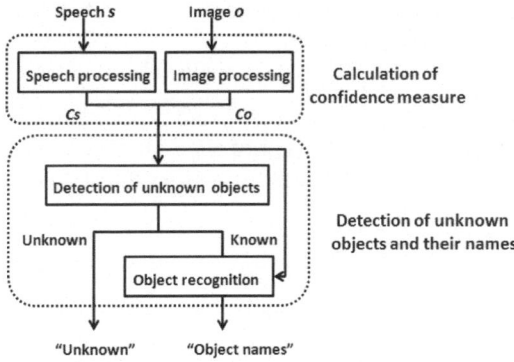

**Fig. 2.** Proposed system configuration diagram

## 2.1  Confidence Measure Integration

The proposed method integrates the confidences of speech recognition results and image recognition results, and the integrated confidence is used in detecting unknown objects and their names.

**Speech Processing.** The features used for speech recognition are Mel-frequency cepstral coefficients ( 12 dimensions ), which are based on short-time spectrum analysis; their delta and acceleration parameters; and the delta of short-time log power. These features ( 37 dimensions ) are obtained by speech recognition software, Julius [7]. The log likelihood of HMMs were calculated by these features and written as follows:

$$P_s(s; \Lambda_i) = \log P(s; \Lambda_i) \tag{1}$$

where $P(s; \Lambda_i)$ is the likelihood of speech and $\Lambda_i$ denotes the word HMM for the name of the $i$-th object. This $P(s; \Lambda_i)$ is used to estimate the confidence. Speech recognition confidence is used to evaluate the reliability of the result of speech recognition and it is obtained by the following formula [8]:

$$C_s(s; \Lambda_i) = \frac{1}{n(s)} \log \frac{P(s; \Lambda_i)}{\max_{u_i \neq i} P(s; \Lambda_{u_i})} \tag{2}$$

where $n(s)$ denotes the number of frames in the input speech, $\Lambda_i$ denotes the word HMM for the name of the $i$-th object, and $u_i$ denotes the best phoneme sequence.

**Image Processing.** The features used in image recognition were L*a*b* components (three dimensions) for the color, complex Fourier coefficients (eight dimensions) of contours for the shape [9], and the area of an object ( one dimension). Gaussian Models were learned using these features with MAP adaptation. The log likelihood of object $P_o(o; g_i)$ is obtained by the following formula [6]:

$$P_o(o; g_i) = \log P(o; g_i) \tag{3}$$

where $P(o; g_i)$ is the likelihood of the object. The confidence of the objects is written as follows:

$$C_o(o; g_i) = \log \frac{P(o; g_i)}{P_{max}} \qquad (4)$$

where $g_i$ denotes the normal distribution of the $i$-th object, and $P_{max} = ((2\pi)^{\frac{d}{2}} | \sum |^{\frac{1}{2}})^{-1}$ denotes the maximum probability densities of Gaussian functions.

## 2.2   Logistic Regression for Modality Integration

The speech recognition confidence measure and object recognition confidence measure are integrated by the following logistic regression function [6]:

$$F_c(C_s, C_o) = \frac{1}{1 + e^{-(\alpha_0 + \alpha_1 C_s + \alpha_2 C_o)}}. \qquad (5)$$

Here $\alpha_0$, $\alpha_1$ and $\alpha_2$ are logistic regression coefficients. In the training of this logistic regression function, the $(i,j)$-th training sample is given as the pair of input signal $(C_s(s_j; \Lambda_i), C_o(o_j; g_i))$ and teaching signal $d_{i,j}$, where $i$ denotes the model index and $j$ denotes the sample index for the model $i$. Thus, the training set T contains ($N$ models and $M$ samples) data.

$$T^{N \times M} = \{C_s(s_j; \Lambda_i), C_o(o_j; g_i), d_{i,j} | i = 1, \cdots, N, j = 1, \cdots, M\} \qquad (6)$$

where $d_{i,j}$ is 0 or 1, depending on whether the object is unknown or known. The likelihood function is written as

$$P(\mathbf{d}|\alpha_0, \alpha_1, \alpha_2) = \prod_{j=1}^{M} \prod_{i=1}^{N} (F_c(C_{s_j}^i, C_{o_j}^i))^{d_{i,j}} (1 - F_c(C_{s_j}^i, C_{o_j}^i))^{1-d_{i,j}} \qquad (7)$$

where $\mathbf{d} = (d_{1,1}, \cdots, d_{N,M})$. Here $C_{s_j}^i$ and $C_{o_j}^i$ are $C_s(s_j; \Lambda_i)$ and $C_o(o_j; g_i)$ respectively for abbreviation. The weights $(\alpha_0, \alpha_1, \alpha_2)$ are optimized by maximum likelihood estimation using Fisher's scoring algorithm [10, 11].

## 3   Detection of Unknown Objects and Their Names

In the detection phase, the input object is classified as an unknown object or a known object using the integrated confidence. When the input object is classified as unknown, it is considered an unknown object is detected and its name is obtained by combining the object image with the input speech. When the input object is classified as known, then the object with its name is output.

### 3.1   Detection of Unknown Objects

Fig. 3 shows the joint distribution of speech recognition confidence and image recognition confidence. It indicates that discriminating unknown and known objects would be possible by using both confidences simultaneously. Given a threshold $\delta$, the object is classified as unknown or known.

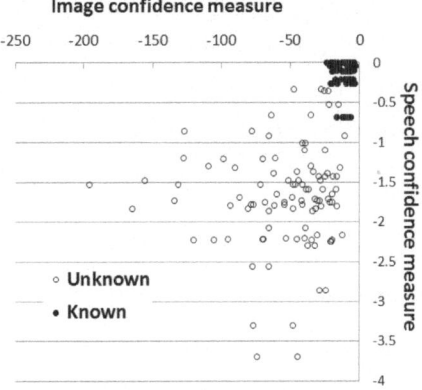

**Fig. 3.** Joint distribution of values of the speech and object confidence

$F_c(C_s, C_o)$ is used for the classification of unknown and known objects. If the following condition is satisfied,

$$\max_i(F_c(C_s(s; \Lambda_i), C_o(o; g_i))) < \delta, \tag{8}$$

the input object is classified as an unknown object, else as a known object.

## 3.2   Object Recognition

When the input object is classified as a known object, it is recognized and its ID is obtained as follows:

$$\hat{i} = \arg\max_i F_c(C_s(s; \Lambda_i), C_o(o; g_i)) \tag{9}$$

Then, the object name is output.

## 3.3   Detection of Multiple Unknown Objects and Their Names

The method for detecting an unknown object was proposed in Section 4.1. This method can be extended to methods which detect multiple unknown objects and their names. The proposed methods are classified into two types. The first type designs one detector for two classes and the other type designs two detectors for three classes.

### Binary Classification

In this section, we propose the binary classification method for the unknown object detection in the case where the input speech is known (Fig.4).

**1)** *Proposed method 1 :*   The method proposed above uses only one detector

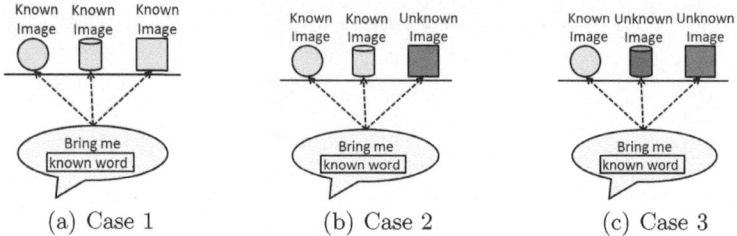

(a) Case 1             (b) Case 2             (c) Case 3

**Fig. 4.** Cases where the input word is known

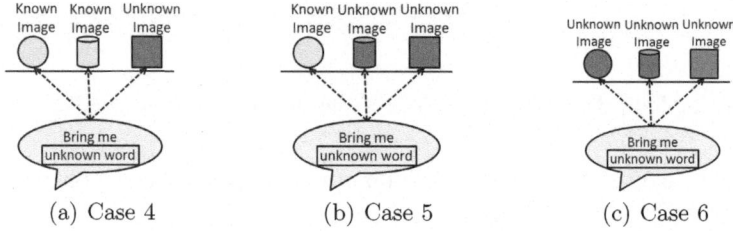

(a) Case 4             (b) Case 5             (c) Case 6

**Fig. 5.** Cases where the input word is unknown

trained using a set of pairs of a known image and a known speech with $d_{i,j} = 1$, and a set of pairs of an unknown image and an unknown speech with $d_{i,j} = 0$. Since the input set of pairs are a known image and speech or an unknown image and speech, this case is suitable for the case where only one object is on a table. This training method is not robust enough to detect multiple unknown objects. **2)** *Proposed method 2* :  In the case where there are multiple objects on a table, the input sets of pairs are not only these sets of pairs used in the proposed method 1, but also the sets of pairs of an unknown image and a known speech, a known image and an unknown speech. From this viewpoint, we propose the second method for unknown detection. In this method, a detector is trained by the set of pairs of a known image and a known speech with $d_{i,j} = 1$, and the sets of others, namely pairs of an unknown image and a known speech, a known image and an unknown speech, and an unknown image and an unknown speech with $d_{i,j} = 0$. Using this detector, the robot can execute the task when the input speech is known (Fig.4) more stably than using the detector proposed first.

The proposed method 1 and 2 can be applied to the cases where the input speech is known in Fig.4, but can not be applied to the cases where the input speech is unknown in Fig.5. In order to apply to the case where the input speech is known, the input sets of pairs of speech and image are needed to be classified into the set of pairs of known speech and known image and other set of pairs. In the case where input speech is unknown , in order to apply to the case, the input sets of pairs of speech and image are needed to be classified into the set of pairs

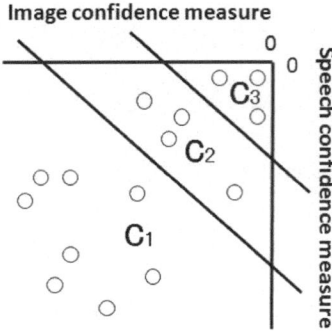

**Fig. 6.** Trinary Classification

of unknown speech and unknown image and other set of pairs. The proposed method 1 and 2 can classify the input sets of pairs of speech and image into the sets of pairs of known speech and known image and other set of pairs, so these methods can not be applied to the case where the input speech is unknown. If the proposed method 1 and 2 are used for the unknown object detection in the case where the input speech is unknown (Fig.5), all the input sets of pairs of image and speech are classified into the same class which consists of the sets of pairs of an unknown image and a known speech, a known image and an unknown speech, and an unknown image and an unknown speech, and the robot can not appliy to the task.

## Trinary Classification

In this section we propose the trinary classification method for the unknown object detection which can be applied to the both cases, the case where the input speech is known and the case where the input speech is unknown (Fig.4 and 5).

*Proposed Method* 3 :  The second proposed method can be applied to cases where the input speech is known, but the method cannot be applied to cases where the input speech is unknown as shown in Fig.5. Since the second method cannot discriminate three sets of pairs; 1) unknown image and speech ($C_1$) and 2) an unknown image and a known speech, and a known image and an unknown speech ($C_2$), 3) known image and speech ($C_3$) shown in Fig.6. To discriminate these sets of pairs, we prepared two detectors. The first detector is trained by the set of pairs of a known image and a known speech confidence measure with $d_{i,j} = 1$, and the set of others as $d_i = 0$. The second detector is trained by the set of pairs of an unknown image and an unknown speech confidence measure with $d_{i,j} = 1$, and the sets of others with $d_{i,j} = 0$. Using these two detectors, the robot can execute the task no matter whether the objects are known or not as shown in Fig.4 and 5.

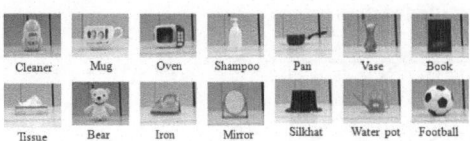 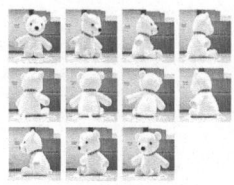

(a) Examples of objects in the home environment

(b) Samples of 11 images of bear taken from 11 directions

**Fig. 7.** Examples of object image used in the experiment

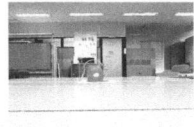 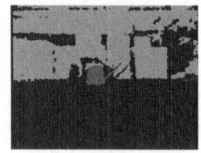 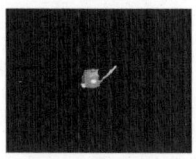

(a) RGB image          (b) Depth map          (c) Extracted object region

**Fig. 8.** Example of information obtained by Kinect

## 4   Experimental Evaluation

We first evaluated the unknown object detection method, and then evaluated object recognition. The coefficients $\alpha_0$, $\alpha_1$, and $\alpha_2$, and threshold $\delta$ were also optimized in the experiment.

Some of the objects used in the experiments are shown in Fig.7. The objects used in the experiments are some of the objects in the home environment since the scene of the task setup in this paper is in the home environment. 50 objects were prepared and for each object, one utterance including its name, and two of the image data sets, data set 1 and data set 2 were prepared. Data set 1 consists of 10 images of each 50 objects which are taken frontally from 10 different positions, respectively. Data set 2 consists of 11 images of each 50 objects which are taken from 11 directions, and examples of these 11 images of bear are shown in Fig. 7.

The size of the image is 640x480 pixels. The RGB image and depth map are taken by Kinect[12], and the object region is automatically extracted by both the RGB image and depth map. Examples of the RGB image, depth map, and extracted object region are shown in Fig. 7. The extracted object regions are used in the experiment.

### 4.1   Evaluation of Unknown Object Detection

The evaluation was performed by leave-one-out cross validation. We investigated (1) if known objects were classified as known objects and then (2) if unknown

**Table 1.** Accuracy of unknown object detection (%)

| Likelihood | Object $P_o$ | Speech $P_s$ | $P_s + P_o$ | SVM | $F_p(P_s, P_o)$ |
|---|---|---|---|---|---|
| Data set 1 | 93.2 | 66.0 | 78.8 | 66.9 | 89.4 |
| Data set 2 | 89.0 | | 72.2 | 65.8 | 85.0 |

| Confidence | Object $C_o$ | Speech $C_s$ | $C_s + C_o$ | SVM | $F_c(C_s, C_o)$ |
|---|---|---|---|---|---|
| Data set 1 | 93.2 | 95.0 | 94.6 | 96.6 | 97.0 |
| Data set 2 | 89.0 | | 93.2 | 94.0 | 94.8 |

objects were classified as unknown objects, and averaged their accuracies. For (1), one image was chosen from each of the 50 objects as test data, and the remaining 450 images were used as training data. For (2), one object was chosen for testing, and the remaining 49 objects were used as training data. We also carried out the experiments for each of the 500 images.

To evaluate the confidence measures, the accuracy of the proposed method using the confidences was compared with that of the method using the log likelihood instead of the confidence. The coefficient set $\{\alpha_0, \alpha_1, \alpha_2\}$ were $\{7.64, 5.22, 5.16e-03\}$ in the proposed method and $\{9.17, 0.02, 0.15\}$ in the log likelihood method. The coefficient $\alpha_2$ of the proposed method using the confidence was much smaller than the coefficients $\alpha_0$ and $\alpha_1$ since the accuracy of the speech data set used in the experiment was high and the speech confidence was mainly used for the unknown object detection in the prepared data set. When the speech data set which accuracy is lower is used in the experiment, the values of the coefficient set $\{\alpha_0, \alpha_1, \alpha_2\}$ varies widely.

The accuracy of the method using polynomial kernel SVM (Support Vector Machine) was compared, too. The accuracy of the unknown detection method using the image and speech separately and their linear combination were also evaluated, too. The optimized threshold $\delta$ of the proposed method was 0.96, and the threshold of the log likelihood based method was 0.98.

The experimental result using the optimized weight set is shown in Table 1. The accuracy of the method using SVM for log likelihoods is low in Table 1, since the accuracy of the method using the speech log likelihood is low. The proposed method $F_c(C_s, C_o)$ is the most efficient in Table 1.

## 4.2   Evaluation of Object Recognition

The evaluation was also performed by leave-one-out cross validation. Under the condition that a known object was input, we chose one image as testing data from each of the 50 objects, and the remaining images were used as training data. The experiment was carried out for all 500 images. The same weight sets described in Section 5.1 were used in this experiment. The experimental result is shown in Table 2. The accuracy of the proposed method and the method using log likelihood is 100%.

The features used in image recognition were L*a*b* components for the color, complex Fourier coefficients of contours for the shape, and the area of an object.

**Table 2.** Accuracy of object detection (%)

| Likelihood | Object $P_o$ | Speech $P_s$ | $P_s + P_o$ | $F_p(P_s, P_o)$ |
|---|---|---|---|---|
| Data set 1 | 98.8 | 96.0 | 99.4 | 100.0 |
| Data set 2 | 88.2 | | 91.6 | 100.0 |

| Confidence | Object $C_o$ | Speech $C_s$ | $C_s + C_o$ | $F_c(C_s, C_o)$ |
|---|---|---|---|---|
| Data set 1 | 98.8 | 96.0 | 99.4 | 100.0 |
| Data set 2 | 88.2 | | 91.6 | 100.0 |

**Table 3.** Accuracy of image recognition for respective feature(%)

| | Lab | Area | Fourier | Lab+Fourier | All |
|---|---|---|---|---|---|
| Data set 1 | 88.0 | 8.4 | 48.4 | 98.2 | 98.8 |
| Data set 2 | 69.6 | 11.4 | 29.2 | 84.8 | 88.2 |

The accuracy of image recognition using each feature is shown in Table 3. From the table, it can be seen that the color and shape information are most effective for object recognition.

### 4.3   Evaluation of Multiple Unknown Objects Detection Method

The evaluation was also performed by leave-one-out cross validation in this section, too. Three proposed methods described in Section 4.3 were carried out for the unknown objects detection. The input sets of the experiment were all combinations namely pairs of known image and speech, a known image and an unknown speech, and an unknown image and a known speech, and unknown image and speech.

Using the proposed method 1 and 2, the task in the case shown in Fig.4 was executed. Since these methods classify the objects into two classes, the sets of a known image and a speech and others were used for training the detector. The accuracy of the unknown object detection method (binary classification method) is shown in Table 4. When the input speech was known, the accuracy of the proposed method 1 and 2 were 75.0% and 90.8% when the data set 1 was used, respectively. The accuracy of the proposed method 2 is 15.8 points higher than that of proposed method 1.

Proposed method 3 can be applied not only to the case shown in Fig.4 but also Fig.5, since the method uses two detectors and classifies the objects into three classes, the sets of a known image and speech, an unknown image and unknown speech, and others were used for training two detectors, detector 1 and 2. Detector 1 classifies the objects into sets of a known image and speech or others, and detector 2 classifies the objects into sets of an unknown image and speech or others. The accuracy of the detectors and the classification are shown in Table 5. The accuracy of the unknown object detection when the input speech was known was 90.8%, the accuracy of the unknown object detection when the input speech was unknown was 76.1%, and the accuracy of the unknown object

**Table 4.** Accuracy of multiple unknown object detection only in the case when the input speech was known(Method1 and 2)(%)

|  | Proposed method 1 | Proposed method 2 |
|---|---|---|
| Data set 1 | 75.0 | 90.8 |
| Data set 2 | 73.8 | 90.4 |

**Table 5.** Accuracy of multiple unknown object detection(Method3)(%)

|  | Detector 1 | Detector 2 | Proposed method 3 |
|---|---|---|---|
| Data set 1 | 90.8 | 76.1 | 82.3 |
| Data set 2 | 90.4 | 72.0 | 81.2 |

detection in the case where the input speech is known or unknown was 83.3% when the data set 1 was used.

The proposed method 1 and 2 can only be applied to the case where the input speech is known (Fig.4), but the proposed method 3 can be applied to all cases (Fig.4 and 5). When the proposed method 1 and 2 are used for the unknown object detection in the case where the input speech is unknown (Fig.5), all the input sets of pairs of image and speech are classified into the same class which consists of the sets of pairs of an unknown image and a known speech, a known image and an unknown speech, and an unknown image and an unknown speech. Therefore, the robot can not excute the task and the accuracy of the unknown object detection become 0%. In the proposed method 3, the accuracy of the unknown object detection when the input speech is known was 90.8% and enough high, but the accuracy of the unknown object detection when the input speech was unknown is 76.1% and low when the data set 1 was used. Consequently, the accuracy of the unknown object detection in the cases when the input speech was known or not (proposed method 3) became lower than that of the unknown object detection in the case when the input speech was known(proposed method 2). In the future work, we propose the method whose accuracy of the unknown object detection in the case where the input speech is unknown is higher.

## 5 Discussion

Let us consider about the implementation of the proposed method on a robot. In the implementation, the task which we set up has multiple objects on a table, and the user tells the robot "bring me OBJECT NAME. " whether the robot knows the objects or not, and the robot responds to the user. When the robot can select the object he is asked to bring, he says gHere you areh while bringing the object to the user. When the robot cannot select the object, it says gI don't know. h, without any actions. The issues which we found crucial in installing the proposed method on robots are as follows:

1. Latency of verbal responses and behaviors (additionally, we must consider the control of the robot interaction)
2. Erroneous motion of the robot
3. Poorer accuracy of the speech recognition (In a real environment, there are environmental noises and the noise by the robot motion is large.)
4. Poorer accuracy of the image recognition (Since the vision camera is fixed at the head of the robot and the angle of the camera depends on the motion of the neck part of the robot, the angle of the camera may be changed at every interaction. )

We confront these issues and implement the robot in the future work.

# 6    Conclusion

Acquiring new knowledge through interactive learning mechanisms is a key ability for robots in a real environment. To acquire new knowledge, the detection and learning of the unknown objects and their names are needed. The proposed method makes it possible for the robot to detect unknown objects and their names online using multimodal information. We will pursue a method for learning unknown objects in a real environment.

# References

1. Araki, T., et al.: Autonomous Acquisition of Multimodal Information for Online Object Concept Formation by Robots. In: IEEE International Conference on Intelligent Robots and Systems (2011)
2. Holzapfel, H., et al.: A Dialogue Approach to Learning Object Descriptions and Semantic Categories. Robotics and Autonomous Systems 56(11), 1004–1013 (2008)
3. Nakano, M., et al.: Grounding New Words on The Physical World in Multi-Domain Human-Robot Dialogues. In: Dialog with Robots: Papers from the AAAI Fall Symposium (2010)
4. Steels, L., Kaplan, F.: AIBO's first words: The social learning of language and meaning. Evolution of Communication 4(1), 3–32 (2002)
5. Skocaj, D., et al.: A basic cognitive system for interactive continuous learning of visual concepts. In: ICRA 2010 Workshop (2010)
6. Zuo, X., et al.: Detecting Robot-Directed Speech by Situated Understanding in Physical Interaction. Journal of Artificial Intelligence 25(25), 670–682 (2010)
7. Julius, http://julius.sourceforge.jp/
8. Jiang, H.: Confidence Measures for Speech Recognition: A survey. Speech Communication 45, 455–470 (2005)
9. Persoon, E., Fu, K.S.: Shape Discrimination Using Fourier Descriptors. IEEE Trans. Accoust. Speech Signal Processing 28(4), 170–179 (1977)
10. Kurita, T.: Interactive Weighted Least Squares Algorithms for Neural Networks Classifiers. In: Proc. Workshop on Algorithmic Learning Theory, pp. 77–86 (1992)
11. Bishop, C.: Pattern Recognition and Machine Learning. Springer Science+Business Media, LLC, New York (2006)
12. Kinect, http://www.microsoft.com/en-us/kinectforwindows/

# Class-Specific Weighted Dominant Orientation Templates for Object Detection

Hui-Jin Lee and Ki-Sang Hong

San 31 Hyojadong Pohang, South Korea POSTECH E.E.
Image Information Processing Lab.

**Abstract.** We present a class-specific weighted Dominant Orientation Template (DOT) for class-specific object detection to exploit fast DOT, although the original DOT is intended for instance-specific object detection. We use automatic selection algorithm to select representative DOTs from training images of an object class and use three types of 2D Haar wavelets to construct weight templates of the object class. To generate class-specific weighted DOTs, we use a modified similarity measure to combine the representative DOTs with weight templates. In experiments, the proposed method achieved object detection that was better or at least comparable to that of existing methods while being very fast for both training and testing.

## 1 Introduction

Object detection is an important, yet challenging vision task. It has many applications, including image retrieval and video surveillance. Template matching is simple and can be applied to different types of objects, and is therefore an attractive object detection method. In this approach, given templates of the object, the task of object detection is to locate in an input image the target object that has properties that are similar to those of the given templates. The template can be represented in various forms such as a raw image, a binary, a set of feature points, or a learned pattern.

In [1,2], the templates are represented as raw intensity or color images, and consider the appearance of the objects. However, appearance templates are too specific to capture general properties of objects. Therefore, binary templates [3,4,5] that represent the contours of the objects are often used to capture information about their shape. The Chamfer distance [6] or Hausdorff distance [7,8] are commonly used to measure the similarity between a binary template and the input image contour; these distances are computed from the Distance Transform (DT) image [9]. Generally, this approach produces many false positives when the background is cluttered, so the magnitudes [10] or orientations [11,12,13] of edges are included as additional information to the DT image. The combination of magnitude and orientation can be used to reduce the number of false positives [14]. However, all DT-based methods have the weakness that contour points must be extracted; the result of this step can be unsatisfactory in images that contain illumination changes and noise.

K.M. Lee et al. (Eds.): ACCV 2012, Part I, LNCS 7724, pp. 97–110, 2013.
© Springer-Verlag Berlin Heidelberg 2013

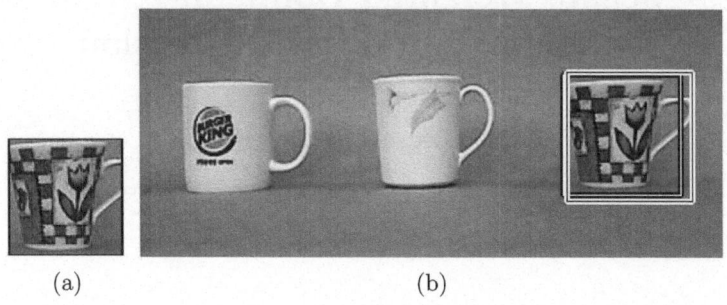

(a)                                    (b)

**Fig. 1.** (a) Target object; (b) Result of template matching using DOT (*white rectangle: detected object in input image*)

To overcome these limitations, the image gradients are considered as the feature constructing templates. The features can be represented [15,16] as rectified responses from an extended set of oriented Haar-like wavelets. PCA-SIFT features, which are variants of SIFT [17], can be obtained by using PCA which projects gradient images onto a basis [18]. Lastly, binary edge-presence voting can be used to assign features into log-polar spaced bins, irrespective of edge orientation [19]. Templates based on these features tend to be sparse, so they may not be suitable for objects that have little texture. Thus, the Histogram of Gradients (HOG) [20] was proposed as a dense image feature. HOG describes the local distributions of image gradients computed on a regular grid, and gives reliable results but tends to be slow due to computational complexity. Thus, all of the existing methods have shortcomings.

Hence, a binary template representation called Dominant Orientation Template (DOT) was introduced [21]. It relies on local dominant orientations instead of local histograms. It is invariant to small translation and at least as discriminant as HOG, while being much faster. However, DOT is somewhat instance-specific, especially when objects are textured. Given the DOT of a cup bearing a flower image (Fig. 1a), DOT detects only that instance, not other cups in the same class of cups (Fig. 1b). Hence, it is more suitable for object recognition than for object detection.

In this paper, we propose a DOT-based template for class-specific object detection to exploit fast DOT, although the original DOT is intended for instance-specific object detection. To accomplish this class-specificity, we form two kinds of templates. One consists of the representative DOTs of an object class; they are automatically selected from DOTs of all training images. The other consists of weight templates of an object class obtained from responses of vertical, horizontal, and diagonal 2D Haar wavelets [22]. To combine the representative DOTs and weight templates, we present a modified similarity measure defined as the product of the representative DOTs and weight templates.

The remainder of this paper is organized as follows: In section 2, we briefly review the concepts of DOT and 2D Haar wavelets and describe the proposed method. In section 3, the experimental results on several classes are shown. In section 4, we conclude the paper.

## 2   The Proposed Method

This section describes Dominant Orientation Templates (DOTs) and 2D Haar wavelets, and how they can be used to generate class-specific weighted DOTs.

### 2.1   DOT

Hinterstoisser et al. [21] retained the orientations of strong gradients based on their magnitude values and considered only the orientations of the gradients where two vectors with 180° separation are regarded as having the same orientation.

Let $I$ be an input image and $O$ be a reference image; each is decomposed into small square regions $R$ over a regular grid. For each $R$, the dominant orientations are considered as features. An operation $DO(O, R)$ returns the set of orientations with strong gradients in region $R$ of $O$ (Fig. 2a, left); a related operation $do(I, c + R)$ returns only one orientation of the strongest gradient in the region at location $c + R$ in $I$ (Fig. 2a, right), where $c$ is a template centered location. Then the obtained orientations are discretized to an integer value $n$ (Fig. 2b). If the gradient magnitude is less than a threshold $\tau$ in a region, it is region is judged to be uniform; the symbol $\perp$ is used to indicate these. Hence, the $DO(.)$ function returns either a set of discretized orientations $[0, n - 1]$ of $k$ strong gradients, or $\{\perp\}$. Similarly, $do(.)$ returns either only one discretized orientation $[0, n - 1]$ of the strongest gradient, or $\{\perp\}$. To measure the similarity between the image $I$ and the template $O$ centered at location $c$ in $I$, the similarity score $\varepsilon(I, O, c)$ can be formalized as:

$$\varepsilon(I, O, c) = \sum_{R \ in \ O} \delta\left(do(I, c + R) \in DO(O, R)\right) \tag{1}$$

where binary function $\delta(P) = 1$ if $P$ is true, and 0 otherwise.

The similarity score $\varepsilon$ can be computed efficiently using a binary representation of $DO(O, R)$ and $do(I, c + R)$. By setting the number $n$ of discretized orientations to 7, $DO(.)$ and $do(.)$ can each be represented as one byte $i.e.$, a 8-bit integer. Each of the first 7 bits corresponds to an orientation; the 8 bit stands for $\perp$. More exactly, bit $0 \leq i \leq 6$ that corresponds to discretized orientation is set to 1; the others are set to 0; if the region is uniform, the $7^{th}$ bit is set to 1. The term $\delta(.)$ in Eq. 1 can be evaluated very quickly by:

$$\delta\left(do(I, c + R) \in DO(O, R)\right) = 1 \ iff \ do(I, c + R) \otimes DO(O, R) \neq 0 \tag{2}$$

where $\otimes$ is the bitwise AND operation.

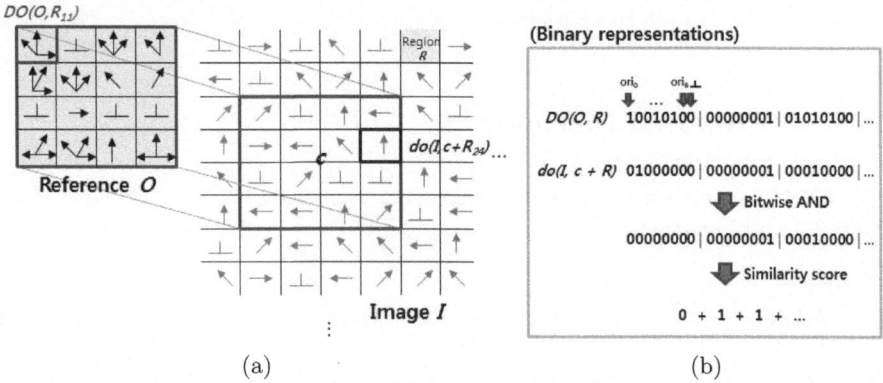

**Fig. 2.** (a) Dominant orientations of input image $I$ and reference image $O$; (b) Similarity score between two images using the bitwise AND operator

## 2.2    2D Haar Wavelets

The Haar wavelet is a sequence of rescaled *square-shaped* functions which together form a wavelet family or basis. The Haar wavelet's mother wavelet function $\psi(t)$ can be described as:

$$\psi(t) = \begin{cases} 1 & 0 \leq t < 1/2 \\ -1 & 1/2 \leq t < 1 \\ 0 & \text{otherwise.} \end{cases} \tag{3}$$

Its scaling function $\phi(t)$ can be described as:

$$\phi(t) = \begin{cases} 1 & 0 \leq t < 1 \\ 0 & \text{otherwise.} \end{cases} \tag{4}$$

The natural extension of wavelets to 2D signals is obtained by taking the tensor product of two 1D wavelet transforms $\psi(t)$ and $\phi(t)$. In [22], three types of wavelets were obtained: one that encodes a difference in the intensity along vertical borders, one that encodes a difference in the intensity along horizontal borders, and one that responds strongly to diagonal boundaries. Therefore, the representation of these wavelets identifies local, oriented intensity difference features at multiple-resolutions and is efficiently computable.

## 2.3    Class-Specific Weighted DOTs

This section presents a method to obtain class-specific weighted DOTs. The original DOT is instance-specific, because it has the information that is specific to a given object to be detected. The goal of class-specific weighted DOTs is to obtain the information that is common to all objects in a given object class.

---

**Algorithm 1. Bottom-up clustering method**

---

**Input**: DOTs obtained from $m$ training images, $T_{i=1,...,m}$
**Output**: Sets $A_{j=1,...,N}$ and cluster templates $C_{j=1,...,N}$ from $N$ clusters

**Clustering**
1. Initialize $y_i = 0$ for all $i = 1, .., m$, where $y_i \in (1,0)$ represents whether $T_i$ belongs to any cluster or not.
2. Repeat for $j = 1, ..., N$:
   a. Create an empty set $A_j$ of $j^{th}$ cluster.
   b. Randomly select a $T_i$ with $y_i = 0$ among $T_{i=1,...,m}$ and put it in $A_j$ and set $y_i = 1$.
   c. Repeat for $k = 1, ..., d$ (where, $d$ is the defined number):
      (a) Obtain $C_j$ using the bitwise OR operation of all DOTs in $A_j$.
      (b) Among $T_{i=1,...,m}$ with $y_i = 0$, select a $T_i$, which has the nearest hamming distance $d_h$ with $C_j$ and put it in $A_j$ and set $y_i = 1$.
3. return $A_{j=1,...,N}$ and $C_{j=1,...,N}$.

---

This goal is achieved by combining representative DOTs and weight templates. The representative DOTs are selected from all DOTs obtained from training images. Weight templates are computed using 2D Haar wavelets (Section 2.2) to obtain the information common to an object class. The modified similarity measure, defined as the product of the representative DOTs and weight templates, is used to get class-specific weighted DOTs.

**Representative DOTs.** Given training images of an object class as reference images, we generate a DOT for each training image (Section 2.1). Conducting template matching using all DOTs obtained from training images would require long run-time and sometimes decrease the accuracy of identification because of redundancy among DOTs. Hence, the representative DOTs of the object class are selected. The overall framework to select them is as follows (Fig. 3).

To remove redundancy among DOTs, we use a bottom-up clustering method [21] (algorithm 1) to gather each group of similar DOTs into a cluster. Because a cluster template $C_j$ contains properties of all DOTs in cluster $A_j$, we assume that in each cluster $A_j$, if a template is more similar to the cluster template $C_j$ than other templates, the template has higher potential as the representative DOT. A representative DOT, $S_j$, in cluster $A_j$ is selected as:

$$S_j = \arg\max_{T_{A_j}} \sum_{R \ in \ C_j} \delta \left( DO(T_{A_j}, R) \in DO(C_j, R) \right) \tag{5}$$

where $T_{A_j}$ is a template in cluster $A_j$. The term $\delta(.)$ in Eq. 5 is defined by

$$\delta \left( DO(T_{A_j}, R) \in DO(C_j, R) \right) = 1 \ \textit{iff} \ d_h(DO(T_{A_j}, R), \ DO(C_j, R)) \geq t \tag{6}$$

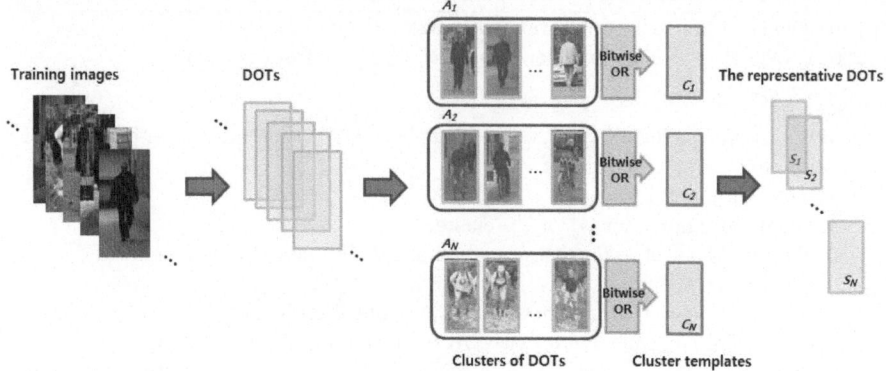

**Fig. 3.** Framework of representative DOT selection

where $d_h$ is the Hamming distance and $t$ is a threshold to decide whether region $R$ of the template coincides with that of the cluster template.

**Weight Templates.** The Haar wavelets encode the difference in average intensity between local regions along different orientations. The responses of wavelets can express visual features of an object class. More specifically, strong response from a particular wavelet indicates the presence of edge at that location in the image, whereas weak response indicates a uniform area. Therefore, by using these wavelets, visually reliable features of class-specific shape can be captured. We use the three types of 2D Haar wavelets (Section 2.2) with the size of $4 \times 4$.

Given the gray-scale training images for an object class, wavelet responses for each training image are computed at every grid point with grid spacing of $4 \times 4$ then nearest-neighbor interpolation of the values of these grid pixels is used assign the values to all other pixels. Then for each orientation, the average responses are computed for all the training images; each average is then normalized to a proportion of maximum average value, resulting in three weight templates: vertical $v(x, y)$, horizontal $h(x, y)$ and diagonal $d(x, y)$.

Training images of cars and pedestrians (Fig. 4b) were used to obtain weight templates (Fig. 4c) that allow identification of significant regions of an object class for each orientations and capture the general property of the object class.

**Class-Specific Weighted DOTs.** To generate class-specific weighted DOTs, the representative DOTs are combined with the weight templates of an object class. To do this, we modify the similarity score (Eq. 1). The modified similarity score $\varphi(I, S_j, c)$ between $I$ and a representative DOT $S_j$ centered at $c$ in $I$ is formalized as:

$$\varphi(I, S_j, c) = \sum_{R_k \ in \ S_j} w(R_k) \cdot \delta \left( do(I, c + R_k) \in DO(S_j, R_k) \right) \qquad (7)$$

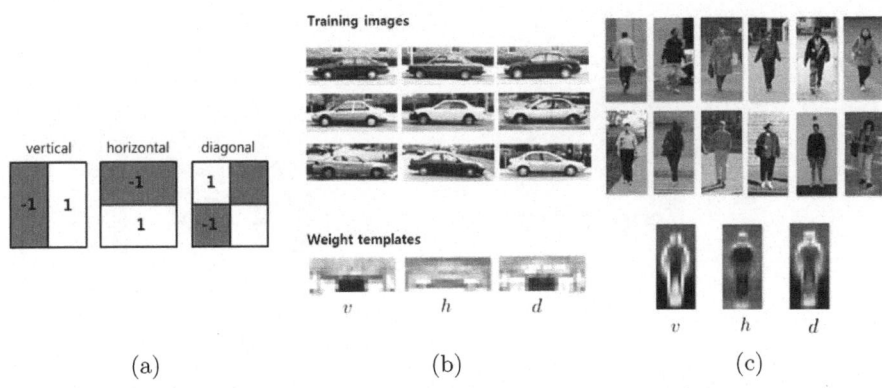

**Fig. 4.** (a) The three types (vertical, horizontal, and diagonal) of 2D Haar wavelets; (b,c) Training images (top) and weight templates (bottom) of cars and pedestrians

where $w(R_k)$ is the weight value of region $R_k$ . If the weight templates are not considered, $w(R_k)$ is set to 1. In this case, $\varphi(.)$ equals the similarity score (Eq.1) of original DOT. If weight templates are considered, $w(R_k)$ is the value of the weight template corresponding to $do(I, c + R_k)$ as follows:

$$w(R_k) = \begin{cases} v(R_k) & do(I, c + R_k) \in \{2^0, 2^6\} \\ h(R_k) & do(I, c + R_k) \in \{2^3\} \\ d(R_k) & do(I, c + R_k) \in \{2^1, 2^2, 2^4, 2^5\} \\ u & do(I, c + R_k) \in \{2^7\} \end{cases} \qquad (8)$$

where $u$ represents a constant weight value of the uniform region. $do(I, c + R_k)$ can be represented as the 8-bit integer (Fig. 5).

For template matching, we scan $I$ with the representative DOTs of the specific class. The best matching template $T^*$ is obtained from:

$$T^* = \arg\max_{S_j} \ \varphi(I, S_j, c) \qquad (9)$$

Once the best matching template $T^*$ is obtained, the similarity score at the location $c$ is stored. Local peaks of these scores represent regions that contain a target object.

To reduce the number of false positives, we use thresholding to derive binary mask images $m_a$ from weight templates, i.e.,

$$m_a(R_k) = \begin{cases} 1 & w(R_k) \geq \tau_{max} \times 0.8 \\ 0 & \text{otherwise.} \end{cases} \qquad (10)$$

where $\tau_{max}$ is the maximum value of the weight template.

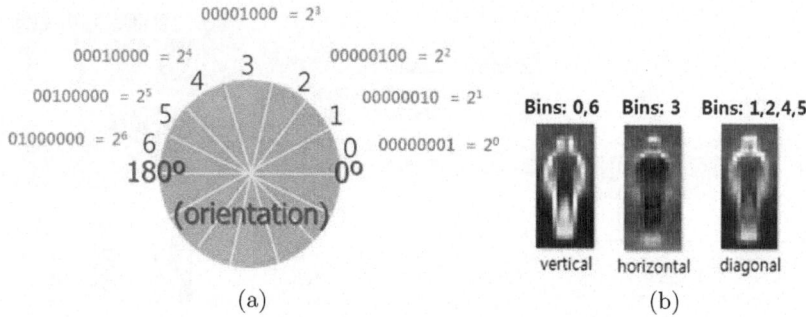

**Fig. 5.** (a) 8-bit representation of each orientation bin; (b) Orientation bin corresponding to each weight template of pedestrians

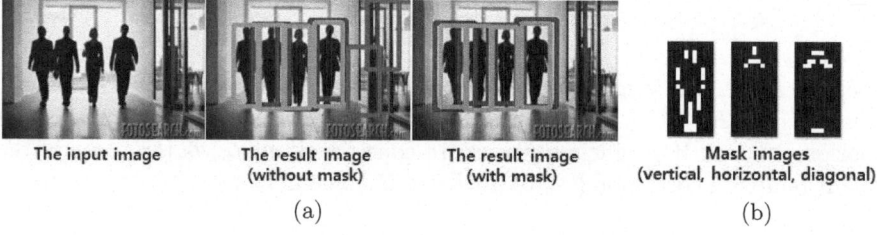

**Fig. 6.** (a) Input image and the detection results of pedestrians without or with mask images (*green rectangle:* ground truth, *blue rectangle:* correct result, *red rectangle:* false positive); (b) Mask images over vertical, horizontal, and diagonal weight templates

Mostly, false positives appear similar to the target object. For instance, because the body shape of a pedestrian is approximately a vertical rectangle, this shape can easily be confused with a background object with a similar shape. To eliminate this type of false positive, we use mask images to verify the detection results. The number $n_{cnt}$ of sub-regions matched with $m_a$ is defined by:

$$n_{cnt} = \sum_{R_k \ in \ S_j} m_a(R_k) \cdot \delta \left( do(I, c + R_k) \in DO(S_j, R_k) \right) \qquad (11)$$

$n_{cnt}$ can reduce the number of false positives by discarding candidate regions in which $n_{cnt}$ is below a threshold, even though they have high similarity score $\varphi(I, T^*, c)$.

Using $m_a$ increases the ability to distinguish a target object from the background (Fig. 6). This approach captures the general property of an object class and ignore unnecessary information inside objects.

# 3  Experimental Results

The proposed method was tested on images of cars (UIUC-single car dataset [1] and CalTech car rear dataset [24]) and pedestrians (USC-A pedestrian test set [23] and INRIA person dataset [20]). For all datasets, the size of decomposed regions $R$ was $4 \times 4$ pixels. In each region, the number $k$ of extracted dominant orientations was 7 in training images and 1 in test images. The detection performance was measured using Equal recall precision Error Rate (1-EER). Detected results were accepted as correct if the intersection area of the detected bounding box and the ground-truth bounding box exceeded 50% of the union of the two boxes. For the comparison, 1-EER was compared with the original DOT [21] to demonstrate the suitability of the proposed method for class-specific object detection, and with different representations of template (contour-based [14] and gradient-based [20]). Experiments were implemented on a quad core CPU operating at 2.6GHz.

## 3.1  Car Detection

**UIUC-Single Car.** This dataset contains side images of cars. The training set consists of 550 car images and 500 non-car images of a fixed size ($100 \times 40$ pixels). The test set consists of 170 images with 200 cars and includes partially-occluded cars and cluttered backgrounds under challenging illumination. In the training step, we used only 550 car images for constructing weight templates and DOTs, among which 20 representative DOTs are selected. In the testing step, the test images were scanned with a step of 4 pixels. Combining weight templates with the original DOTs gave better a result (Fig. 7a) than both the original DOT and the contour-based approach [14] which uses the combination of edge magnitudes and orientations for matching; using mask images further increased the 1-EER (Table 1). For this dataset, the training time was about 4s and the time required to test an image of $189 \times 118$ pixels was 59ms.

**CalTech Car Rear.** This dataset contains images of rear views of cars. For training, the CalTech cars-markus dataset was used; it contains 12 car images obtained in parking lots. From this dataset, we constructed weight templates and DOTs, among which 18 representative DOTs were selected automatically. For testing, the CalTech cars-brad dataset was; it contains 526 car images. Each image in this dataset contains cars on the road; scale variation among the images is significant. Because the test dataset is not annotated, we defined the ground-truth bounding box manually. Therefore, the performance (Fig. 7b) of proposed method can only be compared directly with that of the original DOT, and not with those of other methods. Combining weight templates with the original DOTs significantly improved the true-positive detection rate from 54.56% (using the original DOT) to 82.89%; using mask images further increased the performance increases this rate to 92.02%. In this experiment, the training time was about 3s and in scale space of $360 \times 240$ pixels, the testing time was 400ms.

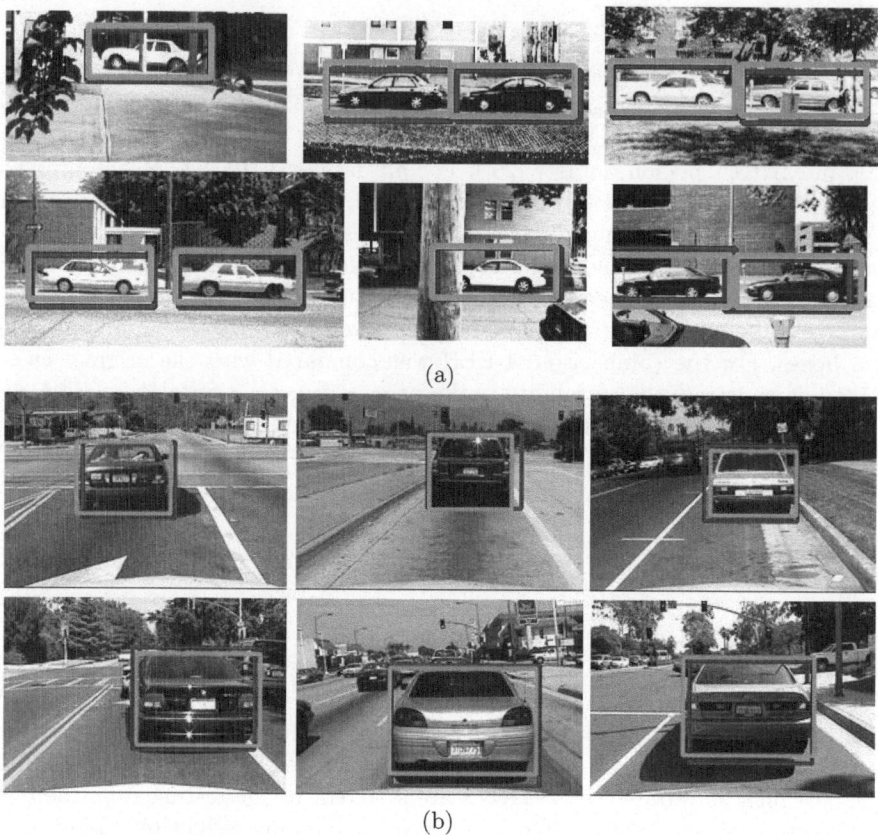

(a)

(b)

**Fig. 7.** Detection results of (a) UIUC car (side); (b) CalTech car (rear) datasets (*green rectangle:* ground truth, *blue rectangle:* detection result)

## 3.2   Pedestrian Detection

**USC-A Pedestrian.** This dataset includes 205 front or rear images of 313 pedestrians in upright standing poses. Ppedestrians are not occluded but the background is cluttered. However, because this dataset consists of a test set only, the MIT pedestrian dataset of 924 training images [15] was used for training, among which 12 representative DOTs were selected. The test images were scanned using $44 \times 88$ window at various scales from 0.6 to 1.2. The detection results were compared with the ground truth given in [23] using the criteria proposed in [2]. Combining weight templates with the original DOTs produced better results (Fig. 8) than using the original DOTs for matching; using mask images considerably improve the performance of detection and provided a result better than that [14] (Table 1). For this dataset, the training time was about 15s. Because we considered the various scales of object for the matching, the testing time to detect all objects in an image was around 350ms.

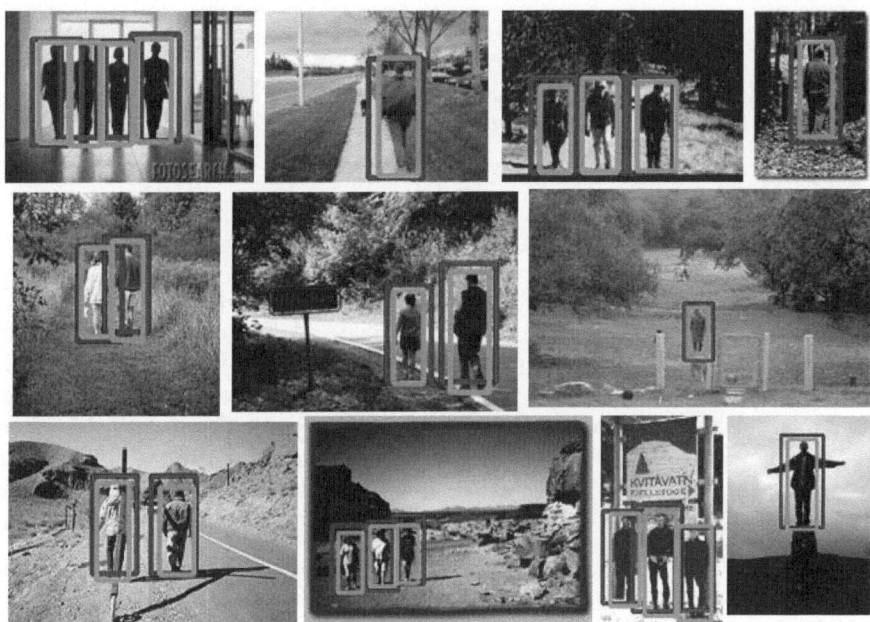

**Fig. 8.** Detection results of the USC-A pedestrian dataset (*green rectangle:* ground truth, *blue rectangle:* detection result of proposed method)

**INRIA Person.** We tested the proposed method on the INRIA person which is more challenging pedestrian dataset. The INRIA person dataset provides both training and testing sets containing positive samples of $64 \times 128$ pixels and negative images that contain no humans. In the training step, we used all 2416 positive training images as training images and selected 18 representative DOTs. We used 1126 positive testing images and negative images obtained by shifting the detection windows by 8 pixels in the negative testing images, all of which are available in the dataset. Positive testing images consist of pedestrians images with the size of $64 \times 128$ cropped from a varied set of personal photos (Fig. 9). The subjects are always upright, but images include some partial occlusions

**Table 1.** 1-EER of original DOT and proposed methods for UIUC-single car and USC-A pedestrian databases

| Methods | | UIUC | USC-A |
|---------|---|------|-------|
| [14] | | 83.0% | 80.0% |
| **Proposed method** | The original DOT [21] | 74.0% | 60.0% |
| | With weight templates (without mask) | 92.0% | 73.8% |
| | With weight templates (with mask) | **93.5%** | **82.4%** |

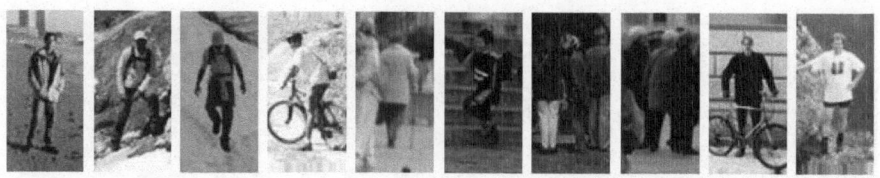

**Fig. 9.** Some sample images from the INRIA person dataset

and a wide range of variations in pose, appearance, clothing, and background. To measure the performance, we used miss rate at $10^{-4}$ False Positives Per Window (FPPW) as a reference point, because it was used in the other methods to compare. The proposed method was significantly better than other feature-based methods, but is comparable to HOG [20] (Table 2). The proposed method is faster than HOG in both training time and testing time: the training time of the proposed method takes several seconds whereas HOG takes several hours. The testing time to process 4000 windows was around 430ms in the proposed method and almost 1s in HOG.

**Table 2.** Miss rate of proposed method and existing methods at $10^{-4}$FPPW for the INRIA person database

| Methods | Miss rate at $10^{-4}$**FPPW(%)** |
|:---:|:---:|
| HOG [20] | 27.0% ~ **11.0%** |
| Wavelet [15,16] PCA-SIFT [17] Shape Context [17] | >> 20.0% |
| **Proposed method** | 17.0% |

## 4   Conclusion

We have introduced a class-specific weighted dominant orientation template (DOT) to construct class-specific templates by combining representative DOTs and weight templates. The representative DOTs of an object class are selected using an automatic selection algorithm, and weight templates are obtained using vertical, horizontal, and diagonal 2D Haar wavelets. A modified similarity measure defined as the product of the representative DOTs and weight templates is used to obtain class-specific weighted DOTs. We compared the performance of the proposed method with existing methods for detecting cars and pedestrians. The results show that the proposed method was more accurate than existing methods and comparably accurate to HOG. Using the concept of DOT enables fast object detection in an input image. Also, generating the representative DOTs and weight templates is rapid because the process is relatively simple.

**Acknowledgement.** This work was supported by the National Research Foundation of Korea(NRF) grant funded by the Korea government(MEST) (No. 2012-0005568).

# References

1. Agarwal, S., Roth, D.: Learning a Sparse Representation for Object Detection. In: Heyden, A., Sparr, G., Nielsen, M., Johansen, P. (eds.) ECCV 2002, Part IV. LNCS, vol. 2353, pp. 113–127. Springer, Heidelberg (2002)
2. Leibe, B., Seemann, E., Schiele, B.: Pedestrian Detection in Crowded Scenes. In: Proc. IEEE Conference on Computer Vision and Pattern Recognition, pp. 878–885 (2005)
3. Gavrila, D., Philomin, V.: Real-Time Object Detection for Smart Vehicles. In: ICCV 1999, pp. 87–93 (1999)
4. Gavrila, D., Dariu, M.: A Bayesian, Exemplar-Based Approach to Hierarchical Shape Matching. IEEE Trans. Pattern Anal. Mach. Intell., 1408–1421 (2007)
5. Thanh, N.D., Ogunbona, P., Li, W.: Human detection based on weighted template matching. In: Proceedings of the 2009 IEEE International Conference on Multimedia and Expo, pp. 634–637 (2009)
6. Barrow, H.G., Tenenbaum, J.M., Bolles, R.C., Wolf, H.C.: Parametric correspondence and chamfer matching: two new techniques for image matching. In: Proceedings of the 5th International Joint Conference on Artificial Intelligence, pp. 659–663 (1977)
7. Huttenlocher, D.P., Klanderman, G.A., Kl, G.A., Rucklidge, W.J.: Comparing Images Using the Hausdorff Distance. IEEE Transactions on Pattern Analysis and Machine Intelligence, 850–863 (1993)
8. Rucklidge, W.J.: Locating objects using the Hausdorff distance. In: Proceedings of the Fifth International Conference on Computer Vision, pp. 457–464 (1995)
9. Borgefors, G.: Hierarchical Chamfer Matching: A Parametric Edge Matching Algorithm. IEEE Trans. Pattern Anal. Mach. Intell., 849–865 (1988)
10. Rosin, P.L., West, G.A.W.: Salience Distance Transforms. Graph. Models Image Process., 483–521 (1995)
11. Gavrila, D.M.: Multi-Feature Hierarchical Template Matching Using Distance Transforms. In: Proceedings of the 14th International Conference on Pattern Recognition, pp. 439–444 (1998)
12. Olson, C.F., Huttenlocher, D.P.: Automatic Target Recognition by Matching Oriented Edge Pixels. IEEE Transactions on Image Processing, 103–113 (1997)
13. Jain, A.K., Zhong, Y., Lakshmanan, S.: Object Matching Using Deformable Templates. IEEE Trans. Pattern Anal. Mach. Intell., 267–278 (1996)
14. Thanh, N.D., Li, W., Ogunbona, P.: An Improved Template Matching Method for Object Detection. In: Zha, H., Taniguchi, R.-i., Maybank, S. (eds.) ACCV 2009, Part III. LNCS, vol. 5996, pp. 193–202. Springer, Heidelberg (2010)
15. Mohan, A., Papageorgiou, C., Poggio, T.: Example based object detection in images by components. IEEE Trans. Pattern Anal. and Machine Intell., 349–361 (2001)
16. Viola, P., Jones, M.J., Snow, D.: Detecting Pedestrians Using Patterns of Motion and Appearance. In: Proceedings of the Ninth IEEE International Conference on Computer Vision, vol. 2, pp. 734–741 (2003)
17. Lowe, D.G.: Distinctive Image Features from Scale-Invariant Keypoints. Int. J. Comput. Vision, 91–110 (2004)

18. Yan, K., Sukthankar, R.: PCA-SIFT: A More Distinctive Representation for Local Image Descriptors. In: CVPR (2) 2004, pp. 506–513 (2004)
19. Belongie, S., Malik, J., Puzicha, J.: Matching Shapes. In: ICCV 2001, pp. 454–461 (2001)
20. Dalal, N., Triggs, B.: Histograms of Oriented Gradients for Human Detection. In: Proc. IEEE Conference on Computer Vision and Pattern Recognition, pp. 886–893 (2005)
21. Hinterstoisser, S., Lepetit, V., Ilic, S., Fua, P., Navab, N.: Dominant Orientation Templates for Real-Time Detection of Texture-Less Objects. In: Proc. IEEE Conference on Computer Vision and Pattern Recognition, pp. 2257–2264 (2010)
22. Papageorgiou, C., Poggio, T.: A Trainable System for Object Detection. Int. J. Comput. Vision, 15–33 (2000)
23. Wu, B., Nevatia, R.: Detection of Multiple, Partially Occluded Humans in a Single Image by Bayesian Combination of Edgelet Part Detectors. In: ICCV 2005, pp. 90–97 (2005)
24. Leibe, B., Leonardis, A., Schiele, B.: Robust Object Detection with Interleaved Categorization and Segmentation. Int. J. Comput. Vision, 259–289 (2008)

# Salient Object Detection via Color Contrast and Color Distribution

Keren Fu, Chen Gong, Jie Yang, and Yue Zhou

Institute of Image Processing and Pattern Recognition,
Shanghai Jiao Tong University, and Key Laboratory of System Control and
Information Processing, Ministry of Education of China, Shanghai 200240

**Abstract.** In this paper, we take the advantages of color contrast and color distribution to get high quality saliency maps. The overall procedure flow of our unified framework contains superpixel pre-segmentation, color contrast and color distribution computation, combination, final refinement and then object segmentation. During color contrast saliency computation, we combine two color systems and then introduce the using of distribution prior before saliency smoothing. It works to select correct color components. In addition, we propose a novel saliency smoothing procedure that is based on superpixel regions and is realized in color space. This processing step leads to total object being highlighted evenly, contributing to high quality color contrast saliency maps. Finally, a new refinement approach is utilized to eliminate artifacts and recover unconnected parts in the combined saliency maps. In visual comparison, our method produces higher quality saliency maps which stress out the total object meanwhile suppress background clutters. Both qualitative and quantitative experiments show our approach outperforms 8 state-of-the-art methods, achieving the highest precision rate 96% (3% improvement from the current highest), when evaluated via one of the most popular data sets [1]. Excellent content-aware image resizing also can be achieved with our saliency maps.

## 1 Introduction

Human usually pay more attention to some parts of a given image. This visual attention mechanism has been extensively studied by researchers, due to it can allow us to allocate our sensory and computational resources to the most valuable information. Salient object detection is one of the most important aspects of such attention mechanism. Various applications have been explored by using saliency detection, such as auto target location and segmentation [2, 3], object based image retrieval [4], content-aware image resizing [5–8] and so on.

Saliency models usually can be divided into two categories, so-called *bottom-up* and *top-down*. Bottom-up model [9–13, 1, 14] simulates our instinctive visual attention mechanism and lots of low-level features like color (intensity), edge (texture) could be adopted. A salient object should be unique or have strong contrast compared to its surroundings on theses features. Among them, color contrast is one low-level feature which may easily draw our attention [15, 16].

K.M. Lee et al. (Eds.): ACCV 2012, Part I, LNCS 7724, pp. 111–122, 2013.
© Springer-Verlag Berlin Heidelberg 2013

Another model called top-down [17–19] is defined in visual perceptual field as using effective memory to process presented saliency information. Via the computer vision techniques, we can realize the top-down model through combining the prior statistical knowledge and learning of classifiers.

In this paper, we take the advantages of color contrast and color distribution to carry out our saliency detection, so our method belongs to bottom-up kind. The previous work which is most related to ours is [10] and recent [11]. The former defines pixel-wise saliency as a pixel's contrast to all other pixels. This is then converted into computation based on color histogram. Also, good results are reported using HC (Histogram Contrast) and RC (Region Contrast) methods in [10]. However, we find that their methods only consider the color contrast but exclude the color distribution, which may also be an important kind of character for salient object. So their HC and RC methods may not get good results on the images in which some parts of background have relatively stronger contrast than the real salient object. Besides, the saliency maps obtained using RC usually highlights some parts of salient object, rather than the overall, and there are also lots of background clutters, as is shown in Fig.3 and Fig.4.

In addition, our work differs from [11] as we perform more processing steps in our color contrast based saliency computation, which are proved to be necessary to improve the final performance in a relative large margin. Moreover, we propose a different approach to refine our saliency maps.

In summary, we propose that a salient object should have the following characters on color feature, in two folds, the color contrast and color distribution.

($i$). The color components belong to a salient object may have strong contrast to their surroundings, which is biologically inspired. (*contrast*)

($ii$). These color components may be located near image center rather than image boundary. It is based on the fact [19] that shows human fixation has much higher probability to fall onto the center of image. (*distribution*)

($iii$). These color components usually distribute compactly. In another word, color components which distribute widely are less likely to belong to a salient object. (*distribution*)

Our method takes the above three characters to perform saliency detection. The experimental results show our algorithm can highlight the whole part of a salient object meanwhile have strong ability to suppress background clutters. As a result, high quality saliency maps can be obtained.

The rest of this paper is organized as follows. Related works are described in Section 2. Our methodology is proposed in Section 3. Experimental results are analyzed in Section 4 while conclusion and future work are drawn in Section 5.

## 2   Related Work

As is mentioned above, the main categories of saliency detection methods are bottom-up and top-down. Because our method belongs to the former, here we only review related bottom-up kind. For top-down kind, we suggest readers to refer to [19].

Among bottom-up kind, as one of the earliest work, Itti *et al* [9] proposed a center-surround operation as local feature contrast in the color, intensity, and orientation of an image. The center-surround operation is realized using DOG (Difference of Gaussians). Then Hou *et al* [12] propose a method based on the spectral residual in the amplitude spectrum of Fourier transform. Zhai *et al* [13] define the saliency of each pixel as its contrast to all other pixels. However, for efficiency, they only consider the luminance channel. Achanta *et al* [1] propose a frequency tuned method which is extremely fast. They define the saliency of a pixel as its distance to the image average. But this algorithm is less promising for images that contain complex background and textures. Goferman *et al* [14] combine local feature and global feature to estimate the patch saliency in multi-scale. This leads to high computational cost. Besides, the use of local feature may cause edges highlighted. Cheng *et al* [10] propose Histogram Contrast based and Region Contrast based methods, called HC and RC respectively, as is mentioned in Section 1. Saliency maps obtained using their methods may contain background clutters and sometimes highlight parts of the object. Although they combine GrabCut [20] and their saliency maps to get good segmentation results, we demonstrate that high quality saliency map is the basis of various post processing. Thus the key point should be focused on how to improve the quality of the obtained saliency map. More recently, Perazzi *et al* [11] combine color contrast and color distribution to perform saliency detection. They show that the complete contrast and saliency estimation can be formulated in a unified way using high dimensional Gaussian filters. However, they only combine basic steps of computing color contrast and distribution.

Furthermore, there are some bottom-up methods which adopt multiple features. Liu *et al* [21] and Alexe *et al* [22] use a sliding window and compute a multiple low-level feature based saliency score for each window. Salient object corresponds to the window with the highest score. Feng *et al* [23] compute the window saliency based on superpixels. They use all the superpixels outside the window to compose the inside ones, thus the global image context is combined.

Our saliency detection method varies from the state-of-the-art bottom-up methods, because our method concentrates on how to produce high quality saliency maps which strongly highlight the total object as well as suppress the background clutters enormously. High quality saliency maps facilitate most post processing like object segmentation and content-aware image resizing, as we will show later.

## 3   Methodology

Fig.1 shows the whole procedure flow of our method, including SLIC superpixel pre-segmentation [24], color contrast and color distribution computation, combination, final refinement and then object segmentation. As high quality saliency maps are produced, using simple thresholding may achieve good segmentation results, as we will show in the final quantitative comparison. Note that an input image is first resized to the size of $(W, H)$, which subjects to $\max(W, H) = 400$. Then all the parameters of our method are tuned on this basic resolution.

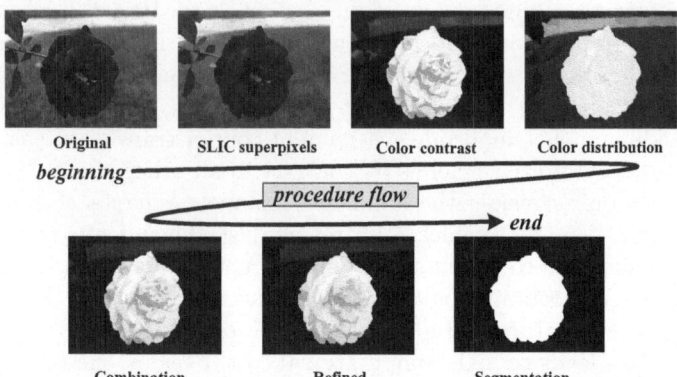

| Original | SLIC superpixels | Color contrast | Color distribution |

*beginning*

procedure flow

→ *end*

| Combination | Refined | Segmentation |

**Fig. 1.** The whole procedure flow of our method, including SLIC superpixel pre-segmentation, color contrast and color distribution computation, combination, final refinement and object segmentation

## 3.1 Pre-segmentation

In order to calculate color contrast of a pixel to all other pixels, a straightforward way is pixel-wise computation, as is mentioned in [13]. However, the computational cost of such algorithms is $O(M^2)$, where $M$ denotes the number of pixels in the input image. An elegant way to speed up and reduce computational cost is histogram based computation [10, 13] or segmenting images into edge-preserving regions, like that in [10, 11, 23]. Pixels in the same region usually have homogenous color component. Computing region based contrast instead of pixel-wise operation enormously pulls down the computational complexity. Thus, we first use SLIC superpixels [24] to decompose an image and generate spatial compact regions $R_i, i = 1, 2, 3...N$. SLIC superpixels are also used in [11] as abstraction technique. Compact SLIC superpixels are generated iteratively using mean-shift clustering based on the initial uniformly distributed region seeds. We use SLIC superpixels in LAB color space, which well characterize human visual perception. For an image with basic resolution, we segment it into about $N = 500$ superpixels, a tradeoff between computational cost and description ability. Here we use $c_i, p_i$ to denote the average color and position of superpixels as

$$c_i = \frac{\sum_{I_m \in R_i} I_m^C}{|R_i|}, \; p_i = \frac{\sum_{I_m \in R_i} I_m^P}{|R_i|} \tag{1}$$

where $I_m^C$ and $I_m^P$ are respectively 6D color vector, constituted by LAB and RGB components (corresponds $c_i^{LAB}$ and $c_i^{RGB}$), and position vector of pixel $I_m$. $|R_i|$ is the sum area of superpixel region $R_i$. Pre-segmenting the image into superpixels eliminates unnecessary details and noises as well.

## 3.2 Color Contrast

According to character $(i)$, we define region's color contrast saliency $S_i^{contrast}$ as

$$S_i^{contrast} = \sum_j D(c_i, c_j)^2 w_{ij}^P \qquad (2)$$

in which $D(c_i, c_j) = ||c_i - c_j||_2$ is Euclidean distance between $c_i$ and $c_j$. That means we first combine both color systems in color contrast computation. This is motivated by one color system does not always work [25]. Note that $c_i$ and $c_j$ is normalized before computation. Here we use quadratic term to suppress the background clutters. $w_{ij}^P = e^{-\alpha||p_i - p_j||^2}$ is spatial constrain, which enhances the effect of nearer neighbors. $\alpha$ controls the weight's sensitivity to spatial distance. When $\alpha \rightarrow 0$, $w_{ij}^P \rightarrow 1$, (2) degrades into global contrast calculation which is similar to that in [10]. In our experiment, we find $5 \times 10^{-5}$ is suitable for $\alpha$.

Besides the color contrast, we also introduce the color distribution prior, which meets character $(ii)$ mentioned in Section 1 and is not considered in [10] and [11]. After combining the distribution prior of region $R_i$, (2) should be rewritten as

$$S_i^{contrast} = D^{prior}(p_i) \sum_j D(c_i, c_j)^2 w_{ij}^P \qquad (3)$$

In (3), $D^{prior}(p_i)$ is the distribution prior at position $p_i$. An advantage of using distribution prior is that we can filter out the background color components which have the similar or even higher contrast than the color components that belong to the real salient object. Notice that in Fig.3, compared with color contrast based methods HC and RC, our approach renders the white road in the background much lower saliency.

According to the fact that human fixation has much higher probability to fall onto the center of the image, $D^{prior}(p_i)$ is larger when $p_i$ is closer to the image center. Here a Gaussian distribution like $D^{prior}(p_i) = e^{-w||p_i-c||^2}$ may be used, in which $c$ denotes image center. However, instead of being puzzled by how to adjust parameter $w$, which controls the probability distribution of salient object's occurrence, a simple but effective statistical approach is used. We compute the average of 1000 ground truth images[1] provided by [1] (Fig.2), noting that ground truth images are first resized to resolution $400 \times 400$. The average image commonly shows where a salient object is most likely to appear. Then it is normalized to have maximum value 1 to form the distribution prior map. In our implementation, the distribution prior map (resolution $400 \times 400$) is resized to the input resolution when it is used, and $D^{prior}(p_i)$ is directly obtained from the resized distribution prior map (Fig.2).

Combining color contrast and distribution prior may highlight some parts of an object, leading to the overall object being ambiguous, as is shown in Fig.3.

---

[1] Actually when we compute the saliency map of an image from this dataset, we should consider the other 999 images' ground truth to calculate the distribution prior. However, the average of 999 images is almost equal to that of 1000 images.

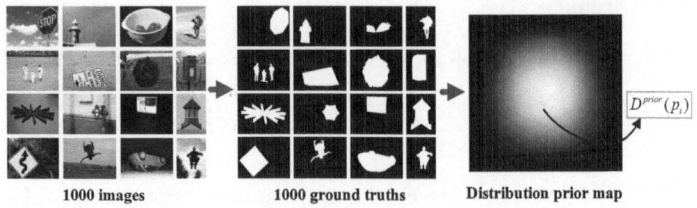

1000 images          1000 ground truths          Distribution prior map

**Fig. 2.** An illustration for obtaining distribution prior map

The color contrast saliency maps produced by RC [10] and SF (called uniqueness in [11]) also have such problem. As a solution, we adopt saliency smoothing in color space to render regions with similar colors the closer saliency values as

$$\overline{S_i^{contrast}} = \sum_j S_j^{contrast} w_{ij}^C \qquad (4)$$

where $\overline{S_i^{contrast}}$ represents the smoothed saliency. $w_{ij}^C = \frac{1}{N^C} e^{-\beta \|c_i^{LAB} - c_j^{LAB}\|}$ is the weight corresponding to color similarity, as LAB is better for smoothing in practice. $N^C = \sum_j e^{-\beta \|c_i^{LAB} - c_j^{LAB}\|}$ is its normalization term that guarantees all weights summed to 1. In our experiment, we find that exponent function works better than Gaussians on smoothing saliency of the whole object. In contrast, Gaussians fall down too sharply and usually highlight parts of object. $\beta$ controls the extent of smoothing. When $\beta \to 0$, $w_{ij}^C \to \frac{1}{N}$, after computing (4), all regions will obtain the same saliency, achieving the most extreme case. When $\beta \to \infty$, output $\overline{S_i^{contrast}}$ equals to $S_i^{contrast}$. Through computing (4), the whole object's saliency becomes more uniform (Fig.3). Here, we set $\beta = 10^{-3}$ for non-normalized LAB color space, which is feasible for highlighting the overall object.

Finally, the smoothed saliency map is normalized to [0, 1] using linear stretch as (5) to get the ultimate color contrast saliency map.

$$\overline{S_i^{contrast}} \leftarrow \frac{\overline{S_i^{contrast}} - \min_j(\overline{S_j^{contrast}})}{\max_j(\overline{S_j^{contrast}}) - \min_j(\overline{S_j^{contrast}})} \qquad (5)$$

### 3.3    Color Distribution

We compute color distribution similarly to [21] to meet character (*iii*), but based on superpixel regions. The distribution of $R_i$ is defined as

$$D_i^{distribution} = \| \sum_j w_{ij}^C p_j^2 - (\sum_j w_{ij}^C p_j)^2 \|_1 \qquad (6)$$

Here, the square of $p_j = (x_j, y_j)^T$ denotes the element square of vector $p_j$, that is $p_j^2 = (x_j^2, y_j^2)^T$. Actually (6) calculates the distribution variance in $x$ and $y$ direction and uses 1-norm to add them up. High distribution variance indicates that the corresponding color components are widely distributed in the

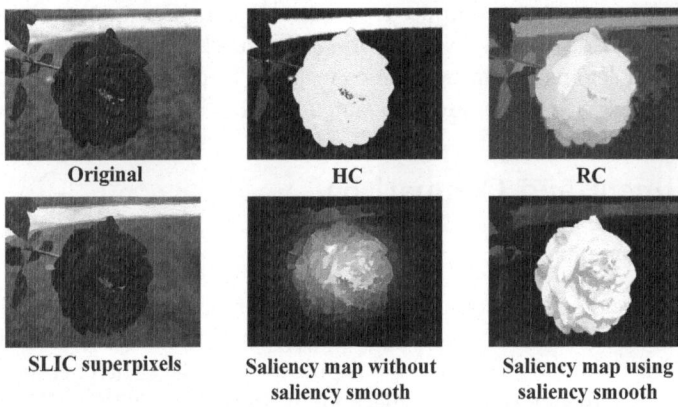

**Fig. 3.** Our smoothing in color space highlights the overall object. The results of contrast based methods HC and RC are also shown. Notice that the road in the background is rendered the highest saliency by HC while RC highlights the flower unevenly.

whole image and are less likely to belong to a salient object, while low variance indicates a spatially compact distribution.

Note that the parameter $\beta$ in $w_{ij}^C$ of (6) is tuned differently from that in (4), resulting in more promising performance in practice. In our implementation, $\beta$ in (6) is set as $10^{-1}$. $D_i^{distribution}$ is then normalized to $[0, 1]$ similarly to (5).

As demonstrated above, regions with high distribution variances should obtain low saliency, so we define the color distribution based saliency as

$$S_i^{distribution} = 1 - D_i^{distribution} \tag{7}$$

### 3.4   Combination and Refinement

We define the final combination as non-linear integration of color distribution saliency and color contrast saliency, as is presented in (8), for we find that such non-linear combination can better pop out salient objects meanwhile suppress background than linear combination.

$$S_i = \overline{S_i^{contrast}} \times S_i^{distribution} \tag{8}$$

After combination, there may still be noises and artifacts due to quantization errors of superpixel segmentation. In order to get high quality saliency maps, we again segment the images into non-compact regions $R'_k, k = 1, 2, 3...N'$ using Mean-shift segmentation [26]. We set fixed parameters $sigmaS = 7, sigmaR = 6.5, minRegion = 240$ for all images. "Non-compact" here means homogenous object surfaces or background will be segmented into one large region. Then the image saliency is refined based on these regions as

$$S_k = \frac{\sum_{I_m \in R'_k} I_m^S}{|R'_k|} \ \ s.t. \ I_m^S = S_i|_{I_m \in R_i} \tag{9}$$

where $I_m^S$ is pixel saliency computed by (8). $|R_k'|$ is the sum area of region $R_k'$. Thanks to this operation, artifacts are eliminated while unconnected parts generated by pre-segmentation become connected. Finally, $S_k, k = 1, 2, 3...N'$ is normalized to $[0, 1]$ to render our final saliency map.

## 4  Experiment and Comparison

### 4.1  Visual Comparison

We test our method on the popular public data set provided by [1], which contains 1000 images as well as the corresponding ground truth images. Each image usually contains one unambiguous salient object. We select the current popular 8 state-of-the-art saliency detection methods including IT [9], SR [12], CA [14], FT [1], LC [13], HC [10], RC [10] and SF [11] for comparison. The saliency maps of previous works excluding SF are provided by [10][2]. The SF [11] saliency maps are obtained from the author's webpage[3]. Fig.4 shows several comparison results. Visually, it can be seen that our method obtains relatively higher quality saliency maps compared with the rest 8 methods, which sometimes highlight parts (RC and SF), corners (IT) or edges (SR and CA) with relatively more background clutters (HC, RC, LC and FT). In contrast, our method performs better on stressing out the complete prominent object while suppressing background. The saliency maps of our method for the 1000 images are provided in the supplementary materials.

### 4.2  Quantitative Comparison

Besides visual comparison, we also implement quantitative comparison. We evaluate the performance of our method by comparing its *precision-recall* rate. For a given threshold $T$, the *precision* and *recall* rate of a certain saliency detection method are defined as

$$Precision(T) = \frac{1}{1000} \sum_{i=1}^{1000} \frac{|M_i(T) \cap G_i|}{|M_i(T)|}, \ Recall(T) = \frac{1}{1000} \sum_{i=1}^{1000} \frac{|M_i(T) \cap G_i|}{|G_i|}$$

(10)

where $M_i(T)$ is the binary mask obtained by directly thresholding the saliency map using threshold $T$ on the $i$th image. $G_i$ is the ground truth. $|\cdot|$ denotes mask's sum area. As we use data set provided by [1], (10) are the averages of 1000 terms. In order to draw the precision and recall curves under different $T$, we use every possible threshold $T$ from 0 to 255. This is similar to the fixed threshold experiment in [10, 11, 1].

The left two in Fig.5 show the precision and recall curves. As can be seen, our method presents the best precision and recall curve. Our maximum precision

---

[2] http://cg.cs.tsinghua.edu.cn/people/~cmm/Saliency/Index.htm
[3] http://www.fedeperazzi.com/saliency_filters/

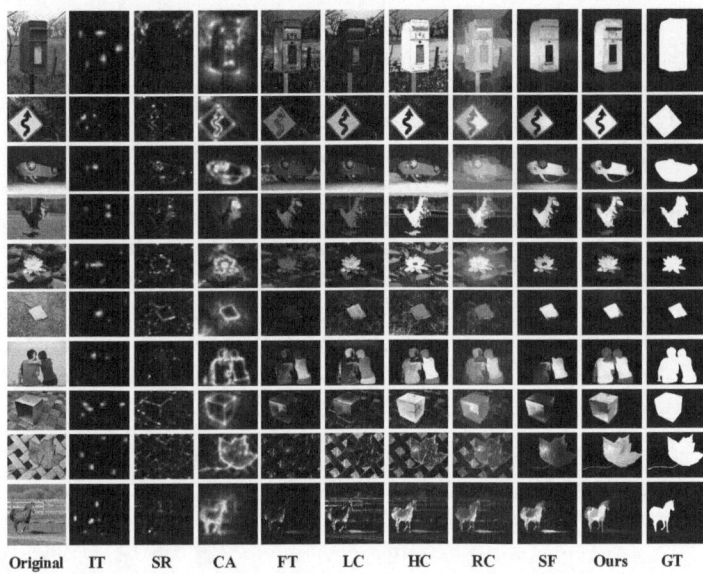

Original  IT  SR  CA  FT  LC  HC  RC  SF  Ours  GT

**Fig. 4.** Visual comparison results between our method and other 8 popular state-of-the-art methods

rate is 96%, with 3% improvement from the second best 93% (SF). Another interesting phenomenon is that our method maintains high precision rate under various recall rate. This is actually consistent with our visual evaluation, which shows our approach provides high quality saliency maps that highlight the whole objects while suppress background, leading to high precision under high recall.

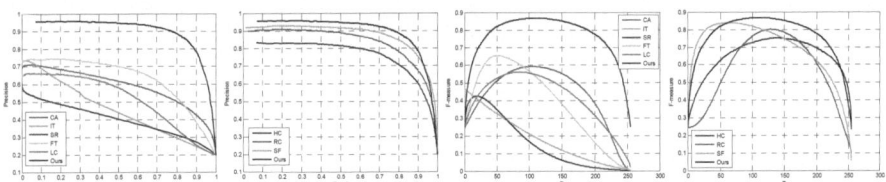

**Fig. 5.** Precision-recall, F-measure curves of 8 state-of-the-art methods including CA, IT, SR, FT, LC, HC, RC, SF as well as our method

In addition to precision-recall curves, we also evaluate the *F-measure*, which is an integrated evaluation criterion that combines precision and recall as

$$F_\beta(T) = \frac{(1+\beta^2)Precision(T) \times Recall(T)}{\beta^2 \times Precision(T) + Recall(T)} \quad (11)$$

where $\beta^2$ is set as 0.3, as is suggested in [10], [11] and [1]. Note that **none of previous works** shows **F-measure curve** varying with threshold $T$. The last two in Fig.5 show our F-measure curves. Compare with other methods, our method achieves the best F-measure curve when $T$ varies from 65 to 240 and second best when $T$ varies from 0 to 65. Notice that under this F-measure criterion, RC sometimes performs less better than HC. This may be attributed to that RC achieves higher precision, but lower recall at the same time, which pulls down the F-measure score to some extent. The same thing also happens on SF. As high quality saliency maps can be obtained using our method, using simple fixed threshold can achieve good segmentation results.

Fig.6 presents the evaluation for individual phase of our algorithm, respectively including only contrast, only distribution, without distribution prior, without saliency smoothing and without refinement. It shows the benefit of combining all steps while adding distribution prior and saliency smoothing really works for enhancing the performance.

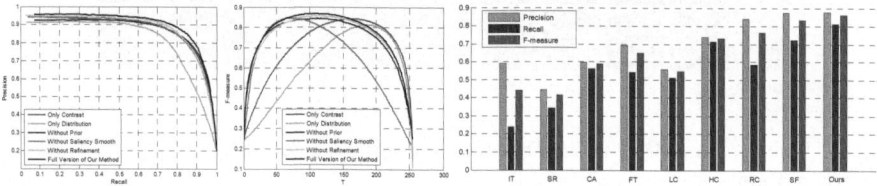

**Fig. 6.** The first two show the individual phase of our algorithm, respectively including only contrast, only distribution, without distribution prior, without saliency smoothing and without refinement. The last histogram shows the evaluation for adaptive threshold experiment.

Besides, an adaptive threshold experiment, similar to that in [11] and [1], is carried out. The adaptive threshold $T_a$ is defined as two times the mean saliency of an obtained saliency map, as is shown in (12).

$$T_a = \min \left\{ 2 \times \frac{\sum_i^M S(I_i)}{M}, T_{max} \right\} \tag{12}$$

where $M$ denotes the number of pixels in the saliency map and $i$ is pixel index. $T_{max}$ is the upper bound for $T_a$ and is set as 255 by us. The last histogram in Fig.6 shows the precision, recall and F-measure in adaptive threshold experiment. It can be seen that in this experiment, RC still achieves high precision but low recall, because RC usually highlights only part of the real salient object. The precision rate of SF is very close to our method, but our method shows the highest recall rate and F-measure score, respectively 81% (9% improvement) and 0.86 (0.03 improvement).

### 4.3    Content-Aware Image Resizing

In content-aware image resizing [5–8], saliency maps are usually used to specify relative importance across image parts. Here we use the framework proposed in

[5] to validate the performance of the saliency maps produced by our method on smart image resizing task. The images are scaled along their $x$-axis. Other cases are straightforward. Fig.7 shows that our method better preserves the whole object than RC and SF during scaling.

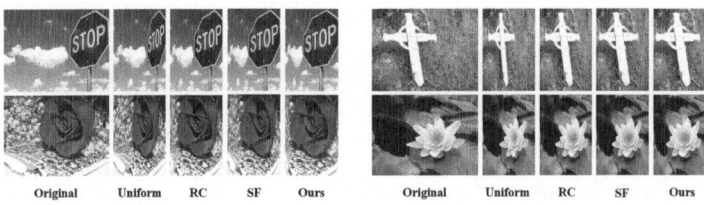

Original    Uniform    RC    SF    Ours          Original    Uniform    RC    SF    Ours

**Fig. 7.** Using saliency maps of RC, SF and ours on content-aware image resizing

## 5    Conclusion and Future Work

In this paper, we show how to combine color contrast and distribution to obtain high quality saliency maps, which highlight overall salient object meanwhile suppress the background. Qualitative and quantitative comparisons show that our method outperforms current popular bottom-up saliency detection methods. Our future work includes mining more low-level features which are effective and combining several high-level features like face and human body detection into our system.

**Acknowledgement.** We thank the anonymous reviewers for their valuable suggestions. This research is partly supported by National Science Foundation, China (No: 61273258).

## References

1. Achanta, R., Hemami, S., Estrada, F., Susstrunk, S.: Frequency-tuned salient region detection. In: CVPR (2009)
2. Rutishauser, U., Walther, D., Koch, C., Perona, P.: Is bottom-up attention useful for object recognition? In: CVPR (2004)
3. Han, J., Ngan, K., Li, M., Zhang, H.: Unsupervised extraction of visual attention objects in color images. IEEE TCSV 16, 141–145 (2006)
4. Chen, T., Cheng, M., Tan, P., Shamir, A., Hu, S.: Sketch2photo: Internet image montage. ACM Trans. Graph. 28, 1–10 (2009)
5. Ding, Y., Jing, X., Yu, J.: Importance filtering for image retargeting. In: CVPR (2011)
6. Pritch, Y., Kav-Venaki, E., Peleg, S.: Shift-map image editing. In: ICCV (2009)
7. Grundmann, M., Kwatra, V., Han, M., Essa, I.: Discontinuous seam carving for video retargeting. In: CVPR (2010)
8. Wolf, L., Guttmann, M., Cohen-Or, D.: Non-homogeneous content driven video-retargeting. In: ICCV (2007)

9. Itti, L., Koch, C., NieBur, E.: A model of saliency-based visual attention for rapid scene analysis. IEEE TPAMI 20, 1254–1259 (1998)
10. Cheng, M., Zhang, G., Mitra, N., Huang, X., Hu, S.: Global contrast based salient region detection. In: CVPR (2011)
11. Perazzi, F., Krahenbul, P., Pritch, Y., Hornung, A.: Saliency filters: Contrast based filtering for salient region detection. In: CVPR (2012)
12. Hou, X., Zhang, L.: Saliency detection: A spectral residual approach. In: CVPR (2007)
13. Zhai, Y., Shah, M.: Visual attention detection in video sequences using spatiotemporal cues. ACM Multimedia, 815–824 (2006)
14. Goferman, S., Zelnik-Manor, L., Tal, A.: Context-aware saliency detection. In: CVPR (2010)
15. Parkhurst, D., Law, K., Niebur, E.: Modeling the role of salience in the allocation of overt visual attention. Vision Res. 42, 107–123 (2002)
16. Einhauser, W., Konig, P.: Does luminance-contrast contribute to a saliency map for overt visual attention? Eur. J. Neurosci. 17, 1089–1097 (2003)
17. Fergus, R., Perona, P., Zisserman, A.: Object class recognition by unsupervised scale-invariant learning. In: CVPR (2003)
18. Parikh, D., Zitnick, C.L., Chen, T.: Determining Patch Saliency Using Low-Level Context. In: Forsyth, D., Torr, P., Zisserman, A. (eds.) ECCV 2008, Part II. LNCS, vol. 5303, pp. 446–459. Springer, Heidelberg (2008)
19. Judd, T., Ehinger, K., Durand, F., Torralba, A.: Learning to predict where humans look. In: ICCV (2009)
20. Rother, C., Kolmogorov, V., Blake, A.: Grabcut- interactive foreground extraction using iterated graph cuts. ACM Trans. Graph. 23, 309–314 (2004)
21. Liu, T., Yuan, Z., Sun, J., Wang, J., Zheng, N.: Learning to detect a salient object. IEEE TPAMI 33, 353–367 (2011)
22. Alexe, B., Deselaers, T., Ferrari, V.: What is an object? In: CVPR (2010)
23. Feng, J., Wei, Y., Tao, L., Zhang, C., Sun, J.: Salient object detection by composition. In: ICCV (2011)
24. Achanta, R., Shaji, A., Smith, K., Lucchi, A., Fua, P., Ssstrunk, S.: Slic superpixels. In: Technical report (2010)
25. Borji, A., Itti, L.: Exploiting local and global patch rarities for saliency detection. In: CVPR (2012)
26. Christoudias, C., Georgescu, B., Meer, P.: Synergism in low level vision. In: ICPR (2002)

# Data Decomposition and Spatial Mixture Modeling for Part Based Model

Junge Zhang, Yongzhen Huang, Kaiqi Huang, Zifeng Wu, and Tieniu Tan

National Lab of Pattern Recognition
Institute of Automation, Chinese Academy of Sciences
{jgzhang,yzhuang,kqhuang,zfwu,tnt}@nlpr.ia.ac.cn

**Abstract.** This paper presents a system of data decomposition and spatial mixture modeling for part based models. Recently, many enhanced part based models (with *e.g.*, multiple features, more components or parts) have been proposed. Nevertheless, those enhanced models bring high computation cost together with the risk of over-fitting. To tackle this problem, we propose a data decomposition method for part based models which not only accelerates training and testing process but also improves the performance on average. Besides, the original part based model uses a strict rigid structural model to describe the distribution of each part location. It is not "deformable" enough, especially for those instances with different viewpoints or poses in the same aspect ratio. To address this problem, we present a novel spatial mixture modeling method. The spatial mixture embedded model is then integrated into the proposed data decomposition framework. We evaluate our system on the challenging PASCAL VOC2007 and PASCAL VOC2010 datasets, demonstrating the state-of-the-art performance compared with other related methods in terms of accuracy and efficiency.

## 1 Introduction

Part based models have been a successful method for representing object categories [1–6]. It was firstly proposed by Fischler and Elschlager [7] in 1973. Later in [8] Marr and Nishihara introduced articulated limb model. In the past several years, Felzenszwalb *et al*'s work [1, 9] significantly advances the original pictorial structure model [7]. Part based models have been widely used in several important computer vision problems such as object detection [1–4, 6, 10, 11], pose estimation [5], action recognition [12] and scene understanding [13].

Part based models consider that an object can be modeled as a collection of local part templates, together with structural constraints. In the past decade, constellation model proposed by Fergus *et al* [11] and pictorial structure model presented by Felzenszwalb *et al* [1, 9] obtained great success. The latter deformable part based model (DPBM) [1] stands out for its outstanding performance on VOC challenges [14]. The use of moving parts can well adapt the learnt model to target image structure. For detection task, this kind of configuration has good property of robustness to deformation and partial occlusion which

K.M. Lee et al. (Eds.): ACCV 2012, Part I, LNCS 7724, pp. 123–137, 2013.
© Springer-Verlag Berlin Heidelberg 2013

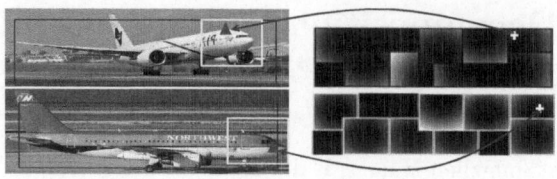

**Fig. 1.** Examples of different viewpoint but the same aspect ratio. The layout of structural constraints should be different.

provides superior performance than rigid template model [15]. However, to our understanding, part based models have two basic limits: 1) the computational complexity is high. 2) The original DPBM is not "deformable" enough.

Recently, there surge many enhanced models through multiple features [3] such as combining Histogram of Oriented Gradients (HOG) and Local Binary Patterns (LBP), more components and parts [5, 16]. These methods obtained very promising results on either detection task or pose estimation. Nevertheless, these models suffer from large computational complexity. Besides, when the length of models becomes longer, they face a higher risk of over-fitting.

The original DPBM [1] uses one unique reference anchor point for each part. This results in that the layout of structural constraints or penalty for each part is all the same and rigid when applying the same component model. We think that each anchor associates a layout of structural constraints. As discussed in [1], the size of each component model is initialized by objects' aspect ratio to avoid bad local minimas. But in practice, two objects with the same aspect ratio may have different viewpoints or poses. As seen from Figure 1, the two aeroplanes share the same aspect ratio but have apparently different viewpoints. In this case, it is inappropriate if we encourage the same layout of structural penalty to both of them.

Motivated by those challenges, this paper tries to address these two limits. Firstly, we propose a method of data decomposition for part based model which not only significantly reduces memory usage and computational cost but also outperforms other related systems. Secondly, we propose a spatial mixture modeling method in which part location is described as mixture distribution learnt from weakly labeled data. Thirdly, we integrate the spatial mixture model into the proposed data decomposition framework and to the best of our knowledge, the presented system achieves the state-of-the-art performance compared with all other related methods from both competition and literature.

The rest of this paper is organized as follows. Section 2 reviews the related work. Section 3 introduces the proposed method. Section 4 gives the experimental results. Section 5 concludes this paper.

## 2    Related Work

As mentioned previously, many enhanced models with multiple features [3, 17], more components or parts [5, 16] are proposed recently. The drawback or limit of these methods is that their models' complexity is too high in terms of computing and memory. Hussain *et al* [17] propose applying partial least squares (PLS) on three different types of visual features. The supervised PLS is performed on each separate root and part filter which requires carefully collecting training data for each root and part model. Besides, how to perform data alignment for such separate learning reductions is difficult. Moreover, it is infeasible for more flexible part models with more features, components and parts.

Patrick *et al* [16] adopt sharing parts across intra and inter categories to reduce the model's complexity. Although sharing parts can reduce the number of parameters, it may face the risk of decreased discrimination of parts. For example, we'd like a car's 'wheel' part has discrimination not only between a car and a person but also between a car and a bus. If the 'wheel' part is shared across car and bus category, its discrimination will certainly decrease when classifying a window as a car or a bus.

Pedersoli *et al* [18] show that the dimensionality of filter and window search space dominate most of the computation time. They propose a coarse-to-fine search strategy to speedup the complex hierarchical part based model. In [19], they propose a selective window sampling strategy via segmentation which makes using multiple features based bag-of-words possible. Those methods indeed reduce search space and speedup training and testing, but they all do not improve models' discrimination. The promising way to improve models' discrimination is building more discriminative appearance feature or modeling strategy.

Yang *et al* [5] extends the DPBM into flexible mixture of parts which is "deformable" enough for pose estimation. They use the relative location between parent node and children node to define the part type. Besides, in DPBM, only one large rigid part is used to describe *e.g.*, a 'leg'. But in [5], a 'leg' is represented by many small flexible rigid parts so that matching articulated pose becomes possible. However, this method requires fully annotated training data and carefully predefined part dependence or part order. Therefore, training a generic class model with weakly labeled training samples is difficult. Besides, compared with larger parts, the discriminability of smaller parts may be decreased.

## 3    Proposed Methods

The proposed system is schematically shown in Figure 2. With the input of different features, we need to perform data calibration for further data decomposition. Then the learnt basis is applied to factorize the feature into lower-dimensional space. Besides, we consider each part's configuration as a spatial mixture model. The structural penalty for each part is more flexible. In the following paragraphs, we will describe the details of the proposed method.

### 3.1    Data Decomposition

As mentioned previously, these enhanced models via multiple features, more components or parts always require huge computation resources. And they also

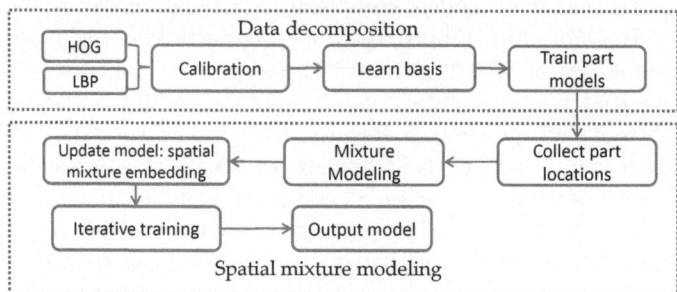

**Fig. 2.** The pipeline of the proposed system, including two parts: data decomposition and spatial mixture modeling

face the higher risk of over-fitting. The first contribution of this paper is reducing part based models' complexity via data decomposition which enables efficient and sufficient training and testing.

Before details, the feature map used in DPBM should be introduced. Cell structured feature map [1] is computed at every scale. This kind of processing enables us to use fast convolution routine for matching. As known that cell filter is the basic unit of either root filter or part filter, therefore, we can perform data decomposition on cell filter.

We know that some cell filters refer to background, while others to objects. Besides, the size of cell filter is usually so small that each cell can not hold sufficient appearance information to represent background or objects. Therefore, the decomposition method should be **unsupervised** or **label independent**. The original feature data (background or objects, and this is why we call our method as data decomposition) can be reconstructed without supervision. This is the basic principle we should follow. Another principle is the decomposition should be **efficient** due to large scale application.

For unsupervised methods, there are *e.g.*, principal components analysis (PCA) and non-negative matrix factorization (NMF). Considering efficiency, PCA rather than NMF is an ideal choice because it benefits from its linear projection. Therefore, we propose using PCA to perform data decomposition. This paper mainly focuses on reducing the complexity of those enhanced models. PCA is already a very useful method to address it. It should be mentioned that this paper considers both training and testing model entirely in the context of multiple features which is different from [1, 20]. [20] considers testing procedure only, while in [1] PCA is used to analyze the basic 36-dim HOG feature and finally they adopt the manually reduced 31-dim HOG feature based on their analysis. Thus, the context and usage of PCA is different.

The problem of PCA is that its results heavily rely on the relative scaling of the original data. If two variables have different units (*e.g.*, kilometers and miles.), the results produced by PCA will be different. Therefore, it is necessary to do data calibration before learning the basis which is in fact very essential for the system.

**Proposed Data Calibration**
Motivated by the promising performance of [3], this paper adopts HOG from [1] and LBP feature with uniform patterns as well. We use $X_1(i)$ and $X_2(j)$ (wherein $i \in [1, 31]$ and $j \in [1, 59]$) to denote HOG and LBP feature and $\eta_1$ and $\eta_2$ for their discriminative ability, respectively. Their relative discriminative ability is defined as: $\lambda = \frac{\eta_1}{\eta_2}$. The average accuracy evaluated on 20 categories from PASCAL VOC2007 reported in [21] is used as their respective discrimination. We don't consider a category dependent discrimination for generalization. The proposed data calibration includes two steps: 1) removing variables with low sample variance; 2) Re-scaling two different sources of data.

As we know, variables with low variance from the same source data indicate low contribution or even damage to discrimination. Therefore, we can remove those variables with very low variance. In [3, 21], the results show that the discrimination of HOG is superior over LBP on average. Motivated by these results, we only remove the variables from LBP. Suppose the variance of $X_2(j)$ is $var_2(j)$ and the 20% lowest variance (it is determined empirically.) is used as threshold $thresh$. Then we remove the variance according to Eq.1.

$$X_2(j) = \begin{cases} 0, & var_2(j) \leq thresh \\ X_2(j), & if\,else \end{cases} \tag{1}$$

The second step is to re-scale the different source data. After removing the variables with low variance from LBP, the mean value of $X_1$ and $X_2$ is computed and denoted as $u_1$ and $u_2$, respectively. $X_1$ is chosen as the reference scale for its better discrimination. Then the relative discriminative ability $\lambda$ is considered into re-scaling problem according to Eq.2.

$$X_2 = \frac{X_2}{\frac{u_2}{u_1} \cdot \lambda} \tag{2}$$

From the statistics, we find that $u_2$ is larger than $u_1$. Thus, we need to re-scale $X_2$ to smaller scale. Besides, the larger $\lambda$ is, the less contribution that $X_2$ gives. Therefore, we divide $X_2$ by $\lambda$ together with $\frac{u_2}{u_1}$ to re-scale the original data to an appropriate relative scale considering both relative mean value and discrimination.

**Implementation Details.** Similar to [1], the models are trained horizontal symmetric. The question is how to find the corresponding relationship between mirrored features in decomposed space or subspace which is another key problem in our detector.

Suppose the extracted low-level feature from one side view image is $f$, then we can get its corresponding symmetric feature $f'$. We use $d$, $d'$ and $g$ to denote their factorized feature in subspace and decomposition function respectively. Then, we get

$$\begin{aligned} d &= g(f) \\ d' &= g(f') \end{aligned} \tag{3}$$

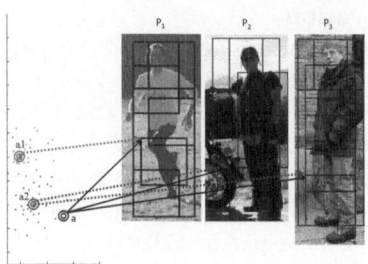

**Fig. 3.** A toy example for illustrating the motivation of spatial mixture modeling

The simplest way of finding their corresponding relationship is regressing $d'$ on $d$. Then it turns to find the transformation matrix $L$ through $d' = g(f') = dL$. In this paper, we adopt PLS which is suitable for multivariate regression.

### 3.2 Spatial Mixture Modeling

We now consider working out the flexible part matching scheme. As we know, the response of each part $p_i$ is simultaneously determined by appearance information and structural penalty.

$$h(p_i) = \max_{s_i \in \zeta} (h_a(s_i) - h_s(s_i))$$ (4)

where $h_a$ and $h_s$ are the appearance and structural response respectively. Part's moving location $s_i : (x_i, y_i)$ (of dimensionality $d$) belongs to the searching space $\zeta$. In the basic DPBM, the structural penalty is achieved by

$$h_s(s_i) = w_i'd(s_i), \quad where \; d(s_i) = \left(dx_i \; dx_i^2 \; dy_i \; dy_i^2\right)$$ (5)

where $w_i'$ and $d(s_i)$ are the deformation coefficients and structural features respectively. In the basic DPBM, only a single layout of structural constraint is used to describe part's distribution. If the viewpoint or pose within the same aspect ratio is the same, a single layout of structural constraints would be sufficient to model the part's spatial distribution. In practice, two objects with the same aspect ratio usually have apparently different viewpoints or poses (*e.g.*,Figure 1 and Figure 3). Therefore, a single layout of structural constraints can not capture such variation and spatial mixture modeling becomes necessary.

In this paper, we assume that the part spatial distribution follows mixture Gaussian distribution. Then we present the spatial mixture modeling based on Gaussian to capture the variations of parts. In this case, the system can make a more "flexible" decision for the structural penalty for each part. Naturally, we define the score of each part as:

$$h(p_i) = \max_{s_i \in \zeta} \left( h_a(s_i) - \sum_{j=1}^{K} \lambda_{i,j} h_{s,j}(s_i) \right)$$ (6)

where $K$ is the number of Gaussian components and $\lambda_j$ is the weight of structural penalty from the $j^{th}$ component. In this case, the structural penalty is weighted accumulated based on the contribution from each Gaussian component. Therefore, when the relative location between the part current moving location and each Gaussian component changes, the layout of structural constraints for that part will change accordingly which makes flexible part matching possible. $\lambda_j$ is obtained through:

$$\lambda_{i,j} = w_{i,j} g\left(s_i | \mu_j, \Sigma_j\right)$$
$$s.t \ \sum_{j=1}^{K} w_{i,j} = 1 \ and \ w_{i,j} \geq 0 \tag{7}$$

where $w_{i,j}$ are the mixture weights, and $g\left(s_i | \mu_j, \Sigma_j\right)$ is the component Gaussian density. $\mu_j, \Sigma_j$ are the mean value and covariance matrix of the $j^{th}$ Gaussian component in the mixture. Each Gaussian probability density is

$$g\left(s_i | \mu_j, \Sigma_j\right) = \frac{1}{(2\pi)^{d/2} |\Sigma_j|^{1/2}} \exp\left\{-\frac{1}{2}(s_i - \mu_j)^T \Sigma_j^{-1} (s_i - \mu_j)\right\} \tag{8}$$

The vector $\phi = (w, \mu, \Sigma)$ is the unknown parameters of the spatial mixture model which needs to be estimated.

There are various algorithms for estimating the parameters of $\phi$. A popular method for maximizing the likelihood of the training data is expectation-maximization (EM). The basic idea of EM algorithm is beginning with initial parameters $\phi$, to evaluate the new parameters $\phi'$, for which we hope the likelihood is larger. The new parameters then become the initial model for the next iteration and the process is repeated until converged. In our system, we use K-means to generate the initial parameters.

**Implementation Details.** Our spatial mixture embedded model starts from training a basic DPBM. Then we collect the part location from those positive samples of 70% overlap with ground truth. After that K-means is applied over each part's location. The mean value and covariance matrix are generated from each cluster. The initial weight for each Gaussian component is determined by the fraction of the number of points in each cluster. With the initial parameters, EM algorithm is executed to find the proper parameters $\phi$. The learnt $\mu$ is then used as the new reference anchor points in the spatial mixture embedded part based model. We use the model with spatial mixture modeling to mine positive and negative training samples for further iteratively training. The score of each part location is determined by Eq.6. The iterative training process terminates at a certain iterations or when the model changes little. The full algorithm is summarized in Algorithm 1.

**Discussions.** The spatial mixture model utilizes mixture layouts of structural constraints and provides a flexible part matching scheme which can well address the problem caused by variations in viewpoint or pose. The superiority of our method can be graphically demonstrated by Figure 3. The locations of the right bottom part (foot part) collected from positive samples are plotted in the left image in Figure 3. The blue point denotes the anchor point in the original DPBM.

---

**Algorithm 1.** Training Spatial Mixture Embedded Model

---

**Input**   : Positive/Negative samples
**Output**: *model*

*1: Train basic DPBM. N: the number of components;*
**for** *component* $i \leftarrow 1$ **to** $N$ **do**
    **for** $k \leftarrow 1$ **to** *iter1* **do**
        Train root model: *model{i}.root*;

    **for** $k \leftarrow 1$ **to** *iter2* **do**
        Train part based model: *model{i}*

*2: Initialize spatial mixture embedded model;*
**for** *component* $i \leftarrow 1$ **to** $N$ **do**
    Apply *model{i}* on positive training samples;
    Collect part locations into $locs_{i,p}$;
    // p is the subscript for each part
    Clustering, generate the initial parameter $\phi_{i,p} = (w_{i,p}, \mu_{i,p}, \Sigma_{i,p})$ for
    each cluster;
    Estimate the parameter $\phi'_{i,p} = \left(w'_{i,p}, \mu'_{i,p}, \Sigma'_{i,p}\right)$ of mixture model
    with EM and $\phi_{i,p}$;
    Initialize spatial mixture model with $\phi'_{i,p}$;

*3: Update model and retrain;*
**for** *component* $i \leftarrow 1$ **to** $N$ **do**
    **for** $i \leftarrow 1$ **to** *iter3* **do**
        Apply updated *model{i}* for collecting training data;
        Part response is determined according to Eq. 6;
        Update parameters and retrain *model{i}*.

---

Apparently, the original DPBM will punish the foot part in $P_2$ and $P_3$ slightly, while punishing that part in $P_1$ heavily which in fact is not desired for that pose. In our system, based on the proposed spatial mixture model, we can match each part more "deformably" or flexibly with mixture layouts of structural penalty (Eq. 6) rather than the original DPBM. Therefore the structural penalty from spatial mixture model can relieve the penalty for the foot part in $P_1$ while still retain slight punishment for that part in $P_2$ and $P_3$. In a word, the proposed method is capable of capturing variations in viewpoint or poses by allowing more flexible part matching. Figure 4 gives an example of learnt deformation model with spatial mixtures. The red cross in each part denotes the learnt anchor for that part. An apparent relative displacement of anchors associated with the same part can be found in Figure 4.

## 4   Experiments

We evaluate the proposed method on challenging PASCAL VOC dataset [14] which is widely recognized as difficult testbed for object detection and most

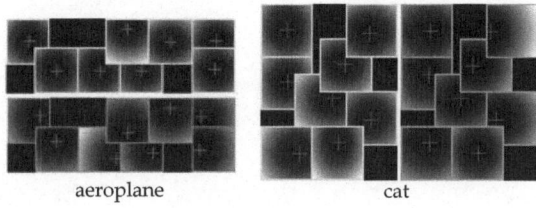

aeroplane                                    cat

**Fig. 4.** Here are two examples of deformation model from spatial mixture modeling: the left one is about aeroplane and the right one is cat

algorithms report their results on this dataset. We use Average Precision (AP) [14] score as the criterion, which is widely adopted in PASCAL VOC challenge. As mentioned in 3.1, HOG and LBP are used as the low-level features. All the models are trained with six components, and each component associates eight parts of cell size $6 \times 6$. The experiments are mainly divided into three subsections: 1) empirical results with data decomposition; 2) experimental results with spatial mixture embedded model; 3) full results on PASCAL VOC2007 and VOC2010 datasets.

## 4.1   Data Decomposition

In this subsection, the experiments include three parts: 1) determining the factorized lower dimensionality; 2) studying the effect of data calibration and 3) training and testing computational cost and accuracy. These experiments on PASCAL VOC2007 are designed for verifying the effectiveness of the proposed methods, hence we only conduct the experiments on several categories. The final complete results will be given in 4.3.

**Determining Dimensionality.** Table 1 illustrates how changing PCA dimension $K$ affects the performance. As seen from Table 1, when $K$ exceeds 30, the performance tends to be stable. Considering the trade-off between efficiency and effectiveness, we set $K$ to 40 which is found performing well on all 20 categories (Note: Before applying PCA, data calibration is performed).

**Table 1.** This table shows how changing PCA dimension $K$ affects the results

| category | K=15 | K=20 | K=25 | K=30 | K=35 | K=40 | K=50 |
|---|---|---|---|---|---|---|---|
| aeroplane | 1.7 | 14.4 | 16.7 | 33.2 | 34.5 | 34.4 | 32.6 |

**Effect of Data Calibration.** The experimental results are shown in Figure 5. Three groups of experiments are conducted: one is the naïve combination which refers to the method concatenating different types of features into a unified feature vector; The second is that we directly perform data decomposition on original data without any calibration; The third is the proposed method.

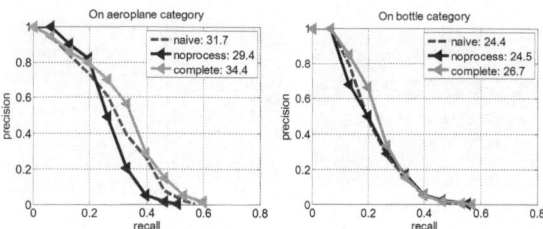

**Fig. 5.** Experimental results of data calibration. naive refers to the naïve combination of HOG and LBP. noprocess denotes the method that perform data decomposition without any calibration. complete represents the proposed data decomposition with data calibration.

As seen from Figure 5, the results of directly applying PCA without any calibration are usually bad. Because the dimensionality and mean value of LBP feature are larger than HOG, the learnt basis from PCA often has bias to LBP which in fact shows poorer discriminability on average than HOG. The results from the complete experiments on aeroplane and bottle verify the positive effect of data calibration via improving noprocess by 5% and 2.2%, respectively.

**Training and Testing Computation Cost and Accuracy.** Table 2 summarizes the quantitive results. All these experiments are conducted on the same computer with the same configuration. The computer is configured with Intel E5520 CPU of 2.27GHz. The training time for cow is all most the same. But the proposed method achieves a speedup, of more than 1.9 times than naïve combination during evaluation. For the cat category, the training time is less than naïve combination, and speedup in evaluation stage is nearly two-fold. The naïve combination requires $O(90)$ (31+59=90) operations at each cell filter while the proposed method requires only $O(40)$ operations. The practical speedup factor is about 1.8 ($1.8 < \frac{90}{40} = 2.25$) which indicates the decomposition costs a bit time but is still very efficient especially for multiple features. The memory consumption is also reduced from original 10G byte to now 4G byte on average during training. We also implement a naïve version of the Boost method according to their description in [3]. We find that the training and testing computational cost is almost the same with naïve combination. Moreover, the proposed method achieves better performance on these two categories than [3]. The improvement over baseline method [1] proves that combining texture feature indeed helps discriminability which has been verified in [3] as well. The improvement over the naïve combination and [3] verifies that data decomposition over the original multiple features can still improve models' discriminability. The reason may be the presented data decomposition suppresses undesired noise and the reduced complexity makes the model can be trained more sufficiently.

## 4.2   Spatial Mixture Modeling

We take a "data-driven" approach to determine the number of mixture components $K$ by analyzing the parts' spatial distribution. Limited by space, we plot

**Table 2.** Training and testing computation cost and accuracy comparison experiments. `Baseline` refers the result from running the provided models [1, 22] in the same environment. `Naïve` stands for naïve combination method. `Boost` refers the method described in [3]. `DD` denotes the proposed system without spatial mixture modeling.

| | Class | Training (hour) | Testing (hour) | AP score |
|---|---|---|---|---|
| Baseline [1, 22] | cow | - | 1.4 | 25.2 |
| | cat | - | 1.3 | 19.3 |
| Naïve | cow | 18.1 | 3.7 | 28.1 |
| | cat | 24.1 | 3.5 | 23.3 |
| Boost[3] | cow | 17.9 | 3.5 | 26.9 |
| | cat | 23.2 | 3.4 | 24.2 |
| DD | cow | 18.0 | **1.9** | **30.4** |
| | cat | 18.3 | **1.8** | **24.6** |

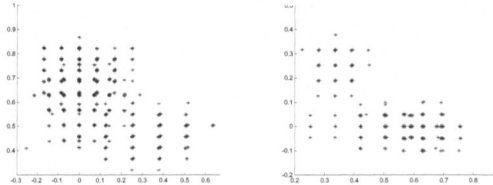

**Fig. 6.** Part spatial distribution. The left one is from `person`'s middle part, and the right one is from `chair`.

only two parts distribution in Figure 6 randomly chosen from `person` and `chair` categories. We can find that the number of peaks is almost 2. Besides, if $K$ is larger, the parameters of the model are more such that it will plague sufficiently training model and efficient testing. Therefore, we set $K$ to 2 generally for all categories on VOC datasets. In this subsection's experiments, we use HOG from [1] without data decomposition. The baseline is the standard DPBM [1, 22]. As seen from Figure 7, the proposed spatial mixture embedded model improves the baseline by 2.4% and 2.8%, respectively. The improvement verifies the effectiveness of the proposed spatial mixture embedded model which provides flexible and more "deformable" part configuration.

### 4.3 Complete Results on PASCAL VOC Datasets

Motivated by the above results, we integrate the proposed spatial mixture embedded model into the data decomposition framework and evaluate the whole system on PASCAL VOC2007 and VOC2010.

**Results on PASCAL VOC2007.** Table 3 gives the results of our detector on PASCAL VOC2007. The results here are without specific context based postprocessing. We compare our method with other related representative methods.

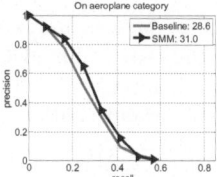 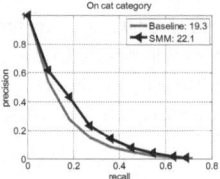

**Fig. 7.** Experimental results of spatial mixture modeling. Baseline is the result from running the provided model [1, 22] on PASCAL VOC2007.

**Table 3.** Full results on PASCAL VOC 2007. DDNoSSM denotes the proposed method without spatial mixture modeling, while DDSSM with spatial mixture modeling. V4 is the popular DPBM proposed by Felzenszwalb *et al*[1, 22]. UCI refers to the method with multi-class layout [23] which wins Marr prize at ICCV2009. LHS stands for the method [4] which shows very competitive performance in recent years. MKL [24] is the winner method at PASCAL VOC2009 challenge, which uses four kinds of multi-level features. LatentCRF is from [2], in which a latent CRF based on a flexible assembly of parts is proposed for object detection. C2F represents the method described in [18]. This paper proposes a coarse-to-fine framework for deformable object detection. SMC denotes the scalable multi-class object detection [25], in which a shared codebook is jointly trained over all classes. PLS refers the method present in [17]. In ParAttr method [26], objects are described using a spatial model based on its constituent parts. HStruct represents the discriminative hierarchical structure model based on multiple features which is described in [27]. ExModel is an interesting method introduced recently in [28]. Boosted refers the winner method [3] in PASCAL VOC2010 challenge. Whether from the number of single class's best score or the mean AP, the proposed method performs best. It should be noted here the proposed method has not be filtered by context information.

| | plane | bicycle | bird | boat | bottle | bus | car | cat | chair | cow | table | dog | horse | mbike | person | plant | sheep | sofa | train | tv | meanAP |
|---|---|---|---|---|---|---|---|---|---|---|---|---|---|---|---|---|---|---|---|---|---|
| V4 [1, 22] | 28.9 | 59.5 | 10.0 | 15.2 | 25.5 | 49.6 | 57.9 | 19.3 | 22.4 | 25.2 | 23.3 | 11.1 | 56.8 | 48.7 | 41.9 | 12.2 | 17.8 | 33.6 | 45.1 | 41.6 | 32.3 |
| UCI [23] | 28.8 | 56.2 | 3.2 | 14.2 | 29.4 | 38.7 | 48.7 | 12.4 | 16.0 | 17.7 | 24.0 | 11.7 | 45.0 | 39.4 | 35.5 | **15.2** | 16.1 | 20.1 | 34.2 | 35.4 | 27.1 |
| LHS [4] | 29.4 | 55.8 | 9.4 | 14.3 | 28.6 | 44.0 | 51.3 | 21.3 | 20.0 | 19.3 | 25.2 | 12.5 | 50.4 | 38.4 | 36.6 | 15.1 | 19.7 | 25.1 | 36.8 | 39.3 | 29.6 |
| MKL [24] | **37.6** | 47.8 | **15.3** | 15.3 | 21.9 | **50.7** | 50.6 | **30.0** | 17.3 | 33.0 | 22.5 | **21.5** | 51.2 | 45.5 | 23.3 | 12.4 | 23.9 | 28.5 | 45.3 | **48.5** | 32.1 |
| LatentCRF [2] | 31.9 | 57.0 | 9.1 | 15.2 | 26.0 | 42.7 | 49.3 | 14.5 | 15.2 | 18.5 | 24.2 | 11.8 | 49.1 | 41.9 | 35.7 | 14.5 | 18.9 | 23.3 | 34.3 | 41.3 | 28.7 |
| C2F [18] | 27.7 | 54.0 | 6.6 | 15.1 | 14.8 | 44.2 | 47.3 | 14.6 | 12.5 | 22.0 | 24.2 | 12.0 | 52.0 | 42.0 | 26.8 | 10.6 | 22.9 | 18.8 | 35.3 | 31.1 | 26.7 |
| SMC [25] | 26.0 | 56.0 | 10.0 | 11.0 | 21.0 | 47.0 | 50.0 | 16.0 | 19.0 | 23.0 | 20.0 | 12.0 | 51.0 | 45.0 | 37.0 | 12.0 | 17.0 | 29.0 | 41.0 | 38.0 | 29.1 |
| PLS [17] | 18.0 | 41.1 | 9.2 | 9.8 | 24.9 | 34.9 | 39.6 | 11.0 | 15.5 | 16.5 | 11.0 | 6.2 | 30.1 | 33.7 | 26.7 | 14.0 | 14.1 | 15.6 | 20.6 | 33.6 | 21.3 |
| ParAttr [26] | 25.6 | 33.0 | 6.8 | 3.2 | 16.3 | 47.7 | 37.9 | 14.0 | 0.9 | 9.6 | 17.0 | 11.5 | 23.3 | 32.5 | 19.8 | 5.3 | **29.9** | 18.0 | 16.7 | 32.1 | 20.1 |
| HStruct [27] | 31.7 | 56.3 | 1.7 | 15.1 | 27.6 | 41.3 | 48.0 | 15.2 | 9.5 | 18.3 | 26.1 | 11.3 | 48.5 | 38.9 | 35.8 | 14.8 | 17.7 | 18.8 | 34.1 | 39.8 | 27.5 |
| ExModel [28] | 20.8 | 48.0 | 7.7 | 14.3 | 13.1 | 39.7 | 41.1 | 5.2 | 11.6 | 18.6 | 11.1 | 3.1 | 44.7 | 39.4 | 16.9 | 11.2 | 22.6 | 17.0 | 36.9 | 30.0 | 22.7 |
| Boosted[3] | 36.7 | 59.8 | 11.8 | **17.5** | 26.3 | 49.8 | 58.2 | 24.0 | **22.9** | 27.0 | 24.3 | 15.2 | 58.2 | 49.2 | 44.6 | 13.5 | 21.4 | 34.9 | 47.5 | 42.3 | 34.3 |
| DDNoSSM | 34.4 | 59.4 | 11.1 | 16.8 | 26.7 | 50.0 | 60.2 | 24.6 | 22.5 | 30.4 | 30.8 | 16.0 | **61.3** | **51.3** | 44.0 | 13.5 | 20.8 | **39.2** | 48.5 | 42.6 | 35.2 |
| DDSSM | 35.8 | **60.4** | 10.9 | 17.3 | **29.9** | 50.1 | **62.6** | 25.5 | 22.8 | **38.2** | **32.1** | 16.1 | 59.9 | 51.1 | **44.8** | 13.2 | 19.8 | 38.5 | **49.5** | 42.6 | **36.0** |

As shown in Table 3, DDSSM (the proposed complete system) obtains the best AP score in 7 of 20 categories. The mean AP score is 36.0%, which is the best among these compared methods. DDNoSSM (the proposed method without spatial mixture modeling.) also obtains best score in 3 categories, and the mean AP is the second best among these methods. The closest approach to us is from [3], our method without spatial mixture modeling exceeds it by 0.9%. The whole system improves [3] by 1.7%. The improvement of DDSSM over DDNoSSM proves that the proposed spatial mixture modeling improves models' discriminability on average. The improvement is promising because the result from [3] is already very challenging. Besides, the proposed system shows advantage over [3] in terms

**Table 4.** Full results on PASCAL VOC2010. V4 is from [22] without context rescoring. sharepart refers the method described in [16]. In [16], certain parts are shared across mutli-class for multi-class object detection. Boosted [3] represents the winner method of PASCAL VOC2010. We run the detector implemented by ourself on PASCAL VOC2010. SegAs is the latest result from [19] which mainly focuses on selecting windows with high "objectness" via segmentation. Their object appearance model is based on bag-of-words. DDNoSSM refers the proposed method without spatial mixture modeling, while DDSSM with spatial mixture modeling.

| | plane | bicycle | bird | boat | bottle | bus | car | cat | chair | cow | table | dog | horse | mbike | person | plant | sheep | sofa | train | tv | meanAP |
|---|---|---|---|---|---|---|---|---|---|---|---|---|---|---|---|---|---|---|---|---|---|
| V4 [1, 22] | 45.4 | 49.8 | 9.5 | 11.9 | 27.5 | 49.0 | 42.4 | 27.7 | 16.8 | 20.3 | 10.2 | 19.2 | 40.0 | 47.0 | 41.8 | 8.7 | 26.1 | 12.2 | 41.4 | 34.3 | 29.1 |
| sharepart [16] | 24.7 | 38.2 | 0.0 | 1.2 | 0.2 | 33.3 | 37.7 | 7.3 | 1.4 | 4.6 | 8.1 | 8.1 | 21.5 | 31.8 | 11.5 | 6.3 | 17.0 | 5.1 | 9.6 | 23.9 | 14.6 |
| Boosted [3] | 49.6 | 51.0 | 12.7 | 15.1 | 26.1 | 50.9 | 44.4 | 30.6 | 17.3 | 25.3 | 15.2 | 22.4 | 42.3 | 51.3 | 43.5 | 8.5 | 28.8 | 20.6 | 43.8 | 36.4 | 31.8 |
| SegAs [19] | **58.2** | 41.9 | **19.2** | 14.0 | 14.3 | 44.8 | 36.7 | **48.8** | 12.9 | 28.1 | **28.7** | **39.4** | 44.1 | 52.5 | 25.8 | **14.1** | **38.8** | **34.2** | 43.1 | **42.6** | 34.1 |
| DDNoSSM | 45.5 | 53.3 | 14.7 | 16.8 | 33.2 | 53.0 | 48.3 | 35.0 | 17.4 | 31.0 | 22.4 | 24.5 | 45.3 | 52.0 | 44.8 | 12.0 | 37.7 | 24.7 | 45.9 | 36.5 | 34.7 |
| DDSSM | 49.9 | **54.9** | 14.9 | **17.0** | **33.6** | **53.6** | **50.6** | 35.4 | **18.1** | 31.4 | 21.7 | 24.5 | **45.8** | **52.6** | **49.2** | 11.6 | 38.2 | 25.5 | **47.4** | 38.3 | **35.7** |

of efficiency. This is currently the state-of-the-art performance without context rescoring and selective window search (e.g., [19]). MKL method with four different features also provides very competitive results, and our system gets better results by nearly 4%. And it is reported [24] that the MKL method takes roughly 67 seconds per image, therefore, the time for evaluating the whole VOC2007 is about 92 hours. Our method not only outperforms it in accuracy but also is very computational efficient. The proposed method takes about 2 hours for evaluation (as we run in different environment, the time here are only for rough comparison). We also noted that the additional experiment of [17] in his thesis [29] shows that they achieved 36.0% which is comparable to us. But our method does not need careful part calibration.

**Results on PASCAL VOC2010.** The complete results on PASCAL VOC2010 are given in Table 4. We compare with other four methods which published their results on PASCAL VOC2010. As seen from Table 4, DDSSM obtains the best score in 11 out of 20 categories and the best mean AP of 35.7% among all these methods. DDNoSSM also obtains the second best mean AP. SegAs [19] focuses on selective window sampling via segmentation. The proposed method exceeds [19] by 1.6% without any selective search. Also the selective search via segmentation is always time consuming. Compared with [3] in which low-level features used are similar to us, the proposed method without spatial mixture modeling improves [3] by nearly 3%, and over 5% improvement which is very challenging on PASCAL VOC datasets is observed on bottle, cow, diningtable and sheep categories. These results indicate that appropriate data decomposition over different sources of data for part based model not only reduces model's training and testing computational cost but also improves the accuracy on average. Besides, spatial mixture modeling improves DDNoSSM by about 1% on average, which further indicates the proposed spatial mixture modeling helps discriminability. In a word, our system obtains the state-of-the-art performance compared with those methods without context rescoring on challenging PASCAL VOC datasets for detection task. Moreover, compared with other related challenging systems, the proposed algorithm requires less memory and computation time both in training and testing phase.

## 5   Conclusion

This paper has presented an enhanced part based model by means of data decomposition and spatial mixture modeling. We have made three major contributions: 1) We have studied the problem of complexity of those enhanced models and address this problem with data decomposition. In practice, we propose the methods for data calibration and finding transformation matrix which are very essential for the whole system. 2) We firstly build a more "deformable" and flexible part based model via spatial mixture modeling without fully annotated training samples. 3) The proposed data decomposition over multiple features for part based model not only reduces the computation requirement but also improves the accuracy and exceeds the previous state-of-the-art algorithms. The integrated system with data decomposition and spatial mixture modeling finally obtains the state-of-the-art performance on PASCAL VOC datasets compared with other methods without context.

Currently, the proposed system is still far from real time. On one hand, we can adopt the strategy such as [18, 19] to reduce the search space. On the other hand, we will continue to study the data decomposition for part based model following the principals described in this paper to reduce the model to a much lower dimensionality. Besides, our future work will also include learning part mixtures as well as the proposed spatial mixtures from weakly labeled data.

**Acknowledgements.** This work is funded by National Natural Science Foundation of China (Grant No. 61175007), the National Key Technology R&D Program (Grant No. 2012BAH07B01), the National Basic Research Program of China (Grant No. 2012CB316302).

## References

1. Felzenszwalb, P., Girshick, R., McAllester, D., Ramanan, D.: Object detection with discriminatively trained part-based models. TPAMI 32, 1627–1645 (2010)
2. Schnitzspan, P., Roth, S., Schiele, B.: Automatic discovery of meaningful object parts with latent crfs. In: CVPR, pp. 121–128 (2010)
3. Zhang, J., Yu, Y., Huang, K., Tan, T.: Boosted Local Structured HOG-LBP for Object Localization. In: CVPR, pp. 1393–1400 (2011)
4. Zhu, L., Chen, Y., Yuille, A.L., Freeman, W.T.: Latent hierarchical structural learning for object detection. In: CVPR, pp. 1062–1069 (2010)
5. Yang, Y., Ramanan, D.: Articulated pose estimation with flexible mixtures-of-parts. In: CVPR, pp. 1385–1392
6. Schnitzspan, P., Fritz, M., Roth, S., Schiele, B.: Discriminative structure learning of hierarchical representations for object detection. In: CVPR, pp. 2238–2245 (2009)
7. Fischler, M., Elschlager, R.: The representation and matching of pictorial structures. IEEE Transactions on Computers C-22, 67–92 (1973)
8. Marr, D., Nishihara, H.K.: Representation and recognition of the spatial organization of three-dimensional shapes. In: Proceedings of the Royal Society of London. Series B, Biological Sciences, pp. 269–294 (1978)
9. Felzenszwalb, P.F., Huttenlocher, D.P.: Pictorial structures for object recognition. Int. J. Comput. Vision 61, 55–79 (2005)

10. Girshick, R., Felzenszwalb, P., McAllester, D.: Object Detection with Grammar Models. In: NIPS (2011)
11. Fergus, R., Perona, P., Zisserman, A.: Object class recognition by unsupervised scale-invariant learning. In: CVPR, pp. 264–271 (2003)
12. Wang, Y., Mori, G.: Hidden part models for human action recognition: Probabilistic versus max margin. TPAMI 33, 1310–1323 (2011)
13. Pandey, M., Lazebnik, S.: Scene recognition and weakly supervised object localization with deformable part-based models. In: ICCV, pp. 1307–1314 (2011)
14. Mark, E., Gool, L., Williams, C.K., Winn, J., Zisserman, A.: The Pascal Visual Object Classes (VOC) Challenge. IJCV, 303–338
15. Dalal, N., Triggs, B.: Histograms of oriented gradients for human detection. In: CVPR, pp. 886–893 (2005)
16. Ott, P., Everingham, M.: Shared parts for deformable part-based models. In: CVPR, pp. 1513–1520 (2011)
17. Hussain, S.U., Triggs, B.: Feature sets and dimensionality reduction for visual object detection, pp. 112.1–112.10. BMVA Press (2010)
18. Pedersoli, M., Vedaldi, A., Gonzalez, J.: A coarse-to-fine approach for fast deformable object detection. In: CVPR, pp. 1353–1360 (2011)
19. van de Sande, K.E.A., Uijlings, J.R.R., Gevers, T., Smeulders, A.W.M.: Segmentation as selective search for object recognition. In: ICCV, pp. 1879–1886 (2011)
20. Felzenszwalb, P.F., Girshick, R.B., Mcallester, D.: Cascade object detection with deformable part models. In: CVPR, pp. 2241–2248 (2010)
21. Zhang, J., Yu, Y., Zheng, S., Huang, K.: An empirical study of visual features for part based model. In: ACPR, pp. 219–223 (2011)
22. Felzenszwalb, P.F., Girshick, R.B., McAllester, D.: Discriminatively Trained Deformable Part Models, Release 4 (2010)
23. Desai, C., Ramanan, D., Fowlkes, C.: Discriminative models for multi-class object layout. In: ICCV, pp. 229–236 (2009)
24. Vedaldi, A., Gulshan, V., Varma, M., Zisserman, A.: Multiple kernels for object detection. In: ICCV, pp. 606–613 (2009)
25. Razavi, N., Gall, J., van Gool, L.: Scalable multi-class object detection. In: CVPR, pp. 1505–1512 (2011)
26. Divvala, S.K., Zitnick, C., Kapoor, A., Baker, S.: Detecting objects using unsupervised parts-based attributes. Technical Report CMU-RI-TR-11-10, Robotics Institute, Pittsburgh, PA (2010)
27. Schnitzspan, P., Fritz, M., Roth, S., Schiele, B.: Discriminative structure learning of hierarchical representations for object detection. In: CVPR, pp. 2238–2245 (2009)
28. Malisiewicz, T., Gupta, A., Efros, A.A.: Ensemble of exemplar-svms for object detection and beyond. In: ICCV, pp. 89–96 (2011)
29. ul Hussain, S.: Machine Learning Methods for Visual Object Detection. PhD thesis, University of Caen (2011)

# Appearance Sharing
# for Collective Human Pose Estimation

Marcin Eichner[1] and Vittorio Ferrari[2]

[1] ETH Zurich, Switzerland
eichner@vision.ee.ethz.ch
[2] University of Edinburgh, United Kingdom
vferrari@staffmail.ed.ac.uk

**Abstract.** While human pose estimation (HPE) techniques usually process each test image independently, in real applications images come in collections containing interdependent images. Often several images have similar backgrounds or show persons wearing similar clothing (foreground). We present a novel human pose estimation technique to exploit these dependencies by sharing appearance models between images. Our technique automatically determines which images in the collection should share appearance. We extend the state-of-the art HPE model of Yang and Ramanan to include our novel appearance sharing cues and demonstrate on the highly challenging Leeds Sports Poses dataset that they lead to better results than traditional single-image pose estimation.

## 1 Introduction

2D articulated human pose estimation (HPE) in still images is a very challenging problem that has received considerable attention in recent years [1–10]. Thanks to the progress in those works, HPE methods can now be applied with some success on uncontrolled still images, without any prior knowledge about poses, the appearance of persons or backgrounds. However, the problem is far from solved. Highly cluttered backgrounds, large scale changes and strong scale variations can cause the failure of even the most recent state-of-the-art methods [10, 9].

A trait common to essentially all approaches [1–10] is to estimate pose *independently* on each image. We believe that this makes the problem harder than its needs to be. In real applications the test images come in *collections*, not one at a time. The user typically runs a pose estimator on a collection and only later inspects the results or inputs them to subsequent stages of a larger system. Importantly, usually there are *dependencies* between the images in a collection. Often some of them show people against a common background, while others show persons wearing very similar clothing (foreground). This happens a lot in sports photography, where both the background (football pitch, gym hall, water pool, tennis court) as well as the foreground recur (different players in the same football team, or even the same athlete in different poses or viewpoints, fig. 1). Images with either foreground or background in common are frequent also in: a) video surveillance (images taken in front of the same background); b) in movies (an actor wearing the same clothes throughout an episode); c) holiday photo collections, where the same person appears in many pictures, often wearing the same clothes and/or repeatedly visiting the same location (e.g. beach, pool, hotel room). Even in pure research

K.M. Lee et al. (Eds.): ACCV 2012, Part I, LNCS 7724, pp. 138–151, 2013.
© Springer-Verlag Berlin Heidelberg 2013

papers with no concrete application, the proposed methods are evaluated on entire test sets [1, 2, 4, 7–9] which feature the dependencies mentioned above. One of the most challenging modern datasets [11], the Leeds Sports Poses (LSP) dataset [7][1] contains numerous images of soccer, baseball, tennis or indoor sports sharing backgrounds or persons wearing very similar outfits (fig. 1a).

In this paper, we propose a novel technique to exploit these phenomena by performing human pose estimation while *sharing appearance* between images. Our method automatically discovers clusters of images with common foreground or background in the collection and thus determines between which images to share appearance (fig. 1a). We robustly estimate color appearance models suitable for all images in a cluster and incorporate them into a state-of-the-art HPE model [10]. Inference on the extended model effectively performs pose estimation jointly over all images in the cluster, guided by the shared appearance models.

Our paper is organized as follows. The next section gives an overview of our approach (sec. 2), followed by a summary of the base HPE model [10] we build on (sec. 3). In sec 4 we present our technique for automatically estimating shared appearance models, and explain how to incorporate them into [10] in sec. 5. We present an extensive experimental evaluation in sec. 6, which demonstrates that our approach for sharing appearance models over images improves performance over [10] run independently on each image.

*Related Works.* Articulated human pose estimation in still images is very challenging due to high variability in person appearance and pose, as well as the presence of background clutter, illumination and self-occlusions. Recent works have addressed these issues with advanced appearance models [1, 4, 3, 12, 7, 5, 10], complex pose priors [7, 5] or non-tree dependencies between body parts [8, 13] or hierarchical models [14]. While the above works build on variants of the Pictorial Structure (PS) model [15], there are also other techniques, e.g. bottom-up body assembling from segmentations [16] or pose estimation by foreground max-covering [17]. A trait common to essentially all approaches is to estimate pose *independently* on each image. In this paper instead we tackle HPE by exploiting multiple images sharing a common appearance.

The importance of good appearance models is reflected by their evolution. Early works employed simple box filters on background subtracted silhouettes [15]. Later, generic appearance models based on image gradients were developed, including generative edge masks [1], discriminatively trained shape-context templates [3], or linear [12] and non-linear [7] HOG templates [18]. In addition to generic templates based on gradients, a few works also employ color appearance models specific to a particular image, like in the iterative image parsing work of [1]. Later [4] extended this idea to transfer color models between body parts of a person, which was also adopted by [6]. In this paper we also propose appearance models based on color, but they are estimated *over multiple images*, following our main spirit of sharing appearance between images.

HPE approaches dedicated to video [19, 20, 2, 21] often employ multi-image models optimizing pose jointly over consecutive video frames. Usually, they exploit pose [2, 21] or appearance [19, 20] consistency over time. In this paper we tackle a different problem. A still image collection lacks temporal continuity and contains many different persons.

---

[1] `http://www.comp.leeds.ac.uk/mat4saj/lsp.html`

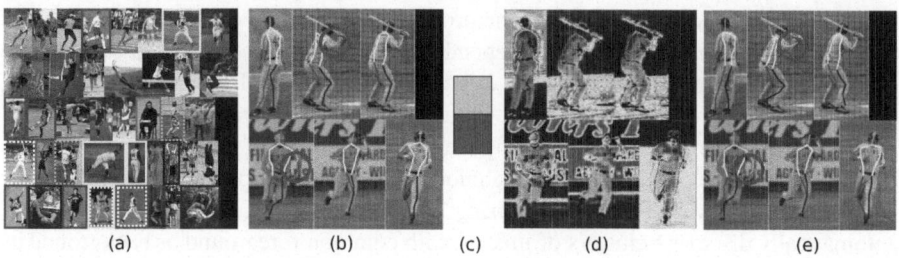

(a)                    (b)              (c)              (d)              (e)

**Fig. 1. Approach overview.** (a) random samples from the LSP dataset with example cluster assignments (solid boxes for background, dashed for foreground; colors depict cluster ids); (b) an automatically discovered foreground cluster with initial pose estimate [10] overlaid; the lower arms in the red circles are incorrectly estimated; (c) two high-weight color bins in the automatically estimated shared foreground model of a lower arm; (d) lower arm foreground likelihood computed according to this appearance model (heat-map); (e) improved pose estimation result produced by our extended HPE model which incorporates the shared appearance model; the lower arms in the red circles are now correctly estimated.

## 2    Overview of our Method

The core idea of our work is to improve HPE by exploiting background and foreground appearance patterns recurring over several images in a large dataset such as *LSP* [7] (fig. 1a). We give here an overview of the processing stages in our pipeline, focusing on the case of foreground appearance. The pipeline for background appearance is analogue. **1)** we run the pose estimator [10] independently for each image (sec. 3). This pose estimator employs person-generic body part appearance models based on gradients. **2)** we group images into clusters likely to have similar foreground appearance in terms of color distribution, based on the initial pose estimates (fig. 1b, sec. 4.2). **3)** for each cluster we robustly estimate a color appearance model *shared across the cluster* by integrating evidence over all images in it (fig. 1c, sec. 4.2). **4)** we use the shared appearance model to derive per-pixel foreground likelihoods for each image in the cluster (fig. 1d, sec. 4.3). **5)** we extend the HPE model of [10] to incorporate these foreground likelihoods as additional unary potentials (sec. 5). **6)** we run inference on the extended model to update the pose estimates in all images (fig. 1e).

Our method exploits the fact that clusters are typically mixed, containing some images with correct and some with wrong pose estimates. Therefore, instead of estimating pose on each image *independently* our method attempts HPE *jointly* over a cluster of images with similar appearance. Stage 3 robustly recovers the underlying shared appearance model, minimizing the impact of incorrect pose estimates. The resulting shared appearance model then helps in stage 6 by guiding the extended HPE towards better pose estimates.

As shown in extensive experiments, our method automatically exploits recurring appearance patters in a large dataset to successfully improve the accuracy of human pose estimation (fig. 1e). Our extended HPE model outperforms the baseline framework of [10] on one of the largest and most challenging HPE datasets available (LSP, sec. 6).

In the remainder of the paper we present each stage of our pipeline in detail.

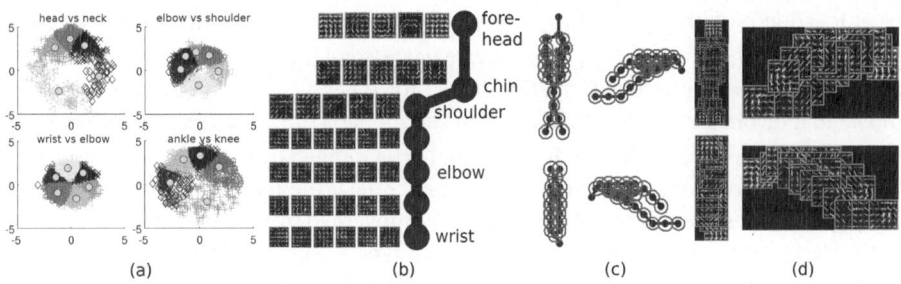

(a)           (b)           (c)           (d)

**Fig. 2. Mixture of pictorial structures model (MoPS) [10].** (a) Clusters of relative joint positions for finding body part types in the LSP training set; (b) a path in the model from the head to the left wrist, along with the HOG appearance templates specialized for each body part and orientation type; (c) visualization of 4 trees drawn out of an exponential number of trees that MoPS can generate; (d) HOG appearance visualization for the trees in (c).

## 3 Base Model [10] (MoPS)[2]

Many human pose estimators build on the pictorial structure model (PS) [1–4, 6–9]. A PS [15] is a conditional random field where nodes explicitly correspond to body parts (e.g. head, torso, left lower arm). The state space of a node is the set of possible $(x, y, \theta)$ positions a part can take in the image. The recent work of [10] introduces a novel representation: a mixture of pictorial structures (MoPS) (fig. 2), where each node represents a body part in a particular orientation. Nodes are now roughly corresponding to joints (e.g. elbow, knee) and midpoints of limbs. Hence, a part is represented as a mixture of axis-aligned templates, one per orientation.

The state space of a node is now only its $(x, y)$ location. However, orientation is implicitly captured by different mixture components. These are estimated from the training data by clustering the relative position between neighboring parts, typically into 5-6 components per part (fig. 2a). This representation is highly flexible and enables to model foreshortening, an effect often responsible for failures of classic PS.

Following the notation of [10], we write $I$ for an image, $p_i$ for the $(x, y)$ location of part $i$ and $t_i$ for its mixture component, where $i \in \{1, ...K\}$, $p_i \in \{1, ...L\}$, and $t_i \in \{1, ...T\}$[3]. Here, $t_i$ is the *type* of part $i$, which implicitly models its orientation. The energy of a body part configuration $(p, t)$ is

$$S(I, p, t) = \sum_i w_i^{t_i} \Phi(I, p_i) + \sum_{ij \in \mathcal{E}} w_{ij}^{t_i, t_j} \Psi(p_i - p_j) + S(t)$$
$$S(t) = \sum_i b_i^{t_i} + \sum_{ij \in \mathcal{E}} b_{ij}^{t_i, t_j} \tag{1}$$

where $\mathcal{E}$ is the set of edges connecting body parts in the kinematic tree. $\Phi(I, p_i)$ is a a feature extracted from image $I$ at $p_i$, so $w_i^{t_i} \Phi(I, p_i)$ is the image likelihood for part $i$ to

---

[2] http://phoenix.ics.uci.edu/software/pose/
[3] We omit the subscript to indicate the set spanned by it (e.g. $t = \{t_1, ...t_K\}$).

be at location $p_i$ with type $t_i$. $\Psi(p_i - p_j) = [dx^2, dx, dy^2, dy]$ is the relative location of parts $i$ and $j$, so $w_{ij}^{t_i,t_j}\Psi(p_i - p_j)$ evaluates a spatial prior defined over locations according to a spring-like deformation model for types $t_i, t_j$; $S(t)$ is a co-occurrence model that favors assigning certain types to certain parts $(b_i^{t_i})$ and certain combinations of types of pairs of parts $(b_{ij}^{t_i,t_j})$. It is a spatial prior defined over types (orientations).

The model components and their parameters reflect the idea of decomposing parts into types. The appearance model $w_i^{t_i}\Phi(I, p_i)$ is governed by parameters $w_i^{t_i}$ representing a HOG template specialized for part $i$ and type $t_i$ (fig. 2b). Hence each part has different templates for different orientations, which helps to capture the multi-modal appearance of body parts [9, 10]. The work of [10] uses a variant of HOG features [22] for $\Phi$. The deformation model $w_{ij}^{t_i,t_j}\Psi(p_i - p_j)$ is a switching spring model controlling the relative placement of two parts. Each spring $w_{ij}^{t_i,t_j}$ is tailored to a particular pair of types $t_i, t_j$. This allows fine-grained control over the amount of deformation tolerable for each pair of part orientations.

*Inference.* Finding the configuration $(p, t)$ that maximizes (1) can be done efficiently because $\mathcal{E}$ forms a tree and the pairwise potentials are quadratic functions. Using dynamic programming and efficient distance transforms [15] exact inference can be performed in complexity $O(KLT^2)$ [10].

*Learning.* The training set contains positive training images $\{I^\rho, p^\rho, t^\rho\}$ labeled by the ground-truth body part configuration on a person, and negative images $I^\eta$ containing no person. Let $z^\rho = (p^\rho, t^\rho)$, with $p^\rho$ the ground-truth joint locations in $I^\rho$ and $t^\rho$ is assigned by clustering $p_i^\rho - p_j^\rho$ over the training set into part type clusters (fig 2a). Note how (1) is linear in the model parameters $\beta = (w, b)$, with $w = (w_1^{t_1}, ...w_K^{t_T}, ...w_{ij}^{t_i,t_j}...)$ and $b = (b_1^{t_1}, b_K^{t_T}, ...b_{ij}^{t_i,t_j}...)$. Hence, it can be rewritten as $S(I, z) = \beta \cdot \Theta(I, z)$, with $\Theta = (\Phi(I, p_1), ..., \Phi(I, p_K), ...\Psi(p_i - p_j), ..., 1, 1, ...1....)$. With this reformulation, the model can be learned with a structured prediction objective function similar to [22]

$$\arg\min_{\beta, \xi_i \geq 0} \quad \frac{1}{2}\beta \cdot \beta + C\sum_\rho \xi^\rho + C\sum_\eta \xi^\eta$$

$$\text{s.t. } \forall \rho \in \text{pos} \quad \beta \cdot \Theta(I^\rho, z^\rho) \geq 1 - \xi^\rho \quad (2)$$

$$\forall \eta \in \text{neg}, \forall z \quad \beta \cdot \Theta(I^\eta, z) \leq -1 + \xi^\eta$$

The constraints state that positive examples (pos) should score at least 1, whereas all possible configurations $z$ of parts in negative images (neg) should score at most -1.

The quadratic program (2) has an exponential number of constraints but it defines a convex problem which can be optimized using a dual coordinate-descent solver [10]. In practice, [10] first trains each body part template independently. These initial templates then serve as a good initialization for training of the entire model using dual coordinate-descent of [10].

## 4   Sharing Appearance

We present here our technique for sharing appearance models between images (stages 2, 3 and 4 in sec. 2). We start by finding clusters of images likely to have similar foreground

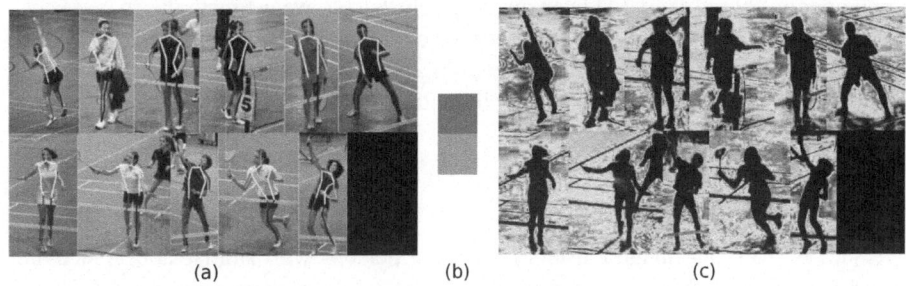

(a)          (b)          (c)

**Fig. 3. Sharing background.** (a) example background cluster automatically found in the LSP dataset with initial pose estimates overlaid; (b) two high-weight color bins from the shared background model $h_{bg}^c$; (c) background likelihood maps $I_{bg}$ computed of all images in the cluster based on $h_{bg}^c$ (visualized as heat maps).

or background appearance (sec. 4.1, 4.2). For each cluster we then estimate appearance models shared by all images in the cluster and derive from them pixel-wise likelihood maps (sec. 4.3). In section 5 we show how to incorporate these likelihood maps as additional unary potentials into the HPE model in order to improve pose estimation performance.

While single-image state-of-the-art HPE techniques typically employ gradients as features [3, 10, 9], our representation is based on color which is better suited to model the appearance of specific backgrounds or clothes.

### 4.1 Sharing Background

The key idea is to exploit images with common backgrounds to generate an informative additional cue for constraining human pose estimation. We start by clustering images according to their background appearance. Next, for every cluster we robustly estimated a shared background appearance model.

*Image Clustering.* For every image $m$ in the input set $\mathcal{I}$, we extract color histograms $h_{bg}^m$ from the entire image except the surface occupied by the initial pose estimate (sec. 2). Even when the initial pose estimate is partially incorrect, the error typically occupies a small portion of the images, so it has a minor influence on the histogram. We then define a pairwise similarity matrix between all images in $\mathcal{I}$ as $W^{mn} = 1 - \frac{\chi^2(h_{bg}^m, h_{bg}^n)}{2}$. Next, we cluster $\mathcal{I}$ according to $W$ using agglomerative clustering (sec. 4.3). This results in disjoint clusters $\mathcal{B}^c \subset \mathcal{I}$, with $\cup_c \mathcal{B}^c = \mathcal{I}$ (fig. 3a).

An advantage of agglomerative clustering over other techniques (e.g. k-means, GMM [23]) is that it does not require the number of clusters as input. Instead, it requires a parameter controlling cluster compactness (i.e. roughly how dissimilar two points can be and yet be in the same cluster). This is desirable in our setting as we want clusters of images with very similar backgrounds, but we do not know how many different types of background there are in the dataset.

*Estimating a Shared Model.* Given an image cluster $\mathcal{B}^c$, we estimate the shared background model $h_{\mathrm{bg}}^c$ by averaging the color histograms $h_{\mathrm{bg}}^m$ of all images $m \in \mathcal{B}^c$ in it. This estimate is robust to incorrect pose estimates in some of the images, as the moderate amount of foreground within their individual histograms is further diminished by averaging over all images (fig. 3b).

## 4.2  Sharing Foreground

We start by forming image clusters containing persons with similar appearance, i.e. wearing similar clothes. In a typical cluster, the initial pose estimation worked correctly on some persons and failed on others (fig. 6). For each body part, the key idea of our method is to robustly recover its correct color model by finding the one which occurs most frequently over the cluster. These *per-part* color models are then used as additional cues to refine the pose estimate (next section). In this manner, our scheme automatically exploits images with correct pose estimates to improve other images where pose estimation failed.

*Image Clustering.* In sec. 4.1 partially incorrect initial pose estimates had little impact, as a wrong limb covers a small portion of the image. Accordingly, the similarity between two images in sec. 4.1 simply ignored this issue. Importantly, in this section we want to find clusters of persons with similar appearance, despite some of them having partially incorrect pose estimates. To succeed we must design a more robust similarity measure that explicitly takes into account partially incorrect poses, as limbs are large relative to the area of a person.

Hence, we define the similarity between images $m, n \in \mathcal{I}$ as follows: $W^{mn} = \sum_i \delta \left(1 - \frac{\chi^2(h_i^m, h_i^n)}{2} > \varrho\right)$, where $h_i^k$ is the color histogram of the patch covered by part $i$ in image $k$, $\varrho$ is a threshold on the similarity of corresponding body parts in the two images (e.g. the left lower arm in each image), and $\delta(\cdot)$ is 1 if the argument is true and 0 otherwise. This similarity measure counts how many body parts have similar appearance in the two images. Again we use agglomerative clustering to partition $\mathcal{I}$ into disjoint image clusters $\mathcal{F}^c$ (sec. 4.3). As fig. 4a shows, the robust similarity measure groups together images of persons wearing similar clothing, despite having errors in the initial pose estimates. These are the right conditions for our approach to make an improvement. As we will see below, the correct pose estimates in the cluster will help to fix the incorrect ones.

*Estimating Shared Models.* Given an image cluster $\mathcal{F}^c$, for each body part $i$ we want to estimate its correct color model $h_i^c$ shared by the persons in the cluster. Simply averaging the color histograms $h_i^m$ of the patches of part $i$ in all images $m \in \mathcal{F}^c$ would not produce a good shared color model. The images where the part is incorrectly estimated would spoil the average (fig. 4a). This is fundamentally different from the background shared model estimation (sec. 4.1). Instead, we propose here a technique for estimating the correct color model which is robust to incorrect initial pose estimates in some images.

We cast the problem as outliers detection. We cluster the patches $\{h_i^m\}_{m \in \mathcal{F}^c}$ using agglomerative clustering (fig. 4b). Then we find the dominant patch cluster $\mathcal{D}_i^c$ (fig. 4b).

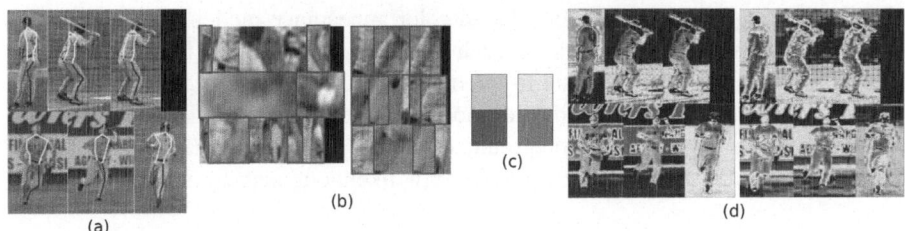

**Fig. 4. Sharing foreground.** (a) example foreground cluster automatically found in the LSP dataset with initial pose estimates overlaid; (b) lower arm (left) and lower leg (right) patches from the initial pose estimates; areas under blue overlays do not belong to the patches; the members of the dominant clusters $\mathcal{D}^c_{\text{lowerarm}}$ and $\mathcal{D}^c_{\text{lowerleg}}$ are marked red; (c) two high-weight color bins in the shared foreground model of the lower arm $h^c_{\text{lowerarm}}$ (left) and lower leg $h^c_{\text{lowerleg}}$ (right), derived from the patches in the dominant clusters $\mathcal{D}^c_{\text{lowerarm}}$ and $\mathcal{D}^c_{\text{lowerarm}}$ respectively; (d) foreground likelihood maps $I_{\text{fg},i}$ for all images in the cluster computed based on $h^c_i$, for $i =$ lower arm (left) and $i =$ lower leg (right).

As the distribution of patch similarities may vary substantially for different kinds of parts $i$ and image clusters $\mathcal{F}^c$, we use the median similarity of patches over all pairs of images in $\mathcal{F}^c$ as the compactness parameter. The key idea behind this dynamic parameter setting is that the similarity of patches within the dominant cluster is higher than the median. Hence, agglomerative clustering will tend to properly form a dominant cluster of highly similar patches, separated from many smaller clusters with other patches (fig. 4b).

Finally, we compute the shared color model $h^c_i$ of part $i$ as the average of the color histograms of the patches in the dominant patch cluster $\mathcal{D}^c_i$ (fig. 4c). This procedure correctly recovers the shared color model although the body part might be incorrectly localized in some images of $\mathcal{F}^c$. In fact it can work when the part is correctly localized even in fewer than 50% of the images, as long as the failures do not have consistent appearance. All it needs is for the correctly localized parts to form a dominant cluster in color space.

### 4.3 Technical Details

*Agglomerative Clustering.* We find background/foreground clusters using agglomerative clustering based on clique partitioning (CP) [24]. We construct a fully-connected graph $G_{\text{CP}}$, where each vertex represents an image $I_m \in \mathcal{I}$ and where edges are weighted according to pairwise similarity matrix $W \in [0, 1] - \tau$, where $\tau$ controls the desired similarity. We partition then $G_{\text{CP}}$ into disjoint cliques using CP. As CP is NP-hard we use the fast approximate clique partitioning technique of [25][4].

Unfortunately, no explicit background/foreground cluster membership annotations are available for the LSP dataset. Therefore, we set the clustering parameters ($\tau_{\text{bg}}$ and $\tau_{\text{fg}}, \varrho$ respectively) empirically using the LSP training set (see 6), such that visually appealing clusters are produced.

---

[4] http://www.robots.ox.ac.uk/~vgg/software/UpperBody/

*Likelihood Maps.* After estimating shared color appearance models, we derive from them a pixel-wise likelihood map for each image in a cluster. The likelihood map is derived by assigning to each pixel its probability according to the color model. In a background cluster $\mathcal{B}^c$, the shared color model $h_{\text{bg}}^c$ yields the same likelihood map $I_{\text{bg}}$ for all body parts (fig. 3c). In a foreground cluster $\mathcal{F}^c$, there is a separate shared color model $h_i^c$ for each part $i$, which yields a different likelihood map $I_{\text{fg},i}$ per part (fig. 4d).

## 5   Extended Model (ExMoPS)

In this section we show how to extend the MoPS model [10] to include the likelihood maps $I_{\text{bg}}, I_{\text{fg},i}$ derived in sec. 4.3 as additional cues to restrict the location of body parts. For this we redefine the base model (1) to have multiple appearance models $a \in \{\text{gen}, \text{bg}, \text{fg}\}$

$$S(I, p, t) = \sum_a \sum_i w_{a,i}^{t_i} \Phi_a(I_{a,i}, p_i) + \sum_{ij \in \mathcal{E}} w_{ij}^{t_i, t_j} \Psi(p_i - p_j) + S(t) \tag{3}$$

gen is the generic HOG appearance model of [10], whereas bg/fg are our foreground / background color appearance models shared over an image cluster (sec. 4).

In (1) there was one appearance template $w_i^{t_i}$ for each body part and type, where in our extended model (3) there are multiple $w_{a,i}^{t_i}$. Each term $w_{a,i}^{t_i} \Phi_a(I_{a,i}, p_i)$ is defined by a kind of template and a feature image $I_{a,i}$. In this notation the original appearance term of [10] is $w_{\text{gen},i}^{t_i} \Phi_{\text{gen}}(I_{\text{gen},i}, p_i)$, based on HOG templates $w_{\text{gen},i}^{t_i}$ applied to a gradient image $I_{\text{gen}}$. We define the new appearance terms $w_{\text{bg},i}^{t_i} \Phi_{\text{bg}}(I_{\text{bg},i}, p_i)$, $w_{\text{fg},i}^{t_i} \Phi_{\text{fg}}(I_{\text{fg},i}, p_i)$, where the templates $w_{\text{bg},i}^{t_i}, w_{\text{fg},i}^{t_i}$ are weight masks applied to background/foreground likelihood maps $I_{\text{bg},i}, I_{\text{fg},i}$ (fig 5). As mentioned in sec. 4.3, the same background likelihood map is used for all body parts $I_{\text{bg},i} = I_{\text{bg}}$, whereas the foreground likelihood map $I_{\text{fg},i}$ is part specific.

*Inference.* Inference in the extended model is analogous to the one for the base model (sec. 3). As we only introduced additional unary terms, the computation complexity of inference remains the same.

*Learning.* Introducing additional appearance terms keeps the model (3) in a form $S(I, z) = \beta \cdot \Theta(I, z)$, but $\beta = (w, b)$ now spans over multiple appearance templates per part and type. This leads to an equivalent learning problem as (2). However, we note that our shared appearance cues are defined only on images that contain persons (sec. 4). Therefore, instead of having a negative training set $I^n$ containing no person [10], we sample negative examples from the positive images $I^p$ (elsewhere than on the ground-truth stickmen).

Analogue to [10], we first train all appearance templates independently, and then use them as initialization to optimize the full model by dual coordinate-descent. This joint optimization of all parameters of the extended model enables to find an optimal balance between all terms, including multiple appearance cues and pose priors. Moreover, different appearance cues may be weighted differently for different body parts. If a cue

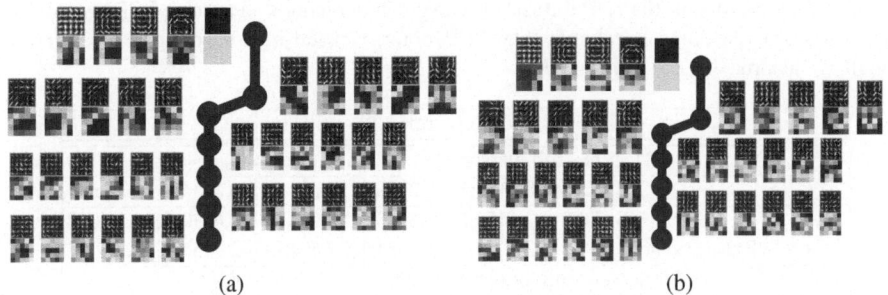

(a)                                                    (b)

**Fig. 5. Extended MoPS appearance templates**. Learned appearance templates for the body parts along the path from forehead to left wrist. (a) appearance templates from the shared background model ExMoPS{gen, bg}; (b) appearance templates from the shared foreground model ExMoPS{gen, bg}. Top rows: generic appearance templates (HOG) defined on image gradients, one per type (orientation). Bottom rows: shared background (a) or foreground (b) appearance models defined on our color likelihood maps. Note how the expected outline of a body part is recognizable in the templates. Also note how the templates for background likelihoods have high weight in regions *around* parts rather than on the parts themselves.

is not informative for a particular body part, it will get a low weight in the extended model. Note how this is different than a simpler solution that would keep the HOG templates $w_{\text{gen},i}^{t_i}$ as pre-trained in the base model, and then trains the new color templates $w_{\text{bg},i}^{t_i}, w_{\text{fg},i}^{t_i}$ on top of them. Fig. 5 shows ExMoPS models with shared foreground and background templates learned by by our method.

*Missing Data.* Not all appearance terms may be available for every training image, e.g. the foreground sharing cue does not make sense on singleton foreground clusters (sec 4.2). One way out would be to train the model only to a subset of images where all appearance cues are available. However, this might lead to over-fitting and at test time it would require applying different models depending on the availability of cues for a particular test image.

Instead, we propose to replace the likelihood maps for the missing cues with null maps filled with a uniform value (e.g. 0 in foreground null maps). The learned model is then able to discard a cue when it is unavailable.

This effectively enables us to train the extended model on the *entire dataset* despite the missing appearance cues. At test time we have a single model which benefits from whatever cues are available for a particular image.

## 6    Experiments

*Dataset.* There are several data-sets for evaluating 2D HPE algorithms [1, 2, 4, 7, 9], some having specific shortcomings: [1] has only a small number of images, while [2, 4] have only moderate pose variability [8]. Hence, we focus the evaluation of our method on the *LSP dataset* [7]. With 2000 images, it is the largest dataset with fully accurate ground-truth annotations (as opposed to the even larger [9]). It is also considered one of the hardest datasets in terms of pose variability and background clutter [11]. The official

**Table 1. PCP results on the LSP dataset.** The **avg** column reports an average PCP over all the body parts. The remaining 10 columns show PCP for torso (t), left-right lower-upper leg-arm (lul, rul, lll, rll, lua, rua, lla, rla) and head (h).

| model | avg | t | lul | rul | lll | rll | lua | rua | lla | rla | h |
|---|---|---|---|---|---|---|---|---|---|---|---|
| LSP testset - full, person-centric annotations (PC) | | | | | | | | | | | |
| [7] | **55.1** | 78.1 | 64.8 | 66.7 | 60.3 | 57.3 | 48.3 | 46.5 | 34.5 | 31.2 | 62.9 |
| MoPS [10] | **50.9** | 82.0 | 53.5 | 55.3 | 50.3 | 52.9 | 43.6 | 38.4 | 30.7 | 26.1 | 75.8 |
| ExMoPS{gen} | **54.2** | 83.5 | 59.5 | 61.4 | 54.1 | 58.5 | 45.3 | 42.7 | 31.3 | 28.7 | 77.1 |
| LSP testset - full, observer-centric annotations (OC) | | | | | | | | | | | |
| MoPS [10] | **60.8** | 84.1 | 69.5 | 69.4 | 64.8 | 66.4 | 53.1 | 51.6 | 37.3 | 34.5 | 77.1 |
| ExMoPS{gen} | **63.7** | 84.9 | 74.0 | 72.3 | 67.9 | 68.6 | 55.7 | 55.9 | 39.9 | 37.3 | 80.1 |
| ExMoPS{gen, bg} 1img | **63.6** | 86.2 | 74.9 | 73.7 | 68.5 | 68.1 | 55.4 | 54.9 | 38.0 | 36.3 | 80.1 |
| ExMoPS{gen, bg} | **64.3** | 86.5 | 75.6 | 74.1 | 68.9 | 69.8 | 57.5 | 55.4 | 38.7 | 36.0 | 80.1 |
| ExMoPS{gen, fg} | **64.2** | 85.6 | 75.2 | 72.5 | 68.3 | 68.0 | 56.6 | 56.6 | 38.4 | 39.7 | 80.4 |
| LSP testset - foreground clusters (141 img), OC annotations | | | | | | | | | | | |
| ExMoPS{gen} | **70.0** | 91.5 | 81.6 | 83.0 | 75.9 | 77.3 | 57.5 | 63.1 | 41.8 | 41.8 | 86.5 |
| ExMoPS{gen, fg} | **72.5** | 91.5 | 84.4 | 81.6 | 80.9 | 79.4 | 58.9 | 70.2 | 40.4 | 47.5 | 90.1 |

protocol [7] has equal test and train splits of 1000 images each, covering various sport activities. This dataset is big enough for our approach to discover clusters of images with common background/foreground appearance.

The annotations in LSP are person-centric (PC), i.e. right/left body parts are marked according to the viewpoint of the person. The right ankle of a person facing the camera is *left* in the image, but it is *right* in the image if the person faces away from the camera. As we do not expect MoPS [10] nor any other state-of-the-art HPE model [1–6, 8, 10, 11] to distinguish between these two situations, we convert all annotations to observer-centric (OC)[5]. Using OC annotations helps reducing confusion during training, e.g. resulting in a more accurate pose prior. Note how OC annotations are by far the most widely used in the 2D HPE community [1–6, 8, 10, 11].

*Evaluation Measure.* We quantify performance using the PCP measure (Percentage of Correctly estimated Parts) introduced by [2] and used in many other works [6, 6, 4, 3, 7, 9, 10, 8, 26, 27]. An estimated part is considered correct if both its segment endpoints lie within 50% of the length of the corresponding ground-truth segment from their annotated location[6].

We follow the typical evaluation protocol used for datasets containing a single person per image [3, 7, 15, 27, 26] and evaluate *only* the MAP solution returned by the HPE model.

*Setup.* Following [10], we use a simplified deformation model for MoPS/ExMoPS with $w_{ij}^{t_i, t_j} = w_{ij}^{t_i}$, i.e. the deformation model depends only on the type of the child part only, not on the parent.

---

[5] We normalize the orientation of the body such that the torso is upright, and then we flip arms/legs according to shoulder/hips annotation points if necessary, so that the left limb is always on the left side of the normalized torso.

[6] [28] noted a discrepancy between PCP measures used across the HPE community, here we exactly follow the PCP measure used in [3, 7].

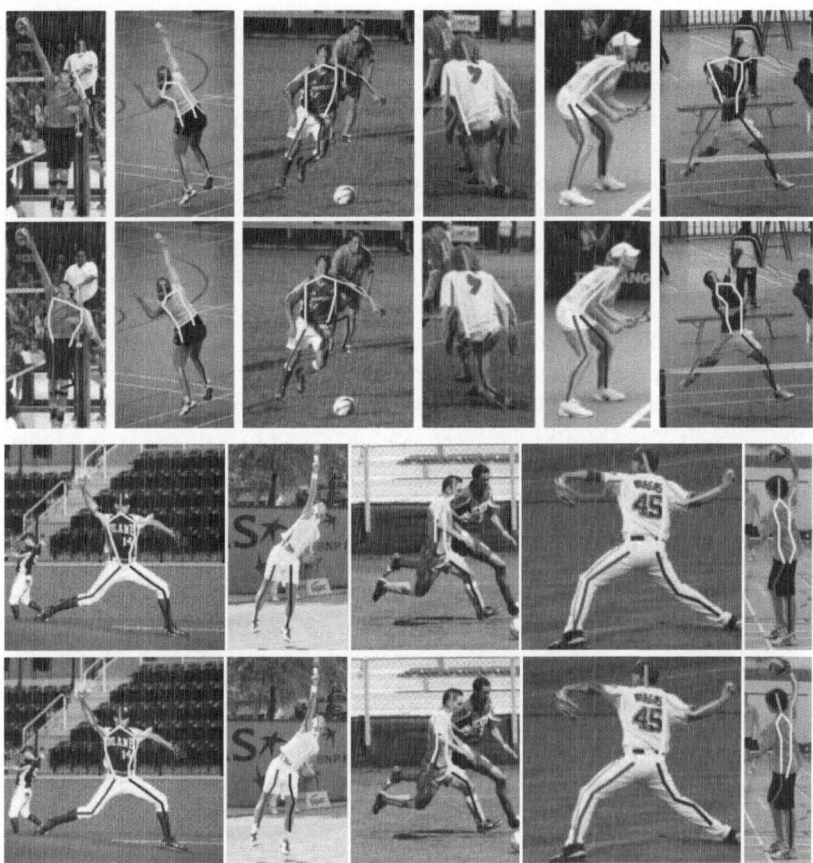

**Fig. 6. Qualitative results on the LSP dataset.** Rows 1 and 3 show the initial pose estimate by MoPS, and rows 2 and 4 show the result of our extended models ExMoPS {gen, bg} or ExMoPS {gen, fg}. Sharing background/foreground appearance models across images help to refine pose in a variety of situations.

The full body MAP output from MoPS/ExMoPS trained/tested on the LSP dataset is a 26 part body configuration (joint locations and midpoints along the kinematic structure except of the head mid-point). As in [10], we convert it to 10 physical parts for PCP evaluation (torso, left-right lower-upper leg-arm and head; abbreviated from now on as t, lul, rul, lll, rll, lua, rua, lla, rla, h).

*Results.* Table 1 reports our results. We start by comparing the base MoPS model [10] to [7, 9]. These are the two works that have published results on LSP before, and they employed the original PC annotations. On these annotations, MoPS performs slightly below [7]. Following [10], MoPS mines negative training examples from negative part of the INRIA pedestrian dataset [18]. Instead, the extended ExMoPS{gen}, mines negative training examples from positive training images. It performs better then MoPS [10] and it is on par with [7]. The method of [9] achieves higher PCP (62.7) but it is not directly comparable as it uses a much larger training set in addition to LSP (10000 images, so 11× more training data). In summary, the baseline model we adopt ExMoPS{gen} already performs on par with the state-of-the-art [7], even without appearance sharing between images.

In all following experiments we employ OC annotations, which we believe are more natural for HPE algorithms relying purely on low-level features [1, 4, 3, 6], as they may not be able to distinguish between front and back views of a person. On these OC annotations, the reference baseline MoPS reaches 60.8% PCP. For a fully transparent comparison, before we investigate the impact of our shared appearance models, we first evaluate MoPS when training from the alternative negative set as above (ExMoPS{gen}). With 63.7%, ExMoPS{gen} achieves higher PCP than MoPS. As both use only the generic HOG appearance term, the difference is completely due the negative examples being better suited for evaluation on the LSP testset.

We are now ready to investigate the improvements brought by incorporating our new shared appearance models. Adding our new background sharing cue yields an improvement to 64.3% PCP (ExMoPS{gen, bg}). An interesting experiment is to remove the sharing element from this cue by enforcing each image to be in its own cluster (ExMoPS {gen, bg} 1img). This degenerates to a technique analogue to [1], where a background color model is estimated from a *single image*, but integrated into MoPS. The performance of this model drops to the level of ExMoPS{gen}, demonstrating that the improvement brought by our background sharing is truly due to *sharing between images*. It supports our claim that collective HPE by sharing background models improve over independent single-image pose estimation, even when augmented with an analogue background term. Importantly, our method discovers between which images to share *fully automatically*.

We now investigate our new foreground sharing, which we apply to foreground clusters with 3 or more images, as foreground sharing is undefined on a single image. These clusters contain 141 of the 1000 test images. On these images, the foreground sharing model ExMoPS{gen, fg} improves PCP performance by +2.5% over the best baseline ExMoPS{gen}. We can also evaluate foreground sharing on the *entire* LSP dataset, by adding a null cue to images in smaller clusters, as described in 5. This also improves performance (64.2%) compared to the best baseline (63.7%), which demonstrates our foreground sharing is a useful new component for HPE. Interestingly, both our newly proposed foreground and background sharing methods achieve similar PCP performance (and they are both equally fully automatic).

Finally, we also investigated a method combining both foreground and background appearance sharing ExMoPS{gen, bg, fg}, its performance however turns out on par with methods using either of the shared components.

*Conclusions.* We have presented a novel technique to perform human pose estimation over multiple images by sharing foreground/background appearance models. As demonstrated on the highly challenging *Leeds Sports Pose* datasets, our collective pose estimation via appearance sharing improves performance over the baseline method [10] applied independently on each image. In future work we plan to share more elements between images, e.g. texture appearance models.

## References

1. Ramanan, D.: Learning to parse images of articulated bodies. In: NIPS (2006)
2. Ferrari, V., Marin-Jimenez, M., Zisserman, A.: Progressive search space reduction for human pose estimation. In: CVPR (2008)

3. Andriluka, M., Roth, S., Schiele, B.: Pictorial structures revisited: People detection and articulated pose estimation. In: CVPR (2009)
4. Eichner, M., Ferrari, V.: Better appearance models for pictorial structures. In: BMVC (2009)
5. Sapp, B., Jordan, C., Taskar, B.: Adaptive pose priors for pictorial structures. In: CVPR (2010)
6. Sapp, B., Toshev, A., Taskar, B.: Cascaded Models for Articulated Pose Estimation. In: Daniilidis, K., Maragos, P., Paragios, N. (eds.) ECCV 2010, Part II. LNCS, vol. 6312, pp. 406–420. Springer, Heidelberg (2010)
7. Johnson, S., Everingham, M.: Clustered pose and nonlinear appearance models for human pose estimation. In: BMVC (2010)
8. Tran, D., Forsyth, D.: Improved Human Parsing with a Full Relational Model. In: Daniilidis, K., Maragos, P., Paragios, N. (eds.) ECCV 2010, Part IV. LNCS, vol. 6314, pp. 227–240. Springer, Heidelberg (2010)
9. Johnson, S., Everingham, M.: Learning effective human pose estimation from inaccurate annotation. In: CVPR (2011)
10. Yang, Y., Ramanan, D.: Articulated pose estimation with flexible mixtures-of-parts. In: CVPR (2011)
11. Andriluka, M., Sigal, L., Black, M.J.: Benchmark Datasets for Pose Estimation and Tracking. Springer (2011)
12. Kumar, M.P., Torr, P.H.S., Zisserman, A.: Efficient discriminative learning of parts-based models. In: ICCV (2009)
13. Jiang, H., Martin, D.R.: Global pose estimation using non-tree models. In: CVPR (2008)
14. Sun, M., Savarese, S.: Articulated part-based model for joint object detection and pose estimation. In: ICCV (2011)
15. Felzenszwalb, P., Huttenlocher, D.: Pictorial structures for object recognition. IJCV (2005)
16. Mori, G., Ren, X., Efros, A., Malik, J.: Recovering human body configurations: Combining segmentation and recognition. In: CVPR (2004)
17. Jiang, H.: Human pose estimation using consistent max-covering. In: ICCV (2009)
18. Dalal, N., Triggs, B.: Histogram of Oriented Gradients for Human Detection. In: CVPR (2005)
19. Bissacco, A., Yang, M.H., Soatto, S.: Fast human pose estimation using appearance and motion via multi-dimensional boosting regression. In: CVPR (2007)
20. Sapp, B., Weiss, D., Taskar, B.: Parsing human motion with stretchable models. In: CVPR (2011)
21. Park, D., Ramanan, D.: N-best maximal decoders for part models. In: ICCV (2011)
22. Felzenszwalb, P., Girshick, R., McAllester, D., Ramanan, D.: Object detection with discriminatively trained part based models. IEEE Trans. on PAMI (2010)
23. Duda, R.O., Hart, P.E., Stork, D.G.: Pattern Classification, 2nd edn. John Wiley and Sons (2001)
24. Graham, R.L., Groetschel, M., Lovasz, L.: Handbook of Combinatorics. Elsevier (1995)
25. Ferrari, V., Tuytelaars, T., Van Gool, L.: Real-time affine region tracking and coplanar grouping. In: CVPR (2001)
26. Tian, T.-P., Sclaroff, S.: Fast Multi-Aspect 2D Human Detection. In: Daniilidis, K., Maragos, P., Paragios, N. (eds.) ECCV 2010, Part III. LNCS, vol. 6313, pp. 453–466. Springer, Heidelberg (2010)
27. Singh, V.K., Nevatia, R., Huang, C.: Efficient Inference with Multiple Heterogeneous Part Detectors for Human Pose Estimation. In: Daniilidis, K., Maragos, P., Paragios, N. (eds.) ECCV 2010, Part III. LNCS, vol. 6313, pp. 314–327. Springer, Heidelberg (2010)
28. Pishchulin, L., Jain, A., Andriluka, M., Thormaehlen, T., Schiele, B.: Articulated people detection and pose estimation: Reshaping the future. In: CVPR (2012)

# Max-Margin Regularization for Reducing Accidentalness in Chamfer Matching

Angela Eigenstetter\*, Pradeep Krishna Yarlagadda\*, and Björn Ommer

Interdisciplinary Center for Scientific Computing, University of Heidelberg, Germany
{aeigenst,pyarlaga,bommer}@iwr.uni-heidelberg.de

**Abstract.** Standard chamfer matching techniques and their state-of-the-art extensions are utilizing object contours which only measure the mere sum of location and orientation differences of contour pixels. In our approach we are increasing the specificity of the model contour by learning the relative importance of all model points instead of treating them as independent. However, chamfer matching is still prone to accidental matches in dense clutter. To detect such accidental matches we learn the co-occurrence of generic background contours to further eliminate the number of false detections. Since, clutter only interferes with the foreground model contour we learn where to place the background contours with respect to the foreground object boundary. The co-occurrence of foreground model points and background contours are both integrated into a single max-margin framework. Thus our approach combines the advantages of accurately detecting objects or parts via chamfer matching and the robustness of a max-margin learning. Our results on standard benchmark datasets show that our method significantly outperforms current directional chamfer matching, thus redefining the state-of-the-art in this field.

## 1 Introduction

Chamfer matching is a widely used technique for object detection. Due to its simplicity and efficiency it has been employed in a variety of applications to match whole object boundaries as well as partial object contours. Despite these advantages chamfer matching has a serious drawback when contours are matched in cluttered image regions. Contour matches in cluttered regions have a high accidentalness which can not be distinguished from matches on the actual object. Recent research made some attempts to improve specificity by including orientation information [1,2] in the distance function. The limitation of these approaches is that the presence of individual model points in a query image is measured independently. As demonstrated by Biederman [3], Attneave [4], and various experiments on illusionary contours, object boundary pixels are not all equally important due to their statistical interdependence. To address this issue we learn the relevance of model points and give higher weight to more

---

\* Both authors contributed equally to this work.

K.M. Lee et al. (Eds.): ACCV 2012, Part I, LNCS 7724, pp. 152–163, 2013.
© Springer-Verlag Berlin Heidelberg 2013

important model points. Furthermore we learn a flexible co-placement of generic background contours to reduce the accidentalness of matches in dense background clutter. We integrated these two learning steps into a single max-margin framework based on the state-of-the-art directional chamfer matching approach of Chellappa et al. [2] and evaluate the gain in performance.

## 2   Related Work

Chamfer matching has been used in a large number of applications in computer vision. It was first introduced by Barrow et al. [5] to match two sets of contour fragments. Since then chamfer matching has been widely applied and has been a successful technique for detecting complete objects or their parts. In [6] hierarchical chamfer matching was suggested where edge points are matched in a coarse-to-fine-manner. Later, chamfer matching was used to build powerful detectors as proposed in [7,8,9]. Leibe et al. [7] combine local features with global shape cues obtained from chamfer matching to verify and refine hypotheses. In [8], Gavrila and Munder have applied chamfer matching for real-time pedestrian detection and tracking. Lin et al. [9] have proposed a hierarchical part-template matching approach for detection and segmentation which measures shape information in terms of chamfer matching scores.

In [10] Thayananthan et al. have compared shape context [11] and chamfer matching of templates for object detection in cluttered images. They reported that chamfer matching is more robust to clutter than shape context. Nevertheless, false positives in cluttered background were still found to be the major downside of chamfer matching.

More recent research has made attempts to address this problem. Shotton et al. [1] suggested an improved matching scheme called oriented chamfer matching (OCM) that takes into account the orientation mismatch between pixels. In [2] an alternative approach for incorporating edge orientation has been proposed which solves the matching problem in an augmented space. It was shown that the suggested directional chamfer matching (DCM) achieves a superior performance compared to oriented chamfer matching. Another improvement was proposed in [12] where manually selected tuples of contour fragments have been used as normalizers for oriented chamfer matching.

[1,2] focus on adding orientation information to improve the matching quality of the foreground template. In both approaches, the score for an object hypothesis is obtained by summing over all the template pixels in the distance transform of the query image. However, an object is more than the mere sum of the distance transformation of each template pixel, considering the evidence from [3,4] which indicates that not all boundary pixels are equally important.

[12] proposed to reduce the chamfer matches in clutter by normalizing template matches with manually combined normalizer contours. These normalizers are placed at the center of the template matches. However, to sufficiently model complex background, it is important to combine simple contours via flexible placement going beyond the manual combinations of normalizers. We measure

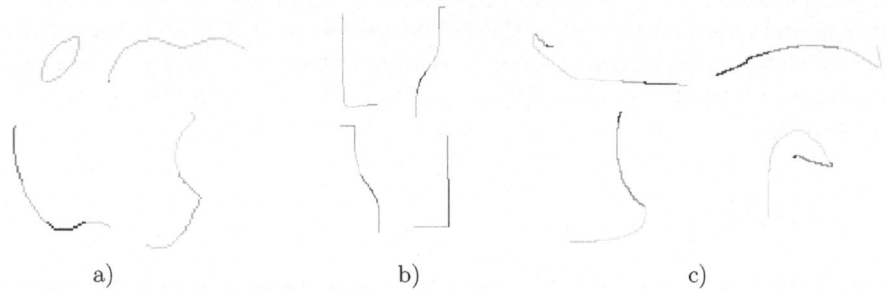

**Fig. 1.** Relative pixels weights for a) applelogos, b) bottles and c) swans learnt with a linear max-margin classifier. Red indicates high weight and blue low weight.

the accidentalness of a match to clutter by learning the co-placement of background contours dependent on the foreground.

We integrate the i) relative importance of different pixels on a foreground template and ii) accidentalness of a template match to clutter into a single discriminative approach. Our final detection system improves the matching performance of a foreground template while suppressing spurious matches in cluttered background using the proposed background regularization.

## 3    Reducing Accidentalness in Chamfer Matching

Our approach is based on the publicly available fast directional chamfer matching approach of [2] which was shown to achieve state-of-the-art performance in chamfer-based matching. Let us now briefly review the fast directional chamfer matching [2] and introduce the required notation. Each object is represented by a collection of contours of its different parts. Let $P = \{\mathbf{p}_i\}$ and $Q = \{\mathbf{q}_j\}$ be the pixels of an object part and query edge maps respectively. Let $\phi(\mathbf{p}_i)$ be the edge orientation of the edge point $\mathbf{p}_i$.

For a given location $\mathbf{x}$ of the object part in the query image, directional chamfer matching aims to find the best $\mathbf{q}_j \in Q$ for each $\mathbf{p}_i \in P$ by minimizing the cost $|(\mathbf{p}_i + \mathbf{x}) - \mathbf{q}_j| + \lambda|\phi(\mathbf{p}_i + \mathbf{x}) - \phi(\mathbf{q}_j)|$. $\lambda$ denotes the weighting factor between location and orientation terms. Thus the directional chamfer distance for placing an object part at location $\mathbf{x}$ is defined as

$$d_{DCM}^{(P,Q)}(\mathbf{x}) = \frac{1}{|P|} \sum_{\mathbf{p}_i \in P} \min_{\mathbf{q}_j \in Q} |(\mathbf{p}_i + \mathbf{x}) - \mathbf{q}_j| + \lambda|\phi(\mathbf{p}_i + \mathbf{x}) - \phi(\mathbf{q}_j)| \qquad (1)$$

### 3.1    Interdependence of Model Points

Not all the pixels on an object part are equally important for detecting objects. Consider for instance the famous Kanizsa triangle. Provided only contour fragments around the corners, the whole triangle can be easily recognized. Similarly, Biederman [3] presents perceptual experiments with degraded contours that demonstrate the varying importance of different points on object contours. Another example is Attneave's cat [4], where for instance, points of high curvature are proposed as the most useful features for recognition. However, we want to automatically learn which parts of the model are important, rather than manually encoding a set of rules that define the importance of contour points. While there is related work, for instance, on saliency [13] and interest point detection [14], we seek a formulation that can be directly integrated into chamfer matching. Moreover, the interest points are detected based on each training image separately whereas we seek important points of an object part based on joint consideration of all the training images.

In chamfer matching, matching costs for an object part are obtained by summing over all the object part pixels in the distance transform of the query image as in Eq. (1). Thus, all the pixels are implicitly considered to be equally important when computing the matching costs. To take into account the fact that not all pixels are equally important, we learn discriminative weights for the co-occurrence of individual points of an object part, i.e., of their matching costs

$$t_i^{(P,Q)}(\mathbf{x}) = \min_{\mathbf{q}_j \in Q} |(\mathbf{p}_i + \mathbf{x}) - \mathbf{q}_j| + \lambda |\phi(\mathbf{p}_i + \mathbf{x}) - \phi(\mathbf{q}_j)| \tag{2}$$

Since adjacent pixels of an object part are statistically dependent, we utilize the line representation for the templates from [2] and learn discriminative weights for each line of the object part. Thus, all the pixels which lie on the same line are assigned the same weight. Let $\bar{t}_l$ denote the matching cost of line $l$ fitted to the object part.

$$\bar{t}_l = \sum_{i \in l} t_i^{(P,Q)}(\mathbf{x}) \tag{3}$$

The discriminative learning algorithm that discovers the weights for the co-occurrences of lines is described in Sect. 3.3. For examples of relative pixel weights see Fig. 1.

## 3.2    Background Contours for Modelling Accidentalness

One of the main drawbacks of chamfer matching is the liability to false positive matches in background clutter. Increasing the specificity of the model contour matches by adding orientation information [2,1] and learning the importance of foreground contour pixels can only partially solve the problems arising from background clutter (see Fig. 4). Consequently we need to measure the accidentalness of an object part matching in the background clutter. To measure such accidentalness, we introduce a set of simple, generic contour segments (see Fig. 2 a) that typically match equally well to background clutter and the correct part contour. We refer to this set of contours as background contours. Since each single background contour segment has a very low specificity we learn discriminative

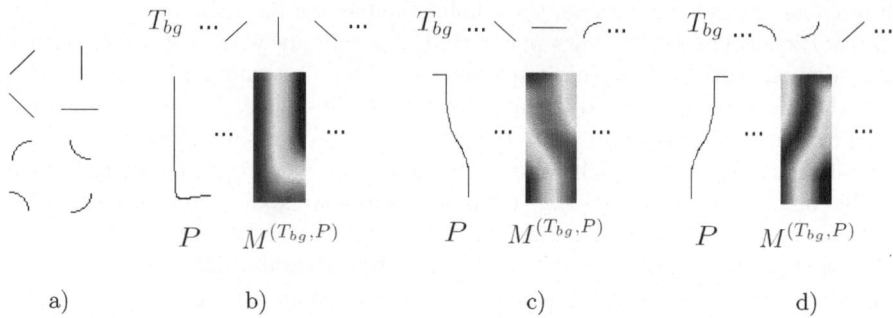

**Fig. 2.** a) shows a set of simple background contours $T_{bg}$. These background contours are used to regularize the chamfer response of a part $P$. b)-d) show the masks $M^{(T_{bg},P)}$ described in Eq. (4) obtained from placing the background contours at the top relative to the object part contour on the left.

co-occurrence patterns which have very low accidentalness. By going for flexible spatial arrangements of background contours, we avoid manually combining tuples of normalizers consisting of one or two contours to form hand designed complex background templates as in [12]. Furthermore, we measure the amount of clutter only in the neighborhood of model contours, where clutter actually interferes with the matching of the model contour while in [12] background contours are placed at a fixed single location (the center of the model contour). The importance of the second point is illustrated by the following example. Consider a U-shaped object part being matched to a query image. Clutter from the query image that is situated within the U does not interfere with the object part. Only clutter that is close to the contour of the U will have an impact. Thus, [12] miss out on measuring the susceptibility of the model contour to clutter and instead measure clutter simply at the center of the object part.

To make sure that background contours $T_{bg}$ are placed on the foreground contour $P$, where accidental matches typically occur, we create a mask for every combination of a foreground part and a background contour

$$M^{(T_{bg},P)}(\mathbf{x}) = 1 - d_{DCM}^{(T_{bg},P)}(\mathbf{x}) \tag{4}$$

These masks give high weight to regions where the background contour matches well on the part contour and low weight otherwise. Figure 2 shows the resultant masks for three different foreground bottle parts in combination with different background contours.

To describe the background matching costs for a hypothesis in a robust way we build weighted histograms over chamfer matching costs. Let $\bar{\mathbf{x}}$ be one specific placement of the foreground object part $P$ on the query image $Q$. Furthermore we define $B(\bar{\mathbf{x}})$ to be the bounding box region of $P$ centered at $\bar{\mathbf{x}}$. For each foreground hypothesis we build weighted histograms $h^{(T_{bg},Q)}$ over the directional chamfer matching costs $d_{DCM}^{(T_{bg},Q)}$ in the corresponding bounding box region. The weights introduced in Eq. (4) are used to weight the histogram votes according to their position relative to the foreground object part. Each histogram consists of $K$ bins where $\mathcal{M}_k$ is the range of the $k$th bin and $k = 1, ..., K$. We define a histogram bin $h_k^{(T_{bg}, Q)}$ as

$$h_k^{(T_{bg}, Q)} = \sum_{\substack{\mathbf{x} \in B(\bar{\mathbf{x}}) \\ d_{DCM}^{(T_{bg}, Q)}(\mathbf{x}) \in \mathcal{M}_k}} M^{(T_{bg}, P)}(\mathbf{x}), \tag{5}$$

for each background contour $T_{bg}$ on a certain position of the foreground object part $P$ in the query image $Q$.

### 3.3   Learning Co-occurrences for Foreground and Background

We combine the twin problems of i) modeling the co-occurrence of points on a foreground object part and ii) modeling the accidentalness of a match by means of co-occurrence patterns of background contours into a single discriminative approach. We regularize directional chamfer matching by learning the characteristic co-occurrence of foreground object part pixels and the joint placement of background contours.

As training data this learning algorithm utilizes the object hypotheses obtained from running the directional chamfer matching code [2] on the training images. A hypothesis $j$ having an overlap greater than 80% with the groundtruth is labeled as positive $y_j = 1$, while a hypothesis with an overlap smaller than 40% is labeled as negative $y_j = -1$. For each object hypothesis we build a feature vector $f_j$ as constructed in Eq. (6).

$$f_j = [\bar{t_1} \ ... \ \bar{t_L} \ h_1 \ ... \ h_K] \tag{6}$$

$L$ denotes the number of line segments fitted to the object part and $K$ denotes the number of background contours.

Let $\mathcal{K}$ be a kernel such that $\mathcal{K}(f_i, f_j)$ represents the similarity between feature vectors $f_i, f_j$. Subsequently, we use the radial basis kernel $\mathcal{K}(f_i, f_j) = \exp\left(-\gamma \|f_i - f_j\|^2\right)$. It is common practice in the field of kernel machines, to interpret the kernel $\mathcal{K}(f_i, f_j)$ as a dot product of transformed features $\psi(f_i), \psi(f_j)$. Here $\psi$ represents the mapping of the feature vector into a higher dimensional space. Due to the seminal 'kernel trick' [15] it is sufficient to define the kernel $\mathcal{K}$ without explicitly representing the mapping $\psi$. We then seek weights $w$ to be applied on $\psi(f_i)$ so that the margin between positive and negative hypotheses in the transformed space is maximized. Since we employ the non-linear RBF kernel, the resulting classifier will learn non-linear relationships between the features and model the joint co-occurrences of foreground and background contours. We need to optimize the following max-margin classification problem to learn the weights $w$.

$$\min_{w, b, \xi} \frac{1}{2} \|w\|_2^2 + C \sum_{j=1}^{N} \xi_j \tag{7}$$

$$\text{subject to :} \qquad y_j(w^T \psi(f_j) + b) \geq 1 - \xi_j \quad \wedge \quad \xi_j \geq 0$$

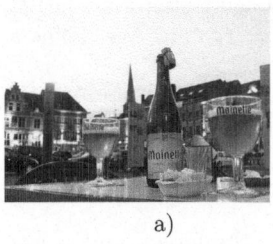
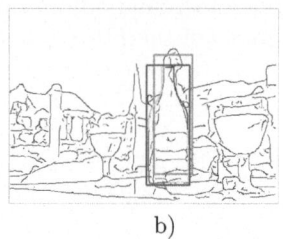
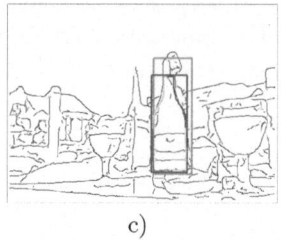

a)                          b)                          c)

**Fig. 3.** Learning discriminative weights for the co-occurrences of $t_i^{(P,Q)}(\mathbf{x})$ improves the matching score of shape template as shown in the example here. The original image, the result obtained from directional chamfer matching and the result obtained from foreground reweighting are shown in panels a,b and c respectively. The groundtruth bounding box is shown in green and the top scoring object hypotheses are shown in red.

where $N$ is the number of training samples, $b$ is the offset, $C$ is the penalty and $\xi_j$ are slack variables allowing for margin violations. Commonly Eq. (7) is converted into its dual form and solved for the dual SVM parameters, the support vectors $S_i$, their coefficients $\alpha_i$ and the offset $b$.

### 3.4   Object Detection Using Regularized Chamfer Matching

In the previous section we have described how the relevance of model points and the accidentalness measured using background contours can be jointly learned. Let us now utilize the combined model of foreground relevance and background accidentalness from Eq. (7) to improve upon the directional chamfer matching cost function Eq. (1). This improved, regularized chamfer distance $d_{RDCM}^{(P,Q)}(\mathbf{x})$ again measures the distortion cost of an object part $f_j$. Let the $j$-th object hypothesis $f_j$, which is described by the feature vector from Eq. (6), be the placement of object part $P$ at location $\mathbf{x}$ in the query image $Q$. Since a non-linear radial basis kernel is employed, the regularized chamfer distance is obtained using the dual SVM parameters, obtained by solving the SVM optimization problem from Eq. (7) in its dual form,

$$d_{RDCM}^{(P,Q)}(\mathbf{x}) = 1 - \left( \sum_i \alpha_i \mathcal{K}(f_j, S_i) + b \right). \qquad (8)$$

Each object part matched to a query image casts a vote with weight $d_{RDCM}$ as computed in Eq. (8) for different placements of the part in the query image. The votes from various parts are collected in a Hough accumulator and non-max suppression is performed to obtain final candidate hypotheses for objects.

## 4   Experimental Evaluation

To demonstrate the utility of the proposed discriminative chamfer regularization, we evaluate our approach on benchmark datasets for chamfer matching. Since we integrated our regularization into the publicly available code of [2], the results reported in [2] have been used as the baseline. To demonstrate the advantage of our regularization over learning the normalization for chamfer distances [12], a comparison is made with the results documented in [12]. We also compare with a sophisticated learning and inference approach applied on object contours [16]. Furthermore, an analysis of the running time overhead caused by discriminative chamfer regularization compared to the running time of the chamfer matching approach of [2] is presented.

To extract the edge maps from input RGB images, we utilize the probabilistic boundary detector of [17]. The weights $w$ in Eq. (7) are learnt using the support vector machine implementation of [18]. To measure the performance of our detection system, we employ the standard PASCAL overlap criterion according to which a detection is correct if the ratio of intersection and overlap between groundtruth and the detection is larger than 50%.

The individual contributions of the proposed foreground and background regularization are presented in Sect. 4.3. We analyze the contribution of reweighting the foreground template pixels as in Eq. (2) and then the performance obtained by the combined foreground and background regularization as in Eq. (7). The gain obtained by these contributions is compared with the baseline obtained by [2]. Sect. 4.4 compares the proposed regularization with other state-of-the-art extensions to chamfer matching such as [12,16].

## 4.1   Datasets

For our experimental evaluation, we use the TUD Pedestrians, TUD Cows and the ETHZ Shape datasets. These are the benchmark datasets for chamfer matching and approaches such as [1,2,12] report their results on one or more of these datasets. The TUD Pedestrian dataset provides two training sets with 210 and 400 side-view pedestrians. Following the protocol of [12], we use 400 images for training, 5 masks from the training images as model shape templates and 250 images for testing. The Cow dataset from the PASCAL Object Recognition Database Collection [19] consists of 111 images in which cows appear with quite different articulation. The protocol from [12] is used to divide the dataset into training and testing sets. Five masks from the training images are obtained as the shape templates. For the ETHZ shape dataset, according to the standard protocol one hand-drawn example provided along with each category is used as a shape template. For the object categories applelogos, bottles and swans,the template is decomposed into four parts while for the categories giraffes and mugs the full template was utilized.

## 4.2   Running Time

To obtain the initial matches for the templates, we run the publicly available directional chamfer matching code of [2] using the default parameters for all the datasets. In our experimental evaluations, we have observed that computing the distance transformation of a query image for each angular quantization is the

**Table 1.** Comparison of **average precision** for three datasets namely, TUD Pedestrians, Cows and the ETHZ Shape classes. We compare DCM [2] which constitutes the basis of our approach with the extension from Sec. 3.1 and our final learning of regularized chamfer matching. All the detections are evaluated based on PASCAL overlap criterion with the groundtruth object annotations.

|                        | Pedestrians | Cows | Applelogos | Bottles | Giraffes | Mugs | Swans |
|------------------------|-------------|------|------------|---------|----------|------|-------|
| DCM [2]                | 3.0         | 88.1 | 60.8       | 85.5    | 27.0     | 10.1 | 33.1  |
| FG Regularization      | 6.8         | 89.2 | 62.0       | 86.9    | 36.3     | **27.3** | 33.8  |
| Combined Regularization| **11.2**    | **91.9** | **81.8** | **90.4** | **43.0** | **27.3** | **47.3** |

most time consuming part in the code of [2]. The proposed chamfer regularization added only a marginal overhead to the computation time. For instance, only 2 second overhead is observed per image from TUD Cow dataset. On the other hand, computations for the baseline performance [2] took about 15 seconds per image. Thus, our approach turns out to be easily integrable into a state-of-the-art chamfer matching approach, without adding significant overhead in terms of running time.

### 4.3   Evaluating Foreground and Background Regularization

Table 1 compares the baseline directional chamfer matching, which constitutes the basis of our approach, with the different components of our discriminative chamfer regularization. In particular, the performance of our foreground regularization method and the performance of our combined detector using foreground and background regularization are evaluated. Figure 1 shows the relative importance of various pixels of the foreground template learnt by using a linear SVM. The experiments show that foreground regularization alone already improves performance in terms of average precision on all of these object categories. Additionally applying the background regularization suppresses even more false positives in cluttered background and, thus, yields a significant further gain.

For the TUD Pedestrian dataset the images in the testing set are provided at a very high resolution which yields very low average precision for the directional chamfer matching which is around 3%. The low baseline can be attributed to the high resolution of the test images, since it is known that chamfer matching is sensitive to all the fine details in the edge map. Our foreground regularization more than doubled the average precision obtained from the baseline. Adding the background regularization brought a further gain of 4.4% in average precision. For the Cow dataset directional chamfer matching yields very good performance around 88% average precision. Nevertheless, our combined detector still improves the performance about 4% by exploiting the advantages of foreground and background regularization. In Fig. 3 one can see how foreground reweighting improves the alignment with the groundtruth. The background normalization becomes particularly useful for categories such as applelogos, bottles and swans where most of the performance gain can be attributed to background regularization.

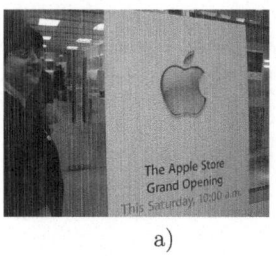
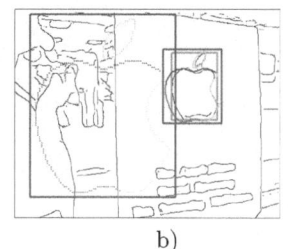
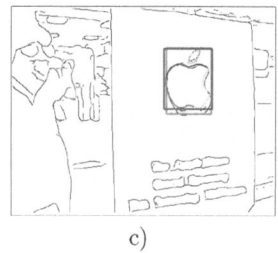

a)                              b)                              c)

**Fig. 4.** This example shows how combined foreground and background regularization Eq. (7) can remove false positive detections which could not be eliminated by foreground reweighting alone. Panel a) shows the original image, b) the result obtained by using foreground reweighting and c) the results from the combined foreground and background regularization. Best viewed in color.

The example in Fig. 4 shows that foreground regularization is not always able to suppress false positives in cluttered background and how background regularization can handle such cases. For a challenging category like giraffes with articulations and background clutter, both foreground and background regularization are found to be equally helpful. For the category of mugs we observed that explaining the foreground more accurately is more important than suppressing false detections in cluttered background. We observe 17.3% improvement in average precision by learning the co-occurrence of template pixels while our combined detector yields results in the same range. All in all our combined detector using foreground and background regularization achieves significant gain on all of the seven categories compared to directional chamfer matching. Additional detection results comparing the regularized chamfer matching to directional chamfer matching are provided in Fig. 5.

### 4.4 Comparison with State-of-the-Art Extensions to Chamfer Matching

We compare our combined foreground and background regularization with other state-of-the-art extensions to chamfer matching such as the normalized oriented chamfer matching by Ma et al. [12] (NOCM) and the hierarchical deformable template model (HDT) by Zhu et al. [16].

[12] have reported results on two datasets: the TUD Pedestrian dataset [20] and the Cow dataset [19]. [16] have evaluated their method on the Cow dataset. Both the approaches report their results in terms of detection rate at 10% precision. In the previous section, we have reported the gain obtained by our regularization in terms of average precision, since it is taking into account the area under the precision recall curve instead of just one point on the performance curve and therefore is a more robust measure. Nevertheless, to compare ourselves with [12,16], we need to report results in terms of detection rate at 10% precision.

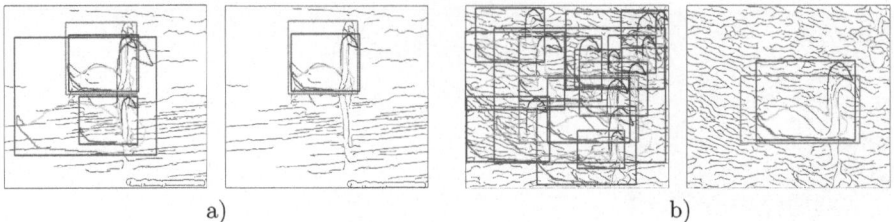

a)                                                    b)

**Fig. 5.** Panel a) and b) show detection results for two examples. The left image of each panel shows results obtained by directional chamfer matching. The right image of each panel shows the improved detection result after applying chamfer regularization. The groundtruth bounding box is shown in green and the top scoring object hypotheses are shown in red. Best viewed in color.

**Table 2.** Comparison in terms of **detection rate** at 10% precision (in %) on the Cow dataset and the TUD Pedestrian dataset with OCM, NOCM and HDT.

|  | Cows | Pedestrians |
|---|---|---|
| OCM [1] | 73.9 | 35.2 |
| NOCM [12] | 91.0 | 70.0 |
| HDT [16] | 88.2 | – |
| Regularized Chamfer Matching | **98.3** | **80.0** |

Table 2 shows the results for the Cow dataset and the TUD Pedestrian dataset. The results indicate that chamfer regularization significantly improves performance on the Cow dataset compared to HDT and NOCM. For TUD Pedestrians we gain 10% in detection rate compared to NOCM. All in all our results confirm that the regularized chamfer matching method significantly improves over state-of-the-art extensions to chamfer matching.

## 5    Conclusion

This contribution extends the well established and widely used chamfer matching technique, particularly by overcoming its susceptibility to clutter. Our results confirm, that learning the co-occurrence of model points is increasing the specificity of the template by supporting the differing relevance of model points instead of treating them as independent and equally important. Furthermore, accidental matches in background clutter can be suppressed by placing our generic contours on the model contour and learning to distinguish the typical co-occurrence of these contours on cluttered background compared to actual objects. These two contributions are integrated in a max-margin learning framework which is based on state-of-the art directional chamfer matching. [1]

[1] This work was supported by the Excellence Initiative of the German Federal Government and the Frontier fund, DFG project number ZUK 49/1.

# References

1. Shotton, J., Blake, A., Cipolla, R.: Multi-scale categorical object recognition using contour fragments. PAMI 30, 1270–1281 (2008)
2. Liu, M., Tuzel, O., Veeraraghavan, A., Chellappa, R.: Fast directional chamfer matching. In: CVPR (2010)
3. Biederman, I.: Recognition-by-components: A theory of human image understanding. Psychological Review 4, 115–147 (1987)
4. Attneave, F.: Some informational aspects of visual perception. Psychological Review 61 (1954)
5. Barrow, H.G., Tenenbaum, J.M., Bolles, R.C., Wolf, H.C.: Parametric correspondence and chamfer matching: Two new techiques for image matching. In: Int. Joint Conf. Artifical Intelligence, pp. 659–663 (1977)
6. Borgefors, G.: Hierarchical chamfer matching: A parametric edge matching algorithm. PAMI 10, 849–865 (1988)
7. Leibe, B., Seemann, E., Schiele, B.: Pedestrian detection in crowded scenes. In: CVPR (2005)
8. Gavrila, D.M., Munder, S.: Multi-cue pedestrian detection and tracking from a moving vehicle. International Journal of Computer Vision 73, 41–49 (2007)
9. Lin, Z., Davis, L.S., Doermann, D., DeMenthon, D.: Hierarchical part template matching for human detection and segmentation. In: ICCV (2007)
10. Thayananthan, A., Stenger, B., Torr, P., Cipolla, R.: Shape context and chamfer matching in cluttered scenes. In: CVPR (2003)
11. Belongie, S., Malik, J., Puzicha, J.: Shape matching and object recognition using shape contexts. PAMI (2002)
12. Ma, T., Yang, X., Latecki, L.J.: Boosting Chamfer Matching by Learning Chamfer Distance Normalization. In: Daniilidis, K., Maragos, P., Paragios, N. (eds.) ECCV 2010, Part V. LNCS, vol. 6315, pp. 450–463. Springer, Heidelberg (2010)
13. Kadir, T., Brady, M.: Saliency, scale and image description. IJCV 45 (2001)
14. Berg, A.C., Malik, J.: Geometric blur for template matching. In: CVPR, pp. 607–614 (2001)
15. Boser, B.E., Guyon, I.M., Vapnik, V.N.: A training algorithm for optimal margin classifiers. In: 5th Annual ACM Workshop on COLT, pp. 144–152 (1992)
16. Zhu, L., Chen, Y., Yuille, A.: Learning a hierarchical deformable template for rapid deformable object parsing. PAMI 99 (2009)
17. Martin, D., Fowlkes, C., Malik, C.: Learning to detect natural image boundaries using local brightness, color and texture cues. PAMI 26, 530–549 (2004)
18. Chang, C.C., Lin, C.J.: LIBSVM: A library for support vector machines. ACM Transactions on Intelligent Systems and Technology 2, 27:1–27:27 (2011)
19. Leibe, B., Leaonardis, A., Schiele, B.: Combined object categroization and segmentation with an implicit shape model. In: ECCV 2004 Workshop on Statistical Learning in Computer Vision (2004)
20. Andriluka, M., Roth, S., Schiele, B.: People-tracking-by-detection and people-detection-by-tracking. In: CVPR (2008)

# Coupling-and-Decoupling: A Hierarchical Model for Occlusion-Free Car Detection

Bo Li[1,2,3], Tianfu Wu[2,3], Wenze Hu[3,4], and Mingtao Pei[1]

[1] Beijing Lab of Intelligent Information, School of Computer Science and Technology, Beijing Institute of Technology, Beijing 100081, P.R.China
[2] BUPT-Seesoft Joint Lab of Visual Computing and Image Communication, Beijing University of Posts and Telecommunications (BUPT), Beijing 100876, P.R.China
[3] Lotus Hill Research Institute, EZhou, P.R.China
[4] Department of Statistics, University of California, Los Angeles
{boli.lhi,tfwu.lhi,wzhu.lhi}@gmail.com, peimt@bit.edu.cn

**Abstract.** Handling occlusions in object detection is a long-standing problem. This paper addresses the problem of X-to-X-occlusion-free object detection (e.g. car-to-car occlusions in our experiment) by utilizing an intuitive coupling-and-decoupling strategy. In the "coupling" stage, we model the pair of occluding X's (e.g. car pairs) directly to account for the statistically strong co-occurrence (i.e. coupling). Then, we learn a hierarchical And-Or directed acyclic graph (AOG) model under the latent structural SVM (LSSVM) framework. The learned AOG consists of, from the top to bottom, (i) a root Or-node representing different compositions of occluding X pairs, (ii) a set of And-nodes each of which represents a specific composition of occluding X pairs, (iii) another set of And-nodes representing single X's decomposed from occluding X pairs, and (iv) a set of terminal-nodes which represent the appearance templates for the X pairs, single X's and latent parts of the single X's, respectively. The part appearance templates can also be shared among different single X's. In detection, a dynamic programming (DP) algorithm is used and as a natural consequence we decouple the two single X's from the X-to-X occluding pairs. In experiments, we test our method on roadside cars which are collected from real traffic video surveillance environment by ourselves. We compare our model with the state-of-the-art deformable part-based model (DPM) and obtain better detection performance.

## 1 Introduction

In the literature of object detection, handling occlusions is very challenging and remains a long-standing problem. The two main reasons are (i) The gap between training and testing. When training an object detector, unoccluded object instances are often collected and used purposely. In testing, however, occlusions are inevitable in real scenarios. As a result, the detection performance will go down significantly as occlusions become severe. And (ii) The lack of common occlusion models. Generally and statistically speaking, it is very difficult to capture and predict occlusions because they can be treated as being uniformly distributed

K.M. Lee et al. (Eds.): ACCV 2012, Part I, LNCS 7724, pp. 164–175, 2013.
© Springer-Verlag Berlin Heidelberg 2013

in the wildest situation. To some extend, that explains, in turn, why the gap between training and testing exists. To address the occlusion problem, among others, hierarchical modeling (e.g. deformable part-based models [5]) has been widely used and shows performance improvement, and a 2-layer model is often adopted for modeling single objects, which can tackle small occlusions implicitly.

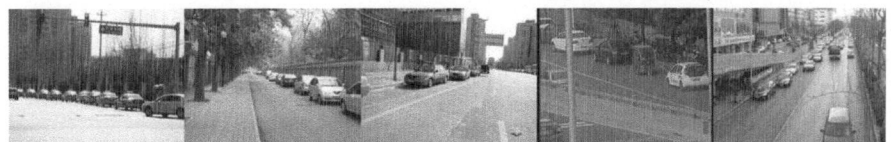

**Fig. 1.** Some examples of roadside cars. There are different types of car-to-car occlusions which challenge the state-of-the-art detectors trained for single cars.

In this paper, we distinguish between two types of occlusions: the X-to-X and X-to-Y occlusions, where "X" and "Y" represent different object categories (e.g. "X" represents car and "Y" person) respectively, and then present a coupling-and-decoupling method for X-to-X occlusion-free object detection without modeling occlusions explicitly. As the running examples, we use roadside cars which are often parked along the curb, leading to the X-to-X occlusions. Occlusion-free roadside car detection can facilitate many important applications in computer vision and intelligent transportation, such as parking violation capturing, license plate detection and parking management. Figure 1 shows some examples of car-to-car occlusions in real traffic video surveillance environment. In the sequel, we concretely use car instead of "X" to present the formulation (but notice that the proposed method is not limited to cars). Our method consists of two stages as follows.

(i) *The "coupling" stage in modeling and learning.* Instead of training a single object detector, we learn hierarchical And-Or directed and acyclic graph (AOG) models for the car-to-car occluding pairs directly to account for the statistically strong coupling. The learned AOG consists of, from the top to bottom, (i) a root Or-node representing different compositions of occluding car-to-car pairs, (ii) a set of And-nodes each of which represents a specific composition of occluding car pairs, (iii) another set of And-nodes representing single cars decomposed from occluding car pairs, and (iv) a set of terminal-nodes which represent the appearance templates for the car pairs, single cars and latent parts of the single cars, respectively. The part appearance templates can also be shared among different single cars. We adopt Histogram of Oriented Gradient (HOG) [2] as the appearance feature as done in DPM [5]. Figure 3 shows the learned AOG for car-to-car pairs (where for clarity only a portion is drawn). We formulate the learning of AOG under the latent structural SVM (LSSVM) framework [13,14,16]. In the training dataset, bounding boxes of car pairs and corresponding two single cars are annotated, and the parts of single cars are treated as latent variables.

(ii) *The "decoupling" stage in detection.* Our AOG model is directed and acyclic and we can utilize the DP algorithm in inference. For detected car pairs, the back-traced bounding boxes for the two single cars are obtained, i.e., decoupled from the car pair. Since the locations and sizes of bounding boxes of the single cars are annotated when jointly training the AOG model, the back-traced ones are the optimal solutions for the two single cars.

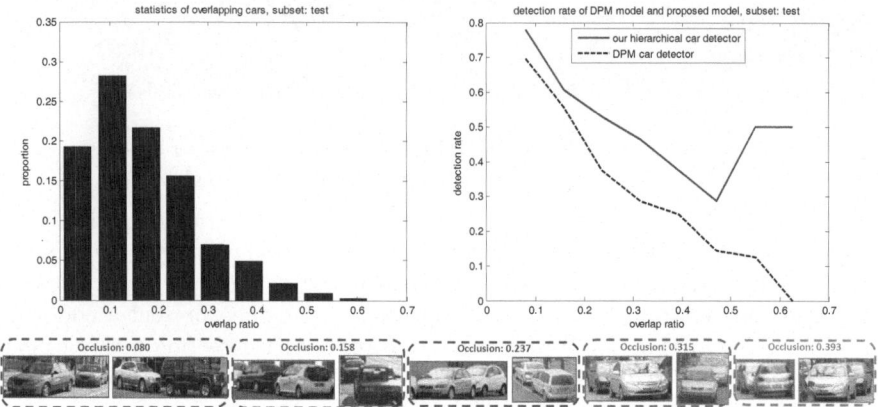

**Fig. 2.** Top-left: The population ratios in the testing set of roadside cars used in this paper. Bottom: Some examples of cropped car-to-car occluding pairs. The occlusion ratio is measured for the back car in the car pairs. Top-right: The plots of detection rates v.s. occlusion ratios, where blue dashed curve is for the state-of-the-art DPM [5] and red curve is for the proposed method. See text for details.

To illustrate the necessity and the advantage of the proposed method in this paper, in Fig. 2, the left figure shows the population ratios of car-to-car pairs with different degrees of occlusions in the testing dataset collected by ourselves from the real traffic video surveillance environment. Some cropped image examples are shown in the bottom. The right figure shows the detection rates against the occlusion ratio for the proposed method (the red curve) and the state-of-the-art DPM [5] (the blue dashed curve). We can observe that,

(i)  The population ratio of car pairs with occlusions being equal or greater than 0.2 is greater than 0.5 (i.e. occlusions become a statistically major factor).

(ii) At the same time, the detection performance of DPM dropped significantly when occlusions go beyond 0.2, while our method can obtain much better performance.

(iii) The detection performance of our method goes up significantly when occlusions are greater than 0.45. This is because that with those severe occlusions, even if DPM could recall the two single cars, their bounding boxes overlap larger than the threshold normally used (e.g. 0.7), and then the one with lower score will be excluded by non-maximum suppressing (NMS) (see the DPM detection results in Fig. 5). Our method can, however, detect those cars correctly by decoupling them from the detected car pairs. More results and final performance comparison are shown in Fig. 5 and Fig .4 respectively.

In the literature of computer vision, car detection for traffic monitoring systems are addressed mainly in single unoccluded situations, such as car type classification [12,8], multiple-view car detection [9,7], or shadow removal from suspicious car regions in images [10]. [1] proposed a method to detect and track multiple cars simultaneously, but they did not address the occlusion problem.

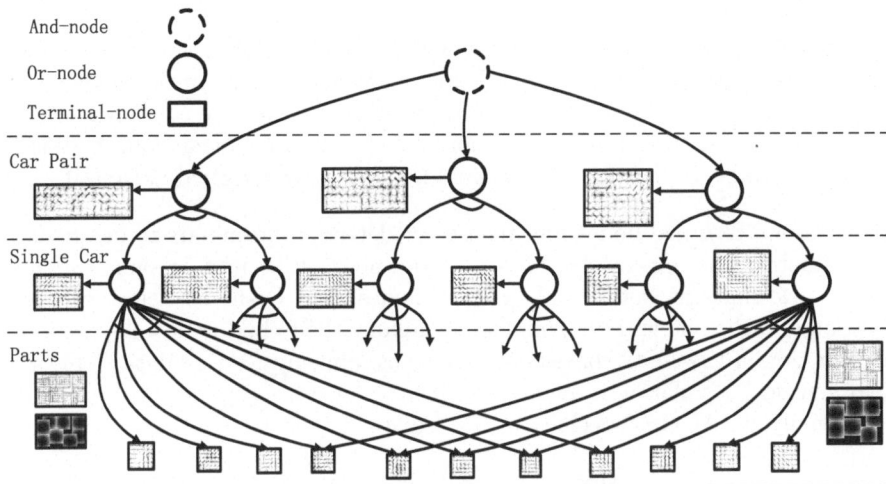

**Fig. 3.** Our AOG Model. First-layer: illustration of car pair And-nodes and their corresponding appearance features. Second-layer: illustration of single car And-nodes and their corresponding appearance features. Third-layer: illustration of car parts Terminal-nodes and their corresponding appearance and deformation features. Parts are shared. For clarity, we just show the parts of two single cars.

## 2    The Model

### 2.1    The AOG

In this section, we specify the AOG hierarchical model used in this paper which is a directed and acyclic graph facilitating the DP algorithm in detection. The learning of AOG will be given in Sec. 4.

By following the framework in [17], our AOG embeds the occluding car pair detection grammars which are embodied by defining three types of nodes:

(i) *The root Or-node O* represents compositional alternatives of the occluding car pairs (e.g., car pairs from different viewpoints or with different degrees of occlusions). The Or-node $O$ has a branching variable, denoted by $\omega(O)$, indicating which child And-node is selected, and $\omega(O)$ will be inferred on-the-fly in detection.

(ii) *A set of And-nodes $V_{And}$.* There are two types of And-nodes: car pairs and single cars. Each car pair And-node represents the decomposition of a specific type of occluding car pair into two single cars (e.g. a frontal view car pair with the back car being occluded by 30% roughly), and each single car And-node represents the decomposition of a single car into a small number of parts.

(iii) *A set of Terminal-nodes $V_T$.* First of all, the And-nodes defined above themselves can terminate directly, creating terminal nodes, when the resolution is low (relative to their own decomposed parts). Secondly, each part is represented by a terminal-node linking to image data. In the model, each terminal-node $t \in V_T$ has its own location, denoted by $l_t$, which will be also inferred on-the-fly in detection. The location for placing an And-node is the same as that for the terminal-node directly terminated from it.

In the AOG, terminal-nodes link the object detection grammars to image data by evaluating the appearance features, And-nodes take into account the geometric deformations between their child nodes, and Or-nodes select the best solution (i.e. the one with maximal score) among their child nodes. So, the scoring function of the AOG consists of two terms: appearance (i.e. data term) and deformation (i.e. relation term).

Formally, an AOG is specified by a 5-tuple,

$$\mathcal{G} = (O, V_{And}, V_T, \Theta^{app}, \Theta^{def}) \qquad (1)$$

where $\Theta^{app}$ are the parameters for the appearance scoring function when placing terminal-nodes in images, and $\Theta^{def}$ the parameters for the deformation cost of a placed terminal-node with respect to its anchor location. They will be learned by LSSVM jointly.

**Part-Sharing in the AOG.** For the child single car And-nodes decomposed from car pair And-nodes, some of them are often with the same type (such as sided view or frontal view cars) but different occlusions. So, they can share part appearance, but might have different deformation models. By sharing-parts, it will supply more data in training the part appearance parameters, and also reduce run-time in detection.

## 2.2   The Scoring Function of an AOG

Let $\Lambda$ be the image lattice and $I_\Lambda$ an image defined on $\Lambda$. In detection, we need to search over scales to detect objects with different sizes. In practice, a feature pyramid of $I_\Lambda$ is generated, denoted by $H$ (e.g. the HOG feature pyramid used in the DPM [5] and our method). When placing an AOG in $I_\Lambda$ at a location $u \in \Lambda$, we have,

(i) The scoring function for evaluating an Or-node $O$ at $u$ is defined by,

$$\text{Score}(O, u) = \max_{A \in ch(O)} \text{Score}(A, u) \qquad (2)$$

where $ch(O) \in V_{And}$ is the set of child And-nodes of the Or-node $O$. We can assign the branching variable $\omega(O) = \arg\max_{A \in ch(O)} \text{Score}(O, u)$.

(ii) The scoring function for computing an And-node $A$ with respect to a placed Or-node $O$ at $u$ is defined by,

$$\text{Score}(A, u | O, u) = <\theta_{t_A}^{app}, \Phi^{app}(H, A, u)> + \sum_{c \in ch(A)} \text{Score}(c | A, u) \qquad (3)$$

where the first term is the appearance score for the terminal-node $t_A$ terminated from And-node $A$ directly, $\theta_{t_A}^{app} \in \Theta^{app}$ is the corresponding appearance parameters, $\Phi^{app}(H, A, u)$ is the features extracted from the feature pyramid, and $ch(A) \in V_{And} \cup V_T$ is the set of child nodes of $A$.

(iii) The scoring function for computing an And-node $A_1$ with respect to a placed And-node $A$ at $u$ is defined by,

$$\text{Score}(A_1 | A, u) = \max_{v \in \Lambda}( <\theta_{t_{A_1}}^{app}, \Phi^{app}(H, A_1, v)> - <\theta_{A_1|A}^{def}, \Phi_{A_1|A}^{def}(v, u)> +$$

$$\sum_{t \in ch(A_1)} \text{Score}(t | A_1, v)) \qquad (4)$$

where $\theta_{\cdot|\star}^{def} \in \Theta^{def}$ is the corresponding deformation parameter for node $\cdot$ (such as $A_1$) with respect to node $\star$ (such as $A$), $\Phi_{\cdot|\star}^{def}(v, u)$ is the deformation feature which we adopt the same quadratic function as used in DPM [5] and we have $\Phi_{\cdot|\star}^{def}(v, u) = [dx^2, dx, dy^2, dy]$ where $(dx, dy)$ is the displacement between $v$ and $u$. The best placed location of node $A_1$ is retrieved by taking $\arg\max_{v \in \Lambda} \text{Score}(A_1 | A, u)$.

(iv) For computing a part terminal-node $t$ with respect to a placed parent And-node $A$ at $u$, the scoring function is defined by,

$$\text{Score}(t | A, u) = \max_{v \in \Lambda}(<\theta_t^{app}, \Phi^{app}(H, t, v)> - <\theta_{t|A}^{def}, \Phi_{t|A}^{def}(v, u)>) \qquad (5)$$

where in practice, we often place node $t$ at twice the spatial resolution relative to node $A$ to capture more detail information.

## 3  The DP Algorithm for Detection

In detection, we first find all the locations in the image pyramid where the scores of the placed AOGs are higher than the estimated threshold $\tau$ . For example, at the original resolution, we have $\{u; \text{Score}(O, u) > \tau, u \in \Lambda\}$. Then, we will utilize the NMS to get final detection results. Since the AOG is directed and acyclic, the AOG scoring function is evaluated in two phases by utilizing the DP algorithm: (i) one bottom-up phase to compute all the appearance scoring maps for terminal-nodes, as well as their transformed maps for different parent nodes which are computed by using the efficient generalized distance transform [6], and then (ii) one top-down phase to retrieve the configurations (i.e., locations of car pair, single cars and parts) for all the locations whose scores are greater than the threshold $\tau$, followed by a post-processing NMS step in practice. We omit the obvious details of the DP algorithm here due to the limited space, which are referred to [5].

By the top-down back-tracing, we can obtain the "decoupled" single cars from detected occluding car pairs. Notice that we may have two inferred locations for a single car which is shared by two adjacent car pairs if the single car appears in the middle of a line of multiple occluding cars. Then, we use the location as the final detection result for the single car which is decoupled from the detected car pair with higher score.

## 4    Learning AOG by Latent Structural SVM

In this section, we formulate the learning of the AOG under the latent structural SVM (LSSVM) framework [13,14,16], which has been widely used in the literature of object detection and machine learning.

*Training Data.* We collect roadside cars from the real traffic video surveillance environment. We annotate the bounding boxes for both occluding car pairs and the corresponding two single cars . When labeling occluded single cars, we annotate their whole bounding boxes. Notice that some cars may be used twice in two adjacent car pairs when they appear in the middle of a line of multiple occluding cars. Those duplicated cars can be treated as bootstrapped ones in learning appearance parameters for single car and parts.

### 4.1    Latent Variables in the AOG

Given the training data specified above, for the AOG defined in Sec. 2.1, we have the latent variables as follows.

**The Branches of the Root Or-Node,** i.e., the mixture components of occluding car pairs. Based on the labeled bounding boxes, we initialize them using $k$-means clustering on the concatenated features ($k = 3$ clusters in our experiment): the aspect ratios of the three annotated bounding boxes and the displacements between the centers of the two single cars relative to that of the car pair (normalized by the size of the car pair bounding box). The aspect ratios of single cars can roughly indicate viewpoints, the displacement have clue on the configuration of car pair and the aspect ratio of car pair can reflect the degree of occlusions. In training, we also incorporate left-right flipped ones as done in [4]. So, we have 6 car pair models in total. We train the initial AOG (consisting of the root Or-node, the six car pair And-nodes, the twelve single car And-nodes, and the corresponding terminal-nodes for the And-nodes) under LSSVM framework by treating the locations and sizes of car pairs and single cars as hidden variables anchored at the annotated bounding boxes. At each step of re-labeling the positive examples (i.e. assigning latent variables) in learning, we force the the assignment of car pair terminal-nodes to overlap more than 0.7 with the ground-truth, and more than 0.8 for single car terminal nodes.

**The Part Configuration for Single Cars and Part-Sharing.** After the initial AOG is trained, we initialize the part configurations for the single cars based on the learned single car template, similar to the greedy pursuit method used in DPM [5]. We used 8 parts of rectangular shape and with equal sizes for each single car. For the part sharing, we use the similar method as done in [11], resulting in 30 part terminal-nodes in total.

## 4.2   Learning by LSSVM

Denote the set of positive training images by $D^+ = \{(I_1, y_1, z_1), \cdots, (I_n, y_n, z_n)\}$, where $y_i = 1$ and $z_i = (\omega_i, B_i, P_i)$ consisting of (i) The Or-node branching variable $\omega_i$ (i.e. the mixture component index); (ii) The labeled three bounding boxes $B_i$ for the car pair and the two single cars respectively; and (iii) The bounding boxes $P_i$ for parts of single cars. $z_i$'s are treated as latent variables during learning with different initialization: $\omega_i$ is initialized by the $k$-mean clustering stated above, $B_i$ by the annotated bounding boxes, and $P_i$ by the greedy pursuit and part-sharing strategy stated above. Let $D^- = \{(I_{n+1}, y_{n+1}), \cdots, (I_N, y_N)\}$ be a set of negative training images (i.e. images without cars appearing) where $y_i = -1$. We first train the initial AOG using $z_i = (\omega_i, B_i)$, and then initialize $P_i$ and learn the full AOG using $z_i = (\omega_i, B_i, P_i)$. Both are done under the LSSVM framework.

Given $z$, the scoring function is a linear function,

$$\text{Score}(I, y, z; \Theta) = <\Theta, \Phi(I, y, z)> \tag{6}$$

where $\Theta = (\Theta^{app}, \Theta^{def})$ and $\Phi(I, y, z) = (\Phi^{app}(I, y, z), \Phi^{def}(y, z))$ specified in Eqn. 3, Eqn. 4 and Eqn. 5.

Under the LSSVM framework, we learn $\Theta$ by solving the following surrogate loss function [14,16],

$$\min_{\Theta} \frac{1}{2}||\Theta||_2^2 +$$

$$\frac{C}{N} \sum_{i=1}^{N} [\max_{y,z}(\text{Score}(I_i, y, z; \Theta) + \Delta(y_i, y, z)) - \max_{z}(\text{Score}(I_i, y_i, z))] \tag{7}$$

where the loss function $\Delta(y_i, y, z) = 1$ if $y_i = y$, 0 otherwise, and $C$ is the tradeoff parameter balancing the first regularization term and the surrogate loss term. The objective function is non-convex, and the concave-convex procedure (CCP) [15,14,16] is used to get a local optimum.

Firstly, Eqn.7 can be re-written as,

$$
\min_{\Theta} \underbrace{\frac{1}{2}\|\Theta\|_2^2 + \frac{C}{N}\sum_{i=1}^{N}\max_{y,z}(\mathrm{Score}(I_i, y, z; \Theta) + \Delta(y_i, y, z))]}_{\triangleq f(\Theta),\ \text{convex function}} +
$$

$$
\underbrace{-\frac{C}{N}\sum_{i=1}^{N}\max_z(\mathrm{Score}(I_i, y_i, z))}_{\triangleq g(\Theta),\ \text{concave function}}
$$

$$(8)$$

Then, at step $t$, based on the current solution $\Theta_t$, The CCCP solves the problem with the two steps as follows.

(i) Bounding $g(\Theta)$ from the upper (since it is concave), i.e., finding hyperplane $p_t$ such that,

$$
g(\Theta) \le g(\Theta_t) + (\Theta - \Theta_t) \cdot p_t
$$

To do that, we first get the best latent variable assignment for each example by solving $z_i^* = \arg\max_{z_i} \mathrm{Score}(I, y_i, z_i)$ using the DP algorithm. Then, $p_t$ is constructed by,

$$
p_t = -\frac{C}{N}\sum_{i=1}^{N}\Phi(I_i, y_i, z_i^*)
$$

(ii) Updating the solution $\Theta_{t+1} = \arg\min_{\Theta}(f(\Theta) + \Theta \cdot p_t)$. The step leads to a standard structural SVM by using different "off-the-shelf" solver such as the cutting plane method. The details are referred to [13,16].

Figure 3 shows a portion of our learned AOG model. The first layer corresponding to car pair, the second layer corresponding to single car, and the third layer corresponding to car parts. Beside each node in the AOG, we visualize the learned appearance and deformation templates.

## 5    Experiments

To evaluate our proposed method, we collected 482 car images from street view scenes and annotated the bounding boxes for both car pairs and single cars. In detail, we obtained 1380 car pairs, 2760 occluded single cars and 702 unoccluded single cars. We randomly select 200 images for training, and use the rest for testing. For the negative set, we use the training negative images from PASCAL VOC 2007 database [3]. We also follow the VOC protocol for reporting results [3]. A putative bounding box is considered correct if the intersection of its bounding box with the ground-truth bounding box is greater than 50% of their union. Multiple detections for the same ground truth are penalized. We compute Precision-Recall (PR) curves and score the average precision (AP) across our test set.

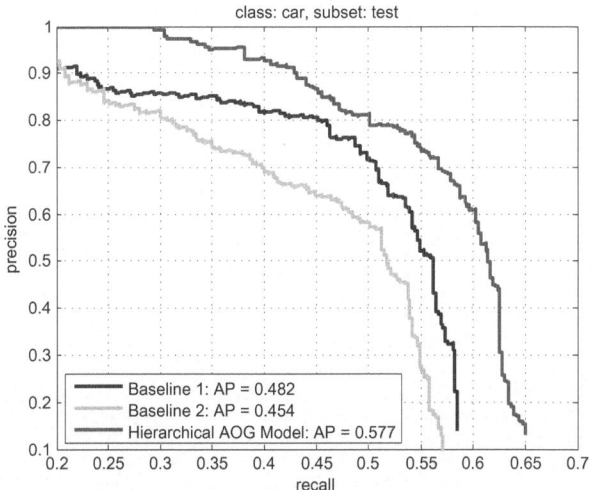

**Fig. 4.** Precision-Recall curves for our model and baseline methods

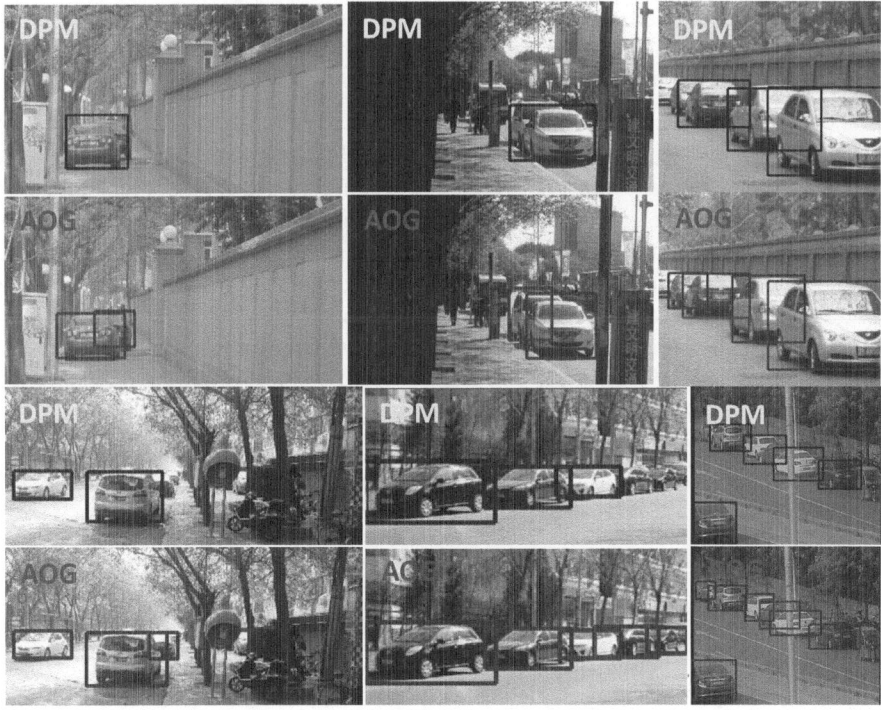

**Fig. 5.** Comparison of DPM car model and our hierarchical AOG model. The first row and the third row show the detection results (blue bounding boxes) of DPM car detector, the second and the fourth row show the detection results (red bounding boxes) of proposed AOG model. Best viewed in color.

In experiments, we compared our AOG with the two baseline DPMs: *Baseline 1.* DPM trained by using occluded single cars in the training set; *Baseline 2.* DPM trained by using all the single cars in the training set. Fig. 4 shows the PR curves of the three methods, where the proposed method outperforms the two baseline DPMs significantly (by 9.5% and 12.3% respectively).

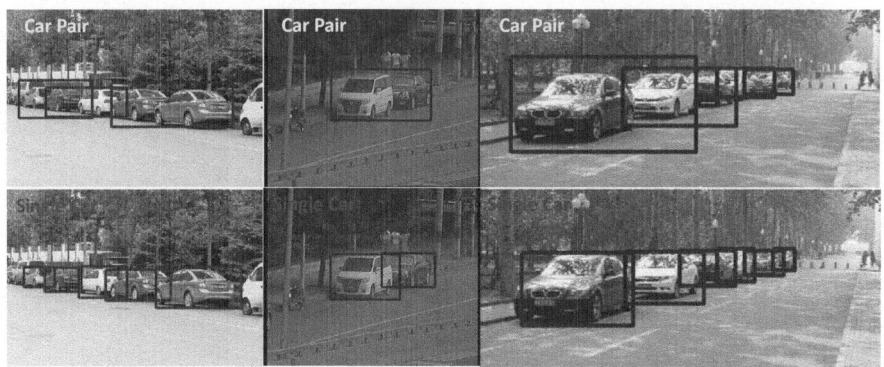

**Fig. 6.** Layered detections of our AOG model. Top: detection results of car pair module by coupling in the first layer. Bottom: detection results of single car module by decoupling in the second layer.

Figure 5 shows detection results of both DPM car model (*Baseline 1* is used since it is better than *Baseline 2* according to the PR curves) and our AOG model. Figure 6 shows some examples of layered detection results of Our AOG model. On the top, we show the detection results of car pair model in our AOG. On the bottom, detection results of single cars are shown by using the full AOG model. Here, we can see that our model can lead to fast coarse-to-fine detection, which we will further investigate in our on-going work.

## 6   Conclusion

In this paper, we proposed a hierarchical And-Or directed acyclic graph (AOG) model to address the problem of X-to-X-occlusion-free object detection. The model is a grammar model. It consists of (i) a root Or-node representing a mixture of different types of occluding X pairs, (ii) a set of And-nodes representing different types of occluding X pairs, (iii) another set of And-nodes representing different types of occluding single X's decomposed from X pairs, and (iv) a set of terminal-nodes representing the appearance templates for the X pairs, single X's and latent parts of the single X's. The part appearance templates can also be shared among different And-nodes of single X's. This model is learned by the latent structural SVM (LSSVM). DP algorithm is used for inference. Our model is a general model, though we only use cars as running examples in this paper, it can be used for other objects potentially.

**Acknowledgement.** We thank the three anonymous reviewers for their helpful comments. This work is supported by China 973 Program under Grant No. 2012CB316300, Natural Science Foundation of China under Grant No.90920009.

# References

1. Choi, J.Y., Sung, K.S., Yang, Y.K.: Multiple Vehicles Detection and Tracking based on Scale-Invariant Feature Transform. In: ITSC, pp. 528–533 (2007)
2. Dalal, N., Triggs, B.: Histograms of Oriented Gradients for Human Detection. In: CVPR, pp. 886–893 (2005)
3. Everingham, M., Van Gool, L., Williams, C.K.I., Winn, J., Zisserman, A.: The PASCAL Visual Object Classes Challenge 2007 (VOC 2007) Results (2007), http://www.pascal-network.org/challenges/VOC/voc2007/workshop/index.html
4. Felzenszwalb, P.F., Girshick, R.B., McAllester, D.: Discriminatively Trained Deformable Part Models, Release 4 (2010), http://people.cs.uchicago.edu/~pff/latent-release4/
5. Felzenszwalb, P.F., Girshick, R.B., McAllester, D.A., Ramanan, D.: Object Detection with Discriminatively Trained Part-Based Models. TPAMI 32, 1627–1645 (2010)
6. Felzenszwalb, P.F., Huttenlocher, D.P.: Distance Transforms of Sampled Functions. Technical report 2004-1963, Cornell University CIS (2004)
7. Gupte, S., Masoud, O., Martin, R.F.K., Papanikolopoulos, N.P.: Detection and Classification of Vehicles. TITS 3, 37–47 (2002)
8. Lai, A.H.S., Fung, G.S.K., Yung, N.H.C.: Vehicle Type Classification from Visual-based Dimension Estimation. In: ITSC, pp. 201–206 (2001)
9. Leotta, M.J., Mundy, J.L.: Vehicle Surveillance with a Generic, Adaptive, 3D Vehicle Model. TPAMI 33, 1457–1469 (2011)
10. Liu, X., Dai, B., He, H.: Real-Time On-Road Vehicle Detection Combining Specific Shadow Segmentation and SVM Classification. In: ICDMA, pp. 885–888 (2011)
11. Ott, P., Everingham, M.: Shared Parts for Deformable Part-based Models. In: CVPR, pp. 1513–1520 (2011)
12. Petrovic, V.S., Cootes, T.F.: Analysis of Features for Rigid Structure Vehicle Type Recognition. In: BMVC, pp. 587–596 (2004)
13. Tsochantaridis, I., Joachims, T., Hofmann, T., Altun, Y.: Large Margin Methods for Structured and Interdependent Output Variables. JMLR 6, 1453–1484 (2005)
14. Yu, C.N.J., Joachims, T.: Learning Structural SVMs with Latent Variables. In: ICML, pp. 1169–1176 (2009)
15. Yuille, A.L., Rangarajan, A.: The Concave-Convex Procedure (CCCP). In: NIPS, pp. 1033–1040 (2001)
16. Zhu, L., Chen, Y., Yuille, A.L., Freeman, W.T.: Latent Hierarchical Structural Learning for Object Detection. In: CVPR, pp. 1062–1069 (2010)
17. Zhu, S.C., Mumford, D.: A Stochastic Grammar of Images. FTCGV 2, 259–362 (2006)

# The Pooled NBNN Kernel:
# Beyond Image-to-Class and Image-to-Image

Konstantinos Rematas[1], Mario Fritz[2], and Tinne Tuytelaars[1]

[1] KU Leuven, ESAT-IBBT
[2] Max Planck Institute for Informatics

**Abstract.** While most image classification methods to date are based on image-to-image comparisons, Boiman *et al.* have shown that better generalization can be obtained by performing image-to-class comparisons. Here, we show that these are just two special cases of a more general formulation, where the feature space is partitioned into subsets of different granularity. This way, a series of representations can be derived that trade-off generalization against specificity.

Thereby we show a connection between NBNN classification and different pooling strategies, where, in contrast to traditional pooling schemes that perform spatial pooling of the features, pooling is performed in feature space. Moreover, rather than picking a single partitioning, we propose to combine them in a multi kernel framework. We refer to our method as the *Pooled NBNN kernel*. This new scheme leads to significant improvement over the standard image-to-image and image-to-class baselines, with only a small increase in computational cost.

## 1 Introduction

When Boiman *et al.* [1] presented their naive Bayes nearest neighbors (NBNN) classifier for multi-class image classification, it was surprising (and confronting) to see how well such a simple algorithm performed as compared to the machine-learning heavy methods used normally. As explained in [1], the success of this method can be attributed to two deviations from the standard approaches: i) the avoidance of a vector quantization step (*i.e.* no visual vocabularies), and ii) the use of image-to-class rather than image-to-image comparisons. While the former is definitely interesting, our focus in this paper goes to the latter aspect.

The NBNN approach combines a naive Bayes assumption together with an approximate Parzen estimate, that results in a very intuitive classification algorithm. The score of each test image with respect to a particular class is determined by how well the set of all features in the class can "reconstruct" the features in the test image. This is measured by summing over the distances to the nearest neighbors. By searching for nearest neighbors over all training images belonging to a class, a new test image is effectively classified by combining bits and pieces of information extracted from different training images. This obviously allows better generalization beyond the original set of training images.

K.M. Lee et al. (Eds.): ACCV 2012, Part I, LNCS 7724, pp. 176–189, 2013.
© Springer-Verlag Berlin Heidelberg 2013

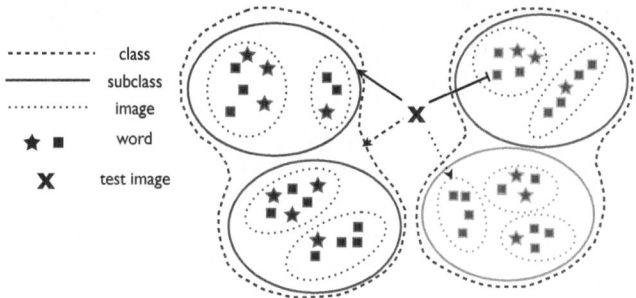

**Fig. 1.** The concept of our framework: For each feature from a given test image we can compute the distances to classes, distances to subclasses, distances to class specific feature clusters, or distances to individual images (= different ways of pooling the reference features in feature space). Summing these distances over all features in the test image (= traditional spatial pooling), we can build various alternative classification schemes in between image-to-image and image-to-class, or combine them for even better performance.

Here we propose to cluster the training images for each class in a number of smaller partitions and/or cluster the features in the reference images of a particular class into class-specific visual words (but without applying any vector quantization). Then a similar scheme as in the work of Boiman *et al.* can be applied (Figure 1), now sharing features within a cluster. This approach makes sense since an object class is defined mostly on semantic grounds, which do not necessarily match with coherence in visual appearance. For instance, different viewpoints typically correspond to different aspects, with completely different feature distributions. As a result, a class can contain different 'modes' or subclasses, where the visual appearance within a subclass is very similar yet can differ a lot between subclasses.

Recently, Tuytelaars *et al.* [2] have proposed a kernelized version of the NBNN framework of [1]. This new scheme keeps the image-to-class comparisons, while at the same time fitting it in the kernel-based line of work popular for image classification. The main advantage is that it allows easy integration with other kernels. Here, we build on the work of [2] and combine different kernels focusing on classes, sub classes and other partitionings at different levels of granularity.

In a sense, this is also reminiscent of the work on the pyramidal match kernel [3] or spatial pyramid [4]. Where they combine different levels of discretization in feature space and in the spatial domain respectively, our work investigates the combination of different levels of discretization along a different dimension, varying class granularity, from specific images over subclasses up to classes. In all these cases, instead of trying to select the one optimal operating point, various modes of operation can be combined into a single scheme for best performance.

*NBNN as pooling along a different dimension.* Most standard algorithms for image classification based on local features consist of the same three consecutive steps: i) feature coding, ii) feature pooling, and iii) classification. Typical examples of the first step (feature coding) include hard or soft assignment to visual words (vector quantization), sparse coding, or Locality-constrained Linear Coding. The second step is usually performed by spatial pooling, *e.g.* resulting in a spatial pyramid, and both sum pooling as well as max pooling have been proposed in this context. For the last step, a support vector machine remains the most popular choice. At first, NBNN or the NBNN kernel do not seem to fit in this scheme. Yet, they also perform various forms of pooling: the nearest neighbor selection can be seen as a max pooling step, while the Naive Bayes classification can be considered as sum pooling. This pooling is a bit extra-ordinary, in that it also pools information along a different dimension (over features extracted from the reference images, rather than features from the test image). We argue that, in other schemes, this type of pooling is also present, yet subsumed in the use of visual words, and therefore not made explicit.

In general, any image classification problem based on local features can be defined as follows: given the features from the training images, predict the correct label for a test image, based on a comparison between training and testing features. Their similarities can be represented by a very large matrix C of size $M \times N$ that contains the pairwise distances from $M$ testing features to the $N$ training features (with $N >> M$). Directly using the matrix C as input for classification doesn't work too well, since i) it's too large (making it impractical in terms of memory usage and sensitive to overfitting), and ii) it depends on the number of features extracted from the test image. So instead, the matrix has to be sparsified (typically achieved by coding) and to be reduced in dimensionality (typically done by pooling). Several methods perform these steps implicitly. For instance, vector quantization pools information from different features observed during training, and hence reduces $N$ to $W$ (the size of the vocabulary). Likewise, the bag-of-words model reduces the number of rows $M$ in C to 1 by pooling information over the entire test image.

In this light, NBNN can be interpreted as follows: a) the NN part reduces the columns of C from N (the number of training features) to the number of classes, by performing max pooling over all the training features belonging to a class, and b) the NB part reduces the rows of C from M (the number of test features) to 1, by sum pooling over all test features. In other words, the Naive Bayes scheme pools information both horizontally as well as vertically. The extension proposed in this paper further considers alternative ways of performing the 'horizontal' max pooling, by partitioning the training data in different ways (into classes, class-specific subclasses and visual words).

*Contributions:* Our main contribution is an exploration of the spectrum between image-to-image and image-to-class distances, that we form in a data-driven manner by building on the recent success of NBNN techniques. We hereby propose a novel series of intermediate object class representations. Combining them, we obtain strong performance on three computer vision benchmark datasets. Moreover, we show a connection between NBNN classification and different pooling strategies, where pooling is performed in feature space.

The remainder of this paper is organized as follows. First, we describe related work (section 2). Then we provide some background information on the NBNN framework of [1] and the kernelized version thereof proposed by [2] (section 3). In section 4, we describe how we extend this framework to explore the full spectrum between image-to-image and image-to-class. Section 5 describes our experimental results and section 6 concludes our paper.

## 2  Related Work

The application of kernel methods to the problem of visual classification has been very successful. From early bag-of-words representations [5] over pyramid schemes [3,4] to recent kernel combinations [6] these methods have greatly advanced the field. The key principle these methods operate on is a similarity measure between data points that is induced by a kernel function. While this unifying view might be perceived as one of the greatest strengths of this approach it comes also with a weakness. Similarities are measured globally between the examples. One direct consequence is that the model cannot easily incorporate any assumptions on the underlying data distribution.

Naive-Bayes-Nearest-Neighbor models (NBNN) [1] on the other hand make one of the most radical assumptions – which is independence between each feature dimension. This is right at the other end of the spectrum when compared with the kernel learning approach as they allow for an explanation of an observation at test time by a recombination of all features in the training using an image-to-class distance. While this approach has a strong generalization performance, it may loose consistency of the prediction as it takes feature sharing to the extreme. In order to balance strength and weaknesses of both approaches recent work aimed at combining both schools of thought [2]. Our work aims at exploring the spectrum in-between these two extremes.

There is a rich literature on employing hierarchies and/or taxonomies to aid classification. Various approaches are based on a semantic ontology as defined by models like wordnet [7,8]. While these ideas appeal on a computational as well as conceptual level, the results often lag behind the expected performance gains.

Apart from hierarchies defined by human domain knowledge, hierarchies and tree structures have a long standing tradition in the machine learning community (e.g. [9,10]). Here, the structure that supports classification is typically build in a data-driven way – and in fact it is unclear in which cases human or data-driven class groupings will give better support for classification. Recent methods followed up on this issue and suggest a relaxed hierarchy that accounts for semantic and classification cost [11]. Our approach follows this line of thought by forming subclasses and feature clusters that still obey the basic category labeling.

Recent work on pooling shows that the classification accuracy can be improved by choosing more carefully the pooling regions. Traditionally the pooling regions were the cells of the spatial pyramid in different levels. The work of [12] introduced spatial regions that do not follow the grid division of spatial pyramid and capture better dataset-specific spatial information. More close to our approach is the work of [13] where they exploit the partitioning in the feature space together with a spatial pyramid partition. However both these methods rely on a visual vocabulary.

## 3  Background

### 3.1  NBNN

For the NBNN classification we use the formulation of [14], which is based on [1]. The sampling of features is motivated by saliency and is similar to how the human eye process an image: starting from a feature $g_1$, the sampling continues to other features $g_t$ based on the saliency distribution $p(g_t|C = k)$ for a specific class $k$. We assume statistical independence between the points given the class label:

$$P(\{g_t\}_1^T|C = k) = \prod_{t=1}^{T} P(g_t|C = k),\qquad(1)$$

with $T$ the number of features. By applying Bayes rule we obtain:

$$P(C = k|\{g_t\}_1^T) = P(C = k) \prod_{t=1}^{T} P(g_t|C = k).\qquad(2)$$

with $P(C = k)$ considered uniform across classes. For the term in the product, the NBNN approach suggests the use of kernel density estimation that is approximated by the 1-nearest-neighbor term as follows [1]:

$$P(g_t|C = k) \propto \max_i \exp(-\|w_{k,i} - g_t\|_2^2),\qquad(3)$$

where $w_{k,i}$, $g_t$ are the original feature vectors of training and test features respectively. As described in [1], the spatial coordinates of each feature can be added to the feature vector, which has shown to improve results for object centered datasets like Caltech 101.

Finally, taking the log of the class posterior leads to the well know sum over minimum distances (nearest neighbors) of NBNN:

$$\log P(C = k|\{g_t\}_1^T) \propto \sum_{t=1}^{T} \max_i(-\|w_{k,i} - g_t\|_2^2)\qquad(4)$$

$$\propto \sum_{t=1}^{T} \min_i \|w_{k,i} - g_t\|_2^2\qquad(5)$$

### 3.2  Kernelized NBNN

In [2], the NBNN formulation has been extended to a discriminative scheme, the *NBNN* kernel. In this way, they were able to introduce the benefits of NBNN in a multiple kernel framework, where it can be combined with other kernels. In this paper we follow their approach for kernelizing the NBNN. However, in this work we focus on the exploitation of the information that is hidden inside the classes themselves and thus, we do not apply the combination with a bag-of-words scheme or phow kernels.

For the implementation of the NBNN kernel, we follow the formulation of [2]. The comparison of two feature sets $X = \{\mathbf{x}\}$ and $Y = \{\mathbf{y}\}$ is based on the *normalized sum match kernel* [15,16,17]:

$$K(X, Y) = \Phi(X)^T \Phi(Y) = \frac{1}{|X||Y|} \sum \sum k(\mathbf{x}, \mathbf{y}). \qquad (6)$$

The local kernel $k(\mathbf{x}, \mathbf{y})$ compares local features $\mathbf{x}$ and $\mathbf{y}$ and is computed as the dot-product between two vectors $\phi(\mathbf{x})$ and $\phi(\mathbf{y})$ with dimension equal to the number of classes and each element focusing on one particular class. $\phi(\mathbf{x})$ is a function of the distances from the feature $\mathbf{x}$ to its nearest neighbors in the different classes $c \in C$:

$$k(\mathbf{x}, \mathbf{y}) = \phi(\mathbf{x})^T \phi(\mathbf{y}), \qquad (7)$$

$$\phi(\mathbf{x}) = [\phi^1(\mathbf{x}) \quad \phi^2(\mathbf{x}) \quad \dots \quad \phi^{|C|}(\mathbf{x})], \qquad (8)$$

$$\phi^c(\mathbf{x}) = d_{\mathbf{x}}^c - d_{\mathbf{x}}^{\bar{c}}, \qquad (9)$$

with $d_{\mathbf{x}}^c$ the distance to the nearest neighbor of $\mathbf{x}$ belonging to class $c$ (calculated using the exponent shown in the right hand side of equation 3) and $d_{\mathbf{x}}^{\bar{c}}$ the distance to the nearest neighbor from all classes except $c$. As shown in equation 9, we follow the suggestion of [2] and do not use the nearest-neighbor distances directly but rather the original distance minus the distance to the nearest other class.

## 4   The pooled NBNN kernel

Our new image representation is based on two observations. First, the NBNN formulation in equation 4 can be understood as first performing max pooling over a code that is formed by computing $L_2$ distances to all features in the training set and then performing spatial sum pooling over all features in the test image. In this paper, we investigate more general pooling strategies for the max operator. While the NBNN approach performs max pooling (finds nearest neighbors) within the features of a certain class, we propose different pooling strategies that are more general. They can be more specific by only pooling over sub-classes or more general by not necessarily obeying class boundaries. The choices that we investigate for such generalized pooled NBNN features are detailed in section 4.1.

Second, while these NBNN features are not necessarily directly useful for classification anymore, we realize that the NBNN kernel [2] uses the class distance as a type of features. Therefore, we propose to include our generalized NBNN features into this kernel learning framework, so that the learning algorithm can exploit the different views on the data. Our experimental results support our claim that our new representation indeed captures complementary information which is useful for visual recognition

Finally, different partitions employed in the pooling scheme can be combined in a multikernel framework, resulting in a new kernel that effectively exploits different levels of granularity (from very specific to very generic). Our experiments show a consistent improvement by incorporating more partitions. Moreover, as we show later, evaluating this kernel is not much more expensive than evaluating the original NBNN kernel.

## 4.1   Partitioning the Feature Space

As described above the NBNN scheme implies a coding of features in terms of $L_2$ distances to the features in the training set. In contrast to the typical spatial pooling employed for visual recognition (which would relate to variations to the sum operator in equation 4), our method targets the max pooling operator in equation 4 that pools in appearance space. The NBNN suggests to pool over all features of the same class. In this section, we propose more general strategies.

The basic *structure* that features belong to is by definition the image, since the feature distribution is populated by features extracted from (training) images. However, we can generalize and assume that in a particular image one or more processes generated the data. This is also the assumption behind the visual word notion: that structures with similar appearance come from the same process.

We derive additional structures at different levels of granularity by clustering the features (or sets of features). In this process, we define an **atom** as an indivisible feature group that a cluster of features builds upon, and the **cluster-level** as the set of features to which the clustering is applied. In case of hierarchical clustering, the atoms correspond to the leaf nodes, while the cluster-level determines the root node. In order to further clarify our framework, we start by describing the image-to-class model for object classification according to our new terminology.

**Image to Class.** In the case of the image-to-class (I2C) distance framework [1], the atoms are images and the cluster-level is the class level. The reason why we consider the images as atoms and not the features directly is because the set of features from a training image can not be separated. In other words, we can not assign features from the same image to different clusters. Note that in this case no clustering algorithm is actually performed and the assignment of atoms to clusters is determined solely based on the annotation (a cluster contains all the features from images with the corresponding class label).

In this paper we focus on two extensions:

1. The atoms are individual images and the cluster-level is the class. This case is similar to the I2C case, but clustering is performed at the class level, resulting in a number of subclasses for each class. We refer to this case as *Image to Subclass* (I2Sub).

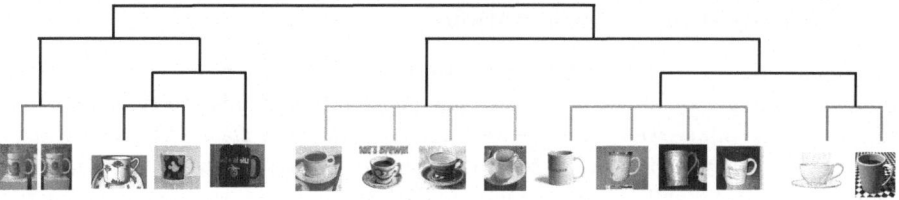

**Fig. 2.** Visualization of the hierarchical partition of class *cup* into 2,4 and 6 subclasses.

2. The atoms are individual features and the cluster-level is the class. The cluster in the feature space can be seen as a large visual word. Therefore, for a new image we calculate the *Image-to-Word* distance (I2Word).

**Image to Subclass.** For the first case, where we are looking in every class separately and the building block is the image, we need to define a measure of similarity between the image feature distributions. Here we use the image-to-image distance, i.e. the sum of the distances of features in image 1 to their nearest neighbors in image 2. This way we obtain a distance matrix of all images belonging to the same class. Based on the distance matrix we apply agglomerative clustering with complete linkage. The result of the clustering shows which images are clustered to the same subclass. Figure 2 illustrates two classes with two of their subclasses from the Caltech-101 dataset.

Each subclass contains images from the original class that are similar in feature space, resulting in a more coherent set of features in feature space. A new test image is then compared to all the subclasses separately. This does not only provide more information to the final classifier, but also reduces the chance of false positives ('accidentally' obtaining a small distance-to-(sub)class is less likely since the subclasses are more compact in feature space). The computation of the distances to subclasses is similar to Eq $(8)^1$.

**Image to Word.** For the second case, we partition our features based on their location in feature space, without imposing features from the same image to be assigned to the same cluster. The cluster level is the class, and therefore features from images of different classes will never end up in the same cluster. As a result, the clusters we obtain are somehow similar to class specific visual words. However, note that we do not perform vector quantization, so this is only a partial analogy. Clusters are created by applying K-means on all features from a class. After that, the original class label is no longer used. For a new image, we then calculate the distance to all class specific "visual-word-like" clusters[2].

---

[1] During training, if a subclass consists of only 1 image, its distance to its own subclass is the average of distances of all images within the class.

[2] But note that the number of clusters is typically kept low, and therefore features within a single cluster show more variability than the variability usually observed in visual words.

## 4.2    Computational Considerations

The clustering of features into subclasses and word clusters is performed once during training. For a new test image the procedure is similar to [1,2]. For each feature in the image we find its nearest neighbor in every class, subclass or word cluster and calculate the distance to that cluster of features using equation (3). Note however that all the partitions of the feature space are performed in the class level. Therefore, we know for each training feature to which partition it belongs (class, subclasses, clusters). Now during testing, the small number of NIMBLE features per image (100) allow us to compute the distance of a test feature to all training features in a class. Thus, by performing a search algorithm we can efficiently find the 1st nn for every semantic partition, without the need for nn search for every kernel case (the nn search time only increases from 7.7 s per image to 9.2 s per image for 15 scenes).

## 5    Experiments

In this section we provide quantitative results for the proposed framework. We investigate different partitions of our feature sets as described in section 4 and combine the resulting kernel representations in a multi-kernel framework. For combining the kernels, we simply use an average kernel as previous results [6] have shown that typical multi-kernel learning schemes tend to results in the same performance range as the average kernel with the cost of additional parameter selection. Our investigations have confirmed this observation for our setting too.

**Datasets.** In order to embed our results in the context of previous methods and compare to the state-of-the-art we have chosen the following three, widely used datasets: Caltech 101 [18], 15 Scenes [4] and Oxford Flowers 17 [19]. Caltech 101 provides a large number of classes and large intra-class variation, which we believe can be captured well by our distance-to-subclass approach (see also figure 2). 15 Scenes dataset on the other hand contains less classes and the intra-class variation is smaller but each class contains a larger number of images, which makes it better suited for svm training. The Oxford Flowers 17 dataset presents high intra-class variation and difficult separation across classes. Moreover, each class contains a large number of images.

**Implementation Details.** We use 4 random train/test splits in order to infer the results presented in this paper (every result is the average over 4 splits). For generating the train/test splits in all datasets we use the framework of [14], that picks random train and test images from each class. Note that, unlike [20,2], we did not add jittered images.

The image representation in our paper is based on the NIMBLE features proposed in [14]. For the experiments reported in this work we use the publicly available code of [14] for extracting the features and the same training/testing setup. We sample 100 features per image, and each of these is described with a 500 dimensional descriptor. This allows for fast and exact nearest-neighbor matching. While NIMBLE features are a convenient choice in the context of

NBNN methods, thanks to their sparsity, we would like to stress that the method proposed in this paper is generic and by no means limited to one particular type of features. The location information was used as additional dimension in the feature vectors similar to [1,14], weighted with a scalar $\alpha$ (1 for Caltech and 17 Flowers and 0.5 for 15 Scenes). We compute the NBNN distances using the code of [21] (FASTANN) for exact nearest neighbor. For training and testing the support vector machines we use the liblinear package [22] with $L_2$-regularized $L_2$-loss support vector classification (primal).

When computing the I2C and I2Subclass distances for the training images, we exclude the image itself from the class set. This way the distance of a training image to the class it belongs to better represents the distance that a testing image will have to the particular class (even if it results in a slightly lower number of class features in those cases, since one image is removed). An alternative could be to remove only the feature under consideration. This approach is followed for the I2Words experiments.

Note that we also report results for vanilla NBNN (i.e., non-kernelized). Since the clusters in our experiments are always class-specific, this is indeed possible, using the following routine: for a new image, we compute the distances to each of the partitions for all features, select the cluster with the smallest cumulative distance, and assign the label of the corresponding class.

| Method | NBNN | NBNN kernel |
|---|---|---|
| I2C (baseline) | 72.0±0.3 | 76.0 ± 0.8 |
| I2Sub-2 | 72.3±1.5 | 76.4 ± 0.4 |
| I2Sub-4 | 68.9±1 | 76.3 ± 2.3 |
| I2Sub-6 | 68.1±3.1 | 76.6 ± 1.0 |
| I2Sub-10 | 66.1±8 | 77.0 ± 0.5 |
| I2Sub-20 | 66.2±1.7 | 76.4 ± 0.4 |
| I2Word-2 | 70.7±0.8 | 74.8 ± 1.3 |
| I2Word-4 | 67.0±0.6 | 74.8 ± 0.5 |
| I2Word-8 | 63.5±1.3 | 75.9 ± 0.3 |
| I2Word-16 | 61.0±0.6 | 74.4 ± 0.7 |
| I2Word-32 | 60.2±3.2 | 71 ± 3 |
| Average Kernel | - | **79.7±1.5** |

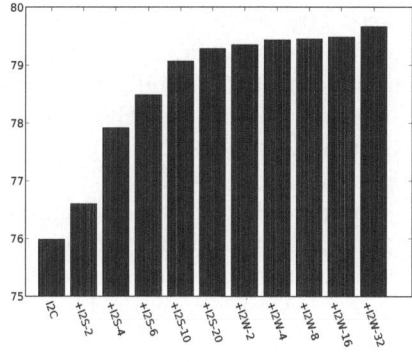

**Fig. 3.** Classification accuracy of NBNN and NBNN kernel for different pooling strategies in 15 Scenes

**Fig. 4.** Performance gain for 15 Scenes when adding kernels. The order of addition is the same order as in Table 3

**15 Scenes.** This dataset contains images from indoor and outdoor scenes belonging to 15 different classes. Both for training and testing we use 100 images. Figure 3 shows the results for the individual partitions as we increase the number of subclasses (I2Sub*) or the number of words (I2Word-*). Using complete agglomerative clustering, we generate for every class 2, 4, 6, 10 and 20 subclasses. For the generation of the word clusters, we use K means with 2, 4, 8, 16 and 32 clusters.

| Method | NBNN | NBNN kernel |
|--------|------|-------------|
| I2C (baseline) | 81.9±1.9 | 83.08±1.5 |
| I2Sub-2 | 81.9±1.9 | 82.9±4.2 |
| I2Sub-4 | 81.1±0.6 | 82.5±1 |
| I2Sub-6 | 79.6±1.6 | 82.6±2 |
| I2Sub-10 | 78.3±3.8 | 82.7±2.1 |
| I2Sub-20 | 77.2±2.1 | 81.7±4.1 |
| I2Word-2 | 80.6±0.1 | 82.3±0.4 |
| I2Word-4 | 77.8±0.8 | 83.5±1.6 |
| I2Word-8 | 72.3±7.5 | 80.3±1 |
| I2Word-16 | 66.9±14 | 82.3±1.2 |
| I2Word-32 | 66.0±11 | 80.8±0.7 |
| Average Kernel | - | **85.3±3.1** |

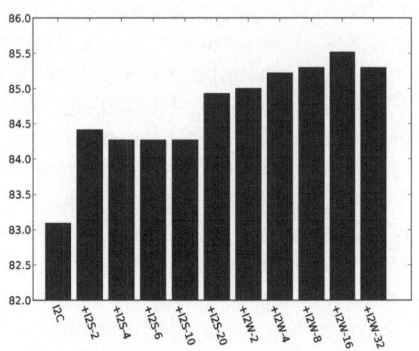

**Fig. 5.** Classification accuracy of NBNN and NBNN kernel for different pooling strategies in 17 Flowers

**Fig. 6.** Performance gain for 17 Flowers when adding kernels. The order of addition is the same order as in Table 5

In accordance with previous findings [2], when using image-to-class comparisons, the NBNN kernel outperforms NBNN in this setting with a performance of 76% versus 72.0%. For NBNN we see a gradual decrease when going to the more fine grained representations. For the NBNN kernel the results seem to be more stable around 75 − 77%. We attribute this to the discriminative training. The kernel framework allows us to further boost performance by combining all the representations in a multi-kernel setting. With a total performance of 79.7% we outperform the best individual kernel by over 2.5% and the NBNN baseline by almost 8%. We consider this as a strong indication that our approach indeed derives representations that capture different aspects of the object classes.

Figure 4 further illustrates the performance gain by adding a single kernel at a time according to the ordering in Table 3 (top to bottom). We observe a consistent improvement by gradually enriching the representation and we achieve strong performance even compared to methods that use a more elaborate spatial model (*e.g.* best results reported in [23,2] rely on a Spatial Pyramid). In 15 Scenes NIMBLE seems not to preform as well as on the other datasets due to the small number of features and saliency map based sampling instead of dense sampling.

**17 Flowers.** This dataset contains 17 different flower classes with each of them consisting of 80 images. For our experiment we use 60 images for training and 20 for testing. The results are summarized in Table 5. Similar to the previous experiment, we observe better performance for the kernelized NBNN compared to NBNN, since the number of training images is large enough.

This experiment is in line with the previous one regarding overall trends and the relative performance of the different kernels. The individual kernels do not exceed the performance of the I2C kernel but their combination again results in an increase in performance. In particular, our final result achieves state-of-the-art results (to the best of our knowledge) compared to other methods that only use one feature. ([24] Color-opponent-SIFT 80%, result taken from [25]).

| Method | NBNN | NBNN kernel |
|---|---|---|
| I2C | 70.6±0.9 | 66.6±0.8 |
| I2Sub-2 | 68.8±1.3 | 67.7±0.9 |
| I2Sub-4 | 66.5±1 | 67.3±1.3 |
| I2Sub-6 | 65.3±1.5 | 67.4±0.1 |
| I2Word-2 | 64.8±0.9 | 68.6±0.6 |
| I2Word-4 | 59.7±2.2 | 68±3 |
| I2Word-8 | 54.5±2 | 61±7 |
| I2Word-16 | 51.0±1 | 43±3 |
| Average Kernel | - | **71.9±0.3** |

**Fig. 7.** Classification accuracy in Caltech 101 (15 images)

| Method | NBNN | NBNN kernel |
|---|---|---|
| I2C | 77.8±0.3 | 76.7±0.5 |
| I2Sub-5 | 73.5±1 | 77.1±1.1 |
| I2Sub-10 | 71.9±1.6 | 77.2±2.6 |
| I2Sub-15 | 71.1±2.2 | 76.2±5.2 |
| I2Word-2 | 72.2±1.3 | 75.3±1.4 |
| I2Word-4 | 67.3±1.8 | 75.4±1.7 |
| I2Word-8 | 61.2±0.6 | 68.8±1.4 |
| I2Word-16 | 57.5±1.6 | 50.8±13 |
| Average Kernel | - | **81.0±1** |

**Fig. 8.** Classification accuracy in Caltech 101 (30 images)

| Method | 15 images | 30 images |
|---|---|---|
| Gehler et al.. [6] | 61.0 ± 0.2 | 69.4 ± 0.4 |
| Griffin et al.. [26] | 59.4 | 67.6 ± 1.4 |
| NBNN [1] | 65.0 ± 1.1 | ~ 72.4 |
| LLE [27] | 65.43 | 73.4 |
| Vedaldi et al.[20] | 66.3 ± 1.1 | - |
| ScSPM [28] | 67.0 ± 0.5 | 73.2 ± 0.5 |
| Pinto et al.. [29] | 61.4 | 67.4 |
| NIMBLE [14] | 70.8±0.7 | 78.5±0.4 |
| NBNN kernel+phow [2] | 69.2 ± 0.9 | 75.2 ± 1.2 |
| GLP+LLC+SPM [23] | 70.3 | **82.6** |
| ours | **71.9±0.3** | 81±1.0 |

**Fig. 9.** Comparison of the proposed method with state-of-the-art (using only one feature type)

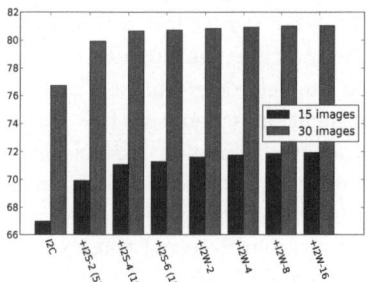

**Fig. 10.** Performance gain for Caltech 101 when adding kernels

**Caltech-101.** Finally, we report results on Caltech-101 [18]. While criticized by many, it is still a widely used dataset, that allows us to compare our method against a wide range of methods in the literature.

First, we study the behavior of different representations derived by our pooled NBNN kernel on Caltech101 using only 15 training images (see figures 7 and 10). For this experiment we investigate 2,4 and 6 subclasses and 2,4,8 and 16 word clusters. We stop at this granularity due to the limited number of training images and hence lack of data in this setting. The findings are consistent with the previous two datasets (adding kernels increase the accuracy, Figure 10). We see a steady decrease in performance for the NBNN method while the NBNN kernel roughly remains constant (or slightly increases). We observe that the NBNN kernel performance at 66.6% is lower than the NBNN baseline at 70.6%. This is an issue already encountered in previous work [2] and is owed to the small number of available samples that makes holding out samples for NBNN representation and classifier learning difficult. However, when combining all the kernels we again manage to (slightly) outperform the NBNN approach with a total performance of 71.9% – even in this unfavorable setting. Hereby, we manage to cure a problem that previous settings were troubled with in the low sample regime. In the second experiment on Caltech 101 we use 30 images for training (Fig. 8). When the number of images is increased the NBNN kernel performs better.

Finally, in Table 9 we compare our best results (the average kernels including I2C, I2Sub and I2Word) to other approaches in the literature using a single feature type, on Caltech 101 with 15/30 images. To the best of our knowledge, for 15 training images our system gives the highest performance among all methods using a single descriptor.

## 6   Conclusion

We have presented a series of object representations that extend previous image-to-image and image-to-class distances to a more general framework that models an object class with a set of distances to partitions of the features space. This representation has an interesting dual interpretation as pooling over features from the reference images. In particular it provides new insights to the NBNN classification scheme in the context of feature coding and pooling. Therefore we call it the pooled NBNN kernel. We explore a variety of partition schemes including subclasses (obeying image constraints and class boundaries) and 'class-specific visual word'-like clusters (obeying class boundaries only) and combine them in a multi-kernel framework.

A combination of all the kernels we derive leads to consistent performance improvements which lets us conclude that the associated representations indeed capture different aspects of the object classes. The resulting kernel achieves strong performance across 3 widely used recognition benchmarks and in particular outperforms the state of the art on Caltech101 and 17 Flowers using a single feature.

**Acknowledgment.** We acknowledge the support from ERC grant Cognimund.

## References

1. Boiman, O., Shechtman, E., Irani, M.: In defense of nearest-neighbor based image classification. In: CVPR (2008)
2. Tuytelaars, T., Fritz, M., Saenko, K., Darrell, T.: The nbnn kernel. In: ICCV (2011)
3. Grauman, K., Darrell, T.: The pyramid match kernel: Efficient learning with sets of features. JMLR 8, 725–760 (2007)
4. Lazebnik, S., Schmid, C., Ponce, J.: Beyond bags of features: Spatial pyramid matching for recognizing natural scene categories. In: CVPR (2006)
5. Csurka, G., Dance, C.R., Fan, L., Willamowski, J., Bray, C.: Visual categorization with bags of keypoints. In: Workshop on Statistical Learning in Computer Vision, ECCV, pp. 1–22 (2004)
6. Gehler, P.V., Nowozin, S.: On feature combination for multiclass object classification. In: ICCV (2009)

7. Marszałek, M., Schmid, C.: Constructing Category Hierarchies for Visual Recognition. In: Forsyth, D., Torr, P., Zisserman, A. (eds.) ECCV 2008, Part IV. LNCS, vol. 5305, pp. 479–491. Springer, Heidelberg (2008)

8. Deng, J., Berg, A.C., Li, K., Fei-Fei, L.: What Does Classifying More Than 10,000 Image Categories Tell Us? In: Daniilidis, K., Maragos, P., Paragios, N. (eds.) ECCV 2010, Part V. LNCS, vol. 6315, pp. 71–84. Springer, Heidelberg (2010)

9. Zhigang, L., Wenzhong, S., Qianqing, Q., Xiaowen, L., Donghui, X.: Hierarchical-support vector machines. In: IGARSS (2005)

10. Xia, S., Li, J., Xia, L., Ju, C.: Tree-Structured Support Vector Machines for Multi-class Classification. In: Liu, D., Fei, S., Hou, Z., Zhang, H., Sun, C. (eds.) ISNN 2007, Part III. LNCS, vol. 4493, pp. 392–398. Springer, Heidelberg (2007)

11. Gao, T., Koller, D.: Discriminative learning of relaxed hierarchy for large-scale visual recognition. In: ICCV (2011)

12. Jia, Y., Huang, C., Darrell, T.: Beyond spatial pyramids: Receptive field learning for pooled image features. In: CVPR (2012)

13. Boureau, Y., Le Roux, N., Bach, F., Ponce, J., LeCun, Y.: Ask the locals: multi-way local pooling for image recognition. In: ICCV (2011)

14. Kanan, C., Cottrell, G.: Robust classification of objects, faces, and flowers using natural image statistics. In: CVPR (2010)

15. Lyu, S.: Mercer kernels for object recognition with local features. In: CVPR (2005)

16. Bo, L., Sminchisescu, C.: Efficient match kernel between sets of features for visual recognition. In: Advances in Neural Information Processing Systems (2009)

17. Haussler, D.: Convolution kernels on discrete structures. In: Technical Report (1999)

18. Fei-Fei, L., Fergus, R., Perona, P.: Learning generative visual models from few training examples: an incremental Bayesian approach tested on 101 object categories. In: Workshop on Generative-Model Based Vision (2004)

19. Nilsback, M.E., Zisserman, A.: A visual vocabulary for flower classification. In: CVPR (2006)

20. Vedaldi, A., Gulshan, V., Varma, M., Zisserman, A.: Multiple kernels for object detection. In: ICCV (2009)

21. Philbin, J., Chum, O., Isard, M., Sivic, J., Zisserman, A.: Object retrieval with large vocabularies and fast spatial matching. In: CVPR (2007)

22. Fan, R.E., Chang, K.W., Hsieh, C.J., Wang, X.R., Lin, C.J.: Liblinear: A library for large linear classification. JMLR 9, 1871–1874 (2008)

23. Feng, J., Ni, B., Tian, Q., Yan, S.: Geometric lp-norm feature pooling for image classification. In: CVPR (2011)

24. van de Sande, K.E.A., Gevers, T., Snoek, C.G.M.: Evaluating color descriptors for object and scene recognition. PAMI 32, 1582–1596 (2010)

25. Fernando, B., Fromont, E., Muselet, D., Sebban, M.: Discriminative feature fusion for image classification. In: CVPR (2012)

26. Griffin, G., Holub, A., Perona, P.: Caltech-256 object category dataset (2007)

27. Wang, J., Yang, J., Yu, K., Lv, F., Huang, T., Gong, Y.: Locality-constrained linear coding for image classification. In: CVPR (2010)

28. Yang, J., Yu, K., Gong, Y., Huang, T.: Linear spatial pyramid matching using sparse coding for image classification. In: CVPR (2009)

29. Pinto, N., Cox, D.D., DiCarlo, J.J.: Why is real-world visual object recognition hard? In: PLoS Computational Biology (2008)

# Local Hypersphere Coding
# Based on Edges between Visual Words

Weiqiang Ren[1], Yongzhen Huang[1], Xin Zhao[2], Kaiqi Huang[1], and Tieniu Tan[1]

[1] National Laboratory of Pattern Recognition, CASIA, China
[2] Department of Automation, University of Science and Technology of China, China
{wqren,yzhuang,xzhao,kqhuang,tnt}@nlpr.ia.ac.cn

**Abstract.** Local feature coding has drawn much attention in recent years. Many excellent coding algorithms have been proposed to improve the bag-of-words model. This paper proposes a new local feature coding method called local hypersphere coding (LHC) which possesses two distinctive differences from traditional coding methods. Firstly, we describe local features by the edges between visual words. Secondly, the reconstruction center is moved from the origin to the nearest visual word, thus feature coding is performed on the hypersphere of feature space. We evaluate our coding method on several benchmark datasets for image classification. The experimental results of the proposed method outperform several state-of-the-art coding methods, indicating the effectiveness of our method.

## 1 Introduction

Local feature coding has been a standard technique in bag-of-words model based image classification. In recent years a large number of coding methods have been designed, achieving state-of-the-art performance on public classification benchmark datasets.

The typical bag-of-words based image classification framework consists of four steps: (1) **Local feature extraction**. Usually local feature descriptors (e.g. SIFT [1], HOG [2]) are densely extracted from each image. (2) **Local feature coding**. In this step, each local feature is encoded with a precomputed dictionary. Coding methods play a vital role in enhancing the discriminative power of image representation. Many recent researches focus on designing more powerful coding methods, from the basic hard quantization [3] to more sophisticated coding methods, e.g. soft quantization [4], sparse coding [5], locality-constraint linear coding(LLC) [6], super vector coding [7],improved fisher kernel [8] [9], etc. (3) **Spatial pooling**. The coding responses of the local features on each visual word are then pooled into a single value, concatenating all these pooled values produces the final image representation. Successful pooling operations include max pooling [5], average pooling [10], weighted average pooling [7], etc. As the standard bag-of-words model does not consider the geometric layout, spatial pyramid matching(SPM) [10] is usually adopted to improve the classification performance. (4) **Classification**. Usually over-complete dictionary is used for

K.M. Lee et al. (Eds.): ACCV 2012, Part I, LNCS 7724, pp. 190–203, 2013.
© Springer-Verlag Berlin Heidelberg 2013

local feature coding, thus the image representation will typically have very high dimensionality. In such case, linear SVM will greatly reduce the training time while obtain even better performance than non-linear classifiers.

As an important step in bag-of-words model, local feature coding can be viewed as a feature space transformation. Local features are transformed from local feature space into a new feature space spanned by a set of precomputed visual words, with higher dimensionality. Traditionally, local feature coding methods are designed based on reconstruction by a linear combination of dictionary bases under different constraints. Sparse coding [11] adds sparsity constraint on reconstruction term, while LLC [6] introduces locality constraint. On the one hand, reconstruction based local feature coding methods retain the most important information by restricting the reconstruction error to be low. On the other hand, they put specific constraint on the solution to obtain discriminative and robust representation. These are also the goal of the proposed coding method in this paper.

As the local feature and visual words are usually $\ell^2$ normalized to unit length, they are all distributed on the surface of a hyperball. Traditional coding methods are carried out in this hyperball, with the local feature described by a linear combination of the visual words. Fig 1-(a) illustrates the reconstruction of local feature $\mathbf{x}$ by a set of visual words. In Fig 1-(a), visual word $\mathbf{d}_1, \mathbf{d}_2$ and $\mathbf{d}_3$ are used for describing local feature $\mathbf{x}$. If $\mathbf{d}_1, \mathbf{d}_2, \mathbf{d}_3$ and $\mathbf{x}$ are coplanar, $\mathbf{x}$ can be perfectly reconstructed by these three visual words. However, in most situations, this assumption does not hold true. Wang $et\ al.$ [6] pointed out that, under certain assumptions, reconstructing local feature with visual words locating on a local smooth manifold produces lower reconstruction error than normal sparse coding. Motivated by the local smooth assumption, we propose to move the origin to the hypersphere and do feature coding on the hypersphere. As shown in Fig 1-(b), rather than reconstruction local feature with visual words, we propose to use the edges connecting the visual words for reconstruction. As a local region on the hypersphere is close to hyperplane, reconstruction on this hypersphere will produce less error than the traditional methods.

We have three main contributions in this paper:

1. Compared with traditional reconstruction based coding methods, we extend the idea of locality and smoothness and perform feature coding on the hypersphere. Moving the origin onto the hypersphere and reconstructing on a local smooth hypersphere obtains better reconstruction and more distinctive representation.

2. The edges between the visual words are utilized for reconstructing the edge from each visual word to the local feature. To the best of our knowledge, this is the first work that encodes local feature with edges between visual words.

3. The proposed new coding scheme can be readily applied to the existing methods. The notion of reconstruction with edges between visual words are general and more regularization can be added to obtain more specialize representation.

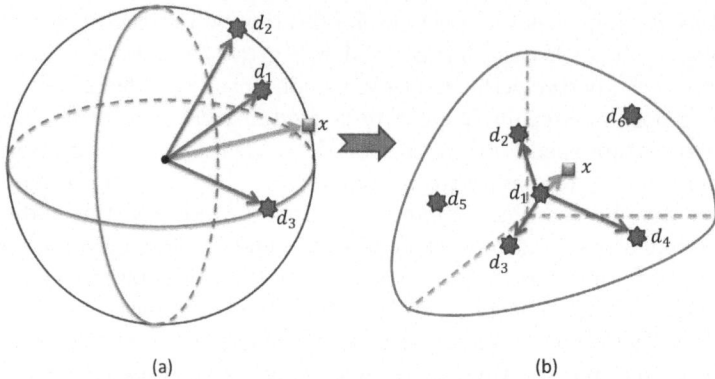

**Fig. 1.** The reconstruction scheme of traditional coding methods and the proposed method. The red stars on the hypersphere are the visual words, while the blue rectangle denotes the local feature to be described. (a) illustrates the reconstruction of traditional reconstruction based coding methods. (b) demonstrates the reconstruction in the proposed method. Note that the coding process is performed on the hypersphere. See text for detail explanation.

The rest of the paper is organized as follows: Section 2 reviews the development of coding method in bag-of-words model. Section 3 presents the proposed feature coding method on hypersphere. In Section 4, we report the experiment results on three widely used benchmark datasets and discuss the parameter settings and its influence on the classification results. And finally in Section 5, we draw the conclusion and discuss the future work.

## 2   Related Work

Over the years there have been a large quantity of novel coding methods proposed for improving the bag-of-words model. These coding methods roughly fall into two categories: (1) reconstruction based coding methods, like hard quantization, sparse coding, LLC, etc. (2) describing the differences between local features and visual words, for example, super vector coding and fisher kernel.

Hard quantization [3] is the basic coding method applied in bag-of-words based image classification. Each local feature votes on the nearest visual words and the final image representation is a histogram of the voting responses.

From the reconstruction point of view, hard quantization only utilizes the nearest visual word. Hard quantization can be viewed as a description of local feature with one single visual word. When dictionary size is small, hard quantization will introduces large quantization error. Soft quantization [4] improves this problem by voting on multiple visual words. Salient coding [12] employs the ratio between local descriptors' nearest code and other codes as the salient representation.

Sparse coding [11] is also reconstruction based method, where sparsity constraint is added. The solution of sparse coding is generally sparse and the responses on most of the visual words are close to zero. Sparse coding achieves better reconstruction than hard quantization and produces more distinctive sparse response. It has been adopted in image classification (See [5]) and achieves state-of-the-art results on several public benchmarks.

However, the $\ell^1$ regularization in sparse coding is not smooth, thus sparse coding might project on totally different visual words for similar local features. Moreover, the $\ell^1$ regularization makes it computationally expensive to do sparse coding. To tackle the problem of sparse coding, LLC [6] replaces the sparsity constraint with locality constraint. It encodes the local feature by projecting each local feature into its local-coordinate system. An approximated version of LLC has more clearly locality constraint and a simpler format than standard LLC. The coding process is performed only on the K-nearest neighbor, where a constraint least square problem can be solved efficiently.

Recently, several more powerful feature coding methods have been proposed, such as code graph [13], fisher kernel [8,9], super vector coding [7], and vector difference coding[14]. Huang et.al [13] propose to improve image classification via exploring the relationship between visual words. Fisher kernel combines the power of both generative model and discriminative model. Rather than explicitly reconstruction of local feature, fisher kernel records the first and second order differences between local features and visual words. Super vector encodes local feature by recording the differences between local feature an visual words. Zhao et.al [14] perform feature coding based on the vector difference in a high-dimensional space via explicit feature maps. Fisher kernel, super vector and vector difference coding representations are about $M$ times larger than other coding methods, such as hard quantization, soft quantization, and LLC. Nevertheless, they achieve state-of-the-art results on several challenging benchmark such as the PASCAL VOC and ImageNet.

## 3   Proposed Method

In this Section, we first briefly review the traditional reconstruction scheme of several classical bag-of-words based coding methods in Section 3.1, then in Section 3.2 we present the proposed local feature coding method in details.

### 3.1   Traditional Reconstruction Scheme of Bag-of-Words Based Coding

Denote $\mathbf{x} \in \mathbb{R}^M$ as a local feature descriptor, e.g., SIFT, HOG, etc., $M$ is the dimensionality of the local feature descriptor. Let $\mathbf{X} = [\mathbf{x}_1, \mathbf{x}_2, \cdots, \mathbf{x}_N] \in \mathbb{R}^{M \times N}$ be the local features extracted from an image. $\mathbf{D} = [\mathbf{d}_1, \mathbf{d}_2, \cdots, \mathbf{d}_K] \in \mathbb{R}^{M \times K}$ is the dictionary with $K$ visual words trained by clustering or dictionary learning. Let $\mathbf{z}$ be the encoded feature. For reconstruction based coding methods, the dimensionality of $\mathbf{z}$ is usually $K$, while for other coding methods the dimensionality may be far more larger than $K$.

For the traditional reconstruction based coding method in bag-of-words model, such as hard quantization, sparse coding, LLC, etc., we can readily put them into an unified framework:

$$\mathbf{z} = \arg\min_{\mathbf{z}} \|\mathbf{x} - \mathbf{Dz}\|_2^2 + \lambda r(\mathbf{z}) \tag{1}$$
$$s.t. \ \mathbf{z} \in \mathcal{C}$$

where $r(\mathbf{z})$ is the regularization term designed from different intuition and $\mathcal{C}$ denote some constraints on the solution.

For hard quantization, $r(\mathbf{z}) = 0$ and $\mathcal{C} = \{\mathbf{z} \mid \|\mathbf{z}\|_0 = 1, \ \mathbf{1}^T\mathbf{z} = 1\}$. The constraint forces the solution to have only one response. This means that hard quantization always produces a coarse reconstruction of $\mathbf{x}$.

For sparse coding, $r(\mathbf{z}) = \|\mathbf{z}\|_1$ and $\mathcal{C} = \mathbb{R}^K$, the $\ell^1$ regularization forces the solution to be sparse. As is pointed by Yang *et al.* [5], sparse coding obtains lower reconstruction and allows the representation to be specialize and salient.

While for LLC, $r(\mathbf{z}) = \sum_i \| \exp(\frac{\text{dist}(\mathbf{x},\mathbf{d}_i)}{\sigma})\mathbf{z}_i\|^2$ and $\mathcal{C} = \mathbb{R}^K$, the regularization term puts locality constraint on the solution so that local feature will have large responses on several closest visual words. For efficient computation, the approximated LLC removes the weighted $\ell^2$ regularization term. It explicitly restricts that only the K nearest visual words are used for reconstruction.

All the reconstruction based coding methods share the same least square error term $\|\mathbf{x} - \mathbf{Dz}\|_2^2$, as shown in Eqn (1). The local feature $\mathbf{x}$ is described as a linear combination of a set of visual words(dictionary), namely,

$$\mathbf{x} \approx \sum_{i=1}^{K} z_i \mathbf{d}_i \tag{2}$$

As shown in Eqn(2), local feature $\mathbf{x}$ is transformed into a new feature space which is spanned by all the visual words in the dictionary. The coefficients $\mathbf{z}$ is the new representation for local feature $\mathbf{x}$, which is more discriminative than the original local feature. Reconstruction term in the objective function restricts the new representation so that most of the important information is preserved. Bad reconstruction loses too much information about the original local feature, which surely leads to bad performance. For example, in hard quantization local feature is described by the nearest visual word, in which quantization error always exists. Soft quantization solves this problem by describing one local feature with multiple visual words, leading to better performance than hard quantization. Sparse coding and LLC take the sparsity and locality constraints into account, respectively. the parameter $\lambda$ in Eqn(1) is used to balance the reconstruction error and the penalty.

## 3.2    Local Hypersphere Coding(LHC)

As demonstrated in Fig 1-(a), in traditional reconstruction based coding algorithms, local feature vector is represented by a set of visual words on the hypersphere. Only the relationships between visual words and local features are considered, ignoring the relationships between visual words. Fig 1-(b) shows that, for one visual word, the edges connecting nearby visual words tend to lie on a local hypersphere approximating a hyperplane. Reconstructing local feature on a hyperplane will produce less error. Motivated by this observation, we propose to do feature coding on local hypersphere to achieve better reconstruction. Rather than reconstructing the raw local feature $\mathbf{x}$, we propose to reconstruct the difference between local feature $\mathbf{x}$ and visual word $\mathbf{d}_i$.

$\mathbf{D} = [\mathbf{d}_1, \mathbf{d}_2, \cdots, \mathbf{d}_K] \in R^{M \times K}$ is a dictionary of size $K$. The directed edge from visual word $\mathbf{d}_i$ to $\mathbf{d}_j$ is denoted as $\mathbf{e}_{ij}$, namely

$$\mathbf{e}_{ij} = \mathbf{d}_j - \mathbf{d}_i \tag{3}$$

The directed edge from visual word $\mathbf{d}_j$ to local feature $\mathbf{x}$ is denoted as $\mathbf{y}_j$, namely

$$\mathbf{y}_j = \mathbf{x} - \mathbf{d}_j \tag{4}$$

As is illustrated in Fig 1-(b), we propose to reconstruct $\mathbf{y}_j$ (the blue arrow) using a subset of the directed edges between visual words(drawn as red arrows). More precisely, denote the set of the $L$ nearest visual words of $\mathbf{d}_j$ as $\mathcal{N}_L(\mathbf{d}_j)$, the subset $\mathbf{D}_e = \{\mathbf{e}_{jk} | k \in \mathcal{N}_L(\mathbf{d}_j)\}$ is retained for reconstruction, see Fig 1-(b). The proposed feature coding method describes $\mathbf{y}_j$ with $\mathbf{z}_j$ by solving the following problem:

$$\arg\min_{\mathbf{z}_j} \|\mathbf{y}_j - \mathbf{D}_e \mathbf{z}_j\|_2^2 \tag{5}$$
$$s.t. \ \mathbf{1}^T \mathbf{z}_j = 1$$

Eqn (5) is a constrained least squares problem, which can be solved efficiently. Denote $\mathbf{Y} = [\mathbf{y}_j, \mathbf{y}_j, \cdots, \mathbf{y}_j] \in R^{M \times L}$, Eqn (5) can be rewritten as

$$\arg\min_{\mathbf{z}_j} \mathbf{z}_j^T \mathbf{C} \mathbf{z}_j \quad s.t. \ \mathbf{1}^T \mathbf{z}_j = 1 \tag{6}$$

where $\mathbf{C}$ is the covariance matrix defined as $\mathbf{C} = (\mathbf{Y} - \mathbf{D_e})^{\mathbf{T}}(\mathbf{Y} - \mathbf{D_e})$.

Eqn (6) can be efficiently minimized by solving the linear system of equations $\mathbf{C}\mathbf{z_j} = \mathbf{1}$, following with a rescaling to make sure the sum-to-one constraint.

The final coded feature of $\mathbf{x}$ is :

$$\beta = [w_1 \mathbf{z}_1^T, w_2 \mathbf{z}_2^T, \cdots, w_K \mathbf{z}_K^T]^T \tag{7}$$

where $w_i$ is a weighting factor indicating the influence of $\mathbf{z}_i$. Here a locality constraint is introduced to ensure that closer visual word contributes more. When visual words are too far away from local feature $\mathbf{x}$, it is justifiable to ignore them and set the corresponding responses to zero.

$$w_i = \begin{cases} \exp(-\frac{\|\mathbf{x} - \mathbf{d}_i\|^2}{\sigma}) & \text{if } i \in \mathcal{N}_S(x) \\ 0 & \text{otherwise} \end{cases} \tag{8}$$

where $\mathcal{N}_S(x)$ is the index set of the $S$ nearest visual words of $\mathbf{x}$. $\sigma$ is a smooth factor. Unlike normal coding methods that produce only one response on each visual word, our method produces a vector of $L$-dimensional on each visual word.Thus the final representation for each local feature is $KL$-dimensional.

### 3.3  Properties of Local Hypersphere Coding (LHC)

The proposed feature coding algorithm has three desirable properties:

- **Better Reconstruction.** As can be seen from Fig 1-(b), reconstruction on local hypersphere with edges between visual words is more likely coplanar than traditional coding methods, which will naturally do better reconstruction.

- **Distinctive Representation.** There have been a couple of works considering the distinctiveness of feature, such as SIFT, LLC, as well as salient coding. The proposed coding method produces distinctive representation, in the sense that, by considering both locality and visual words ambiguity, dissimilar features are more easily distinguished from each other. For example, on the one hand, two features with different nearest neighbours will have totally different responses using LHC. On the other hand, we produce similar responses for similar local features and retain most of the important information.

- **Efficient Implementation.** As the proposed feature coding can be reformatted as a linear system of equations, it has very simple computation and can be efficiently solved. This is especially desirable for large scale problems where efficient feature coding is extremely important. We list the time cost of each methods with codebook size 64 for processing one image: HQ(0.31s), SQ(0.46s), LHC(3.27s), LLC(5.17s), SC(52.23s).

## 4  Experiments

In this Section, we first introduce the general experimental settings in Section 4.1. Then in the next several sections we present the performance of the proposed method on three benchmark datasets: Caltech-101 [15], 15-Scenes [16,17,10] and PASCAL VOC 2007 [18].

### 4.1  Experimental Settings

For all the experiments we present, a single local feature descriptor, SIFT , is used. The 128-dimensional SIFT descriptors are densely extracted from each image, with step size of 4 pixels and three scales: $16 \times 16$, $24 \times 24$, $32 \times 32$. For one image, there are roughly 10k to 20k SIFT descriptors extracted. The dictionary is generated using standard K-means clustering algorithm. For all the experiments on the same dataset with same dictionary size, we used the same dictionary trained with $2,000,000$ patches randomly sampled from the training images. After coding the local features with different coding methods, the encoded features are pooled over subregions with spatial pyramid matching(SPM) [10].

We adopted $1 \times 1$, $2 \times 2$, $4 \times 4$ sub-regions SPM on 15-Scenes and Caltech-101 dataset, while on PASCAL VOC 2007 we used $1 \times 1$, $2 \times 2$, $3 \times 1$ sub-regions for SPM. As the focus of this paper is concentrated on the coding methods for local feature description, we choose max-pooling[1] for all the coding methods. Finally for classifier, we use linear kernel as most of the recent works in the literature. We utilized the widely used SVM software-LIBLINEAR [20] for image classification.

To verify the effectiveness of the proposed method, we compare our method with four representative coding methods:

- HQ: the basic hard quantization [3]. We implement hard quantization ourselves following the original paper.
- SQ: soft quantization [4]. We implement a "localized" version of soft quantization ourselves following [19]. We only consider the 5 nearest visual words.
- SC: sparse coding. We use the public available source code from ScSPM [5]. The regularization term $\lambda$ in sparse coding is set to 0.15.
- LLC: locality-constraint linear coding. We use the implementation supplied by the author [6]. The approximated LLC is used throughout the evaluation. The parameter K is set to 5, which means that we use the 5 nearest visual words for reconstruction.
- LHC: The proposed local hypersphere coding method . the parameter $S = 10$, $L = 5$ is used for all the experiments. In Section 4.5 we will study the impact of $S$ and $L$ in details. $\sigma$ in Eqn (8) is set to 0.1.

This paper focuses on the evaluation of the effectiveness of the proposed local feature coding method. Rather than comparing to the results published in the literature, we decided to put them in the same framework with same dictionary, and same SPM and classifier parameters for all the experiments for fair comparison, the only difference is the coding methods.

## 4.2 Caltech-101

The Caltech-101 dataset [15] is composed of 101 classes and a background class. There are totally 9144 images and the number of images in each class ranges from 31 to 800. Following the literature, we random sampled a fixed number of images from each class for training and used the rest images for testing. For each experiment settings, we repeat for 5 times with different splitting of training set and testing set. We reported the mean and standard deviation as the final experiment results.

Table 1 shows the experimental results on Caltech-101 with 30 training images per class, under dictionary size of 64, 128, 256, 512 and 1024. As shown, our coding methods achieves the best performance on compared with the listed methods. The differences of the performance results became small as larger dictionary is used. This is consistent with what we have observed from results on 15-Scenes. We also compare our result with several published results in Table 2.

---

[1] Theoretical analysis [19] and experimental results show that max pooling generally demonstrates higher performance than sum pooling and average pooling.

**Table 1.** Classification rate(%) comparison on Caltech-101 with 30 training image per class using different dictionary sizes

| K | 64 | 128 | 256 | 512 | 1024 |
|---|---|---|---|---|---|
| HQ | 57.8 ± 0.7 | 64.9 ± 0.6 | 69.2 ± 0.4 | 71.1 ± 0.8 | 73.1 ± 1.1 |
| SQ | 59.7 ± 0.5 | 66.8 ± 0.9 | 70.5 ± 1.1 | 73.9 ± 0.4 | 75.1 ± 0.8 |
| SC | 63.0 ± 1.5 | 67.3 ± 1.0 | 69.4 ± 0.5 | 72.4 ± 0.9 | 73.7 ± 1.0 |
| LLC | 63.7 ± 0.9 | 66.5 ± 1.5 | 69.5 ± 1.4 | 70.2 ± 0.7 | 71.3 ± 0.6 |
| **LHC** | **69.0 ± 0.8** | **71.2 ± 1.3** | **73.5 ± 1.3** | **74.9 ± 0.9** | **75.5 ± 1.2** |

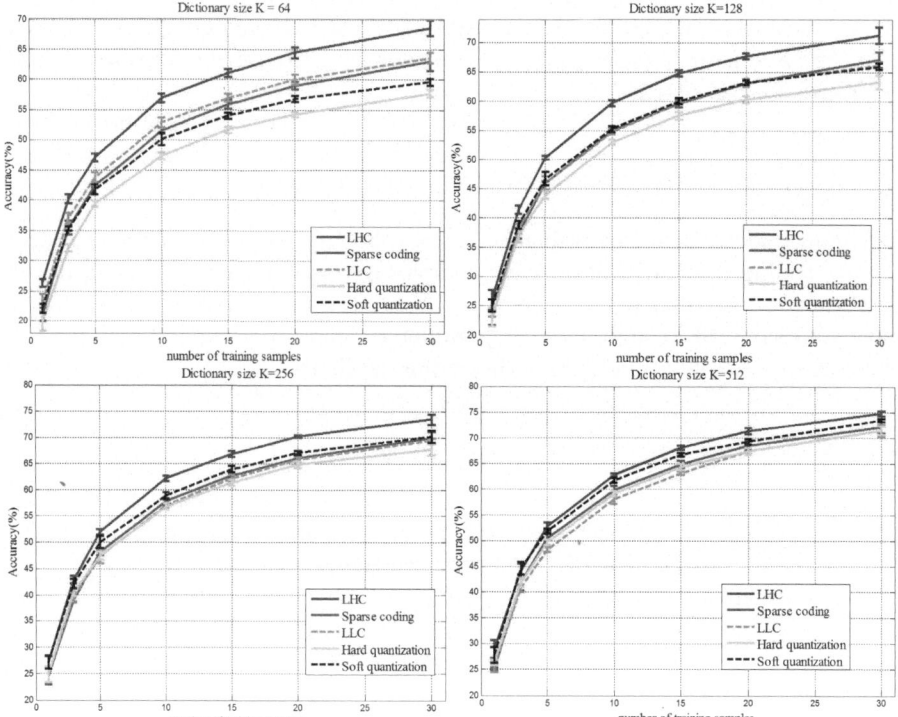

**Fig. 2.** The mean classification accuracy and standard deviation of different coding methods on Caltech-101, using different number of training samples. We choose 1, 3, 5, 10, 15, 20 and 30 training samples per class for training and use the rest for testing. The dictionary sizes used are 64, 128, 256, 512, respectively. For each setting, we repeat for 5 times with randomly split training set and testing set.(Please view in color.)

For both 15 training and 30 training, our proposed coding method achieves the best performance. Note that for [21] we list the result of linear kernel, since we do not use non-linear kernels in our experiments.

**Table 2.** Classification rate(%) comparison on Caltech-101 with results from the literature

| Algorithms | 15 training | 30 training |
|---|---|---|
| Jain *et al.* [22] | 61.0 | 69.6 |
| ScSPM [5] | 67.0±0.45 | 73.2±0.54 |
| LLC [6] | 65.43 | 73.44 |
| Boureau *et al.* [21] | - | 75.1±0.9 |
| LHC | **68.44 ± 0.54** | **75.49 ± 1.24** |

To see the influence of the number of training images on the performance, we report the results with 1, 3, 5, 10 , 15, 20, 30 training images per class, using dictionary size $K = 64, 128, 256$, and 512. The experimental results are presented in Fig 2. When dictionary size $K = 64$, it is clear that the proposed method outperforms other coding methods by a large margin. As more images are used for training, the performance keeps growing, this is a common result in all coding methods. We can also see that when dictionary size becomes larger, we always obtain better performance. At the same time, the performance differences between different coding methods become smaller. This is natural as there are more visual words used for reconstruction.

## 4.3 15-Scenes

The 15-Scenes dataset [10] is an expansion of previously published datasets [16,17]. This dataset consists of 4485 images out of 15 categories of natural scenes and indoor scenes. Each category contains 200 to 400 images with a resolution of about $300 \times 250$ pixels. Following the standard evaluation process in the literature, we randomly sampled 100 images per category for training and used the rest images for testing. For each setting we repeat for 5 times with different splitting of the training set and testing set.

We reported the mean and standard deviation as the final experiment result in Table 3. For different dictionary size, we present the performance of HQ, SQ, SC, LLC, as well as the proposed coding method. As shown, the proposed method significantly outperforms other coding methods. Especially when dictionary size is small, our method outperforms HQ by more than 11 percent, SQ by more than 8 percent, SC by more than 5 percent, and LLC by 3.9 percent. The remarkable performance improvement shows the discriminative power of the proposed method. We again note that as the dictionary size grows larger, the performance differences between different coding methods become smaller. Nevertheless, our proposed coding method still manages to outperform the best of the four other methods by 1.4 percent.

**Table 3.** Classification rate(%) comparison on 15-scenes with different dictionary sizes

| K | 32 | 64 | 128 | 256 | 512 | 1024 |
|---|----|----|-----|-----|-----|------|
| HQ | 62.2 ± 0.8 | 69.4 ± 0.4 | 74.1 ± 0.3 | 76.4 ± 0.7 | 78.5 ± 0.3 | 79.9 ± 0.4 |
| SQ | 65.3 ± 0.4 | 71.6 ± 0.8 | 75.4 ± 0.7 | 77.4 ± 0.3 | 79.8 ± 0.3 | 80.4 ± 0.6 |
| SC | 68.1 ± 0.4 | 71.8 ± 0.7 | 74.6 ± 0.2 | 77.5 ± 0.2 | 78.9 ± 0.5 | 80.7 ± 1.1 |
| LLC | 70.0 ± 0.7 | 73.1 ± 0.1 | 75.1 ± 0.6 | 76.4 ± 0.5 | 78.0 ± 0.4 | 78.6 ± 0.3 |
| LHC | **73.9 ± 0.7** | **76.1 ± 0.4** | **78.1 ± 0.7** | **80.2 ± 0.5** | **80.1 ± 0.3** | **82.1 ± 0.4** |

## 4.4 Pascal VOC 2007

**Table 4.** Comparison of different coding methods on PASCAL VOC 2007, with dictionary size 1024

| AP(%) | HQ | SQ | SC | LLC | LHC | Improvement |
|-------|----|----|----|-----|-----|-------------|
| aeroplane | 63.87 | 66.64 | 68.93 | 67.15 | **69.68** | +0.75 |
| bicycle | 46.69 | 51.46 | 53.98 | 52.76 | **56.65** | +2.67 |
| bird | 30.06 | 34.28 | 36.45 | 34.51 | **42.25** | +5.80 |
| boat | 57.69 | 61.08 | 61.09 | 61.97 | **62.68** | +0.71 |
| bottle | 13.91 | 16.87 | 21.06 | 19.50 | **22.00** | +0.94 |
| bus | 43.42 | 49.27 | 51.25 | 46.95 | **58.26** | +7.01 |
| car | 68.78 | 71.57 | 72.78 | 72.15 | **76.13** | +3.35 |
| cat | 46.47 | 50.60 | 45.12 | 45.78 | **52.84** | +2.24 |
| chair | 43.35 | 47.42 | 49.75 | 47.54 | **50.16** | +0.41 |
| cow | 35.10 | 36.16 | 33.60 | 35.60 | **39.91** | +3.75 |
| diningtable | 31.39 | 34.03 | 36.99 | 35.96 | **38.63** | +1.64 |
| dog | 32.56 | 35.50 | 36.19 | 32.45 | **38.05** | +1.86 |
| horse | 67.29 | 69.20 | 73.17 | 71.80 | **73.92** | +0.75 |
| motorbike | 48.57 | 53.06 | 52.03 | 51.91 | **58.45** | +5.39 |
| person | 77.35 | 78.82 | 78.21 | 77.96 | **81.19** | +2.37 |
| pottedplant | 14.61 | 17.45 | 15.95 | 15.42 | **18.75** | +1.30 |
| sheep | 32.82 | 34.99 | 35.67 | 37.21 | **38.80** | +1.59 |
| sofa | 42.76 | 45.91 | 43.40 | 42.68 | **49.02** | +3.11 |
| train | 65.63 | 68.37 | 63.55 | 67.83 | **70.87** | +2.50 |
| tvmonitor | 41.70 | 46.78 | 47.56 | 45.88 | **48.68** | +1.12 |
| average | 45.20 | 48.47 | 48.84 | 48.15 | **52.35** | +2.46 |

We also evaluate our algorithm on PASCAL VOC 2007 [18], which consists of 9963 images from 20 classes. The dataset is divided into three subsets: a training set with 2501 images, a validation set with 2510 images, and a testing set with 4952 images. PASCAL VOC 2007 is one of the most challenging benchmark datasets for classification task as there are large in-class divergence, including variation on scale, illumination, view, deformation, as well as severe object occlusions.The classification performance is measured by average precision(AP), which indicates the area under precision/recall curve. This measure favours both high precision and recall.

We used both the training set and validation set for training and report the average precision(AP) for each class on the testing set. Table 4 shows the 20 scores obtained by our method as well as other coding method with dictionary size 1024.

As shown, the proposed coding method achieves 52.35% mean AP score. Our method significantly outperforms other methods by 3.5% to more than 7%. For single class AP, the proposed method performs better than the other four methods for all 20 classes. The last column of Table 4 presents the improvement of the proposed coding method over the best of the four other coding methods. We achieve a performance improvement of 2.46% in average. There are also three classes that achieve more than 5 percent improvement(bird:+5.8%, bus:+7.0% and motorbike: +5.4%).

### 4.5  The Impact of $S$ and $L$ on the Performance

There are two important KNN parameters in the proposed method, $L$ from Eqn (5) and $S$ from Eqn (8). $L$ controls the number of bases used for reconstruction the edge from visual word to local feature. This parameter has a direct affection to the dimensionality of the final representation. $S$ dominates contribution of each visual word to the local feature to be described. It also controls the sparsity of the encoded feature.

In this Section, we study the impact of $S$ and $L$ on the final classification accuracy in the proposed method. We carry out experiments with a small dictionary size 32. For different combinations of $S$ and $L$, we repeat the experiments for 5 times and report the mean and standard deviation. The results are demonstrated in Table 5.

**Table 5.** The impact of $S$ and $L$ on the performance on 15-Scenes, with dictionary size 32.

| $S$ \ $L$ | 5 | 10 | 15 | 20 |
|---|---|---|---|---|
| 5 | 73.5±0.7 | 74.3±0.7 | 73.1±0.6 | 74.7±0.6 |
| 10 | 73.9±0.7 | 73.9±0.9 | 73.5±0.2 | 74.2±0.6 |
| 15 | 73.4±0.7 | 73.9±0.5 | 74.2±1.1 | 74.3±0.8 |
| 20 | 73.6±0.8 | 73.9±0.6 | 73.4±0.5 | 74.8±0.7 |

When the parameters $S$ and $L$ change, the classification accuracy only has a minor change. This indicates that the proposed coding method is not sensitive to the two parameters. In practice, choosing small $L$ is sufficient and more efficient, since larger $L$ means higher dimensional feature vector. That's why we fix $S = 10$ and $L = 5$ in our experiments.

## 5    Conclusion

In this paper, we have analyzed traditional reconstruction based coding methods in bag-of-words model and shown that reconstruction on the hypersphere performs better. Based on our observation and analysis, we have proposed a new local feature coding method called local hypersphere coding (LHC). It performs feature coding on the hypersphere of the feature space and describes local feature with the edges between visual words. Experiments on three benchmark datasets shown that the proposed coding method significantly outperforms other reconstruction based coding methods, indicating the effectiveness of the proposed method.

The proposed coding scheme is general and can be extended easily. In the proposed coding method, coding of local feature $\mathbf{x}$ starts by calculating the directed edge $\mathbf{y}_j$ from visual word $\mathbf{d}_j$ to $\mathbf{x}$ (See Fig 1-(b)), followed with a decomposition of $\mathbf{y}_j$ by the edges $\mathbf{D}_e = \{\mathbf{e}_{jk}|k \in \mathcal{N}_L(\mathbf{d}_j)\}$ between visual words. The second step is a reconstruction of $\mathbf{y}_j$ with $\mathbf{D}_e$, where any other reconstruction based regularization can be added. In fact, we can adopt some existing coding methods here to do the decomposition. In future, we will study other coding methods under the proposed reconstruction scheme. Our interests are obtaining more compact and discriminative image representation.

**Acknowledgement.** This work is funded by National Natural Science Foundation of China (Grant No. 61175007), the National Basic Research Program of China (Grant No. 2012CB316302), the National Key Technology R&D Program (Grant No. 2012BAH07B01).

## References

1. Lowe, D.G.: Distinctive image features from scale-invariant keypoints. Int. J. Comput. Vision 60, 91–110 (2004)
2. Dalal, N., Triggs, B.: Histograms of oriented gradients for human detection. In: IEEE Computer Society Conference on Computer Vision and Pattern Recognition, CVPR 2005, vol. 1, pp. 886–893 (2005)
3. Csurka, G., Dance, C.R., Fan, L., Willamowski, J., Bray, C.: Visual categorization with bags of keypoints. In: Workshop on Statistical Learning in Computer Vision, ECCV, pp. 1–22 (2004)
4. van Gemert, J.C., Geusebroek, J.M., Veenman, C.J., Smeulders, A.W.M.: Kernel Codebooks for Scene Categorization. In: Forsyth, D., Torr, P., Zisserman, A. (eds.) ECCV 2008, Part III. LNCS, vol. 5304, pp. 696–709. Springer, Heidelberg (2008)
5. Jianchao, Y., Kai, Y., Yihong, G., Huang, T.: Linear spatial pyramid matching using sparse coding for image classification. In: IEEE Conference on Computer Vision and Pattern Recognition, CVPR 2009, pp. 1794–1801 (2009)
6. Jinjun, W., Jianchao, Y., Kai, Y., Fengjun, L., Huang, T., Yihong, G.: Locality-constrained linear coding for image classification. In: 2010 IEEE Conference on Computer Vision and Pattern Recognition, CVPR, pp. 3360–3367 (2010)

7. Zhou, X., Yu, K., Zhang, T., Huang, T.S.: Image Classification Using Super-Vector Coding of Local Image Descriptors. In: Daniilidis, K., Maragos, P., Paragios, N. (eds.) ECCV 2010, Part V. LNCS, vol. 6315, pp. 141–154. Springer, Heidelberg (2010)

8. Perronnin, F., Dance, C.: Fisher kernels on visual vocabularies for image categorization. In: IEEE Conference on Computer Vision and Pattern Recognition, CVPR 2007, pp. 1–8 (2007)

9. Perronnin, F., Sánchez, J., Mensink, T.: Improving the Fisher Kernel for Large-Scale Image Classification. In: Daniilidis, K., Maragos, P., Paragios, N. (eds.) ECCV 2010, Part IV. LNCS, vol. 6314, pp. 143–156. Springer, Heidelberg (2010)

10. Lazebnik, S., Schmid, C., Ponce, J.: Beyond bags of features: Spatial pyramid matching for recognizing natural scene categories. In: 2006 IEEE Computer Society Conference on Computer Vision and Pattern Recognition, vol. 2, pp. 2169–2178 (2006)

11. Olshausen, B.A., Fieldt, D.J.: Sparse coding with an overcomplete basis set: a strategy employed by v1. Vision Research 37, 3311–3325 (1997)

12. Huang, Y., Huang, K., Yu, Y., Tan, T.: Salient coding for image classification. In: 2011 IEEE Conference on Computer Vision and Pattern Recognition, CVPR, pp. 1753–1760. IEEE (2011)

13. Huang, Y., Huang, K., Wang, C., Tan, T.: Exploring relations of visual codes for image classification. In: 2011 IEEE Conference on Computer Vision and Pattern Recognition, CVPR, pp. 1649–1656. IEEE (2011)

14. Zhao, X., Yu, Y., Huang, Y., Huang, K., Tan, T.: Feature coding via vector difference for image classification. In: IEEE International Conference on Image Processing, ICIP (2012)

15. Fei-Fei, L., Fergus, R., Perona, P.: Learning generative visual models from few training examples. In: Workshop on Generative-Model Based Vision, IEEE Proc. CVPR (2004)

16. Oliva, A., Torralba, A.: Modeling the shape of the scene: A holistic representation of the spatial envelope. Int. J. Comput. Vision 42, 145–175 (2001)

17. Fei-Fei, L., Perona, P.: A bayesian hierarchical model for learning natural scene categories. In: IEEE Computer Society Conference on Computer Vision and Pattern Recognition, CVPR 2005, vol. 2, pp. 524–531 (2005)

18. Everingham, M., Van Gool, L., Williams, C.K.I., Winn, J., Zisserman, A.: The PASCAL Visual Object Classes Challenge 2007 (VOC 2007) Results (2007)

19. Liu, L., Wang, L., Liu, X.: In defense of soft-assignment coding. In: 2011 IEEE International Conference on Computer Vision, ICCV, pp. 2486–2493 (2011)

20. Fan, R.E., Chang, K.W., Hsieh, C.J., Wang, X.R., Lin, C.J.: Liblinear: A library for large linear classification. J. Mach. Learn. Res. 9, 1871–1874 (2008)

21. Boureau, Y.L., Bach, F., LeCun, Y., Ponce, J.: Learning mid-level features for recognition. In: 2010 IEEE Conference on Computer Vision and Pattern Recognition, CVPR, pp. 2559–2566 (2010)

22. Jain, P., Kulis, B., Grauman, K.: Fast image search for learned metrics. In: IEEE Conference on Computer Vision and Pattern Recognition, CVPR 2008, pp. 1–8 (2008)

# Spatially Local Coding
# for Object Recognition

Sancho McCann and David G. Lowe

Department of Computer Science, University of British Columbia

**Abstract.** The spatial pyramid and its variants have been among the most popular and successful models for object recognition. In these models, local visual features are coded across elements of a visual vocabulary, and then these codes are pooled into histograms at several spatial granularities. We introduce spatially local coding, an alternative way to include spatial information in the image model. Instead of only coding visual appearance and leaving the spatial coherence to be represented by the pooling stage, we include location as part of the coding step. This is a more flexible spatial representation as compared to the fixed grids used in the spatial pyramid models and we can use a simple, whole-image region during the pooling stage. We demonstrate that combining features with multiple levels of spatial locality performs better than using just a single level. Our model performs better than all previous single-feature methods when tested on the Caltech 101 and 256 object recognition datasets.

## 1 Introduction

Models based on histograms of visual word frequencies have been quite successful for object recognition, delivering good results on varied datasets. The spatial pyramid was introduced by Lazebnik *et al.* [1] to allow the representation to account for the spatial distribution of these visual features. In this model, visual features are coded across elements of a visual vocabulary, and these codes are pooled into histograms at several spatial granularities.

Many improvements have been made to the original spatial pyramid model. These include replacing nearest neighbor vector quantization with sparse coding [2] or localized soft assignment [3] and replacing average pooling with max-pooling in each spatial bin [4,5,3,2]. Boureau *et al.* [4] analyzed the various choices available during the coding and pooling stages: hard assignment vs. soft assignment, average pooling vs. max-pooling, and the linear kernel vs. the histogram intersection kernel.

It is useful to view these approaches in the context of how each method attends to spatial locality and appearance locality. Prior to spatial pyramids, the bag-of-features method [6] enforced appearance locality in the coding step by its nearest-neighbor vector quantization. Using only a whole-image pooling region, it did not enforce any spatial locality. The spatial pyramid introduced spatial locality using a spatially hierarchical pooling stage. The sparse coding spatial

K.M. Lee et al. (Eds.): ACCV 2012, Part I, LNCS 7724, pp. 204–217, 2013.
© Springer-Verlag Berlin Heidelberg 2013

pyramid method [2] takes a different approach to appearance locality that can select very different bases for patches that are visually similar [7]. Boureau *et al.* [5] re-instated stricter appearance locality by modifying the pooling stage to enforce to appearance locality. Table 1 presents a taxonomy of these methods based on how they attend to appearance and spatial locality.

**Table 1.** A taxonomy of histogram-based recognition models focusing on how they attend to appearance and spatial locality. Spatially local coding moves spatial locality into the coding step.

| Method | Appearance locality | Spatial locality |
|---|---|---|
| Bags-of-features [6] | Coding | - |
| Spatial pyramid [1] | Coding | Pooling |
| Sparse coding [2] | Sparse coding | Pooling |
| LLC [7] | Local coding | Pooling |
| "Ask-the-locals" sparse coding [5] | Sparse coding + Pooling | Pooling |
| Spatially local coding (this work) | Coding | Coding |

In contrast to the spatial pyramid approaches, we explore moving the task of enforcing spatial locality into the coding step. We first present more detail about the related spatial pyramid methods. Then we present our method, tuning and implementation details, and finally, experimental results on Caltech 101 and Caltech 256.

## 2    Related Methods

### 2.1    The Coding/Pooling Pipeline

As our method relates closely to the previous bag-of-features and spatial pyramid approaches, we will explain our method in the context of these other methods. This will facilitate comparisons with these approaches in Section 6.

We adopt the coding/pooling framework of Boureau *et al.* in which all the bag-of-features and spatial pyramid methods can be seen as various choices for a coding and pooling step. Given an image $\mathcal{I}$, we first do feature extraction: $\Phi(\mathcal{I}) : \mathcal{I} \mapsto \{(\phi_1, x_1, y_1), (\phi_2, x_2, y_2), \ldots (\phi_{n_\mathcal{I}}, x_{n_\mathcal{I}}, y_{n_\mathcal{I}})\}$. The features $\phi_i$ are typically local image descriptors (SIFT, for example) and they vary in number from image to image ($n_\mathcal{I}$). The pixel location at which feature $i$ is centered is $(x_i, y_i)$.

After we extract features, we code them using some coding function $g((\phi_i, x_i, y_i))$. In previous work, this coding function has included nearest neighbor vector quantization, sparse coding, soft assignment, and localized soft assignment. In bags-of-features and spatial pyramid methods, the coding has been limited to the appearance portion of the descriptor $\phi_i$, such that $g((\phi_i, x_i, y_i)) = (\hat{g}(\phi_i), x_i, y_i)$. That is, the extracted descriptor's appearance is converted into a coded version, still associated with the original pixel location.

We'll now give some concrete examples of the appearance coding function $\hat{g}$ for the coding methods just mentioned. In these examples, assume that we have constructed a dictionary $\mathbf{D}$ of $k$ appearance elements. This is often referred to as a codebook, and the elements called codewords.

For nearest neighbor vector quantization, we use a 1-of-$k$ coding:

$$\hat{g}(\phi_i) = [u_{i1}, u_{i2}, \ldots, u_{ik}]: \qquad u_{ij} = \begin{cases} 1 \text{ if } j = \text{argmin}_a \|\phi_i - \mathbf{D}_a\|, \\ 0 \text{ otherwise} \end{cases} \qquad (1)$$

For soft assignment, demonstrated by van Gemert $et$ $al.$ [8], a feature is coded across many codebook elements instead of just one:

$$\hat{g}(\phi_i) = [u_{i1}, u_{i2}, \ldots, u_{ik}]: \qquad u_{ij} = \frac{\exp(-\beta\|\phi_i - \mathbf{D}_j\|^2)}{\sum_{a=1}^{k} \exp(-\beta\|\phi_i - \mathbf{D}_a\|^2)} \qquad (2)$$

where $\beta$ is a parameter controlling how widely the assignment distributes the weight across all the codewords. A small $\beta$ gives a broad distribution, while a large $\beta$ gives a peaked distribution, more closely approximating hard assignment.

This is further improved by Liu $et$ $al.$ [3], who use localized soft assignment. Instead of distributing the weight across all codebook elements, they confine the soft assignment to a local neighborhood around the descriptor being coded. Let $\text{NN}_{(\kappa)}(\phi_i)$ be the set of $\kappa$ nearest neighbors to $\phi_i$ in $\mathbf{D}$. Then, the localized soft assignment coding is:

$$\hat{g}(\phi_i) = \mathbf{u}_i = [u_{i1}, u_{i2}, \ldots, u_{ik}]: \qquad u_{ij} = \frac{\exp(-\beta d(\phi_i, \mathbf{D}_j)}{\sum_{a=1}^{k} \exp(-\beta d(\phi_i, \mathbf{D}_a))} \qquad (3)$$

$$d(\phi_i, \mathbf{D}_j) = \begin{cases} \|\phi_i - \mathbf{D}_j\|^2 & \text{if } \mathbf{D}_j \in \text{NN}_{(\kappa)}(\phi_i) \\ \infty & \text{otherwise} \end{cases}$$

Sparse coding ([2], [4]) codes a descriptor by using the coefficients of a linear combination of the codewords in $D$, with a sparsity-promoting $l_1$ norm:

$$\hat{g}(\phi_i) = \mathbf{u}_i = \underset{\mathbf{u} \in \mathbb{R}^k}{\text{argmin}} \|\phi_i - \mathbf{D}\mathbf{u}\|_2^2 + \lambda\|\mathbf{u}\|_1 \qquad (4)$$

Locality constrained linear coding (LLC) is similar, but adds a penalty for using elements of the codebook that have a large Euclidean distance from the descriptor being coded [7].

After choosing one of the above coding functions for $\hat{g}$, we obtain the coding for every descriptor extracted from an image: $g((\phi_i, x_i, y_i)) = (\mathbf{u}_i, x_i, y_i)$.

The pooling stage combines these coded features within an image region into a histogram. This histogram $\mathbf{h}_m$ associated with spatial pooling region $\mathcal{S}_m$ is obtained using a pooling function:

$$\mathbf{h}_m = f(\{\mathbf{u_i}|(x_i, y_i) \in \mathcal{S}_m\}). \qquad (5)$$

The structure of the spatial pooling regions $\mathcal{S}$ varies between methods. In the bag-of-features approach of Csurka *et al.* [6], there is just a single spatial pooling region—one comprising the entire image. In the spatial pyramid, there are several spatial pooling regions—one comprising the entire image and additional regions that split the image into quadrants and even finer subdivisions.

Previous work has chosen between two options for the pooling function: average-pooling and max-pooling. Average-pooling produces a histogram that represents the average value of $\mathbf{u}$ within a spatial pooling region. Max-pooling instead takes the maximum value of each dimension of $\mathbf{u}$ within a spatial pooling region.

$$\mathbf{h}_{\text{avg}\,m} = \frac{\sum_{\{i | (x_i, y_i) \in \mathcal{S}_m\}} \mathbf{u}_i}{|\{(x_i, y_i) \in \mathcal{S}_m\}|} \tag{6}$$

$$\mathbf{h}_{\max m} = [h_{m1}, h_{m2}, \ldots, h_{mk}] \quad \text{where}$$

$$h_{mj} = \max\{u_{ij} | (x_i, y_i) \in \mathcal{S}_m\} \tag{7}$$

The final image representation used by the classifier is a concatenation of those histograms $\mathbf{h}_m$:

$$\mathbf{H} = [\mathbf{h}_1 \mathbf{h}_2 \ldots \mathbf{h}_M] \tag{8}$$

## 2.2    Other Spatial Models

We present in Section 3 perhaps the simplest approach for adding spatial information to the local features, but first, we outline relevant previous work that has attempted to account for the spatial layout of visual features.

Boiman *et al.*, in their Naive Bayes nearest neighbor work [9], append a weighted location to the feature vectors, which matches our approach. However, in contrast with the coding/pooling pipeline, they do not quantize features using a codebook. They instead maintain an index of all features extracted from the training data.

Zhou *et al.* [10] use a mixture of Gaussians to model visual appearance, followed by spatially hierarchical pooling of the local features' membership in each of the mixture's components. This is essentially a variant of the spatial pyramid model where soft codeword assignment is performed via a Gaussian mixture model, and better results have been achieved by spatial pyramids using localized soft assignment coding and max-pooling [3].

Krapac *et al.* [11] introduced a compact Fisher vector coding to encode spatial layout of features. They first learn an appearance codebook using k-means or a mixture of Gaussians. Then, for each appearance component, they learn a mixture of Gaussians to represent its spatial distribution. While their representation is more compact, their evaluation shows marginal (if any) improvement over SPM in terms of classification accuracy.

Oliveira *et al.* introduced a method called *sparse spatial coding* [12]. In their work, they code a descriptor using sparse codebook elements nearby in descriptor space. In this sense, it is very close to LLC [7]. In contrast to our work, despite their method's name, sparse spatial coding is local in *descriptor* space, not *pixel* space. As a separate contribution, they introduce a new learning stage called Orthogonal Class Learning that results in better performance than the standard SVM classifier. However, that work is complementary to the work improving the coding/pooling pipeline. Their results using the standard SVM classifier are inferior to LLC [7], NBNN [9], and sparse coding SPM [2].

## 3   Spatially Local Coding

Our method differs from the previous coding/pooling methods in that we choose a coding function $g$ that directly handles spatial locality, and use a single, whole-image pooling region during the pooling stage. Instead of choosing $g(\phi_i, x_i, y_i) = (\hat{g}(\phi_i), x_i, y_i)$, we simultaneously code $\phi_i$ and the location $(x_i, y_i)$. In the standard models, $\phi_i = [\phi_{i1}, \phi_{i2}, \ldots, \phi_{id}]$. In spatially local coding, we introduce use a location-augmented descriptor: $\phi_i^{(\lambda)} = [\phi_{i1}, \phi_{i2}, \ldots, \phi_{id}, \lambda x_i, \lambda y_i]$. Where $\lambda \in \mathbb{R}$ is a location weighting factor giving the importance of the location in feature matching.

For example, hard assignment, nearest neighbor vector quantization becomes:

$$g(\phi_i, x_i, y_i) = \mathbf{u}_i : \qquad u_{ij} = \begin{cases} 1 \text{ if } j = \text{argmin}_a \, \|[\phi_i^{(\lambda)} - \mathbf{D}_a^{(\lambda)}\|, \\ 0 \text{ otherwise} \end{cases} \qquad (9)$$

where we have constructed the codebook $\mathbf{D}^{(\lambda)}$ by k-means clustering over a set of location-augmented descriptors and locations extracted from the training data.

All of the coding functions presented in Section 2 can use the location-augmented descriptors in place of the standard appearance-only descriptors.

In summary, spatially local coding uses location-augmented feature vectors, and a single, whole-image spatial pooling region, because the features themselves already carry sufficient spatial information. We have moved the task of maintaining spatial locality into the coding stage. Previously, this has been left for the pooling stage.

One advantage of spatially local coding is that we avoid having to commit to artificial grid boundaries to define the spatial pooling regions. Other authors have had to work around this by experimenting with alternate binning geometries to engineer one that performs well for their problem [13], or supervised learning of optimal pooling regions from an over-complete set of rectangular bins [14]. Both of these methods keep the responsibility for spatial locality in the pooling stage.

Instead, our $\lambda$ parameter defines a receptive field associated with each codebook element.

### 3.1   Multi-level Spatially Local Coding

The $\lambda$ parameter plays an important role in our model. If we set $\lambda = 0$, we revert to the standard bag-of-features representation. If we set $\lambda$ to be high, we learn features that are very strictly localized. Figure 1 shows that it is possible to determine a somewhat optimal setting for $\lambda$ (approximately 1.5 for the Caltech 101 dataset). However, the specific $\lambda$ may depend on the particulars of the dataset. Instead of committing to a single $\lambda$, we build several codebooks, each with a different $\lambda$, and code image features across all of the codebooks simultaneously. This is similar in spirit to having multiple levels in the spatial pyramid, with each level dividing space into finer and finer regions. Table 2 shows that this combination is beneficial.

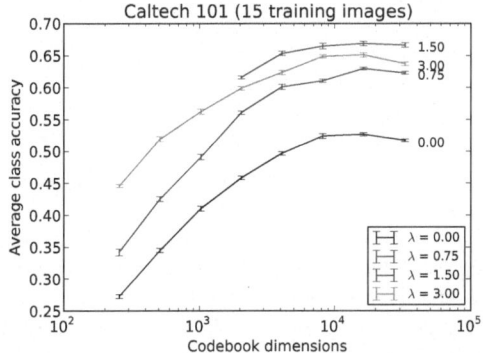

**Fig. 1.** The performance of single-codebook SLC is dependent on the choice of $\lambda$. Regardless of the choice of $\lambda$, the optimal codebook dimensionality is similar. Based on this observation, we can choose to use the same dimensionality across all of the codebooks in a multi-$\lambda$ model.

**Table 2.** The experimental setting of these results is explained in detail in Section 6. This shows that the combination of multiple codebooks, each with a different $\lambda$-weighting, produces higher classification accuracy than any of the codebooks individually.

| Codebook (8192D) | Caltech 101 (15 training) |
|---|---|
| $\lambda = 0.00$ | $52.4 \pm 0.4$ |
| $\lambda = 0.75$ | $61.1 \pm 0.2$ |
| $\lambda = 1.50$ | $66.5 \pm 0.5$ |
| $\lambda = 3.00$ | $64.9 \pm 0.3$ |
| 4-level (linear kernel) | $68.4 \pm 0.2$ |

Figure 2 shows the types of features learned by our system. For this visualization, we choose a particular category and determine the per-codeword weights derived from the linear SVM model (the SVM training is described further in Section 6). These are the codewords that most signal the presence of the object of interest. We show the distribution of features found in the training images that match the top-weighted codewords. The SVM can choose between unlocalized and highly localized features.

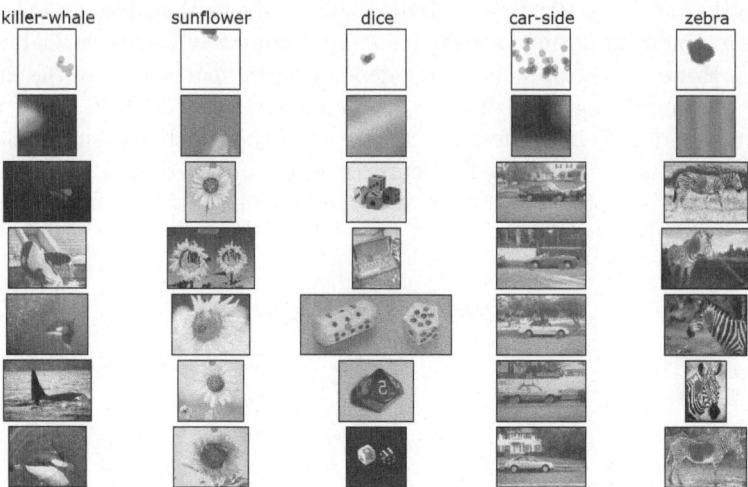

**Fig. 2.** Visualization of top-ranked features (hand-picked from among the top ten) for five of the object categories. The top row is the spatial distribution of each codeword and the second row is the average appearance of each codeword (as in Fig. 3). The subsequent rows show where occurrences of the codewords are centered in particular training images. Looking down each column shows that these codewords tend to be associated with particular parts or textures.

## 4    Optimal Codebook Size and Model Size

In [1], Lazebnik *et al.* reported their model reached optimal performance for Caltech 101 with approximately 200-400 codewords. We verify that in Fig. 4. We also confirm that localized soft assignment coding [3] achieves superior performance and can effectively make use of more codebook elements. Our model performs even better, but requires more codebook elements (for this figure, we used 4-codebook SLC with $\lambda = 0, 0.75, 1.5, 3.0$, localized soft assignment, and max-pooling).

These results may seem counter to those reported by Chatfield *et al.* in [15], who report performance of spatial pyramid methods never decreasing on Caltech 101 as codebook size grew up to 8,000 dimensions. However, those results were shown for a much denser SIFT sampling density than used in our experimental setups. We extract single-scale SIFT every 8 pixels. Chatfield *et al.* extracted SIFT at 4 scales every 2 pixels, resulting in approximately 64× the descriptors as in our experimental setting. In Section 6, we show some results at higher extraction densities and note that at higher densities, the optimal codebook dimensionality is higher. We hypothesize that Chatfield *et al.* had not reached that optimal dimensionality for their extremely dense extraction setting.

Our results match those by Boureau *et al.* [4] who reported that on Caltech 101, optimal codebook size is relatively low for hard assignment coding, higher for soft assignment coding, and higher when extraction densities increase. These trends are also observed by van Gemert *et al.* [8].

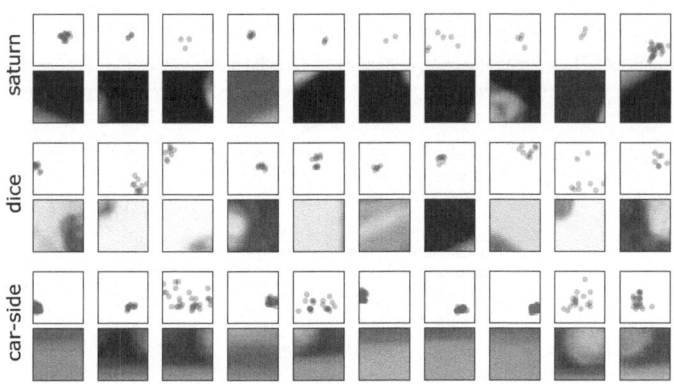

**Fig. 3.** Each pair of rows is a visualization of the top ten features from an object category. The scatter-plots show the spatial distribution of each codeword, while the grey-scale snippets show their average appearance.

Comparing the required codebook size is useful, as it points to a potential increase in the computational cost of the coding phase, but comparing the resulting *model* size is also useful, as this affects the computational cost of learning and testing. In 3-level spatial pyramid models, the model dimensionality is $21\times$ the size of the codebook. This is due to the 21 spatial pooling regions (1 whole-image region, $2 \times 2$ regions in the second level, and $4 \times 4$ regions at the third level). Figure 4 also compares the methods based on their model dimensionality, not just their codebook size. 4-codebook SLC produces better classification accuracy than a state-of-the-art spatial pyramid at comparable *model* dimensionalities.

## 5   Efficient Codebook Construction

As highlighted in the previous section, the codebook size used by our model is significantly larger than those used by spatial pyramid methods. Efficient codebook construction becomes important. The standard algorithm for k-means takes $O(nkd)$ per iteration, where $n$ is the number of data points (SIFT features) being clustered into $k$ clusters and $d$ is the data dimensionality. We used two approximations in our implementation of k-means to achieve efficient clustering.

First, we use FLANN (Fast Library for Approximate Nearest Neighbors) [16] to perform approximate assignment of data points to clusters during each iteration of k-means. FLANN automatically selects and tunes its approximate nearest neighbor search algorithm to the particulars of the dataset in order to achieve a specified accuracy with maximum efficiency. This is similar to the approximate k-means described by Philbin *et al.* in [17], but with more precise control of the approximation error. Figure 5 shows how classification performance and construction time is affected by changing FLANN's approximation accuracy.

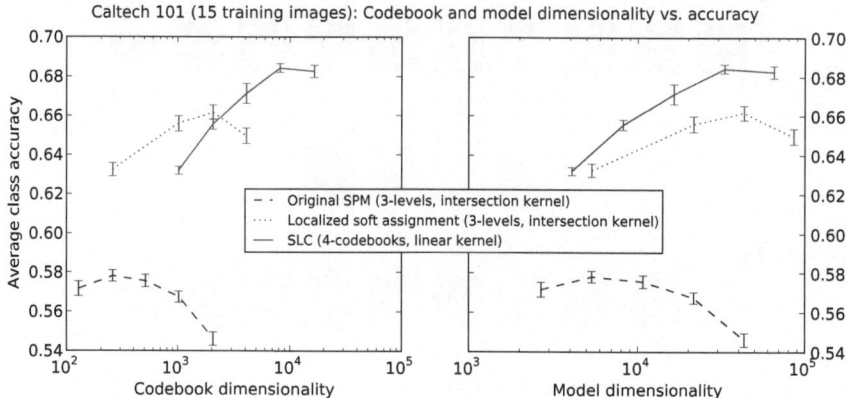

**Fig. 4.** We compare the performance of the original spatial pyramid model with the localized soft assignment variant and our SLC model. The localized soft assignment performs better than the original and requires larger codebook sizes for optimal performance. Our SLC model achieves even better performance, but requires even more codebook dimensions. When comparing the model dimensionalities ($21\times$ the size of the codebook to account for the spatial pyramid bins, or $4\times$ the size of the codebook to account for our 4-codebook SLC), SLC outperforms the others at the equivalent model dimensionalities.

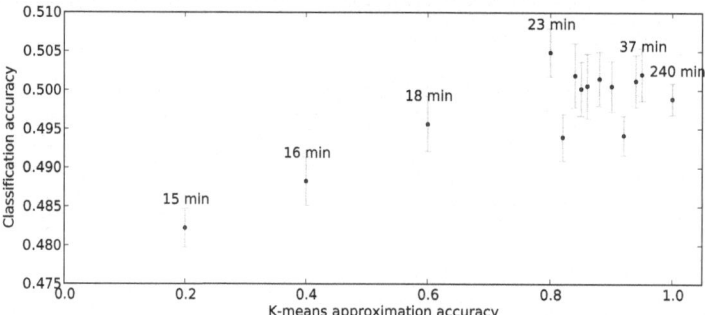

**Fig. 5.** Codebooks produced by approximate k-means give similar classification accuracies as codebooks produced by the exact k-means algorithm. The construction time for several data points is shown. In this experiment, we clustered 1,000,000 features into 4096 codewords to use in a bag-of-features model. Initialization was with kmeans++. The dataset was Caltech 101, using 15 training images per category. (Dataset details are in Section 6.)

Second, we have observed a small improvement in classification accuracy by using the kmeans++ [18] initialization method rather than random initialization. However, this initialization method is expensive, so we use a subsampled kmeans++ initialization that does not significantly affect our results. Instead of performing kmeans++ initialization using all descriptors being clustered, we do kmeans++ initialization using a random 10% of the descriptors. This gives the benefit of an improved initialization at a fraction of the cost. When using subsampled kmeans++ initialization instead of full kmeans++ initialization, construction time (clustering 1,000,000 descriptors into a 4096-dimensional codebook) with 95% accuracy drops from 37 minutes to 20 minutes. At 80% accuracy, the construction time drops from 23 minutes to 12 minutes. Note that exact kmeans using full kmeans++ initialization requires approximately 240 minutes in this setting (see Fig. 5). We use 90% target accuracy and subsampled kmeans++ in all of our following experiments.

## 6    Experiments

We compare spatially local coding against a variety of state-of-the-art spatial pyramid variants on Caltech 101 [19] and Caltech 256 [20].[1]

We resize Caltech 101 and Caltech 256 images to fit inside a $300 \times 300$ pixel square. This is consistent with the published results we compare against. We compared methods using 15 and 30 training images per category for Caltech 101, and using 30 training images per category for Caltech 256, all common points of reference from the literature.

We first learn a codebook using a random subsampling of 1,000,000 descriptors from the training set. This is an appearance-only codebook for all of the spatial pyramid methods. For our SLC method, we learn multiple spatially local codebooks, with $\lambda = \{0, 0.75, 1.50, 3.00\}$.

Then, we form the spatial pyramid or SLC representations of the training images. For our implementation of the original spatial pyramid, we use nearest-neighbor vector quantization and average pooling in three spatial pyramid levels, as in [1]. For our implementation of the localized soft assignment spatial pyramid, we use soft assignment over the ten nearest codebook elements, and max-pooling in three spatial pyramid levels as in [3]. For our SLC model, we also use soft assignment over the ten nearest codebook elements from each $\lambda$-level, and max-pooling over a global spatial pooling region. In [3], they showed results motivating a small neighborhood, with ten neighbors being the optimal for Caltech 101. We confirmed that this still holds in our codebooks.

We learn for each class a one-vs-all SVM (using the LibSVM library), selecting the regularization parameter via cross-validation. For each run of the experiment, we record the average class accuracy over 101 or 256 classes (ignoring the background class as suggested by [20]).

---

[1] Code is available at http://www.cs.ubc.ca/projects/spatially-local-coding for ease of comparison.

We experimented with both the linear SVM and histogram intersection kernels SVM, but found that the linear SVM outperforms the histogram intersection kernel for our model (see Fig. 6). Thus, in Table 3, the results shown for our SLC model are obtained using a linear SVM.

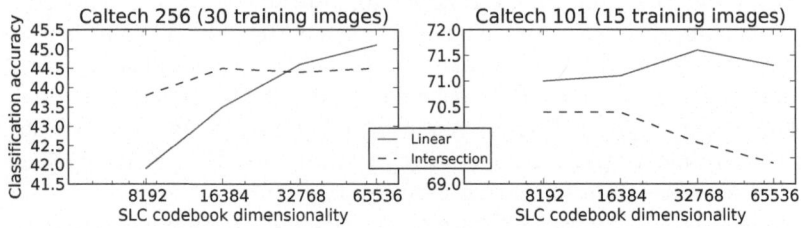

**Fig. 6.** Our model yields best results with a linear SVM. Only at low dimensionalities on Caltech 256, where the performance of both SVM types is low, does the intersection kernel outperform the linear SVM. At optimal codebook dimensionalities, our model's performance using a linear SVM dominates the performance of the histogram intersection kernel.

All of our reported numbers are based on 10 repetitions of the experiment, each time selecting a different training/testing split, building new codebooks, and learning new models. We report the mean and standard error of the mean.

The methods we compare against have generally published their results based on single-scale 16x16 SIFT features [21] using the VLFeat implementation [22] extracted every 8 pixels [1,3,4,2]. We perform the majority of our comparisons at this setting as well. We re-implement the original spatial pyramid method [1] and the best performing state-of-the-art variant, localized soft assignment [3] so as to provide a head-to-head comparison based on our extracted features. To report the classification accuracy achieved by our re-implementations, we ran them at various dimensionalities, since their performance is dependent on codebook dimensionality, and we report the highest result we could achieve with the other methods. Despite our results on SLC being obtained at higher *codebook* dimensionalities, this comparison is fair, since the *model* dimensionalities are comparable (see Fig. 4), and performance only deteriorates for the other methods as we increase their codebook size.

Table 3 shows that spatially local coding achieves better classification accuracy than all previous alternatives using single-scale SIFT features on Caltech 101 and Caltech 256.

Boureau *et al.* [5] have reported higher accuracy than any of the other previous methods. However, they achieve these results using a denser SIFT sampling (every 4 pixels), and use a feature based on the concatenation of 4 individual SIFT features within a small region which they call *macrofeatures*. We set these results aside from the rest of the reported numbers to highlight this difference, and run a separate comparison where we also extract SIFT every 4 pixels (however, we don't construct their macrofeatures). Spatially local coding again achieves a higher classification accuracy.

**Table 3.** Results on Caltech 101 (using 15 and 30 training examples per class) and 256 (using 30 training examples per class). We compare our SLC method against previously published figures and against re-implementations of the original spatial pyramid and localized soft assignment tested on our feature set. The numbers we report for our re-implementations of previous methods are the best results we could achieve from among a range of codebook dimensionalities. Bold method names show our experiments; the others are from the literature.

| | Cal. 101 (15) | Cal. 101 (30) | Cal. 256 (30) |
|---|---|---|---|
| | | Single-scale SIFT features extracted every 8 pixels | |
| Original SPM [1] | 56.4 | $64.6 \pm 0.8$ | - |
| **Original SPM (ours)** | $57.8 \pm 0.3$ | $65.2 \pm 0.4$ | $30.0 \pm 0.4$ |
| Localized soft assignment [3] | - | $74.21 \pm 0.81$ | - |
| **Localized soft assignment (ours)** | $66.2 \pm 0.4$ | $72.2 \pm 0.3$ | $37.2 \pm 0.2$ |
| Sparse Coding SPM [2] | $67.0 \pm 0.45$ | $73.2 \pm 0.54$ | $34.02 \pm 0.35$ |
| Sparse Coding SPM [4] | - | $71.8 \pm 1.0$ | - |
| **SLC [8192d × 4]** | $\mathbf{68.4 \pm 0.2}$ | $75.5 \pm 0.4$ | $38.9 \pm 0.3$ |
| **SLC [16384d × 4]** | $68.3 \pm 0.3$ | $\mathbf{75.7 \pm 0.4}$ | $\mathbf{40.0 \pm 0.2}$ |
| | | Multi-scale features extracted every 8 pixels | |
| LLC [7] (HOG) | 65.43 | 73.44 | 41.19 |
| Localized soft assignment [3] (SIFT) | - | $76.48 \pm 0.71$ | - |
| **SLC [8192d × 4]** | $71.4 \pm 0.4$ | $78.0 \pm 0.4$ | $41.8 \pm 0.3$ |
| **SLC [16384d × 4]** | $\mathbf{72.5 \pm 0.3}$ | $\mathbf{79.2 \pm 0.2}$ | $43.4 \pm 0.2$ |
| **SLC [32768d × 4]** | $70.9 \pm 0.4$ | $77.2 \pm 0.6$ | $\mathbf{44.3 \pm 0.1}$ |
| **SLC [65536d × 4]** | $69.6 \pm 0.3$ | $77.5 \pm 0.4$ | $43.4 \pm 0.3$ |
| | | Single-scale SIFT features extracted every 4 pixels | |
| Boureau *et al.* [5] | - | $77.3 \pm 0.6$ | $41.7 \pm 0.8$ |
| **SLC [8192d × 4]** | $71.0 \pm 0.3$ | $77.6 \pm 0.2$ | $41.9 \pm 0.2$ |
| **SLC [16384d × 4]** | $71.1 \pm 0.3$ | $78.9 \pm 0.2$ | $43.5 \pm 0.3$ |
| **SLC [32768d × 4]** | $\mathbf{71.6 \pm 0.4}$ | $\mathbf{79.6 \pm 0.8}$ | $44.6 \pm 0.2$ |
| **SLC [65536d × 4]** | - | - | $\mathbf{45.1 \pm 0.2}$ |
| | | Multi-scale SIFT features extracted every 4 pixels | |
| **SLC [65536d × 4]** | $\mathbf{72.7 \pm 0.4}$ | $\mathbf{81.0 \pm 0.2}$ | $\mathbf{46.6 \pm 0.2}$ |

Wang *et al.* [7] use another slightly different feature set for their experiments on locality constrained linear coding. They extract multiscale features (HOG) every 8 pixels at three different sizes. We again set these reported results aside from the rest and run a separate comparison.

While the above comparisons are sufficient to demonstrate SLC's superior performance as compared to state-of-the-art spatial pyramids, we provide an additional evaluation at an even denser extraction setting, extracting multiscale SIFT every 4 pixels.

These experiments show that spatially local coding outperforms all previous spatial pyramid methods for object recognition on Caltech 101 and Caltech 256. We have shown this in the setting of single-scale and multi-scale SIFT features, at two different extraction densities. In addition, we have provided a detailed survey and comparison of the previously published results, making clear how they are comparable with each other or not.

To the best of our knowledge, any previous work reporting higher accuracy than ours combines together multiple complimentary feature types.

### 6.1    Notes on Timing

Codebook construction scales logarithmically with the number of codebook dimensions, because we use approximate matching at each k-means step. SLC's multiple codebook construction can be multi-threaded, giving elapsed real time for codebook construction that scales logarithmically with the number of codebook dimensions.

Vector quantization also scales logarithmically with the number of codebook dimensions and linearly with the number of codebooks. To code 7680 training images (for Caltech 256), 1024D SPM required 2 minutes. SLC using four 16384D codebooks takes 11 minutes. That is 5.5x the compute time, despite the model size being 64x as large.

SVM training is the bottleneck regardless of the approach. This time is unaffected by switching from local soft assignment SPM to SLC. Both use soft assignment across a small number of nearest neighbors, giving sparse feature vectors. Gram matrix construction for Caltech 256's 7680 training images took 55 minutes using local soft assignment SPM with 8192D, and 50 minutes under SLC using four 8192D dictionaries. Doubling the SLC dimensionality to 16384D increased the gram matrix construction time to 65 minutes.

## 7    Conclusion

Spatially local coding is a simpler and more flexible way to enforce spatial locality in histogram-based object models than previous approaches. By simultaneously coding appearance and location, we remove the necessity of a complicated pooling stage to adequately model the spatial locations of visual features. We have shown that a combination of location-augmented codebooks gives better classification accuracy than spatial pyramid models.

The large codebook dimensionality required by our models potentially poses extra computational cost, but we have shown approximations that speed up the codebook construction process and an evaluation of the effect of those approximations on classification accuracy.

We have presented these results alongside a useful survey of previously published results and our re-implementations of previous results. To the best of our knowledge, we have shown the highest classification accuracy achieved on Caltech 101 and Caltech 256 using a single visual feature type.

## References

1. Lazebnik, S., Schmid, C., Ponce, J.: Beyond Bags of Features: Spatial Pyramid Matching for Recognizing Natural Scene Categories. In: CVPR (2006)
2. Yang, J., Yu, K., Gon, Y., Huang, T.: Linear spatial pyramid matching using sparse coding for image classification. In: CVPR (2009)
3. Liu, L., Wang, L., Liu, X.: In Defense of Soft-assignment Coding. In: ICCV (2011)
4. Boureau, Y.L., Bach, F., LeCun, Y., Ponce, J.: Learning mid-level features for recognition. In: CVPR (2010)

5. Boureau, Y.L., Le Roux, N., Bach, F., Ponce, J., LeCun, Y.: Ask the locals: multi-way local pooling for image recognition. In: ICCV (2011)
6. Csurka, G., Dance, C., Fan, L., Willamowski, J., Bray, C.: Visual categorization with bags of keypoints. In: Workshop on Statistical Learning in Computer Vision, ECCV (2004)
7. Wang, J., Yang, J., Yu, K., Lv, F., Huang, T., Gong, Y.: Locality-constrained linear coding for image classification. In: CVPR (2010)
8. van Gemert, J.C., Veenman, C.J., Smeulders, A.W.M., Geusebroek, J.M.: Visual word ambiguity. PAMI 32, 1271–1283 (2010)
9. Boiman, O., Shechtman, E., Irani, M.: In defense of nearest-neighbor based image classification. In: CVPR (2008)
10. Zhou, X., Cui, N., Li, Z., Liang, F., Huang, T.S.: Hierarchical Gaussianization for Image Classification (2009)
11. Krapac, J., Verbeek, J., Jurie, F.: Modeling spatial layout with Fisher vectors for image categorization. In: ICCV (2011)
12. Oliveira, G.L., Nascimento, E.R., Vieira, A.W., Campos, M.F.: Sparse Spatial Coding: A Novel Approach for Efficient and Accurate Object Recognition. In: ICRA (2012)
13. Laptev, I., Marszalek, M., Schmid, C.: Learning realistic human actions from movies. In: CVPR (2008)
14. Jia, Y., Huang, C.: Beyond Spatial Pyramids: Receptive Field Learning for Pooled Image Features. In: NIPS 2011 Workshop on Deep Learning and Unsupervised Feature Learning (2011)
15. Chatfield, K., Lempitsky, V., Vedaldi, A.: The devil is in the details: an evaluation of recent feature encoding methods. In: BMVC (2011)
16. Muja, M., Lowe, D.: Fast approximate nearest neighbors with automatic algorithm configuration. In: VISSAPP (2009)
17. Philbin, J., Chum, O., Isard, M., Sivic, J., Zisserman, A.: Object retrieval with large vocabularies and fast spatial matching. In: CVPR (2007)
18. Arthur, D., Vassilvitskii, S.: K-means ++: The Advantages of Careful Seeding. In: Eighteenth Annual ACM-SIAM Symposium on Discrete Algorithms, SODA, New Orleans, Louisiana, pp. 1027–1035. Society for Industrial and Applied Mathematics (2007)
19. Fei-Fei, L., Fergus, R., Perona, P.: Learning generative visual models from few training examples: An incremental Bayesian approach tested on 101 object categories. In: Workshop on Generative-Model Based Vision, CVPR (2004)
20. Griffin, G., Holub, A., Perona, P.: Caltech-256 Object Category Dataset. Technical report, California Institute of Technology (2007)
21. Lowe, D.G.: Distinctive Image Features from Scale-Invariant Keypoints. IJCV 60, 91–110 (2004)
22. Vedaldi, A., Fulkerson, B.: VLFeat: An open and portable library of computer vision algorithms (2008), www.vlfeat.org

# Semantic Segmentation with Millions of Features: Integrating Multiple Cues in a Combined Random Forest Approach*

Björn Fröhlich, Erik Rodner, and Joachim Denzler

Computer Vision Group, Friedrich Schiller University Jena, Germany
http://www.inf-cv.uni-jena.de

**Abstract.** In this paper, we present a new combined approach for feature extraction, classification, and context modeling in an iterative framework based on random decision trees and a huge amount of features. A major focus of this paper is to integrate different kinds of feature types like color, geometric context, and auto context features in a joint, flexible and fast manner. Furthermore, we perform an in-depth analysis of multiple feature extraction methods and different feature types. Extensive experiments are performed on challenging facade recognition datasets, where we show that our approach significantly outperforms previous approaches with a performance gain of more than 15% on the most difficult dataset.

## 1 Introduction

Recognition of semantic categories in images is an important field in computer vision and especially labeling each pixel of an image is a challenging structural task. Solving this task requires to take several different cues into account, such as color, shape, and texture. Furthermore, contextual information, like probable constellations and positions of categories in an image, is essential to achieve consistent and accurate results [16].

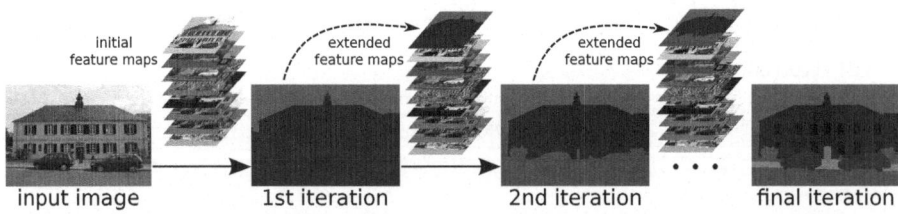

**Fig. 1.** Basic idea of our approach: features are added and updated incrementally to the set of available features to refine the semantic segmentation result

* Sponsored by the Graduate School on Image Processing and Image Interpretation, TMBWK ProExzellenz program.

K.M. Lee et al. (Eds.): ACCV 2012, Part I, LNCS 7724, pp. 218–231, 2013.
© Springer-Verlag Berlin Heidelberg 2013

In this paper, we present a powerful semantic segmentation framework, which handles different information cues and features in a combined manner. In contrast to previous work [16,22,23], where contextual constraints are integrated after a local classification step, our approach allows for learning them directly and jointly together with other feature types. This is done by estimating contextual cues in an iterative manner based on the output of the classifier built in a previous step.

Features, whether or not contextual, are calculated with feature extraction methods performed on so called feature maps, which contain a value for each pixel of the original image. The number of possible combinations of all parameters leads to millions of possible features and we show how to handle them with random decision forests in an efficient manner. The approach can be easily extended and adapted to other application areas, simply by extending the set of feature maps. Another advantage is that due to the iterative and combined nature of our approach, the trade-off between accuracy and computation time for learning and testing can be controlled. With slightly modifications and a loss of accuracy the introduced method has anytime capabilities which has be shown in [8].

***Related Work on Semantic Segmentation.*** We incorporate context knowledge by using the output of previous levels of a decision tree classifier as features for a new one. This strategy is similar to the one used by Fink and Perona [6] for their mutual boosting approach, where they train a set of object detectors simultaneously. In each round of the Boosting method, features are added derived from the results of the current classifier.

Our work is also related to the approach of Shotton *et al.* [16], where a two stage segmentation technique is proposed. Their idea is to first train a random forest using basic local features and then to train a second random forest using context features calculated using the first forest. In contrast, we learn a single random forest and incrementally add context features derived from coarser levels. This allows for handling the problem in a combined manner, where dependencies between contextual features and non-contextual features are exploited directly. Considering image and context features jointly is beneficial, because it reflects more the inherent dependency between both types. For example, blue might be a typical color for a car, but only when we know that there is no building underneath, which would give a good hint for a sky region. Those situations can not be modeled by considering contextual after color features. Typically, context information is modeled by time consuming random field approaches [11,13,22,23]. For a good overview of other semantic segmentation approaches, we refer the reader to Arbelaez *et al.* [1].

***Related Work on Facade Recognition.*** The application considered in this paper is semantic segmentation for facade recognition based on standard color images. The task is to estimate the position and size of various structural (*e.g.* "window", "door") and non-structural elements (*e.g.* "sky", "road", "building") in a given image of a building or street scene. This recognition task has gained interest in recent years [9], which is mainly due to the growing need to store the appearance of buildings in large 3D city models [9]. For example, an efficient representation of already labeled images with a grammar based compression scheme [15] allows for reducing each facade image to a few parameters. Furthermore, by incorporating a large amount of prior knowledge, the recognition of facade elements also allows for estimating the rough 3D structure of buildings [9].

The work of Fröhlich et al. [7] propose an approach, which classifies local color features with a random decision forest and further refines the result by fusing with an unsupervised segmentation. In contrast to our approach, they do not incorporate contextual information and the feature set is strictly limited. Yang and Förstner [23] use a conditional Markov random field (CRF), in which the unary potentials are computed by applying a random forest classifier. A subsequent work of the same authors [22] improves this method by considering a hierarchical CRF that exploits region segmentations on multiple image scales. Our approach takes high-order dependencies of multiple pixels into account and integrates classification and contextual inference in a combined approach. Furthermore, the approach does not incorporate any prior model-based knowledge about facades as utilized in Teboul et al. [18].

**Outline.** The remainder of this paper is structured as follows. In Section 2, we introduce a new flexible framework for semantic segmentation based on random decision forests including feature extraction and classification with respect to spatial context. Several high-level cues and feature types that are integrated in our approach are presented in Section 3. Extensive experiments and an analysis of the results are done in Section 4. A summary of our findings and a discussion of future research directions conclude the paper.

## 2    Semantic Segmentation with Iterative Context Forests

Our semantic segmentation approach, named Iterative Context Forests (ICF), is based on the massive use of random decision forests and the computation of several basic as well as high-level contextual features during learning.

**Random Decision Forest.** Random decision forests (RDF) are an extension of the well known decision trees. The main disadvantage of decision trees is the high risk of over-fitting and the high computation time during learning. Breiman [2] showed how to circumvent both aspects with different kinds of randomization. RDFs use multiple decision trees in which each tree is trained with a different random and balanced subset of the training data. Furthermore, in an inner node of a tree, only a random subset $S \subseteq U$ with $\tau$ features is used to find the best binary split of the training data, which is done by maximizing the information gain. A huge benefit of this idea is that not all available features have to be computed in each inner node, which is an essential property for our approach. To treat every feature equally, independent of its number of possible parameter

**Table 1.** List and description of feature extraction methods

| abbr. | description | abbr. | description |
|-------|-------------|-------|-------------|
| PP1 | diff. of two random pixel | RA2 | centered rectangle |
| PP2 | absolute diff. of two random pixel | RA3 | diff. of two centered rectangles |
| PP3 | sum of two random pixel | HL1 | horizontal Haar features |
| PP4 | value of a single random pixel | HL2 | vertical Haar features |
| RP1 | relative x-position of the pixel | HL3 | diagonal Haar features |
| RP2 | relative y-position of the pixel | HL4 | 3 rows of horizontal Haar features |
| RA1 | random rectangle | HL5 | 3 columns of vertical Haar features |

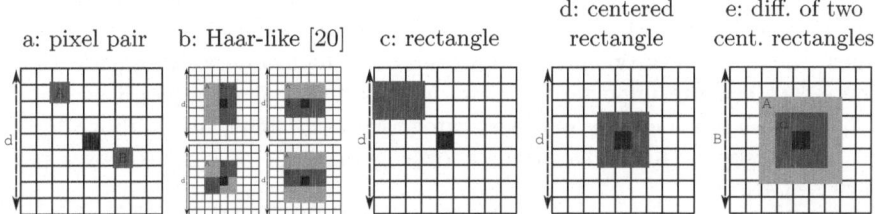

a: pixel pair    b: Haar-like [20]    c: rectangle    d: centered rectangle    e: diff. of two cent. rectangles

**Fig. 2.** Feature extraction methods applied to feature maps: features are computed in a window of size $d$ around the current pixel position (blue pixel). Depending on the type of a feature one or two pixels [16] (a) or one (c and d) or two areas (b and e) are randomly selected. Every parameter $\theta$ is selected randomly (the size of an area, the position of the area, etc.) under some constraints, *e.g.*, for (d) the rectangle is centered. For features utilizing areas, the mean values of the areas are used.

values, we first sample the feature type uniformly and then sample the parameter vector (*e.g.* position and size of the region) in a second step.

For classification, a new example finds its path through each decision tree and the average of the empirical distribution in the reached leaves is used as an estimate for class-wise probabilities.

***Generating Millions of Features.*** The question remains how the set $\mathcal{U}$ of all available features is defined. Our approach is based on extracting large sets of features of very different characteristics from an input image $\mathcal{I}$. This is done by first computing several feature maps $(\mathcal{M}_i)_{i=1}^{m}$, which are matrices that store a value for each pixel of the input image. For example, one very simple feature map is the red channel of the image. After computing these maps, we apply several feature extraction methods $g_\theta$ to the feature maps to actually compute feature values. Those feature extraction methods are parameterized by a vector $\theta$ including the index of the feature map used and parameters for the exact position. A list of the feature extraction methods used in this paper is given in Table 1 and illustrated in Fig. 2.

Due to the large number of possible locations and feature maps, the set of available features $\mathcal{U}$ goes up to several million features. For example, for only one feature extraction method on a window of a size of $d = 50$ pixel, the number of possible feature pairs is $6.25 \cdot 10^6$. Due to the reason that we have many different feature extraction methods for many channels the real number of possible features increases dramatically. However, the randomization techniques of the RDF classifier allow us to handle these sets in an efficient manner by only computing a small random selection of them.

***Auto Context Features.*** Estimating semantic labels for each image pixel is a structured task requiring the usage of context knowledge to exploit the intrinsic dependencies between different parts of the image. A common approach is to use conditional Markov random fields with a pairwise potential modeling dependencies between two pixels. However, often high-order contextual cues are required to capture important context information. For example, if we like to model the relative locations of object categories, *e.g.*, "building" is above "road" but below "sky". This sort of prior knowledge can not be captured by a plain pairwise CRF.

Therefore, we use a concept known as *auto-context* [19], where features are computed based on previous classification results. Shotton *et al.* [16] used this technique in a two stage manner, where a first RDF was built on color features only and a second RDF used the results of the first one as auxiliary features. Our approach was inspired by this technique but extends it by applying auto context in an iterative manner. We built and traverse the trees always in a breadth-first manner, which allows us to use the results of a previous level as a source for additional features. In our case, we compute probability maps for the whole image in each level of a decision tree and use them as additional feature maps. This allows for extracting high-level contextual features. For example, the rectangle feature extraction method RA1 (see Table 1) evaluated in a region above a pixel yields a feature giving a cue whether a certain class is present on top of the current one.

## 3   High-level Cues for Semantic Segmentation

In this section, we present how to compute feature maps and how to incorporate them in our framework. Besides simple operations like the conversion of the image from the RGB color space to the HSI color space and the computation of gradient images we are using an unsupervised segmentation [3], 3D geometric context features [10], and a high-level color transformation [21]. We call the set of all used feature maps the feature pool. The feature extraction methods from the previous section are applied on these feature maps to extract features for each pixel.

***Unsupervised Segmentation.*** In previous approaches an unsupervised segmentation is used to smooth the results to get one label for homogeneous regions [4,7,22,23]. There are two common ways in literature to incorporate the regions.

d: unsupervised

a: RGB image          b: hue          c: saturation          segmentation

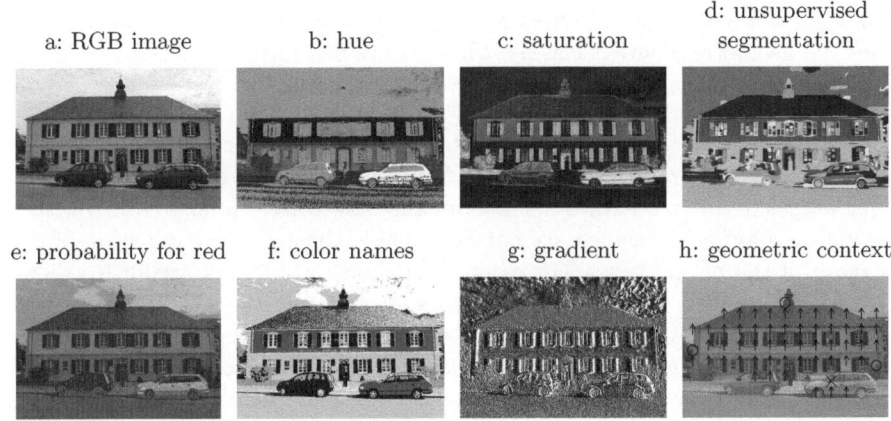

e: probability for red    f: color names          g: gradient          h: geometric context

**Fig. 3.** Overview of the algorithms used to compute feature maps: a: input RGB image, b: color hue, c: color saturation, d: unsupervised segmentation result, where each area is encoded by a different color, e: probability map for class red, the right car is highlighted in this map, f: most probable color for each pixel based on the probability maps from image e, g: gradient image of the RGB image, h: geometric context features, for details we refer to [10].

The first way is to annotate every pixel with the most probable class of one region after all other steps are finished [4,7]. Furthermore, the second way is to utilize the regions in an early step to initialize a graph for a CRF were each region is a node and the neighborhood of two regions is modeled as an edge [22,23]. In our framework, we found a third way to integrate region information. We propose to use the segmentation result as an additional feature added to the feature pool. After each iteration we compute the mean probability for each class in each region. Consequently, we have for each pixel the information about the previous classification result of all classes in the region where the pixel belongs to. We decided to utilize one of the most used unsupervised segmentation method, which is the mean-shift segmentation introduced by [3]. Please note that there are many alternative unsupervised segmentation methods like the very fast graph based segmentation introduced by Felzenszwalb and Huttenlocher [5].

***3D Geometric Context Features.*** A human is using 3D context features not only for classifying objects in the real world, but also for objects in 2D images. Of course, there is no direct 3D information in a 2D image without any additional knowledge. An important aspect is the Manhattan world assumption which says that most of the man-made environments are based on objects perpendicular to each other. Hoiem *et al.* [10] tries to learn such information from some hand labeled images, where they differ between the three main classes: "ground plane", "surfaces at roughly right angles to the ground plane" and "sky". These surfaces are split into "planar" and "non planar" surfaces. Furthermore, the "non planar" surfaces are split up into "solid" and "porous'" and "planar" is subdivided into planar surfaces facing "left", "right", or "centered" towards the camera. Following this method, we can extract seven probability maps, one for each of these 3D geometric context classes, which are added directly as features to our feature pool.

**Color Names.** An interesting idea to transform RGB color features to another feature space is introduced by van de Weijer *et al.* [21]. They describe these color names as linguistic labels that humans attach to colors. Therefore, they use eleven main colors which are not describable through a combination of two or more of the other colors. For example, nobody would say "reddish yellow" instead of "orange". To learn a transformation between the L*a*b*-color space and the color names the authors use a set of annotated images, where in each image one object of a specific color is masked. The color space is partitioned into $10 \times 20 \times 20$ bins for each channel of the L*a*b*-space. The distribution of each bin is calculated by counting pixels of each color ending up in a specific bin. With this it is possible to transform each RGB value into pseudo probabilities for each color name.

## 4   Experiments

In the following, we evaluate our methods on some facade datasets. The analysis concentrates on recognition performance as well as time needed for labeling a single image.

**Experimental Setup.** For feature extraction, we use a window with a size of $d = 50$ pixels for the non-context features and $d = 200$ pixels for the auto context features. The random forest contains five trees with a maximum depth of 15 levels and a random subset of $\tau = 400$ features is used in each node during learning. Computation times are evaluated on an Intel®Core$^{TM}$i7 CPU 930 with 2.8GHz with four cores. We differentiate between the average recognition rate over all classes and pixel-wise accuracy, which we refer to as overall recognition rate. The different modifications of the ICF are illustrated by additional letters. $H$ represents the use of the geometric context features, $G$ the usage of the gradient image and $W$ the color representation of van de Weijer [21]. Furthermore, mean-shift [3] is used as an unsupervised segmentation method providing optional feature for the feature pool ($S+$), or for post processing ($S$-). For example, ICFHG represents an Iterative Context Forest using the geometric context features and gradient images besides the HSI channel and the auto context features.

**Facade Recognition.** For our experiments, we use the eTRIMS dataset originally introduced by Korč and Förstner [12]. We use ten different random splits of the data into 40 images for training and 20 images for testing similar to [22,23]. Furthermore, the LabelMeFacade dataset introduced in [7], which contains 100 images for training and 845 images for testing, is used as a second more challenging dataset. Both datasets consists of the eight classes shown in Fig. 4 and

**Table 2.** Recognition rates of our experiments with different classifiers in comparison to previous work. In contrast to [7], we used random splits of training and testing for the eTRIMS dataset to allow for fair comparison with [22,23]. ICF represents our proposed approach including auto-context and the HSI color channels. An additional letter shows the usage of the feature channels: $H$ in the name represents the usage of the geometric context features of Hoiem *et al.* [10], $W$ the usage of the color names from van de Weijer *et al.* [21], $S+$ the direct incorporation of the mean-shift segmentation [3] and $S-$ the usage of mean-shift as a post-processing step.

| dataset | approach | average recognition rate | overall recognition rate |
|---|---|---|---|
| eTRIMS | CRF [23] | 49.75% | 65.80% |
| | HCRF [22] | 61.63% | 69.00% |
| | 3-Layer [14] | 63.25% | **81.94%** |
| | SIFT/RDF [7] | 62.81% (±1.58) | 64.00% (±3.28) |
| | SIFT/SLR [7] | 65.57% (±2.47) | 71.18% (±2.69) |
| | ICF | 68.61% (±1.71) | 70.81% (±1.32) |
| | ICFwoC | 64.07% (±1.72) | 61.11% (±1.59) |
| | ICFHGW | 71.47% (±1.25) | 72.59% (±1.06) |
| | ICFHGWS+ | 68.94% (±1.48) | 73.65% (±1.07) |
| | ICFHGWS- | 72.22% (±2.17) | 75.09% (±1.60) |
| | ICFHS- | **72.26%** (±3.25) | 76.10% (±1.24) |
| | ICFHGS- | 72.23% (±1.76) | 77.22% (±1.22) |
| LabelMeF | SIFT/RDF [7] | 44.08% (±0.45) | 49.06% (±0.52) |
| | SIFT/SLR [7] | 42.81% (±0.89) | 48.46% (±1.58) |
| | ICF | 49.39% (±0.48) | 60.68% (±0.72) |
| | ICFwoC | 47.66% (±0.06) | 43.97% (±0.03) |
| | ICFHGW | 56.95% (±0.28) | 61.93% (±0.65) |
| | ICFHGWS+ | 56.61% (±0.32) | **67.33%** (±0.67) |
| | ICFHGWS- | 57.11% (±0.20) | 66.08% (±1.68) |
| | ICFHS- | **57.82%** (±0.19) | 64.76% (±0.78) |
| | ICFHGS- | 57.35% (±0.51) | 66.86% (±0.41) |

an additional background class named "unlabeled". For trivial decision rules or random guessing the average recognition rate for both datasets is 12.5% and the overall recognition rate is less than 35% (all pixels labeled as building).

Table 2 and Fig. 4 shows some results on the eTRIMS and the LabelMeFacade datasets using different methods for semantic segmentation. First of all, one can see that we outperform all previous state-of-the-art approaches on these datasets significantly. All previous approaches from [7,22,23] are based on SIFT features, which need to be fully computed in advance. The Iterative Context Forest (ICF) only using simple color features (HSI) and the auto context features is as good as previous state-of-the-art results. Furthermore, incorporating additional features improves the results significantly. The usage of the gradients, the unsupervised segmentation as an post-processing step and the geometric context from Section 3 improves the recognition rate obviously. Unfortunately, the utilization of the color names does not bring any improvement of the results, but a decrease in performance. We also did experiments with the MSRC21 dataset achieving an

original      ground-truth      ICFwoC          ICF          ICFHGS-

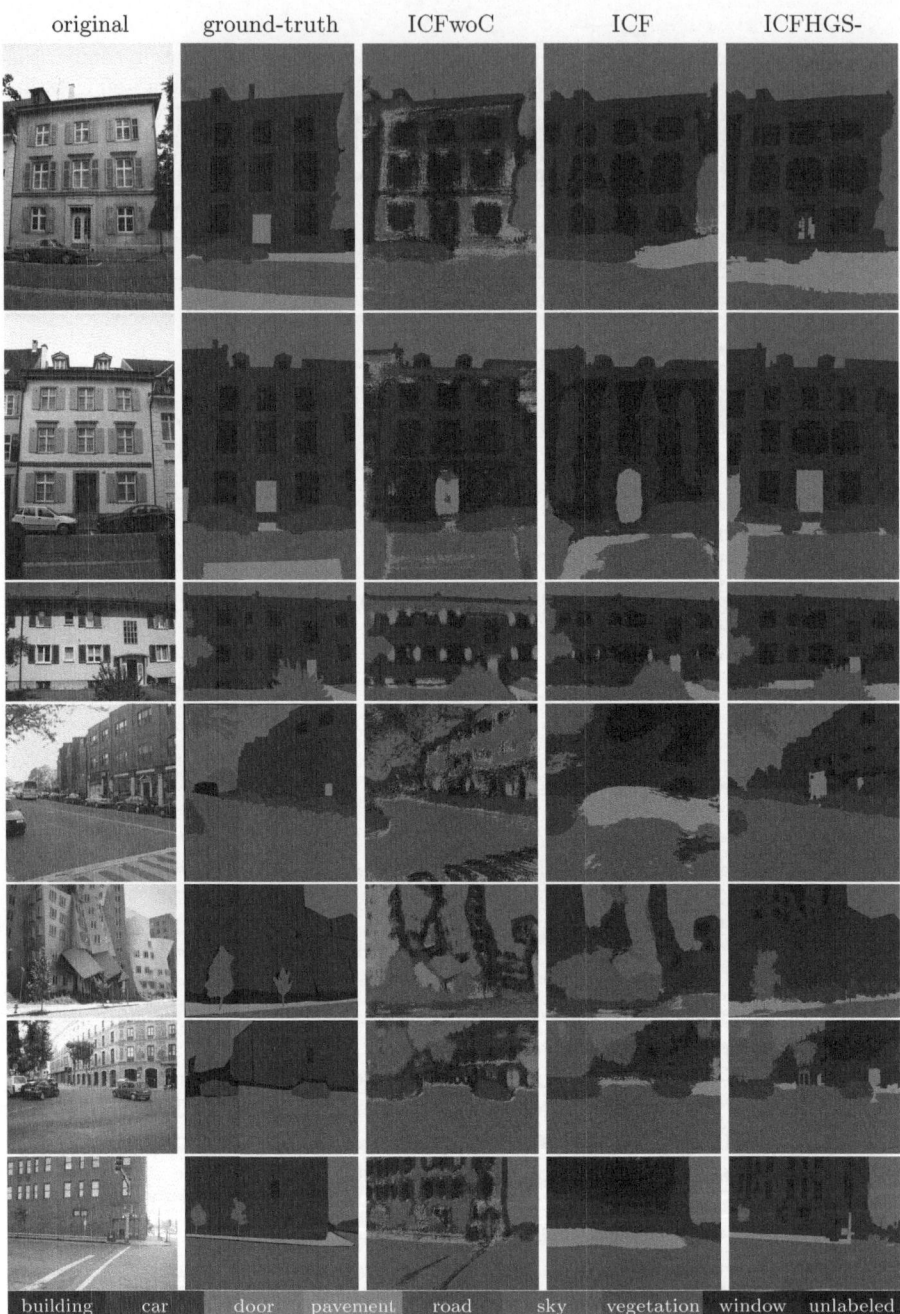

building    car    door    pavement    road    sky    vegetation    window    unlabeled

**Fig. 4.** Example images from eTRIMS (first three rows) and LabelMeFacade database (last four rows). The corresponding results obtained by a decision tree without any auto context (ICFwoC), Iterative Context Forests using only color features (ICF), and Iterative Context Forests using color, gradients, 3D geometric context and an unsupervised segmentation (ICFHGS-) are shown.

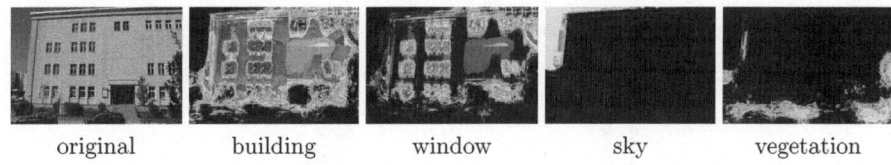

| original | building | window | sky | vegetation |

**Fig. 5.** Probability maps of some classes for a specific image. Warm colors correspond to areas with high probability.

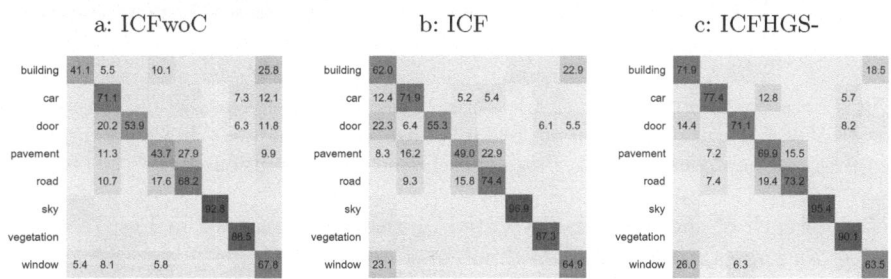

a: ICFwoC          b: ICF          c: ICFHGS-

**Fig. 6.** Confusion matrices for one run in the eTRIMs dataset using the same settings as shown in Fig. 4

overall accuracy of 67.2% using ICFHGWS-. The accuracy increases with each iteration until it converges. We point to [8] for further results of the different iterations.

The computation time depends on the usage of the feature channels. The ICF using auto-context and the HSI color channels needs $\approx 3s$ per image. Computing the 3D geometric context features increases the time by $\approx 10s$, the segmentation $\approx 3s$ and the color names $\ll 1s$. Therefore, it is possible to adjust between a fast computation of the result or a high accuracy by choosing different types of features and by selecting parameters like the amount of trees and the depth of each tree.

Some samples for the auto context feature maps are shown in Fig. 5. Each of these channels is computed after each iteration and used for computing the splits in the next level of the forest (see Section 2).

The confusion matrices for three different settings of our framework are presented in Fig. 6. Incorporating context features increases the recognition rate for the classes "building", "road", and "sky" significantly. Furthermore, using the additional features increases the recognition rates for "building","car", "door", "pavement" and "vegetation" clearly. All proposed methods still have problems with the confusion of "window" and "building" as well as "pavement" and "road".

***Evaluation of Feature Usage.*** As mentioned above, we use a huge amount of different feature extraction methods. In this section, we want to analyze the

a: feature extraction method relevance     b: Usage of raw vs. context features

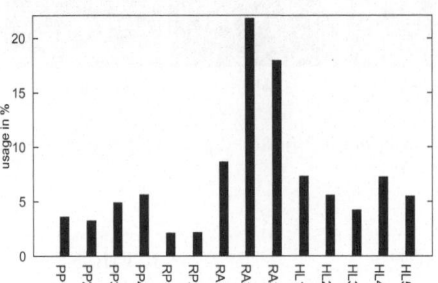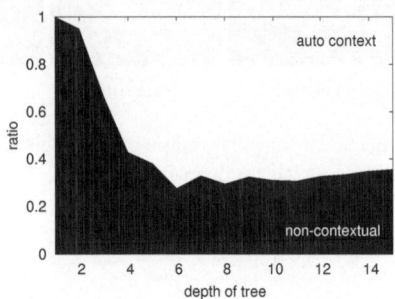

**Fig. 7.** Statistical analysis of used features types and feature extraction methods. a: Usage of each feature extraction method in a learned decision forest, b: Usage of context features and non-contextual features for each level of the decision trees.

usage of each of the methods presented in Table 1. As shown in Fig. 7a by far the most important features are different kinds of rectangle features (*cf.* [17]), led by the single window centered at the current pixel position, followed by the difference of two windows centered in the middle and a rectangle with a random position relative to the current position. More than 48% of all decisions over all trees are done using these three feature extraction types. Another 30% of the decisions are done using some of the Haar features. The pixel-pair respectively the single pixel features are chosen in about 17% of all cases and only 4% of all decisions are based on the relative position of a pixel in an image. This is more or less what we have expected. Relative positions should not be that important, due to a high risk of over-fitting, but it is still an useful information for some classes like "sky". Pixel-pair features are much more sensitive against image noise compared to rectangle features.

In Fig. 7b the usage of non-contextual versus auto context features is plotted. In the first level of a tree it is not possible to use any auto context features, but from the second level of a tree the influence of the contextual features is slowly increasing. Beginning at a depth of about six levels the ratio converges at about 60% auto context features and about 40% non-contextual features. This shows that both feature types are important to train an ICF and that the importance of the auto context features increases with the quality of previous outputs.

***Looking Beyond the Current Horizon.*** As we have seen in the previous sections, our method is able to remarkably outperform state of the art approaches for semantic segmentation. However, we discovered several special cases, where our proposed method failed during evaluations. We visualized exemplary images in Fig. 8 showing problematical details of the classification results from Fig. 4. (1) Untypical positions like the windows on the roof are underrepresented in the training data. Obviously, these problems can be solved by adding more images to the training data. (2) Another problem are badly labeled images as shown in the second row of Fig. 8. This is a twofold problem. First of all, during training the

original          ground-truth          ICFHGS-

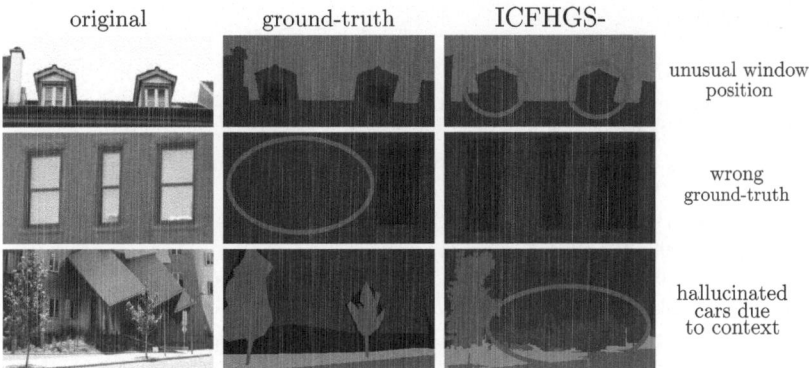

unusual window
position

wrong
ground-truth

hallucinated
cars due
to context

**Fig. 8.** Detailed analysis of the results of our approach

classifier learns the class "building" based on noisy data leading to disturbed classification models. On top of that, evaluations are negatively skewed since test images are counted as wrongly classified in these regions due to the missing ground truth data. (3) As shown in the last row of Fig. 8 in some special cases objects are identified which are not in the image but would have been expected to be based on contextual assumptions. In this example the ICF tries to fit the class "car" between "pavement" and "building" instead of "vegetation". Apparently the classifier was not sure how to classify these regions. Although this may be due to missing training data for this constellation of classes, it would be interesting to regularize the influence of context in such scenarios.

## 5   Conclusion and Further Work

In this work, we presented a new approach for incorporating context features and multiple other features in a single framework for semantic segmentation. We have shown that our approach is very flexible and can simply be adjusted between fast evaluation and high accuracy. In extensive experiments, we have shown that our approach significantly outperforms other state of the art methods including time consuming conditional random field techniques. Furthermore, we have shown that extending the set of available features can increase the recognition rate. Especially 3D geometric context features lead to a high performance gain for the challenging LabelMeFacade dataset.

For future work, we plan to adapt the random sampling to allow for integration of prior knowledge about feature relevance. The current approach samples uniformly from the set of available feature types and does not differentiate between them. Furthermore, the sampling could be also tuned towards sampling easy-computable features with high probability. This strategy would lead to trees with a lower average computation time for classifying a new test input.

# References

1. Arbelaez, P., Hariharan, B., Gu, C., Gupta, S., Bourdev, L., Malik, J.: Semantic segmentation using regions and parts. In: CVPR (2012)
2. Breiman, L.: Random forests. Machine Learning 45(1), 5–32 (2001)
3. Comaniciu, D., Meer, P.: Mean shift: a robust approach toward feature space analysis. PAMI 24(5), 603–619 (2002)
4. Csurka, G., Perronnin, F.: An efficient approach to semantic segmentation. IJCV 95(2), 198–212 (2011)
5. Felzenszwalb, P.F., Huttenlocher, D.P.: Efficient graph-based image segmentation. IJCV 59(2), 167–181 (2004)
6. Fink, M., Perona, P.: Mutual boosting for contextual inference. In: NIPS, vol. 16, pp. 1515–1522 (2003)
7. Fröhlich, B., Rodner, E., Denzler, J.: A fast approach for pixelwise labeling of facade images. In: ICPR, pp. 3029–3032 (2010)
8. Fröhlich, B., Rodner, E., Denzler, J.: As Time Goes by—Anytime Semantic Segmentation with Iterative Context Forests. In: Pinz, A., Pock, T., Bischof, H., Leberl, F. (eds.) DAGM/OAGM 2012. LNCS, vol. 7476, pp. 1–10. Springer, Heidelberg (2012)
9. Gool, L.J.V., Zeng, G., den Borre, F.V., Müller, P.: Towards mass-produced building models. In: Photogrammetric Image Analysis, pp. 209–220 (2007)
10. Hoiem, D., Efros, A.A., Hebert, M.: Geometric context from a single image. In: ICCV, vol. 1, pp. 654–661. IEEE (October 2005)
11. Kohli, P., Ladicky, L., Torr, P.: Robust higher order potentials for enforcing label consistency. In: CVPR, pp. 1–8 (2008)
12. Korč, F., Förstner, W.: eTRIMS image database for interpreting images of man-made scenes. Tech. Rep. TR-IGG-P-2009-01, University of Bonn (2009)
13. Ladický, Ľ., Russell, C., Kohli, P., Torr, P.H.S.: Associative hierarchical crfs for object class image segmentation. In: ICCV, pp. 739–746 (2009)
14. Martinović, A., Mathias, M., Weissenberg, J., Van Gool, L.: A Three-Layered Approach to Facade Parsing. In: Fitzgibbon, A., Lazebnik, S., Perona, P., Sato, Y., Schmid, C. (eds.) ECCV 2012, Part VII. LNCS, vol. 7578, pp. 416–429. Springer, Heidelberg (2012)
15. Ripperda, N., Brenner, C.: Evaluation of Structure Recognition Using Labelled Facade Images. In: Denzler, J., Notni, G., Süße, H. (eds.) DAGM 2009. LNCS, vol. 5748, pp. 532–541. Springer, Heidelberg (2000)
16. Shotton, J., Johnson, M., Cipolla, R.: Semantic texton forests for image categorization and segmentation. In: CVPR, pp. 1–8 (2008)
17. Shotton, J., Winn, J., Rother, C., Criminisi, A.: TextonBoost: Joint Appearance, Shape and Context Modeling for Multi-class Object Recognition and Segmentation. In: Leonardis, A., Bischof, H., Pinz, A. (eds.) ECCV 2006. LNCS, vol. 3951, pp. 1–15. Springer, Heidelberg (2006)
18. Teboul, O., Simon, L., Koutsourakis, P., Paragios, N.: Segmentation of building facades using procedural shape priors. In: CVPR, pp. 3105–3112 (2010)
19. Tu, Z., Bai, X.: Auto-context and its application to high-level vision tasks and 3d brain image segmentation. PAMI 32(10), 1744–1757 (2010)

20. Viola, P., Jones, M.: Robust real-time object detection. IJCV 57, 137–154 (2002)
21. van de Weijer, J., Schmid, C.: Applying color names to image description. In: ICIP, vol. 3, pp. 493–496 (2007)
22. Yang, M.Y., Förstner, W.: A hierarchical conditional random field model for labeling and classifying images of man-made scenes. In: ICCV Workshops, pp. 196–203 (2011)
23. Yang, M.Y., Förstner, W.: Regionwise Classification of Building Facade Images. In: Stilla, U., Rottensteiner, F., Mayer, H., Jutzi, B., Butenuth, M. (eds.) PIA 2011. LNCS, vol. 6952, pp. 209–220. Springer, Heidelberg (2011)

# Semi-Supervised Learning on a Budget: Scaling Up to Large Datasets

Sandra Ebert, Mario Fritz, and Bernt Schiele

Max Planck Institute for Informatics
Saarbrucken, Germany

**Abstract.** Internet data sources provide us with large image datasets which are mostly without any explicit labeling. This setting is ideal for semi-supervised learning which seeks to exploit labeled data as well as a large pool of unlabeled data points to improve learning and classification. While we have made considerable progress on the theory and algorithms, we have seen limited success to translate such progress to the large scale datasets which these methods are inspired by. We investigate the computational complexity of popular graph-based semi-supervised learning algorithms together with different possible speed-ups. Our findings lead to a new algorithm that scales up to 40 times larger datasets in comparison to previous approaches and even increases the classification performance. Our method is based on the key insights that by employing a density-based measure unlabeled data points can be selected similar to an active learning scheme. This leads to a compact graph resulting in an improved performance up to 11.6% at reduced computational costs.

## 1 Introduction

Research on semi-supervised learning (SSL) aims to leverage unlabeled data to support learning and classification tasks. A key assumption is that the underlying data distribution carries valuable information about the class distribution. In combination with the limited amount of available labeled data one can achieve better performance than with labeled data alone. This idea is also fueled by the availability of vast sources of unlabeled images from the web.

Due to the active research on semi-supervised learning, the understanding of theory and algorithms in this area have greatly improved. One of the most promising frameworks is graph-based label propagation which leads to many insights [1] as well as high performance algorithms [2,3]. However, those algorithms typical come with a quadratic complexity that is contradictory to the initial goal to scale up to large datasets. The "the-more-data-the-better" strategy that usually increases the performance of SSL [4] can often be not applied due to the prohibitive time and space complexity.

In this work, we question this strategy and show that we can indeed increase the performance with a more careful selection of *unlabeled* data. As a result we get similar or even better performance with only a fraction of all unlabeled data. This advantage becomes particularly evident when using large datasets like

K.M. Lee et al. (Eds.): ACCV 2012, Part I, LNCS 7724, pp. 232–245, 2013.
© Springer-Verlag Berlin Heidelberg 2013

ILSVRC 2010 with 1,000 categories and more than a million images. In contrast to previous selection approaches [5,6] that are only applicable to mid-sized data collections with up to 30,000 data points, we are able to handle 40 times larger datasets. A further advantage of our selection method is that we can efficiently combine label propagation with active learning to further improve performance. In the context of active learning graph size plays a crucial role and thus our effective selection of unlabeled data becomes even more advantageous.

**Contributions.** First, we introduce two selection strategies (Sec. 3). We compare these criteria to previous methods and show on mid-sized datasets that we improve these approaches when we consider more realistic datasets with occlusions, truncations, and background clutter (Sec. 6). After that, we illustrate on a subset of ILSVRC 2010 with 100 classes that we get better performance when using only a representative subset of all images instead of all unlabeled data. We also show that our approach is able to process the entire ILSVRC 2010 dataset with 1,000 classes and more than one million images. Finally, we conclude our work in Sec. 7 by applying graph propagation in combination with active learning resulting in increased performance.

## 2    Related Work

Large-scale computer vision has become more and more prominent in recent research. There is many work utilizing vast amount of images from the internet in order to improve one specific object category [7], to generate new datasets within an active learning framework [8], or to use it for image retrieval [9]. For image classification, ILSVRC 2010 [10] with 1,000 classes and more than one million images is currently one of the most difficult datasets according to size and number of classes. Although, there are many approaches addressing this dataset most of them focus more on faster and better image description [11], analyze semantic similarities [12], or evaluate the scalability of knowledge transfer [13]. However, there are surprisingly few works that consider more advanced classification schemes beyond linear classifiers.

In contrast, semi-supervised learning (SSL) in particular graph-based methods are made to leverage labeled as well as unlabeled data to improve performance of classification. We observe a large progress towards algorithmic contributions [14,15]. More recently, there is also a focus on improving graph construction – the most critical part of these algorithms. Previous works propose a better weighting function [16,17], make use of discriminative algorithms like SVM [18], or remove noise of the data [1]. But although there is a common believe that more unlabeled data helps for learning, there is almost no work that address the scalability issue to take advantage of this huge available amount.

Main problem is that graph-based algorithms come with a quadratic runtime and space complexity. Previous work proposes methods to reduce the dimensionality of the used image descriptors [19], or classify with an approximation [20]. Other works reduce the amount of unlabeled data to approximate the distance matrix [21,22], or to construct a smaller graph that represents the entire data

data distribution [5,6,23]. In this work, we build on this idea. But instead of representing the entire data space we focus on the data regions that are more relevant for our image classification task.

# 3   General SSL-Framework

This section briefly introduces our SSL setup consisting of label propagation [14] extended with active learning [24] to further improve the performance.

## 3.1   Label Propagation (LP)

Given $n = l + u$ data point with $l$ labeled examples $L = \{(x_1, y_1), ..., (x_l, y_l)\}$ and $u$ unlabeled ones $x_{l+1}, ..., x_n$ with $x \in \mathbb{R}^d$ the features, $y \in \mathcal{L} = \{1, ..., c\}$ the labels, and $c$ the number of classes. We build a symmetric $k$-nearest neighbor graph with the L1 distance and use a Gaussian kernel to get the final weighted graph $W$. Based on this graph a normalized graph Laplacian is computed

$$\mathcal{S} = D^{-1/2}WD^{-1/2} \quad \text{with} \quad D_{ij} = \begin{cases} \sum_j W_{ij} & \text{if } i = j \\ 0 & \text{otherwise} \end{cases} \tag{1}$$

We use an iterative procedure [14] to propagate labels through this graph

$$Y_m^{(t+1)} = \alpha \mathcal{S} Y_m^{(t)} + (1 - \alpha) Y_m^{(0)} \quad \text{with } 1 \leq m \leq c, \tag{2}$$

with $Y_m^*$ the limit of this sequence. The initial label vector is set as follows $Y_m^{(0)} = (y_1^m, ..., y_l^m, 0, ..., 0)$ with $y_i^m \in \{1, -1\}$ for the labeled data and zero otherwise. Parameter $\alpha \in (0, 1]$ controls the overwriting of the original labels. Finally, the prediction of the data $\hat{Y} \in \mathcal{L}$ is obtained by $\hat{Y} = \text{argmax}_{1 \leq m \leq c} Y_m^*$.

## 3.2   Active Learning (AL)

Similar to [24], we combine uncertainty (exploitation) and density (exploration) criteria. For uncertainty, we use entropy over the class posterior $P(\tilde{y}_{ij}|x)$ by normalizing the prediction values from Eq. 2:

$$\mathcal{H}(x_i) = -\sum_{j=1}^{c} P(\tilde{y}_{ij}|x_i) \log P(\tilde{y}_{ij}|x_i). \tag{3}$$

For the density-based sampling, we employ the graph density criteria introduced by [24]. This criteria make use of the symmetric $k$-NN graph to find dense regions and is defined by the sum of all neighboring nodes divided by the number of neighbors

$$\mathcal{D}(x_i) = \frac{\sum_j W_{ij}}{\sum_j P_{ij}}, \tag{4}$$

with an adjacency matrix $P$ and the weight matrix $W$. To make both criteria comparable, we compute a ranking for each criteria separately such that high entropies or dense regions are mapped to small ranking values. These numbers are used to combine both criteria $s(x_i) = \beta \mathcal{H}(x_i) + (1 - \beta)\mathcal{D}(x_i)$ with parameter $\beta \in [0, 1]$. Finally, we query the label with the smallest score $s$ and add this sample to our labeled set.

# 4    Graph Enhancement Techniques

As motivated above, graph-based SSL-techniques are quadratic in the number of data samples. Therefore, we are interested in techniques that benefit from more unlabeled data while simultaneously minimizing the runtime. After reviewing previous techniques (Sec. 4.1) we propose two novel techniques (Sec. 4.2) that can be scaled to 40 times larger datasets than any previous techniques that we aware of due to their lower computational complexity (Sec. 4.3).

## 4.1    Previous Techniques

Several approaches have been proposed to enrich a given dataset. The simplest one is to add unlabeled data randomly with a uniform distribution either from an already existing dataset or from the internet. To have a stronger baseline for our experiments, we enrich our data distribution with already existing datasets to exclude wrong annotated and thus misleading images that are an integral part of web sources. We call this baseline *random*.

There are several other approaches that propose a graph construction with a representative unlabeled subset called anchor graph. In [6] *k-means* cluster centroids are used as anchor points which can be advantageous when the clusters represent one class each. Otherwise they introduce many shortcuts between different classes. We show experimentally that *k-means* works well for datasets with a smooth manifold structure but fails for more difficult data collections.

The second approach [5] finds representative unlabeled data in a *greedy* fashion by repeatedly selecting the sample that is farthest from the current subset $S$ consisting of the training set $L$ and the already selected unlabeled data $Z$: $\arg\min_{j \in Z \setminus S} \sum_{i \in L \cup S} W_{ij}$, with $W$ a similarity matrix for all images using L1 distance and a Gaussian weighting function. This method covers the entire data space without introducing redundant information and works well as long as there are not too many outliers in the data collection.

All methods aim to represent the entire unlabeled data space independently from the task itself. If the unlabeled data is representative for the test data as it is the case for ETH80 (Sec. 5), these methods work well. However, when the ratio between test samples and unlabeled data is very small as it is often the case for large datasets, these approaches fail to focus on the relevant part of the distribution thus not achieving optimal performance.

## 4.2   Novel Techniques to Enrich Graph Structure

In this work, we propose two novel selection criteria called *dense* and *NN* that focus on the classification task at hand but in a completely unsupervised way. Our goal is to enrich the area around a given set $T$ consisting of training and test data with unlabeled data. The idea behind this is that we want to benefit from unlabeled where it is most needed and helpful. Additionally, for large-scale datasets we cannot apply "the-more-data-the-better" strategy due to the time and space complexity issues.

We consider three scenarios for extension: 1) training set only; 2) test set only; and 3) training+test set. The first scenario leads only to local improvements because of the small amount of labeled data. Additionally, this approach becomes problematic if the neighborhoods around the labels are sparse as it leads to many false neighbors. Enhancing the area around the test data only improves the results for the same reasons. Experimentally, we observed that enriching the neighborhood of both training and test works best so that we report only results for this setting in the following.

**(i) *Dense*.** Our first criteria uses the previously introduced graph structure to find dense and thus representative regions. Of course, these regions can be anywhere in the unlabeled data space. Therefore, we look only in the immediate neighborhood of $T$ for high density nodes. More specifically, we select the $k$ nearest neighbors for each $x_i \in T$ so that we have a pool of at least $|Z_{pool}| + c$ samples with $|Z_{pool}| + c \gg |Z|$, i.e.,

$$Z_{pool} \leftarrow \{x_j\} \text{ with } x_j \text{ the k nearest neighbors of } x_i \in T. \tag{5}$$

We order these data points by their graph density $\mathcal{D}$ from Eq. 4

$$r(x_i) = m_i, \quad \text{where} \quad m_i \leq m_j \Leftrightarrow \mathcal{D}(x_i) \geq \mathcal{D}(x_j) \tag{6}$$

with $x_i, x_j \in Z_{pool}$. Finally, we select the first $|Z|$ data points with the smallest score $r(x_i)$,

$$Z \leftarrow \{x_i\} \text{ where } r(x_i) \text{ belongs to the } |Z| \text{ smallest scores} \tag{7}$$

Usually, the chosen data points are more representative for a group of samples so that propagation is more reliable. In the experimental part, we will see this positive behavior in particular for a small set of $Z$. The larger $|Z|$ becomes, the more redundant nodes are selected.

**(ii) *NN*.** Beside this positive behavior regarding our set $T$, this method still does not scale well to large datasets (see Sec. 4.3) as we have to calculate the entire distance matrix. For this reason, we propose a second criteria *NN* that can be seen as an approximation of *dense*. This selection technique needs only the distances between $x_i \in T$ to all unlabeled data $x_i \in U$ with $U = N \setminus T$ and all data $N$. Usually, we have $|T| \ll |U|$ so that the runtime is moderate. To enhance $T$, we select the first $k$ nearest neighbors for each $x_i \in T$, i.e.,

$$Z_{pool} \leftarrow \{x_{i_k}\} \text{ with } x_{i_k} \text{ the k nearest neighbors of } x_i \in T \tag{8}$$

This procedure ensures that each point in $T$ is separately enriched. For the case that $|Z_{pool}| > |Z|$ we randomly subsample this set until we achieve our selection size $|Z|$.

### 4.3    Runtime Complexity

In the following, we briefly analyze the runtime complexity of all introduced graph enhancement techniques and then compare their runtime behavior in the context of label propagation (see Fig. 1). Given $|N| = |T| + |U|$ images with $T$ the original dataset consisting of training and test set and $U$ the pool of unexplored and unlabeled data. The runtime of $k$-means is directly linked to the number of clusters, i.e., $O(|Z||U|m)$ with $|Z|$ the number of anchor points ($\sim$ number of added data) and $m$ the dimensionality of the image descriptor. With increasing unlabeled data volume, memory and and runtime requirements increase disproportionately as can be seen in Fig. 1 (left).

For *greedy*, we have to compute all distances between the current point set $L \cup Z^{(t)}$ at time $1 \le t \le |Z|$ to all remaining unlabeled data $U \setminus Z$, i.e., $O(|Z||T||U|m)$. This iterative procedure is the most time-consuming part. Depending on the dataset size and $|Z|$, it is faster to compute the entire distance matrix once $(O(|N|^2m))$. But for large pools of unlabeled data with more than one million data, the full matrix does not fit into memory so that we have to deal with approximations instead.

For our *dense* criteria, we require $O(|N|^2m)$ to compute all distances and $O(|N|^2 \log(|N|))$ to sort these distances for each image separately. Graph construction and calculation of graph density is considered a linear operation. Advantage of this method is the small memory requirement because we can split $|N|$ into smaller pieces $N_i \ll |N|$ so that we need at most $N_i \times |N|$ space. Finally, we are only interested in the first $k$ nearest neighbor, i.e., we disregard all other distances. In our case, we set $k = 1,000$. We have to compute this distance matrix only once because we can reuse it for label propagation itself or for different training and test sets.

As mentioned before, *NN* serves as a good approximation of *dense*. Instead of computing the entire distance matrix over $|N|$, we only need to calculate all distances between $T$ and all unlabeled data $U$. Additionally, we also have to sort $T$ times the according distances. Finally, we get a runtime complexity of $O(|T||U|m + |T||U| \log(|U|))$.

To run LP, we have to construct the $k$-NN graph thus requiring $O((|T| + |Z|)^2m)$ to compute all distances for the set $T \cup Z$, and $O((|T| + |Z|)^2 \log(|T| + |Z|))$ to sort these. LP itself needs $O((|T|+|Z|)^2C)$ with $C$ the number of classes. The calculation of the graph Laplacian $\mathcal{S} = D^{-1/2}WD^{-1/2}$ is fast because $D$ is a diagonal matrix and the graph structure $W$ is sparse so that we do not observe any memory problems.

Fig. 1 visualizes on the left side the runtime of the several graph enhancement methods including the *random* baseline for the dataset IM100 introduced in the next section. This is a subset of ILSVRC 2010 with 100 classes and approx. $130,000$ images. We plot number of added images against the expected runtime.

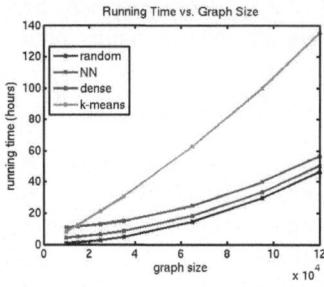 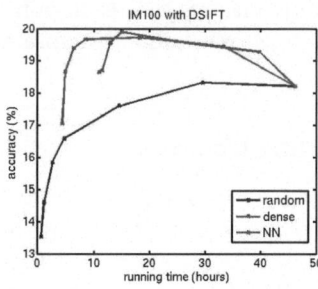

**Fig. 1.** Left: Complexity for selecting $|S|$ unlabeled data $x \in U$ with $m$ dimensions of the image descriptor given a fixed training and test set $|T|$ and label propagation. Right: Complexity against performance of IM100 (see Sec. 5) for DSIFT.

To approximate the runtime, we run one experiment 5 times under almost ideal conditions, i.e., only one process per time and scale this value to all other points in this plot given our complexity analysis. Note, the values of *k-means* are optimistic because it assumes that the algorithm converges after one iteration which is usually not the case.

*Greedy* is not shown in this figure because it does not fit on the y-axis: For the first point, i.e., adding 10,000 unlabeled images we need approx. 80 hours. *k-means* needs only 8 hours and is slightly faster than our *dense* criteria with 10.9 hours but slower than *NN* with 4.4 hours. To increase the dataset size by 25,000 unlabeled data points, *k-means* needs 21.1 hours while *NN* requires only 6.4 hours and *dense* needs 12.9 hours. For *random*, we would need 2.7 hours.

On the right side of Fig. 1, we plot runtime against classification performance for the same dataset. *k-means* and *greedy* cannot be applied on this large unlabeled pool due to the runtime and space complexity. Most interestingly we see for a given time budget that we achieve better performance than *random*. For example if we look at 20 hours for *random* that corresponds to a graph size of 65,000 images, we get a performance of 17.6%. In contrast, *dense* and *NN* need only a graph size of 25,000 to get a higher performance with 19.9% and 19.6% respectively. This emphasizes our claim that we are not only faster but also obtain better performance with a more representative subset of the unlabeled data. Although "the-more-data-the-better" strategy actually leads to a mostly consistent improvement (blue curve) the final performance is clearly below the results achieved with our methods (red and green curve). This loss of performance is often a consequence of added images that connect many images from different classes bringing them mistakingly close together.

## 5    Dataset and Image Representation

In our experiments, we analyze four different datasets with increasing dataset size and number of classes. Example images are shown in Fig. 2. ETH80 [25]

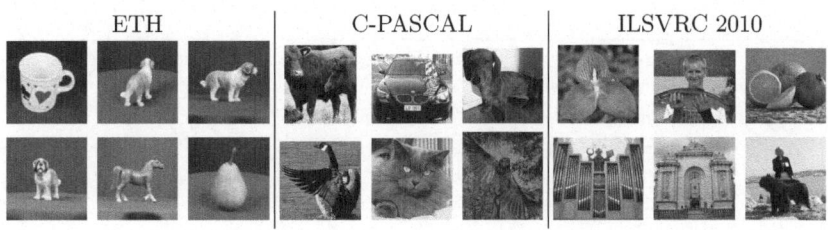

| ETH | C-PASCAL | ILSVRC 2010 |

**Fig. 2.** Example images for ETH (left), C-PASCAL (middle), and ILSVRC 2010 (right)

contains 3,280 images divided in 8 object classes with 10 instances per class. Each instance is imaged from 41 viewpoints in front of a uniform background.

Cropped PASCAL (C-PASCAL) is introduced in [4]. Bounding box annotations of the PASCAL VOC challenge 2008 training set are used to extract the objects such that classification can be evaluated in a multi-class setting. In this paper, we use the larger PASCAL VOC challenge 2011 with 8,900 images of aligned objects from 20 classes but with varying object poses, challenging appearances, background clutter, and truncation.

IM100 is subset of the ILSVRC 2010 challenge one of the state-of-the-art datasets for large-scale image classification. IM100 contains 100 classes with approx. 130,000 images. Finally, we show also results on ILSVRC 2010 with 1,000 categories and approx. 1.26 million images. Objects can be anywhere in an image and images contain background clutter, occlusions, or truncations.

For all datasets, we evaluate three different image descriptors to show that our insights generalize to several settings. Gist (960 dimensions) is computed by using the code of [26]. Dense SIFT (DSIFT) and spatial dense SIFT (SpDSIFT) are extracted with the implementation VLFeat proposed by [27]. SIFT features are calculated on a regular grid and quantized into 1000 visual words. For SpDSIFT, we use a subdivision of $4 \times 4$ that are concatenated to a final histogram representation with 9,000 dimensions.

## 6  Experiments

In our experiments, we select randomly 5 training samples and 45 test samples per class that serves as the original dataset $T$. This setting exactly corresponds to the classical semi-supervised setting with 10% labeled data [2,16,4]. The remaining images of these datasets are considered as the data pool $U$ from which we select unlabeled data to enrich $T$. We run all experiments 5 times with 5 different sets $T$ and evaluate the performance on the test set only. Therefore, we are able to compare our results independently from the amount of added data. In the following, we analyze each dataset separately.

**ETH80.** Fig. 3 shows for all three image descriptors graph quality (GQ, first row) and accuracy after label propagation (second row) without (solid lines) and with (dashed lines) active learning (AL). Graph quality denotes the average

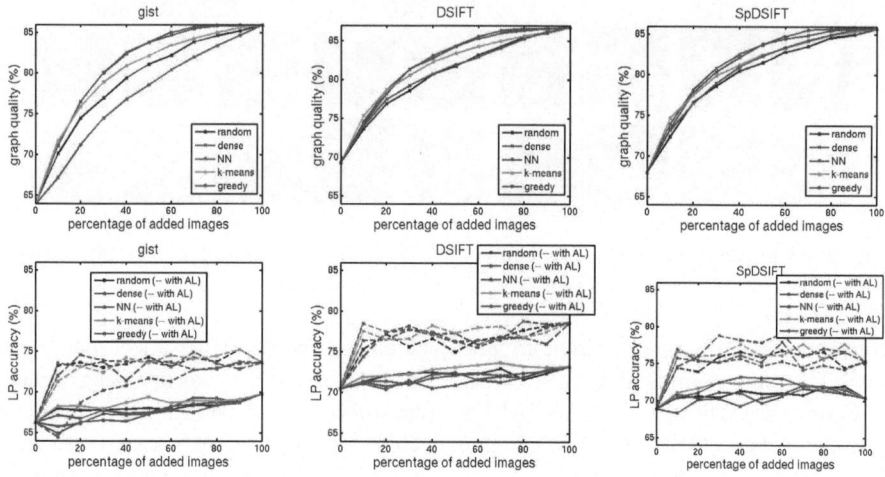

**Fig. 3.** Graph quality (first row) and LP accuracy (second row) for ETH80 with (dashed lines) and without (solid lines) active learning for different number of added images: Gist (left), dense SIFT (middle), and spatial dense SIFT (right)

number of correct nearest neighbors in our symmetric $k$-NN graph structure for the training and test data and serves only as a theoretic measure as we need to know all labels for this evaluation. For AL, we start with one training example per class randomly selected from our fixed training set of 5 samples per class, and request in average 4 labels per class from the remaining training set plus the additional unlabeled set.

We observe that the graph quality starts saturating after 60% to 70% added data. The performance of all selection methods is similar including the *random* baseline. This can be explained by the smooth manifold structure of the dataset. There are almost no outliers in this dataset so that our test set benefits from almost all images equally. For LP, we see a consistent improvement when active learning is used[1]. Tab. 1 shows graph quality (GQ) and accuracies with 50% ($\approx 1500$) additional unlabeled data. For DSIFT with *NN* selection we improve LP without AL from 72.4% to 77.3% with AL. *k-means* performs slightly better for LP without AL. The cluster centers seem to be good anchor points for the test data. Our density selection criteria shows on average slightly worse performance for LP without AL probably due to the oversampling of dense regions (e.g. apples and tomatoes are high density regions which are preferred by this criteria).

**C-PASCAL.** This dataset corresponds to a more difficult classification problem with many outliers and overlapping classes. We observe for both GQ and LP (Fig. 4) a large performance gap between our selection methods and previous methods. For SpDSIFT and DSIFT, *k-means* and *greedy* are even worse than the

---

[1] as this is true also for all other datasets we show only the performance for active learning in the following.

**Table 1.** Graph quality (GQ) and LP accuracy without and with (+AL) active learning for ETH80 after adding 50% unlabeled images

| method | Gist | | | DSIFT | | | SpDSIFT | | |
|---|---|---|---|---|---|---|---|---|---|
| | GQ | LP | +AL | GQ | LP | +AL | GQ | LP | +AL |
| random | 81.5 | 68.0 | **74.3** | 82.1 | 72.33 | 75.0 | 82.3 | 70.9 | 75.9 |
| dense | 83.0 | 67.2 | 73.8 | 84.1 | 70.9 | 76.3 | 83.0 | 70.3 | 74.7 |
| NN | **83.3** | 67.4 | 73.7 | **84.1** | 72.4 | **77.3** | **83.5** | 69.7 | 75.2 |
| k-means [6] | 82.5 | **69.4** | 73.6 | 83.6 | **73.1** | **77.3** | 82.9 | 72.7 | 76.1 |
| greedy [5] | 78.1 | 67.3 | 71.7 | 81.7 | 72.1 | 76.2 | 82.2 | **73.1** | **77.8** |

**Table 2.** Graph quality (GQ) and LP accuracy without and with (+AL) active learning for C-PASCAL after adding 50% unlabeled images

| method | Gist | | | DSIFT | | | SpDSIFT | | |
|---|---|---|---|---|---|---|---|---|---|
| | GQ | LP | +AL | GQ | LP | +AL | GQ | LP | +AL |
| random | 21.1 | **21.1** | 21.4 | 21.7 | 19.0 | 21.8 | 28.9 | 27.3 | 28.3 |
| dense | 23.8 | 20.8 | 22.1 | **26.1** | **20.3** | **24.3** | **33.4** | 29.0 | 32.2 |
| NN | **23.9** | 20.9 | **22.7** | 25.9 | 20.0 | 24.0 | 33.1 | **29.0** | **32.9** |
| k-means | 20.5 | 20.8 | 21.6 | 21.6 | 19.1 | 21.2 | 24.0 | 25.0 | 20.1 |
| greedy | 19.4 | 20.6 | 21.3 | 20.1 | 19.8 | 19.5 | 25.4 | 26.2 | 23.5 |

random baseline, e.g., LP+AL decreases for SpDSIFT from 28.3% with *random* to 20.1% with *k-means*, and to 23.5% with *greedy*. For *k-means*, this drop is a direct consequence of the used cluster centroids. Many clusters contain more than one class so that these clusters connect all examples of those classes and bring them closer together. In contrast, *greedy* focus more on outliers.

*NN* and *dense* perform similarly well. Furthermore, we observe a decrease in graph quality as well as LP accuracy when using all unlabeled data. For SpDSIFT, we get best performance for 50% ($\approx 4,600$) added images with 33.4% GQ, and 29.0% LP accuracy. These values drop to 29.8% GQ and 28.4% LP+AL when using all data. This is an important insight because it demonstrates that there is no need to use an arbitrary large number of unlabeled data. As a consequence we are able to reduce the amount of unlabeled data drastically without loss of performance. Note, the decrease of the GQ is a side effect of the symmetric graph structure. The more data the more unrelated samples connect to our training and test data. Although the graph quality of a non-symmetric graph shows better performance, label propagating through this graph structure consistently leads to worse results (up to 5%, see supplementary material).

**IM100.** In the following, we analyze a subset of ILSVRC 2010 with approx. $130,000$ images. This subset is large enough to increase the amount of unlabeled data by a factor of 25 but also small enough to run SSL on the entire dataset. *k-means* and *greedy* cannot be applied to this dataset due to their time and space complexities (see Sec. 3). Similar to all previous subsections, we show GQ and

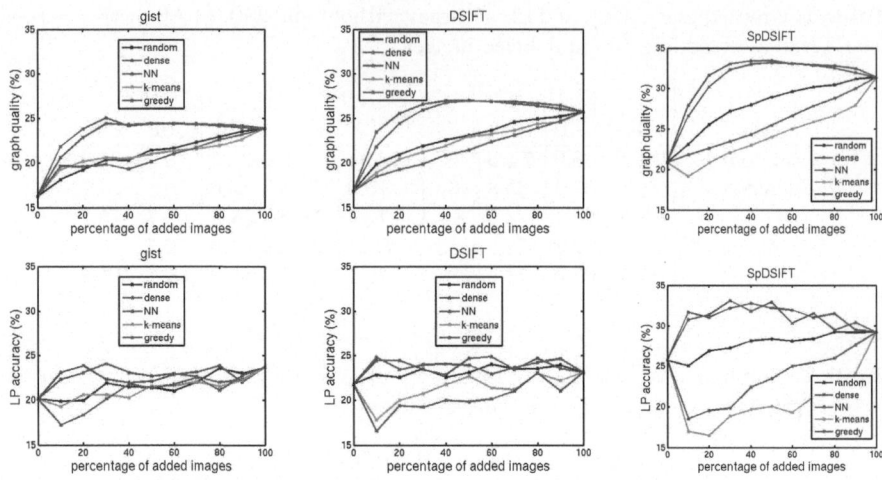

**Fig. 4.** Graph quality (first row) and LP accuracy (second row) for C-PASCAL with (dashed lines) and without (solid lines) active learning for different number of added images: Gist (left), dense SIFT (middle), and spatial dense SIFT (right)

**Table 3.** Graph quality (GQ) and LP accuracy without and with (+AL) active learning for IM100 after adding 30,000 unlabeled images ($\approx 23\%$)

| method | Gist GQ | LP | +AL | DSIFT GQ | LP | +AL | SpDSIFT GQ | LP | +AL |
|---|---|---|---|---|---|---|---|---|---|
| random | 15.7 | 11.6 | 14.9 | 17.0 | 12.2 | 16.6 | 20.4 | 16.4 | 21.1 |
| dense | **23.2** | 12.6 | **17.7** | 24.0 | **13.0** | **19.9** | **30.5** | 17.9 | **27.0** |
| NN | 22.0 | **12.7** | 17.3 | **24.1** | **13.0** | 19.7 | 30.2 | **18.0** | 26.2 |

LP+AL in Fig. 5 for different numbers of added data (graph size), and Tab. 3 contains results when adding 20% unlabeled data.

Again, we observe a significant improvement of our selection methods over *random*. For SpDSIFT, we increase GQ from 20.4% with *random* to 30.5% with *dense* and to 30.2% with *NN*, and LP+AL from 21.1% to 27.0%. Similar to C-PASCAL, our performance is with 20% to 30% additional data better than using all unlabeled data. For SpDSIFT, we observe a decrease of GQ from 31.2% with *dense* and 30% unlabeled data to 27.6% with all data.

**ILSVRC 2010.** Finally, we run LP on the entire ILSVRC 2010 challenge with 1,000 classes. We start with our set $T$ given by 5 training samples and 45 test sample per class, i.e., 50,000 images (Tab. 4, first line). After that, we continuously add 50,000 unlabeled data from the pool of the remaining 1.2 million images. Tab. 4 shows graph quality (GQ), top 1, and top 5 accuracy for LP+AL and the difference to *random* selection. For computational reason, we apply only *NN*. To further increase the speed of AL, we use batch active learning with a batch size of 100 labels per query. So that we request 400 times a batch of 100 labels to get in average 5 labels per class.

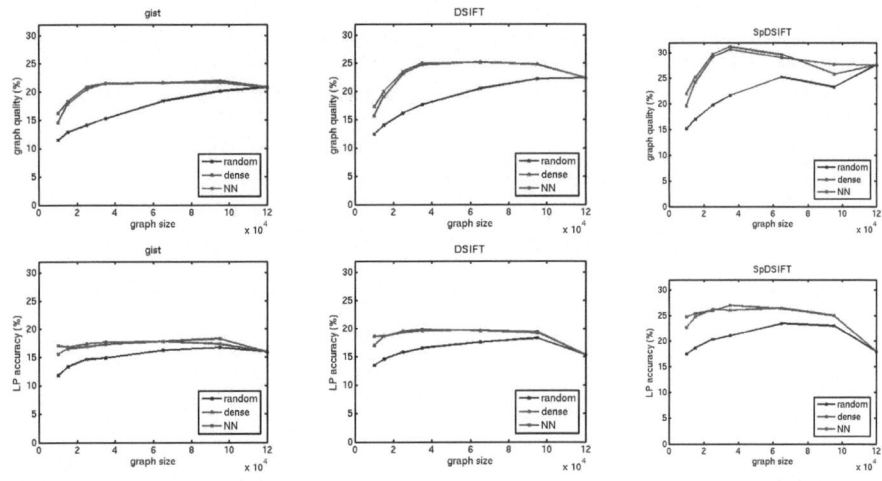

**Fig. 5.** Graph quality (first row) and LP accuracy (second row) for IM100 with active learning for different number of added images: Gist (left), dense SIFT (middle), and spatial dense SIFT (right)

**Table 4.** ILSVRC 2010 with *random* and *NN* enrichment for DSIFT: graph quality (GQ), top 1 and top 5 accuracy after LP with AL, and the difference to *random*

| added data | random | | | NN selection | | | | | |
|---|---|---|---|---|---|---|---|---|---|
| | GQ | top 1 | top 5 | GQ | diff | top 1 | diff | top 5 | diff |
| 0 | 2.4 | 2.8 | 7.1 | 2.4 | | 2.8 | | 7.1 | |
| 50,000 | 3.5 | 3.9 | 8.4 | 5.3 | +1.7 | 5.0 | +1.2 | 9.4 | +1.0 |
| 100,000 | 4.3 | 4.1 | 8.7 | 7.2 | +2.9 | 5.4 | +1.3 | 9.7 | +1.0 |
| 150,000 | 4.8 | 4.2 | 8.8 | 8.5 | +3.7 | 5.5 | +1.3 | 9.9 | +1.1 |
| 200,000 | 5.3 | 4.5 | 9.0 | 9.5 | +4.1 | 5.7 | +1.2 | 10.0 | +1.0 |
| 250,000 | 5.8 | 4.5 | 9.1 | 10.1 | +4.4 | 5.7 | +1.2 | 10.0 | +1.0 |

For comparison, we run also a linear SVM on the base setting with $50,000$ images and with different parameters. The best performance we observe is $0.22\%$ averaged over 5 different runs. In contrast with LP without enrichment we get $2.8\%$ top 1 accuracy. This large difference can be explained by the additional graph structure we used in SSL. According to the selection criteria, we improve increasingly our graph quality (GQ). For $50,000$ additional unlabeled images we note a difference between *random* and *NN* of $+1.7\%$ while for $250,000$ added images this difference increase to $+4.4\%$. We also observe an improvement for LP. For $150,000$ additional images, we increase LP from $4.2\%$ with *random* to $5.5\%$ with *NN*. However, LP benefits only limited from this improving structure. One explanation might be that we run a batch AL instead of a single AL. Usually these batch AL show worse performance in comparison to single AL.

**Table 5.** IM100: baseline (5 training + 45 test images per class), 25,000 randomly added data without and with AL (row 2-3), with 25,000 *NN* selections without and with AL (row 4-5), and using all unlabeled data without and with AL (row 6-7)

| | gist | | DSIFT | | SpDSIFT | |
|---|---|---|---|---|---|---|
| | acc | gain | acc | gain | acc | gain |
| LP | 11.2 | | 11.4 | | 14.7 | |
| +25,000 random | 11.8 | +0.6 | 12.2 | +0.8 | 16.6 | +2.0 |
| +AL | 14.5 | +3.3 | 16.3 | +4.8 | 21.4 | +6.7 |
| +25,000 NN | 12.2 | +1.0 | 13.0 | +1.6 | 17.8 | +3.1 |
| +AL | **17.9** | **+6.8** | **19.7** | **+8.3** | **26.3** | **+11.6** |
| using all data | 12.4 | +1.2 | 12.8 | +1.4 | 16.7 | +2.0 |
| +AL | 16.3 | +5.1 | 16.1 | +4.7 | 20.6 | +5.9 |

# 7 Conclusion

In this paper, we enhance the graph structure for graph-based algorithms with more unlabeled data and address the scalability of these approaches. These algorithms come with a quadratic runtime so that "the-more-data-the-better" strategy does not scale to large datasets like ILSVRC 2010 with 1,000 classes and over one million of images. We propose two selection criteria for enriching a dataset and to improve the graph structure. These criteria drastically reduce the amount of unlabeled data in comparison to the "the-more-data-the-better" strategy while still achieving better performance than using all unlabeled data. Moreover, given a fixed time budget we show significant improvements on four different datasets with less unlabeled data in contrast to previous approaches.

Tab. 5 summarizes our main insights from this paper on the dataset IM100. First of all, we see a consistent improvement when adding more unlabeled data. For SpDSIFT, we increase from 14.7% to 16.6% with randomly added 25,000 unlabeled data points to finally 16.7% when adding all available data. But these results are clearly below the performance of 17.8% that we achieve with our novel criteria *NN*. This fact becomes even more obvious in combination with active learning where we improve SpDSIFT with our new criteria by 11.6% to 26.3% while we increase this performance only by 5.9% when applying "the-more-data-the-better" strategy.

This summary shows once more that a careful selection of unlabeled data leads to better results as well as to a more compact graph that scales also to large datasets such as the complete ILSVRC 2010 dataset containing over a million images.

# References

1. Hein, M., Maier, M.: Manifold Denoising. In: NIPS (2006)
2. Zhou, D., Huang, J.: Learning from Labeled and Unlabeled Data on a Directed Graph. In: ICML (2005)

3. Liu, W., Chang, S.: Robust multi-class transductive learning with graphs. In: CVPR (2009)
4. Ebert, S., Larlus, D., Schiele, B.: Extracting Structures in Image Collections for Object Recognition. In: Daniilidis, K., Maragos, P., Paragios, N. (eds.) ECCV 2010, Part I. LNCS, vol. 6311, pp. 720–733. Springer, Heidelberg (2010)
5. Delalleau, O., Bengio, Y., Le Roux, N.: Efficient non-parametric function induction in semi-supervised learning. In: AISTATS (2005)
6. Liu, W., He, J., Chang, S.: Large graph construction for scalable semi-supervised learning. In: ICML (2010)
7. Schroff, F., Criminisi, A., Zisserman, A.: Harvesting Image Databases from the Web. In: ICCV (2007)
8. Collins, B., Deng, J., Li, K., Fei-Fei, L.: Towards Scalable Dataset Construction: An Active Learning Approach. In: Forsyth, D., Torr, P., Zisserman, A. (eds.) ECCV 2008, Part I. LNCS, vol. 5302, pp. 86–98. Springer, Heidelberg (2008)
9. Kulis, B., Grauman, K.: Kernelized locality-sensitive hashing for scalable image search. In: ICCV (2009)
10. Deng, J., Dong, W., Socher, R., Li, L.-J., Li, K., Fei-Fei, L.: ImageNet: A large-scale hierarchical image database. In: CVPR (2009)
11. Perronnin, F., Liu, Y., Sánchez, J.: Large-scale image retrieval with compressed Fisher vectors. In: CVPR (2010)
12. Deselaers, T., Ferrari, V.: Visual and Semantic Similarity in ImageNet. In: CVPR (2011)
13. Rohrbach, M., Stark, M., Schiele, B.: Evaluating Knowledge Transfer and Zero-Shot Learning in a Large-Scale Setting. In: CVPR (2011)
14. Zhou, D., Schölkopf, B., Bousquet, O., Lal, T.N., Weston, J.: Learning with Local and Global Consistency. In: NIPS (2004)
15. Sindhwani, V., Niyogi, P., Belkin: Beyond the point cloud: from transductive to semi-supervised learning. ML (2005)
16. Zhu, X., Ghahramani, Z., Lafferty, J.: Semi-supervised learning using gaussian fields and harmonic functions. In: ICML (2003)
17. Wang, F., Zhang, C.: Label propagation through linear neighborhoods. TKDE 1, 55–67 (2007)
18. Zhang, Z., Wang, J., Zha, H.: Adaptive Manifold Learning. TPAMI, 1–14 (2011)
19. Torralba, A., Fergus, R., Weiss, Y.: Small codes and large image databases for recognition. In: CVPR (2008)
20. Fergus, R., Weiss, Y., Torralba, A.: Semi-supervised learning in gigantic image collections. In: NIPS (2009)
21. Zhang, Z., Zha, H., Zhang, M., Tech, G.: Spectral Methods for Semi-supervised Manifold Learning. In: CVPR (2008)
22. Zhang, K., Kwok, J.T., Parvin, B.: Prototype vector machine for large scale semi-supervised learning. In: ICML (2009)
23. Li, Y.F., Zhou, Z.H.: Towards Making Unlabeled Data Never Hurt. In: ICML (2011)
24. Ebert, S., Fritz, M., Schiele, B.: Reinforced Active Learning: An Object Class Learning-By-Doing Approach. In: CVPR (2012)
25. Leibe, B., Schiele, B.: Analyzing Appearance and Contour Based Methods for Object Categorization. In: CVPR (2003)
26. Oliva, A., Torralba, A.: Modeling the shape of the scene: A holistic representation of the spatial envelope. IJCV (2001)
27. Vedaldi, A., Fulkerson, B.: VLFEAT: An Open and Portable Library of Computer Vision Algorithms (2008)

# One-Class Multiple Instance Learning
# via Robust PCA for Common Object Discovery

Xinggang Wang[1,*], Zhengdong Zhang[2],
Yi Ma[2], Xiang Bai[1], Wenyu Liu[1], and Zhuowen Tu[2,3]

[1] Huazhong University of Science and Technology
[2] Visual Computing Group, Microsoft Research Asia
[3] Lab of Neuro Imaging and Department of Computer Science, UCLA
{wxghust,zhangzdfaint}@gmail.com, mayi@microsoft.com
{xbai,liuwy}@hust.edu.cn, ztu@loni.ucla.edu

**Abstract.** Principal component analysis (PCA), as a key component in statistical learning, has been adopted in a wide variety of applications in computer vision and machine learning. From a different angle, weakly supervised learning, more specifically multiple instance learning (MIL), allows fine-grained information to be exploited from coarsely-grained label information. In this paper, we propose an algorithm using the robust PCA (RPCA) [1] in a iterative way to perform simultaneous common object discovery and model learning under a one-class multiple instance learning setting. We show the advantage of our method on common object discovery and model learning, which needs no fine/coarse alignment in the input data; in addition, it achieves comparable results with standard two-class MIL learning algorithms but our method is learning from one-class data only.

## 1 Introduction

Principal component analysis (PCA) has been adopted in a wide variety of domains [2], enjoying its simplicity and effectiveness. A robust principal component analysis model (RPCA) [1] was recently proposed along the line of increasingly popular sparsity and robust measures (e.g. the $\ell_1$ norm) [3]. Unlike the $\ell_2$ norm used in the standard PCA approach, RPCA encourages a low-rank part in the data matrix while having the $\ell_1$ norm on the residual, allowing the robust handling of data corruption and missing entries. The general assumption of PCA and RPCA though depends on well-aligned input data. However, this requirement is often too strong, especially for data of high dimension, which is particularly problematic in computer vision; for example, even well-studied frontal faces are hard to be perfectly aligned due to their intrinsic ambiguity. A so-called robust alignment by sparse and low-rank decomposition (RASL) algorithm [4] was very recently developed based on RPCA to deal with the local transformation/alignment. However, RASL only works on image data with small deformations; it is hard to apply RASL in more general cases without high quality initializations.

---

* This work was done while the author was an intern in Microsoft Research Asia.

K.M. Lee et al. (Eds.): ACCV 2012, Part I, LNCS 7724, pp. 246–258, 2013.
© Springer-Verlag Berlin Heidelberg 2013

From a different angle, weakly supervised learning, more specifically multiple instance learning (MIL) [5–8], allows fine-grained information to be exploited from coarsely-grained label supervision. In MIL, a training set consists of many bags (images in our case); each bag consists of a number of instances (patches in our case); only bag-level labels are given in training; the instance-level labels are therefore unknown in the training stage; the training algorithm then automatically explores instance-level and bag-level models to best fit the given bag labels. One promising aspect of MIL is that it allows for the automatic model learning and instance-level label prediction at the same time. In the end, a discriminative classifier is learned with the simultaneous label predictions on the instances. Thus, MIL seems to be on the complementary side of PCA and RPCA in removing the restrictions on having well-aligned input data. However, existing MIL methods are mostly focused on learning discriminative models requiring both the positive and negative data; essentially, the instance–level labels for the negative bags are known to us since we assume the presence of positive instances only in the positive bags. Here, we assume no given negative bags and we want to learn a PCA-like generative model for the instance-level data of interest; this represents many practical situations which are hard to be handled by the existing MIL methods.

Another recent active research area in computer vision is unsupervised/weakly-supervised object discovery [8–11]. However, the existing approaches either separate the task of object discovery from model learning or are formulated in a standard MIL setting. Different the other approaches try to discovery multi-class objects, e.g. [10], we focus on *common* object discovery. Thus, we requires all images come from the same class; no negative/irrelevate images are needed.

In this paper, we propose a new algorithm using robust principal component analysis (RPCA) to perform simultaneous object discovery and model learning within a one-class multiple instance learning framework. In the experiments, we show the advantage of our method on several applications to discover e.g. frontal faces of large variations; it also achieves comparable results as the standard two-class MIL learning algorithms with models learned from one-class data only.

## 2   Related Work

A robust principal component analysis (RPCA) was recently proposed in [1] for video surveillance and face recognition; there has been also immediate work adopting RPCA: further optimization approach was engaged to enhance the results of RPCA [12]; in [4], robust alignment by sparse and low-rank decomposition (RASL) was applied for face alignment. RASL aims to align multiple images of an object class of interest to a canonical template and it assumes that the degree of initial misalignment is not too large. In our problem, as stated before, we allow for objects of unknown locations and scales with possibility in severe occlusions.

Multiple instance learning (MIL) has recently received a lot of attentions. The diverse density (DD) method [13] tackles MIL by finding regions in the instance space with instances from many different positive bags and few instances from negative bags. In [6] learning algorithm of DD is refined using expectation maximization (EM). MI-SVM and MILBoost are proposed in [14] and [8] in which they train SVM and boosting classifier for instances respectively. Our method only models the positive instances without the negative bags. We use a EM-like algorithm to learn our generative model which is similar to [6]. Similar to MI-SVM and MIL-Boost, our model maintains a latent selection of most positive instance with a bag. However, our model is generative studying the instances of interest directly and explicitly.

Object discovery is a recent active research area [15–20]; although their results on benchmark datasets are promising, these existing methods are for specific purposes built with complicated systems. Here, we focus on a simple but general framework to discover objects and learn a PCA model from images known to contain an object class of interest. Therefore, we only focus on rigid objects which can be modeled by a PCA-like model. It alleviates the burden in having negative bags, as required by many MIL approaches. Our method shows its particular robustness in handling occlusions and outliers. Other methods such as 'co-segmentation' method in [21] and the detecting and sketching the common method in [22] do not require negative images for detection. However, they work on two (or a few) images only with no explicit model learning in an integrated framework.

# 3  Notation and Problem Formulation

In this section, we first give a brief introduction to the notation that will be used throughout this paper. Then a detailed discussion about the formulation of our problem will follow.

## 3.1  Notation

Suppose we are given $N$ bags of instances. Each instance is represented by a $d$-dimensional vector $x \in \mathbb{R}^d$, and the $k$-th bag contains $n_k$ instances. We name all the instances for the $k$-th bag as $x_1^k, x_2^k, \ldots, x_{n_k}^k$, and by putting them together we get a representing matrix $X_k = \left[ x_1^k, x_2^k, \ldots, x_{n_k}^k \right] \in \mathbb{R}^{d \times n_k}$ for each of the bags. Each instance $x_i^k$ belongs to either the positive or the negative category. So we label it with a binary variable $z_i^k \in \{0, 1\}$, where $z_i^k = 1$ indicates positiveness and vice versa. Each bag is also associated with a binary label $Z_k$ based on the labels of its instances: $Z_k = \bigvee_{i=1}^{n_k} z_i^k$. Intuitively speaking, a bag is positive if and only if some of its instances is positive.

For convenience we define a new operator $x \circ z$ as follows:

$$x \circ z = \begin{cases} x & \text{if } z = 1 \\ 0 & \text{otherwise} \end{cases}$$

Moreover, we generalize this operation to the bag level:

$$X^k \circ Z^k = \left[ x_1^k \circ z_1^k, \ldots, x_{n_k}^k \circ z_{n_k}^k \right].$$

Following the convention, $\| \cdot \|_*$ stands for nuclear norm of a matrix(sum of the singular values), and $\| \cdot \|_1$ means $l_1$-norm(sum of the magnitude of entries) for both vectors and matrices, $\|\cdot\|_0$ counts the number of non-zero entries in a vector and matrix. Moreover, $[n]$ denotes the set of positive integers less than or equal to $n$: $\{1, 2, \ldots, n\}$.

## 3.2    One-Class Multiple Instance Learning via Robust Rank Minimization

As has stated in Section 1, traditional settings of the Multiple Instance Learning problem requires both positive bags and negative bags to be available. Also in the training stage we must know exactly which bags are positive and which are not. In this paper, we will study how to tackle this challenging problem under a totally different setting. Basically it is assumed that we only have access to the positive bags, *without* any touch on the rest negative bags. Specifically, in our notation, $\forall k \in [N]$, we have $Z_k = \bigvee z_i^k = 1$.

Hence, by throwing away negative bags, we also disable ourselves from seeking discriminative information to separate positive and negative bags. Therefore, to make the problem tangible, some special assumptions on the intrinsic structure of positive and negative bags must be made. Below is the one of our choice.

> *Assumption 1: All the positive instances lie in a subspace $\Omega$ with extremely low dimensionality. Meanwhile, all the negative instances lies in another high-dimensional subspace that is incoherent with $\Omega$.*

This assumption is in fact pretty reasonable in practice. For example, let us examine the scenario of single common object discovery in images. If we align the common objects together, they actually form a rank 1 subspace $\Omega$. Background patches and other uncommon objects naturally lie on another subspace which, compared with $\Omega$, is of much higher dimensionality, since they are by definition uncommon between images.

Under this assumption, we have turned our task into the following form:

> *From each bag, pick out several positive instances, such that when we put all these instances together as a whole into a matrix, that matrix is of the lowest-rank possible.*

Mathematically, we are trying to solve the following optimization.

$$\min_{z_i^k \in \{0,1\}} rank\left([X_1 \circ Z_1 | X_2 \circ Z_2 | \ldots | X_N \circ Z_N]\right) \quad s.t. \quad \forall k \in [N], Z_k = \bigvee_{i=1}^{n_k} z_i^k = 1$$

(1)

For simplicity, we abbreviate $([X_1 \circ Z_1 | X_2 \circ Z_2 | \ldots | X_N \circ Z_N])$ into $X \circ Z \in R^{d \times (n_1 + \ldots + n_N)}$. Unfortunately, even though the ground-truth positive instances may satisfy this strict low-rank assumption, the observed versions of them seldom meet this requirement. One cause of this is due to quantization errors, changes on illumination, noise and even occlusions. Apart from these, a small fraction of the positive instances may turn out to be wrongly labeled, i.e., they come from negative categories. To handle these in a uniform framework, we model all of the corruption and outliers as sparse error added to the clean data. In other words, the observation $X \circ Z$ is a superposition of a low-rank component $L$ and sparse error matrix $S$:

$$X \circ Z = L + S$$

Here $\Omega = span(L)$. In the following sections of the paper, by a slight abuse of notation, we will not distinguish between $\Omega$ and $L$. Thus (1) is reshaped into:

$$\min_{z_i^k \in 0,1,L,S} rank(L) + \lambda_0 \|S\|_0, \quad s.t. \ X \circ Z = L + S, \forall k \in [N], Z_k = \bigvee_{i=1}^{n_k} z_i^k = 1 \quad (2)$$

$\lambda_0$ here is a weight that balances the low-rankness of $L$ and the sparsity of $S$.

## 4    Solution via Iterative Robust PCA

Notice that the highly combinatorial nature of (2) on binary variables $z_i^k \in \{0, 1\}$ makes it difficult to tackle. So we borrow the idea of iterative minimization from k-means to design an approximate solution. Specifically we would like to fix the guess of instance labels $Z$ and estimate the low-dimensional subspace $L$ despite corruption $S$. Then with the estimated $L$ and $S$ we update the instance labels $Z$ under certain strategy. We keep iterating the above two steps until convergence. The algorithm is summarized in Algorithm 4.2.

### 4.1    Estimate the Low-Rank Subspace by Robust Principal Component Analysis

With $Z$ fixed, the constraints of (2) is already linear with respect to $L$ and $S$. So we just need to address the non-convex function $rank(\cdot)$ and $\|\cdot\|_0$. As proposed in [1], replacing the intangible operator $rank$ and $\| \cdot \|_0$ with their convex surrogate nuclear norm($\| \cdot \|_*$) and $l_1$-norm($\| \cdot \|_1$) actually will not affect the global optimal solution under mild conditions. Based on this fact, we transform (2) into the following form:

$$\min_{L,S} \|L\|_* + \lambda \|S\|_1, \quad s.t. \ X \circ Z = L + S \quad (3)$$

Notice that here $\lambda = 1/\sqrt{\min(d, N)}$ guarantees the global convergence to the desired solution under reasonable assumptions [1]. This convex optimization problem exactly obeys the form of the Robust PCA and can be solved efficiently utilizing the Augmented Lagrangian Multiplier method proposed in [12].

### 4.2    Update Instance Labels through $l_1$ Regression

Once the low-rank subspace $L$ is retrieved, to update the guess of labels of each instance $x$, we need to test how well $x$ fits into the subspace $L$. This can be measured by the $l_1$ regression error $e$ of $x$ over $L$ , which is defined as follows:

$$e = \min_w \|x - Lw\|_1 \quad (4)$$

This regression can also get efficiently solved via [23]. Because each bag contains at least one positive instance, we sort the instances $x_i^k$ by $e_i^k$ in an ascent order, pick the best $\rho$ instances to be positive and set the rest negative.

---

**Algorithm 1.** Iterative RPCA for One-Class Multiple Instance Learning

---

**Input**: Positive bags $X$, initialized instance labels $Z_0$, weight $\lambda$, parameter $\rho$.
**Initialize**: $L = 0$, $Z = Z_0$.
**While** not converged **Do**
    **Step 1.** Fix labels $Z$, update $L$ via Robust PCA:
        $(L^*, S^*) \leftarrow \arg\min_{L,S} \|L\|_* + \lambda\|S\|_1, \quad s.t. \quad X \circ Z = L + S.$
        $L \leftarrow L^*$
    **Step 2.** Update the label based on $L$.
        **For** each bag $X_k$
            **For** each instance $x_i^k$ in $X_k$
                Get the reconstruction error by $l_1$-regression:
                    $e_i^k = \min_w \|x_i^k - Lw\|_1$
            **EndFor**
            **If** $e_j^k$ is within the $\rho$-th smallest among all $e_i^k, i \in [n_k]$,
                Set $z_j^k = 1$
            **Else**
                Set $z_j^k = 0$
            **EndIf**
        **EndFor**
**EndWhile**
**Output**: The learned low-dimensional subspace $L$ and the instance labels $Z$.

---

### 4.3    Implementation Details

*Construction of bags/instances.* In the common object discovery task, we run saliency detection method in [24] on all the images to get a set of salient patches, each with a score indicating the saliency degree. Each image is considered as a bag, and the salient patches detected by saliency detector described using HoG feature in [25] are considered as instances; number of instances is determined by the output of [24].

*Initialization of Labels.* Different strategies applies to different scenarios. For the task of common object discovery in images, we choose the patch with the highest saliency score to be positive and set the rest negative. For other tasks such as multiple instance learning on existing online published datasets, the saliency based method could not apply since we only have access to the well-prepared instance points and bags. In this situation, we just randomly pick out a few instances from each bag as positive. Then we turn to RANSAC, repeating the estimation independently a few times and selecting out the best model. Often the bags in these datasets do not contains many instances, thus this random initialization strategy has a fairly large chance of success provided repeated enough times.

*Choice of $\lambda$ in (3).* Although $\lambda = 1/\sqrt{\min(d, N)}$ has already given (3) a lot of nice properties, in practice we sometimes still need to tune it to further improve the results. For instance, in single common object discovery in images, we lower $\lambda$ to $1/\sqrt{2\min(d, N)}$ to make sure that $rank(L) = 1$. However, setting $\lambda$ out of the range $\left[1/2\sqrt{\min(d, N)}, 2/\sqrt{\min(d, N)}\right]$ will not make the algorithm produce anything meaningful at least empirically.

*Choice of ρ.* For single common object discovery, since the positive subspace has the property that $rank(L) = 1$, $\rho = 1$ is definitely the best choice. And typically $\rho = 1$ will not make the algorithm go wrong in most of the situations. However, if there are multiple objects that presents simultaneously in the same image or the common object is represented by multiple instances that almost do not overlap, then we have to set $\rho$ to larger values. In the experiments on MIL benchmark datasets, we don't know number of positive instances in each bag, so we find the best value of $\rho$ by running cross validation on training data.

## 5    Experiments

In this part, we carry out the object discovery experiments on image datasets and test our RPCA-based one-class MIL algorithm on standard MIL benchmark. As the baseline of comparison, we would like to slightly change our method in Algorithm 4.2 by replacing the Robust PCA component to classical PCA which is not robust to corruptions but is optimal provided no outliers exist. By slight abuse of notation, we denote the original algorithm using RPCA by *RPCA-based learning method* (for short, RPCA method) and the modified version is named *PCA-based learning method* (for short, PCA method). To compare PCA with RPCA fairly, we set the number of projection dimension of PCA to the rank of $L$ in RPCA. In the following experiments, we will demonstrate the advantages of RPCA method over the PCA method. We also compare RPCA method to other related state-of-the-art methods. We do not aim at developing a system to over-perform the state-of-the-art methods. Instead, we just want to highlight that RPCA model truthfully reflect the existing outliers or corruptions that is massively existing in the data of real world.

### 5.1    Occluded Face Discovery

We collect a face image dataset which contains 50 face images with many occluded faces at different sizes from web and the LFW image dataset [26]. Some of the images in the dataset are shown in Fig. 1. As is shown there, faces are occluded by different kinds of objects, ranging from sunglass, tennis, to hands etc. Aside from this, expressions on faces and background of faces in images also vary a lot.

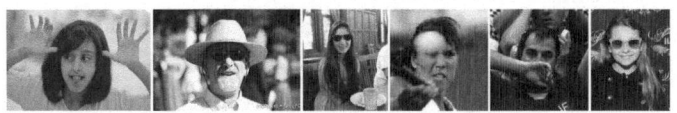

**Fig. 1.** Some face images in the face image dataset

In Fig. 2, we show the image patches for initialization (in the first column among each group), face discovery results of PCA method (in the second column among

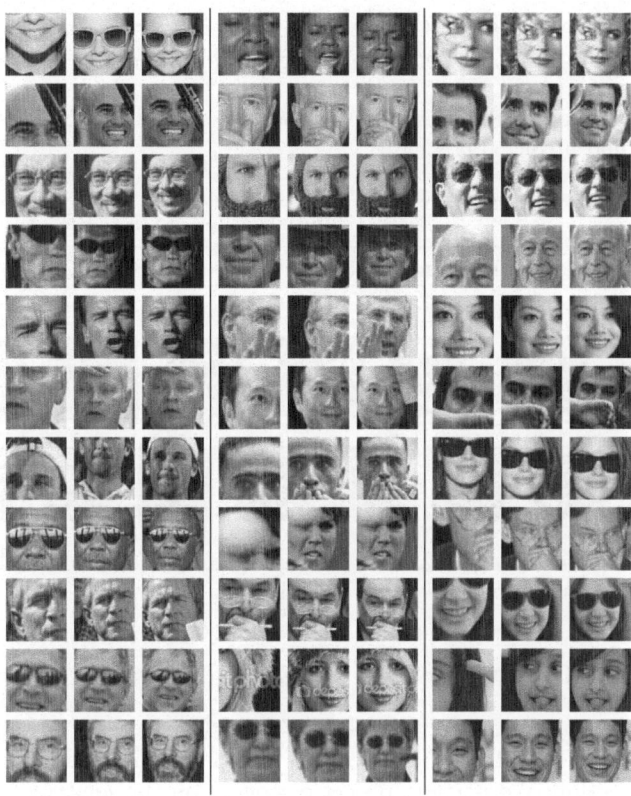

**Fig. 2.** Face discovery results: the first column among each group shows image patches for initialization, the second column shows results of PCA method, the third column shows results of RPCA method

each group) and face discovery results of RPCA method (in the third among each column) for 33 of all 50 images. Fig. 2 shows that image patches used for initialization are extremely challenging. Only part of the faces are present in each patch. What's worse is that even the present patches are not consistent across different images. Notice that here we do not use the raw pixels but rather extract some HoG features from each patch to represent every instance. As is observed in Fig. 2: Faces discovered by PCA method are not well aligned, most of which shift away from centers due to occlusion; while RPCA method align these discovered faces pretty well. Quantitative results are in Table 1 which also shows that RPCA can significantly outperform PCA in this occluded face discovery experiment.

Our conclusion of this experiment is that RPCA method outperforms PCA method on this occluded face discovery task due to the fact that RPCA in [1] is designed to handle large sparse error on data, and in this case, the large sparse error corresponds to the occlusion on face images.

Fig. 3 visualizes the learned low-rank subspace in HoG feature space in every iteration for both PCA method and RPCA method. The visualization method is from [25]. It shows that RPCA method can iteratively get the sketch of face, while PCA method can not converge to a good face model.

**Table 1.** The overlap percentages between ground-truth and initialized box, predicted box by PCA, and predicted box by RPCA

|  | Initialization | PCA | RPCA |
| --- | --- | --- | --- |
| Overlap with ground-truth | 40.94% | 65.88% | **79.28%** |

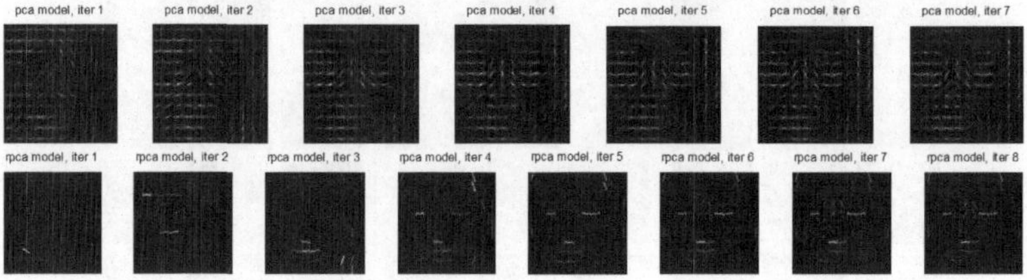

**Fig. 3.** Visualization of the PCA model (above) and the RPCA model (below) in every iteration. For better viewing, please see the original pdf file.

## 5.2 Common Object Discovery on ETHZ Dataset

In this experiment, we use RPCA method and PCA method for object discovery on the challenging ETHZ dataset [27] which is widely used for supervised objection detection. We perform object discovery on the *applelogos* and *bottles* classes separately. There are 40, 48 images in the *applelogos* and *bottles* classes respectively. Images in the two classes have significant intra-class variation, scale change, and illumination difference; some of images have very clustered background. Because HoG template cannot handle large deformation in the other three classes in ETHZ dataset, we don't work on them.

A discovered window is correct if it intersects with a groundtruth object by more than half of their union (PASCAL criteria). Object discovery performance is evaluated by 1) precision-recall curves, generated by varying the score threshold, 2) average precision (AP), computed by averaging multiple precisions corresponding to different recalls at regular internals and 3) detection rate against the number of false-positives averaged over all images with the class (FPPI).

We first compare RPCA method to PCA method, and the salient object detection (SD) method in [24]. Precision-recall curves and average precision in Fig. 4 illustrate the performance of RPCA method, PCA method, and SD method. Both RPCA method and PCA method outperform SD method significantly, and RPCA method works better then PCA method. We then compare RPCA method to a supervised object detection method [28] in which half of the images with bounding boxes in each class are used for training. Detection rates at 0.3/0.4 FPPI of [28] and RPCA method are listed in Table 2. It illustrates that RPCA method is comparable to the supervised object detection method [28] on *applelogos* and *bottles* classes. Fig. 5 shows the most confident detection

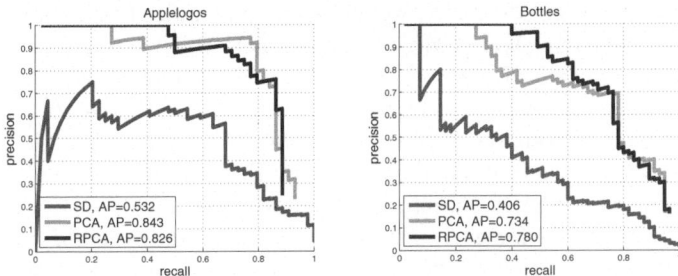

**Fig. 4.** Precision-recall curves for RPCA method (in blue), PCA method (in green) and SD method in [24] (in red) on ETHZ *applelogos* class (left) and *bottles* class (right).

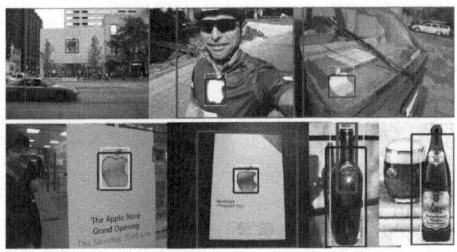

**Fig. 5.** The most confident detection hypothesises given by SD method in [24] (in red) and RPCA method (in blue), groundtruth objects are in yellow on ETHZ dataset.

hypothesis given by SD method and RPCA method in some of images in the dataset. As shown in this figure, using the objects in red boxes as initialization, our RPCA method can iteratively find the true object locations marked in blue. The salient object detection result on the other three classes of ETHZ dataset are too bad, so we have not tested the performance of the proposed method on the other three classes.

**Table 2.** Comparison of detection rates of the supervised object detection method [28] and RPCA method at 0.3/0.4 FPPI on ETHZ *applelogos* class and *bottles* class.

| classes | *applelogos* | *bottles* |
|---|---|---|
| Ferrari et al. [28] | 0.777/0.832 | 0.798/0.816 |
| RPCA | 0.800/0.864 | 0.709/0.763 |

### 5.3 Classification on MIL Benchmark Dataset

Until now, we have demonstrated a lot about the power of Robust PCA method for solving one class Multiple Instance Learning Problem without any information about negative bags. In this experiment, we will show that utilizing the learned model, with simple modification, our method can actually do the same two classes bag classification tasks. Moreover, we will show that indeed this simple modification would grant our algorithm with similar performance compared with the popular discriminative MIL method, e.g., the mi-SVM method.

Specifically, suppose we have learned the low-rank subspace $L$ for positive instances from the given positive training data. But after this we now have additional access to some other negative bags. Utilizing the new negative bags and $L$, we can train a SVM classifier as follows: Upon each bag $X_k$, no matter its positive or negative, for each instance $x_i^k$ in this bag, we build a histogram $h_k$ to show the distribution of the $l_1$ reconstruction error $e_i^k$, and use $h_k$ as the final representation for $X_k$. Then we train a simple linear SVM classifier using $h_k$ as training bags to accomplish the bag classification task. To compare the proposed RPCA method with standard two-class MIL learning algorithms, we evaluate RPCA method on four benchmark datasets [14] that are very popularly in studies of multiple instance learning, including *Musk1, Elephant, Fox and Tiger*. For each dataset, first we use the random initialization strategy described in the previous sections to set up the algorithm. Then RPCA model and PCA model are learned only using positive bags according to Algorithm 4.2. Then classifiers are trained based on all these. Following the standard verification convention, experiments are performed in a 10-fold cross-validation manner and per-fold average test classification performance is reported in Table 3.

**Table 3.** Results on MIL benchmark datasets. Bag classification accuracies (%) of RPCA method and PCA method on four MIL benchmark datasets compared to the state-of-the-art. The results of the upper part are taken from respective papers.

| Datasets | *Musk1* | *Elephant* | *Fox* | *Tiger* |
|---|---|---|---|---|
| MI-SVM [14] | 77.9 | 81.4 | 59.4 | 84.0 |
| mi-SVM [14] | 87.4 | 82.0 | 58.2 | 78.9 |
| EM-DD [6] | 84.8 | 78.3 | 56.1 | 72.1 |
| PPMM Kernel [29] | **95.6** | 82.4 | 60.3 | 80.2 |
| MIGraph [30] | 90.0±3.8 | 85.1±2.8 | 61.2±1.7 | 81.9±1.5 |
| miGraph [30] | 88.9±3.3 | **86.8±0.7** | 61.6±2.8 | **86.0±1.6** |
| MI-CRF [7] | 87.0 | 85.0 | **65.0** | 79.5 |
| PCA | 85.7±1.4 | 73.0±1.5 | 60.8±1.4 | 75.8±2.0 |
| RPCA | 82.9±2.8 | 78.3±1.1 | 61.0±1.4 | 76.9±0.9 |

In Table 3, we have compared RPCA method to PCA method, some popular MIL methods and the state-of-the-art methods, such as [6, 7, 14, 29, 30] are also listed. RPCA method outperforms PCA method in 3 of the 4 datasets (mark in red color), which shows that RPCA method is more practical than PCA method in general data. Only positive bags are used for learning the model in our proposed RPCA method. However, the performance of RPCA method is comparable to discriminative mi-SVM method in [14]. This good property makes the proposed RPCA method can be more widely used, such as unsupervised object detection without any negative training images in section 5.1. In the state-of-the-art face detection approach in [31], it need about 10000 non-face images for training.

# 6    Conclusion and Future Work

In this paper we proposed a new one-class multiple instance learning method based on Robust PCA [1] without negative bags. The algorithm achieves comparable robustness to both corruption on data and wrongly categorized instances, thus can work in some situations that PCA doesn't work well. We also show that with slight modification our method can achieve comparable performance to some popular methods that leverage discriminative information. In the future, we will develop composition model for object representation, rather than the current simple HoG template, to discover more complex objects in images.

**Acknowledgement:** The work was supported by NSF CAREER award IIS-0844566, NSF award IIS-1216528, and by the National Natural Science Foundation of China (NSFC) Grants 60903096, 61173120 and 61222308.

# References

[1] Candes, E., Li, X., Ma, Y., Wright, J.: Robust principal component analysis? Journal of the ACM 58 (2011)
[2] Jolliffe, I.T.: Principal component analysis. Springer (1986)
[3] Candes, E., Tao, T.: Near-optimal signal recovery from random projections: universal encoding strategies. IEEE Trans. Inform. Theory 52, 5406–5425 (2005)
[4] Peng, Y., Ganesh, A., Wright, J., Xu, W., Ma, Y.: Rasl: Robust alignment by sparse and low-rank decomposition for linearly correlated images. In: CVPR, pp. 763–770 (2010)
[5] Dietterich, T.G., Lathrop, R.H.: Solving the multiple-instance problem with axis-parallel rectangles. Artificial Intelligence 89, 31–71 (1997)
[6] Zhang, Q., Goldman, S.A.: Em-dd: An improved multiple-instance learning technique. In: Advances in Neural Information Processing Systems, pp. 1073–1080. MIT Press (2001)
[7] Deselaers, T., Ferrari, V.: A conditional random field for multiple-instance learning. In: Proceedings of the 26th International Conference on Machine Learning (2010)
[8] Viola, P., Platt, J.C., Zhang, C.: Multiple instance boosting for object detection. In: Advances in Neural Information Processing Systems, pp. 1419–1426. MIT Press (2006)
[9] Russell, B.C., Efros, A.A., Sivic, J., Freeman, W.T., Zisserman, A.: Using multiple segmentations to discover objects and their extent in image collections. In: IEEE Conference on Computer Vision and Pattern Recognition (2006)
[10] Lee, Y.J., Grauman, K.: Shape discovery from unlabeled image collections. In: IEEE Conference on Computer Vision and Pattern Recognition (2009)
[11] Deselaers, T., Alexe, B., Ferrari, V.: Localizing objects while learning their appearance. ETHZ TR No 276, Eidgenossische Technische Hochschule Zurich (2011)
[12] Lin, Z., Chen, M., Wu, L., Ma, Y.: The augmented lagrange multiplier method for exact recovery of corrupted low-rank matrices. UIUC Technical Report UILU-ENG-09-2215 (2009)

[13] Maron, O., Lozano-Prez, T.: A framework for multiple-instance learning. In: Advances in Neural Information Processing Systems, pp. 570–576. MIT Press (1998)

[14] Andrews, S., Tsochantaridis, I., Hofmann, T.: Support vector machines for multiple-instance learning. In: Advances in Neural Information Processing Systems, pp. 561–568. MIT Press (2003)

[15] Fergus, R., Perona, P., Zisserman, A.: Object class recognition by unsupervised scale-invariant learning. In: IEEE Conference on Computer Vision and Pattern Recognition (2003)

[16] Chum, O., Zisserman, A.: An exemplar model for learning object classes. In: IEEE Conference on Computer Vision and Pattern Recognition (2007)

[17] Vijayanarasimhan, S., Grauman, K.: Keywords to visual categories: Multiple-instance learning for weakly supervised object categorization. In: IEEE Conference on Computer Vision and Pattern Recognition (2008)

[18] Lee, Y.J., Grauman, K.: Object-graphs for context-aware category discovery. IEEE Transactions on Pattern Analysis and Machine Intelligence, TPAMI (2011)

[19] Zhu, L(L.), Lin, C., Huang, H., Chen, Y., Yuille, A.L.: Unsupervised Structure Learning: Hierarchical Recursive Composition, Suspicious Coincidence and Competitive Exclusion. In: Forsyth, D., Torr, P., Zisserman, A. (eds.) ECCV 2008, Part II. LNCS, vol. 5303, pp. 759–773. Springer, Heidelberg (2008)

[20] Wu, Y.N., Si, Z., Gong, H., Zhu, S.C.: Learning active basis model for object detection and recognition. International Journal of Computer Vision 90, 198–235 (2010)

[21] Rother, C., Minka, T.P., Blake, A., Kolmogorov, V.: Cosegmentation of image pairs by histogram matching - incorporating a global constraint into mrfs. In: IEEE Conference on Computer Vision and Pattern Recognition, pp. 993–1000 (2006)

[22] Bagon, S., Brostovski, O., Galun, M., Irani, M.: Detecting and sketching the common. In: IEEE Conference on Computer Vision and Pattern Recognition (2010)

[23] Yang, A., Ganesh, A., Sastry, S., Ma, Y.: Fast l1-minimization algorithms and an application in robust face recognition: A review. Technical Report UCB/EECS-2010-13, EECS Department, University of California, Berkeley (2010)

[24] Feng, J., Wei, Y., Tao, L., Zhang, C., Sun, J.: Salient object detection by composition. In: International Conference on Computer Vision (2011)

[25] Felzenszwalb, P., Girshick, R., McAllester, D., Ramanan, D.: Object detection with discriminatively trained part based models. IEEE Transactions on Pattern Analysis and Machine Intelligence 32 (2010)

[26] Huang, G.B., Ramesh, M., Berg, T., Learned-Miller, E.: Labeled faces in the wild: A database for studying face recognition in unconstrained environments. Technical Report 07-49, University of Massachusetts, Amherst (2007)

[27] Ferrari, V., Tuytelaars, T., Van Gool, L.: Object Detection by Contour Segment Networks. In: Leonardis, A., Bischof, H., Pinz, A. (eds.) ECCV 2006. LNCS, vol. 3953, pp. 14–28. Springer, Heidelberg (2006)

[28] Ferrari, V., Jurie, F., Schmid, C.: From images to shape models for object detection. International Journal of Computer Vision 87, 284–303 (2010)

[29] Wang, H., Yang, Q., Zha, H.: Adaptive p-posterior mixture-model kernels for multiple instance learning. In: Proceedings of the 26th International Conference on Machine Learning (2008)

[30] Zhou, Z., Sun, Y., Li, Y.: Multi-instance learning by treating instances as noni.i.d. samples. In: Proceedings of the 26th International Conference on Machine Learning (2009)

[31] Viola, P., Jones, M.: Robust real-time face detection. International Journal of Computer Vision 57, 137–154 (2004)

# Online Semi-Supervised Discriminative Dictionary Learning for Sparse Representation

Guangxiao Zhang, Zhuolin Jiang, and Larry S. Davis

University of Maryland, College Park, MD, 20742
{gxzhang,zhuolin,lsd}@umiacs.umd.edu

**Abstract.** We present an online semi-supervised dictionary learning algorithm for classification tasks. Specifically, we integrate the reconstruction error of labeled and unlabeled data, the discriminative sparse-code error, and the classification error into an objective function for online dictionary learning, which enhances the dictionary's representative and discriminative power. In addition, we propose a probabilistic model over the sparse codes of input signals, which allows us to expand the labeled set. As a consequence, the dictionary and the classifier learned from the enlarged labeled set yield lower generalization error on unseen data. Our approach learns a single dictionary and a predictive linear classifier jointly. Experimental results demonstrate the effectiveness of our approach in face and object category recognition applications.

## 1 Introduction

Learning dictionaries for sparse coding has recently led to state-of-art performances in many computer vision tasks [1–4]. The performance of image classification, in particular, has been further improved by learning discriminative dictionaries for sparse coding. Consider an input signal $\mathbf{x} \in \mathbb{R}^n$. It can be represented as a linear combination of a few atoms from a dictionary $D = \{d_1...d_K\} \in \mathbb{R}^{n \times K}$, *i.e.*, $\mathbf{x} = D\mathbf{z}$. The vector $\mathbf{z} \in \mathbb{R}^K$ is called the sparse code of $\mathbf{x}$ with respect to $D$. The resulting $\mathbf{z}$ is discriminative when $D$ has discriminative power.

Some discriminative dictionary learning approaches have been proposed recently for classification [5–10]. However, most of them are based on iterative batch procedures [5, 9, 11, 12], which access the whole dataset at each iteration and optimize over all data. For large scale datasets, this becomes a big challenge due to memory requirements and computational complexity. Although some online dictionary learning algorithms [13, 14] have been proposed for image restoration purpose recently, incorporating the discriminative information in online dictionary learning for discriminative tasks has not been fully explored.

Learning a discriminative dictionary usually requires sufficient labeled training data, which is expensive and difficult to obtain. Insufficient labeled training data yields a dictionary with potentially bad generalization power. By exploiting the information provided by the vast quantity of inexpensive unlabeled data, we aim to develop an online algorithm to learn a dictionary which is more representative and discriminative than a dictionary trained using only a limited number

K.M. Lee et al. (Eds.): ACCV 2012, Part I, LNCS 7724, pp. 259–273, 2013.
© Springer-Verlag Berlin Heidelberg 2013

of labeled samples in a batch procedure [15]. More importantly, we show how to identify those 'important' unlabeled data points, such as the points located near the decision boundary in sparse feature space, or points representing items very different from those we have seen before, and manually label those points in an active learning setting [16].

In this paper, we propose an online, semi-supervised dictionary learning algorithm that integrates dictionary learning and classifier training. We introduce a novel objective function which includes terms representing the reconstruction error of both labeled and unlabeled data, the discriminative sparse-code error, and the classification error. Compared to supervised dictionary learning approaches, our approach improves the representation power of the dictionary by exploiting the unlabeled data. It takes the reconstruction error of the unlabeled data to account in the objective function, and treats the unlabeled points with high confidence in label prediction as 'labeled' points. In addition, it identifies the unlabeled points with the most uncertainty in label prediction for manually labeling. Our approach learns a single over-complete dictionary and an optimal linear classifier jointly. Our main contributions are:

- We propose an online framework of discriminative dictionary learning for classification tasks, which is suitable for large data sets or dynamic training.
- The dictionary learns from labeled samples for discrimination as well as a large number of unlabeled samples. Learning from unlabeled data further increases its representative power.
- Our approach actively identifies the hard classified samples to be manually labeled and selects the easily classified samples as labeled data, using a probabilistic model of the sparse code of an input signal. In this way, unlabeled data also contribute to learning discriminative dictionaries with minimal human supervision.

### 1.1 Related Work

Discriminative dictionary learning for sparse coding has received a lot of attention recently. Some approaches treat dictionary learning and classifier training as two separate processes as in [8, 18–21]. The sparse codes associated with the dictionary trained in the first step are later fed into classifiers such as SVMs as feature attributes. For those methods, the discrimination power comes from either the sophisticated classifiers in the later stage, or learning multiple category-specific dictionaries [8, 20, 22], which might not be suitable when there are a large number of classes. Some other approaches incorporate category label information into the dictionary training process [5–9, 12, 23]. The dictionaries are learned by optimizing a unified objective function combining reconstructive and discriminative terms. In general, the optimization processes are iterative batch procedures: [6] alternates between dictionary construction and classifier design, and [7–9] alternate between supervised sparse coding and dictionary update. However these existing approaches cannot handle very large training sets.

To address these issues, several incremental learning or online learning algorithms [13, 14, 17, 24] have been proposed recently. [24] utilizes first-order

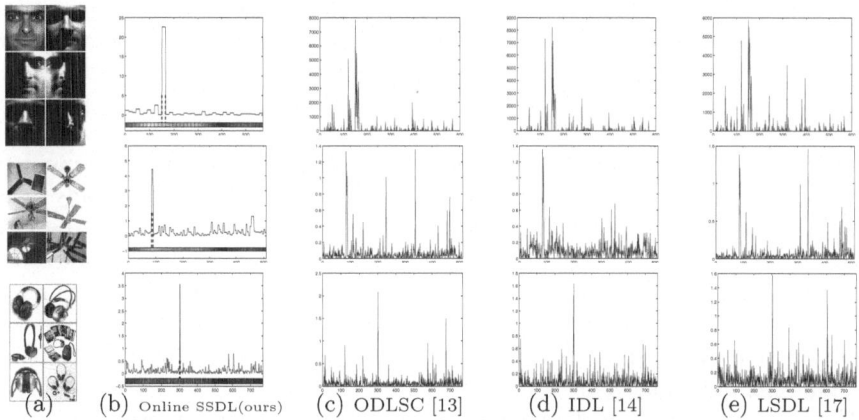

**Fig. 1.** Examples of sparse codes using dictionaries learned by different approaches on the Extended YaleB, Caltech101, and Caltech256 datasets. Each waveform indicates a sum of absolute sparse codes for different testing images from the same class. The 1st, 2nd, and 3nd row correspond to class 11 (28 testing frames) in Extended YaleB, class 18 (61 testing frames) in Caltech101, and class 101 (123 testing frames) in Caltech256 respectively. (a) are sample images from these classes. Each color from the color bar in (b) represents one class for a subset of dictionary items. The black dashed lines indicate that the curves are highly peaked in one class. (c) Online Dictionary Learning for sparse coding (ODLSC) [13], (d) Incremental Dictionary Learning (IDL) [14], (e) Large Scale Dictionary Learning (LSDL) [17]. The figure is best viewed in color and 600% zoom in.

stochastic gradient descent with projections on the constraint set for dictionary learning. [13] efficiently minimizes a quadratic surrogate function of the empirical cost over the set of constraints at each step. [14] utilizes locality constraints to project each descriptor into its local-coordinate system so that the objective function can be optimized analytically. The dictionary is then updated incrementally in a gradient descent fashion. Unfortunately, all of these techniques focus on minimizing the reconstruction error, which is good for reconstruction tasks but not for discrimination tasks such as classification. One of the major difficulties here is that we cannot afford to obtain sufficient labeled training samples. Therefore, learning a discriminative dictionary in an online fashion with minimal human supervision becomes an interesting problem.

## 2    Sparse Representation and Dictionary Learning

Consider a set of N input signals $X = [\mathbf{x}_1...\mathbf{x}_N] \in \mathbb{R}^{n \times N}$. Given a dictionary $D$ of size $K$, the sparse representations $Z = [\mathbf{z}_1...\mathbf{z}_N] \in \mathbb{R}^{K \times N}$ for $X$ can be obtained by:

$$Z = \arg\min_{Z} ||X - DZ||_2^2, \quad s.t. \forall i, \quad ||\mathbf{z}_i||_0 \leq \varepsilon \tag{1}$$

where $\|\mathbf{z}_i\|_0 \leq \varepsilon$ is a sparsity constraint. The performance of sparse representation highly depends on $D$. Traditional dictionary learning for sparse coding is achieved by minimizing the empirical reconstruction error:

$$< D, Z > = \arg\min_{D,Z} \|X - DZ\|_2^2, \quad s.t. \forall i, \quad \|\mathbf{z}_i\|_0 \leq \varepsilon \tag{2}$$

where $D = [d_1...d_K] \in \mathbb{R}^{n \times K}$ is the learned dictionary. In general, the number of training samples is larger than the size of $D$ ($N \gg K$), and $\mathbf{x}_i$ only uses a few dictionary items out of total $K$ for its reconstruction under the sparsity constraint. K-SVD [11] is an efficient algorithms to solve (2); it alternates between dictionary construction and sparse coding while keeping the other fixed until convergence is achieved. However, K-SVD only focuses on minimizing the reconstruction error. In addition, for a large training set, batch optimization techniques may be impractical.

There are two classes of algorithms that solve the optimization problems in (2) even with large training sets. One is classical projected first-order stochastic gradient descent [17, 24]. With an appropriate selection of a learning rate, the dictionary is sequentially updated by:

$$D_t = \Pi_c \left[ D_{t-1} - \frac{\rho}{t} \nabla_D l(\mathbf{x}_t, D_{t-1}) \right], \tag{3}$$

Another class of algorithms does not require explicit learning rate tuning; instead, they exploit the structure of the problem based on the second-order stochastic approximation [13]. The new dictionary $D_t$ is computed by minimizing the following cost function over the convex set $\mathcal{C} = \{D \in \mathbb{R}^{n \times K}, s.t. \forall j = 1, ..., K, \mathbf{d_j}^T \mathbf{d_j} \leq 1\}$

$$D_t = \arg\min_{D \in \mathcal{C}} \frac{1}{t} \sum_{i=1}^{t} \frac{1}{2} \|\mathbf{x}_i - D\mathbf{z}_i\|_2^2 + \lambda \|\mathbf{z}_i\|_0$$

$$= \arg\min_{D \in \mathcal{C}} \frac{1}{t} \left( \frac{1}{2} Tr(D^T D \sum_{i=1}^{t} \mathbf{z}_i \mathbf{z}_i^T) - Tr(D^T \sum_{i=1}^{t} \mathbf{x}_i \mathbf{z}_i^T) \right)$$

$$= \arg\min_{D \in \mathcal{C}} \frac{1}{t} \left( \frac{1}{2} Tr(D^T D A_t) - Tr(D^T B_t) \right) \tag{4}$$

With some simple algebra, it is easy to show that algorithm 1 (below) gives the solution to the convex optimization problem with respect to the $j$-th column while keeping the others fixed. Here matrices $A = \sum_{i=1}^{t} \mathbf{z}_i \mathbf{z}_i^T$ and $B = \sum_{i=1}^{t} \mathbf{x}_i \mathbf{z}_i^T$ propagate information from the past. This efficient online algorithm outperforms its batch counterpart in natural image experiments [13].

Unfortunately, these online algorithms are not explicitly designed for classification tasks. To further enhance the discrimination power of the dictionary, we propose an online semi-supervised dictionary learning algorithm which will be discussed in the next section.

# 3 Online Semi-Supervised Dictionary Learning

## 3.1 Problem Statement

To improve the discriminative power of a dictionary, we follow [9] and combine two discriminative term- the 'discriminative sparse-code error' and the 'classification error'- with the reconstruction error term to form an objective function for dictionary learning. In this way, the dictionary and the classifier are learned jointly. To take advantage of the large number of inexpensive unlabeled data, the reconstructive term consists of two parts: one from labeled training data and the other from unlabeled training data. To be concrete, the objective function for our dictionary learning is defined as:

$$< D, G, W, Z > = \arg \min_{D,G,W,Z} \alpha \|X^u - DZ^u\|_2^2 + \beta \|X^l - DZ^l\|_2^2$$

$$+ \gamma \|Q - GZ^l\|_2^2 + \|H - WZ^l\|_2^2 \quad s.t. \forall i, \quad \|\mathbf{z}_i\|_0 \leq \varepsilon \qquad (5)$$

The superscripts $u$ and $l$ specify whether the sample is from the unlabeled set or the labeled set. The first two terms are the reconstruction errors, while the last two terms are the discrimination errors. Parameters $\alpha, \beta, \gamma$ control the relative weight of these terms. In the $\|Q - GZ^l\|_2^2$ term, $Q = [\mathbf{q}_1^l, ..., \mathbf{q}_N^l]$ is a label-consistency matrix of size $K \times N^l$, with $N^l$ being the number of the labeled training samples. Each dictionary item in our approach is attached to a specific class label. Each column $\mathbf{q}_j \in \mathbb{R}^K$ is a discriminative sparse code corresponding to $\mathbf{x}_j$. $\mathbf{q}_j(i) = 1$ only when dictionary item $d_i$ and the training point $\mathbf{x}_j$ share the same class label; otherwise $\mathbf{q}_j(i) = 0, i = 1...K$. $G \in \mathbb{R}^{K \times K}$ is a linear transformation matrix that projects the sparse codes $\mathbf{z}$ to a discriminative sparse feature space $\mathbb{R}^K$.

The term $\|H - WZ^l\|_2^2$ measures the classification error. Suppose we have $m$ classes in the classification task. A linear predictive classifier $f(z; W) = Wz$ is employed, where $W \in \mathbb{R}^{m \times K}$ is the classifier parameters. A column $h_i$ of $H = [h_1, ..., h_N] \in \mathbb{R}^{m \times N}$ is the label vector for $\mathbf{x}_i$, where non-zero position indicates the category label of $\mathbf{x}_i$. The classifier $W$ is learned jointly with the transformation matrix $G$ and the dictionary $D$ by solving (5).

A major consideration in choosing a suitable optimization method is that since our problem is to be solved in an online learning setting, we cannot separate the labeled set and the unlabeled set in advance. Supervised learning and the unsupervised learning interleave as new data comes in; thus we require an adaptive strategy.

## 3.2 Optimization

Our algorithm alternates between sparse coding and dictionary updating as the input signals arrive sequentially. We rewrite the objective function in (5) as:

$$\min_{D,G,W,Z} \sum_{i=1}^{N_u} \left\{ \alpha \|\mathbf{x}_i^u - D\mathbf{z}_i^u\|_2^2 \right\} + \sum_{i=1}^{N_l} \left\{ \beta \|\mathbf{x}_i^l - D\mathbf{z}_i^l\|_2^2 + \gamma \|\mathbf{q}_i - G\mathbf{z}_i^l\|_2^2 + \|\mathbf{h}_i - W\mathbf{z}_i^l\|_2^2 \right\},$$

$$s.t. \forall i, \|\mathbf{z}_i\|_0 \leq \varepsilon \qquad (6)$$

where $N_u$ and $N_l$ are the number of unlabeled and labeled training samples respectively.

**Initialization.** We assume that, initially, we have a small labeled data set spanning all classes. To meet the requirement that each dictionary item is associated with a class label, we learn multiple class-specific dictionaries separately using K-SVD and then combine their dictionary items together. For simplicity we allocate equal number of dictionary items to each class, and the class labels attached to the dictionary items remain the same no matter how we update them throughout the training process. The initialization process is completely supervised.

---

**Algorithm 1:** Dictionary Update

**Input**: current dictionary $D_{t-1}$;
$\qquad A_t = \sum_{i=1}^{t} \mathbf{z}_i \mathbf{z}_i^T = [\mathbf{a}_1 ... \mathbf{a}_t]$,
$\qquad B_t = \sum_{i=1}^{t} \mathbf{x}_i \mathbf{z}_i^T = [\mathbf{b}_1 ... \mathbf{b}_t]$;
**Output**: updated dictionary $D_t$.
**repeat**
$\quad$ **for** $j = 1, 2, ....., K$ **do**
$\qquad$ Update the $j$-th column
$\qquad\qquad \mathbf{u}_j \leftarrow \frac{1}{A_{j,j}}(\mathbf{b}_j - D\mathbf{a}_j) + \mathbf{d}_j$.
$\qquad\qquad \mathbf{d}_j \leftarrow \frac{1}{\max ||\mathbf{u}_j||_2, 1} \mathbf{u}_j$.
$\quad$ **end for**
**until convergence**
**Return**

---

**Online Sparse Coding.** At time $t$, given that the dictionary $D$, the label-consistency transformation matrix $G$, and the label matrix $H$ are all fixed, the task is to find the sparse code $\mathbf{z}_t$ for the signal $\mathbf{x}_t$.

– For unlabeled $\mathbf{x}_t$, the sparse coding problem simply takes this standard form: $\mathbf{z}_t = \arg\min_{\mathbf{z} \in \mathbb{R}^K} ||\mathbf{x}_t - D\mathbf{z}||_2^2, s.t. ||\mathbf{z}||_0 \leq \varepsilon$. The orthogonal matching pursuit (OMP) algorithm is adopted here for its efficiency.
– For labeled $\mathbf{x}_t$, first construct the label-consistency vector $\mathbf{q}_t$ and label vector $\mathbf{h}_t$. The sparse coding problem becomes:

$$\mathbf{z}_t = \arg\min_{\mathbf{z} \in \mathbb{R}^K} \beta||\mathbf{x}_t - D\mathbf{z}||_2^2 + \gamma||\mathbf{q}_t - G\mathbf{z}||_2^2 + ||\mathbf{h}_t - W\mathbf{z}||_2^2, s.t. ||\mathbf{z}||_0 \leq \varepsilon, \quad (7)$$

which can be rewritten as,

$$\mathbf{z}_t = \arg\min_{\mathbf{z} \in \mathbb{R}^K} \left\| \begin{pmatrix} \sqrt{\beta}\mathbf{x}_t \\ \sqrt{\gamma}\mathbf{q}_t \\ \mathbf{h}_t \end{pmatrix} - \begin{pmatrix} \sqrt{\beta}D \\ \sqrt{\gamma}G \\ W \end{pmatrix} \mathbf{z} \right\|_2^2 = \arg\min_{\mathbf{z} \in \mathbb{R}^K} ||\tilde{\mathbf{x}}_t - \tilde{D}\mathbf{z}||_2^2, \quad (8)$$

With definition of augmented input signal $\tilde{\mathbf{x}}_t = [\sqrt{\beta}\mathbf{x}_t^T, \sqrt{\gamma}\mathbf{q}_t^T, \mathbf{h}_t^T]^t$ and augmented dictionary $\tilde{D} = [\sqrt{\beta}D^T, \sqrt{\gamma}G^T, W^T]^T$, the sparse code of the labeled $\mathbf{z}_t$ can be solved by OMP as for the unlabeled case.

**Dictionary Update.** Once the sparse code for $\mathbf{x}_i$ is obtained, we perform the dictionary update motivated by [13]. First, the coefficient matrix $B_t = \sum_{i=1}^{t} \mathbf{x}_i \mathbf{z}_i^T$, which carry all the information from the past sparse codes $\mathbf{z}_1, ..., \mathbf{z}_t$, is augmented to $\tilde{B}$ as the $\mathbf{x}_i$'s are augmented to $\tilde{\mathbf{x}}_i = [\sqrt{\beta}\mathbf{x}_i^T, \sqrt{\gamma}\mathbf{q}_i^T, \mathbf{h}_i^T]^T$. Note that $\tilde{B}$ is iteratively updated by both labeled data and unlabeled data. In the latter case, only the first $n$ rows which correspond to $\mathbf{x}_i$'s are updated. In essence, the first $n$ rows in $\tilde{B}$ record the past information of all training data, and the remaining $K + m$ rows (the dimension of $\mathbf{q}_i$ plus $\mathbf{h}_i$) reflect only the history of the labeled data. Second, the dictionary is updated either by itself or with $G$ and $W$ jointly in the augmented $\tilde{D}$, depending on whether the signal is labeled or not in that iteration. Given sparse codes $\mathbf{z}_i, i = 1...t$, the updated dictionary using algorithm 1 is the solution to (4) stated in section 2.

Note that algorithm 1 can also be applied to solve (4) with the augmented dictionary simply by replacing $\mathbf{x}_i$ with the augmented $\tilde{\mathbf{x}}_i = [\sqrt{\beta}\mathbf{x}_i^T, \sqrt{\gamma}\mathbf{q}_i^T, \mathbf{h}_i^T]^T$.

### 3.3   Learning from Unlabeled Data

So far we have discussed our online dictionary learning strategy with a mixture of labeled and unlabeled training samples. In practice, it still remains unclear how to choose which input data to label. After labeling the first few samples for the initial dictionary learning, we wish to keep the manual labeling effort minimum without sacrificing discriminative capability. In this section we propose a selection criterion based on a probabilistic model from the signal's sparse code.

Consider the sparse representation $\mathbf{z} = [z_1...z_K]^T$ of an input signal $\mathbf{x}$. Since once a dictionary element has its class determined, that can never change, the sparse coefficients $z_j$ associated with item $d_j$ can be used to compute the probability of signal $\mathbf{x}$ being in the same class as dictionary item $d_j$. If we sum up the absolute sparse codes associated with dictionary items from the same class and normalize them, we obtain the class probability distribution of the signal. Concretely, suppose we have an $m$-class classification problem, where each class is represented by $k$ dictionary items, $k \times m = K$. The class probability of an input signal $\mathbf{x}$ with $\mathbf{z} = [z_1...z_K]^T$ being in class $l$, given $D$, is computed as:

$$p_l(\mathbf{x}) = Pr(\mathcal{L}(\mathbf{x}) = l | D) = \frac{\sum_{j:\mathcal{L}(d_j)=l} |z_j|}{\sum_j |z_j|}, \tag{9}$$

where $\mathcal{L}$ maps a data point or a dictionary item to a specific class label $l \in \{1...m\}$. The class probability distribution $P(\mathbf{x})$ for signal $\mathbf{x}$ is calculated by $P(\mathbf{x}) = [p_1(\mathbf{x})...p_m(\mathbf{x})]^T$.

The probability distribution informs us how well the dictionary discriminates the input signal. To quantify the confidence level of the discriminability of an input signal, we compute the entropy of its sparse code:

$$ent(\mathbf{x}) = -\sum_{l=1}^{m} p_l(\mathbf{x}) \log p_l(\mathbf{x}). \tag{10}$$

Intuitively if the dictionary is highly discriminative to an input signal, we expect the large values of the sparse code to concentrate at certain dictionary items, and thus the class distribution should be peaked at the most likely class. Quantitatively, we set two thresholds on the entropy of the probability distribution.

Any entropy value smaller than a lower bound indicates a 'good' input signal with respect to the current dictionary, and we are fairly confident about our maximum likelihood class label prediction of this signal. Such points can thus be automatically added to the labeled set for dictionary learning with no human cost.

An entropy value higher than an upper bound tells us one of two things: it could be a difficult or uncertain input signal, or the current dictionary cannot represent Here it well. These points are critical to the dictionary learning because this highly uncertain point might be located near the decision boundary in the feature space, or might be new data unlike any we have seen before. In both situations, manual labeling will have its greatest impact.

**Parameter Selection.** The values of parameter $\phi_{low}$ and $\phi_{high}$ are chosen empirically. Here we use the sparse codes of the training data using the initial dictionary to approximate the class distributions of the training data, and then generate a distribution of the entropy values as a basis to determine the values of the thresholds. $\phi_{high}$ can be roughly estimated according to the budget of the manual labeling, while the best $\phi_{low}$ can be determined by five-fold cross validation on the training set. $\alpha, \beta,$ and $\gamma$ are also determined via cross validation.

To summarize the discussions above, we propose the following semi-supervised learning strategy. The initial dictionary is learned under full supervision. As the unlabeled training data sequentially arrives, we compute the probability distribution of the sparse codes given the current dictionary, and evaluate the confidence level of the data. If the entropy value is lower than the lower bound, then we automatically label the point as the dominating class, and treat it as labeled data. If, in rare cases, the entropy value exceeds our upper threshold the user will be requested to label it. For those falling in between, we leave them as unlabeled data.

Algorithm 2 presents the pseudocode of our approach. The normalization step at the end of the dictionary update for the labeled data completes the iteration. Note that the columns of $D$, $G$ and $W$ are $L_2$-normalized in $\tilde{D}$ jointly, i.e., $\forall j, \| \left[ d_j^T, g_j^T, w_j^T \right]^T \|_2 = 1$. The desired dictionary $\hat{D}$, the transformation matrix $\hat{G}$, and the classifier $\hat{W}$ can be computed as [5]:

$$\hat{D} = \left[ \frac{d_1}{||d_1||_2} \cdots \frac{d_K}{||d_K||_2} \right]; \hat{G} = \left[ \frac{g_1}{||d_1||_2} \cdots \frac{g_K}{||d_K||_2} \right]; \hat{W} = \left[ \frac{w_1}{||d_1||_2} \cdots \frac{w_K}{||d_K||_2} \right]; \quad (11)$$

### 3.4   Classification Approach

Once we obtain the discriminative $\hat{D}$, $\hat{G}$ and $\hat{W}$ from Algorithm 2, we need to recompute the sparse codes $Z_l$ of the labeled data $X_l$ to re-estimate $\hat{W}$, which includes the original labeled data, the automatically labeled data, and the manually labeled data. Given $Z_l$, the classifier $\hat{W}$ is estimated by using the multivariate ridge regression model with quadratic loss and $L_2$ norm regularization:

$$\arg\min_W \|H - WZ^l\|_2^2 + \lambda\|W\|_2^2, \quad (12)$$

which yields the analytic solution: $\hat{W} = HZ^T(ZZ^T + \lambda I)^{-1}$. When a testing point $\mathbf{x}^{test}$ comes in, we first compute its sparse code $\mathbf{z}^{test}$, and then compute $\hat{W}\mathbf{z}^{test}$.

The label for $\mathbf{x}_j$ is assigned by the position corresponding to the largest value in the label vector: $\chi = \hat{W}\mathbf{z}^{test}$, where $\chi \in \mathbb{R}^m$.

---

**Algorithm 2:** Online Semi-Supervised Dictionary Learning (Online SSDL)

---

**Input**: input signals $X = \{\mathbf{x}_1...\mathbf{x}_N\}$ and their labels, if any; regularization
      constant $\alpha$, $\beta$ and $\gamma$; lower bound $\phi_{low}$ and upper bound $\phi_{high}$
**Output**: $D$, $G$, and $W$.
**Initialization**: Compute $D_0$, $G_0$, and $W_0$ via LC-KSVD
                $A_0 \leftarrow 0; \tilde{B}_0 \leftarrow 0$
**for** $t = 1, 2, ...., N$ **do**
    Draw $\mathbf{x}_t$ from the sequence;
    *Sparse coding*: compute sparse code $\mathbf{z}_t$ using (1);
    **if** $\mathbf{x}_t$ is unlabeled,
        Compute the entropy $ent(\mathbf{x}_t)$ using (10);
        **if** $ent(\mathbf{x}_t) \leq \phi_{high}$ and $ent(\mathbf{x}) \geq \phi_{low}$;
        % dictionary update with unlabeled data
            $A_t \leftarrow A_{t-1} + \alpha\mathbf{z}_t\mathbf{z}_t^T$;
            $B_t \leftarrow \tilde{B}_{t-1}(1:n,:); B_t \leftarrow B_t + \alpha\mathbf{x}_t\mathbf{z}_t^T$;
            *Dictionary update* by unlabeled data:
                update $D_t$ using algorithm 1 with $D_{t-1}$, $A_t$, and $B_t$;
        **continue**;
        **elseif** $ent(\mathbf{x}_t) < \phi_{low}$
        % automatical labeling on the confident point
            $\mathcal{L}(\mathbf{x_t}) = \arg\max_j p_j(\mathbf{x})$;
        **else** $ent(\mathbf{x}_t) > \phi_{high}$
        % manual labeling on the difficult point
            $\mathcal{L}(\mathbf{x_t}) = l$;
        **endif**
    **endif**
    % dictionary update with labeled data
    Construct $\tilde{\mathbf{x}}_t = [\sqrt{\beta}\mathbf{x}_t^T; \sqrt{\gamma}\mathbf{q}_t^T; \mathbf{h}_t^T]^T$, and $\tilde{D}_{t-1} = [\sqrt{\beta}D_{t-1}^T; \sqrt{\gamma}G_{t-1}^T; W_{t-1}^T]^T$;
    $A_t \leftarrow A_{t-1} + \mathbf{z}_t\mathbf{z}_t^T$;    $\tilde{B}_t \leftarrow \tilde{B}_{t-1} + \tilde{\mathbf{x}}_t\mathbf{z}_t^T$;
    *Dictionary update* by labeled data:
        update $\tilde{D}_t$ using algorithm 1 with $\tilde{D}_{t-1}$, $A_t$, and $\tilde{B}_t$;
    obtain $D$, $G$ and $W$ from $\tilde{D}_t$ and normalize them by (11).
**end for**
**Return** $D$, $G$, and $W$.

---

## 4   Experiments

We evaluate our approach on three popular datasets: Extended YaleB database [25], Caltech101 [26], and Caltech256 [27]. We compare our results with two competing supervised dictionary learning algorithms: D-KSVD [8], LC-KSVD [9], as well as three online dictionary learning algorithms including Online Dictionary Learning for Sparse Coding (ODLSC) [13], Incremental Dictionary Learning (IDL) [14] and Large Scale Dictionary Learning (LSDL) [17], and some other benchmark algorithms such as K-SVD [11].

Since the number of labeled samples varies with our selection of $\phi_{low}$ and $\phi_{high}$ and the classification accuracy depends on the number of labeled training samples, it is tricky to do a fair comparison with other methods unless we fix our settings. To address this issue, we conducted the experiments in two folds: (1) Split the training set into labeled set and unlabeled set. We want to demonstrate the effect of the number of labeled samples on our performance in comparison with others. While our method takes advantage of both sets due to our learning strategy, the competing methods can only take the labeled set for training since the unlabeled samples are useless to them. (2) To compare our best recognition rate with the state-of-the-arts, we assumed all the training samples are labeled. We'd like to point out two facts: (a) our method adopts a simple classifier jointly learned with the dictionary, whereas other methods take advantage of sophisticated classifiers such as SVM; (2) although the advantage is not too obvious in terms of recognition rate in case of which all the training samples are labeled, the benefit of our method can be signified when the labeled samples are few, which is demonstrated at the starting points of all curves (see Fig. 2(a), 3(a), and 3(b)).

### 4.1   Extended YaleB Database

The extended YaleB database [25] contains $2,414$ images of 38 human frontal faces under about 64 illumination conditions and expressions. The images were chopped to $192 \times 168$ pixels. Each face was projected to a 504-dimensional random space by multiplying a random matrix introduced in [3, 5]. The entries of the matrix follow a zero-mean Gaussian distribution. We randomly selected 32 faces per person as training data, and the rest 32 are for testing. We report the results from the average of ten such random splits of the training and testing images.

To make the initial dictionary discriminative, we trained 38 dictionaries of six items for each person with eight samples using K-SVD, and combine them as our initial dictionary of 228 items. The remaining $24 \times 38$ training samples are randomly permutated as sequential input signals to our online algorithm. The dictionary size and the item labels are fixed during the learning process. We conducted two experiments on this dataset for the purpose discussed previously.

**Experiment 1.** We compare our approach with two supervised methods: LC-KSVD and D-KSVD. We fixed $\phi_{low} = 4.5$ for automatic labeling, and incrementally tune $\phi_{high}$, each value corresponding to a set of selected samples for manual labeling. The same number of manually labeled samples are used as training set for D-KSVD and LC-KSVD. Figure 2(a) shows that the recognition rate goes up as the number of labeled samples increases as expected. Our approach takes all the training samples regardless of whether they are labeled or unlabeled, and thus achieves a higher recognition rate even with few manually labeled data (the left end of the curve).

To demonstrate the impact of the lower threshold, we present another set of curves in Figure 2(b). Each curve corresponds to recognition rate growing with the number of manually labeled samples for a given value of the lower threshold. All curves are obtained with the same set of parameters ($\alpha$, $\beta$ and $\gamma$) and the same set of higher thresholds.

From the curves we clearly see that a higher $\phi_{low}$, i.e. more automatic labels, is most beneficial to the case when manual labels are scarce (the left end of the curves). When the number of manual labels increase, the recognition rates with different lower thresholds tend to converge. In addition, the curve with $\phi_{low} = 4.5$ in Figure 2(b) is different from the curve in Figure 2(a) due to different parameter settings.

**Table 1.** Recognition results using random face features on the Extended YaleB. We obtained the accuracies of LSDL, OSCDL, and IDL by running the codes, while the accuracies of the other methods are copied from the references.

| Method | K-SVD [11] | D-KSVD [5] | SRC [3] | LLC [14] | LC-KSVD [9] |
|--------|-----------|-----------|---------|----------|-------------|
| Acc. | 93.1 | 94.1 | 80.5 | 82.2 | 94.5 |

| Method | LSDL [17] | ODLSC [13] | IDL [14] | Online SSDL | |
|--------|-----------|------------|----------|-------------|--|
| Acc. | 90.5 | 91.4 | 89.6 | **94.7** | |

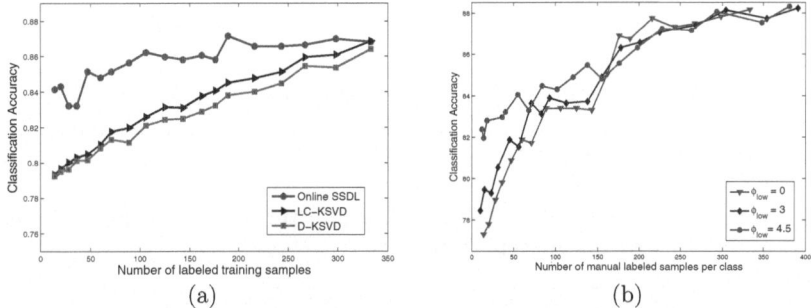

(a)                                             (b)

**Fig. 2.** Recognition performance on the Extended YaleB. (a) Recognition performance with varying number of labeled samples, where $K = 6 \times 38$ and $N = 24 \times 38$; (b) An illustration of the effect of the lower bound. The curves are obtained with the same set of parameters: $\alpha$, $\beta$, $\gamma$ and the same set of higher entropy thresholds.

**Experiment 2.** In the second experiment, we compare with other online dictionary learning approaches: ODLSC [13], IDL [14] and LSDL [17], and some state-of-art dictionary learning approaches [3, 5, 9, 11, 14]. Here we set $\phi_{low} = \phi_{high} = 0$, i.e. we get an online dictionary learning algorithm in which all new samples are labeled, as opposed to supervised algorithm in batch mode (LC-KSVD) and unsupervised online algorithms such as ODLSC, IDL, LSDL. As shown in Table 1, our approach (referred to as Online SSDL) has the best performance.

## 4.2   Caltech101 Dataset

The Caltech101 dataset [26] contains $9,144$ images of 102 categories (101 categories of objects and a 'background' category). There are about 40 to 800 images per category. All images are resized to be smaller than $300 \times 300$ pixels. We extract sift descriptor with 128 dimension from $16 \times 16$ patches. Then we extract the spatial pyramid features with three grids of size $1 \times 1$, $2 \times 2$ and $4 \times 4$, and reduce them to $3,000$ dimensions by PCA. Similarly, we conducted two experiments: one is the recognition versus the number of manual labels (seen in Figure 3(a)), and the other is a comparison with the state-of-art methods, using 5, 10, 15, 20, 25 and 30 training samples per category. The results are summarized in Table 2. The training samples are randomly selected from each category, and the remaining images are used for testing. We repeated this sampling process to get ten splits and report their average. Following the experimental settings for other

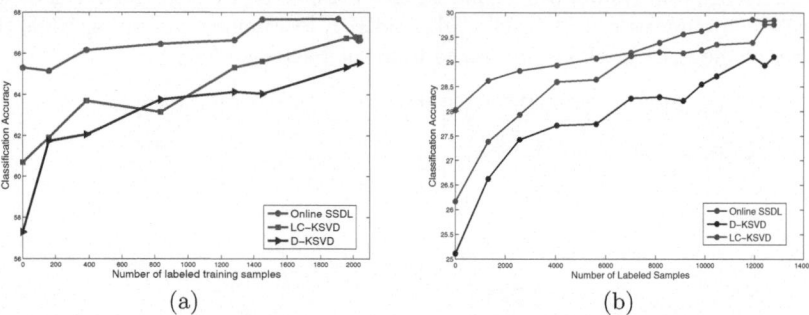

(a)                                                                    (b)

**Fig. 3.** Recognition rate on Caltech101 and Caltech256 with varying number of labeled samples. (a) Caltech101 with $K = 10 \times 102$ and $N = 20 \times 102$; (b) Caltech256 with $K = 3 \times 256$ and $N = 50 \times 102$;

**Table 2.** Recognition results using spatial pyramid features on the Caltech101. The accuracies of the other results are copied from the references.

| Training Images | 5 | 10 | 15 | 20 | 25 | 30 |
|---|---|---|---|---|---|---|
| Malik [28] | 46.6 | 55.8 | 59.1 | 62.0 | - | 66.20 |
| Lazebnik [29] | - | - | 56.4 | - | - | 64.6 |
| Griffin [27] | 44.2 | 54.5 | 59.0 | 63.3 | 65.8 | 67.60 |
| Irani [30] | - | - | 65.0 | - | - | 70.40 |
| Grauman [31] | - | - | 61.0 | - | - | 69.10 |
| Venkatesh [6] | - | - | 42.0 | - | - | - |
| Gemert [32] | - | - | - | - | - | 64.16 |
| Yang [2] | - | - | 67.0 | - | - | 73.20 |
| Wang [14] | 51.15 | 59.77 | 65.43 | 67.74 | 70.16 | 73.44 |
| SRC [3] | 48.8 | 60.1 | 64.9 | 67.7 | 69.2 | 70.7 |
| K-SVD [11] | 49.8 | 59.8 | 65.2 | 68.7 | 71.0 | 73.2 |
| D-KSVD [5] | 49.6 | 59.5 | 65.1 | 68.6 | 71.1 | 73.0 |
| IDL [14] | 51.2 | 61.5 | 65.7 | 68.4 | 71.6 | - |
| LSDL [17] | 52.8 | 61.5 | 65.7 | 68.4 | 71.5 | - |
| ODLSC [13] | 52.8 | 61.5 | 65.6 | 68.5 | 71.3 | 72.4 |
| LC-KSVD [9] | 54.0 | 63.1 | 67.7 | 70.5 | 72.3 | 73.6 |
| **Online SSDL** | **55.0** | **62.6** | **67.2** | **69.6** | **72.4** | **74.3** |

methods, we trained dictionaries of the same size as the training samples, *i.e.*, $K = 510, 1020, 1530, 2040, 2550, 3060$. Again, by setting $\phi_{low} = \phi_{high} = 0$, we essentially label all the training data, and this yields the best performance compared to the competition. As shown in Table 2, our approach is comparable to LC-KSVD but outperforms the other methods because we take the discriminative error into account.

### 4.3   Caltech256 Dataset

The Caltech256 dataset [27] contains $30,607$ images of 256 categories. There are at least 80 images per category. Compared to Caltech101 dataset, it is much more difficult due to the variability in object location, pose and size, etc. In contrast to Caltech101, here we extract HOG descriptors from each patch at three scales, $16 \times 16$, $25 \times 25$ and $31 \times 31$. The dimension of each HOG descriptor is 128. We extracted the spatial pyramid features using $4 \times 4$, $2 \times 2$ and $1 \times 1$ sub-regions. Finally we

**Table 3.** Recognition results using spatial pyramid features on the Caltech256. The accuracies in the first three rows are copied from the references, and the rest are obtained from our implementations. In our own implementation, dictionary size is fixed to be $3 \times 256 = 768$)

| Training Images | 15 | 30 | 45 | 60 |
|---|---|---|---|---|
| Griffin [27] | 28.30 | 34.10 | - | - |
| Gemert [32] | - | 27.17 | - | - |
| Yang [2] | 27.73 | 34.02 | 37.46 | 40.14 |
| IDL [14] | 19.9 | 21.7 | 23.9 | 26.3 |
| LSDL [17] | 23.3 | 25.6 | 28.4 | 30.5 |
| ODLSC [13] | 19.3 | 21.3 | 23.6 | 26.1 |
| LC-KSVD [9] | 24.6 | 28.6 | 30.3 | 34.9 |
| **Online SSDL** | **27.9** | **31.9** | **34.4** | **36.7** |

reduce the dimension of the features to 305 using PCA. We used 15, 30, 45 and 60 training samples per class for dictionary learning. Again, training images are randomly selected from each category and all are manually labeled. But unlike the common setup, where the dictionary size equals the number of training samples, we trained dictionaries that contains only 3 items per class. Also, consistent with our previous experiments, we used low-dimensional features and a simple linear classifier instead of sophisticated features and discriminative classifiers such as SVMs. As shown in Table 3, our approach achieves good performance even with a simple classifier and significantly smaller dictionary sizes. Note that the accuracies in the first three rows (group 1) are copied from the references, and the rest (group 2) are obtained from our implementation. The differences in experimental settings might account for the average drop in performance of group 2. The recognition performances with varying number of labeled samples perclass are presented in Figure 3(b). The advantage of our method is shown especially when the manual labels are few.

## 5   Conclusion

We proposed an online semi-supervised dictionary learning approach for classification. It's particularly suitable for large scale datasets where batch mode doesn't work well. Moreover, by using a probabilistic model of the sparse codes, our algorithm actively seeks for the critical points for labeling, and identifies the easily classified points as labeled data. In this way we reduce the manual labeling effort to the minimum without sacrificing the performance too much. The fact that the dictionary and the classifier are jointly learned further enhances the discriminative power. Experimental results showed that our approach achieves state-of-art performance. Possible future work includes updating the learned discriminative dictionary for input signals from a new category.

**Acknowledgement.** This work was supported by the Army Research Office MURI Grant W911NF-09-1-0383.

# References

1. Elad, M., Aharon, M.: Image denosing via sparse and redundant representations over learned dictionaries. IEEE Trans. Img. Proc. 54, 3736–3745 (2006)
2. Yang, J., Yu, K., Gong, Y., Huang, T.: Linear spatial pyramid matching using sparse coding for image classification. In: CVPR (2009)
3. Wright, J., Yang, M., Ganesh, A., Sastry, S., Ma, Y.: Robust face recognition via sparse representation. TPAMI 31, 210–227 (2009)
4. Bradley, D., Bagnell, J.: Differential sparse coding. In: NIPS (2008)
5. Zhang, Q., Li, B.: Discriminative k-svd for dictionary learning in face recognition. In: CVPR (2010)
6. Pham, D., Venkatesh, S.: Joint learning and dictionary construction for pattern recognition. In: CVPR (2008)
7. Mairal, J., Bach, F., Ponce, J., Sapiro, G., Zisserman, A.: Supervised dictionary learning. In: NIPS (2009)
8. Mairal, J., Bach, F., Ponce, J., Sapiro, G., Zisserman, A.: Discriminative learned dictionaries for local image analysis. In: CVPR (2008)
9. Jiang, Z., Lin, Z., Davis, L.: Learning a distriminative dictionary for sparse coding via label consistent k-svd. In: CVPR (2011)
10. Qiu, Q., Jiang, Z., Davis, L.: Sparse dictionary-based representation and recognition of action attributes. In: ICCV (2011)
11. Aharon, M., Elad, M., Bruckstein, A.: K-svd: An algorithm for designing overcomplete dictionries for sparse representation. IEEE Trans. on Signal Processing 54, 4311–4322 (2006)
12. Yang, J., Yu, K., Huang, T.: Supervised translation-invariant sparse coding. In: CVPR (2010)
13. Marial, J., Bach, F., Ponce, J., Sapiro, G.: Online dictionary learning for sparse coding. In: ICML (2009)
14. Wang, J., Yang, J., Yu, K., Lv, F., Huang, T., Gong, Y.: Locality-constrained linear coding for image classification. In: CVPR (2010)
15. Raina, R., Battle, A., Lee, H., Packer, B., Ng, A.: Self-taught learning: Transfer learning from unlabeled data. In: ICML (2007)
16. Zeng, H., Wang, X., Chen, Z., Lu, H., Ma, W.: Clustering based text classification requiring minimal labeled data. In: ICDM (2003)
17. Xie, B., Song, M., Tao, D.: Large-scale dictionary learning for local coordinate coding. In: BMVC (2010)
18. Boureau, Y., Bach, F., LeCun, Y., Ponce, J.: Learning mid-level features for recognition. In: CVPR (2010)
19. Grosse, R., Raina, R., Kwong, H., Ng, A.Y.: Shift-invariant sparse coding for audio classification. In: Conf. on Uncertainty in AI (2007)
20. Zhang, W., Surve, A., Fern, X., Dietterich, T.: Learning non-redundant codebooks for classifying complex objects. In: ICML (2009)
21. Rodriguez, F., Sapiro, G.: Sparse representations for image classification: Learning discriminative and reconstructive non-parametric dictionaries. IMA Preprint 2213 (2007)
22. Yang, L., Jin, R., Sukthankar, R., Jurie, F.: Unifying discriminative visual codebook genearation with classifier training for object category recognition. In: CVPR (2008)
23. Lian, X.-C., Li, Z., Lu, B.-L., Zhang, L.: Max-Margin Dictionary Learning for Multiclass Image Categorization. In: Daniilidis, K., Maragos, P., Paragios, N. (eds.) ECCV 2010, Part IV. LNCS, vol. 6314, pp. 157–170. Springer, Heidelberg (2010)

24. Aharon, M., Elad, M.: Sparse and redundant modeling of image content using an image-signaturedictionary. SIAM J. Imaging Sciences 1, 228–274 (2008)
25. Georghiades, A., Belhumeur, P., Kriegman, D.: From few to many: Illumination cone models for face recognition under variable lighting and pose. TPAMI 23, 643–660 (2001)
26. FeiFei, L., Fergus, R., Perona, P.: Learning generative visual models from few training samples: An incremental bayesian appoach tested on 101 object categories. In: CVPR Workshop on Generative Model Based Vision (2004)
27. Griffin, G., Holub, A., Perona, P.: Caltech-256 object category dataset. CIT Technical Report 7694 (2007)
28. Zhang, H., Berg, A., Maire, M., Malik, J.: Svm-knn: Discriminative nearest neighbor classification for visual category recognition. In: CVPR (2006)
29. Lazebnik, S., Schmid, C., Ponce, J.: Beyond bags of features: Spatial pyramid matching for recognizing natural scene categories. In: CVPR (2007)
30. Boiman, O., Shechtman, E., Irani, M.: In defense of nearest-neighor based image classification. In: CVPR (2008)
31. Jain, P., Kullis, B., Grauman, K.: Fast image search for learned metrics. In: CVPR (2008)
32. van Gemert, J.C., Geusebroek, J.-M., Veenman, C.J., Smeulders, A.W.M.: Kernel Codebooks for Scene Categorization. In: Forsyth, D., Torr, P., Zisserman, A. (eds.) ECCV 2008, Part III. LNCS, vol. 5304, pp. 696–709. Springer, Heidelberg (2008)

# Efficient Discriminative Learning
# of Class Hierarchy for Many Class Prediction

Lin Chen[1], Lixin Duan[2], Ivor W. Tsang[1], and Dong Xu[1]

[1] School of Computer Engineering, Nanyang Technological University
[2] SAP Research Singapore
{chen0631,ivortsang,dongxu}@ntu.edu.sg, lxduan@gmail.com

**Abstract.** Recently the maximum margin criterion has been employed
to learn a discriminative class hierarchical model, which shows promising
performance for rapid multi-class prediction. Specifically, at each node
of this hierarchy, a separating hyperplane is learned to split its associated classes from all of the corresponding training data, leading to a
time-consuming training process in computer vision applications with
many classes such as large-scale object recognition and scene classification. To address this issue, in this paper we propose a new efficient
discriminative class hierarchy learning approach for many class prediction. We first present a general objective function to unify the two state-
of-the-art methods for multi-class tasks. When there are many classes,
this objective function reveals that some classes are indeed redundant.
Thus, omitting these redundant classes will not degrade the prediction
performance of the learned class hierarchical model. Based on this observation, we decompose the original optimization problem into a sequence
of much smaller sub-problems by developing an adaptive classifier updating method and an active class selection strategy. Specifically, we iteratively update the separating hyperplane by efficiently using the training
samples only from a limited number of selected classes that are well
separated by the current separating hyperplane. Comprehensive experiments on three large-scale datasets demonstrate that our approach can
significantly accelerate the training process of the two state-of-the-art
methods while achieving comparable prediction performance in terms of
both classification accuracy and testing speed.

## 1 Introduction

Multiclass classification has attracted growing attention in the computer vision
community because of its broad application in large-scale object recognition [1]
and scene classification [2]. Given $c$ classes, conventional strategies such as one-
versus-one (1vs1) and one-versus-rest (1vsR), convert the multiclass problem to
$\frac{c(c-1)}{2}$ and $c$ binary class classification tasks, respectively, and all the learned
binary classifiers are involved to predict the class label of each test sample.
However, typical computer vision tasks such as object recognition may involve
millions of test samples and the number of classes $c$ can also be very large, thus
the prediction process using those conventional methods becomes intractable.

K.M. Lee et al. (Eds.): ACCV 2012, Part I, LNCS 7724, pp. 274–288, 2013.
© Springer-Verlag Berlin Heidelberg 2013

In the past few years, class hierarchy learning has been proposed to reduce the testing complexity to be sub-linear with respect to the number of classes [3–6]. The class hierarchy is assumed to be a tree structure in these methods, which is learned by recursively partitioning the classes (associated with an internal node of the tree) into two disjoint subsets (associated with the child nodes of the internal node). Recently, Yang and Tsang [6] borrowed the maximum margin criterion from support vector machines (SVMs) and proposed a maximum separating margin model (MSM) to determine the child nodes of any internal node. Their method can ensure that the classes associated with two child nodes are most separable, and it has achieved better performance than [3–5]. However, the training process of MSM involves an alternating optimization by iteratively using the cutting plane method [7–10] and solving the multi-kernel learning (MKL) problem [11], which is quite time-consuming when the training set is large. In [12], Gao and Koller proposed a method (referred to as SVMRH here), which solves a problem similar to [6]. The learning process of SVMRH also involves an alternating optimization by solving the Quadratic Programming (QP) and the Integer Programming (IP) problems. However, this Mixed Integer Programming (MIP) problem is NP hard. As a result, they employed multiple initializations in SVMRH so as to obtain a robust solution. In order to achieve a better tradeoff between classification accuracy and testing speed, they also introduced the Relaxed Hierarchy (RH) strategy [13], where the decisions for the confused classes are postponed to the next level when learning the class hierarchy. However, both MSM and SVMRH iteratively solve a QP problem (MKL also needs to solve a QP problem), thus they are quite slow in the training process when the training set is large.

In this paper, we propose an efficient and scalable discriminative class hierarchy learning approach for many class prediction. Our objective is to achieve comparable prediction performance to MSM and SVMRH in terms of both classification accuracy and testing speed, while significantly accelerating the training process. In contrast to the previous works in [6][12] which use the training samples from all the associated classes to train the separating hyperplane at each node of the class hierarchy, we observe that the performance of the learned class hierarchical model omitting redundant classes will not be degraded. Based on this observation, we therefore propose a many-to-few decomposition approach to decompose the original optimization problem into a sequence of much smaller sub-problems by developing an adaptive classifier updating method and an active class selection strategy. Specifically, we iteratively update the separating hyperplane by efficiently using the training samples from only a small subset of the selected classes. Since the optimal partition of the classes is to be learned, we propose to select the most confident classes from the remaining ones based on the current separating hyperplane. The updating process is repeated until the stopping criteria is met.

The main contribution of this paper is a new approach for efficient discriminative class hierarchy learning. To the best of our knowledge, this is the first work to significantly accelerate the training process of discriminative hierarchy learning while achieving comparable prediction performance.

## 2   Related Works

In this section, we review some existing methods for multiclass classification. The most popular approach is to convert the multiclass problem into several binary classification tasks, such as the 1vs1 and 1vsR strategies. Although the training process of each classifier in the 1vs1 strategy is quite fast by using the training samples only from two classes when learning each classifier, there are totally $\frac{c(c-1)}{2}$ classifiers to be learned and all of them are involved to predict the class label of each test sample. While 1vsR only performs $c$ predictions, it takes much longer training time as the training samples from all the classes are used to train each classifier. Besides 1vs1 and 1vsR, other methods include various output coding and decoding schemes [14], and the decision directed acyclic graph (DDAG) [15], in which the 1vs1 classifiers are organized in a directed acyclic graph in order to discard many class labels during the testing process. However, the number of classifier evaluations in these methods is still no less than $c$, which can be very slow for applications where the data come from many classes.

On the other hand, the class hierarchy learning methods attempt to learn an optimal class hierarchy in order to achieve sub-linear testing speed with only $\mathcal{O}(\log c)$ predictions for each test sample. For instance, the Filter Tree (FT) method [4] uses a randomly generated binary tree structure, which leads to a fast training process but degrades the prediction performance. To learn a better class hierarchy, Conditional Probability Tree (CPT) [3] employs an online learning method to update the tree structure by assuming the training samples arrive one by one. Specifically, if the label of newly coming sample has been seen before, the corresponding nodes containing this label along a path from the root node to the leaf node are updated; otherwise, a new leaf node for this label is inserted into the tree. Generally, CPT achieves better prediction performance than FT, but it is still worse than 1vsR or 1vs1 in terms of classification accuracy. The Label Embedded Tree (LET) method [5] constructs a tree by recursively performing graph cut [16] based on the label confusion matrix from the 1vsR method. However, as discussed in [6], its prediction performance heavily depends on the results from 1vsR classifiers. Recent work [17] extended LET to learn a more balanced tree by additionally introducing an ambiguity measure.

Recently, Yang and Tsang [6] proposed the MSM method to learn a better class hierarchical model than FT, CFT and LET. However, the training process of MSM is inefficient because it involves time-consuming operations for solving a set of MKL problems. Gao and Koller [12] proposed to directly optimize a similar problem without solving the MKL problem. They also introduced the Relaxed Hierarchy (RH) to efficiently balance classification accuracy and testing speed. However, a set of SVMs are iteratively trained in order to obtain a robust solution in [12], which is also very time-consuming when the training set is large. These methods can generally achieve sub-linear predictions for each test sample with the tradeoff of a certain amount of sacrifice in classification accuracy. In summary, MSM and SVMRH generally achieve the state-of-the-art performance for multiclass prediction, but their training complexity is very high for computer vision tasks like large-scale object recognition and scene classification. In this work, we focus on the acceleration of the training process of both methods, while still achieving comparable prediction performance.

## 3 Maximum Separating Margin Model

Note that existing works [5, 6, 12] can be formulated as a set of internal node splitting problems. Without loss of generality, we focus on the splitting of a specific internal node in the remainder of this paper. We define $\mathcal{S} = \{(\mathbf{x}_i, y_i)\}_{i=1}^n$ as the training set, where $\mathbf{x}_i \in \mathcal{R}^m$ and $y_i \in \mathcal{C} = \{1, ..., c\}$. Let $\boldsymbol{\mu} = [\mu_1, ..., \mu_c]^\top$ and $\boldsymbol{z} = [z_1, ..., z_n]^\top$ be the partition indicator vectors of the $c$ classes and $n$ samples, respectively. Then we have $z_i = \mu_{y_i}$. The notation $\odot$ denotes the element-wise product operator between two vectors or matrices. And $|S|$ is the cardinality of the set $S$. We also define $\mathbb{1}(\cdot)$ as an indicator function. Moreover, we denote $\mathbf{1}_n$ and $\mathbf{0}_n$ as two $n \times 1$ vectors of all ones and all zeros, respectively.

To measure the goodness of the partition, Yang and Tsang [6] borrowed the maximum margin criteria from SVM. Intuitively, the larger the separating margin, the more discriminative the partition is. Based on this criterion, they proposed MSM to learn such an optimal partition by solving the following optimization problem:

$$\min_{\boldsymbol{z}, \mathbf{w}, \xi_i} \frac{1}{2}\|\mathbf{w}\|^2 + \frac{C}{2}\sum_{i=1}^n \xi_i^2, \tag{1}$$
$$s.t. \quad z_i \in \{-1, 1\}$$
$$z_i \mathbf{w}^\top \phi(\mathbf{x}_i) \geq 1 - \xi_i, \ i = 1, ..., n,$$

where $C$ is a tradeoff parameter. Moreover, more constraints for $\boldsymbol{z}$ (i.e. $\mathcal{Z} = \{\boldsymbol{z} | - \eta \leq \boldsymbol{z}^\top \mathbf{1}_n \leq \eta, \eta \geq 0; \ z_i = z_j; \ \text{if } y_i = y_j\}$) are introduced to enforce a balanced partition and ensure that all the samples from the same class are assigned to the same partition. The problem in (1) is solved by exploring its dual form with respect to $\mathbf{w}$ and $\xi_i$'s as follows:

$$\min_{\boldsymbol{z} \in \mathcal{Z}} \max_{\boldsymbol{\alpha} \in \mathcal{A}} -\frac{1}{2}\boldsymbol{\alpha}^\top \left(K \odot (\boldsymbol{z}\boldsymbol{z}^\top) + \frac{1}{C}I\right)\boldsymbol{\alpha} + \mathbf{1}_n^\top \boldsymbol{\alpha}, \tag{2}$$

where $\boldsymbol{\alpha} = [\alpha_1, ..., \alpha_n]^\top$ is a vector of dual variables, $\mathcal{A} = \{\boldsymbol{\alpha} | \boldsymbol{\alpha} \geq \mathbf{0}_n\}$ is the domain of $\boldsymbol{\alpha}$, $K \in \mathcal{R}^{n \times n}$ is the kernel matrix with $K_{ij} = \phi(\mathbf{x}_i)^\top \phi(\mathbf{x}_j)$ being the kernel function defined by the feature mapping $\phi$. Note that (2) is a mixed integer programming (MIP) problem. To make it more tractable, Yang and Tsang [6] further relaxed (2) as an MKL problem by replacing $K \odot (\boldsymbol{z}\boldsymbol{z}^\top)$ with $\sum_{k:\boldsymbol{z}^k \in \mathcal{Z}} d_k K \odot (\boldsymbol{z}^k \boldsymbol{z}^{k\top})$, where the linear combination coefficients $d_k$'s are to be learned by using SimpleMKL [11].

Gao and Koller [12] solved a similar optimization problem by additionally introducing the relaxed hierarchy [13]. Specifically, they introduced an additional term and arrived at the following optimization problem[1]:

$$\min_{\boldsymbol{\mu},\mathbf{w},\xi_i} \frac{1}{2}\|\mathbf{w}\|^2 + \frac{C}{2}\sum_{i=1}^{n}|\mu_{y_i}|\xi_i^2 - A\sum_{i=1}^{n}|\mu_{y_i}|, \tag{3}$$

$$s.t. \ \mu_{y_i} \in \{-1, 0, +1\}, \ y_i \in \{1, ..., c\},$$

$$\mu_{y_i}\mathbf{w}^\top\phi(\mathbf{x}_i) \geq 1 - \xi_i, \ i = 1, ..., n,$$

where $A$ is a tradeoff parameter. Also, some additional constraints for $\boldsymbol{\mu}$ are introduced to enforce a balanced partition and to avoid a trivial solution, *i.e.* $-B \leq \sum_{k=1}^{c}\mu_k \leq B$, $\sum_{k=1}^{c}\mathbb{1}\{\mu_k > 0\} \geq 1$, and $\sum_{k=1}^{c}\mathbb{1}\{\mu_k < 0\} \geq 1$. Note that when $\mu_k = 0$, the $k$-th class will not be considered in the training process and it will be freely assigned to both child nodes. Moreover, the last term in the objective function of (3) encourages all $|\mu_k|$ to be 1. (3) is also an MIP problem. Gao and Koller directly optimized (3) by iteratively solving $\boldsymbol{\mu}$ and an SVM problem, rather than relaxing the MIP problem as in MSM [6]. However, the MIP problem is NP hard. Their method also involves iteratively solving the QP problem and the training process is slow when the training set is large. Because this method uses the relaxed hierarchy [13] and involves solving an SVM problem, we refer to it as SVMRH.

## 4    A Many-to-Few Approach for Many Class Prediction

In this section, we first present a general objective function to unify the discriminative hierarchy learning methods such as [6, 12]. Formally, we present the general formulation by using the square hinge loss function as follows:

$$\min_{\boldsymbol{\mu},\mathbf{w},\xi_i} \frac{1}{2}\|\mathbf{w}\|^2 + \frac{C}{2}\sum_{i=1}^{n}\xi_i^2 - A\sum_{i=1}^{n}|\mu_{y_i}|, \tag{4}$$

$$s.t. \ \xi_i \geq |\mu_{y_i}|\left(1 - \mu_{y_i}\mathbf{w}^\top\phi(\mathbf{x}_i)\right), \tag{5}$$

$$y_i \in \{1, ..., c\}, \ i = 1, ..., n.$$

Note that when $\mu_{y_i} = -1$ or 1, each inequality constraint in (5) can be rewritten as $\mu_{y_i}\mathbf{w}^\top\phi(\mathbf{x}_i) \geq 1 - \xi_i$; and when $\mu_{y_i} = 0$, the constraint becomes $\xi_i \geq 0$. In the general forumulation, if we define $\boldsymbol{\mu} \in \{-1, 1\}^c$, we have $|\mu_{y_i}| = 1$, $\forall i$, and the last term in (4) can be directly removed from the objective function. Recall that we have $z_i = \mu_{y_i}$. (4) then becomes (1) which is exactly the formulation of MSM [6]. On the other hand, if $\boldsymbol{\mu} \in \{-1, 0, 1\}^c$, (4) is equivalent to (3) (*i.e.* the formulation of SVMRH [12]).

However, (4) is still an MIP problem, and its computational complexity is related to the exponential number of candidates of $\boldsymbol{\mu}$. If the length of $\boldsymbol{\mu}$ is very large (*i.e.* $c$ is very large), it will be computationally intractable to solve the MIP problem in (4).

---

[1] Note that the hinge loss function was used in [12]. To present a general objective function to unify MSM and SVMRH, we instead use the square hinge loss function in this work which achieves very similar results to those using the hinge loss function.

---

**Algorithm 1.** The Many-to-Few Approach

---

1: **input:** Training data $\mathcal{S} = \{(\mathbf{x}_i, y_i)\}_{i=1}^n$, $\mathcal{C} = \{1, .., c\}$, the number of selected active classes per iteration $n_{inc}$.
2: **initialization:** $\tau \leftarrow 0$, $\mathcal{C}_\tau = \emptyset$, $\mathcal{C}_{rest} \leftarrow \mathcal{C}$.
3: $\mathcal{C}_\tau \leftarrow$ two well separated classes from $\mathcal{C}_{rest}$;
4: $\mathcal{C}_{rest} \leftarrow \mathcal{C}/\mathcal{C}_\tau$;
5: Train an initial classifier $f^\tau$ by using the training samples from the classes in $\mathcal{C}_\tau$;
6: **repeat**
7:    Predict the training samples from the classes in $\mathcal{C}_{rest}$ by using $f^\tau$;
8:    $\mathcal{C}_\tau \leftarrow n_{inc}$ most confident classes from $\mathcal{C}_{rest}$ by active class selection;
9:    $\mathcal{C}_{rest} \leftarrow \mathcal{C}_{rest}/\mathcal{C}_\tau$;
10:   Train $f^{\tau+1}$ by using $f^\tau$ and the training samples from the classes in $\mathcal{C}_\tau$;
11:   $\tau \leftarrow \tau + 1$;
12: **until** $|\mathcal{C}_{rest}| < n_{inc}$ or all the training data are well separated by the current hyperplane subject to the balance constraints for the two partitions.

---

Note that, when there are many classes (as discussed in this work), it is very likely that the square hinge loss of the training samples (*i.e.* $(\max\{0, 1 - \mu_{y_i}\mathbf{w}^\top\phi(\mathbf{x}_i)\})^2$) from some classes will be large. As a result, the $\mu_{y_i}$'s for those classes are encouraged to be zeros such that the $\xi_i$'s for the corresponding training samples will become zeros. In this work, we refer to such classes as *redundant* classes, as they will not affect the optimal solution to (4).

Since the corresponding constraints for redundant classes are inactive and can be omitted in (4), (4) can be simplified by fixing $\mu_k = 0$ for the classes that are likely to be redundant. After that, we further propose to decompose the original optimization problem in (4) into a sequence of much smaller sub-problems, each of which has only a few classes (referred to as the few class problem). Specifically in this work, we first follow [12] to select a pair of well separated classes from all the $c$ classes. The samples from the two classes are then used to train an initial classifier $f^0$. After that, based on the prediction from $f^0$, we construct a class set $\mathcal{C}_1$ by selecting the $n_{inc}$ most confident classes from the set of remaining classes $\mathcal{C}_{rest}$ (see Section 4.2 for details on how to actively select the most confident classes). Then, we learn an updated classifier $f^1$ which is adapted from the initial classifier $f^0$ with the adaptation error learned by using the data only from the $n_{inc}$ selected most confident classes (see Section 4.1 for details on how to update the classifier in an adaptive manner). Again, we use the classifier $f^1$ to construct a class set $\mathcal{C}_2$ by selecting another $n_{inc}$ most confident classes for the consecutive iterations. We repeat this process until the stopping criterion is met. The whole algorithm is detailed in Algorithm 1.

Note that MSM with relaxed hierarchy (MSMRH) and SVMRH can be readily incorporated into our many-to-few approach. We then refer to MSMRH and SVMRH after employing the adaptive process as AMSMRH and ASVMRH, respectively.

## 4.1    Adaptive Classifier Updating

Based on the decomposition of the optimization problem in (4) into a sequence of few class problems, we develop a method to adaptively update the classifier, which can significantly accelerate MSM and SVMRH.

Formally, given the classifier $f^\tau$ from the $\tau$-th sub-problem, we learn an updated classifier $f^{\tau+1}$ at time $\tau+1$ by using $f^\tau$ and the training samples from the selected $n_{inc}$ most confident classes in the $\tau$-th sub-problem, i.e. $\{(\mathbf{x}_{j_m}, y_{j_m})\}$, where $j_m \in \mathcal{I}^\tau$ and $\mathcal{I}^\tau = \{j_m | m = 1, \ldots, n_\tau, 1 \leq j_1 < \cdots < j_{n_\tau} \leq n\}$ is the index set of the $n_\tau$ training samples in the selected $n_{inc}$ active classes at time $\tau$. Inspired by [18], we define the classifier $f^{\tau+1}$ as follows:

$$f^{\tau+1}(\mathbf{x}) = f^\tau(\mathbf{x}) + \Delta f^\tau(\mathbf{x}) = f^\tau(\mathbf{x}) + \mathbf{w}^{\tau\top}\phi(\mathbf{x}),  \quad (6)$$

where $\Delta f^\tau(\mathbf{x}) = \mathbf{w}^{\tau\top}\phi(\mathbf{x})$ can be considered as a perturbation function which models the adaptation error from time $\tau$ to time $\tau+1$. Both MSM and SVMRH can be used to solve the $\tau$-th few class problem. Here we first take MSM as an example and propose to find $\mathbf{w}^\tau$ by using the training samples from the $n_{inc}$ selected active classes in $\mathcal{C}_\tau$ as follows:

$$\min_{\mathbf{z}^\tau \in \mathcal{Z}^\tau, \mathbf{w}^\tau, \xi_{j_m}} \frac{1}{2}\|\mathbf{w}^\tau\|^2 + \frac{C}{2}\sum_{m=1}^{n_\tau}\xi_{j_m}^2,  \quad (7)$$

$$s.t.  \quad z_m^\tau f^{\tau+1}(\mathbf{x}_{j_m}) \geq 1 - \xi_{j_m},  \quad m = 1, \ldots, n_\tau.  \quad (8)$$

where $\mathbf{z}^\tau = [z_1^\tau, \ldots, z_{n_\tau}^\tau]^\top$, and $\mathcal{Z}^\tau = \{\mathbf{z}^\tau | -\eta \leq \mathbf{z}^{\tau\top}\mathbf{1}_{n_\tau} \leq \eta, \eta \geq 0; z_p^\tau = z_q^\tau, \text{ if } y_{j_p} = y_{j_q} \text{ and } j_p, j_q \in \mathcal{I}^\tau\}$ is the domain of $\mathbf{z}^\tau$ for the training samples at time $\tau$.

By introducing the Lagrange multipliers $\alpha_i$'s for the inequality constraints in (8), we arrive at the dual problem with respect to $\mathbf{w}$ and $\xi_{j_m}$'s as follows:

$$\min_{\mathbf{z}^\tau \in \mathcal{Z}^\tau} \max_{\boldsymbol{\alpha} \in \mathcal{A}} -\frac{1}{2}\boldsymbol{\alpha}^\top\left(K \odot (\mathbf{z}^\tau\mathbf{z}^{\tau\top}) + \frac{1}{C}I\right)\boldsymbol{\alpha} + \boldsymbol{\alpha}^\top\left(\mathbf{1}_{n_\tau} - \mathbf{z}^\tau \odot \boldsymbol{f}^\tau\right),  \quad (9)$$

where $\boldsymbol{\alpha} = [\alpha_1, \ldots, \alpha_{n_\tau}]^\top$ is a vector of the dual variables, $\mathcal{A} = \{\boldsymbol{\alpha} | \boldsymbol{\alpha} \geq \mathbf{0}_{n_\tau}\}$ is the feasible set of $\boldsymbol{\alpha}$, $K \in \mathcal{R}^{n_\tau \times n_\tau}$ is the kernel matrix with $K_{pq} = \phi(\mathbf{x}_{j_p})^\top\phi(\mathbf{x}_{j_q})$, and $\boldsymbol{f}^\tau$ is a $n_\tau \times 1$ vector with its $m$-th element as $f^\tau(\mathbf{x}_{j_m})$.

**Enumeration on $\boldsymbol{\mu}$:** For each few class problem, we only have a small number of classes. Therefore, we propose to find the exact solution to the problem in (9). Here we show some cases (i.e. $n_{inc} = 2, 4$ and $6$) of the few class problem. Note we only use those even numbers in order to construct a balanced class hierarchy (i.e. $\sum_{k: k \in \mathcal{C}_\tau} \mathbb{1}\{\mu_k > 0\} = \sum_{k: k \in \mathcal{C}_\tau} \mathbb{1}\{\mu_k < 0\} = \frac{1}{2}n_{inc}$). In this case, the additional constraints for $\boldsymbol{\mu}$ to avoid a trivial solution in (4) are naturally satisfied. Considering that the elements in $\mathbf{z}$ and $\boldsymbol{\mu}$ satisfy the constraint $z_i = \mu_{y_i}$, we only analyze those cases based on $\boldsymbol{\mu}$.

When $|\mathcal{C}_\tau| = 2$, we have $\binom{2}{1} = 2$ choice for $\boldsymbol{\mu}$, i.e. $\boldsymbol{\mu} = \{[1, -1]^\top, [1, -1]^\top\}$. In this case, we only need to train two SVM classifiers to solve (9) and select the one with the smaller objective value. When $|\mathcal{C}_\tau| = 4$, we have $\binom{4}{2} = 6$ choices for $\boldsymbol{\mu}$, i.e. $\boldsymbol{\mu} \in \{[1, 1, -1, -1]^\top, [1, -1, 1, -1]^\top, [1, -1, -1, 1]^\top, [-1, -1, 1, 1]^\top, [-1, 1, -1, 1]^\top, [-1, 1, 1, -1]^\top\}$. So, to solve (9), we train six SVM classifiers and select the one with the smallest objective value. Due to space limitations, we do not list the $\binom{6}{3} = 20$ candidates of $\boldsymbol{\mu}$ for $|\mathcal{C}_\tau| = 6$. As $|\mathcal{C}_\tau|$ is small, we enumerate all possible $\boldsymbol{z}^\tau \in \mathcal{Z}^\tau$ in order to find the exact solution to (9). Generally, we can achieve better accuracy but slower training speed when using a larger $n_{inc}$. Observing that the accuracy is generally saturated when setting $n_{inc} \geq 6$, we empirically fix it to 6 in the experiments.

Recall that we only use the training data from the selected active classes to solve the $\tau$-th few class problem. For ASVMRH, we just need to solve the problem as in (7) by fixing $\boldsymbol{z}^\tau$ with the labels determined by the active class selection (see Section 4.2).

**Classifier Updating:** After obtaining the optimal $\boldsymbol{z}^\tau$ and $\boldsymbol{\alpha}$ by solving (9), we can rewrite the perturbation function as follows:

$$\Delta f^\tau(\mathbf{x}) = \sum_{m:\, \alpha_m \neq 0} \alpha_m z_m^\tau k(\mathbf{x}_{j_m}, \mathbf{x}). \tag{10}$$

Therefore, the classifier $f^{\tau+1}$ for the $(\tau+1)$-th few class problem can be obtained by substituting $\Delta f^\tau(\mathbf{x})$ in (10) into (6).

### 4.2   Active Selection of the Most Confident Classes

In our many-to-few approach, we propose to iteratively select the active classes that are most confident for the $\tau$-th few class problem. Specifically at time $\tau$, based on our proposed general formulation in (4), we employ the classifier $f^\tau$ to partition the data from the classes in $\mathcal{C}_{rest}$ by solving the following integer programming problem:

$$\min_{\boldsymbol{\mu}} \quad \sum_{k:\, k \in \mathcal{C}_{rest}} n_k |\mu_k| \left( \frac{1}{n_k} \sum_{i:\, y_i = k} \frac{\xi_i^2}{2} - \frac{A}{C} \right), \tag{11}$$

$$s.t. \quad \xi_i = \max\{0, 1 - \mu_{y_i} f^\tau(\mathbf{x}_i)\}, \quad \mu_k \in \{-1, 0, 1\},$$

$$\sum_{k:\, k \in \mathcal{C}_{rest}} \mathbb{1}\{\mu_k > 0\} = \frac{1}{2} n_{inc}, \quad \sum_{k:\, k \in \mathcal{C}_{rest}} \mathbb{1}\{\mu_k < 0\} = \frac{1}{2} n_{inc}, \tag{12}$$

where $n_k$ is the number of training samples from the $k$-th class, and $\frac{1}{n_k} \sum_{i:\, y_i = k} \frac{\xi_i^2}{2}$ can be thought of as the average square hinge loss of the $k$-th class. An intuitive explanation of the above problem is that we automatically select $n_{inc}$ active classes from $\mathcal{C}_{rest}$ with the minimal square hinge loss. In other words, the less confused classes (i.e. with smaller average square hinge loss) will be selected at early iterations, while the more confused classes (i.e. with larger average square hinge loss) will wait to be selected later. Then, the set of selected most confident classes is $\mathcal{C}_\tau = \{k \mid \mu_k \neq 0, \ k \in \mathcal{C}_{rest}\}$.

Note that (11) is an integer programming problem, which is similar to that in solving SVMRH (see (3)) except for the constraints on $\boldsymbol{\mu}$. Specifically, at each node of the class hierarchy, SVMRH tries to find the optimal partition for all classes associated with that node. In contrast, our approach ignores the redundant classes and actively identifies the $n_{inc}$ most confident classes by solving (11) subjected to the constraints in (12) to update the separating hyperplane. Due to the differences in constraints, we solve (3) for the purpose of active class selection, which is not considered in [12].

### 4.3 Complexity Analysis

We analyze the computational complexity of our proposed approach by taking AMSMRH as an example and it is also applicable to SVMRH. We compare the complexity of AMSMRH with MSM at the root node of the hierarchy which contains all classes. The complexity of AMSMRH at other internal nodes can be similarly derived.

MSM involves solving a set of MKL problems, each of which requires the alternating optimization between an SVM problem and a linear programming problem to find the kernel combination coefficients. Because the main cost in MSM for each iteration is from solving the SVM problem with the worst case complexity as $\mathcal{O}(n^3)$, the total complexity for solving MSM is thus $\mathcal{O}(T_1 n^3)$, where $T_1$ is a constant. For AMSMRH, we first assume that the number of samples from each class in the training set is the same, which is actually the setting used in our experiments. Then we have $n/c$ samples from each class. At each iteration in AMSMRH, we use the $n_{inc}$ most confident classes for training. And the exact solution requires training of $\binom{n_{inc}}{\frac{n_{inc}}{2}}$ SVMs. Therefore, the complexity for each iteration is $\mathcal{O}\left(\binom{n_{inc}}{\frac{n_{inc}}{2}}(\frac{n}{c}n_{inc})^3\right)$. Moreover, the number of iterations required by AMSMRH is bounded by $\lceil \frac{c}{n_{inc}} \rceil$. Thus, the total complexity of AMSMRH is $\mathcal{O}\left(\frac{c}{n_{inc}}\binom{n_{inc}}{\frac{n_{inc}}{2}}(\frac{n}{c}n_{inc})^3\right)$. Since we set $n_{inc} = 6$ in the experiments (*i.e.* $n_{inc} \ll c$), the acceleration magnitude of the training process of AMSMRH over MSM is $\mathcal{O}(c^2)$. Even if we use the empirical complexity $\mathcal{O}(n^{2.3})$ for solving the SVM problem [15], the acceleration magnitude is still $\mathcal{O}(c^{1.3})$. If we assume the numbers of samples and classes for MSM and AMSMRH are the same at other corresponding nodes, the analysis is also applicable to other nodes with only different values of $c$.

## 5 Experiments

We evaluate our proposed methods AMSMRH and ASVMRH on three large-scale datasets with many classes (*i.e.* sector [19], Caltech-256 [1] and SUN-397 [2]). Specifically, we compare our methods with the one-versus-one strategy (1vs1), the one-versus-rest strategy (1vsR), Filter Tree (FT) [4], Conditional Probability Tree (CPT) [3], Label Embedded Tree (LET) [5], Maximum Separating Margin (MSM) [6] and SVMRH [12].

**Table 1.** Summarization of the datasets used in the experiments

| Dataset | # training samples | # test samples | # classes | # feature dim. |
|---|---|---|---|---|
| sector | 2100 | 7519 | 105 | 55197 |
| Caltech-256 | 10240 | 10240 | 256 | 43008 |
| SUN-397 | 19850 | 19850 | 397 | 6300 |

Following [12], we evaluate the experimental results of each method based on the following evaluation metrics: classification accuracy, testing speed and training speed. The classification accuracy is defined as the mean of per-class accuracies over all classes [1]. For the evaluation of testing speed, we report the mean number of classifier evaluations for the linear kernel and report both the mean number of classifier evaluations and the mean number of kernel evaluations for the non-linear kernel [12], over all the test samples. For the training speed, we report the recorded CPU time during the training process for each method. All the experiments are conducted on a DELL server with 64G RAM and multi-core 3.07GHz processors.

### 5.1   Datasets and Experimental Setup

In the experiments, we use three large-scale datasets for performance evaluations (also see the summarization in Table 1):

- **Sector [19]:** It contains a total number of 9619 documents from 105 classes. We adopt the linear kernel on this dataset, because the dimension of the term frequency features is very high and the linear kernel is commonly used for document classification. For each class, we randomly sample 20 documents as the training data, and the remaining documents are used for testing.
- **Caltech-256 [1]:** It consists of 30607 images from 256 categories. Following [20], we extract the so-called ScSPM feature from each image. Specifically, we first resize each image to fit inside a $300 \times 300$ region by keeping the same aspect ratio. We then extract the dense SIFT descriptors from $16 \times 16$ patches over a grid with a spacing of 4 pixels. And then we employ the sparse representation and maximum pooling based techniques in [20] to extract the ScSPM feature, in which we use a codebook of size 2048 and three-level pyramids. Finally, each image is represented as a 43008 dimensional feature vector. We also use the linear kernel because the feature dimension is very high and the linear kernel was used in existing work [20]. We randomly sample 40 training images and 40 testing images for each class.
- **SUN-397 [2]:** It contains 397 well sampled scene categories. For image feature representation, we adopt the HOG pyramid feature with the histogram intersection kernel, because this combination achieves the best results among all the single feature based methods as reported in [2]. We randomly sample 50 training images and 50 testing images for each class.

For all the datasets, we randomly sample the training data five times and report the mean performance over five rounds in terms of classification accuracy, testing speed and training speed. For fair comparison, we set the tradeoff parameter $C$ (like in SVM) to 10 for all the methods by using cross validation for 1vsR. For 1vs1, the final prediction is based on decision values from $\binom{c}{2}$ classifiers. For 1vsR, we classify each test sample to the class whose classifier gives the largest decision value among the $c$ decision values. Note that the multiclass methods (*i.e.* FT, CPT, LET and MSM) do not consider the relaxed hierarchy strategy [13]. So for each of those methods, we adjust the hierarchy levels from 2 to 5 and use the 1vsR method for each leaf node associated with more than 2 classes. We only report the results of MSM on the sector dataset, because it is computationally prohibitive to train the classifier on the other two larger datasets (*i.e.* Caltech-256 and SUN-397). For SVMRH and our methods AMSMRH and ASVMRH, the relaxed hierarchy strategy is adopted, and we set the number of hierarchy levels to be 5 (*resp.* 8) for the sector and Caltech-256 datasets (*resp.* the SUN-397 dataset). For SVMRH and our methods AMSMRH and ASVMRH, we vary the fraction $\frac{A}{C}$ (*i.e.* $\rho$ in [12]) within the range of [0.5, 1] in order to show the tradeoff between classification accuracy *vs.* testing speed and the training speed *vs.* the testing speed. For SVMRH, we directly use their implementation[2] and follow their settings in [12].

## 5.2  Results

**Classification Accuracy *vs.* Testing Speed:** Fig. 1 shows the classification accuracy of different methods with respect to the testing speed in terms of the number of classifier evaluations on the three datasets. As the testing speed of 1vs1 in terms of classifier evaluations is extremely slow, we do not put its results in the figures. The number of classifier evaluations (*resp.* classification accuracy) of 1vs1 are 5460 (*resp.* 79.78%), 32640 (*resp.* 43.81%) and 78606 (*resp.* 24.64%) on sector, Caltech-256 and SUN-397, respectively. From the results, we have the following observations. Firstly, the computational costs of the conventional classification strategies 1vs1 and 1vsR in the testing process are very high, although they have good classification accuracies. Secondly, the maximum margin based methods (*i.e.* MSM, SVMRH, AMSMRH and ASVMRH) are generally much better than non-margin based methods (*i.e.* FT, CPT and LET) in terms of both classification accuracy and testing speed, which shows the effectiveness of this criteria in learning the class hierarchical model. Thirdly, we observe that our methods AMSMRH and ASVMRH generally achieve comparable prediction performance to SVMRH on the three datasets and to MSM on the sector dataset, demonstrating the effectiveness of our proposed many-to-few approach in learning the class hierarchical model. Recall that the histogram intersection kernel is used on the SUN-397 dataset. As suggested in [12], we also report the classification accuracy of different methods with respect to the mean number of kernel evaluations on the SUN-397 dataset in Fig. 3(a), in which we cache the kernel computations from different binary classifiers and reuse them whenever possible. Again, the maximum margin based methods are generally much better than the non-margin based methods and our proposed method AMSMRH is comparable to SVMRH. It is worth noting that the behavior of the curves in Fig. 3(a) is different from those in Fig. 1 due to the caching of the kernel computations, and similar results can be found in [12].

---

[2] http://www.stanford.edu/~tianshig/software

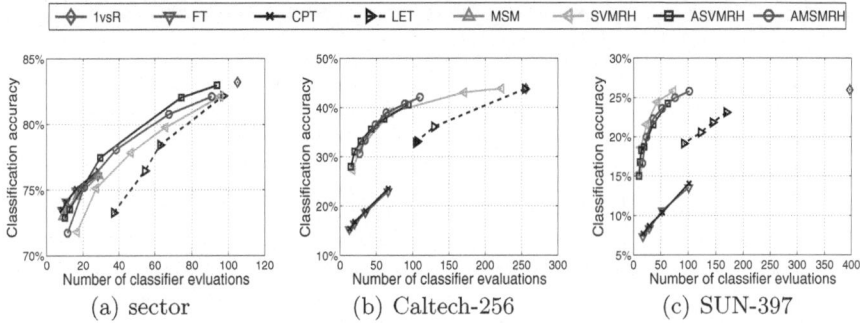

**Fig. 1.** Classification accuracy *vs.* testing speed using different methods on the three datasets. The testing speed is evaluated by using the number of classifier evaluations.

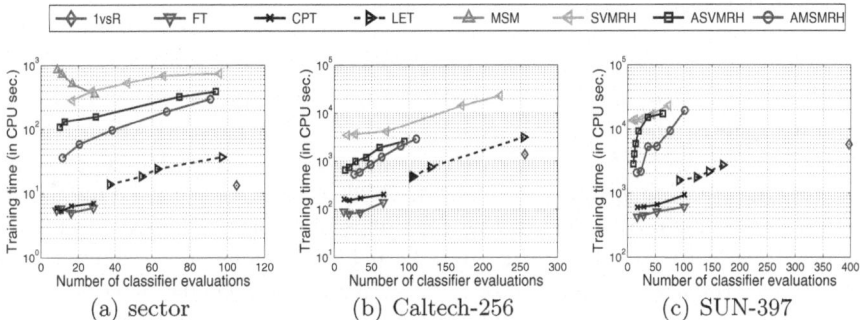

**Fig. 2.** Training speed (in log scale) *vs.* testing speed using different methods. The testing speed is evaluated by using the number of classifier evaluations.

**Training Speed *vs.* Testing Speed:** In Fig. 2, we show the comparisons of different methods in terms of training speed (in log scale) with respect to testing speed in terms of number of classifier evaluations on the three datasets. Again, we do not include the results of 1vs1 in the figures. The training time of 1vs1 is 0.60 sec., 17.37 sec. and 63.87 sec. on sector, Caltech-256 and SUN-397, respectively. We observe that the non-margin based methods (*i.e.* FT, CPT and LET) are very fast in training. An explanation is that FT is based on random partitions and CPT adopts an online learning method to learn the class hierarchy. Though they have fast training speed, their prediction performance in terms of both classification accuracy and testing speed are very poor, as shown in Fig. 1 and Fig. 3(a). And the calculation time of the label confusion matrix are 64, 3997 and 21553 CPU seconds on sector, Caltech-256 and SUN-397, respectively. We also observe that the training process of the maximum margin based methods MSM and SVMRH is quite slow, as they require computationally expensive optimization procedures to solve their learning problems. However, our methods AMSMRH and ASVMRH are generally much faster than MSM and SVMRH when using the same number of classifier evaluations or kernel evaluations, which demonstrates the efficiency of our proposed approach to decompose the optimization problem into a set of sub-problems by using the developed adaptive classifier updating method and active class selection strategy. AMSMRH is up

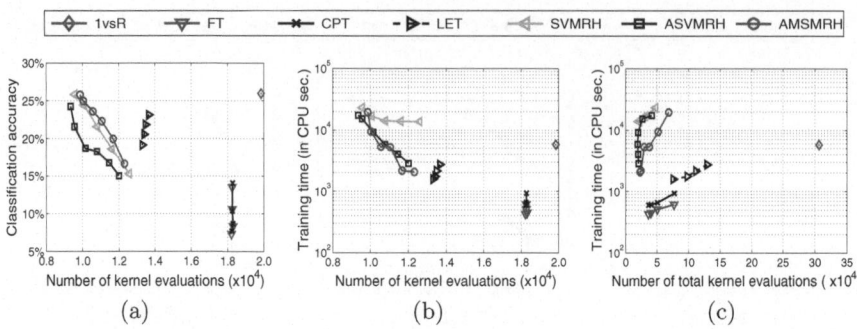

**Fig. 3.** Performance comparison of different methods on the SUN-397 dataset. (a) Classification accuracy *vs.* testing speed. (b) Training time *vs.* testing speed in terms of number of kernel evaluations with kernel caching strategy. (c) Training time *vs.* number of total kernel evaluations without kernel caching strategy.

to 22 times faster than MSM and ASVMRH is up to 4 times faster than SVMRH. More importantly, the prediction performance of AMSMRH and ASVMRH are also comparable to MSM and SVMRH, respectively, as shown in Fig. 1. We also show the training speed of different methods with respect to the number of kernel evaluations on SUN-397 in Fig. 3(b). It is interesting to observe that the training time decreases when using more kernel evaluations. The explanation is that we cache the kernel computations in Fig. 3(b), which means the kernel value between any two training samples will be computed only once and may be reused in other classifiers. If we count the number of total kernel evaluations without using the kernel caching strategy (see Fig. 3(c)), the training time will increase when using more kernel evaluations, similarly as in Fig. 2(c). However, how to develop a class hierarchy learning method to encourage the reuse of cached kernel values will be investigated in the future.

**Table 2.** Means and Standard deviations of training time (in CPU seconds) at the root node of four methods

| | MSM [6] | SVMRH [12] | AMSMRH | ASVMRH |
|---|---|---|---|---|
| sector | $130.43 \pm 23.37$ | $95.73 \pm 8.32$ | $75.38 \pm 2.90$ | $37.91 \pm 3.09$ |
| Caltech-256 | - | $1448.90 \pm 64.64$ | $29.75 \pm 1.31$ | $95.36 \pm 14.23$ |
| SUN-397 | - | $7449.53 \pm 223.60$ | $82.40 \pm 1.91$ | $280.76 \pm 9.09$ |

**Training Speed at the Root Node:** As the root node contains all the classes, it is a good choice for us to more precisely compare the training time of the maximum margin based methods MSM, SVMRH, AMSMRH and ASVMRH. We then report the means and standard deviations of training time over five rounds of experiments on the three datasets from each of these methods when learning the classifier at the root node in Table 2. Again, we only report the results of MSM on sector, because it is computationally prohibitive to train its classifier on the other two larger datasets (*i.e.* Caltech-256 and SUN-397). We can see that the training process of our proposed methods AMSMRH and ASVMRH is much faster than MSM and SVMRH, and the improvement is more significant when using a larger dataset. On Caltech-256, AMSMRH and ASVMRH are 48 times and 14 times faster than SVMRH, respectively; and on SUN-397, AMSMRH and ASVMRH are 89 times and 26 times faster than SVMRH, respectively. The results clearly demonstrate the efficiency of the proposed approach.

## 6  Conclusion

We have proposed an efficient discriminative class hierarchy learning framework for many class prediction. In our framework, we decompose the original many class problem into a sequence of much smaller sub-problems by developing an adaptive classifier updating method and an active class selection strategy. Specifically, we iteratively update the separating hyperplane by efficiently using the training samples only from a few selected classes. And based on our developed active class selection strategy, those selected classes are guaranteed to be well separated by the current separating hyperplane in the iterative updating procedure. Using this approach, we developed AMSMRH and ASVMRH to significantly accelerate the training process of the existing methods MSM [6] and SVMRH [12]. Comprehensive experimental results on three large-scale datasets clearly demonstrate that our proposed methods AMSMRH and ASVMRH can significantly accelerate the training process of MSM and SVMRH, while still achieving comparable prediction performance.

**Acknowledgement.** This study is supported by the National Research Foundation Singapore under its Interactive & Digital Media (IDM) Public Sector R&D Funding Initiative (Grant No. NRF2008IDM-IDM004-018) and administered by the IDM Programme Office.

## References

1. Griffin, G., Holub, A., Perona, P.: Caltech-256 object category dataset. Technical Report 7694, California Institute of Technology (2007)
2. Xiao, J., Hays, J., Ehinger, K., Oliva, A., Torralba, A.: Sun database: Large-scale scene recognition from abbey to zoo. In: CVPR (2010)
3. Beygelzimer, A., Langford, J., Lifshits, Y., Sorkin, G., Strehl, A.: Conditional probability tree estimation analysis and algorithms. In: UAI, pp. 51–58 (2009)
4. Beygelzimer, A., Langford, J., Ravikumar, P.: Error-Correcting Tournaments. In: Gavaldà, R., Lugosi, G., Zeugmann, T., Zilles, S. (eds.) ALT 2009. LNCS, vol. 5809, pp. 247–262. Springer, Heidelberg (2009)
5. Bengio, S., Weston, J., Grangier, D.: Label embedding trees for large multi-class tasks. In: NIPS, pp. 163–171 (2010)
6. Yang, J., Tsang, I.W.: Hierarchical maximum margin learning for multi-class classification. In: UAI, pp. 753–760 (2011)
7. Li, Y.F., Tsang, I.W., Kwok, J.T., Zhou, Z.H.: Tighter and convex maximum margin clustering. In: AISTATS, pp. 344–351 (2009)

8. Li, W., Duan, L., Xu, D., Tsang, I.W.: Text-based image retrieval using progressive multi-instance learning. In: ICCV, pp. 2049–2055 (2011)
9. Duan, L., Li, W., Tsang, I.W., Xu, D.: Improving web image search by bag-based re-ranking. T-IP 20, 3280–3290 (2011)
10. Li, W., Duan, L., Tsang, I.W., Xu, D.: Batch mode adaptive multiple instance learning for computer vision tasks. In: CVPR, pp. 2368–2375 (2012)
11. Rakotomamonjy, A., Bach, F., Canu, S.: SimpleMKL. JMLR 9 (2008)
12. Gao, T., Koller, D.: Discriminative learning of relaxed hierarchy for large-scale visual recognition. In: ICCV, pp. 2072–2079 (2011)
13. Marszałek, M., Schmid, C.: Constructing Category Hierarchies for Visual Recognition. In: Forsyth, D., Torr, P., Zisserman, A. (eds.) ECCV 2008, Part IV. LNCS, vol. 5305, pp. 479–491. Springer, Heidelberg (2008)
14. Escalera, S., Pujol, O., Radeva, P.: Error-correcting ouput codes library. Journal of Machine Learning Research 11, 661–664 (2010)
15. Platt, J.: Fast training of support vector machines using sequential minimal optimization. In: Advances in Kernel Methods: Support Vector Learning, pp. 185–208. MIT Press (1999)
16. Luxburg, U.: A tutorial on spectral clustering. Statistics and Computing 17, 395–416 (2007)
17. Deng, J., Satheesh, S., Berg, A., Fei-Fei, L.: Fast and balanced: Efficient label tree learning for large scale object recognition. In: NIPS (2011)
18. Duan, L., Tsang, I.W., Xu, D., Luo, J.: Visual event recognition in videos by learning from web data. In: CVPR, pp. 1959–1966 (2010)
19. McCallum, A., Nigam, K.: A comparison of event models for naive bayes text classification. In: AAAI Workshop on Learning for Text Categorization (1998)
20. Yang, J., Yu, K., Gong, Y., Huang, T.: Linear spatial pyramid matching using sparse coding for image classification. In: CVPR, pp. 1794–1801 (2009)

# Grouping Active Contour Fragments
# for Object Recognition

Wei Zheng[1,2], Songlin Song[1,2], Hong Chang[1], and Xilin Chen[1]

[1] Key Lab of Intelligent Information Processing of Chinese Academy of Sciences
(CAS), Institute of Computing Technology, CAS, Beijing, 100190, China
[2] Graduate School of the Chinese Academy of Sciences, Beijing, 100039, China
{wei.zheng,songlin.song,hong.chang,xilin.chen}@vipl.ict.ac.cn

**Abstract.** In this paper, we try to address the challenging problem of combining local shape features to describe long and continuous shape characteristics. To this end, we firstly propose a novel type of local shape feature, namely Active Contour Fragment (ACF), to encode the shape deformation in a local region. An ACF is automatically learnt from the contours of a specific object class and capable to describe the intra-class shape characteristics based on the point distribution model. Secondly, we combine multiple ACFs into a group, namely Active Contour Group (ACG), to describe the long shape characteristics .We model the ACFs in an ACG using an undirected chain model and estimate the parameters of the chain model in a subspace for accelerating the learning and matching processes of ACGs. Finally, we discriminatively train the classifiers based on ACFs and ACGs in a boosting framework for localizing objects as well as delineating object boundaries. Both qualitative and quantitative evaluations show that our approach is capable of describing long shapes and the proposed recognition algorithm achieves promising performance on the public datasets.

## 1 Introduction

Shape-based object recognition has been extensively studied [1] [2], since shape is an informative and stable cue to distinguish the target objects from background.

Lots of local shape templates [3] [4] [5] can provide an explicit, effective and efficient representation for shapes, thus they are widely utilized for localizing and delineating objects in real-scene images. Ideal shape features should be both descriptive to fit the object boundaries and discriminative to reject the non-object shapes. Therefore, the local shape templates should be deformable in case they are misaligned with the object boundaries as shown in Fig. 1 (a). However, deformable local shape templates may falsely match to the inner parts or cluttered background since they ignore shape constraints in larger regions. In Fig. 1 (a), we show three local shape templates (red fragments) and their matching results (green fragments). These local shape templates are deformable, and their matching results are in the inner or background edges according to some matching algorithm (to be discussed in Sec. 3.2). The knowledge from perceptual grouping inspires us to group the local shape templates and jointly match them

K.M. Lee et al. (Eds.): ACCV 2012, Part I, LNCS 7724, pp. 289–301, 2013.
© Springer-Verlag Berlin Heidelberg 2013

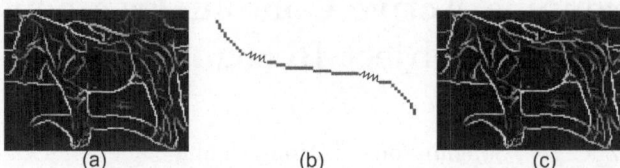

**Fig. 1.** Comparing matching results with and without chain constraint. (a) Deformable shape templates may fit to inner edges or cluttered background. (b) Bundling shape templates with spring-like connections to describe long shapes. (c) Chained shape templates match to long boundary of horse back.

to images. We believe that the matching results of neighboring shape templates should preserve the continuation property if they match to the same object, i.e., they may simultaneously match to a long and continuous contour instead of scattered ones. Intuitively, we add a spring-connection between the neighboring templates and group the shape templates into a long chain to guarantee the continuation property (see Fig. 1 (b)). The three templates may match to the long boundary of the horse back with the spring-connections as shown in Fig. 1.

Our motivation is to encode the local deformations using deformable shape templates and then group them to describe the long and continuous shape characteristics. We highlight this paper from three folds. Firstly, we propose a novel type of local shape feature, namely, Active Contour Fragment (ACF). An ACF encodes the deformation based on the Point Distribution Model (PDM), which can be learnt from weakly labelled data. Secondly, we combine different ACFs into one group, namely, Active Contour Group (ACG), to describe long and continuous shapes with an undirected chain model. We propose an efficient inference algorithm for the chain model by estimating the parameters in a linear subspace that is learnt from training data. Then, we present an incremental learning algorithm to group the ACFs into ACGs based on an efficient inference algorithm. Finally, we demonstrate the performance of ACGs for object recognition in a boosting framework. The object classifiers can not only localize the objects with bounding boxes but also delineate object boundaries.

We evaluate the proposed approach on Weizmann Horses dataset [5] and ETHZ shape dataset [6]. Experiments show that ACGs can fit to the object boundaries well. The object classifiers based on ACFs and ACGs achieve promising performance on object detection and boundary localization.

## 2    Related Works

We review the related works from the following two aspects, namely, shape representation and perceptual grouping.

Shape representation has been extensively studied recently. Some researchers represent shapes with a group of local shape templates [3] [4] [5] or descriptors [7] [8], while others represent shapes with a global shape model. One merit of local shape features is that they may be robust to the occlusions and T-junctions in the real-scenes. For many local shape templates, there are two additional merits: 1) they describe shapes explicitly with contour segments; 2) they are efficient in computation. Therefore, many researchers utilize the local shape templates

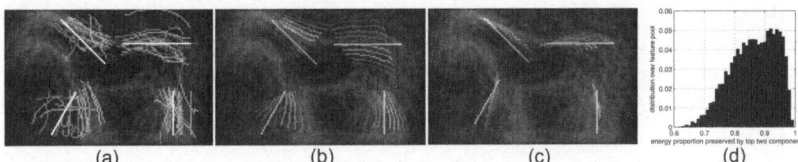

**Fig. 2.** Learnt ACFs. (a) Shape bases (white line fragments) and best matching contours (color fragments). (b) (c) First and second principal components. (d) Distribution of energy proportion preserved by top two principal components over feature pool.

for object detection, such as edgelet [4], strip [3], contour fragments [5] and boundary fragments [9]. However, the local shape features ignore the global shape constraint and susceptible to background clutter, thus many researchers propose lots of global shape models, such as hand-drawn skeleton or silhouette [10] [11], boundary structure model [12], Shape Boltzmann Machine (SBM) [13] and Point Distribution Model (PDM) [14] [1]. Our approach is different from the above local shape features and global shape models. On one side, the proposed ACGs encode the long and continuous part of shapes instead of the global shape characteristics. On the other side, the proposed ACGs encode more shape constraints than the local shape features.

Perceptual grouping is a hot topic in the area of computer vision. The basic assumption behind these works is that the contour fragments that are related by some perceptually properties should belong to the same object. The perceptual properties include continuation [15], parallelism [16], closure [17] and so on. Such properties may be the driving force for designing feature bundle [18] or learning shape model [8]. Some recent works [1] [6] group $k$ Adjacent Segments ($k$AS) to represent generic shapes. Different from $k$AS, the proposed ACGs are class-specific and thus may be more suitable for object recognition of a specific class.

## 3   Active Contour Fragments

We firstly propose to automatically learn ACFs from the weakly unsegmented training data. Then, we present the matching algorithm of ACFs.

### 3.1   Learning ACFs from Contours

For a specified object class, we label the training objects with bounding boxes and normalize them into an object window of a specific size (see Table 1). To obtain the contours of objects, we extract the edge maps using the Berkeley edge detector [19] and link the edgels (edge pixels) [20]. The $j^{th}$ object can be represented by a *contour set* as

$$\mathbf{C}_j = \{\mathbf{c}_{j,1}, \mathbf{c}_{j,2}, ..., \mathbf{c}_{j,|\mathbf{C}_j|}\}, \tag{1}$$

where $\mathbf{c}_{j,k}$ is a contour (represented by a list of edgels). As shown in Fig. 2 (a), the horse backs have simple translation variance while the horse legs have both large articulation and non-rigid deformations. Such shape characteristics can be described by the contour fragments. We propose to encode the deformation from the contour fragments. Our approach consists of two steps, i.e., grouping contour fragments and learning the deformation from the contour fragments.

To group the contour fragments, we utilize a set of shape bases $\{\mathbf{b}_i\}_{i=1,...,N}$. The shape bases are generated by uniformly sampling line segments of 12~48 pixels in the object window (see Table 1). We match each shape basis to the contour set of training images and find the best matching results according to

$$\mathbf{f}_{i,j}^* = \underset{|\mathbf{f}_{i,j}|=|\mathbf{b}_i|,\mathbf{f}_{i,j}\subseteq\mathbf{c}_{j,k},\mathbf{c}_{j,k}\in\mathbf{C}_j}{argmin} \Phi(\mathbf{b}_i,\mathbf{f}_{i,j}), \qquad (2)$$

where $\mathbf{f}_{i,j}$ is a *contour fragment* that has the same number of edgels with $\mathbf{b}_i$ on $\mathbf{c}_{j,k}$ and $\Phi(\bullet)$ represents the following distance function

$$\Phi(\mathbf{b}_i,\mathbf{f}_{i,j}) = \sum_{p=1}^{|\mathbf{b}_i|} \|\mathbf{b}_i(p) - \mathbf{f}_{i,j}(p)\|_D, \qquad (3)$$

where $\mathbf{b}_i(p)$ represents the $p^{th}$ edgel of $\mathbf{b}_i$ and we use the same notation in the following. We measure the distance $\| \bullet \|_D$ between two edgels as

$$\|\mathbf{e}_i - \mathbf{e}_j\|_D = \beta((x_i - x_j)^2 + (y_i - y_j)^2)) + (\theta_i - \theta_j)^2, \qquad (4)$$

where an edgel $\mathbf{e}_i$ is represented by its coordinates $(x_i, y_i)$ and normal orientation $\theta_i$. The factor $\beta$ is a constant that balances the importance of position and rotation. We let $\beta$ equal to $25/A$, where $A$ is the area of the object window. In Fig. 2 (a), we visualize four shape bases and the matched contours on 20 horses.

Based on the matched contour fragments, we adopt the PDM to model the shape deformation. Suppose the matched contour fragments $\mathbf{f}_{i,j}^*$ distribute in a $2|\mathbf{f}_{i,j}^*|$-dimensional space, the shape model can be obtained by Principal Component Analysis (PCA). The $i^{th}$ ACF $\psi_i$ generated by $\mathbf{b}_i$ is formulated as

$$\psi_i : \mathbf{t}_i^{\alpha_{i,1},...,\alpha_{i,K}} = \bar{\mathbf{s}}_i + \sum_{k=1}^{K}\alpha_{i,k}\mathbf{v}_{i,k}, s.t.|\alpha_{i,k}| \leq 2\sqrt{\lambda_{i,k}}, \qquad (5)$$

where $\bar{\mathbf{s}}_i$ is the averaged contour of $\{\mathbf{f}_{i,j}^*\}_{j=1,..,M}$, $\{\mathbf{v}_{i,k}, \lambda_{i,k}\}_{k=1,,K}$ are the top $K$ eigenvectors and eigenvalues returned by PCA and $\mathbf{t}_i^{\alpha_{i,1},...,\alpha_{i,K}}$ is a reasonable shape generated by the shape model. The eigenvectors encode the deformation and the eigenvalues reflect the importance of deformation. Fig. 2 (b) and (c) show the deformation described by the top two components. The white line fragments are shape bases and the blue ones are averaged contour fragments. We vary the first coordinate from $-2\sqrt{\lambda_{i,k}}$ to $2\sqrt{\lambda_{i,k}}$ , and the shape deforms from dark red to bright red then from bright green to dark green. Fig. 2 (d) shows that most of ACFs preserve more than 80% energy by the top two principal components.

### 3.2   Matching ACFs to Images

Hereby, we give the matching algorithm for ACFs. As discussed in Sec. 3.1, most of ACFs can be briefly represented by only two coordinates as in Eqn. 5. Then, the matching energy of the ACF $\psi_i$ is defined as

$$E_{\psi_i}(\mathbf{E}) = \underset{\alpha_{i,1},\alpha_{i,2}}{min} \sum_{p=1}^{|\mathbf{t}_i^{\alpha_{i,1},\alpha_{i,2}}|} \underset{\mathbf{e}_p\in\mathbf{E}}{min} \|\mathbf{t}_i^{\alpha_{i,1},\alpha_{i,2}}(p) - \mathbf{e}_p\|_D, \qquad (6)$$

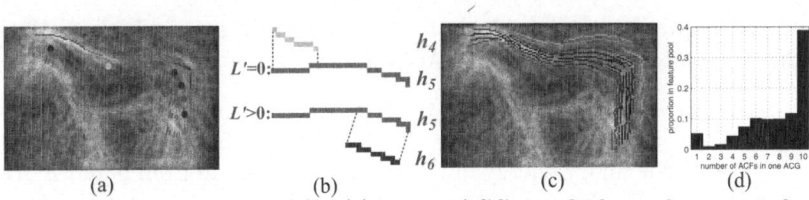

**Fig. 3.** Illustration of learnt ACGs. (a) Learnt ACG on which numbers are indexes of ACFs. (b) Pairwise energy is measured by connected segments of same length when two neighboring ACFs are of different lengths. (c) First principal component of learnt ACG. (d) Distribution of ACF numbers in each ACG over feature pool.

where $\mathbf{e}_p$ is an edgel of the edge map $\mathbf{E}$. When fixing $\alpha_{i,1}$ and $\alpha_{i,2}$, the energy can be fast calculated via look-up table based on the distance transform as discussed in [5]. To match ACFs to images, we should minimize Eqn. 6 over $\alpha_{i,1}$ and $\alpha_{i,2}$. We quantize $\alpha_{i,1}$ into $N_1 = 11$ values from $-2\sqrt{\lambda_{i,1}}$ to $2\sqrt{\lambda_{i,1}}$ and $\alpha_{i,2}$ into $N_2 = 7$ values from $-2\sqrt{\lambda_{i,2}}$ to $2\sqrt{\lambda_{i,2}}$. Once we find the best configuration $(\alpha_{i,1}^*, \alpha_{i,2}^*)$, we obtain the matching curve $\mathbf{t}^*$ according to Eqn. 5.

## 4   Active Contour Groups

We firstly model multiple ACFs with an undirected chain model to describe longer shapes. Then, we give the matching and learning algorithms for ACGs.

### 4.1   Chain Model for ACGs

We define an *Active Contour Group (ACG)* as a group of ACFs as

$$\Psi_h = \{\psi_{h_1}, \psi_{h_2}, .., \psi_{h_{|\Psi_h|}}\}, \tag{7}$$

where the $i^{th}$ element of the $h^{th}$ ACG corresponds to an ACF. In this paper, we suppose the ACFs in an ACG are organized under an undirected chain model as shown in Fig. 3 (a). Each vertex of the chain corresponds to an ACF and each edge of the chain describes the pairwise relationship of two neighboring ACFs. Formally, we define the neighborhood system of the chain model as

$$\mathbf{N} = \{(\psi_{h_i}, \psi_{h_j}) | \psi_{h_i} \in \Psi_h, \psi_{h_j} \in \Psi_h, |i - j| = 1\}, \tag{8}$$

Our objective is to use the chain model to encode long and continuous shape characteristics, thus we require the neighboring ACFs to preserve the continuation property. Two neighboring ACFs should satisfy the following two conditions

$$\begin{aligned} \|\bar{\mathbf{s}}_{h_i}(|\bar{\mathbf{s}}_{h_i}|) - \bar{\mathbf{s}}_{h_{i+1}}(1)\|_2 &\leq \Gamma, \\ \|\bar{\mathbf{s}}_{h_i}(1) - \bar{\mathbf{s}}_{h_{i+1}}(|\bar{\mathbf{s}}_{h_{i+1}}|)\|_2 &\geq \max(|\bar{\mathbf{s}}_{h_i}|^2, |\bar{\mathbf{s}}_{h_{i+1}}|^2), \end{aligned} \tag{9}$$

where $\bar{\mathbf{s}}_{h_i}$ is the average contour fragment of $\psi_{h_i}$. $\Gamma$ is a constant that is set as 4 in our experiments. Taking the two neighboring ACFs (e.g., $\psi_{h_1}$ and $\psi_{h_2}$) in Fig. 3 (a) as an example, $\psi_{h_1}$ should be connected with $\psi_{h_2}$ on one end and should not be connected with $\psi_{h_2}$ on the other end. In the learning process (see

Sec.4.2), we require that the neighboring ACFs should satisfy Eqn. 9. Hereby, we define the matching energy of an ACG as

$$E_{\Psi_h}(\mathbf{E}) = \sum_{\psi_{h_i} \in \Psi_h} E_{\psi_{h_i}}(\mathbf{E}) + \sum_{(\psi_{h_i}, \psi_{h_j}) \in \mathbf{N}} E_N(\psi_{h_i}, \psi_{h_j}), \qquad (10)$$

where $E_{\psi_{h_i}}(\bullet)$ is the unary energy of the $i^{th}$ ACF defined in Eqn. 6 and $E_N(\bullet, \bullet)$ is the pairwise energy of two neighboring ACFs, which is defined as

$$E_N(\psi_{h_i}, \psi_{h_{i+1}}) = \sum_{p=1}^{L} \|(\mathbf{t}_{h_i}^{\alpha_{h_i,1}, \alpha_{h_i,2}}(L' + p) - \bar{\mathbf{s}}_{h_i}(L' + p)))$$
$$- (\mathbf{t}_{h_{i+1}}^{\alpha_{h_{i+1},1}, \alpha_{h_{i+1},2}}(p) - \bar{\mathbf{s}}_{h_{i+1}}(p))\|_D, \qquad (11)$$

where the symbols are the same with Eqn. 5, $L = \min(|\mathbf{t}_{h_i}|, |\mathbf{t}_{h_{i+1}}|)$ and $L' = \max(|\mathbf{t}_{h_i}| - |\mathbf{t}_{h_{i+1}}|, 0)$. As shown in Fig. 3, we pick up two connected segments of the same length from $\psi_{h_i}$ and $\psi_{h_{i+1}}$ when the neighboring ACFs are of different lengths. Then, we calculate the pairwise energy by accumulating the deformation differences of the two connected segments. For a good matching result, the pairwise energy should be small since the neighboring segments should have similar deformations. As shown in Fig. 3, $h_5$ and $h_6$ match to the back of the same horse, thus they should deform to high position or low position simultaneously. Since the neighboring ACFs are connected and have similar deformations in the chain model, the deformable ACG may always preserve the continuation property.

## 4.2 Learning ACGs from ACFs

To match ACGs to images, we should minimize Eqn. 10 over a $2|\Psi_h|$-dimensional parameter space $\{\alpha_{h_1,1}, \alpha_{h_1,2}, ..., \alpha_{h_{|\Psi_h|},1}, \alpha_{h_{|\Psi_h|},2}\}$ but solving the minimization problem is computational prohibitive. For an ACG that consists of 10 ACFs, the computation complexity of the brute-force search is $O((N_1 N_2)^{10})$ if we use the same quantization criterion for $\alpha_{h_i,1}, \alpha_{h_i,2}$ as dicussed in Sec.3.2. Although there are some fast inference approaches (e.g., belief propagation [21]), the computation complexity is still too high. Hereby, we propose an efficient matching algorithm that reduces the computation complexity from $O(N_1 N_2)^{10}$ to $O(N_1 N_2)$. Then, we present an incremental learning algorithm of ACGs based on the efficient matching algorithm.

The basic idea of the proposed matching algorithm is to constrain the parameter space of Eqn. 10 using the training data. Supposing that $\Psi_h$ is an ACG that is defined in Sec. 4.1, the matching result of $\Psi_h$ on the $j^{th}$ training sample is represented as a $2|\Psi_h|$-dimensional vector

$$\Theta_{h,j}^* = \{\alpha_{h_1,1,j}^*, \alpha_{h_1,2,j}^*, \alpha_{h_2,1,j}^*, \alpha_{h_2,2,j}^*, \ldots, \alpha_{h_{|\Psi_h|},1,j}^*, \alpha_{h_{|\Psi_h|},2,j}^*\}. \qquad (12)$$

$\Theta_{h,j}^*$ can be obtained according to Eqn. 14 (to be discussed later). Once we have the matching results of training samples, we can derive a linear subspace using PCA. Then, we estimate the matching parameters of $\Psi_h$ according to

$$\Psi_h : \Theta_h^{\gamma_{h,1}, \ldots, \gamma_{h,K}} = \bar{\mathbf{d}}_h + \sum_{k=1}^{K} \gamma_{h,k} \mathbf{u}_{h,k}, s.t. |\gamma_{h,k}| \le 2\sqrt{\eta_{h,k}}, \qquad (13)$$

where $\bar{\mathbf{d}}_h$ is the averaged vector of the matching results over the training set and $\{\mathbf{u}_{h,k}, \eta_{h,k} | k = 1, ..., K\}$ are the top K eigenvectors and eigenvalues returned by

PCA. We only consider the top two principal components. To find the best $\gamma_{h,1}$ and $\gamma_{h,2}$, we quantize $\gamma_{h,1}$ into $N_1 = 11$ values from $-2\sqrt{\eta_{h,1}}$ to $2\sqrt{\eta_{h,1}}$ and $\gamma_{h,2}$ into $N_2 = 7$ values from $-2\sqrt{\eta_{h,2}}$ to $2\sqrt{\eta_{h,2}}$ as discussed in Sec. 3.2. Then, we match ACGs to the images by minimizing Eqn. 10 over $\gamma_{h,1}$ and $\gamma_{h,2}$ and the computational complexity is $O(N_1 N_2)$. After obtaining the best parameters $\gamma_{h,1}^*$ and $\gamma_{h,2}^*$, we can derive the matching curve according to Eqn. 13 and Eqn. 5.

Hereby, we give the learning algorithm based on Eqn.13 and explain how to calculate $\Theta_{h,j}^*$ in Eqn. 12. Every ACG starts from one ACF and grows into a long chain. At first, we select an ACF as the seed of the chain, which is considered as the initial ACG. Then, we find all the candidate ACFs that are neighboring with the head or the tail of the ACG according to Eqn. 9. Supposing that a candidate ACF $\psi_c$ is neighboring with the head of the ACG $\Psi_h$, we add $\psi_c$ in front of the current ACG's head. For the new ACG, the matching energy on the $j^{th}$ training sample $\mathbf{E}_j$ can be calculated incrementally according to

$$E_{\{\psi_c, \Psi_h\}}(\mathbf{E}_j) = E_{\Psi_h}(\mathbf{E}_j) + E_{\psi_c}(\mathbf{E}_j) + E_N(\psi_c, \psi_{h_1}), \tag{14}$$

We can obtain the new matching result $\{\alpha_{c,1,j}^*, \alpha_{c,2,j}^*, \Theta_{h,j}^*\}$ by minimizing Eqn. 14. To this end, we search the solution over the solution space $\{\alpha_{c,1,j}, \alpha_{c,2,j}, \Theta_{h,j}\}$. Since $\Theta_{h,j}$ can be estimated using the linear subspace according to Eqn. 13, the computation complexity of minimizing Eqn. 14 exhaustively is $O((N_1 N_2)^2)$ if we use the same quantization strategy over the solution space as discussed before. For each candidate ACF, we sum the minimized energy in Eqn. 14 over the training set and select the one with the minimum energy. Finally, we add the selected ACF as the head of the chain and update the subspace in Eqn. 13. When the candidate ACF $\psi_c$ is connected with the tail of the ACG $\Psi_h$, we can grow the ACG in a similar way. We repeat the growing process until the subspace cannot preserve minimum energy or the number of ACFs in one ACG exceeds the maximum number. We set the minimum energy as 95% of the total energy and the maximum number of ACFs as 10.

Each ACF can grow into an ACG according to the above algorithm. Fig. 3 (a) shows one learnt ACG. In Fig. 3 (c), we show the first principal component of the learnt subspace. In Fig. 3 (d), we can see that most of ACGs have more than 1 ACF. To be mentioned, it is difficult to directly learn long ACFs from images, since the T-junctions and occlusions of the edges may destroy the long shape characteristics. However, the proposed algorithm can group the short shape templates (i.e., ACF) into long shape templates(i.e., ACG).

## 5    Recognition Algorithm

We utilize ACFs or ACGs as shape features for object recognition in a boosting framework. Similar to [4] [5] [9], we match the ACFs or ACGs to images by minimizing the energy function (Eqn. 6 for ACFs and Eqn. 10 for ACGs) and use the minimum energy as feature scores. Then, we select ACFs or ACGs from feature pools into a cascaded classifier using RealBoost [22]. For acceleration, we use Histogram of Oriented Gradients (HOG) in the first 10 stages (see [23] for detials). We give an evaluation for the HOG filter in Sec. 6.2.

**Table 1.** Sizes of detection window and feature pools of ACFs and ACGs

|  | Horses | Applelogos | Bottles | Giraffes | Mugs | Swans |
|---|---|---|---|---|---|---|
| Detection window | $150 \times 100$ | $80 \times 80$ | $50 \times 120$ | $150 \times 150$ | $90 \times 70$ | $120 \times 60$ |
| Feature pool | 10315 | 6627 | 4070 | 14815 | 6137 | 7052 |

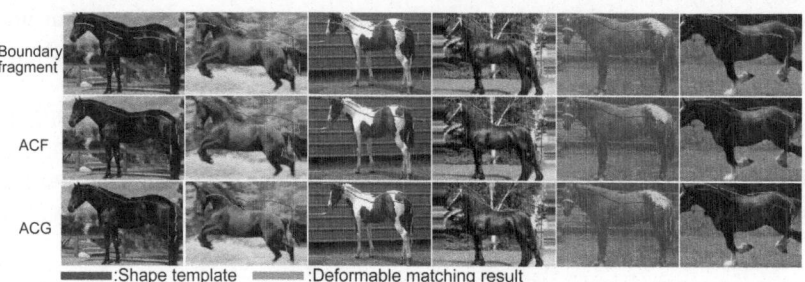

**Fig. 4.** Comparing matching curves of boundary fragments,ACFs and ACGs

The boundary localization is only conducted on the object windows. An object is identified when a detection window is classified as positive at a false positive rate of $10^{-5}$. The final boundary localization results can be obtained by averaging the results of multiple sliding windows in all the scales. To this end, we give the voting algorithm in one detected window. For each ACF (or ACG), we can obtain a matching curve after minimizing Eqn. 6 (or Eqn. 10). Each point $\mathbf{m}$ on the matching curve casts a vote for the detection window according to

$$P(b_{\mathbf{x}} = 1) = \sum_{b_{\mathbf{m}}=0,1} P(b_{\mathbf{x}} = 1|b_{\mathbf{m}})P(b_{\mathbf{m}}) \quad = \mathrm{I}(\mathbf{x} == \mathbf{m})\frac{W_{f_{\mathbf{m}}}^{+}}{W_{f_{\mathbf{m}}}^{+} + W_{f_{\mathbf{m}}}^{-}}, \quad (15)$$

where $\mathbf{x}$ represents any point in the detection window, $b_{\mathbf{x}}$ identifies whether the point $\mathbf{x}$ is a boundary ($b_{\mathbf{x}} = 1$) or not ($b_{\mathbf{x}} = 0$), $P(b_{\mathbf{x}} = 1|b_{\mathbf{m}} = 0)$ is supposed to be 0, $\mathrm{I}(\mathbf{x} == \mathbf{m})$ equals to 1 if $\mathbf{x} == \mathbf{m}$ or else equals to 0, $f_{\mathbf{m}}$ is the matching score corresponding to the matching point $\mathbf{m}$, $W_{f_{\mathbf{m}}}^{+}$ (or $W_{f_{\mathbf{m}}}^{-}$) is the proportion of positive (or negative) samples when the feature response equals to $f_{\mathbf{m}}$. $W_{f_{\mathbf{m}}}^{+}$ and $W_{f_{\mathbf{m}}}^{-}$ can be efficiently derived using look-up table since $f_{\mathbf{m}}$ is calculated in the detection process. Fig. 8 shows some boundary localization results.

## 6    Experiments

We show the effectiveness and efficiency of the proposed matching approach in this section. In Table 1, we list the sizes of detection windows and feature pools of ACFs and ACGs for each object class used in our experiments.

### 6.1   Comparing Matching Approaches on Weizmann Horses Dataset

We adopt Weizmann Horses dataset to evaluate the proposed matching approach. We use the training-testing split (100 horses for training and 456 images

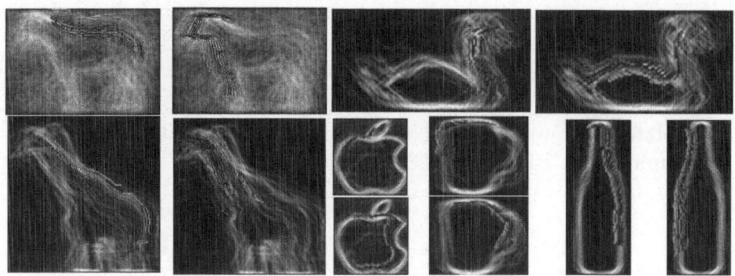

**Fig. 5.** Top two selected ACGs capture long and salient shape characteristics

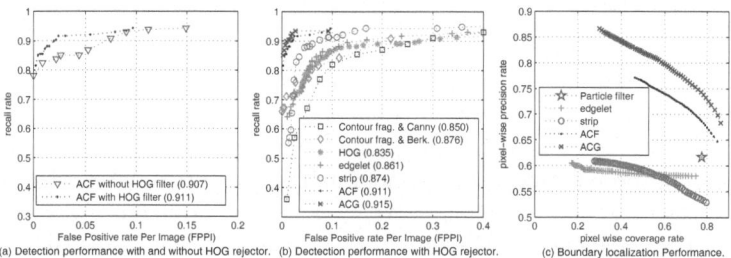

(a) Detection performance with and without HOG rejector.   (b) Dectection performance with HOG rejector.   (c) Boundary localization Performance.

**Fig. 6.** Detection and boundary localization performance on Weizmann Horses

including 228 horse images for testing) as in [5] [24].We learn ACFs and ACGs from the 100 horses and match them to the testing horses. We compare the matching results of ACFs, ACGs and boundary fragments [9]. The boundary fragments use the averaged contour fragments of ACFs as templates and match to images by translating the templates in a local region of $10 \times 10$ pixels. We omit the quantitative comparison due to space limit, but present some qualitative comparison in Fig.4. It can be seen that both ACFs and ACGs can fit to the object boundaries more accurately than the boundary fragment. Furthermore, ACGs do not only fit the object boundaries well, but also preserve the continuation of the shape. We also show the top two features that are selected by the boosting algorithm in Fig. 5. Apparently, these features capture the long and salient shapes and delineate the major shapes for each object class.

## 6.2   Recognition Results on Weizmann Horses Dataset

We evaluate our method on object detection using PASCAL IoU 50% criterion [25]. In Fig. 6 (a) (b), we plot the recall rate against False Positives Per Image (FPPI) and give the Average Precision (AP) in the legend for each approach. We give a quantitative evaluation for the 10-stage HOG filter proposed in Sec.5. We implement two cascaded classifiers using ACFs: one uses 10-stage HOG filter and the other uses only ACFs. We can see that the one with HOG filter is slightly better than the other, and the HOG filter can also accelerate the search process. Thus, we use the 10-stage HOG filer in the following experiments. We compare our approach with other shape-based approaches, namely, *contour fragment* [5],

**Table 2.** Comparing APs of different approaches on ETHZ shape dataset

| Shape classes | Applelogos | Bottles | Giraffes | Mugs | Swans |
|---|---|---|---|---|---|
| Fan shape model [2] | 0.866 | **0.975** | **0.832** | 0.843 | 0.828 |
| Many-to-one [8] | 0.845 | 0.916 | 0.787 | **0.888** | **0.922** |
| Grouping with PF [28] | 0.844 | 0.641 | 0.617 | 0.643 | 0.798 |
| OB+GB [29] | 0.675 | 0.781 | 0.585 | 0.559 | 0.661 |
| Dominant Set [18] | 0.705 | 0.761 | 0.687 | 0.625 | 0.773 |
| kAS [6] | 0.351 | 0.733 | 0.391 | 0.476 | 0.273 |
| TPS-RPM [1] | 0.689 | 0.643 | 0.333 | 0.585 | 0.390 |
| Ours (ACFs) | 0.910 | 0.847 | 0.791 | 0.853 | 0.674 |
| Ours (ACGs) | **0.920** | 0.864 | 0.782 | 0.856 | 0.653 |

*edgelet* [4] and *strip* [3]. We use 10-stage HOG filer in the cascaded classifiers with ACFs and ACGs. For contour fragment, we report two results, which are based on Canny edge (referred from [5]) and Berkeley edge (implemented by ourselves). The proposed approach uses deformable shape templates while contour fragment uses fixed shape template, which is the only difference between these two approaches. We can see the deformation algorithm improves the detection performance by $3\% \sim 4\%$. Our approach outperforms the other shape features since ACFs and ACGs are capable of learning the deformation of horses before the matching process. Recently, some approaches [24] [26] achieve even better performance than our approach. These approaches combine shape features with texture and color features, while our approach only uses shape features.

To quantitatively evaluate our method on boundary localization, we show the coverage-against-precision curves [1] averaged over correct detections when the false positive rate equals $10^{-5}$ and the curves are obtained by varying the threshold of boundary probability. In Fig. 6 (c), We compare our approach with *particle filter* [27], *edgelet* [4] and *strip* [3]. For particle filter, we refer to the reported result. For other approaches, we vote for boundary probability according to Eqn. (15). Apparently, our approach outperforms all the other approaches. Compared with ACFs, ACGs do not obviously improve the detection performance but they improve the boundary localization performance. The possible reason is that ACGs can capture long and salient shape characteristics and suppress the false matches on the background clutter.

### 6.3    Recognition Results on ETHZ Shape Dataset

We evaluate our approach in detection and boundary localization on the ETHZ shape dataset. This dataset includes 5 classes, namely, *applelogo*, *bottle, giraffe*, *mug* and *swan*. We follow the same training and testing splits suggested by [6].

For object detection, we report the results of our approach and some related methods in Table 2. For *kAS* and *TPSRPM*, we estimate the APs from [1]. Obviously, both ACFs and ACGs achieve competitive performance. For evaluating boundary localization, we compare the results of our approach with those of *TPSRPM* and *Bounding Boxes (B.B.)* reported in [1] in Fig. 7. Apparently, both

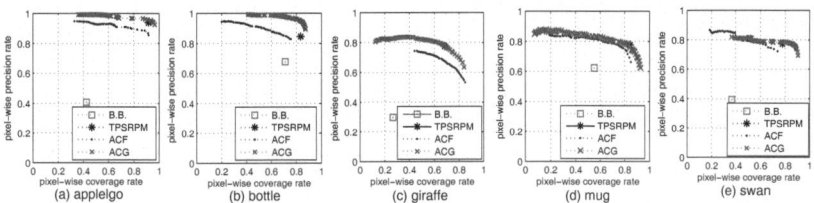

**Fig. 7.** Quantitative evaluation of boundary localization using coverage-against-precision curves on ETHZ shape dataset

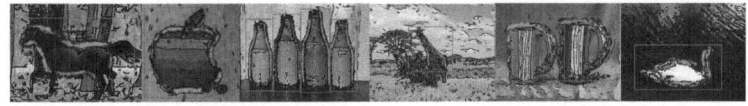

**Fig. 8.** Recognition examples. Black points are edgels while green points indicate boundary probability. Bright green means higher confidence and vice versa.

ACFs and ACGs substantially outperform the *B.B.* especially for the less rectangular objects, i.e., swans and giraffes. ACGs achieve similar or better performance comparing with *TPSRPM*. Comparing with ACFs, ACGs achieve better precision in most cases, as ACGs can suppress many false matches on the inner or background edges. Fig. 8 shows some recognition examples.

## 7 Conclusion and Future Works

This paper proposes a novel type of local shape features (i.e., ACFs) and an algorithm to group the local shape features together (i.e., ACGs) for object recognition. The proposed features encode the local deformation based on the PDM and the grouping algorithm combines multiple local shape features to describe long and continuous shapes. We assemble ACFs and ACGs under the boosting framework for localizing objects as well as delineating object boundaries. Qualitative and quantitative experiments show that the proposed approach is effective and efficient for object detection and boundary localization. Furthermore, the proposed approach does not require segmented data in the training process.

The ACGs are still not global shape features although they can describe long and continuous shape characteristics. We will consider some other perceptual properties (e.g., closure and symmetry) in the grouping process to make ACGs more global and further improve the performance of object recognition. Furthermore, ACGs might be promising for foreground segmentation based on the shape information. We will pursue this possibility in the future.

**Acknowledgement.** This work is partially supported by Natural Science Foundation of China (NSFC) under contract Nos. 61025010, 60832004, and 61001193; and Beijing Natural Science Foundation (New Technologies and Methods in Intelligent Video Surveillance for Public Security) under contract No. 4111003.

# References

1. Ferrari, V., Jurie, F., Schmid, C.: From images to shape models for object detection. International Journal of Computer Vision 87, 284–303 (2010)
2. Wang, X., Bai, X., Ma, T., Liu, W., Latecki, L.: Fan shape model for object detection. In: CVPR (2012)
3. Zheng, W., Liang, L.: Fast car detection using image strip features. In: CVPR (2009)
4. Wu, B., Nevatia, R.: Detection and tracking of multiple, partially occluded humans by bayesian combination of edgelet based part detectors. International Journal of Computer Vision 75, 247–266 (2007)
5. Shotton, J., Blake, A., Cipolla, R.: Multiscale categorical object recognition using contour fragments. IEEE Transactions on Pattern Analysis and Machine Intelligence 30, 1270–1281 (2008)
6. Ferrari, V., Fevrier, L., Jurie, F., Schmid, C.: Groups of adjacent contour segments for object detection. IEEE Transactions on Pattern Analysis and Machine Intelligence 30, 36–51 (2008)
7. Belongie, S., Malik, J., Puzicha, J.: Shape matching and object recognition using shape contexts. IEEE Transactions on Pattern Analysis and Machine Intelligence 24, 509–522 (2002)
8. Srinivasan, P., Zhu, Q., Shi, J.: Many-to-one contour matching for describing and discriminating object shape. In: CVPR (2010)
9. Opelt, A., Pinz, A., Zisserman, A.: A Boundary-Fragment-Model for Object Detection. In: Leonardis, A., Bischof, H., Pinz, A. (eds.) ECCV 2006, Part II. LNCS, vol. 3952, pp. 575–588. Springer, Heidelberg (2006)
10. Bai, X., Wang, X., Latecki, L., Liu, W., Tu, Z.: Active skeleton for non-rigid object detection. In: ICCV (2009)
11. Ferrari, V., Tuytelaars, T., Van Gool, L.: Object Detection by Contour Segment Networks. In: Leonardis, A., Bischof, H., Pinz, A. (eds.) ECCV 2006, Part III. LNCS, vol. 3953, pp. 14–28. Springer, Heidelberg (2006)
12. Toshev, A., Taskar, B., Daniilidis, K.: Object detection via boundary structure segmentation. In: CVPR (2010)
13. Eslami, S., Heess, N., Unit, G., Winn, J.: The shape boltzmann machine: a strong model of object shape. In: CVPR (2012)
14. Cootes, T., Taylor, C., Cooper, D., Graham, J., et al.: Active shape models-their training and application. Computer Vision and Image Understanding 61, 38–59 (1995)
15. Rothwell, C., Zisserman, A., Forsyth, D., Mundy, J.: Planar object recognition using projective shape representation. International Journal of Computer Vision 16, 57–99 (1995)
16. Lowe, D.: Three-dimensional object recognition from single two-dimensional images. Artificial Intelligence 31, 355–395 (1987)
17. Ming, Y., Li, H., He, X.: Connected contours: a new contour completion model that respects the closure effect. In: CVPR (2012)
18. Yang, X., Liu, H., Latecki, L.J.: Contour-based object detection as dominant set computation. In: ACCV (2010)
19. Martin, D., Fowlkes, C., Malik, J.: Learning to detect natural image boundaries using local brightness, color, and texture cues. IEEE Transactions on Pattern Analysis and Machine Intelligence 26, 530–549 (2004)

20. Suzuki, S., et al.: Topological structural analysis of digitized binary images by border following. Computer Vision, Graphics and Image Processing 30, 32–46 (1985)
21. Pearl, J.: Probabilistic reasoning in intelligent systems: networks of plausible inference. Morgan Kaufmann (1988)
22. Schapire, R., Singer, Y.: Improved boosting algorithms using confidence-rated predictions. Machine Learning 37, 297–336 (1999)
23. Zhu, Q., Yeh, M., Cheng, K., Avidan, S.: Fast human detection using a cascade of histograms of oriented gradients. In: CVPR (2006)
24. Gall, J., Yao, A., Razavi, N., Van Gool, L., Lempitsky, V.: Hough forests for object detection, tracking, and action recognition. IEEE Trans. Pattern Anal. Mach. Intell. 33, 2188–2202 (2011)
25. Everingham, M., Zisserman, A., Williams, C., Van Gool, L.: The pascal visual object classes challenge 2006 (voc 2006) results (2006)
26. Shotton, J., Blake, A., Cipolla, R.: Efficiently combining contour and texture cues for object recognition. In: BMVC (2008)
27. Yang, X., Latecki, L.J.: Weakly Supervised Shape Based Object Detection with Particle Filter. In: Daniilidis, K., Maragos, P., Paragios, N. (eds.) ECCV 2010, Part V. LNCS, vol. 6315, pp. 757–770. Springer, Heidelberg (2010)
28. Lu, C., Latecki, L., Adluru, N., Yang, X., Ling, H.: Shape guided contour grouping with particle filters. In: ICCV (2009)
29. Schlecht, J., Ommer, B.: Contour-based object detection. In: BMVC (2010)

# Detecting Partially Occluded Objects with an Implicit Shape Model Random Field

Paul Wohlhart, Michael Donoser, Peter M. Roth, and Horst Bischof

Graz University of Technology, Institute for Computer Graphics and Vision
{wohlhart,donoser,pmroth,bischof}@icg.tugraz.at

**Abstract.** In this paper, we introduce a formulation for the task of detecting objects based on the information gathered from a standard Implicit Shape Model (ISM). We describe a probabilistic approach in a general random field setting, which enables to effectively detect object instances and additionally identifies all local patches contributing to the different instances. We propose a sparse graph structure and define a semantic label space, specifically tuned to the task of localizing objects. The design of the graph structure then allows to define a novel inference process that efficiently returns a good local minimum of our energy minimization problem. A key benefit of our method is, that we do not have to fix a range for local neighborhood suppression, as necessary for instance in related non maximum suppression approaches. Our inference process implicitly is capable to separate even strongly overlapping object instances. Experimental evaluation compares our method to state-of-the-art in this field on challenging sequences showing competitive and improved results.

## 1   Introduction

Localizing instances of arbitrary categories in cluttered scenes is one of the main challenges in computer vision. In general, most methods learn appearance and spatial relation models of the categories from labeled training images and use the obtained models to localize previously unseen instances in test images.

Currently, mainly two different approaches can be distinguished: (a) sliding window based and (b) part based methods. Sliding window based methods like [1,2] evaluate powerful classifiers on windows at all possible image locations, analyzing discriminative local descriptors like the histogram-of-gradients [3]. Although, these approaches have shown to provide excellent results for rectangular shaped categories, they yield limited performance for deformable objects. Thus, recently part based models have become more popular. The notion of parts has a long history in computer vision, starting from the Pictorial Structures model [4], where each object is represented as an assembly of local parts and flexible spatial relations between them. While early work in this field manually identified semantically meaningful parts, recent research [5,6] focused on how to automatically select discriminative parts from training data.

Part-based models mainly differ in the way the spatial relations between the individual parts are defined, ranging from fully connected models, where each

K.M. Lee et al. (Eds.): ACCV 2012, Part I, LNCS 7724, pp. 302–315, 2013.
© Springer-Verlag Berlin Heidelberg 2013

part is connected to all other parts (constellation model [7]), to models without any spatial relation (bag-of-words model [8]). Thus, they mainly differ concerning their inference complexity, where a constellation model for example is only able to handle a few parts and additionally has to significantly reduce the number of part candidates in each test image.

Recently, tree models have become the most popular spatial model for part-based recognition due to the highly efficient inference possibilities for tree structures. Such tree models for example have led to the deformable part model [6], one of the most successful algorithms on the PASCAL Visual Object Class (VOC) challenge.

One of the first tree-shaped models for the task of object detection focussed on a specific sub-type, the star shaped model, where each part is only connected to a centroid part. The underlying representation was denoted as the *Implicit Shape Model* (ISM) [9], which constituted the basis for several extensions in the following years [10]. The ISM represents objects as a collection of a potentially large number of prototype patches, that in general exhibit a much denser coverage of the object area.

The ISM requires bounding box annotated training data to learn the model. The first step is to build a visual codebook, representing prototypical patch appearances. For each visual word the likelihood of having an object of the target class at the corresponding location is estimated by counting how often it is found on the object versus in the background. Additionally, for each occurrence on a positive training sample, the relative location of the object's centroid is stored. This information defines the spatial and the appearance model and is used to localize instances in previously unseen test images. During testing all local features are assigned to the most similar visual word. All object features vote for the object centroid locations and these votes, weighted by their foreground probability, are finally analyzed for providing detection hypotheses.

Despite the simplicity of this approach, the ISM has become one of the most popular object detection approaches due to some important properties. First, it has shown to yield excellent performance, mainly explained by the fact that a large number of local features contribute to each hypothesis. Second, it implicitly handles occlusions using a highly local and part based approach. Third, it has the possibility to combine parts from the whole range of positive training images and thus enables detection of object instance configurations never seen during training. Finally, inference is quite efficient since all features independently vote for the centroid. Variants of the ISM mainly differ in the way the visual vocabulary is built and how a local feature in an image is assigned to a visual word.

The final step of an ISM is to infer object location hypotheses from the provided centroid voting information. In this field mainly two dominant approaches emerged. The first approach, as proposed in [9], is based on applying mean shift over the voting space to estimate the probability density for the correct object location. Afterwards, a Minimum Description Length (MDL) criterion is analyzed aiming at resolving ambiguities between neighboring hypotheses. The second approach is to accumulate the weighted centroid votes in a Hough voting manner (Generalized Hough Voting), where afterwards local maxima are identified by some type of non-maximum suppression, that discards the less confident of every sufficiently overlapping detection pair [5]. Although this summing of probabilities does not have a sound probabilistic interpretation, this simple accumulation process works quite well in practice.

All these methods have in common that they iteratively detect instances and they cannot enforce that patches are only assigned to a single object. Thus they all show quite limited performance if objects-to-be-detected are significantly overlapping. This was also pointed out in [11], where a probabilistic formulation of the object detection task based on the generalized Hough transformation was presented. This approach can be seen as a principled non-maximum suppression procedure, where the theoretical foundations for an improved analysis of the generalized Hough space were introduced. The algorithm has shown to especially improve results if detections overlap, as it frequently happens, *e.g.*, in human detection tasks.

In this work, we propose a novel random field based probabilistic formulation of the object detection task, based on the aforementioned ISM concept. Our method is most closely related to the work presented in [11], but, in contrast, we introduce a novel graph structure and adapt the semantics of the considered labels. This allows us to formulate our problem as a Markovian random field (MRF), which is one of the most popular models for structured inference. Considering object detection as application, we are able to define a novel semantic label space and a quite sparse graph structure. This structure enables a novel, efficient inference algorithm to search for a strong, local minimum of the random field energy function. In such a way, we find a common, global solution, where patches can be reassigned during the inference process. The final result of our method is a set of detection hypotheses, and for each detection the corresponding local patches that have voted for it. The proposed approach has several important properties: (a) we provide a joint, global solution for all object locations and individual pixel assignments, (b) we do not have to fix a range for local neighborhood suppression, (c) we maintain the results of standard NMS approaches in non-overlapping cases, while (d) implicitly separating even strongly overlapping object instances yielding (e) significantly improved detection scores.

## 2   A Random Field for Object Detection

The goal of this work is to provide a framework for object detection based on an Implicit Shape Model (ISM). Thus, as starting point, we assume that we are given a codebook consisting of several visual words, and that we can assign local features of a test image (*e.g.*, a dense set of patches) to the individual visual words. Additionally, each visual word stores a set of training samples (patches) that were assigned to it. These patches carry a label indicating if they appeared somewhere in the background (negative training set) or somewhere on a positive training sample (positive training set). Those from positive training samples additionally

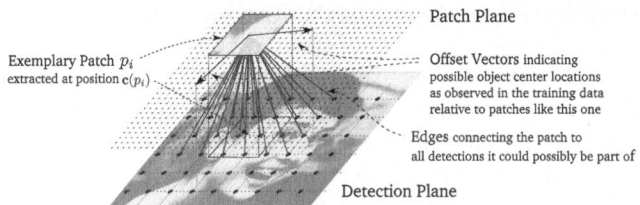

**Fig. 1.** Constructing a random field for object detection: The graph consists of a set of nodes positioned at patches extracted at each pixel in the image (the patch plane) and a coarser grid of nodes defining possible locations of detection centroids (detection plane). Each patch node is connected to the detection nodes it could be part of, where offset vectors stored in the implicit shape model define the connections' likelihood. Our novel inference process jointly solves the problems of detecting all objects and uniquely assigning contributing patch nodes to them.

store a relative offset vector to the corresponding object centroid. Given this information, our Implicit Shape Model is able to provide pixel-wise probabilities $p(y|x_i)$ for having a part of an object of category $y$ at location $i$ and a list of relative offset vectors to the object centroid.

The overall goal of our method is to fuse the provided information of the ISM in a probabilistically meaningful way, which jointly decides where in a test image instances of the learned category are depicted and which local features are part of the individual detections. Our method is based on a random field formulation. We first introduce the underlying graph structure in Sec. 2.1. An important part is our novel definition of a semantic label space tuned to the specific task of localizing objects based on an ISM, which is described in Sec. 2.2. Finally, we define our random field energy minimization problem in Sec. 2.3.

### 2.1 Two-Layer Graph Structure

The core idea of this work is to take the probabilistic formulation of [11], and reformulate it to better fit the special case of object detection with Implicit Shape Models. One of the key insights of [11] was the following: an element in the ISM can vote for multiple objects at different positions in the image, because it was seen in training images on different locations relative to the object centroid. In one particular input image, however, each of the pixels is only part of exactly one object. Thus, when solving the detection task we ultimately have to decide for each patch to which detection it belongs (or implicitly do so). Contrary to the generic formulation in [11], we make use of the fact that in an ISM an element cannot vote for every detection hypothesis, but only for those that are reachable with an offset vector. The offset vectors define a fixed set of detection nodes a patch can interact with, relative to its position.

We thus define a two-layer graph structure, as illustrated in Fig. 1. The Graph $\mathcal{G} = (\mathcal{V}, \mathcal{E})$ is defined by a set of nodes $\mathcal{V}$ and edges $\mathcal{E}$ connecting the nodes. The set of nodes $\mathcal{V}$ consists of patch nodes $\mathcal{P}$ at an image layer and detection nodes

$\mathcal{D}$ at a detection layer (*i.e.*, $\mathcal{V} = \mathcal{P} \cup \mathcal{D}$). The patch nodes $\mathcal{P} = \{p_0, \ldots, p_{wh}\}$ form a grid spanning the whole input image, with one node per extracted, local feature for the ISM. In our case, this is the dense grid of pixels of the input image, *i.e.*, $w, h$ are width and height of the image. The set of detection nodes $\mathcal{D} = \{d_0, \ldots, d_{uv}\}$ defines a coarser grid of size $u \times v$, where each $d_j$ specifies the center of a potential object detection.

Each patch node $p_i$ is connected by an edge $e_{p_i, d_j} \in \mathcal{E}$ to every node $d_j$ that defines a detection that $p_i$ could potentially be part of. This means, if the pixel coordinates of patch $p_i$, which we will denote as $\mathbf{c}(p_i)$, lie within a hypothetical detection bounding box centered at $\mathbf{c}(d_j)$, then there is an edge $e_{p_i, d_j}$ connecting them. This is illustrated in Fig. 1 for one exemplary patch node.

Note that in this graph there are no connections between detection nodes. We initially intended to add such relations to implement local neighborhood suppression, but found that this is unnecessary in our framework. Since patch nodes are not allowed to contribute to more than one detection in the inference process, stronger detections pull away evidence from nearby detections automatically. Thus, our method does not require to fix a range for local neighborhood suppression as necessary in non maximum suppression methods, but implicitly is capable to separate even strongly overlapping object instances.

Using the graph $\mathcal{G}$, we define the random field, by associating a random variable with each node (which we also denote as $p_i$ and $d_j$ for simpler notation). Each random variable can be assigned one of the labels of the label set $\mathcal{L} = \{l_{\mathrm{bg}}, l_{\mathrm{fg}}, l_0, \ldots, l_n\}$. We will denote the label currently assigned to node $v$ as $l_v$ and the set of assignments to all patch and detection nodes as $l_{\mathbf{p}}$ and $l_{\mathbf{d}}$ respectively.

## 2.2   Defining the Label Set

The semantics of assigning one of the labels to a node, which is the essential characteristic of our formulation, is defined in the following way. Assigning the background label $l_{\mathrm{bg}}$ to a detection node (*i.e.*, $d_j = l_{\mathrm{bg}}$) means that there is no detection at this position. Likewise, a configuration having $d_j = l_{\mathrm{fg}}$ specifies that there is an object centered at $\mathbf{c}(d_j)$. For a patch node $p_i = l_{\mathrm{bg}}$ signifies that at the center of the patch $\mathbf{c}(p_i)$ there is no object, but background. This does not imply that none of the detection nodes connected to $p_i$ can be set to $l_{\mathrm{fg}}$, since the bounding box of a detection might well contain some background pixels.

The crucial point of our framework is the meaning of the labels $l_0, \ldots, l_n$. Assigning one of these labels to a patch node indicates that this patch is part of a detection centered on a specific detection node, specified as follows. As shown in Fig. 2, the detection node with the closest pixel coordinates to the patch (printed in dark blue) defines the origin of a coordinate system of relative offsets in the detection grid. From the training data, we can determine the maximal range of the offset vectors, stored with the codebook entries. This range defines a fixed rectangular area of detection nodes that a patch could potentially vote for with its offset vectors. Within this area we reserve a separate label for each detection node. Assigning this label to the patch means that it is part of the corresponding

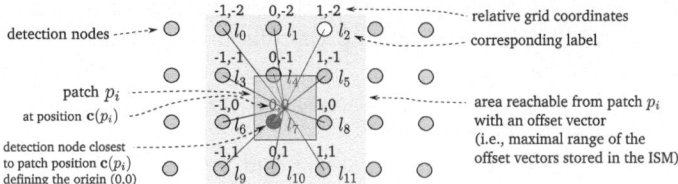

**Fig. 2.** A patch $p_i$ centered at pixel $\mathbf{c}(p_i)$ is connected to all detections it could potentially be part of. The relative position on the grid defines the semantics of the labels for this patch. *E.g.*, assigning label $l_2$ to the patch would mean that it is part of (votes for) a detection centered at the detection node (white) at position $(1,-2)$ relative to its closest detection node (dark blue).

detection. For an example, see Fig. 2. Note that the set of labels is the same for all patch nodes. However, the semantic meaning of label assignments is spatially varying, since the label implicitly defines an assignment to different object hypotheses depending on the location of the patch. For notational convenience, we will denote the label that specifies that the patch at $p_i$ is part of the object centered on detection node $d_j$ as $\hat{l}_{i,j}$.

## 2.3  Energy Function

Given an input image $I$ and the graph structure as defined in Section 2.1, the probability of an assignment of labels to all nodes, *i.e.*, a total configuration of the random field, can be written as

$$p(l_{\mathbf{p}}, l_{\mathbf{d}}|I) = \prod_{p_i \in \mathcal{P}} p(l_{p_i}|I) \prod_{d_j \in \mathcal{D}} p(l_{d_j}|I) \prod_{e_{p_i,d_j} \in \mathcal{E}} p(l_{p_i}, l_{d_j}|I). \tag{1}$$

Taking the log of Eq. (1) leads to the formulation of the energy function to be minimized:

$$E(l_{\mathbf{p}}, l_{\mathbf{d}}) = \sum_{p_i \in \mathcal{P}} \psi_{p_i}(l_{p_i}) + \sum_{d_j \in \mathcal{D}} \psi_{d_j}(l_{d_j}) + \sum_{e_{p_i,d_j}} \psi_{i,j}(l_{p_i}, l_{d_j}), \tag{2}$$

where $\psi_{p_i}(l_{p_i}) = -\log(p(l_{p_i}|I))$ is the unary cost of assigning the label $l_{p_i}$ to node $p_i$, $\psi_{d_j}(l_{d_j})$ is the equivalent for detection node $d_j$ and $\psi_{i,j}(l_{p_i}, l_{d_j})$ is the resulting pairwise cost. With these definitions, finding the objects in the image amounts to finding the assignment of labels to all nodes that minimizes Eq. (2).

*Definition of Unary Potentials.* Starting with the first term in Eq. (1), $p(l_{p_i}|I)$ represents the probability of assigning the label $l_{p_i}$ to node $p_i$, given the image data. Let $x_i$ be the appearance of the local feature extracted around $\mathbf{c}(p_i)$. By making the same independence assumption as in [11], namely that the probability of a label on a patch only depends on its appearance $x_i$, we can define the posterior probability of the labeling of a patch node by $p(l_{p_i}|I) = p(l_{p_i}|x_i)$. This probability can be derived from the statistics collected in the ISM as follows.

In order to get an estimate of how likely a detection at a certain position is, given one patch, we have to sum up the offset vectors that point from the patch to that detection. Since, as in [5], we want to allow the patch to move slightly around its original offset position, all voting vectors are aggregated by a Gaussian centered at the detection.

This summing up of evidence for an object center around a detection node also has a different interpretation. In order to achieve the tolerance for small shifts of the patch, we could also resample the training set and insert additional offset vectors pointing to positions around the original centroid location, giving the same effect as the smoothing with a Gaussian. Unfortunately, this smoothing or resampling introduces additional virtual samples that change the ratio of positive to negative samples in the ISM statistics. Thus, it is not possible to directly take the summed up voting weights at each detection node as probabilities for the labels. Correcting for this bias would be a tedious task since the amount of virtually introduced samples depends on the density of the detection grid and the distribution of offset vectors. Additionally, the statistics stored with the codebook are not completely reliable, as for instance an entry with no single negative training patch would indicate zero probability for a patch with this appearance to appear somewhere in the background. This almost certainly does not reflect truth but is an artifact of insufficient training data.

Barinova $et\ al.$ [11] bypass these problems, by setting the probability for assigning background to a patch node to a constant chosen on a validation set. We take a different approach, trying to make more use of the inexact but nonetheless valuable information stored with the codebook entries. We take the probability of being foreground ($pfg_{p_i}$) estimated from the original ratio of training samples stored in the ISM and estimate $p(p_i = l_{\text{bg}}|x_i)$ by taking it as input to the shifted sigmoidal function:

$$p(p_i = l_{\text{bg}}|x_i) = 1 - \frac{pfg_{\max}}{1 + \exp(-\alpha(pfg_{p_i} - \beta))}. \tag{3}$$

All parameters of this function can be estimated once on a validation set and are kept fixed at $pfg_{\max} = 0.95, \alpha = 10, \beta = 0.4$. This procedure of limiting the foreground probability to a maximum value of $pfg_{\max}$ can also be seen as combining the estimated distribution with a uniform Dirichlet prior. The probabilities for the labels $l_0, \ldots, l_n$ are then defined by taking the evidence gathered above for each detection node and scaling it such that the maximum reaches $1 - p(p_i = l_{\text{bg}}|x_i)$.

The second term of Eq. (1), $p(l_{d_j}|I)$, encodes the probability for a label on a detection node. This can be used to express a prior probability for a detection. However, in practice we do not make assumptions about the distribution or frequency of detections and thus set $p(d_j = l_{\text{bg}}) = p(d_j = l_{\text{fg}}) = 0.5$. Detection nodes can thus be seen as auxiliary variables, collecting the information of its connected patch nodes via the pairwise relations. All other labels $l_0, \ldots, l_n$ are invalid for detection nodes, so their probability is set to 0.

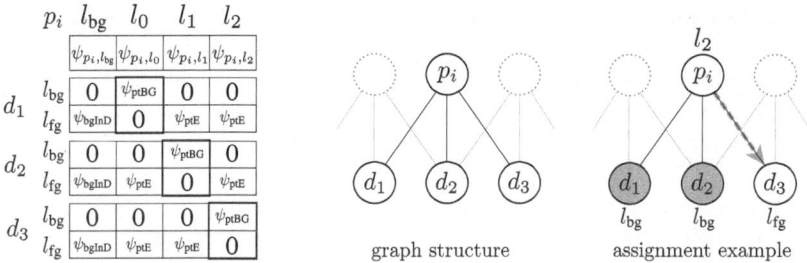

**Fig. 3.** A simple 2D example: each patch node connects to three detection nodes. The table on the left shows all unary (first row) and binary costs for all possible labeling combinations for one patch node $p_i$ and its associated detection nodes. Example shown on the right: Let $p_i = l_2$ (*i.e.*, patch $p_i$ votes for detection $d_3$) and the detection nodes are set to $d_1 = l_{bg}, d_2 = l_{bg}, d_3 = l_{fg}$; the total cost of the configuration is $\psi_{p_i}(l_2) + \psi_{i,1}(l_2, l_{bg}) + \psi_{i,2}(l_2, l_{bg}) + \psi_{i,3}(l_2, l_{fg}) = \psi_{p_i, l_2} + 0 + 0 + 0$.

*Definition of Pairwise Potentials.* The pairwise costs $\psi_{i,j}(l_{p_i}, l_{d_j})$ reflect the semantics of the labels for the relationship between patch nodes and detection nodes. Fig. 3 shows a simple example with one exemplary patch node connected to three detection nodes. The tables on the left list the costs for all different kinds of label configurations for one patch and its neighboring detection nodes. The first row contains the unary cost for assigning each label to the patch node $\psi_{p_i}(l_{p_i})$, as defined above. The three separate tables below show the pairwise costs for combinations of label assignments to the patch and each detection node. Each has one row for the costs of assigning $l_{bg}$ and $l_{fg}$ to the detection node respectively. The blue frames mark the column with the costs for assigning label $\hat{l}_{i,j}$ to the patch, which means that the patch $p_i$ is part of the corresponding detection $d_j$.

If detection and patch are both assigned to background, this is a valid combination and the cost is 0. The same is true if a detection $d_j = l_{bg}$ and the patch is set to anything else but $\hat{l}_{i,j}$, or $d_j = l_{fg}$ and $p_i = \hat{l}_{i,j}$ (*i.e.*, the detection is switched on and the patch is part of it). A patch being part of a detection at an inactive detection node (*i.e.*, $p_i = \hat{l}_{i,j} \wedge d_j = l_{bg}$) is an invalid configuration resulting in a cost of $\psi_{ptBG}$, which we can set to $\infty$ (or in practical implementations to a very high cost). Conversely, a patch assigned to background $p_i = l_{bg}$, in the range of an active detection $d_j = l_{fg}$, adds a fixed cost $\psi_{bgInDet}$, derived from the probability that a pixel inside a detection rectangle might be background, which can be estimated from the training data. This expresses the fact that objects in the training and test data do not completely fill the bounding box they are annotated with. This parameter also controls how much of an object must be visible (not occluded) for a valid detection. Finally, from the point of view of the detection, there is no difference if the patch is assigned to background or to any other detection close by, so $\psi_{ptE} = \psi_{bgInDet}$.

## 3   Inference

Since our defined pairwise costs fulfill the conditions of *regularity* [12], we could, *e.g.*, apply standard graphcut-based inference methods such as alpha expansion or alpha/beta swap [13] to solve the labeling problem. However, generic solving algorithms fail for our particular graph structure and definition of potentials. The main problem is that trying to change a single node, or even all nodes, to exactly one new label can almost never result in a lower energy.

For example, as can be seen from Fig. 3, if all nodes are assigned the background label $l_{\mathrm{bg}}$, switching a patch node to any different label will result in adding the very high cost $\psi_{\mathrm{ptBG}}$ at one binary relation. Switching a single detection node to $l_{\mathrm{fg}}$ will not change the unary cost for this node but increase the total energy of each pairwise edge that connects this detection node to any patch node by the cost $\psi_{\mathrm{bgInDet}}$. Thus, setting every node to $l_{\mathrm{bg}}$ results in a strong local minimum of the energy and thus, inference approaches like alpha-expansion that only consider changing nodes to a single, new label per iteration, immediately fail.

For this reason, we propose an inference approach tuned to our specific graph structure and label semantics. The core idea is a novel move making strategy, which is described in detail in Section 3.1. The corresponding inference process is outlined in Section 3.2, while Section 3.3 discusses the overall characteristics of our inference approach.

### 3.1   Moves

We propose to use a different kind of move, specialized for our problem setup, that changes the labels of several nodes simultaneously. The central observation, that was also already pointed out in [11], is that given a labeling of the detection nodes, the optimal label for each patch can be determined independently, since the graph is bipartite. Careful inspection of our setup reveals that we can efficiently compute the new optimal assignment for each patch node when a single detection node changes its label in $O(1)$, if we know the previously optimal assignment and cost. This allows us to construct an efficient inference algorithm that is described in the following paragraphs.

The prerequisite of a starting point with known optimal assignments of the patch nodes and total costs is easily fulfilled by setting all detection nodes to $l_{\mathrm{bg}}$. The optimal label for each patch is then also $l_{\mathrm{bg}}$, because any other label would add $\psi_{\mathrm{ptBG}}$ to the total cost. The total energy of this configuration amounts to the sum of unary costs for $l_{\mathrm{bg}}$ of all detection and patch nodes (all pairwise costs are 0). The sum of costs for each label at each patch node, that we will need later in the process, is its unary cost plus, for each label other than $l_{\mathrm{bg}}$, one binary cost of $\psi_{\mathrm{ptBG}}$.

Then, we consecutively turn on one detection $d_j$ after the other, and find the optimal configuration of patch node labels for the new situation, to discover which one lowers the total energy most. To compute the total energy of a new configuration we need to keep track of the change of energy $\Delta E$ for each node that changes its label during the process, and affected edges. The change in unary cost for the detection node is $-\psi_{d_j}(l_{\mathrm{bg}}) + \psi_{d_j}(l_{\mathrm{fg}})$. Since none of the connected patch nodes can have pointed to $d_j$ before (since it was background), all pairwise relations switch from 0 cost to $\psi_{\mathrm{bgInDet}}$ or $\psi_{\mathrm{ptE}}$ (which are equal).

Now we have to check for each patch node $p_i$ connected to the currently tested detection node $d_j$, for the new best label. The optimal label for a patch node depends on the patch's unary cost for the label, plus the pairwise to all detection nodes it is connected to. To find the label with lowest energy in a brute force manner, we would have to go over all labels and for each of them sum up the binary costs of all the edges of the patch. Despite our sparse graph structure in which a patch is not connected to all detection nodes, this would require $O(|L|^2)$. But, in fact, for every label the only change in energy is in the pairwise connection between the patch and the changed detection $d_j$, so we can update them incrementally. Additionally, we do not even have to go over all labels to find the new best, since we know that the label currently assigned to $p_i$ was the best one before the current move and looking at Fig. 3 we see that only switching to $\hat{l}_{i,j}$ can possibly result in a decrease of the energy. So the only possibility we have to check is, if the total cost of the patch's old label is now bigger than the cost for $\hat{l}_{i,j}$. We keep track of the total change of costs for the better of those two possibilities. This is an $O(1)$ operation for each patch.

### 3.2 Overall Inference Process

Thus, in total, calculating the change in energy for switching on a single detection hypothesis and finding the optimal configuration of patch labels is a fast operation. Therefore, we can afford to test every single detection hypothesis and take the best one, without having to rely on a heuristic to propose potentially good hypotheses. After the new best detection hypothesis is found, we switch the corresponding detection node $d_j$ to $l_{\mathrm{fg}}$ and each patch node, for which this results in a better energy, to $\hat{l}_{i,j}$, to associate it with the new detection, and update the costs for each label. This is only done once per newly found detection and only for the patches connected to the new detection. The whole process is repeated until no move lowers the total energy.

### 3.3 Discussion

Note that the decision of finally taking the most probable detection in each iteration is greedy. However, the greedy decision is based on the evaluation of every single possible move that switches on one detection node and finds the new optimal configuration of all patch nodes. Even after the move is taken, the patch nodes that were switched to the new detection in this iteration, are not fixed to this decision, but can switch to a different detection found later, if this again decreases the total energy.

Additionally, the order of configurations checked by the algorithm assures fast convergence to a good minimum of the energy by making use of domain knowledge. For instance, in a generic solver it would be hard to exploit the fact that switching on lots of detection nodes at once is very unlikely to give a low energy, or encode the knowledge which set of labels to apply to the corresponding patch nodes.

As a final remark we would like to point out that after the first iteration not all possible remaining hypotheses have to be checked again to find the next best detection. The total benefit (reduction of cost) for each hypothesis can only become smaller with the new detection from the last iteration now switched on and adding pairwise costs to every patch node not pointing towards it. Thus, we do not have to check those hypotheses that already did not have a negative $\Delta E$ in the last run. Since even for a crowded scene the number of objects is way lower than the number of detection nodes, this again dramatically reduces the search space.

## 4    Experiments

To create the codebook for the ISM, we use Random Forests, trained as proposed in [5]. The smoothing kernel's sigma is set to $\sigma = 3.0$ to allow for small shifts of the patches, with respect to the object center. Derived from this, we set the resolution of the detection grid to $8 \times 8$. A coarser grid would miss detections, because the patches can only vote for detection sites within the range of the Gaussian. A denser grid would linearly increase computation time with the number of detection nodes. The only parameter left to set is $\psi_{\mathrm{bgInDet}}$. Basically, it defines how much of an object must be visible in order to create a positive detection. Since we want to detect highly overlapping instances, we set it quite low, to a value of 0.4. Conversely this implies a high probability of about $e^{-0.4} \approx 67\%$ of a patch to be background within a valid detection.

To get multi-scale detection results, we first process each scale individually, but afterwards, according to our localization principle, ensure that also over scales each patch only votes for a single detection. From the final configurations of the random fields per scale, we obtain all detections and the corresponding set of patches assigned to them, which defines a pixel-wise voting mask per detection (see Fig. 5). We collect these masks over all scales and resize them to a reference frame. Then we sort all detections by their confidences and, starting with the most confident, accept only detections that do not overlap (considering the voting masks) with those already taken. Thus, we again ensure that also over scales each patch is only assigned to a single detection. Thereby, we effectively suppress lower scoring redetections in nearby scales and obtain a unified solution for multi-scale analysis.

Similar to [5], we report rectangles of mean aspect ratio (estimated from the training data) centered at each active detection node. The confidence of each reported detection is set to the absolute value of the decrease in energy that was recorded during testing the corresponding detection node.

## 4.1   Datasets

The choice of evaluation datasets is motivated by several factors. First we want to have a direct comparison to the most closely related approach [11]. The publicly available implementation comes with its own set of random forests, trained for detection of side views of pedestrians. Thus, we also focus on this task, although our method is not specifically tailored towards it and potentially handles arbitrary object categories.

Another aspect is the resolution of the objects in the images. Part based approaches, like ISMs, can only capitalize on their strengths if the objects are depicted at a resolution where the parts are distinguishable. Thus we require the smallest category instances to have at least about 100 pixels in height.

Since for non overlapping object instances our proposed method reaches the same decisions as standard NMS (as was tested and assured in evaluations on single scale datasets like UIUC cars), we are especially interested in testing the capability of our algorithm to resolve detections of strongly overlapping objects. Thus, we evaluate it on the *TUD crossing* and *TUD campus* sequences [14], also used in [11], where both datasets require the ability to locally decide for each patch to which detection it belongs in a reasonable manner. Additionally, we evaluate all approaches on the PETS 2009 dataset, also featuring close to side views of a large number of pedestrians with heavy overlaps.

The *TUD campus* and *TUD crossing* datasets contain two sequences of images showing pedestrians in street side scenarios. In *TUD campus* there are 71 images of highly overlapping persons walking along a side walk. This sequence especially features large changes in scale, as well as strong occlusions. The *TUD crossing* sequence contains 201 images of a relatively crowded scene, showing profile views of pedestrians crossing a street. We use the extended ground truth from [15].

The PETS 2009 Benchmark Data [16] includes several datasets of which we take View001 of sequence S1.L1 to further evaluate the performance of our method. This sequence shows several groups of people walking closely and thus heavily occluding each other. In total the groundtruth annotation contains 4348 persons.

As training data for all experiments we use the training set of the *TUD-pedestrian* dataset, consisting of 400 images of mostly side views of pedestrians.

## 4.2   Results

We directly compare our results to the two most related approaches: the Hough Forests using standard non maximum suppression [5] and the probabilistic framework of Barinova *et al.* [11]. Detections are considered as valid analyzing the standard PASCAL-VOC overlap criterion, with the threshold set to 50%. For both methods compared, we used the publicly available source codes and associated configuration files as published by the respective authors. For training the Hough Forests we used exactly the same data as for our method.

Fig. 4 shows precision-recall curves for all three methods on all three databases. As can be seen, our method significantly improves over [5] and also outperforms [11] on all three datasets, gaining about 10% recall, at precision levels

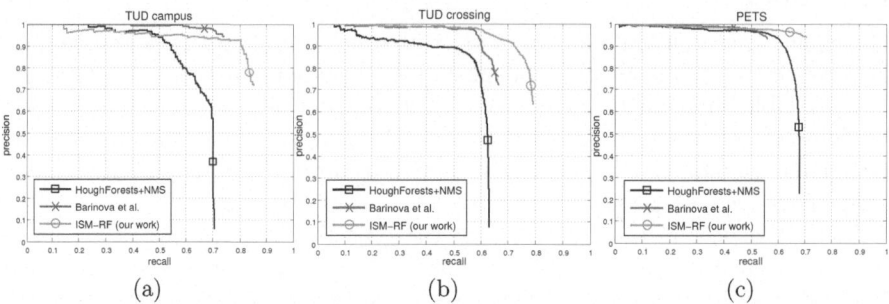

(a)                                    (b)                                    (c)

**Fig. 4.** Precision/Recall curves on (a) *TUD campus*, (b) *TUD crossing* and (c) PETS 2009 S1.L1 sequence for all three methods

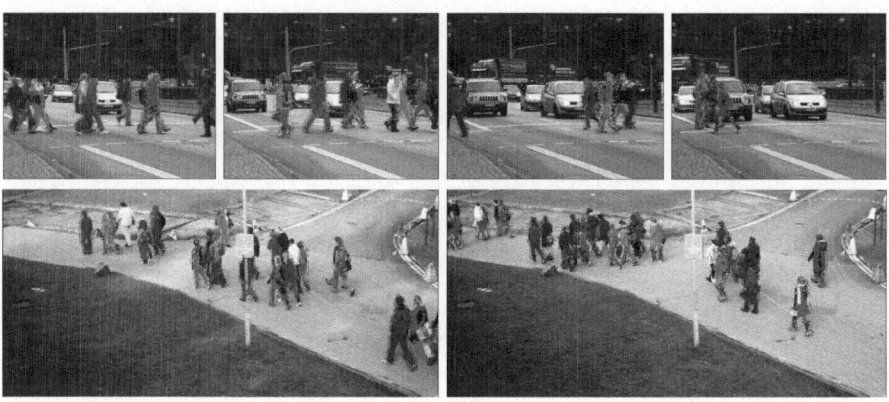

**Fig. 5.** Sample detections on the TUD crossing sequence (top row) and PETS 2009 (bottom row). For each detection the uniquely assigned patches are plotted in a different color. Note how closely walking pedestrians, overlapping each other, are correctly separated.

above 90%. Fig. 5 additionally visualizes detection results and all local patches that were assigned to each detected instance by our inference process in different colors. Note how even strongly overlapping persons are correctly separated from each other.

## 5   Conclusion

In this work, we have proposed a new formulation for the task of detecting objects based on the information gathered in an Implicit Shape Model. We formulated the dual problem of detecting a set of object hypotheses and assigning local patches to the detections in a random field manner using a significantly sparser graph structure than in related approaches. Furthermore, the specific graph structure allowed to define a novel, fast inference algorithm to solve our defined energy minimization problem. Our method does not require to fix a range for local neighborhood suppression as it is necessary in related methods, but implicitly is capable to separate even strongly overlapping object instances. Experiments demonstrated that we are able to accurately detect object hypotheses and their local support patches on challenging data sets achieving competitive or even improved results in comparison to state-of-the-art in this field.

**Acknowledgement.** This work was supported by the Austrian Science Foundation (FWF) project Advanced Learning for Tracking and Detection in Medical Workflow Analysis (I535-N23) and by the Austrian Research Promotion Agency (FFG) project SHARE (831717) in the IV2Splus program.

# References

1. Viola, P., Jones, M.: Robust real-time face detection. IJCV 57, 137–154 (2004)
2. Lampert, C.H., Blaschko, M.B., Hofmann, T.: Efficient subwindow search: A branch and bound framework for object localization. IEEE Trans. on PAMI 31, 2129–2142 (2009)
3. Dalal, N., Triggs, B.: Histograms of oriented gradients for human detection. In: Proc. CVPR (2005)
4. Fischler, M., Elschlager, R.: The representation and matching of pictorial structures. IEEE Trans. on Computers C-22, 67–92 (1973)
5. Gall, J., Lempitsky, V.: Class-specific Hough forests for object detection. In: Proc. CVPR (2009)
6. Felzenszwalb, P.F., Girshick, R.B., McAllester, D., Ramanan, D.: Object detection with discriminatively trained part-based models. IEEE Trans. on PAMI 32, 1627–1645 (2010)
7. Fergus, R., Perona, P., Zisserman, A.: Weakly supervised scale-invariant learning of models for visual recognition. IJCV 71, 273–303 (2007)
8. Sivic, J., Zisserman, A.: Video Google: A text retrieval approach to object matching in videos. In: Proc. ICCV (2003)
9. Leibe, B., Leonardis, A., Schiele, B.: Combined object categorization and segmentation with an implicit shape model. In: Proc. ECCV (2004)
10. Lehmann, A., Leibe, B., Gool, L.V.: PRISM: PRincipled Implicit Shape Model. In: Proc. BMVC (2009)
11. Barinova, O., Lempitsky, V., Kohli, P.: On the detection of multiple object instances using Hough transforms. In: Proc. CVPR (2010)
12. Kolmogorov, V., Zabin, R.: What energy functions can be minimized via graph cuts? IEEE Trans. on PAMI 26, 147–159 (2004)
13. Boykov, Y., Veksler, O., Zabih, R.: Fast approximate energy minimization via graph cuts. IEEE Trans. on PAMI 23, 1222–1239 (2001)
14. Andriluka, M., Roth, S., Schiele, B.: People-tracking-by-detection and people-detection-by-tracking. In: Proc. CVPR (2008)
15. Riemenschneider, H., Sternig, S., Donoser, M., Roth, P.M., Bischof, H.: Hough Regions for Joining Instance Localization and Segmentation. In: Fitzgibbon, A., Lazebnik, S., Perona, P., Sato, Y., Schmid, C. (eds.) ECCV 2012, Part III. LNCS, vol. 7574, pp. 258–271. Springer, Heidelberg (2012)
16. Ferryman, J., Shahrokni, A.: PETS2009: Dataset and challenge. In: PETS (2009)

# Relative Forest for Attribute Prediction

Shaoxin Li[1,2], Shiguang Shan[1], and Xilin Chen[1]

[1] Key Lab of Intelligent Information Processing of Chinese Academy of Sciences
(CAS), Institute of Computing Technology, CAS, Beijing, 100190, China
[2] Graduate University of Chinese Academy of Sciences, Beijing 100049, China
{shaoxin.li,shiguang.shan,xilin.chen}@vipl.ict.ac.cn

**Abstract.** Human-Namable visual attributes are promising in leveraging various recognition tasks. Intuitively, the more accurate the attribute prediction is, the more the recognition tasks can benefit. Relative attributes [1] learns a ranking function per attribute which can provide more accurate attribute prediction, thus, show clear advantages over previous binary attribute. In this paper, we inherit the idea of learning ranking function per attribute but propose to improve the algorithm in two aspects: First, we propose a *Relative Tree* algorithm which facilitates more accurate nonlinear ranking to capture the semantic relationships. Second, we develop a *Relative Forest* algorithm which resorts to randomized learning to reduce training time of *Relative Tree*. Benefiting from multiple tree ensemble, *Relative Forest* can achieve even more accurate final ranking. To show the effectiveness of proposed method, we first compare *Relative Tree* method with Relative Attribute on PubFig and OSR dataset. Then to verify the efficiency of *Relative Forest* algorithm, we conduct age estimation evaluation on FG-NET dataset. With much less training time compared to Relative Attribute and *Relative Tree*, proposed *Relative Forest* achieves state-of-the-art age estimation accuracy. Finally, experiments on the large scale SUN Attribute database show the scalability of proposed *Relative Forest*.

## 1 Introduction

Recently, computer vision researchers have proposed to explore human-namable visual attribute as a valuable semantic cue to boost the performance of traditional recognition tasks [2–5] or enable various new applications [6–10]. While visual attribute shows encouraging capacity in enhancing the robustness of real-world face [2], human [3] and object [4, 5] recognition, the ever growing interest in attribute-centric modeling is even more popularized by its intuitive appeal to facilitate nature image describing [6–8] and knowledge transferring [9, 10].

Notwithstanding the great potential of attribute-centric modeling, few works are devoted to generate informative attribute predictions. Most of existing work [2–10] modeled attribute as binary property and predicted its presence. Although binary prediction is adequate for some attributes, such as having horn and wearing glasses, it is too restrictive and unnatural for a large variety of other attributes, such as human age and object size. As indicated in [1], describing

K.M. Lee et al. (Eds.): ACCV 2012, Part I, LNCS 7724, pp. 316–327, 2013.
© Springer-Verlag Berlin Heidelberg 2013

using relative visual properties is a much more informative and effective way for humans to recognize specific objects. Even for properties which are commonly regarded as binary, relative description can provide more information about the image. For example, it is better to describe a scene of country road as "more manmade than a scene of mountains but more natural than tall building" than simply categorize it as natural or manmade. To model such relationship of a given attribute between different classes, Relative Attribute learns a ranking function for each attribute. By estimating a continuous ranking score rather than a binary presence, Relative Attribute can provide much more informative description to enhance subsequence recognition or other tasks. However, since only a linear hyperplane is learned as ranking function, Relative Attribute may not be capable in handling high dimensional nonlinear data.

In this paper, we focus on efficiently generating informative attribute predictions. Inheriting the elegant idea of learning ranking function per attribute with ordered or similar constraints, we propose to improve Relative Attribute in two aspects: 1) Facilitates more accurate nonlinear ranking to cope with high dimensional visual features lying on nonlinear manifold; 2) Reduces time complexity to handle large scale data set. To achieve the first goal, we employ Relative Attribute as base ranking function to construct a Relative Tree according to maximal information gain criterion [11]. Due to the hierarchical tree structure, the proposed Relative Tree can efficiently capture the complex nonlinear structure of feature manifold and generate a piecewise linear ranking function to rank the nonlinear data accurately. Although only linear ranking function is employed, our method can automatically discover the intrinsic nonlinear structure of the data manifold and adapt to arbitrary data distributions. To accomplish the second goal, which is essential for scaling the algorithm up to handle more realistic dataset such as [12] and [13], we first resort to randomized learning to significantly reduce the complexity of building single *Relative Tree*. Then borrowing the idea of random forest [14], we combine multiple randomized *Relative Tree* to construct a *Relative Forest* which can further boosts the ranking accuracy with much less training time.

## 2 Brief Review of Relative Attribute

Before presenting proposed method, we briefly review Relative Attribute [1]. Unlike most existing attribute-based methods, Relative Attribute learns a ranking function rather than binary prediction per attribute. The key idea is to learn a linear ranking direction to maximize rank margin between given pairs of examples.

Given a set of training samples $X = \{x_k | k = 1, 2, ... , K\}$, where $K$ is the number of training samples. For each attribute, an ordered constraint set $O = \{o_n | o_n = (k_{n1}, k_{n2}), n = 1, 2, ..., N\}$ and an similar constraint set $S = \{s_m | s_m = (k_{m1}, k_{m2}), m = 1, 2, ..., M\}$ are provided to depict the relationships between pairs of samples. Where $N$ is the number of ordered constraints and M is the number of similar constraints. Each ordered constraint $o_n \in O$ indicates that $k_{n1} \succ k_{n2}$, i.e. sample $k_{n1}$ has a higher presence of given attribute than $k_{n2}$, while each similar constraint $s_n \in S$ indicates that $k_{m1} \sim k_{m2}$, i.e. sample $k_{m1}$ has similar attribute presence with sample $k_{m2}$. Intuitively, the optimal linear ranking direction $w$ should satisfy the ordered and similar constraints as many as possible. As this problem is NP-hard, non-negative slack variables $\xi_n, \gamma_m$ proposed in [15] are introduced to relax the problem to the final objective of Relative Attribute:

$$\underset{w}{\arg\min} \quad (\frac{1}{2} \parallel w \parallel_2^2 + C(\sum_{n=1}^{N} \xi_n^2 + \sum_{m=1}^{M} \gamma_m^2))$$

$$s.t. \quad w^T(x_{k_{n1}} - x_{k_{n2}}) \geq 1 - \xi_n; \; \forall o_n \in O \qquad (1)$$

$$|w^T(x_{k_{m1}} - x_{k_{m2}})| \leq \gamma_m; \; \forall s_m \in S$$

$$\xi_n, \gamma_m \geq 0,$$

where $C$ is used to trade off between large rank margin and number of satisfied constraints. By considering all margins between closest pairs of ordered samples, the learned linear function $w$ is much more suitable for ranking the data than linear classification hyperplane learned from nearest binary-labeled samples. It is important to note that the relative constraint used in Relative Attribute is also more natural to depict some attribute which are hard to be quantized, such as "smile face" and "open scene".

## 3   Relative Tree

In this section, we propose to extend linear ranking algorithm, i.e. Relative Attribute, to deal with nonlinear ranking. As introduced in [16], a set of tree structured projections can hierarchically partition data into pieces in a manner that is provably sensitive to low dimensional manifold structure. Inspired by this idea, in section 3.1, we propose a method to facilitate hierarchical nonlinear ranking by constructing a *Relative Tree*, in which Relative Attribute serves as base ranking function(also referred to as splitting function) in each tree node. Then in section 3.2 we present how to predict attribute with the constructed *Relative Tree*.

### 3.1   Tree Construction—Hierarchical Ranking

The basic idea of *Relative Tree* is to learn a set of hierarchical ranking functions. Then by traversing down the tree, a test sample can obtain gradually finer ranking score. Although it is also possible to apply kernel trick to equation (1) for nonlinear ranking, our method bears certain intuitive appeal that the data-driven tree construction involves non hypothesis about data distribution. And all leaf nodes actually consist a global piecewise linear ranking on origin data manifold. Thus our proposed *Relative Tree* can cope with arbitrary data distribution and automatically learns a set of piecewise linear ranking functions according to the intrinsic structure. We show a sample of construction procedure

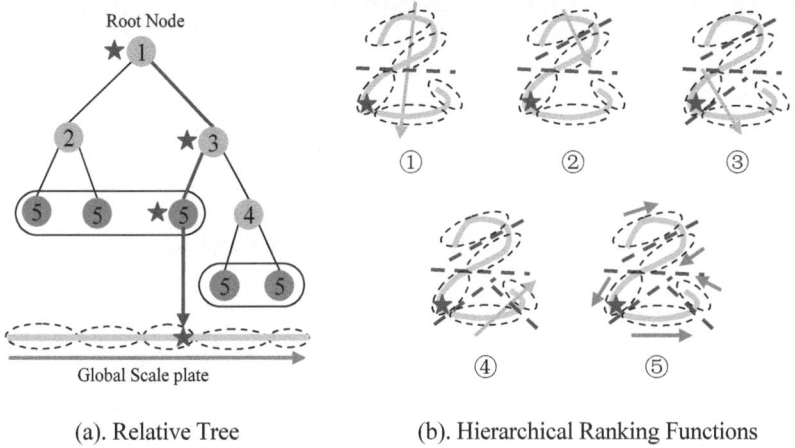

(a). Relative Tree                    (b). Hierarchical Ranking Functions

**Fig. 1.** Learning procedure of Relative Tree(a) on a "S-shape" nonlinear manifold and its corresponding set of Hierarchical Ranking Functions(b). Numbers in the circle indicate train step index. Green color indicates non-leaf nodes while blue color indicates leaf nodes. Ranking functions of all leaf nodes can be normalized to a global "scale-plate" and generate final unified ranking score.

of proposed *Relative Tree* on a "S-shape" manifold in Fig. 1, where Fig. 1(a) is the learned hierarchical *Relative Tree* and Fig. 1(b) shows the learning steps. The "S-shape" nonlinear manifold can be quantized into 5 approximate linear part. Each of them falls in a dotted elliptical outline in Fig. 1(b). The ranking function learned in the root node(See Fig.1(a)) is actually the result of Relative Attribute algorithm [1]. As is shown, this ranking function(see Fig.1(b): ①) gives almost highest ranking score to the test sample indicated by the purple star. Unlike Relative Attribute, besides of the global coarse ranking function, *Relative Tree* automatically learns finer local ranking functions according to the intrinsic structure of data. As a result, it can predict accurate ranking position of the purple star localizing in the end of the third dotted elliptical outline.

For further clarification, we present the pseudo code of the tree construction procedure in Algorithm. 1, in which there are two key problems remain to be solved: 1) Whether the chosen node is divisible(Algorithm 1 Line: 1); 2) How to find best split(Algorithm Line: 4).

**Divisibility.** If the presence of attribute is quantifiable, the ordered label can be assigned to samples. In this circumstance, if all the data fall in a node have the same label then this node is strictly indivisible. However, strictly indivisible is almost impossible. Therefore, in our algorithm, we determine a node as indivisible if the entropy of the data falling in this node is less than a given threshold. Once the threshold is small enough the performance will be satisfiable. On the other hand, if only some relative pairs of attribute presence degree are provided, we determine a node as strictly indivisible when there is no ordered pairs between training samples fall in this node. In real world case, when the

---

**Algorithm 1. Relative Tree Construction**

---

**Input:**
    Training features: $X$;
    Ordered constraint set: $O$;
    Similar constraint set: $S$.
**Output:**
    Relative Tree: $T$.
1: **if** size($X$)>Minimal Node size and $X$ is divisible **then**
2:    Calculate Relative Attribute: $W = $ RelativeAttribute($X, O, S$);
3:    Calculate ranking score: $R = W^T X$;
4:    Find best splitting threshold $b$;
5:    T.Data $= (R, W, b)$;
6:    Split training data: $X^{(L)} = \{x_k | R_k < b\}$, $X^{(R)} = \{x_k | R_k > b\}$;
7:    Split ordered constraint set:
        $O^{(L)} = \{o_n | x_{k_{n1}}, x_{k_{n2}} \in X^{(L)}\}$; $O^{(R)} = \{o_n | x_{k_{n1}}, x_{k_{n2}} \in X^{(R)}\}$;
8:    Split similar constraint set:
        $S^{(L)} = \{s_m | x_{k_{m1}}, x_{k_{m2}} \in X^{(L)}\}$; $S^{(R)} = \{s_m | x_{k_{m1}}, x_{k_{m2}} \in X^{(R)}\}$;
9:    Save left node $(T.LeftNode, X^{(L)}, O^{(L)}, S^{(L)})$ as a splitting candidate $P$;
10:   Save right node $(T.RightNode, X^{(R)}, O^{(R)}, S^{(R)})$ as a splitting candidate $P$;
11:   Find best splitting node (T,X,O,S) in pool $P$;
12:   Repeat steps 1–15;
13: **else**
14:   $T = NULL$;
15: **end if**
16: **return** $T$;

---

ratio of ordered samples which is at least relate to another sample under ordered constraint exceeds a given threshold, we determine this node as divisible.

**Split Criterion.** Once the node is determined as divisible, we need to find the best split to partition the data. To achieve this goal, we first employ Relative Attribute algorithm [1] to learn a linear ranking direction. If ordered label is available, similar to [11], we calculate optimal splitting threshold $b$ to split the data based on maximal information gain criterion:

$$argmin_b \Delta E(b) = E(X) - frac|X^{(L)}||X|E(X^{(L)}) - \frac{|X^{(R)}|}{|X|} E(X^{(R)}), \quad (2)$$

where $E(X)$ is the Shannon entropy of the classes in the set of samples X. $X^{(L)}/X^{(R)}$ is the sample data partitioned to the Left/Right child node. If only partial relative pairwise constraints are available, we choose optimal splitting threshold $b$ which separates maximal number of ordered pair and maintains maximal number of similar pair:

$$argmin_b \Delta I(b) = I(O, S) - \frac{|X^{(L)}|}{|X|} I(O^{(L)}, S^{(L)}) - \frac{|X^{(R)}|}{|X|} I(O^{(R)}, S^{(R)}), \quad (3)$$

where $I(O, S) = |O| - |S|$, $|O|$ is the number of ordered constraint on $X$ and $|S|$ is the number of similar constraint on $|X|$. Intuitively, the more the ordered pairs and less similar pairs, the more uncertain the data is. In other words, $I(O, S) \propto E(X)$. It is true that more complex and accurate approximation of $E(X)$ can be made with $O$ and $S$. In this paper, we simply use the heuristic approximation given out by equation (3).

At last, we analyze time complexity of proposed *Relative Tree*. As mentioned in the last paragraph of section 2, the time complexity of Relative Attribute is $O(K^3)$. For proposed *Relative Tree*, in the best case, i.e. we get a complete binary tree and at each node the data is equally distributed to left and right nodes, the complexity is $\sum_{i=0}^{\log_2^K} 2^i O((\frac{K}{2^i})^3) = O(K^3)$. Indeed, if the training data do not severely biased or ordered constraint are uniformly distribute on samples, our method tends to choose balanced split. In our experiments, consuming time of constructing a *Relative Tree* is approximately 3.5 times of training a Relative Attribute in average.

## 3.2   Tree Prediction—Ranking Score Normalization

With the learned *Relative Tree*, a test sample get gradually finer ranking by traversing down the tree(see Fig. 1(a)). Unlike classical decision tree, which averaging(regression) or voting(classification) training data's labels falling in leaf nodes to generate predictions of test samples, the relative tree will calculate ranking score of the test sample using the leaf node's ranking function. However, the ranking score calculated in different leaf nodes(see Fig. 1) is incomparable since these functions are trained with disjoint subsets of original training set, thus we need to normalize the ranking results obtained by different ranking functions in a *Relative Tree*. The basic idea is to normalize all the ranking score with a unique global "scale plate". If the ordered label is available, the unique global "scale plate" can be directly set as the corresponding label of the data, then the normalization parameter of given ranking function can be obtained by:

$$\arg\min_{s,b} \sum \|l_i - s \cdot (r_i - b)\|_2^2, \tag{4}$$

where $l$ is the ordered label vector and $r$ is the ranking score vector obtained in training step(see Algorithm 1 Line: 3). $s$ and $b$ are normalization parameters which are used to map local rank value to global "scale plate". For the situation when only partial ordered pairwise constraints are given, we can set the unique global "scale plate" as $[0, 1]$. We show detailed normalization in Algorithm 2.

After score normalization, the proposed *Relative Tree* algorithm can generate a global ranking score, thus facilitate adaptive piecewise linear ranking on nonlinear data.

## 4   Relative Forest

Although *Relative Tree* facilitate more accurate nonlinear ranking, it may suffer from over-fitting and is time consuming. In this section, we propose *Relative Forest* algorithm based on *Relative Tree*. Resorting to randomized and ensemble

**Algorithm 2. Relative Tree Prediction without Ordered Label**

**Input:**
    Relative Tree: $T$;
    Test sample: $x$.

**Output:**
    Ranking score of give sample: $R_x$.

1: $b_{inf} = 0$; $b_{sup} = 1$
2: **while** T!=NULL **do**
3:    $(R, W, b) = T.Data$
4:    Calculate ranking score of test sample: $r_x = W^T x$
5:    Normalize training set ranking score to global unique "scale plate":
        $R \Rightarrow [b_{inf}, b_{sup}]$, accordingly $b = Norm\_b$, $r_x = Norm\_r_x$
6:    **if** $r_x < b$ **then**
7:        $T = T.LeftNode$; $b_{sup} = Norm\_b$
8:    **else**
9:        $T = T.RightNode$; $b_{inf} = Norm\_b$
10:   **end if**
11: **end while**
12: $R_x = Norm\_r_x$
13: **return** $R_x$;

learning, compared to *Relative Tree*, the proposed *Relative Forest* obtain even more accurate prediction of attribute while consuming significantly less training time.

## 4.1   Randomized Learning

In original random forest algorithm [14] and its extending works [11, 17, 18] Randomness usually injected at three aspects during training: 1) bootstrap subset of training data to grow each random relative tree; 2) choose subset of feature dimensions for calculating splitting function $f$; 3) use random splitting threshold $b$. In the proposed *Relative Forest*, we employ first two randomization strategies but select a optimal splitting threshold $b$ based on equation (2) or (3).

Additionally, we develop a specific randomized learning strategy for Relative Attribute which serve as node splitting function. As mentioned in the last paragraph of section 2, the total number of relative constraints is $O(K^2)$. When $K$ is large, the number of pairwise constraints becomes untractable. We propose to randomly pick a subset of constraints for optimizing equation (1). Intuitively, we want every sample at least related to another sample with one order constraint and one similar constraint. Suppose that there are $c$ different ordered levels for a given attribute, and in each level $n$ samples are given. Thus totally $K = cn$ samples are provided. In this case, there are totally $|O| = \frac{c(c-1)}{2}n^2$ ordered constrains, in which totally $|O_i| = (c - 1)n$ ordered constraints are related to a given sample $i$. Then by randomly selecting $mK$ ordered constraints, it is easy to see that when $K \gg 1$, the probability that none ordered constraints include sample $i$ is selected is $[1 - \frac{|O_i|}{|O|}]^{mK} \approx e^{-2m}$. For similar constraints, the same criterion also holds. Thus in our experiments, we set $m = 2$, in other words, only randomly choose $2K$ ordered and similar constraints respectively. And the corresponding probability for each sample to be selected in at least one ordered (or similar) constraint is $1 - e^{-4} = 0.9817$. As only $O(K)$ comparing to original $O(K^2)$ constraints are used, when $K$ is very large this strategy can significantly reduce the number of used constraints. These randomized learning strategies not only speed up the training procedure but also reduce over-fitting [19].

### 4.2   Tree Ensemble

With randomized learning strategies we can build a *Relative Tree* much more faster. However, the ranking accuracy will degrade to some extent. To further boost the performance, we average the ranking score obtained from different randomized *Relative Tree* to generate the final prediction As all the rank scores are normalized to a unique global "scale plate". The average step can be directly applied. Due to the randomization, ranking results of different trees are independent. Thus the ensemble of different random *Relative Tree* improves the estimation accuracy notably as the tree number increase.

## 5   Experiments

We conduct comprehensive experiments on four datasets: (1) Outdoor Scene Recognition (OSR) Dataset [20] containing 2688 images from 8 categories; (2) A subset of the Public Figure Face (PubFig) Database [2] containing 800 images from 8 random identities (100 images each); (3) FG-NET Face Aging (FG-NET) Dataset [21] containing 1002 images form 82 individuals; (4) Sun Attribute Dataset [12]. For OSR and PubFig dataset, we use exactly the same attributes and data introduced in [1] with exactly the same feature and training\test distribution. For FG-NET, we simply use age as ordered label and conduct leave-one-out experiments according to the evaluation protocol, and for Sun Attribute database We use all 87 attributes collecting in 'asymmetric' splits, but reorganize the train/test split to demonstrate the capability of *Relative Forest* in large scale scenario. For each attribute, we use all image data which receive at least 2 votes as the positive data and randomly select data which receive 0/1 vote as the negative data. We set $N_0 = N_1 = N_2 + N_3$ ($N_0, N_1, N_2$ and $N_3$ are the numbers of selected samples receiving 0, 1, 2, 3 vote(s) respectively). Then 5 fold cross validation is constructed for evaluation.

### 5.1   Relative Tree vs. Relative Attribute

We use the data provided by authors of [1] to conduct experiments in this subsection. For an image pair $(i, j)$ in a test set (2648 images for OSR, 560 for PubFig), we compare ranking scores obtained by different methods namely B-SVM(binary SVM), SVR, RA(Relative Attribute) and RT(Relative Tree). If $R(x_i) > R(x_j)$ we predict $i \succ j$ else $i \prec j$, then this prediction are compared to the ground-truth

**Table 1.** Relative Accuracy on OSR Dataset(%)

|  | Natural | Open | Perspective | Large | Diagonal | Close |
|---|---|---|---|---|---|---|
| B-SVM | 91.10 | 86.06 | 78.98 | 65.01 | 80.77 | 87.20 |
| SVR | 94.01 | 90.42 | 85.51 | 86.17 | 86.87 | 87.34 |
| RA [1] | 94.40 | 91.01 | 85.08 | 86.39 | 87.52 | 88.71 |
| RT | 95.24 | 92.39 | 87.58 | 88.34 | 89.43 | 89.54 |

**Table 2.** Relative Accuracy on PubFig Dataset(%)

|  | Masculine | White | Young | Smiling | Chubby | Forhead |
|---|---|---|---|---|---|---|
| B-SVM | 70.12 | 64.64 | 75.49 | 66.97 | 59.37 | 76.50 |
| SVR | 75.36 | 69.98 | 76.25 | 76.58 | 72.34 | 85.79 |
| RA [1] | 81.00 | 77.31 | 81.05 | 79.66 | 76.14 | 87.91 |
| RT | 85.33 | 82.59 | 84.41 | 83.36 | 78.97 | 88.83 |
|  | Eyebrow | Eye | Nose | Lips | Face |  |
| B-SVM | 69.05 | 74.90 | 66.29 | 74.52 | 74.25 |  |
| SVR | 75.22 | 77.08 | 69.14 | 71.86 | 74.23 |  |
| RA [1] | 78.89 | 80.72 | 74.84 | 78.07 | 80.46 |  |
| RT | 81.84 | 83.15 | 80.43 | 81.87 | 86.31 |  |

relative ordering. The accuracy of predictions is shown in Table 1 (OSR) and Table 2 (PubFig). As seen, the proposed *Relative Tree* outperform all competitive algorithms in all given attributes.

As mentioned in section 3.2, once ordered label is given, we regard it as unique global "scale plate" and normalize the ranking score according to it. In this circumstance, the normalized ranking score of test sample can be directly compared with given ordered label of each individual using Euclidean distance in order to recognize it. With this simple method, recognition accuracy using attribute prediction of *Relative Tree* is 84.37% and 70.24% on the OSR and PubFig datasets, respectively, as compared to 77.40% and 65.54% if using ranking score obtained by Relative Attribute.

## 5.2    Relative Forest vs. Relative Tree

We compare *Relative Forest* to *Relative Tree* in two aspects: Prediction Accuracy and Time Consumption. The evaluation is conducted on the FG-NET data set. Images of the first person (15 images) in this data set are used as the test set, and images of all the other person (987 images) are used for training. Mean Absolute Error(MAE) is used to evaluate the estimation accuracy. The evaluation results are shown in Fig. 2. The dotted green line is the results of Relative Attribute with the score normalization using equation (4). The dotted blue line is the results of *Relative Tree* and the solid red line is the results of *Relative Forest*. In *Relative Forest*, we randomly bootstrap 40% samples with replacement for each tree. In tree construction step, 30% features are randomly selected to train splitting function, i.e. Relative Attribute. We try 10 times and select the best

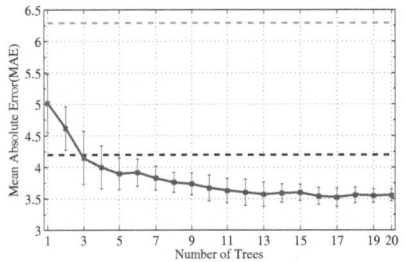

**Fig. 2.** Age estimation result of *Relative Forest* as the tree number increases

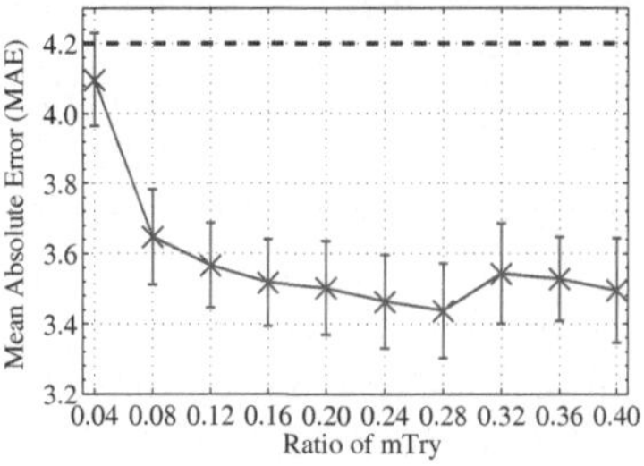

**Fig. 3.** Analysis of selected feature number of *Relative Forest*

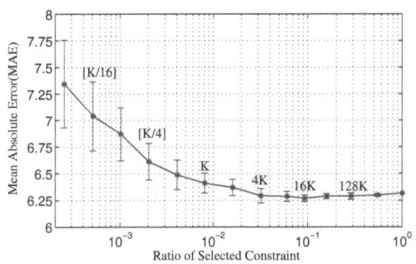

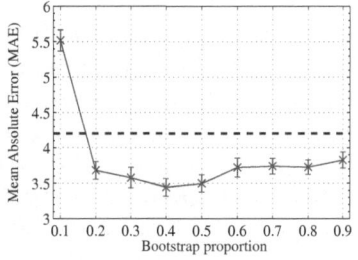

**Fig. 4.** Analysis of selected constraints number of Relative Attributes [1]

**Fig. 5.** Analysis of bootstrap sample number of *Relative Forest*

based on information gain criterion [11]. When the size of forest grows larger than 5, *Relative Forest* performs consistently better than *Relative Tree*. For each method, we repeat the algorithm 10 times and calculate mean consumption time. The consumption times are 121.8s and 417.7s for Relative Attribute and *Relative Tree* respectively. When the number of tree is 20, *Relative Forest* consumes 60.3s.

We also analyze effect of three kinds of randomization introduced in subsection 4.1. The corresponding key parameters are: 1)number of bootstrap samples for training each single tree (see Fig. 5); 2)selected dimensions for training Relative Attribute in node splitting step (see Fig. 3); 3)selected number of constraints used in training Relative Attribute (see Fig. 4). Note that the default parameters of tree number, bootstrap proportion, mTry Ratio and constraint number are 20, 40%, 30% and $2K$ respectively. When analyzing one parameter, we fix the other three.

### 5.3   Relative Forest for Age Estimation

We conduct facial age estimation on FG-NET dataset. Similar to [22], we first use OLPP [23] to extract informative feature from gray scale face image, then use proposed *Relative Forest* to predict age of subjects. The MAE results of our method and state-of-the-art age estimation methods [22, 24–26] are shown in Table 3. With the same features used in [22], our method achieve the best MAE

**Table 3.** MAEs Comparison on FG-NET aging database

| Methods | OHRanker [24] | MTWGP [25] | MHR [26] | LARR [22] | SVR [27] | Relative Forest |
|---|---|---|---|---|---|---|
| MAEs | 4.48 | 4.83 | 4.87 | 5.07 | 5.79 | **4.45±0.02** |

result on FG-NET database. With the same feature we used, MAE result of Support Vector Regression(SVR) is also shown in Table 3 for more clear comparison.

### 5.4  Relative Forest for Large Scale Attribute Prediction

We also present results on the SUN attribute database [12]. GIST feature is used. All three comparison methods predict continuous label. We set an attribute as present if predicted label is larger than 0.5. We calculate all 87*5 prediction accuracies, and the mean accuracies are: $Acc_{SVR} = 67.78$; $Acc_{RA} = 68.29$; $Acc_{RF} = 69.57$;. Note that for Relative Attribute method we simply sample part of the data and part of positive and negative constraints to train ranking function, or it cannot scale to such large scale testing.

## 6  Conclusion

Human-Namable visual attribute bears intuitive appeal in strengthening object recognition, facilitating zero shot learning, enabling knowledge transfer and image describing, which make the accurate estimation of attribute in large scale scenario especially important. Aiming at efficiently predicting accurate relative attribute, we first propose *Relative Tree* to facilitate more precise nonlinear ranking, and then propose *Relative Forest* to further boost the performance while significantly reducing training time.

**Acknowledgements.** This work is partially supported by Natural Science Foundation of China (NSFC) under contract Nos. 61025010, 61173065, and 60833013; and Beijing Natural Science Foundation (New Technologies and Methods in Intelligent Video Surveillance for Public Security) under contract No. 4111003.

## References

1. Parikh, D., Grauman, K.: Relative attributes. In: ICCV, pp. 503–510 (2011)
2. Kumar, N., Berg, A., Belhumeur, P., Nayar, S.: Attribute and simile classifiers for face verification. In: ICCV, pp. 365–372 (2009)
3. Yao, B., Jiang, X., Khosla, A., Lin, A., Guibas, L., Fei-Fei, L.: Human action recognition by learning bases of action attributes and parts. In: ICCV, pp. 1331–1338 (2011)

4. Wang, J., Markert, K., Everingham, M.: Learning models for object recognition from natural language descriptions. In: BMVC (2009)
5. Wang, G., Forsyth, D.: Joint learning of visual attributes, object classes and visual saliency. In: ICCV, pp. 537–544 (2009)
6. Farhadi, A., Endres, I., Hoiem, D., Forsyth, D.: Describing objects by their attributes. In: CVPR, pp. 1778–1785 (2009)
7. Bourdev, L., Maji, S., Malik, J.: Describing people: A poselet-based approach to attribute classification. In: ICCV, pp. 1543–1550 (2011)
8. Siddiquie, B., Feris, R., Davis, L.: Image ranking and retrieval based on multi-attribute queries. In: CVPR, pp. 801–808 (2011)
9. Fergus, R., Bernal, H., Weiss, Y., Torralba, A.: Semantic Label Sharing for Learning with Many Categories. In: Daniilidis, K., Maragos, P., Paragios, N. (eds.) ECCV 2010, Part I. LNCS, vol. 6311, pp. 762–775. Springer, Heidelberg (2010)
10. Lampert, C., Nickisch, H., Harmeling, S.: Learning to detect unseen object classes by between-class attribute transfer. In: CVPR, pp. 951–958 (2009)
11. Shotton, J., Johnson, M., Cipolla, R.: Semantic texton forests for image categorization and segmentation. In: CVPR, pp. 1–8 (2008)
12. Patterson, G., Hays, J.: Sun attribute database:discovering, annotating, and recognizing scene attributes. In: CVPR, pp. 2751–2758 (2012)
13. Xiao, J., Hays, J., Ehinger, K., Oliva, A., Torralba, A.: Sun database: Large-scale scene recognition from abbey to zoo. In: CVPR, pp. 3485–3492 (2010)
14. Breiman, L.: Random forests. Machine Learning, 5–32 (2001)
15. Joachims, T.: Optimizing search engines using clickthrough data. In: SIGKDD, pp. 133–142 (2002)
16. Freund, Y., Dasgupta, S., Kabra, M., Verma, N.: Learning the structure of manifolds using random projections. In: NIPS, pp. 473–480 (2007)
17. Geurts, P., Ernst, D., Wehenkel, L.: Extremely randomized trees. Machine Learning, 3–42 (2006)
18. Bosch, A., Zisserman, A., Muoz, X.: Image classification using random forests and ferns. In: ICCV, pp. 1–8 (2007)
19. Amit, Y., Geman, D.: Shape quantization and recognition with randomized trees. Neural Computation, 1545–1588 (1997)
20. Oliva, A., Torralba, A.: Modeling the shape of the scene: A holistic representation of the spatial envelope. IJCV, 145–175 (2001)
21. FGNET: The fg-net aging database (2002), http://sting.cycollege.ac.cy/~alanitis/fgnetaging/index.html
22. Guo, G., Fu, Y., Dyer, C., Huang, T.: Image-based human age estimation by manifold learning and locally adjusted robust regression. TIP, 1178–1188 (2008)
23. Cai, D., He, X., Han, J., Zhang, H.: Orthogonal laplacianfaces for face recognition. TIP, 3608–3614 (2006)
24. Chang, K., Chen, C., Hung, Y.: Ordinal hyperplanes ranker with cost sensitivities for age estimation. In: CVPR, pp. 585–592 (2011)
25. Zhang, Y., Yeung, D.: Multi-task warped gaussian process for personalized age estimation. In: CVPR, pp. 2622–2629 (2010)
26. Qin, T., Zhang, X., Wang, D., Liu, T., Lai, W., Li, H.: Ranking with multiple hyperplanes. In: SIGIR, pp. 279–286 (2007)
27. Chang, C., Lin, C.: Libsvm: a library for support vector machines. TIST 27 (2011)

# Discriminative Dictionary Learning
# with Pairwise Constraints

Huimin Guo*, Zhuolin Jiang*, and Larry S. Davis

University of Maryland, College Park, MD, 20742
{hmguo,zhuolin,lsd}@umiacs.umd.edu

**Abstract.** In computer vision problems such as pair matching, only binary information - 'same' or 'different' label for pairs of images - is given during training. This is in contrast to classification problems, where the category labels of training images are provided. We propose a unified discriminative dictionary learning approach for both pair matching and multiclass classification tasks. More specifically, we introduce a new discriminative term called 'pairwise sparse code error' for the discriminativeness in sparse representation of pairs of signals, and then combine it with the classification error for discriminativeness in classifier construction to form a unified objective function. The solution to the new objective function is achieved by employing the efficient feature-sign search algorithm. The learned dictionary encourages feature points from a similar pair (or the same class) to have similar sparse codes. We validate the effectiveness of our approach through a series of experiments on face verification and recognition problems.

## 1 Introduction

Different from many classification problems where the specific class label of each image is given during training, only binary information such as same/different or relevant/irrlevant is provided for training data in applications such as face verification (given a *target* and a *query* image, determine whether they are from the same person), pair matching, image retrieval, etc. Typically, a discriminative similarity measure is learned through metric learning [1–4] from pairs of training images labeled as 'same' or 'different'; this provides less specific information than known classes - category labels. In this paper, we propose a framework to learn a discriminative dictionary satisfying pairwise constraints. The learned dictionary is suitable for pair matching problems with the pairwise constraints from the binary similarity or dissimilarity information; in addition, it is also suitable for classification problems given pairwise constraints about category information.

Sparse coding [5] approximates a signal $y$ as a linear combination of a few atoms from a learned dictionary $A$, *i.e.*, $y = Ax$, and leads to good performance in numerous applications. The learned dictionary $A$ is critical to performance. K-SVD [6] minimizes a reconstruction error to learn an over-complete dictionary. However, despite its many successful applications, K-SVD is not suitable for classification, where the dictionary should be not only representative, but also

---

* Indicates equal contributions.

K.M. Lee et al. (Eds.): ACCV 2012, Part I, LNCS 7724, pp. 328–342, 2013.
© Springer-Verlag Berlin Heidelberg 2013

discriminative. Hence, some supervised dictionary learning approaches incorporate classification error into the objective function to construct a dictionary with discriminative power. However, such frameworks consider only discriminativeness in the classifier construction, but do not guarantee the discriminativeness in the sparse representations of input signals. The discriminative capability of a dictionary usually comes from category label information. We will show that considering the pair similarity/dissimilarity constraints without category labels during dictionary learning can also improve the discriminative power of a dictionary; no existing dictionary learning approach has fully explored this property. Our dictionary learning approach explicitly integrates pairwise constraints for sparse codes of input signals and a linear predictive classifier into one objective function. The learned dictionary encourages signals from the same class (or a similar pair) to have similar sparse codes, and signals from different classes (or a dissimilar pair) to have dissimilar sparse codes, illustrated in Figures 1 and 2. The similarity can be thresholded to yield a binary decision of same/different (face verification), or it can be used to find the most similar face in a gallery (face recognition). The main contributions of this paper are:

- We present a dictionary learning framework with explicit pairwise constraints, which unifies the discriminative dictionary learning for pair matching and classification problems.
- Our framework furthermore integrates the pairwise constraints for sparse codes of input signals and a linear predictive classifier into the objective function for dictionary learning, which addresses the desirable properties of discriminativeness in the sparse representations of signals, and the discriminativeness in classifier construction.
- The objective function can be optimized via the efficient feature-sign search algorithm [7].
- Our approach is validated on various public face verification and recognition benchmarks.

## 1.1 Related Work

Metric learning (ML) aims at learning a discriminative similarity measure between different images [1–4]. An appropriate distance metric plays a very important role in many learning problems. Most work in metric learning, including LDML [1], MkNN [1], ITML [2], CSML [3], etc, relies on learning a Mahalanobis distance to map the feature space into a target space [4]. Less work, however, has been done for face verification using dictionary learning with pairwise similarity and dissimilarity constraints on input training examples.

[5] used sparse representations for face recognition (1:N matching problem which finds a nearest neighbor of a given *probe* in a *gallery* face set) by relating the problem of finding the most similar face to noiseless signal reconstruction. Since then, many other researchers have developed methods for face recognition using sparse representations or dictionary learning [5, 9–14]. Although many of these existing algorithms have been shown to perform well in classification

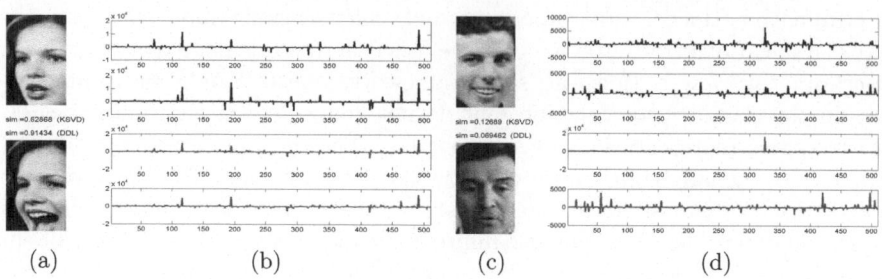

**Fig. 1.** An example of sparse codes (HoG feature) and similarity scores obtained by K-SVD dictionary learning and our proposed discriminative dictionary learning with pairwise constraints. Image pairs are from test set 1 of the LFW [8] dataset. (a) Original faces of the 'same' pair and their similarity scores obtained by 'K-SVD' and 'DDL'. (b) Sparse codes for the 'same' pair obtained from 'K-SVD'(blue) and 'DDL'(red), respectively. (c) Original faces of a 'different' pair. (d) Sparse codes for the 'different' pair. It can be seen that our dictionary encourages a pair from 'same' person to have similar sparse codes while a pair from 'different' persons to have dissimilar sparse codes.

(e.g. face recognition) applications, most of them do not explicitly deal with dictionary learning with pairwise constraints - when only binary information such as same/different or relevant/irrelevant is given in the training stage (e.g. face verification). Our dictionary learning framework is more general since it deals with face verification and face recognition problems simultaneously.

To enhance discrimination power, our dictionary learning framework explicitly integrates pairwise constraints for sparse codes of input signals and a linear predictive classifier into the objective function during training. Most previous approaches treat dictionary learning and classifier training as two separate processes, such as [15–20]. In these approaches, a dictionary is typically learned first and then a classifier is trained based on it. There are also sophisticated approaches [13, 21–23] combining dictionary learning and classifier training in a mixed reconstructive and discriminative formulation. Our approach falls into this category. We learn a single dictionary and an optimal classifier jointly.

Laplacian Sparse Coding [24] explicitly introduces a locality preserving constraint among similar local features in the sparse coding step to preserve the consistence of the sparse codes. This is different since our approach is to learn a dictionary which encourages signals from a similar pair (or the same class) to have similar sparse codes. Furthermore, our approach integrates a linear predictive classifier into the objective function to learn the dictionary and the classifier simultaneously while [24] learns the dictionary and the classifier separately.

## 2  Sparse Coding and Dictionary Learning

### 2.1  Sparse Coding

Let $Y = [\boldsymbol{y}_1, \boldsymbol{y}_2, ... \boldsymbol{y}_N] \in \mathbb{R}^{n \times N}$ be the data matrix of $N$ input signals, where $y_i \in \mathbb{R}^n$ denotes the $i$-th input signal with $n$-dimensional feature description.

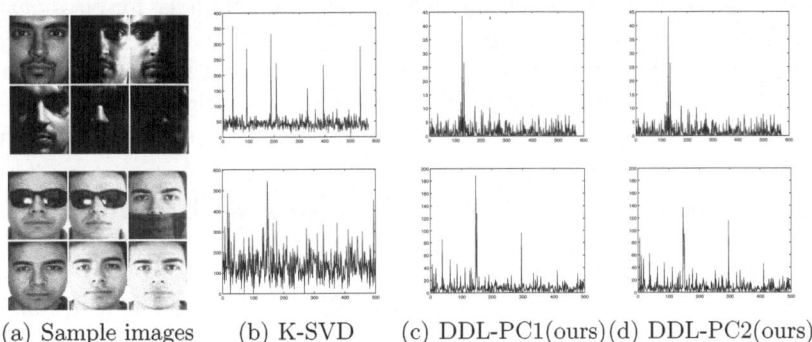

(a) Sample images     (b) K-SVD     (c) DDL-PC1(ours) (d) DDL-PC2(ours)

**Fig. 2.** Examples of sparse codes using dictionaries learned by K-SVD and our approaches on the Extended YaleB [25] and AR [26] databases. X axis indicates the dimensions of sparse codes. Y axis indicates the average of absolute sparse codes for different testing images from the same class. The first and second row correspond to class 9 in Extended YaleB (32 images) and class 30 in AR database (6 images), respectively. The consistency of sparse codes of signals from the same class should have low entropy (*i.e.*, less high values) of these average sparse codes.

Given a dictionary $A = [a_1, a_2, ..., a_K] \in \mathbb{R}^{n \times K}$, where $a_i$ is the $i$-th dictionary atom ($l_2$-normalized), sparse coding [5] with $l_1$ regularization computes the sparse representations $X = [x_1, x_2, ..., x_N] \in \mathbb{R}^{K \times N}$ of the input signals $Y$, through solving the following $l_1$-minimization problem,

$$X^* = \arg\min_X \sum_{i=1}^{N} (\|y_i - Ax_i\|_2^2 + \gamma \|x_i\|_1) \qquad (1)$$

where constant $\gamma$ is a sparsity constraint factor and the term $\|y_i - Ax_i\|_2^2$ denotes the reconstruction error. Each input signal $y_i$ can be represented as a sparse linear combination of a few dictionary atoms. The feature-sign search algorithm [7] is an efficient algorithm that can be used to solve (1).

## 2.2 Dictionary Learning

The goal of dictionary learning is to find optimized dictionaries that provides a succinct representation for most statistically representative input signals. The learning procedure can be formulated as solving the following problem [7],

$$< A^*, X^* > = \arg\min_{A,X} \sum_{i=1}^{N} (\|y_i - Ax_i\|_2^2 + \gamma \|x_i\|_1) \qquad (2)$$

The optimization problem is convex in $A$ (while holding $X$ fixed) and convex in $X$ (while holding $A$ fixed), but not convex in both simultaneously. Usually, the above objective is iteratively optimized in a two stage manner, by alternatively optimizing with respect to $A$ (bases) and $X$ (coefficients) while holding the other fixed. The formulation (2) only focuses on minimizing the reconstruction error and does not consider the discriminative power of a dictionary for classification tasks. Hence, some supervised approaches [12, 13, 21–23] have been proposed to improve the discriminative power of dictionary, by integrating the category label information into the objective function of dictionary learning. However, most of them do not explicitly deal with dictionary learning with pairwise constraints.

# 3   Discriminative Dictionary Learning with Pairwise Constraints (DDL-PC)

In this section, we present our Discriminative Dictionary Learning with Pairwise Constraints algorithm which takes into account the relationships of each pair of learned sparse codes $(\boldsymbol{x}_i, \boldsymbol{x}_j)$. Here, the intuition is to encourage signals from a similar pair to have similar sparse codes. We subsequently focus on the effects of adding a discriminative term, and a classification error term into the objective function in (2). We refer to them as DDL-PC1 and DDL-PC2, respectively.

## 3.1   DDL-PC1

To obtain discriminative sparse codes $\boldsymbol{x}$ with the pairwise constrained dictionary $A$, the objective function for dictionary construction is defined as:

$$
\begin{aligned}
< A^*, X^* > &= \arg\min_{A,X} \sum_{i=1}^{N} (\|\boldsymbol{y}_i - A\boldsymbol{x}_i\|_2^2 + \gamma\|\boldsymbol{x}_i\|_1) + \frac{\beta}{2} \sum_{i,j=1}^{N} (\|\boldsymbol{x}_i - \boldsymbol{x}_j\|_2^2 M_{ij}) \\
&= \arg\min_{A,X} \sum_{i=1}^{N} (\|\boldsymbol{y}_i - A\boldsymbol{x}_i\|_2^2 + \gamma\|\boldsymbol{x}_i\|_1) + \beta(Tr(X^T X D) - Tr(X^T X M)) \\
&= \arg\min_{A,X} \sum_{i=1}^{N} (\|\boldsymbol{y}_i - A\boldsymbol{x}_i\|_2^2 + \gamma\|\boldsymbol{x}_i\|_1) + \beta(Tr(X^T X L))
\end{aligned}
\tag{3}
$$

where the constants $\gamma$ and $\beta$ control the relative contribution of the corresponding terms. The first term $\|\boldsymbol{y}_i - A\boldsymbol{x}_i\|_2^2$ is the *reconstruction error term*, which evaluates the reconstruction error of the approximation to the input signals. The second term $\|\boldsymbol{x}_i\|_1$ is the *regularization term* for sparsity. The last term, which is new and proposed here, is the *discrimination term* called 'pairwise sparse code error' based on pairwise constraints which are encoded in matrix $M$. $D = diag\{d_1, ...d_N\}$ is a diagonal matrix whose diagonal elements are the sums of the row elements of $M$ (see below), $d_i = \sum_{j=1}^{N} M_{ij}$. $L = D - M$ is the Laplacian matrix. Matrix $M$ has different forms depending on the problems being considered. For example, in face verification, the relationship of a pair $(\boldsymbol{y}_i, \boldsymbol{y}_j)$ is given as same/different. Thus, given the sets of 'same' and 'different' pairs $\mathcal{S}$ and $\mathcal{D}$, we define matrix $M$ to encode the (dis)similarity information as

$$
M_{ij} = \begin{cases} +1, & \text{if } (\boldsymbol{y}_i, \boldsymbol{y}_j) \in \mathcal{S} \\ -1, & \text{if } (\boldsymbol{y}_i, \boldsymbol{y}_j) \in \mathcal{D} \\ 0, & \text{otherwise} \end{cases}
\tag{4}
$$

## 3.2 DDL-PC2

Although (3) can already be used for classification by defining $M$ based on the pairwise similarity constraints with category labels (see Sec. 3.4), the classification error can be further included as an additional term in the objective function in (3). Here we use a linear predictive classifier $f(\boldsymbol{x}; W) = W\boldsymbol{x}$. The objective function for learning a pairwise constrained dictionary $A$ with both reconstructive and discriminative power can then be defined as follows:

$$< A^*, X^*, W^* >= \underset{A,X,W}{\arg\min} \sum_{i=1}^{N} (\|\boldsymbol{y}_i - A\boldsymbol{x}_i\|_2^2 + \gamma\|\boldsymbol{x}_i\|_1)$$

$$+\frac{\beta}{2} \sum_{i,j=1}^{N} (\|\boldsymbol{x}_i - \boldsymbol{x}_j\|_2^2 M_{ij}) + \alpha \sum_{i=1}^{N} (\|\boldsymbol{h}_i - W\boldsymbol{x}_i\|_2^2 + \lambda\|W\|_2^2) \qquad (5)$$

The new term $\|\boldsymbol{h}_i - W\boldsymbol{x}_i\|_2^2 + \lambda\|W\|_2^2$, where $\|\boldsymbol{h}_i - W\boldsymbol{x}_i\|_2^2$ represents the classification error and $\|W\|_2^2$ is the regularization penalty term, supports learning an optimal linear predictive classifier. $\boldsymbol{h}_i = [0, 0, ...1...0, 0]^T \in \mathbb{R}^m$ ($m$: number of classes) is a label vector corresponding to an input signal $\boldsymbol{y}_i$, where the non-zero position indicates the class label of $\boldsymbol{y}_i$.

## 3.3 Optimization Procedure

In this section, we only describe the optimization procedure for DDL-PC2 since DDL-PC1 utilizes the same procedure except that $\alpha = 0$ in (6)(7)(8) and the classifier $W$ update step is not considered during dictionary learning. Solving (5) is a challenging task because the objective function is not convex for $A$, $X$ and $W$ simultaneously; but fortunately, it is convex in one variable when the other two variables are fixed. In [7], (2) was solved by an efficient feature-sign search algorithm. Motivated by [7], we optimize $A$, $X$ and $W$ alternatively. Algorithm 1 presents the pseudocode of algorithm DDL-PC2.

**Computing Sparse Codes $X$ with Fixed $A$ and $W$.** When $A$ and $W$ are fixed, we optimize $\boldsymbol{x}_i$ alternately and fix other $\boldsymbol{x}_j(j \neq i)$ for other signals. Optimizing (5) is equivalent to:

$$\min_{\boldsymbol{x}_i} \mathcal{L}(\boldsymbol{x}_i) + \gamma\|\boldsymbol{x}_i\|_1 \qquad (6)$$

where $\mathcal{L}(\boldsymbol{x}_i) = \|\boldsymbol{y}_i - A\boldsymbol{x}_i\|_2^2 + \beta(2\boldsymbol{x}_i^T(XL_i) - \boldsymbol{x}_i^T\boldsymbol{x}_i L_{ii}) + \alpha(\boldsymbol{x}_i^T W^T W\boldsymbol{x}_i - 2\boldsymbol{x}_i^T W^T \boldsymbol{h}_i)$, $L_i$ is the $i^{th}$ column of $L$ and $L_{ii}$ is the $(i, i)$ element of $L$. (6) is exactly the problem that the feature-sign search algorithm in [7] solves. [7] iteratively searches for the coefficient sign vector $\boldsymbol{\theta}$ for $\boldsymbol{x}_i$, then (6) reduces to a standard, unconstrained quadratic optimization problem (QP). To compute the analytical solution, we calculate the gradient of $\mathcal{L}(\boldsymbol{x}_i)$ with respect to $\boldsymbol{x}_i$:

$$\frac{\partial \mathcal{L}(\boldsymbol{x}_i)}{\partial \boldsymbol{x}_i} = 2A^T(A\boldsymbol{x}_i - \boldsymbol{y}_i) + 2\beta(XL_i) + 2\alpha(W^T W\boldsymbol{x}_i - W^T \boldsymbol{h}_i) + \gamma\boldsymbol{\theta} \qquad (7)$$

Finally the analytic solution of $\boldsymbol{x}_i$ can be obtained when we have $\frac{\partial \mathcal{L}(\boldsymbol{x}_i)}{\partial \boldsymbol{x}_i} = 0$:

$$\boldsymbol{x}_i^* = (A^T A + 2\beta L_{ii} I + 2\alpha W^T W)^{-1} (A^T \boldsymbol{y}_i + 2\alpha W^T \boldsymbol{h}_i - 2\beta \sum_{k \neq i} \boldsymbol{x}_k L_{ki} - \gamma \boldsymbol{\theta}) \quad (8)$$

In practice, a very small $\beta$ is chosen to guarantee the Hessian matrix ($A^T A + 2\beta L_{ii} I$) to be positive semidefinite, hence (3) is convex.

**Updating Dictionary $A$ with Fixed $X$ and $W$.** Given $X$ and $W$, we use the Lagrange dual in [7] to optimize the following objective function:

$$\min_A \sum_{i=1}^N \|\boldsymbol{y}_i - A\boldsymbol{x}_i\|_2^2 \quad s.t. \|\boldsymbol{a}_j\|_2^2 \leq c, \quad \forall j = 1...K. \quad (9)$$

The analytical solution of $A$ can be computed as: $A^* = YX^T(XX^T + \Lambda)^{-1}$, where $\Lambda$ is a diagonal matrix constructed from all the dual variables.

**Updating Classifier $W$ with Fixed $X$ and $A$.** Given $X$ and $A$, we employ the multivariate ridge regression model [22] to update $W$, with the quadratic loss and $l_2$ norm regularization:

$$\min_W \sum_{i=1}^N \|\boldsymbol{h}_i - W\boldsymbol{x}_i\|_2^2 + \lambda\|W\|_2^2, \quad (10)$$

which yields the following solution: $W^* = HX^T(XX^t + \lambda I)^{-1}$.

---

**Algorithm 1.** Discriminative Dictionary Learning with Pairwise Constraints-2 (DDL-PC2)

---

**Input**: input signals $Y$, Laplacian matrix $L$, label matrix $H$, regularization constant $\gamma$, $\beta$ and $\alpha$, iteration number $\hat{T}$
**Output:** learned dictionary $A$, classifier $W$ and sparse code $X$.
**Initialization:** Compute initial $A_0$ via K-SVD, initial $X_0$, $W_0$ using (1), (10)
    **for** $t = 1, 2, ...., \hat{T}$ **do**
        Sparse Coding: compute sparse code $X$ using (6);
        Dictionary Update: update dictionary $A$ using (9);
        Classifier Update: update classifier $W$ using (10).
    **end for**

---

### 3.4   Matching Approach

**Face Verification.** In face verification or pair matching problems, a similarity measure is typically learned from pairs of training images labeled as 'same' or 'different'; this provides less specific information than known identities - image labels. Given a training set of pairs, we first construct matrix $M$ with their pairwise relationships. For example, suppose three pairs of feature vectors are given - $(\boldsymbol{y}_1, \boldsymbol{y}_2)$ are features vectors from the same person, $(\boldsymbol{y}_3, \boldsymbol{y}_4)$ are also features vectors from the same person and $(\boldsymbol{y}_5, \boldsymbol{y}_6)$ are features vectors from different persons. Matrix $M$ would then be:

$$
M = \begin{array}{c}
\phantom{y1} \\ y1 \\ y2 \\ y3 \\ y4 \\ y5 \\ y6
\end{array}
\begin{bmatrix}
y1 & y2 & y3 & y4 & y5 & y6 \\
0 & 1 & 0 & 0 & 0 & 0 \\
1 & 0 & 0 & 0 & 0 & 0 \\
0 & 0 & 0 & 1 & 0 & 0 \\
0 & 0 & 1 & 0 & 0 & 0 \\
0 & 0 & 0 & 0 & 0 & -1 \\
0 & 0 & 0 & 0 & -1 & 0
\end{bmatrix}
$$

With the given training set of pairs and the corresponding matrix $M$, an optimized discriminative dictionary $A$ (initialized by K-SVD algorithm [6]) can be learned using DDL-PC1. Then, when a new test pair $\boldsymbol{y}_i$ and $\boldsymbol{y}_j$ comes in, we can compute the optimized sparse codes $\boldsymbol{x}_i$ and $\boldsymbol{x}_j$ with dictionary $A$ by solving (1). Finally, the cosine similarity [3, 27] of the two sparse codes is used as the similarity metric between the image pair. This similarity is thresholded to yield a binary decision of same/different.

**Face Recognition.** In face recognition, class labels are given for each image in the training set. The pair relationships are derived from the category labels. If $\boldsymbol{y}_i$ and $\boldsymbol{y}_j$ belong to the same class, we define $M_{ij}$ as 1; otherwise we set it to 0. Matrix $M$ encoding the (dis)similarity information can be defined as

$$
M_{ij} = \begin{cases} 1, \text{ if } (\boldsymbol{y}_i, \boldsymbol{y}_j) \in c_k, k = 1...m \\ 0, \text{ otherwise} \end{cases} \tag{11}
$$

There are two ways to construct the classifier $W$ here. For DDL-PC1, we obtain $A$ and $X$ first and then the matrix $W$ is trained separately using (10). For DDL-PC2, we obtain $A$ and $W$ jointly using Algorithm 1.

Then, when a new test sample $\boldsymbol{y}_i$ comes in, we compute its sparse code $\boldsymbol{x}_i$ with respect to $A$ by solving (1). Finally we simply use $W$ to estimate a class label vector for $\boldsymbol{y}_i$: $l = W\boldsymbol{x}_i$, where $l \in \mathbb{R}^m$. The label of $\boldsymbol{y}_i$ is assigned as the index $j$ where $l_j$ is the largest element of $l$.

## 4   Experimental Results

We evaluate the proposed algorithm on the LFW dataset [8] for face verification task, and the Extended YaleB database [25] and AR face database [26] for face recognition task.

### 4.1   Face Verification

**LFW Database.** The Labeled Faces in the Wild (LFW) dataset was recently introduced as a challenging benchmark for face verification in unconstrained environments. Real-world images in the LFW dataset exhibit visual variations caused by pose, facial appearance, age, lighting, expression, occlusion, scale, camera, misalignment hairstyle, etc.

The dataset comes with a division of 10 splits/folds (disjoint subject identities) for cross validation with three evaluation protocols: unsupervised, image-restricted, and image-unrestricted protocols [8]. We only consider the most common protocol called 'image-restricted': in this setting, it is known whether an image pair belongs to the same person or not, but identity information of the images is not provided. The aligned version lfw-a is used in all experiments.

In our evaluations, for each independent fold, we randomly choose 500 pairs of 'same' and 500 pairs of 'different' from the training set (other 9 splits, 5400 image pairs) to learn an optimal dictionary through DDL-PC1. The learned dictionary consists of 510 atoms. $\gamma$ is set to be 30 and $\beta$ is set to be 0.1.

**Experimental Setup.** All the faces are cropped and rescaled to $80 \times 148$. According to [28–31], combining multiple similarities from different descriptors usually boosts performance. In our experiments, the intensity, HoG, LBP, and Gabor features are used. Finally, the four scores for different features are fused by averaging (no training) or training SVM. For extracting HoG and LBP features, we divide the faces into blocks of $20 \times 20$ and extract the 16-bin HoG feature and the 59-bin uniform LBP feature for each block. For Gabor features, we adopt five scales and eight orientations of the Gabor filters. The final Gabor feature vector is obtained by concatenating the responses at every 10 pixels in order to reduce the dimensionality of the feature vector to manageable size.

Fig.3 shows some examples (5 'same' and 5 'different') of testing image pairs from the LFW dataset. The similarity scores obtained from KSVD dictionary learning and our DDL-PC1 are listed under each pair. As it shows, compared to KSVD, higher similarity scores for the 'same pairs' and lower similarity scores for 'different' pairs are obtained by our discriminative dictionary learning.

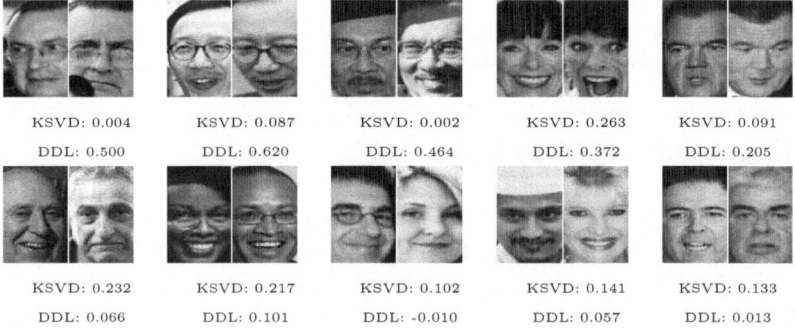

**Fig. 3.** Examples of some image pairs from the LFW dataset and the similarity scores obtained from KSVD dictionary learning and proposed DDL-PC1 respectively. Top row: Five examples of '**same**' pairs; Bottom row: Five examples of '**different**' pairs.

Table 1 summarizes the performances of our method with individual feature and their fusion. The first column shows the face verification accuracy (at equal error rate) obtained from using the Euclidean distance of the original feature vector pairs as similarity measure. The second column shows the accuracy from the dictionary learned by K-SVD (followed by the $l_1$ based sparse coding) and the third column shows those from the proposed DDL-PC1. The combined scores are the results from fusing the four scores for all features by averaging (no training) or training SVM. Clearly, DDL-PC1 works best in all situations comparing to 'Euclidean' and 'K-SVD'.

**Table 1.** Mean ($\pm$ standard error) verification accuracy at equal error rate of different feature descriptors and their fused scores on LFW dataset. Euclidean, dictionaries learned by K-SVD and the proposed DDL-PC1 are compared.

| Descriptor | Euclidean | K-SVD | DDL-PC1 |
|---|---|---|---|
| Intensity | 0.7140±0.0056 | 0.7424±0.0051 | 0.7870±0.0048 |
| HoG | 0.6803±0.0046 | 0.7524±0.0049 | 0.8030±0.0037 |
| LBP | 0.6763±0.0054 | 0.7433±0.0052 | 0.7876±0.0032 |
| Gabor | 0.6920±0.0041 | 0.7646±0.0047 | 0.7996±0.0052 |
| Combined (Avg) | 0.7013±0.0045 | 0.8056±0.0045 | 0.8410±0.0041 |
| Combined (SVM) | 0.7216±0.0047 | 0.8196±0.0036 | 0.8603±0.0033 |

**Comparison with the State-of-the-art Methods.** Table 2 shows the face verification accuracy of our method compared with recent methods with the Image-Restricted protocol. The 'flip' means that when comparing image pair $I$ and $J$, we also compare $I$ and the horizontally flipped image of $J$ to reduce the effects of pose variation. Then, the average of the two scores is taken as the final similarity score. Figure 4 contains the ROC curve of our approach (dotted red line), along with the ROC curves of selected recent state-of-the-art methods with the Image-Restricted protocol for presentation clarity.

The results show that the verification accuracy of our approach is comparable with the state-of-the-art methods on the LFW benchmark in the challenging image-restricted protocol. Moreover, the methods marked by '*' use training data outside of LFW for facial point detection or pose/illumination classification and so on. Those can have a significant impact on verification accuracy, thus not directly comparable. Kumar [32] achieved excellent results, marginally lower than ours. However, the work of Kumar requires expensive training of high-level classifiers incorporating a huge volume of images outside of the LFW dataset. The LE method [30] relies on facial feature point detectors. Predict-Associate [33] not only relies on facial feature point detectors, but also uses the Multi-PIE dataset with identities covering 7 poses and 4 illumination conditions as prior knowledge. For other methods we are in the same category with, [31] is most comparable. Wolf [31] also combines multiple descriptors; their method adds up several layers of information and leverages metric learning [33]. Moreover, one disadvantage of Wolf's method is that it requires background samples (a fixed set

**Table 2.** Mean (± standard error) verification accuracy on the LFW dataset, image-restricted protocol using the proposed DDL-PC1, and the same model except the addition of the 'flipped' image idea. '*' denotes methods using outside training data.

| Method | Accuracy |
|---|---|
| LDML [1] | 0.7927±0.0060 |
| Hybrid [29] | 0.8398±0.0035 |
| Combined b/g samples based [31] | 0.8683±0.0034 |
| *Attribute and Simile classifiers [32] | 0.8529±0.0123 |
| Single LE + holistic [30] | 0.8122±0.0053 |
| *Multiple LE + comp [30] | 0.8445±0.0046 |
| *Predict-Associate [33] | 0.9057 ±0.0056 |
| LARK + OSS [34] | 0.8512 ±0.0037 |
| **DDL-PC1** | **0.8603 ±0.0033** |
| **DDL-PC1 (flip)** | **0.8710 ±0.0035** |

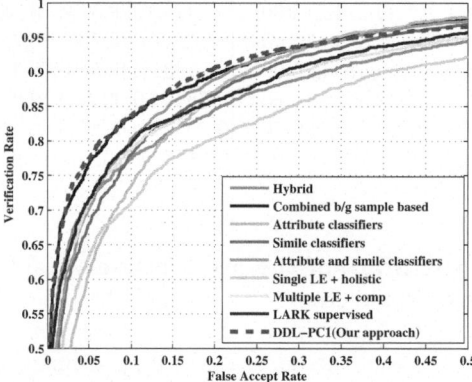

**Fig. 4.** ROC curves for View 2 of the LFW dataset (Image-Restricted protocol). Only shown with the selected **best** results that recently reported for clarity.

of 'negative' examples) that have similar properties as the faces being compared and do not contain faces from any person who might subsequently appear in a pair to be compared. It learns models for each pair being compared on-the-fly, which might not be desirable in practical applications. Overall, our DDL-PC1 achieves competitive accuracy without local feature identification or any other additional information.

## 4.2   Face Recognition

**Extended YaleB Database.** The Extended YaleB database [25] contains 38 persons under 64 illumination conditions, $2,414$ frontal-face images. The original images are cropped to $192 \times 168$. We used the random face features [5, 13] to represent the face images. Following [12, 13], we project each face image into a 504-dimensional feature vector using a random matrix of zero-mean normal distribution. Each row of the random matrix is $l_2$ normalized. We randomly sample 32 images per person for training and taking the rest as testing. We repeated 10 times such this sampling process and report their average as the recognition accuracy. The parameter $\gamma$ is set to 20; $\beta$ and $\alpha$ are set to 2.0 and $\lambda$ is 1.0 here.

We fix the dictionary size of 570 atoms as in [12, 13] and evaluate our approach. We compare the recognition accuracy with K-SVD [6], D-KSVD [13], SRC [5], LLC [35] and recently proposed LC-KSVD [12]. We obtain the original implementations of LC-KSVD [1] from the authors [12]. A D-KSVD is implemented by eliminating the label consistent term in LC-KSVD. For SRC, we randomly select the average of dictionary size per person from each person and report the best result we achieved. For LLC, we perform the experiment with 30 local bases, which determines the sparsity of the LLC codes. The results are summarized in Table 3. Our approaches achieve better results than K-SVD, D-KSVD, SRC and LLC and are comparable to LC-KSVD.

We also evaluate our approach using random-face features and dictionary sizes 190, 380, 570 and 760. Then we compare the classification accuracy with state-of-art approaches including LC-KSVD, D-KSVD, K-SVD, SRC and LLC which use the same features and dictionary sizes. As shown in Figure 5, our approach has higher accuracy than K-SVD, D-KSVD, SRC and LLC, and is comparable to LC-KSVD.

**Table 3.** Recognition results using random-face features on the Extended YaleB.

| Method | K-SVD[6] | D-KSVD[13] | SRC[5] | LLC[35] | LC-KSVD[12] | **DDL-PC1** | **DDL-PC2** |
|---|---|---|---|---|---|---|---|
| Acc. (%) | 90.5 | 94.1 | 88.6 | 82.3 | 95.0 | **94.5** | **95.3** |

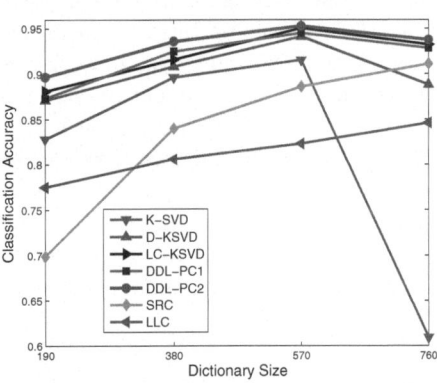

**Fig. 5.** Recognition performance on the Extended YaleB with varying number of dictionary sizes

**AR Face Database.** The AR face database [26] contains over 4,000 color face images of 126 persons taken during two sessions, with 26 images per person. The main characteristic of the AR database is that it includes frontal views of faces

---

[1] LC-KSVD here is the approach LC-KSVD2 in [12].

with different facial expressions, lighting conditions and occlusion conditions. All the faces are cropped to $165 \times 120$. Following the standard evaluation protocol, we use a subset of the database consisting of $2,600$ images from 50 males and 50 females. For each person, we randomly select 20 images for training and the other six for testing. We report the results from the average of ten such random splits. Each face image is projected into the 540-dimensional feature vector with a randomly generated matrix as in [12, 13]. The feature descriptors used here are random face features. The parameter $\gamma$ is set to be 30, $\beta$ is 0.5, $\alpha$ and $\lambda$ are 1.0.

We evaluate our approach with a dictionary of size 500 and compare with state-of-art approaches [5, 6, 12, 13, 35]. As shown in Table 4, both DDL-PC1 and DDL-PC2 obtain better results than K-SVD, D-KSVD, SRC, LLC and LC-KSVD. DDL-PC2 obtains a 2% improvement over DDL-PC1.

**Table 4.** Recognition results using random face features on the AR face database

| Method | K-SVD[6] | D-KSVD[13] | SRC[5] | LLC[35] | LC-KSVD[12] | **DDL-PC1** | **DDL-PC2** |
|---|---|---|---|---|---|---|---|
| Acc. (%) | 87.2 | 88.8 | 74.5 | 88.7 | 93.7 | **94.0** | **96.0** |

## 5  Conclusions

We presented a novel dictionary learning approach that tackles the pair matching and classification problem in a unified framework. We introduced a discriminative term called 'pairwise sparse code error' based on pairwise constraints and combined it with the classification error term to form the objective function of dictionary learning for better discriminating power. The objective function can be optimized by employing the efficient feature-sign search algorithm. The effectiveness of our approach was evaluated on both face verification and face recognition tasks. Experimental results on face verification demonstrated that our approach is competitive with existing techniques without using facial feature point detectors or other additional information. We also compared our approach with several recently proposed dictionary learning methods on two well-known face databases. Our approach can obtain comparable face recognition performance to state-of-art on both databases.

**Acknowledgement.** This work was supported by the Army Research Office MURI Grant W911NF-09-1-0383.

## References

1. Guillaumin, M., Verbeek, J., Schmid, C.: Is that you? metric learning approaches for face identification. In: ICCV (2009)
2. Davis, J.V., Kulis, B., Jain, P., Sra, S., Dhillon, I.S.: Information-theoretic metric learning. In: ICML (2007)

3. Nguyen, H.V., Bai, L.: Cosine Similarity Metric Learning for Face Verification. In: Kimmel, R., Klette, R., Sugimoto, A. (eds.) ACCV 2010, Part II. LNCS, vol. 6493, pp. 709–720. Springer, Heidelberg (2011)

4. Nowak, E., Jurie, F.: Learning visual similarity measures for comparing never seen objects. In: CVPR (2007)

5. Wright, J., Yang, A.Y., Ganesh, A., Sastry, S.S., Ma, Y.: Robust face recognition via sparse representation. IEEE Trans. Pattern Anal. Mach. Intell. 31 (2009)

6. Aharon, M., Elad, M., Bruckstein, A.: K-svd: An algorithm for designing overcomplete dictionries for sparse representation. IEEE Trans. on Signal Processing 54, 4311–4322 (2006)

7. Lee, H., Battle, A., Raina, R., Ng, A.Y.: Efficient sparse coding algorithms. In: NIPS (2007)

8. Huang, G.B., Ramesh, M., Berg, T., Learned-Miller, E.: Labeled faces in the wild: A database for studying face recognition in unconstrained environments. Technical report, University of Massachusetts, Amherst (2007)

9. Nagesh, P., Li, B.: A compressive sensing approach for expression-invariant face recognition. In: CVPR (2009)

10. Yang, M., Zhang, L.: Gabor Feature Based Sparse Representation for Face Recognition with Gabor Occlusion Dictionary. In: Daniilidis, K., Maragos, P., Paragios, N. (eds.) ECCV 2010, Part VI. LNCS, vol. 6316, pp. 448–461. Springer, Heidelberg (2010)

11. Gao, S., Tsang, I.W.-H., Chia, L.-T.: Kernel Sparse Representation for Image Classification and Face Recognition. In: Daniilidis, K., Maragos, P., Paragios, N. (eds.) ECCV 2010, Part IV. LNCS, vol. 6314, pp. 1–14. Springer, Heidelberg (2010)

12. Jiang, Z., Lin, Z., Davis, L.: Learning a discriminative dictionary for sparse coding via label consistent k-svd. In: CVPR (2011)

13. Zhang, Q., Li, B.: Discriminative k-svd for dictionary learning in face recognition. In: CVPR (2010)

14. Yang, M., 0006, L.Z., Feng, X., Zhang, D.: Fisher discrimination dictionary learning for sparse representation. In: ICCV (2011)

15. Huang, K., Aviyente, S.: Sparse representation for signal classification. In: NIPS (2007)

16. Boureau, Y., Bach, F., LeCun, Y., Ponce, J.: Learning mid-level features for recognition. In: CVPR (2010)

17. Grosse, R., Raina, R., Kwong, H., Ng, A.Y.: Shift-invariant sparse coding for audio classification. In: Conf. on Uncertainty in AI (2007)

18. Mairal, J., Leordeanu, M., Bach, F., Hebert, M., Ponce, J.: Discriminative Sparse Image Models for Class-Specific Edge Detection and Image Interpretation. In: Forsyth, D., Torr, P., Zisserman, A. (eds.) ECCV 2008, Part III. LNCS, vol. 5304, pp. 43–56. Springer, Heidelberg (2008)

19. Zhang, W., Surve, A., Fern, X., Dietterich, T.: Learning non-redundant codebooks for classifying complex objects. In: ICML (2009)

20. Rodriguez, F., Sapiro, G.: Sparse representations for image classification: Learning discriminative and reconstructive non-parametric dictionaries (2007); IMA Preprint 2213

21. Yang, J., Yu, K., Huang, T.: Supervised translation-invariant sparse coding. In: CVPR (2010)

22. Pham, D., Venkatesh, S.: Joint learning and dictionary construction for pattern recognition. In: CVPR (2008)

23. Mairal, J., Bach, F., Ponce, J., Sapiro, G., Zisserman, A.: Supervised dictionary learning. In: NIPS (2009)

24. Gao, S., Tsang, I.W., Chia, L.T., Zhao, P.: Local features are not lonely - laplacian sparse coding for image classification. In: CVPR (2010)
25. Georghiades, A., Belhumeur, P., Kriegman, D.: From few to many: Illumination cone models for face recognition under variable lighting and pose. IEEE Trans. Pattern Anal. Mach. Intelligence 23, 643–660 (2001)
26. Martinez, A.M., Benavente, R.: The AR Face Database. Technical report (1998)
27. Yan, S., Wang, H., Tang, X., Huang, T.: Exploring feature descritors for face recognition. In: ICASSP (2007)
28. Wolf, L., Hassner, T., Taigman, Y.: Descriptor based methods in the wild. In: ECCV (2008)
29. Taigman, Y., Wolf, L., Hassner, T.: Multiple one-shots for utilizing class label information. In: BMVC (2009)
30. Cao, Z., Yin, Q., Tang, X., Sun, J.: Face recognition with learning-based descriptor. In: CVPR (2010)
31. Wolf, L., Hassner, T., Taigman, Y.: Similarity Scores Based on Background Samples. In: Zha, H., Taniguchi, R.-i., Maybank, S. (eds.) ACCV 2009, Part II. LNCS, vol. 5995, pp. 88–97. Springer, Heidelberg (2010)
32. Kumar, N., Berg, A.C., Belhumeur, P.N., Nayar, S.K.: Attribute and Simile Classifiers for Face Verification. In: ICCV (2009)
33. Yin, Q., Tang, X., Sun, J.: An associate-predict model for face recognition. In: CVPR (2011)
34. Seo, H.J., Milanfar, P.: Face verification using the lark representation. IEEE Transactions on Information Forensics and Security 6, 1275–1286 (2011)
35. Wang, J., Yang, J., Yu, K., Lv, F., Huang, T., Gong, Y.: Locality-constrained linear coding for image classification. In: CVPR (2010)

# Adaptive Unsupervised Multi-view Feature Selection for Visual Concept Recognition

Yinfu Feng[1], Jun Xiao[1], Yueting Zhuang[1], and Xiaoming Liu[2]

[1] School of Computer Science, Zhejiang University, Hangzhou 310027, P.R.China
[2] Department of Computer Science and Engineering, Michigan State University, USA

**Abstract.** To reveal and leverage the correlated and complemental information between different views, a great amount of multi-view learning algorithms have been proposed in recent years. However, unsupervised feature selection in multi-view learning is still a challenge due to lack of data labels that could be utilized to select the discriminative features. Moreover, most of the traditional feature selection methods are developed for the single-view data, and are not directly applicable to the multi-view data. Therefore, we propose an unsupervised learning method called Adaptive Unsupervised Multi-view Feature Selection (AUMFS) in this paper. AUMFS attempts to jointly utilize three kinds of vital information, i.e., data cluster structure, data similarity and the correlations between different views, contained in the original data together for feature selection. To achieve this goal, a robust sparse regression model with the $l_{2,1}$-norm penalty is introduced to predict data cluster labels, and at the same time, multiple view-dependent visual similar graphs are constructed to flexibly model the visual similarity in each view. Then, AUMFS integrates data cluster labels prediction and adaptive multi-view visual similar graph learning into a unified framework. To solve the objective function of AUMFS, a simple yet efficient iterative method is proposed. We apply AUMFS to three visual concept recognition applications (i.e., social image concept recognition, object recognition and video-based human action recognition) on four benchmark datasets. Experimental results show the proposed method significantly outperforms several state-of-the-art feature selection methods. More importantly, our method is not very sensitive to the parameters and the optimization method converges very fast.

## 1 Introduction

Owing to the increasingly powerful computational capabilities and the rapid development of feature selection techniques, objects are often represented by multiple heterogenous features from various representations in many visual concept recognition tasks [1–3]. Each representation of feature characterizes these objects in one specific feature space and has particular physical meaning and statistic property. Conventionally this type of data is named as multi-view data to distinguish from the single-view data. One typical example is that a color image can be represented by multiple heterogeneous visual features, such as global

K.M. Lee et al. (Eds.): ACCV 2012, Part I, LNCS 7724, pp. 343–357, 2013.
© Springer-Verlag Berlin Heidelberg 2013

features [1] (e.g., color, texture and shape) and local features (e.g., SIFT [4], LBP [5] and GLOH [6]). Similarly, human action is often associated with multiple visual features, which can be either appearance features (e.g., color, texture, edge) or motion features (e.g., motion history and optical flow) [3].

Since different views of features characterize different aspects of the objects and have different intrinsic discriminative power, an intuitive idea is to combine them to improve the recognition performance. However, most traditional data mining and machine learning methods are developed for the single-view data scenario, and they may not be applied to the multi-view data directly [7]. To tackle this problem, a straightforward solution is to concatenate features of all views and transform a multi-view data into a single-view data. However, this solution disregards the underlying correlations between different views, and moreover, it also lacks of physical meaning. On the other hand, it has shown extensively in prior research that leveraging information contained in multiple views can dramatically improve the learning performance [7–9]. As a result, multi-view learning research has been continuing to flourish in recent years. A great deal of efforts have been carried out in this field with a wide variety of applications, such as dimensionality reduction [7], clustering [8] and classification [9].

To the best of our knowledge, little progress has been made on multi-view feature selection, whereas it plays a crucial role in learning more compact and accurate feature representation from the original multiple high-dimensional features. In general, feature selection has twofold advantages [10]: 1) the learned feature subset has lower dimensionality than the original one, making the subsequential computation more efficient; 2) most relevant features can be selected, thus irrelevant and noisy features are discarded, potentially leading to more accurate results.

Based on whether the data labels are available, existing feature selection methods can be broadly divided into two categories, i.e., supervised feature selection methods and unsupervised feature selection methods. The former methods usually select discriminative features according to labels of the training data, such as Fisher Score [11] and sparse multi-output regression [12]. While the latter ones, such as Laplacian Score [13], Feature Ranking [14] and Multi-Cluster Feature Selection [15], select features best preserve the data similarity or manifold structure derived from the whole feature set. It is well known that, in many real world applications, labeled data are limited while unlabeled data are ample. Also, the unlabeled data are much easier to obtain than the labeled ones. Consequently, there is a growing need for effective and efficient unsupervised learning approaches.

However, most of the existing unsupervised learning methods are also developed for the single-view data, and thus they fail to leverage the correlated and complementary information between different views when they are applied to the multi-view data. Furthermore, in addition to exploit data similarity or manifold structure information, some researchers recently suggested to utilize data cluster labels to select discriminative features in the unsupervised scenario [10, 16]. But, both [10] and [16] are devised for the single-view scenario, so they still suffer from the aforementioned problem. Meanwhile, the cluster label prediction functions used in [10, 16] are not robust, which will be discussed in Section 2.

In light of this, we propose an unsupervised multi-view learning method called Adaptive Unsupervised Multi-view Feature Selection (AUMFS) algorithm in this paper. The flowchart of AUMFS is illustrated in Fig.1. AUMFS integrates three kinds of vital information, i.e., data cluster structure, data similarity and the correlations between different views, together for the unsupervised multi-view feature selection. Specifically, an improved robust sparse regression model with the $l_{2,1}$-norm penalty is adopted to predict data cluster labels based on data cluster structure. At the same time, multiple view-dependent visual similar graphs are constructed to flexibly model the visual similarity in each view and then these learned graphs are united with a non-negative view-weight vector to form the objective function of adaptive multi-view visual similar graph learning, which leverages the correlations between different views and establishes adaptive weights for each view. Finally, we integrate data cluster labels prediction and adaptive multi-view visual similar graph learning into a unified framework. Based on this framework, we can simultaneously estimate data cluster labels, adaptive view weights, and feature selection matrix. We apply AUMFS to three visual concept recognition tasks and compare it with several state-of-the-art methods. Our extensive experiments on four benchmark datasets show that AUMFS has very competitive performance with state-of-the-art feature selection methods. More importantly, AUMFS is not very sensitive to the parameters and the optimization method converges very fast.

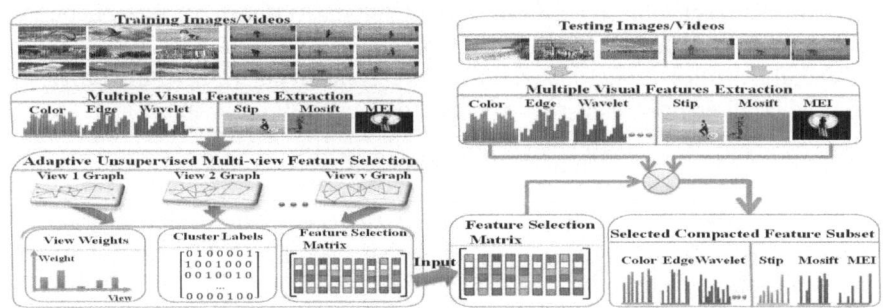

**Fig. 1.** The flowchart of proposed AUMFS

## 2   Proposed Methodology

### 2.1   Notations

To better present the details of AUMFS, we provide some important notations used in the rest of this paper. Capital letters, e.g., $X$, represent matrices or sets. $X_{ij}$ is the $(i,j)$th entry of $X$ and $X_{i:}$ denotes the $i$th row of $X$. Lower case letters, e.g., $x$, represent vectors or scale values, and $x_i$ is the $i$th element of vector $x$. Superscript $(i)$, e.g., $X^{(i)}$ and $x^{(i)}$, represents datum from the $i$th view. Throughout this paper, $I_c$ denotes the $c \times c$ identity matrix. $\|X\|_F$ denotes the Frobenius norm of matrix $X$ and for an arbitrary matrix $X \in R^{p \times q}$, its $l_{2,1}$-norm is defined as $\|X\|_{2,1} = \sum_{i=1}^{p} \sqrt{\sum_{j=1}^{q} X_{ij}^2}$.

## 2.2   The Objective Function

Given a centered multi-view data set which consists of $n$ objects from $m$ views, we denote this set as $\mathcal{X} = \{x_1, \ldots, x_n\}$, wherein $x_i = [(x_i^{(1)})^T, \ldots, (x_i^{(m)})^T]^T \in R^{(\sum_{v=1}^{m} d_v) \times 1}$ is the $i$th multi-view datum and $x_i^{(v)} \in R^{d_v \times 1}$ is its $v$th view feature. Thus, the feature data matrix of $v$th view and all views can be denoted as $X^{(v)} = [x_1^{(v)}, \ldots, x_n^{(v)}]^T$ and $X = [X^{(1)}, \ldots, X^{(m)}]^T \in R^{d \times n}$ respectively, wherein $d = \sum_{v=1}^{m} d_v$.

To select the compact and relevant feature subset, we argue that the utilization of three kinds of vital information, which are data cluster structure, data similarity and the correlations between different views, can boost the performance. The reason is that the first one reflects the discriminative information contained in different clusters, the second one holds the data geometric structure in the original high dimensional feature space and the third one may enhance or correct the weak views. Meanwhile,

Now, we first elaborate on how to utilize the data cluster structure information and define a scaled data cluster label matrix $F = [f_1, \ldots, f_n]^T \in R^{n \times c}$, which can be regarded as pseudo class labels, wherein $c$ is the data cluster number and $f_i$ is the estimated label of $x_i \in X$ by a prediction function $p(x)$. Clearly, $F$ represents the discriminative information of the data. Hence we now encounter a problem: how to construct or learn the prediction function $p(x)$? By assuming $F$ is available, to learn $p(x)$ based on $F$, a reasonable choice is to minimize the total prediction error of $p(x)$ with respect to $F$ over all data samples:

$$\min \sum_{i=1}^{n} loss(p(x_i), f_i). \tag{1}$$

In [10], the authors implicitly assumed that there is a "hard" linear transformation between features and pseudo labels, i.e., $p(x_i) = W^T x_i$. However, this transformation is likely to be nonlinear in real-world applications [17]. To mitigate this problem, an explicitly "soft" linear constrained transformation has been adopted in [16] by using a $l_{2,1}$-norm regularized least square loss function, which can be rewritten in a matrix form:

$$\min \|X^T W - F\|_F^2 + \beta \|W\|_{2,1}, \tag{2}$$

where $W \in R^{d \times c}$. We denote this loss function as $LS\_L21$. Thus, the relationship between data features and data cluster labels are specified by Eq.(2). More importantly, the data cluster structure information has utilized via $F$ which reflects the discriminative information of the data.

Because the error of each data sample used in Eq.(2) is squared residue error in the form of $\|W^T x_i - f_i\|^2$, a few outliers with large errors can easily dominate the objective function. Therefore, the above loss function is well-known to be unstable w.r.t. noise and outliers [18, 19]. Unfortunately, many real-world data are likely to contain noise and outliers. Moreover, the data cluster label matrix $F$ is normally learned via clustering methods, and tends to contain some labeling errors. For this reason, a robust loss function for learning data cluster label prediction function is desired. Inspired by [19, 20], we assume that the mapping from data features to data labels can be approximated by a robust sparse regression model with the $l_{2,1}$-norm penalty, which can be formulated as:

$$\min \|X^T W - F\|_{2,1} + \beta \|W\|_{2,1}. \tag{3}$$

In this robust formulation, we replace the Frobenius norm on the regression term with a $l_{2,1}$-norm, which brings twofold benefits: 1) since the residue error has changed to be not squared, the large errors due to outliers do not dominate the loss function; 2) the $l_{2,1}$-norm constraint results in row sparseness property, which is consistent with the ideal feature selection matrix $W$. We denote this improved robust loss function as $L21\_L21$.

We use a 2D toy data experiment to illustrate the robustness of $L21\_L21$ in Fig.2. In this experiment, two classes of artificial data samples are generated. Ten randomly selected data samples are assigned labels, wherein three samples contain the error labels. We use these labeled data samples to train $LS\_L21$ and $L21\_L21$ respectively and then use the learned $W$ to predict cluster labels for all data. To make the comparison fair, we tune $\beta$ from $\{10^{-4}, 10^{-2}, 1, 10^2, 10^4\}$ and report the best prediction results for each model. From Fig. 2(c) and Fig.2(b), we observe that $L21\_L21$ is much more robuster than $LS\_L21$.

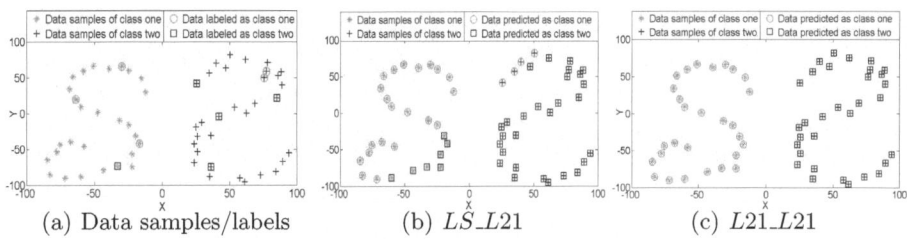

(a) Data samples/labels          (b) $LS\_L21$          (c) $L21\_L21$

**Fig. 2.** 2D toy data for label prediction. (a) shows the original data samples and the selected labeled samples. (b) and (c) show the prediction results by $LS\_L21$ and $L21\_L21$ respectively.

Recent studies [7, 13, 14, 21] have shown that in many practical applications, data samples lie on a low-dimensional manifold embedding in a high dimensional abient space. Hence, it is necessary to consider the data similarity or data geometric structure in feature selection. For any particular $v$th view data $X^{(v)}$, a view-depended visual similar graph $A^{(v)}$ is constructed according to the $v$th view features, whose element $A_{ij}^{(v)}$ reflects the visual similarity between the two features $x_i^{(v)}$ and $x_j^{(v)}$. There exist two popular ways for the graph construction:

one is the $k$-nearest-neighbor method, and the other is the $\epsilon$-ball based method. To reduce the number of parameters, we adopt the former one and define $A^{(v)}$ as follows:

$$A_{ij}^{(v)} = \begin{cases} 1 \text{ if } x_i^{(v)} \text{ is among the } k\text{-nearest-neighbors of } x_j^{(v)} \text{ and vice versa,} \\ 0 \text{ otherwise.} \end{cases}$$

To preserve the data geometric structure, it is essential to preserve the local consistency that similar data should have high probability to be clustered into the same class. To achieve this goal, we minimize the following objective function for the $v$th view:

$$\min \frac{1}{2} \sum_{l=1}^{c} \sum_{i,j=1}^{n} (F_{il} - F_{jl})^2 A_{ij}^{(v)} \qquad s.t. \quad F^T F = I_c. \qquad (4)$$

Note that

$$\sum_{l=1}^{c} \sum_{i,j=1}^{n} (F_{il} - F_{jl})^2 A_{ij}^{(v)} = \sum_{i,j=1}^{n} A_{ij}^{(v)} (f_i^T f_i + f_j^T f_j - 2f_i^T f_j)$$
$$= 2tr(F^T (D^{(v)} - A^{(v)})F) = 2tr(F^T L^{(v)} F), \quad (5)$$

where $tr(\cdot)$ denotes the trace operator, $D^{(v)}$ is a diagonal matrix with $D_{ii}^{(v)} = \sum_{j=1}^{n} A_{ij}^{(v)}$, and $L^{(v)} = D^{(v)} - A^{(v)}$ is the geometric laplacian matrix. Thus, Eq.(4) can be reformulated as:

$$\min tr(F^T L^{(v)} F) \qquad s.t. \quad F^T F = I_c. \qquad (6)$$

Because different views of features characterize different aspects of the objects, the intrinsic difference of each view leads to different contribution to the final recognition results [7]. Meanwhile, the underlying correlated and complemental information between different views may be exploited to enhance or correct the weak views. Thus, we are motivated to exploit these information. By combining all of the view-dependent geometric laplacian matrices using an adaptive non-negative view-weight vector $\lambda = [\lambda_1, \ldots, \lambda_m]^T \in R^{m \times 1}$, we obtain the adaptive multi-view visual similar graph learning objective function as follows:

$$\min_{F,\lambda} \sum_{v=1}^{m} \lambda_v tr(F^T L^{(v)} F) = \min tr(F^T \sum_{v=1}^{m} \lambda_v L^{(v)} F)$$
$$s.t. \quad F^T F = I_c, \sum_{v=1}^{m} \lambda_v = 1, \lambda_v \geq 0. \qquad (7)$$

Also, the intrinsic discriminative ability of each view is revealed by $\lambda$.

To leverage aforementioned three kinds of vital information simultaneously, we integrate data cluster labels prediction and adaptive multi-view visual similar graph learning into a unified framework:

$$\min_{F,\lambda,W} tr(F^T \sum_{v=1}^{m} \lambda_v L^{(v)} F) + \alpha\|X^T W - F\|_{2,1} + \beta\|W\|_{2,1}$$
$$s.t. \quad F^T F = I_c, \sum_{v=1}^{m} \lambda_v = 1, \lambda_v \geq 0. \qquad (8)$$

However, there still remains two issues of Eq.(8). The first one is regarding the sign of $F$. Like most clustering algorithms, we impose the orthogonal constraint on $F$. While it is still likely to have mixed signs in the final result of $F$ and it may severely deviate from the ideal solution that only 0 and 1 are contained in $F$. Moreover, since $F$ is defined as the data cluster label matrix, negative entries in $F$ not only are lack of clear physical meaning but also make it difficult to assign the cluster labels. Recently, Yang $et\ al.$[22] declared explicitly imposing non-negative constraint on $F$ would make result much closer to the idea solution. So, it is necessary to impose non-negative constraint on $F$. The second one is why we adopt the linear weight $\lambda$ on each view? In fact, the solution of $\lambda$ in Eq.(7) is $\lambda_v = 1$ corresponding to the minimum $tr(F^T L^{(v)} F)$ over different views, and other entries in $\lambda$ equal to 0. It means that only one view is selected by this method. To handle this problem, we adopt a trick utilized in [7, 21], i.e., we set $\lambda_v \leftarrow \lambda_v^r$ with $r > 1$. Thus, the improved objective function of AUMFS can be formulated as:

$$\min_{F,\lambda,W} tr(F^T \sum_{v=1}^m \lambda_v^r L^{(v)} F) + \alpha\|X^T W - F\|_{2,1} + \beta\|W\|_{2,1}$$

$$s.t. \quad F^T F = I_c, F \geq 0, \sum_{v=1}^m \lambda_v = 1, \lambda_v \geq 0. \tag{9}$$

From the definition of the $l_{2,1}$-norm, we can see that when the penalty $\beta$ increases, many rows of $W$ will shrink (or be closer) to zeros. Consequently, for a datum $x$, $\tilde{x} = W^T x$ can be treated as a new representation after feature selection wherein only the most relevant feature subset remains. In other words, we can rank all feature components $c_i|_{i=1}^d$ according to the $\|W_{i:}\|$ in descending order and select top ranked components in a batch mode.

## 2.3  Optimization Method

Clearly, Eq.(9) is a nonlinearly constrained nonconvex optimization problem. In the following, we introduce an iterative approach based on coordinate descent to solve it. Firstly, we relax the orthogonal constraint by adding a large enough penalty term $\gamma\|F^T F - I_c\|_F^2$ (e.g., $\gamma = 10^8$ in our experiment.) and rewrite it as follows:

$$\min_{F,\lambda,W} tr(F^T \sum_{v=1}^m \lambda_v^r L^{(v)} F) + \alpha\|X^T W - F\|_{2,1} + \beta\|W\|_{2,1} + \gamma\|F^T F - I_c\|_F^2$$

$$s.t. \quad F \geq 0, \sum_{v=1}^m \lambda_v = 1, \lambda_v \geq 0. \tag{10}$$

Let $\mathcal{J}$ denote the objective function in Eq.(10). We initialize $\lambda_v = \frac{1}{m}$, set $F$ using the clustering result obtained by K-means and set $W$ with a random matrix. Then, we iteratively update $W$, $F$ and $\lambda$ individually, while holding the other variables constant.

**Optimize $W$ for Fixed $F$ and $\lambda$.** For the fixed $F$ and $\lambda$, the part of $\mathcal{J}$ that involves $W$ is

$$\min_W \alpha\|X^T W - F\|_{2,1} + \beta\|W\|_{2,1}, \tag{11}$$

which is further equivalent to [20]:

$$\min_{W,E} \|E\|_{2,1} + \|W\|_{2,1}, \quad s.t. \quad X^T W + \frac{\beta}{\alpha} E = F. \tag{12}$$

Let $B = \begin{bmatrix} X^T & \frac{\beta}{\alpha}I \end{bmatrix}$ and $U = \begin{bmatrix} W \\ E \end{bmatrix}$, then Eq.(12) is equivalent to:

$$\min_{U} \|U\|_{2,1} \quad s.t. \quad BU = F. \tag{13}$$

We introduce the Lagrange multiplier $\psi \in R^{n \times c}$ and the Lagrange function is:

$$\mathscr{L}(U, \psi) = \|U\|_{2,1} - tr(\psi^T (BU - F)). \tag{14}$$

Setting $\frac{\partial \mathscr{L}(U,\psi)}{\partial U} = 0$, we obtain:

$$2PU - B^T \psi = 0, \tag{15}$$

where $P$ is a diagonal matrix with the $i$th diagonal element as $P_{ii} = \frac{1}{2\|U_{i:}\|_2}$ [1]. Left multiplying the two sides of Eq.(15) by $BP^{-1}$, and using the constraint $BU = F$, we have [20]:

$$2BU - BP^{-1}B^T \psi = 0 \Rightarrow \psi = 2(BP^{-1}B^T)^{-1}F. \tag{16}$$

By substituting Eq.(16) into Eq.(15), we obtain:

$$U = P^{-1}B^T(BP^{-1}B^T)^{-1}F. \tag{17}$$

Since Eq.(13) is a convex problem, $U$ is a global optimum solution to the problem if and only if Eq.(17) is satisfied. Therefore, if we iteratively update $U$ and the corresponding $P$, we can get the global optimum solution of $U$. Because of $U = \begin{bmatrix} W \\ E \end{bmatrix}$, $W$ can also be directly obtained from $U$.

**Optimize $F$ for Fixed $W$ and $\lambda$.** Similarly, given $W$ and $\lambda$, we update $F$ to decrease the value of $\mathcal{J}$. Let $L = \sum_{v=1}^{m} \lambda_v^r L^{(v)}$, then $\mathcal{J}$ becomes:

$$\min_{F} tr(F^T LF) + \alpha \|X^T W - F\|_{2,1} + \gamma \|F^T F - I_c\|_F^2 \quad s.t. \quad F \geq 0. \tag{18}$$

Since $F \geq 0$, we introduce the Lagrange multiplier $\Phi \in R^{n \times c} \geq 0$, thus, the Lagrange function is:

$$\mathscr{L}(F, \Phi) = tr(F^T LF) + \alpha \|X^T W - F\|_{2,1} + \gamma \|F^T F - I_c\|_F^2 - tr(\Phi^T F). \tag{19}$$

---

[1] In practice, $\|U_{i:}\|_2$ could be close to zero but not zero. When $\|U_{i:}\|_2 = 0, P_{ii} = 0$ is a subgradient of $\|U\|_{2,1}$. However, we can not set $P_{ii} = 0$ when $\|U_{i:}\|_2 = 0$, otherwise the derived algorithm for updating $U$ can not be guaranteed to converge [20].So, we regularize $P_{ii} = \frac{1}{2\sqrt{U_{i:}^T U_{i:} + \epsilon}}$, where $\epsilon$ is a very small constant.

Setting $\frac{\partial \mathscr{L}(F,\Phi)}{\partial F} = 0$, we get:

$$\frac{\partial \mathscr{L}(F,\Phi)}{\partial F} = 2LF + 2\alpha Q(X^T W - F) + 4\gamma F(F^T F - I_c) - \Phi = 0$$

$$\Rightarrow \Phi = 2LF + 2\alpha Q(X^T W - F) + 4\gamma F(F^T F - I_c), \qquad (20)$$

where $Q$ is a diagonal matrix with the $i$th diagonal element as $Q_{ii} = \frac{1}{2\|(X^T W - F)_{i:}\|_2}$. Using the Karush-Kuhn-Tucker condition [23] $\Phi_{ij} F_{ij} = 0$, we have:

$$(LF + \alpha Q(X^T W - F) + 2\gamma F(F^T F - I_c))_{ij} F_{ij} = 0. \qquad (21)$$

Eq.(21) leads to the following updating formula:

$$F_{ij} = F_{ij} \frac{(\alpha Q F + 2\gamma F)_{ij}}{(LF + \alpha Q X^T W + 2\gamma F F^T F)_{ij}}. \qquad (22)$$

Finally, we normalize $F$ such that $(F^T F)_{ii} = 1, i = 1, ..., c$.

**Optimize $\lambda$ for Fixed $F$ and $W$.** Now, we decrease the objective function with respect to $\lambda$ given $F$ and $W$. The objective function $\mathcal{J}$ degenerates into the following equation:

$$\min_{\lambda} tr(F^F \sum_{v=1}^m \lambda_v^r L^{(v)} F) \quad s.t. \sum_{v=1}^m \lambda_v = 1, \lambda_v \geq 0. \qquad (23)$$

By using a Lagrange multiplier $\xi$ to take the constraint $\sum_{v=1}^m \lambda_v = 1$ into consideration, we get the Lagrange function as follows [7]:

$$\mathscr{L}(\lambda,\xi) = tr(F^F \sum_{v=1}^m \lambda_v^r L^{(v)} F) - \xi(\sum_{v=1}^m \lambda_v - 1). \qquad (24)$$

Setting the derivative of $\mathscr{L}(\lambda,\xi)$ with respect to $\lambda_v$ and $\xi$ to zero, we have:

$$\begin{cases} \frac{\partial \mathscr{L}(\lambda,\xi)}{\partial \lambda_v} = r\lambda_v^{r-1} tr(F^T L^{(v)} F) - \xi = 0, \\ \frac{\partial \mathscr{L}(\lambda,\xi)}{\partial \xi} = \sum_{v=1}^m \lambda_v - 1 = 0. \end{cases} \qquad (25)$$

Solving Eq.(25), the updating formula for $\lambda_v$ can be obtained:

$$\lambda_v = \frac{(1/tr(F^T L^{(v)} F))^{1/(r-1)}}{\sum_{v=1}^m (1/tr(F^T L^{(v)} F))^{1/(r-1)}}. \qquad (26)$$

The updating rules for $F$, $W$ and $\lambda$ should be recursively applied until the convergence is achieved. Then, local optimum solution of $F$,$W$ and $\lambda$ to the objective function $\mathcal{J}$ can be obtained. Following the aforementioned feature selection rule with respect to $W$, the desired compact and relevant feature subset can be selected. Due to the space limitation, the convergence proof of the proposed optimization method is omitted. Similar proof can be found in [7, 10, 16, 22].

## 3    Experiments

In this section, we evaluate the performance of AUMFS by applying it to three visual concept recognition applications, including social image concept recognition, object recognition and video-based human action recognition, on four public datasets.

### 3.1    Experiment Setup

Two image datasets (i.e., Corel5K [24] and NUS-WIDE-OBJECT [25]) and two video datasets (i.e., Weizmann [26] and KTH [27]) are used in our experiments. For image datasets, we extract five types of features, i.e., color histogram (64d), color auto-correlogram (144D), edge direction histogram (73D), wavelet texture (128D) and block-wise color moments (225D), following [25]. For video datasets, holistic features and space-time local features are combined in these experiments. We use the frame differencing to compute holistic features, avoiding background substraction and object tracking [2]. Based on single differencing frames and motion energy images, two kinds of holistic features are computed with Zernike moments and Hu moments respectively. Because the single differencing frame contains spatial pattern of an action and the motion energy image represents the temporal pattern of it, both spatial and temporal patterns are considered. We adopt stip [28] and mosift [29] features as the space-time local features. After extracting all of these features from all videos, k-means clustering is applied to product the bag-of-words descriptor for each kind of features. Then, each kind of moment features and space-time local features of an video are quantized into 50 dimensional and 500 dimensional features respectively. Table 1 summarizes the detailed information of these datasets used in our experiments. We compare the performance of AUMFS with six state-of-the-art unsupervised feature selection methods: All Features (A baseline where all features are used for recognition), Max Variance, Laplacian Score [13], Feature Ranking [14], Multi-Cluster Feature Selection (MCFS) [15] and Nonnegative Discriminative Feature Selection (NDFS) [16]. For image datasets, we randomly select 1000 samples as training data and the remainder samples are served as testing data. For video datasets, we perform leave-one-out cross-validation to evaluate all the methods. To fairly compare all the methods, we fix the nearest neighborhood value $k$ to 5 for graph-based methods such as Laplacian Score, MCFS, NDFS and AUMFS. For AUMFS, we empirically set $\gamma$ to $10^8$ and $r$ to 4 and tune $\alpha$ and $\beta$ from $\{10^{-5}, 10^{-3}, 10^{-1}, 1, 10, 10^3, 10^5\}$. Because the dimensionality of image

**Table 1.** Data set description

| Name | Size | # of concept | # of feature | Data Type |
|------|------|------|------|------|
| Corel5K | 5000 | 50 | 64+144+73+128+225= 634 | Image |
| NUS-WIDE-OBJECT | 30000 | 31 | 64+144+73+128+225= 634 | Image |
| Weizmann | 90 | 10 | $50 \times 4 + 500 \times 2 = 1200$ | Video |
| KTH | 600 | 6 | $50 \times 4 + 500 \times 2 = 1200$ | Video |

data is 634 and video data is 1200, we set the selected feature dimensionality as $\{20 : 20 : 600\}$ for image datasets and $\{100 : 100 : 1200\}$ for video datasets. For the other algorithms, we tune the algorithm dependent parameters and adopt the best setting. Also, we repeat all the experiments 10 times in the image datasets and due to using the leave-one-out rule, experiments on Weizmann and KTH have repeated 9 and 25 times. The average accuracy results are reported for all the algorithms.

We have reason to believe that good features should yield high recognition accuracy. To exclude the factor of classifiers, we use the nearest neighbor classifier (NCC) and SVM to evaluate the performance. NNC is a simple and non-parameter classifier, while SVM is a robust and sophisticated classifier. For the image dataset, we use SVM with the RBF kernel and tune both of its parameters $\mathcal{C}$ and $\gamma$ in the range of $[2^{-5}, 2^{-4}, \ldots, 2^4, 2^5]$ using 5-fold cross-validation to select the best parameters. Because the dimension of video features is very high while the number of instances is small, especially in Weizmann dataset, the linear kernel is adopted for video datasets following [30].

In addition to the comparison of different algorithms, we also study the sensitiveness of parameters and the convergence of AUMFS. We have evaluated $\alpha$, $\beta$ and $r$ except $\gamma$ which has already been empirically fixed to $10^8$. As declared in [7] that the optimal value of $r$ is data set dependent. Therefore, we tune $r$ from $\{2, 4, 6, 8, 10\}$ and randomly select 10,20,30 and 50 concepts from Corel5K dataset to construct dataset with different size for testing $r$. Also, the selected feature number has fixed to 300 and 600 for image datasets and video datasets respectively in these parameter-related experiments.

## 3.2   Experimental Results

Figure 3 and Fig.4 show the recognition results of different algorithms on four data sets. It is clear that our method almost consistently outperforms other methods on these four data sets, especially when the number of selected feature is relatively low, which is likely to be the operational point in practices. The superiority of our method may arise in the twofold: 1) AUMFS simultaneously leverages the underlying three kinds of vital information,i.e., data cluster structure, data similarity and the correlations between different views; 2) the no-negative constraint on $F$ and the $l_{2,1}$-norm constraint on the loss function $L21\_L21$ are incorporated in the final objective function, making more reasonable and the robust formulation which contributes to more faithful results. Besides, AUMFS performs better than using all features in the video datasets. Meanwhile, we notice that although feature selection methods can not guarantee to consistently improve the performance in some cases, they can achieve almost the same recognition accuracy while merely using less than 50% of the original features. From Fig. 5 and Fig. 6, we can see that AUMFS is not very sensitive to the parameters $\alpha$, $\beta$ and $r$. In Fig.6(b), the optimal value of $r$ is 8, 6, 8 and 2 with respect to 10, 20, 30 and 50 concepts respectively, which demonstrates the conclusion given by [7]: the optimal value of $r$ is dataset dependent.

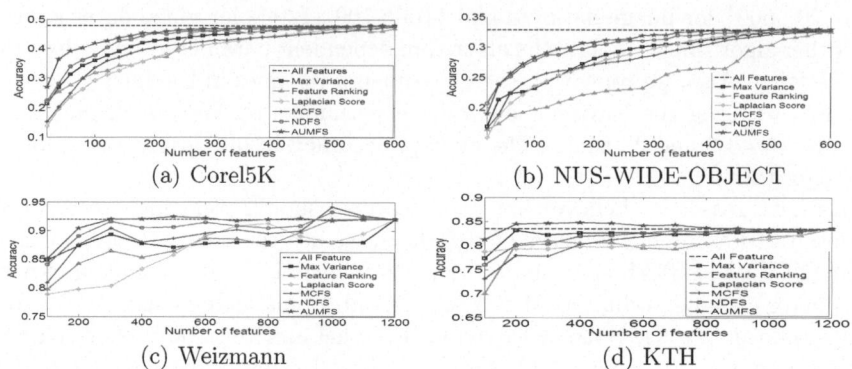

**Fig. 3.** Performance comparison on four popular datasets using NNC

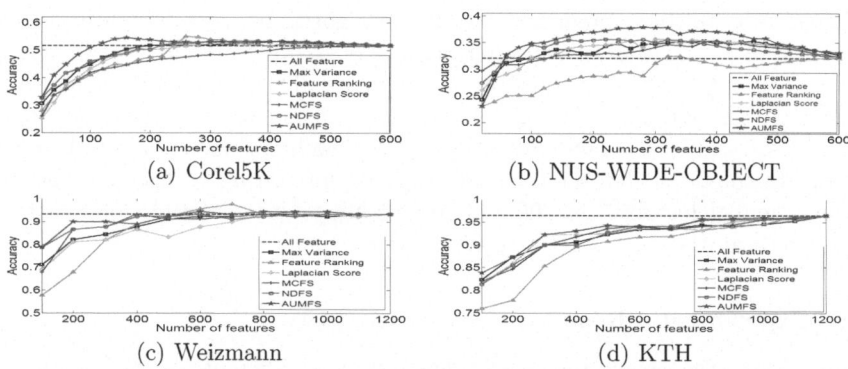

**Fig. 4.** Performance comparison on four popular datasets using SVM

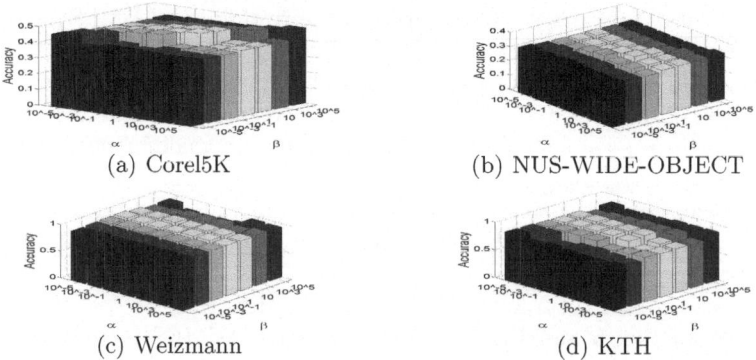

**Fig. 5.** Performance variations of AUMFS on four datasets with fixed $r = 4$ and different $\alpha$ and $\beta$

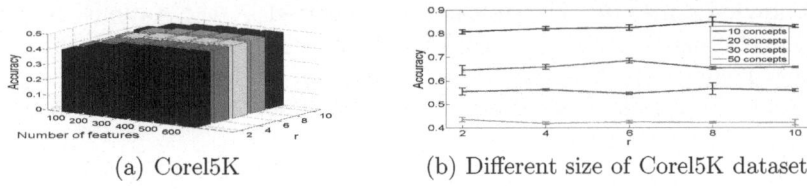

(a) Corel5K

(b) Different size of Corel5K dataset

**Fig. 6.** Performance variations of AUMFS with fixed $\alpha = 10$, $\beta = 10$ and different parameter $r$

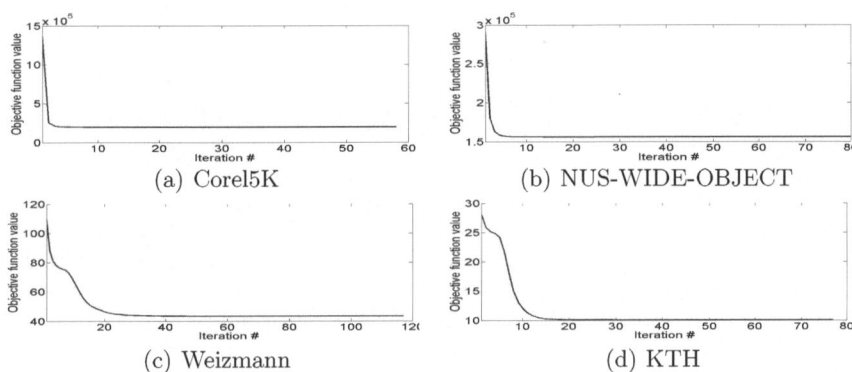

(a) Corel5K

(b) NUS-WIDE-OBJECT

(c) Weizmann

(d) KTH

**Fig. 7.** Illustration of the convergence of AUMFS on four datasets

Figure 7 shows the convergence curves of AUMFS over four datasets. It provides empirical evidences on the convergency of AUMFS. We observe that the proposed optimization method for AUMFS always converges very fast, well within 100 iterations.

## 4 Conclusion

In this paper, we propose an unsupervised learning method, called Adaptive Unsupervised Multi-view Feature Selection (AUMFS) to handle multi-view feature selection problem in the unsupervised learning scenario. An efficient iterative optimization method for AUMFS is also proposed. Experiments with three visual concept recognition applications demonstrate the advantages of our method. More importantly, empirical results show that AUMFS is not very sensitive to the parameters and the corresponding optimization method converges very fast, which suggest that our method can be applied to a wide range of practical problems.

**Acknowledgements.** This research is supported by the National Key Basic Research Program (973) of China (No. 2012$CB$316400), the National Natural Science Foundation of China (No. 60903134) and the National High Technology Research and Development Program (863) of China (No. 2012$AA$011502).

# References

1. Lisin, D., Mattar, M., Blaschko, M., Learned-Miller, E., Benfield, M.: Combining local and global image features for object class recognition. In: IEEE Workshop on Learning in CVPR (2005)
2. Sun, X., Chen, M., Hauptmann, A.: Action recognition via local descriptors and holistic features. In: CVPR Workshops, pp. 58–65. IEEE (2009)
3. Cao, L., Tian, Y., Liu, Z., Yao, B., Zhang, Z., Huang, T.S.: Action detection using multiple spatial-temporal interest point features. In: ICME, pp. 340–345 (2010)
4. Lowe, D.: Distinctive image features from scale-invariant keypoints. J. of CV 60, 91–110 (2004)
5. Ahonen, T., Hadid, A., Pietikainen, M.: Face description with local binary patterns: Application to face recognition. J. of TPAMI 28, 2037–2041 (2006)
6. Mikolajczyk, K., Schmid, C.: A performance evaluation of local descriptors. J. of TPAMI 27, 1615–1630 (2005)
7. Xia, T., Tao, D., Mei, T., Zhang, Y.: Multiview spectral embedding 40, 1438–1446 (2010)
8. Bickel, S., Scheffer, T.: Multi-view clustering. In: ICDM, pp. 19–26 (2004)
9. Okun, O., Priisalu, H.: Multiple views in ensembles of nearest neighbor classifiers. In: ICML Workshop on Learning with Multiple Views (2005)
10. Yang, Y., Shen, H., Ma, Z., Huang, Z., Zhou, X.: L21-norm regularized discriminative feature selection for unsupervised learning. In: IJCAI (2011)
11. Duda, R., Hart, P., Stork, D.: Pattern Classification, 2nd edn. Wiley-Interscience, Chichester (2001)
12. Zhao, Z., Wang, L., Liu, H.: Efficient spectral feature selection with minimum redundancy. In: AAAI (2010)
13. He, X., Cai, D., Niyogi, P.: Laplacian score for feature selection. In: NIPS (2005)
14. Zhao, Z., Liu, H.: Spectral feature selection for supervised and unsupervised learning. In: ICML, pp. 1151–1157 (2007)
15. Cai, D., Zhang, C., He, X.: Unsupervised feature selection for multi-cluster data. In: KDD, pp. 333–342 (2010)
16. Zechao, L., Yi, Y., Jing, L., Xiaofang, Z., Hanqing, L.: Unsupervised feature selection using nonegative spectral analysis. In: AAAI (2012)
17. Shi, J., Malik, J.: Normalized cuts and image segmentation. J. of TPAMI 22, 888–905 (2000)
18. Piepel, G.: Robust regression and outlier detection. Technometrics 31, 260–261 (1989)
19. Kong, D., Ding, C., Huang, H.: Robust nonnegative matrix factorization using $l_{21}$-norm. In: CIKM, pp. 673–682 (2011)
20. Nie, F., Huang, H., Cai, X., Ding, C.: Efficient and robust feature selection via joint $l_{2,1}$-norms minimization. NIPS 23, 1813–1821 (2010)
21. Wang, M., Hua, X.S., Yuan, X., Song, Y., Dai, L.R.: Optimizing multi-graph learning: Towards a unified video annotation scheme. In: ACM MM, pp. 862–870 (2007)

22. Yang, Y., Shen, H.T., Nie, F., Ji, R., Zhou, X.: Nonnegative spectral clustering with discriminative regularization. In: AAAI (2011)
23. Boyd, S., Vandenberghe, L.: Convex optimization. Cambridge Univ. Pr. (2004)
24. Duygulu, P., Barnard, K., de Freitas, J.F.G., Forsyth, D.: Object Recognition as Machine Translation: Learning a Lexicon for a Fixed Image Vocabulary. In: Heyden, A., Sparr, G., Nielsen, M., Johansen, P. (eds.) ECCV 2002, Part IV. LNCS, vol. 2353, pp. 97–112. Springer, Heidelberg (2002)
25. Chua, T.S., Tang, J., Hong, R., Li, H., Luo, Z., Zheng, Y.T.: Nus-wide: A real-world web image database from national university of singapore. In: CIVR (2009)
26. Blank, M., Gorelick, L., Shechtman, E., Irani, M., Basri, R.: Actions as space-time shapes. In: ICCV, pp. 1395–1402 (2005)
27. Schuldt, C., Laptev, I., Caputo, B.: Recognizing human actions: A local SVM approach. In: ICPR, vol. 3, pp. 32–36. IEEE (2004)
28. Laptev, I.: On space-time interest points. J. of IJCV 64, 107–123 (2005)
29. Chen, M., Hauptmann, A.: Mosift: Recognizing human actions in surveillance videos. In: CMU-CS-09-161 (2009)
30. Chang, C.C., Lin, C.J.: LIBSVM: A library for support vector machines. J. of ACM TIST 2, 1–27 (2011)

# Iris Recognition
# Using Consistent Corner Optical Flow

Aditya Nigam and Phalguni Gupta

Department of Computer Science and Engineering,
Indian Institute of Technology Kanpur, India-208016
{naditya,pg}@cse.iitk.ac.in

**Abstract.** This paper proposes an efficient iris based authentication system. Iris segmentation is done using an improved circular hough transform and robust integro-differential operator to detect inner and outer iris boundary respectively. The segmented iris is normalized to polar coordinates and preprocessed using $LGBP$ (Local Gradient Binary Pattern). The corners features are extracted and matched using dissimilarity measure $CIOF$ (Corners having Inconsistent Optical Flow). The proposed approach has been tested on publicly available CASIA 4.0 Interval and Lamp databases consisting of $2,639$ and $16,212$ images respectively. It has been observed that the segmentation accuracy of more than $99.6\%$ can be achieved on both databases. This paper also provides error classification for wrong segmentation and also determines influential parameters for errors. The proposed system has performed with $CRR$ of $99.75\%$ and $99.87\%$ with an $EER$ of $0.108\%$ and $1.29\%$ on Interval and Lamp databases respectively.

## 1   Introduction

Biometrics can be an alternative to any token-based as well as knowledge based traditional methods as they are easier to use and harder to circumvent. The state of the art identification systems are mainly based on fingerprint, face [16,17], iris [5,22,21,2,12,14] and palmprint as major biometric traits along with some minor traits such as finger-knuckle [18], gait *etc*. But each biometric trait has its own set of challenges and trait specific issues. Thin circular diaphragm between cornea and lens is called as iris which have abundance of micro-textures as crypts, furrows, ridges, corona, freckles and pigment spots. These textures are randomly distributed; hence they are believed to be unique [10]. Iris texture is stable between subjects and even between right and left eye of the same subject [7]. Iris is a well-protected biometric trait as compared to the other traits and it is also invariant to age.

Huge amount of work is done in the field of iris recognition. In [5], gabor wavelet responses are quantized to generate feature vector and matching is done using hamming distance. In [22], hough transform is used for iris localization and Laplacian of Gaussian ($LOG$) is used for matching. In [12], vanishing and appearing of important image structures are considered as key local variations and

K.M. Lee et al. (Eds.): ACCV 2012, Part I, LNCS 7724, pp. 358–369, 2013.
© Springer-Verlag Berlin Heidelberg 2013

dyadic wavelets are used to transform 2D image signals into 1D signals for unique features. There are some significant contributions like application of Principle Component Analysis ($PCA$) and Independent Component Analysis ($ICA$) on iris recognition in [4,9]. In [8], gabor wavelet with elastic graph matching is used for iris recognition. In [15], Discrete Cosine Transform ($DCT$) coefficients are quantized that are extracted from non-overlapping rectangular angular blocks and matched using hamming distances. In [14], phase only correlation ($POC$) and band limited phase only correlation ($BLPOC$) are used for accurate iris recognition. In [21], compact and highly efficient ordinal measures are applied for iris recognition. In [19], variational model is applied to localize iris while modified contribution selection algorithm ($MCSA$) is used for iris feature ranking. A comprehensive iris literature survey is presented in [3].

Iris recognition systems consist of several steps: *Image acquisition, Iris Segmentation, Iris Normalization, Preprocessing, Feature extraction* and *Matching.* Each step affects overall performance of the system, but segmentation is the most critical step. Wrong segmentation would render the subsequent steps meaningless. In this paper some new steps are proposed in iris segmentation making it efficient and accurate followed by a novel iris enhancement, transformation and recognition method. The paper is organized as follows: Section 2 describes the proposed system. Section 3 presents the experimental results followed by the last section that presents the concluding remarks.

## 2   Proposed System

In this paper two state of the art techniques (Integro-differential and Hough transformation) are applied in a way such that they can compliment each other for efficient and accurate iris segmentation. The iris texture is enhanced by the proposed local enhancement method. A novel $LGBP$ transformation (*i.e. Local Gradient Binary Pattern*) that uses $x$ and $y$ direction gradient information is proposed to get robust image information representation (*i.e. vcode* and *hcode*). Corner Features are extracted from *vcode* and *hcode* by calculating the eigen values of Hessian matrix at every pixel. Iris recognition is performed by tracking corner features in the corresponding *vcode* and *hcode* considering the consistent optical flow and using $CIOF$ (*i.e. Corners having Inconsistent Optical Flow*) dissimilarity measure.

### 2.1   Iris Segmentation

The proposed iris segmentation approach involves two major steps: (A) Inner boundary localization followed by (B) Outer boundary localization of iris images.

[A] **Inner Boundary Localization:** An iris image $I$ is first *thresholded* to filter out the dark pupil pixels. The resultant binary image is *flood-filled* to remove specular reflection, so that it does not affect the boundary detection as shown in Fig. 1(b). For inner boundary detection strong edges are detected by applying vertical and horizontal Sobel filters.

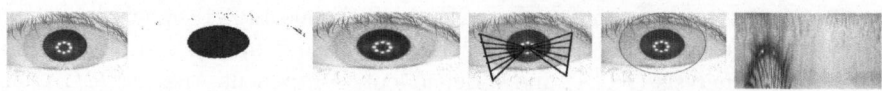

(a) Original (b) Thresholded (c) Seg. Pupil (d) Angle (e) Seg. Iris (f) Nor. Iris

**Fig. 1.** Automatic Iris Segmentation

Standard hough transform extracts circle in an image by searching the optimal parameters in the whole three dimensional parametric space of abscissa and ordinate of center and radius $i.e$ 3-tuple $<x, y, r>$ . It has been improved by using the orientation of each pixel to reduce the search space from $3D$ to $1D$ of the radius only. The improved Hough transform can efficiently detect the circle without reducing the accuracy as shown in Fig. 1(c). It makes use of the key observation that *"if an edge point lies on a circle, then the center of circle should lie on the normal to the edge direction (orientation) at that point"*. Thus, for an edge point $(x, y)$ in an image and for a radius $r$, the center coordinates $(c_1^x, c_1^y)$ and $(c_2^x, c_2^y)$, for two circles (one to its left and other to right half) can be computed as:

$$(c_1^x, c_1^y) = (x + r \cdot \sin\left(\theta(x,y) - \frac{\pi}{2}\right), \quad y - r \cdot \cos\left(\theta(x,y) - \frac{\pi}{2}\right)) \tag{1}$$

$$(c_2^x, c_2^y) = (x - r \cdot \sin\left(\theta(x,y) - \frac{\pi}{2}\right), \quad y + r \cdot \cos\left(\theta(x,y) - \frac{\pi}{2}\right)) \tag{2}$$

**[B] Outer Boundary Localization:** The robust circular integro-differential operator as defined in [6], is applied over two non-occluded sectors which are selected empirically. Inner boundary localization of iris is used to guide the outer boundary localization. A simple heuristic which is used to make process efficient is that *"iris inner and outer boundaries have centers which are not necessarily concentric, but within a certain small window (W) of each other"*. Thus, candidate center points of outer boundary are generated within a window of the inner center. Each of these candidates $(c^x, c^y)$ and radius $r$ defines a circle for the the outer iris boundary. The standard integro-differential operator sums the pixel intensity values over this circle and calculates the change in the summation over a neighbor concentric circle. The candidate circle with the maximum change per unit circumference gives the outer iris boundary. To prevent noise due to eyelids and lashes the circular summation is done over empirically selected two non-occluded sectors of $\alpha_{range} = (-\pi/4, \pi/6)^c \cup (5\pi/6, 5\pi/4)^c$ as shown in Fig. 1(d). Finally segmented iris image is shown in Fig. 1(e).

## 2.2   Iris Normalization

After iris is segmented from the image, it is transformed to polar coordinates in order to overcome the dimensional inconsistencies between eye images as suggested in [6]. In this paper, the segmented iris images are unwrapped into normalized images of $40 \times 256$ size as shown in Fig. 1(f).

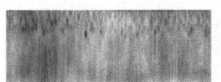  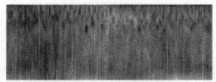 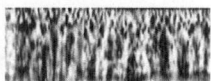

(a) Original Iris     (b) Estimated Illum.     (c) Uniform Illum.     (d) Weiner Filtering

**Fig. 2.** Iris Texture Enhancement

## 2.3   Iris Recognition

The texture of normalized iris images are enhanced and transformed to robust representation *i.e vcode, hcode* that can tolerate illumination variations. To achieve some robustness against affine transformations KL-tracking, that is constrained by some statistical and geometrical parameters is used for matching.

**[A] Iris Enhancement:**   The texture of unwrapped iris images are enhanced so as to make the information more discriminative using the proposed local enhancement method. The iris image is divided into blocks of size $8 \times 8$ and the mean of these blocks are considered as the coarse illumination of that block. This mean is expanded to the original size of the iris as shown in Fig. 2(b). Smaller block size produces almost same estimate of illumination as that of the original image and bigger will produce improper estimates. Non-uniform illumination is compensated by subtracting estimated illumination from the original image to obtain uniformly illuminated iris image as shown in Fig. 2(c). Then the contrast of uniformly illuminated image is enhanced using Contrast Limited Adaptive Histogram Equalization (CLAHE). It removes the artificially induced borders of tiles using bilinear interpolation and enhances the contrast of image without introducing any external noise. Finally, wiener filter is applied for reducing constant power additive noise to obtain enhanced texture iris image as shown in Fig. 2(d). It can be observed that the texture of enhanced image Fig. 2(d) is much better than Fig. 2(a). The proposed enhancement method has shown encouraging recognition performance boost-up as discussed in Section 3.2 and shown in Fig. 6(a).

**[B] *LGBP* Transformation:**   It transforms normalized and enhanced noisy iris images into *vcode* and *hcode* respectively so as to obtain robust features. The gradient of any edge pixel will be positive if it lies on an edge created due to light to dark shade (*i.e. high to low gray value*) transition else it will be having negative gradient value. Hence all the edge pixels can be divided into two classes of $+ve$ and $-ve$ gradient values as shown in Fig. 3. The *sobel* kernel lacks rotational symmetry hence more consistent *scharr* kernels which are obtained by minimizing angular error is applied. The *scharr* $x$-direction kernel of size $3 \times 3$ and $9 \times 9$ are applied to get Fig. 3(b), 3(c) respectively. Bigger size kernel produces coarse level features as shown in Fig. 3(c). This gradient augmented information of each edge pixel can be more discriminative and robust. The proposed transformation precisely uses this information to calculates a 8-bit code for each pixel using $x$ and $y$-direction derivatives of its 8 neighboring pixels to obtain *vcode* and *hcode* respectively.

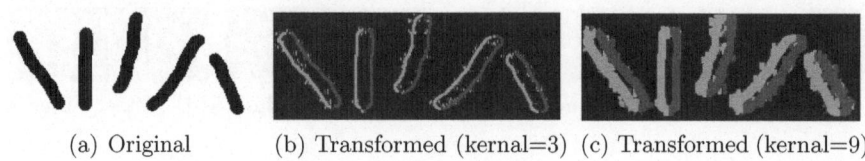

(a) Original        (b) Transformed (kernal=3)   (c) Transformed (kernal=9)

**Fig. 3.** *LGBP* Transformation (Red: -ve gradient;Green: +ve grad.;Blue: zero grad.)

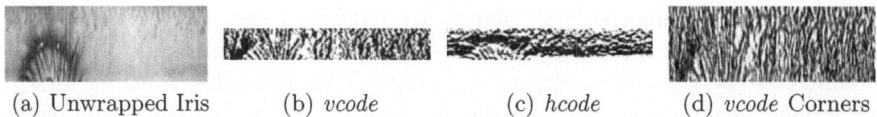

(a) Unwrapped Iris        (b) *vcode*        (c) *hcode*        (d) *vcode* Corners

**Fig. 4.** Iris Recognition Steps

Let $P_{i,j}$ be the $(i,j)^{th}$ pixel of an iris image $P$ and $Neigh[l], l = 1, 2, ...8$ are the gradients of 8 neighboring pixels centered at pixel $P_{i,j}$ obtained by applying *scharr* kernel, then the $k^{th}$ bit of the 8-bit code (termed as *lgbp_code*) is given by

$$lgbp\_code[k] = \begin{cases} 1 & \textbf{if } Neigh[k] > 0 \\ \\ 0 & \textbf{otherwise} \end{cases} \qquad (3)$$

In *vcode* or *hcode* every pixel is represented by its *lgbp_code* as shown in Fig. 4(b), 4(c) respectively. The pattern of edges within a neighborhood can be assumed to be robust; hence each pixel's *lgbp_code* is considered which is just an encoding of edge pattern in its 8-neighborhood. Also *lgbp_code* of any pixel considers only the sign of the derivative within its specified neighborhood hence ensures the robustness of the proposed transformation in illumination variation.

**[C] Feature Extraction Using KLT Corner Detector [20]:** Corners in *vcode* and *hcode* are robust features that can be tracked accurately even in varying illumination because they have two high derivatives in orthogonal directions. The eigen analysis of Hessian matrix of size $2 \times 2$, for each pixel is done and two possible eigen values $\lambda_1$ and $\lambda_2$ such that $\lambda_1 \geq \lambda_2$ are obtained. Like [20], all pixels having $\lambda_2 \geq T$ (smaller eigen value greater than a threshold) are considered as corner feature points as shown in Fig. 4(d).

**[D] Matching Using KL Tracking [11]:** Let $Iris_a$ and $Iris_b$ are two normalized enhanced iris images that have to be matched and $I_A^v$, $I_B^v$ and $I_A^h$, $I_B^h$ are their corresponding *vcode* and *hcode* respectively. KL tracking [11] has been used for matching between $Iris_a$ and $Iris_b$. It is assumed that the tracking performance of KL algorithm is good while tracking between features of same subject (genuine matching) and degrades substantially for others (imposter matching).

**KL Tracking [11]:** Let us assume a corner at spatial location $(x, y)$ in an image $I$ with intensity $I(x, y, t)$ at some time instance $t$. KL Tracking can be used to estimate sparse optical flow at time instance $t + \delta t$. This estimate is based on three assumptions; [1] Brightness consistency, [2] Temporal persistence and [3] Spatial coherency as defined below:

[1] **Brightness Consistency:** It assumes little change in brightness for the small value of $\delta t$.

$$I(x, y, t) \approx I(x + \delta x, y + \delta y, t + \delta t) \qquad (4)$$

[2] **Temporal Persistence:** Small feature movement for small $\delta t$. One can get Eq. (5) for each corner feature.

$$I_x V_x + I_y V_y = -I_t \qquad (5)$$

where $V_x, V_y$ are the respective components of the optical flow velocity for feature at pixel $I(x, y, t)$ and $I_x, I_y$ and $I_t$ are the local image derivatives in $x$, $y$ and $t$ directions respectively.

[3] **Spatial Coherency:** Estimating unique flow vector from Eq. (5) for every feature point is an ill-posed problem. Hence KL tracking estimates the motion of any feature by assuming local constant flow (*i.e* a patch of pixels moves coherently).

The tracking performance depends on how well these three assumptions are satisfied. However, all tracked corner features may not be the true matches because of noise, local non-rigid distortions in iris and also less difference in inter class and more in intra class matching.

**Consistent Optical Flow:** It can be noted that true matches have the optical flow which can be aligned with the actual affine transformation between the two images. The estimated optical flow direction is quantized into eight directions and the most consistent direction is selected as the one which has most number of successfully tracked corner features. Any corner matching having optical flow direction other than the most consistent direction is considered as false matching. A dissimilarity measure $CIOF$ (Corners having Inconsistent Optical Flow) has been proposed to estimate the KL-tracking performance by evaluating some geometric and statistical quantities that are defined as:

[a] **Proximity Constraints**: Euclidean distance between any corner and its estimated tracked location should be less than or equal to an empirically selected threshold $TH_d$. The parameter $TH_d$ depends upon the amount of translation and rotation in the sample images. High $TH_d$ signifies more translation and vise-versa.

[b] **Patch Dissimilarity**: Tracking error defined as pixel-wise sum of absolute difference between a local patch centered at current corner and that of its estimated tracked location patch should be less than or equal to an empirically selected threshold $TH_e$. The parameter $TH_e$ ensures that the matching corners must have similar neighboring patch around it.

**Matching Algorithm:** Given two *vcode* $I_A^v$, $I_B^v$ and two *hcode* $I_A^h$, $I_B^h$, Algorithm 1 has been presented which can be used to compare $Iris_a$ with $Iris_b$

---

**Algorithm 1.** $CIOF(Iris_a, Iris_b)$

---

**Require:** The two $vcode$ $I_A^v, I_B^v$ and two $hcode$ $I_A^h, I_B^h$ of normalized and enhanced iris images $Iris_a, Iris_b$ respectively.
$N_a^v$, $N_b^v$, $N_a^h$ and $N_b^h$ are the number of corners in $I_A^v, I_B^v, I_A^h$, and $I_B^h$ respectively.

**Ensure:** Return the symmetric function $CIOF(Iris_a, Iris_b)$.

1: Track all the corners of $vcode$ $I_A^v$ in $vcode$ $I_B^v$ and that of $hcode$ $I_A^h$ in $hcode$ $I_B^h$.

2: Calculate the number of successfully tracked corners in $vcode$ tracking (*i.e.* $stc_{AB}^v$) and $hcode$ tracking (*i.e.* $stc_{AB}^h$) that have their tracked position within $TH_d$ and their local patch dissimilarity under $TH_e$.

3: Similarly calculate successfully tracked corners of $vcode$ $I_B^v$ in $vcode$ $I_A^v$ (*i.e.* $stc_{BA}^v$) as well as $hcode$ $I_B^h$ in $hcode$ $I_A^h$ (*i.e.* $stc_{BA}^h$).

4: Quantize optical flow direction for each successfully tracked corners into only eight directions (*i.e.* at $\frac{\pi}{8}$ interval) and obtain 4 histograms $H_{AB}^v, H_{AB}^h, H_{BA}^v$ and $H_{BA}^h$ using $stc_{AB}^v, stc_{AB}^h, stc_{BA}^v$ and $stc_{BA}^h$ respectively.

5: For each histogram, out of 8 bins the bin (*i.e.* direction) having the maximum corners is considered as the consistent optical flow direction. The maximum value obtained from each histogram is termed as corners having consistent optical flow represented as $cof_{AB}^v, cof_{AB}^h, cof_{BA}^v$ and $cof_{BA}^h$.

6: $ciof_{AB}^v = 1 - \frac{cof_{AB}^v}{N_a^v}$;  $ciof_{BA}^v = 1 - \frac{cof_{BA}^v}{N_b^v}$;[Cor. with Inconsis. Opti. Flow (*vcode*)]

7: $ciof_{AB}^h = 1 - \frac{cof_{AB}^h}{N_a^h}$;  $ciof_{BA}^h = 1 - \frac{cof_{BA}^h}{N_b^h}$;[Cor. with Inconsis. Opti. Flow (*hcode*)]

8: **return** $CIOF(Iris_a, Iris_b) = \frac{ciof_{AB}^v + ciof_{AB}^h + ciof_{BA}^v + ciof_{BA}^h}{4}$;[SUM RULE]

---

using $CIOF$. The $vcode$ $I_A^v$, $I_B^v$ are matched while $hcode$ $I_A^h$, $I_B^h$ are matched. Final score $CIOF(Iris_a, Iris_b)$ is obtained by using sum rule fusion of horizontal and vertical matching scores. Such a fusion is very useful and boost-up the performance of the proposed system because some of the images are having more discrimination in vertical direction while others have it in horizontal direction. Any corner is considered as tracked successfully if the euclidean distance between itself and its estimated tracked location and the local patch-wise sum of absolute difference is less than $TH_d$ and $TH_e$ respectively. Out of all the successfully tracked corners ($stc_{AB}^v, stc_{AB}^h$) those that are having inconsistent optical flow are considered as false matches. In order to make measure symmetric the average of $ciof_{AB}$ and $ciof_{BA}$ is used.

## 3   Experimental Results

**Database:** The proposed system is tested on two publicly available CASIA V4 Interval and Lamp iris databases. Interval database contains 2,639 iris images collected from 249 subjects having 395 distinct irises and about 7 images per iris. On the other hand Lamp is huge database consisting of 16,212 images collected from 411 subjects having 819 distinct irises and 20 images per iris. Interval images are taken in two session under indoor environment while Lamp images are taken in only one session under indoor environment with lamp on/off. Iris images in Lamp database are more challenging because of nonlinear deformation

**Table 1.** Parameters: $p_{r_{min}}$, $p_{r_{max}}$, $i_{r_{min}}$ and $i_{r_{max}}$ are Pupil and Iris radius range

| Default parameters | | | | | | | | |
|---|---|---|---|---|---|---|---|---|
| Database | $s(scale)$ | $t$ | $p_{r_{min}}$ | $p_{r_{max}}$ | $i_{r_{min}}$ | $i_{r_{max}}$ | $W$ | $\alpha_{range}(radians)$ |
| Interval | 0.5 | 0.41 | 20 | 90 | 80 | 130 | 15 | $(-\pi/4, \pi/6) \cup (5\pi/6, 5\pi/4)$ |
| Lamp | 0.5 | 0.125 | 16 | 70 | 65 | 120 | 11 | $(-\pi/3, 0) \cup (\pi, 4\pi/3)$ |

**Table 2.** Segmentation Error. (Last row: errors occurred in Interval, Lamp databases)

| Eyelid | Eyelash | Spec.Reflection | Pupil Noise | Bright image | Dark image |
|---|---|---|---|---|---|
| | | | | | |
| 4,300 | 15,288 | 5,68 | 71,160 | 11,1 | 39,53 |

due to variations of visible illumination. Also, it is a challenge to get good results on any huge database because number of false acceptances grows very fast with the database size [1].

### 3.1 Segmentation Accuracy

The segmentation accuracy of the proposed system is found to be 94.5% and 94.63% for Interval and Lamp database respectively using the default parameters as shown in Table 1. The erroneous segmentations are critically analyzed and are corrected by adjusting few parameters. This adjustment helps to achieve an accuracy of more than 99.6% on both databases. Some very critically occluded images are segmented manually ($< 0.4\%$). The error analysis along with some of the example images where the proposed segmentation has been failed are shown in Table 2. There are only two critical parameters viz. threshold ($t$) and angular range ($\alpha_{range}$) (as defined in Section 2.1) that are required to be adjusted as suggested in Table 3 for accurate segmentation.

**Table 3.** Statistics and the suggested variations for $t$ and $\alpha_{range}$

| Threshold parameter ($t$) value | | | | | Suggested Variation | |
|---|---|---|---|---|---|---|
| Sub-Category | Mean | Min | Max | Std Devi. | ($t$) value | $\alpha_{range}$ |
| Eyelid | 0.39 | 0.36 | 0.41 | 0.022 | - | ↓ |
| Eyelash | 0.39 | 0.3 | 0.43 | 0.040 | ↓- | ↓ |
| Specular Reflection | 0.44 | 0.36 | 0.5 | 0.066 | ↑ | - |
| Pupil Boundary Noise | 0.4 | 0.26 | 0.5 | 0.056 | ↑↓ | - |
| Bright image | 0.46 | 0.35 | 0.52 | 0.06 | ↑ | - |
| Dark image | 0.36 | 0.25 | 0.51 | 0.052 | ↓ | - |

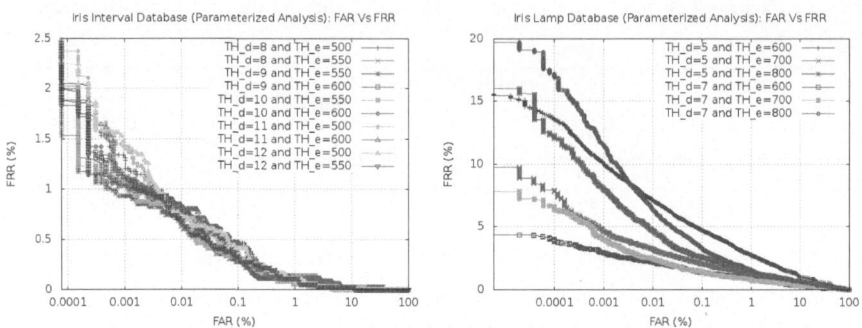

**Fig. 5.** ROC of proposed system for different set of parameters (only *vcode* matching)

## 3.2   Recognition Accuracy

This subsection analyses the recognition performance of the proposed system. In all of the graphs *vcode* represents results using only *vcode* matching and similar representation for *hcode* and fusion is used. In order to test the system on Interval database, iris images of first session are taken as training while remaining are taken as testing. For Lamp database, first 10 image are considered as training and rest are taken as testing images. Hence a total of $3,657$ genuine and $1,272,636$ imposter matchings are considered for Interval database testing while $78,300$ genuine and $61,230,600$ imposter matchings are considered for Lamp database. The performance of the system is measured using correct recognition rate ($CRR$) in case of identification and equal error rate ($EER$) for verification. The $CRR$ (*i.e.* the **Rank 1** accuracy) of any system is defined as the ratio of the number of correct (Non-False) top best match of iris ROI and the total number of iris ROI in the query set. At any given threshold, the probability of accepting the impostor, known as false acceptance rate ($FAR$) and probability of rejecting the genuine user known as false rejection rate ($FRR$) are obtained. Equal error rate ($EER$) is the value of FAR for which FAR and FRR are equal.

$$EER = \{FAR|FAR = FRR\} \qquad (6)$$

**Parameterized Analysis:** The proposed $CIOF$ dissimilarity measure is primarily parameterized by two parameters $TH_e$ and $TH_d$. The system is tested using these parameters as input and their values are selected so as to maximize the performance of the system by considering only first 100 subjects from each database and using only *vcode* matching. The parameter values for which system has found to be performing with maximum $CRR$ and minimum $ERR$ are $TH_e = 600$ with patch size of $5 \times 5$ and $TH_d = 7$ for Lamp while $TH_e = 600$ with patch size of $5 \times 5$ and $TH_d = 10$ for Interval databases as shown in Fig. 5. This parametric analysis inferred that Interval has more translation in iris images of same subject than Lamp database.

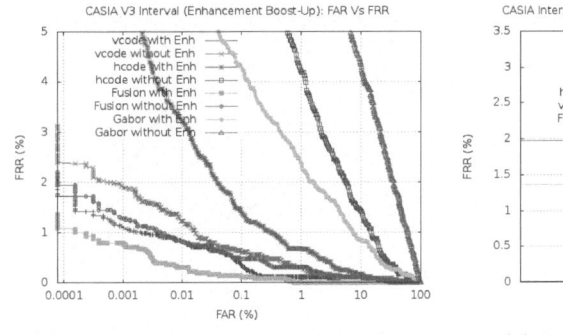

(a) Enhancement based Per. boost-up

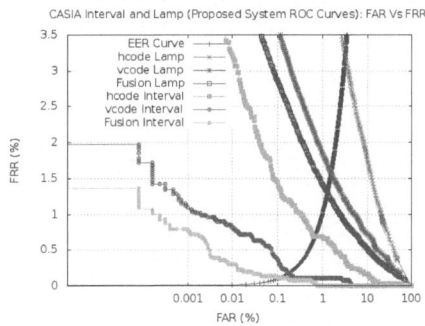

(b) ROC for Interval and Lamp

**Fig. 6.** Receiver Operating Characteristic Curves for the Proposed System

**Table 4.** Comparative Performance Analysis

| Systems | Interval | | | Lamp | | |
|---------|----------|------|------|------|------|------|
| | DI | CRR% | EER% | DI | CRR% | EER% |
| Daugman | 1.961 | 99.46 | 1.881 | 1.2420 | 98.90 | 5.59 |
| Li Ma [19] | - | 95.54 | 2.07 | - | - | - |
| Masek | 1.99 | 99.58 | 1.09 | - | - | - |
| K. Roy [19] | - | 97.21 | 0.71 | - | - | - |
| **Proposed** | **2.35** | **99.75** | **0.108** | **2.22** | **99.87** | **1.29** |

**Enhancement Based Performance Boost-Up:** The proposed local enhancement method significantly improves the random micro level iris texture as it is evident from the graph shown in Fig. 6(a). For *vcode*, *hcode*, fusion or even gabor approach [5], the performance of the system is significantly improved after enhancement.

The proposed system has been compared with state of the art iris recognition systems [5,12,13,19]. For comparing with [5,13] we have coded their systems and with [12,19] we have used the results as stated in [19]. It is found that the $CRR$ (**Rank 1** accuracy) of the proposed system is more than 99.77% for both databases. The comparison of the proposed system with other state of the art systems is shown in Table 4. Further, its $EER$ is 0.108% for Interval and that for Lamp is 1.29% which is better than the reported systems. For both databases, Receiver Operating Characteristics (ROC) curves are shown in Fig. 6(b) for the proposed system. The ROC curves comparing proposed system with the open source Masek system (Log-Gabor) [13] as well as Daugman system (Gabor) [5] are shown in Fig. 7. Masek's system cannot be tested on Lamp database as the optimal parameters are not known and with default set of parameters its performance is very poor. The decidability index $(d')$ measures separability between imposter and genuine matching scores is defined as:

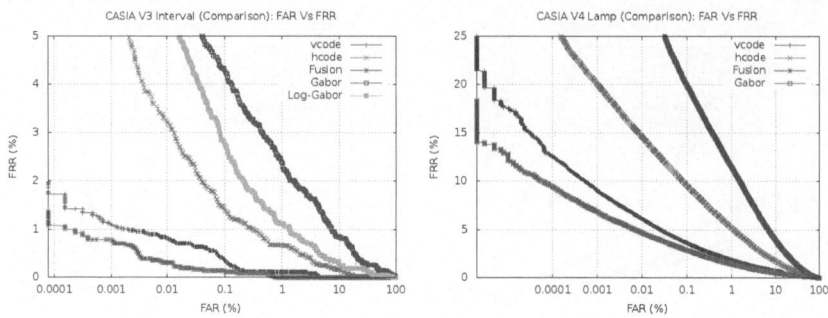

**Fig. 7.** Comparing Proposed System

$$d^{'} = \frac{|\mu_G - \mu_I|}{\sqrt{\frac{\sigma_G^2 + \sigma_I^2}{2}}} \tag{7}$$

where $\mu_G$ and $\mu_I$ are the mean, and $\sigma_G$ and $\sigma_I$ are the standard deviation of the genuine and imposter scores respectively. The decidability index $(d^{'})$ are found to be 2.35 and 2.22 for Interval and Lamp databases respectively.

## 4    Conclusion

In this paper an efficient iris based authentication system has been proposed. Inner iris boundary is segmented using the improved circular hough transform while outer boundary is detected using integro-differential operator. Texture of the normalized iris images are enhanced using the proposed local enhancement method. The segmented and enhanced iris images are transformed using local gradient binary pattern $(LGBP)$ so as to get robust image information representation (*i.e.* vcode, hcode). The corner features are matched using a dissimilarity measure Corners having Inconsistent Optical Flow $(CIOF)$ that tracks corners using KL tracking. The proposed system has been tested on publicly available CASIA 4.0 Interval and Lamp databases consisting of 2, 639 and 16, 212 images respectively. The segmentation accuracy of 99.6% has been achieved with little bit of parameter tuning on both databases. The errors in segmentation are classified into six classes and parameterized segmentation analysis is also carried out to infer the influence of parameters towards errors. The system has achieved $CRR$ of 99.75% with an $EER$ of 0.108% on Interval and $CRR$ of 99.87% with an $EER$ of 1.29% on Lamp databases.

## References

1. Amit, S.C., Mhatre, J., Palla, S., Govindaraju, V.: Efficient search and retrieval in biometric databases. In: Proc. SPIE, vol. 5779, pp. 265–273 (2005)
2. Bendale, A., Nigam, A., Prakash, S., Gupta, P.: Iris Segmentation Using Improved Hough Transform. In: Huang, D.-S., Gupta, P., Zhang, X., Premaratne, P. (eds.) ICIC 2012. CCIS, vol. 304, pp. 408–415. Springer, Heidelberg (2012)

3. Bowyer, K.W., Hollingsworth, K., Flynn, P.J.: Image understanding for iris biometrics: A survey. Computer Vision and Image Understanding 110(2), 281–307 (2008)
4. Cui, J., Wang, Y., Huang, J., Tan, T., Sun, Z.: An iris image synthesis method based on pca and super-resolution. In: Proceedings of the 17th International Conference on Pattern Recognition (ICPR), vol. 4, pp. 471–474. IEEE (2004)
5. Daugman, J.: High confidence visual recognition of persons by a test of statistical independence. IEEE Transactions on Pattern Analysis and Machine Intelligence (1993)
6. Daugman, J.: How iris recognition works. In: International Conference on Image Processing (ICIP), pp. 33–36 (2002)
7. Daugman, J., Downing, C.: Epigenetic randomness, complexity and singularity of human iris patterns. In: Proceedings of Royal Society London Biological Sciences (2001)
8. Farouk, R.: Iris recognition based on elastic graph matching and gabor wavelets. Computer Vision and Image Understanding 115(8), 1239–1244 (2011)
9. Huang, Y., Luo, S., Chen, E.: An efficient iris recognition system. In: Proceedings of the International Conference on Machine Learning and Cybernetics, vol. 1, pp. 450–454. IEEE (2002)
10. Jain, A., Pankanti, S., Prabhakar, S., Hong, L., Ross, A.: Biometrics: A grand challenge. In: Proceedings of the 17th International Conference on Pattern Recognition (ICPR), vol. 2, pp. 935–942. IEEE (2004)
11. Lucas, B.D., Kanade, T.: An Iterative Image Registration Technique with an Application to Stereo Vision. In: International Joint Conference on Artificial Intelligence (IJCAI), pp. 674–679 (1981)
12. Ma, L., Tan, T., Wang, Y., Zhang, D.: Efficient iris recognition by characterizing key local variations. IEEE Transactions on Image Processing 13(6), 739–750 (2004)
13. Masek, L., Kovesi, P.: Matlab source code for a biometric identification system based on iris patterns. M.Tech Thesis (2003)
14. Miyazawa, K., Ito, K., Aoki, T., Kobayashi, K., Nakajima, H.: An effective approach for iris recognition using phase-based image matching. IEEE Transactions on Pattern Analysis and Machine Intelligence 30(10), 1741–1756 (2008)
15. Monro, D., Rakshit, S., Zhang, D.: Dct-based iris recognition. IEEE Transactions on Pattern Analysis and Machine Intelligence 29(4), 586–595 (2007)
16. Nigam, A., Gupta, P.: A new distance measure for face recognition system. In: International Conference on Image and Graphics (ICIG), pp. 696–701 (2009)
17. Nigam, A., Gupta, P.: Comparing human faces using edge weighted dissimilarity measure. In: International Conference on Control, Automation, Robotics and Vision (ICARCV), pp. 1831–1836 (2010)
18. Nigam, A., Gupta, P.: Finger Knuckleprint Based Recognition System Using Feature Tracking. In: Sun, Z., Lai, J., Chen, X., Tan, T. (eds.) CCBR 2011. LNCS, vol. 7098, pp. 125–132. Springer, Heidelberg (2011)
19. Roy, K., Bhattacharya, P., Suen, C.Y.: Iris recognition using shape-guided approach and game theory. Pattern Analysis and Applications 14(4), 329–348 (2011)
20. Shi, J., Tomasi: Good features to track. In: Computer Vision and Pattern Recognition, pp. 593–600 (1994)
21. Sun, Z., Tan, T.: Ordinal measures for iris recognition. IEEE Transactions on Pattern Analysis and Machine Intelligence 31(12), 2211–2226 (2009)
22. Wildes, R.: Iris recognition: an emerging biometric technology. Proceedings of the IEEE 85(9), 1348–1363 (1997)

# Face Recognition in Videos – A Graph Based Modified Kernel Discriminant Analysis

Gayathri Mahalingam and Chandra Kambhamettu

Video/Image Modeling and Synthesis Laboratory (VIMS),
Dept. of Computer and Information Sciences,
University of Delaware, Newark, DE 19711
{mahaling,chandrak}@udel.edu

**Abstract.** Grassmannian manifolds have been an effective way to represent image sets (video) which are mapped as data points on the manifold. Recognition can then be performed by applying the Discriminant Analysis (DA) on such manifolds. However, the local structure of the data points are not exploited in the DA. This paper proposes a modified Kernel Discriminant Analysis (KDA) approach on Grassmannian manifolds that utilizes the local structure of the data points on the manifold. The KDA exploits the local structure using between-class and within-class adjacency graphs that represent the between-class and within-class similarities, respectively. The maximum correlation from within-class and minimum correlation from between-class is utilized to define the connectivity between points in the graph thus exploiting the geometrical structure of the data. The discriminability is further improved by effective feature representation using LBP which can discriminate data across illumination, pose, and minor expressions. Effective recognition is performed by using only the cluster representatives extracted by clustering the frames of a video sequence. Experiments on several video datasets (Honda, MoBo, ChokePoint, NRC-IIT, and MOBIO) show that the proposed approach obtains better recognition rates, in comparison with the state-of-the-art approaches.

## 1   Introduction

Face recognition algorithms proposed in the past decades can be categorized into two categories: 1. Face recognition from single face image and 2. Face recognition using video sequences (image sets). Face recognition in video sequences has gained more attention in the past decade due to its direct application in real-world scenarios such as video surveillance and video retrieval. These applications require a reliable recognition due to the presence of variations such as pose, expressions, illumination, age, etc. in the video sequences.

Face recognition on image sets has been explored in the past decade due to its advantages over image-based recognition [1],[2],[3],[4],[5],[6]. A complete evaluation of the current methods are given in [7]. The major advantage is the availability of temporal information of faces which can improve the recognition task.

K.M. Lee et al. (Eds.): ACCV 2012, Part I, LNCS 7724, pp. 370–381, 2013.
© Springer-Verlag Berlin Heidelberg 2013

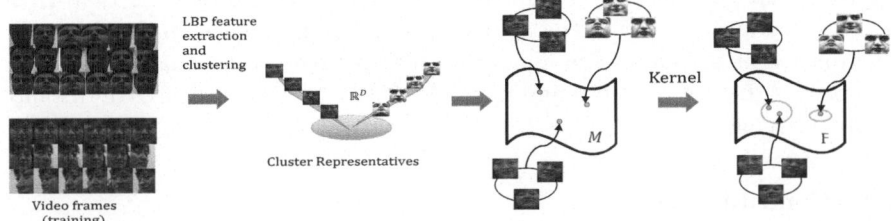

**Fig. 1.** An overview of the proposed approach. The LBP features are extracted from the image sets and are clustered. The cluster representatives for each image set are represented in $\mathcal{R}^D$ by linear subspaces. The LBP features of the cluster representatives are mapped on to the Grassmannian manifold $\mathcal{M}$ as points $X_i$. The kernel discriminant tranform that uses the adjacency graphs to represent the topology of the points in the manifold $\mathcal{M}$ is applied to map the points to the feature space $\mathcal{F}$. Matching is performed by computing the nearest neighbor distances between the points $Y_i$ and $Y_j$ on the feature space $\mathcal{F}$.

It has been shown that an improved performance can be achieved when the high-dimensional image sets are modeled using linear subspaces [8]. Hakan and Triggs [5] proposed an approach in which the image sets are represented as affine and convex subspaces.

The concept of canonical correlation has recently gained attention for image set matching and has been proposed in [9] and [10]. Kim *et al.* [11] used a linear discriminant function that maximizes the canonical correlations of within-class sets and minimizes the canonical correlations of between-class sets. Semi-supervised learning approaches [12], [6] exploit the properties of a face data manifold using a computationally inexpensive graph-based Discriminant Analysis (DA). The graph-based DA is based on the framework proposed by Yan *et al.* [13].

The above approaches draw holistic face representation. Discriminative approaches has been suggested by Mian [14], which computes image descriptors at interest points in the image.

The conventional DA suffers from the discrimination of data within and between classes i.e. the local structure of the data [15]. This can be overcome by discriminating the topology of the data mapped as points on a Grassmannian manifold ([6], [13]). Motivated by these facts, we propose a modified kernel based discriminant analysis which utilizes the discriminant power of image descriptors (LBP) and the topology of the data points on the Grassmannian manifold. The advantage of the proposed approach is on its discrimination of data at the high dimensional space using discriminative features and also at the manifold space by exploiting its local structure through a graph based representation.

The proposed KDA utilizes the local structure (unlike traditional LDA) by means of the within-class and between-class adjacency graphs which can improve the discrimination accuracy. The novelty lies in the effective mapping of the data points to another manifold using the kernel which maps the intra-class points closer while mapping the inter-class points farther to each other. Besides, our approach has the advantage of having higher projection directions than LDA and also performs a more general DA since no assumption is made about the distribution of the data. The main difference between traditional DA and our approach is the use of graphs and manifolds instead of vector spaces in distance metric learning.

## 1.1   Contributions

We summarize our contributions below;

- We propose to use exemplars from videos, which are extracted by clustering using their LBP descriptors that can discriminate across pose and illumination variations. Our experimental results indicate the superior performance of using only the exemplars in recognition.
- We propose a modified KDA that improves the discrimination of data in manifold space using the adjacency graphs.
- We provide an empirical analysis by evaluating the proposed approach using datasets with varied video resolutions and input conditions.

The motivation behind constructing between-class and within-class adjacency graphs (for both our work and [6]) is inspired from LDA which uses between-class and within-class scatter matrices for discrimination. However, there are main algorithmic differences between our work and [6], which are listed below.

The primary difference between our work and [6] is in the construction of the adjacency graphs, which play a major role in discrimination of the data. In [6], the neighbors of a node are those that have the same class label as the node. Whereas, in our work, the neighbors of a node are determined by their distance to the node in the projected space, in addition to the class labels. This provides better discrimination of the data as the neighbors are decided based on their similarity in the feature space. The second difference is that [6] considers only $v$ neighbors for a node, whereas in our approach we restrict the number of neighbors based on their distance with the node in feature space. This generates a graph with nodes similar in features connected with each other, thus intrinsically representing the local structure of the data in feature space. The measure of similarity and the projection distance is effectively represented by the LBP features, which can well discriminate various pose changes and data from different classes. This ensures that videos that are similar in class and pose are mapped closer in feature space. This in turn allows for effective adjacency graph construction.

The paper is organized as follows. Section 2 discusses the extraction of LBP feature descriptors, the clustering process and the extraction of cluster representatives for each image set. Section 2.2 discusses the generation of Grassmannian manifolds using the LBP feature descriptors of the cluster representatives. Section 3 discusses the proposed kernel discriminant transform that utilizes the adjacency graphs generated using the Gram matrix (kernel matrix). The experimental results are presented in Section 4. Finally, we present the conclusions in Section 5.

## 2    Feature Extraction and Clustering

Each frame of the video sequence is described by computing the Local Binary Pattern (LBP) descriptors for the face region of the frame. The face region is divided into blocks and the LBP operator is applied to each block to extract a feature histogram. The final LBP feature descriptor is obtained by concatenating the individual LBP histograms.

The LBP operator with $P$ sampling points on a circle of radius $R$ is given by,

$$LBP_{P,R} = \sum_{p=0}^{P-1} s(g_p - g_c)2^p,$$

(1)

where

$$s(x) = \begin{cases} 1 \text{ if } x \geq 0 \\ 0 \text{ if } x < 0 \end{cases}$$

(2)

where $g_c$ corresponds to the grey value of the center pixel of the local neighborhood pixels with grey values $g_p$, $p = 0, ..., P - 1$. For our experiments, we use $LBP_{8,1}^{u2}$ operator, which is a uniform LBP operator with 8 sampling points around a radius of 1.

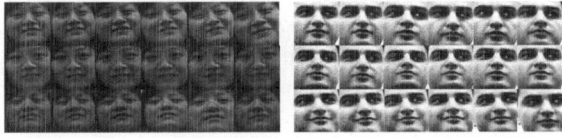

**Fig. 2.** The clusters generated by k-means clustering process using LBP features. Each row of the image shows sample images from each cluster.

### 2.1    Clustering and Cluster Representatives Extraction

Kruger and Zhou [16] and Hadid and Pietikainen [17] have used *exemplars* (cluster representatives) in recognition from videos and have shown that face sequence length affects the joint spatio-temporal representation and exemplars offer to learn the probabilistic settings of each individual from a gallery video. Also, the exemplars provide a compact and robust representation with and without the presence of the temporal dynamics of the video.

In our approach, the exemplars are extracted by clustering the frames of a video sequence and extracting a frame closest to the mean of the cluster. The distance between two LBP features is measured using the cosine similarity measure. The images are clustered using the k-means algorithm [18] which utilizes the LBP features extracted from the image sets for clustering. The motivation behind using the LBP features is due to its invariance to illumination and expression variations ([19], [20]). Also, the face is comprised of micro-patterns which are well captured by LBP. The use of LBP for face description is mainly driven by the need for achieving better accuracy and robustness across challenges such as pose variations, misalignment, etc. A video sequence of a subject can include frames with varied pose of the face of the subject. Intuitively, the linear space that represents the image set from the video sequence should span the entire set of pose variations of the face. Hence, the LBP features extracted from the image set should be capable of discrimination across pose of the face. Figure 2 shows sample images from each cluster of the video sequences of two subjects. From the figure, it can be seen that the LBP is capable of discriminating even minor pose variations.

## 2.2   Grassmannian Manifolds

Manifold analysis has received great attention in recent years. This is due to the ability of manifolds to capture the image variability and provide more information than a single image. A manifold represents the local structure exhibited by the image sets. Conceptually, image sets can be described in $\Re^D$ by linear subspaces. The linear subspaces in $\Re^D$ can be represented as points on the Grassmannian manifold $\mathcal{M}$. The problem of matching sets comprising $m$ images reduces to point classification problem on the Grassmannian manifold.

The Grassmannian manifold $\mathcal{G}(m, D)$ is defined as the set of $m$-dimensional linear subspaces of the $\Re^D$. An element of $\mathcal{G}(m, D)$ is represented by an orthonormal matrix $X$ of size $D \times m$. The matrix representation of two points is not unique and hence two points are said to be equivalent if the $span(X_1) = span(X_2)$, where $X_1$ and $X_2$ are the orthogonal matrices of the two points. Principal angles between the subspaces have been used in the past ([6], [9]) to measure the distances between image sets.

Recent approaches [21], [22], [23] proposed to treat the Grassmannian space as a Euclidean space by the use of Grassmannian kernels. Also, the non-linear property of the image sets makes it difficult to directly compute the discriminating features between two classes of image sets. Hence, by defining a non-linear mapping from the input space to a high-dimensional feature space, a linearly separable distribution in the feature space can be obtained. Thus, the kernel allows for a non-linear mapping enabling convenient computations in the input space. In our approach, we use Grassmannian kernels to perform non-linear mapping of points on a Grassmannian manifold.

The distance between two points on a Grassmannian manifold can be measured using the Grassmann kernels. Grassmann kernels are positive definite and are used to measure the similarity between two image sets. In our approach, projection kernel is used to compute the similarity score between two points on the Grassmannian manifold. The projection kernel is defined as follows:

$$K_p(X_i, X_j) = \left\| X_i^T X_j \right\|_F^2 . \tag{3}$$

Hamm and Lee [21], [22] has shown that a linear combination of positive definite kernels is also a positive definite kernel and can be used in the computation of similarity between two image sets.

For each image set $X_i$, a kernel representation $K$ and the projection matrix $P$ is obtained using the above explained procedure. The final mapping is obtained using the equation $Y = P^T K$. For recognition purposes, the kernel matrices for the training set and the testing are obtained and are then used to project the points on the Grassmannian manifold to the feature space. Matching is then performed using the nearest neighbor approach.

## 3   Modified Kernel Discriminant Analysis

The traditional Laplacian eigenmaps [24] perform dimensionality reduction by constructing a weighted graph with the points on the manifold as nodes of the graph, and a set of edges connecting a point with its closest neighbors. It also imposes the optimization problem

$$X^* = \underset{X^T D X = 1}{\arg\min} \ X^T L X. \tag{4}$$

where, $L = D - W$ is the Laplacian matrix of the graph $G$ given by the weighted adjacency matrix $W$, and the diagonal matrix $D$ such that, $D_{ii} = \sum_{j \neq i} W_{ij}$. The advantage of constructing a weighted graph is geometrically motivated, as it retains the topological relationship between the points. However, the generated weighted graph fails to discriminate between the between-class and within-class similarities of the points on the manifold. Hence, it becomes necessary to represent the between-class and within-class relationships topologically through individual adjacency graphs in order to improve the discriminatory power of the mapping function.

A transformation function that utilizes the discriminant information from the points on the manifold can optimally transform all subspaces of image sets to another space by providing maximal correlation within the same class and minimal correlation between different classes. This motivates the use of the Kernel Discriminant Analysis (KDA) [25] with the adjacency graphs and utilize it in finding a non-linear projection through eigen-analysis.

Hence, our proposed approach can be treated as a modified Laplacian Eigenmap which utilizes the concept of within-class and between-class similarities and the kernel-trick to find the optimal non-linear projection.

Given $n$ points $\{X_1, \ldots, X_n\}$ from the underlying Grassmannian manifold $\mathcal{M}$, where $X_i \in \Re^{D x m}$ ($m$ - the number of cluster representatives) and each $X_i$ belonging to the class $c_i$, the kernel similarity score between two points on the manifold is given by,

$$k_{ij} = \langle X_i, X_j \rangle, \tag{5}$$

where $\langle . \rangle$ denotes the inner product. In this paper, $k_{ij}$ is the projection kernel defined later in this section. The adjacency graphs for between-class and within-class is given by,

$$S_b(i,j) = \begin{cases} 1, & \text{if } k_{ij} \geq \epsilon \text{ and } c_i \neq c_j \\ 0, & \text{otherwise} \end{cases} \tag{6}$$

$$S_w(i,j) = \begin{cases} 1, & \text{if } k_{ij} \leq \epsilon \text{ and } c_i = c_j \\ 0, & \text{otherwise} \end{cases} \tag{7}$$

where, $S_b$ is the between-class adjacency graph, $S_w$ is the within-class adjacency graph, and $c_i$ and $c_j$ are the class labels for $X_i$ and $X_j$, respectively. The reasoning behind defining the connectivity based on the threshold $\epsilon$ is due to a better geometrical representation of the local structure of the points in the manifold when compared with a graph in which each node has exactly $k$ number of neighbors.

The kernelization in KDA allows to map the data from the original input space to a high-dimensional Hilbert space as $\phi : X_i \mapsto Y_i$. The matching between two points $Y_i$ and $Y_j$ can then be computed using the Euclidean distance measures. The optimal embedding by $\phi$ should allow the connected points from the same class to map to points as close as possible in the feature space, while separating the points between classes as far as possible in the feature space. The embedding provided by Laplacian Eigenmap minimizes the following objective function.

$$\min \sum_{i,j} (Y_i - Y_j)^2 W_{ij}. \tag{8}$$

and can be written as,

$$\min \frac{1}{2} \sum_{i,j} (Y_i - Y_j)^2 W_{ij} = Y^T L Y, \tag{9}$$

where $W$ is the weight matrix constructed using the adjacency graph, $L = D - W$. The aim of our approach is to maximize the distance between points of different classes and minimizing the distance between points of the same class in the feature space. Hence, we provide the following objective functions based on the Equation 9.

$$\min \frac{1}{2} \sum_{i,j} (Y_i - Y_j)^2 S_w(i,j) = Y^T L_w Y, \tag{10}$$

and

$$\max \frac{1}{2} \sum_{i,j} (Y_i - Y_j)^2 S_b(i,j) = Y^T L_b Y, \tag{11}$$

where $L_w = D_w - W_w$ and $L_b = D_b - W_b$. The minimization problem from Equation 10 can be written as follows.

$$\min \sum_{i,j} (Y_i^2 + Y_j^2 - 2Y_iY_j)S_w(i,j) = 2Y^T L_w Y. \tag{12}$$

It can be seen that this calculation shows that $L_w$ is positive semi definite. Equation 12 can be written as,

$$\arg\min_Y 2Y^T L_w Y. \tag{13}$$

$$= \arg\min_Y (2Y^T D_w Y - 2Y^T W_w Y). \tag{14}$$

$$= \arg\min_Y (1 - Y^T W_w Y) \text{ subject to } Y^T D_w Y = 1. \tag{15}$$

The constraint $Y^T D_w Y = 1$ removes the arbitrary scaling factor in the embedding. The minimization problem from Equation 15 can be re-written as a maximization problem as follows.

$$\begin{aligned} \arg\max_Y \quad & (Y^T W_w Y), \\ \text{subject to} \quad & Y^T D_w Y = 1. \end{aligned} \tag{16}$$

Similarly, the maximization problem from Equation 11 becomes,

$$\arg\max_Y (Y^T L_b Y). \tag{17}$$

Combining Equations 16 and 17, we get,

$$\begin{aligned} \arg\max_Y \quad & (Y^T L_b Y + Y^T \beta W_w Y). \\ = \arg\max_Y \quad & (Y^T (L_b + \beta W_w)Y), \\ \text{subject to} \quad & Y^T D_w Y = 1. \end{aligned}$$

where $\beta$ is the regularization parameter. Converting Equation 3 to a generalized eigenvalue problem, we get,

$$Y^T (L_b + \beta W_w)Y = \lambda Y^T D_w Y. \tag{18}$$

Defining the solution $Y = P^T K$, where $P$ is the desired projection matrix and $K$ is the kernel matrix, $P$ can be obtained by substituting the value of $Y$ in Equation 18 and maximizing it as follows:

$$\frac{K^T D_w K}{K^T (L_b + \beta W_w)K}. \tag{19}$$

Equation 19 refers to the Rayleigh quotient whose eigenvectors are the eigenvectors of the projection matrix $P$.

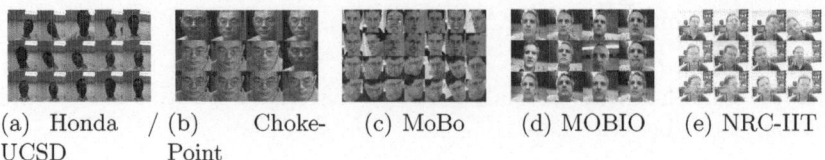

(a) Honda  / (b)      Choke-    (c) MoBo    (d) MOBIO    (e) NRC-IIT
UCSD         Point

**Fig. 3.** Sample video frames from various datasets

## 4    Experiments

**Experimental Setup:** For each video frame, the face region is cropped using the Viola-Jones [26] face detector. Since LBP is illumination invariant, no illumination normalization is performed on the images. The cropped face region is resized to $150 \times 150$ pixels. The $D$ dimensional LBP features are computed using uniform LBP with 8 sampling points and a radius of 1 pixel. The LBP features of each image set are clustered using k-means with $k$ being 20 in our experiments. Cluster representatives are then selected to form a $D \times m$ data matrix $X$. Orthogonal bases are computed for each image set using Singular Value Decomposition (SVD) on $X_i$ to represent each training subspace. The error in orthogonalization is avoided by reorthogonalizing the bases using SVD. The Gram matrix $K$ (kernel matrix) is computed using the projection kernel. The adjacency graphs $S_b$ and $S_w$ are computed using $K$, which are in turn used in kernel discriminant transform. The projection matrix $P$ is obtained by maximizing the Rayleigh equation (Equation 19) by Eigen decomposition.

**Datasets:** In order to show the effectiveness of the proposed approach, face recognition experiments are conducted using I. The Honda/UCSD video database [27], II. The ChokePoint dataset [28], III. The CMU MoBo database [29], IV. NRC-IIT Facial video database [30] (videos taken using webcam), and V. MOBIO database [31] (videos taken using mobile phones). The statistics on these datasets are provided in Table 1. Figures 3 show sample video frames from all the datasets.

**Table 1.** Statistics of the video datasets used in the experiments

| Dataset | # Videos (#training, #testing) | # Subjects | Resolution | Variations (pose, occlusion, scale) |
|---|---|---|---|---|
| Honda [27] | 56 (33, 23) | 20 | $640 \times 480$ | yes |
| ChokePoint [28] | 434 (218, 216) | 25 | $160 \times 120$ | yes |
| MoBo [29] | 96 (72, 24) | 25 | $640 \times 480$ | yes |
| NRC-IIT [30] | 22 (11, 11) | 11 | $160 \times 120$ | yes |
| MOBIO [31] | 1790 (895, 895) | 152 | varies | yes |

**Experimental Evaluation:** In order to evaluate the proposed approach, face recognition experiments are conducted on four different datasets and compared with two state-of-the-art approaches proposed by Cevikalp and Triggs [5] and Harandi *et al.* [6]. To illustrate the effectiveness of the cluster representatives based recognition, we performed face recognition using all the frames of the video sequences in addition to the proposed approach.

## 4.1 Experimental Results

The face recognition accuracies from the proposed approach (using cluster representatives), a variant of the proposed approach (using all frames of the video), the Kernel AHISD [5] approach, the GGDA [6] approach, and the traditional Kernel DA [25] for all the four datasets are summarized in Table 2. The results indicate that the proposed modified kernel DA provides a better recognition performance when compared with the traditional DA. This shows the effectiveness of the adjacency graphs in discriminating the data between classes and within a class. The results also indicate the effectiveness of using the cluster representatives as it can be seen that the recognition accuracy is improved when compared with those in which all the frames of the video sequences are used. In addition, it can be seen that the proposed approach without clustering process (row 4 of table 2) provides a better recognition accuracy for low resolution videos when compared with other approaches (Kernel AHISD and GGDA) in spite of using all the frames of the video sequences.

The results indicate that the proposed approach provides a better performance for varying image resolutions. In particular, the performance is superior to other state-of-the-art approaches in case of low resolution image sets (ChokePoint, NRC-IIT, and MOBIO), which is the most natural setting for video sequences obtained from surveillance.

**Table 2.** Face recognition accuracies of various approaches on different datasets

|  | Honda | ChokePoint | MoBo | NRC-IIT | MOBIO |
|---|---|---|---|---|---|
| Kernel DA [25] | 56.27% | 32.64% | 53.67% | 42.33% | 41.63% |
| Kernel AHISD [5] | 100% | 74.92% | 91.66% | 53.33% | 63.64% |
| GGDA [6] | 65.22% | 48.28% | 66.67% | 46.67% | 44.81% |
| Proposed (no clustering) | 95.65% | 76.39% | 87.50% | 58.33% | 70.41% |
| Proposed (cluster reps.) | **100%** | **97.22%** | **94.25%** | **83.33%** | **74.52%** |

The experiments on all the datasets were performed with the same set of parameter values. For example, the value for the regularization parameter $\beta$ from Equation 19 is set to 5 (optimally chosen using images across datasets) for the experiments on all the datasets. Also, the cropped face images are resized to $150 \times 150$ pixels in order to retain uniformity in the computation of the LBP from the face images across datasets.

# 5   Conclusions

In this work we proposed a modified kernel discriminant analysis for recognizing faces from video sequences. The modified KDA utilizes the adjacency graphs which represent the between-class and within-class similarities of the video sequences. Effective recognition is performed with minimal set of key frames extracted from the video sequence by clustering the video frames. Exemplars are extracted for each video frame by clustering them based on their LBP descriptors and are mapped as points on the Grassmannian manifold. Recognition is performed in the projected space using the nearest neighbor approach. Experiments on various datasets illustrate the effectiveness of the proposed approach across various challenges. In future, it is interesting to apply the approach for general object recognition.

# References

1. Fukui, K., Yamaguchi, O.: Face recognition using multi-viewpoint patterns for robot vision. In: International Symposium of Robotics Research (2003)
2. Fan, W., Yeung, D.Y.: Locally linear models on face appearance manifolds with application to dual-subspace based classification. In: Computer Vision and Pattern Recognition (2006)
3. Wang, R., Shan, S., Chen, X., Gao, W.: Manifold-manifold distance with application to face recognition based on image sets. In: Computer Vision and Pattern Recognition (2008)
4. Lee, K.C., Mo, J., Yang, M.H., Kriegman, D.: Video-based face recognition using probabilistic appearance manifolds. In: Computer Vision and Pattern Recognition (2003)
5. Cevikalp, H., Triggs, B.: Face recognition based on image sets. In: Computer Vision and Pattern Recognition (2010)
6. Harandi, M.T., Sanderson, C., Shirazi, S., Lovell, B.C.: Graph embedding discriminant analysis on grassmannian manifolds for improved image set matching. In: Computer Vision and Pattern Recognition Workshop (2011)
7. Poh, N., Rua, E.A., Struc, V.: An evaluation of video-to-video face verification. IEEE Trans. of Information Forensics and Security 5 (2010)
8. Arandjelovic, O., Shakhnarovich, G., Fisher, J., Cipolla, R., Darrell, T.: Face recognition with image sets using manifold density divergence. In: Proc. of Computer Vision and Pattern Recognition, vol. 1, pp. 581–588 (2005)
9. Yamaguchi, O., Fukui, K., Maeda, K.: Face recognition using temporal image sequence. In: Proc. Automatic Face and Gesture Recognition, pp. 318–323 (1998)
10. Nishiyama, M., Yamaguchi, O., Fukui, K.: Face Recognition with the Multiple Constrained Mutual Subspace Method. In: Kanade, T., Jain, A., Ratha, N.K. (eds.) AVBPA 2005. LNCS, vol. 3546, pp. 71–80. Springer, Heidelberg (2005)
11. Kim, T.K., Kittler, J., Cipolla, R.: Discriminative learning and recognition of image set classes using canonical correlations. IEEE Trans. on Pattern Anal. Mach. Intell. 29, 1005–1018 (2007)
12. Kokiopoulou, E., Froddard, P.: Video face recognition with graph-based semi-supervised learning. In: Proc. ICME, pp. 1564–1565 (2009)

13. Yan, S., Xu, D., Zhang, B., Zhang, H.J., Yang, Q., Lin, S.: Graph enbedding and extensions: A general framework for dimensionality reduction. IEEE Trans. Pattern Anal. Mach. Intell. 29, 40–51 (2007)
14. Mian, A.: Unsupervised learning from local features for video-based face recognition. In: IEEE Int. of Conf. Automatic Face Gesture Recognition, pp. 1–6 (2008)
15. Chen, J., Ye, J., Li, Q.: Integrating global and local structures: A least squares framework for dimensionality reduction. In: Proc. Computer Vision and Pattern Recognition, pp. 1–8 (2007)
16. Kruger, V., Zhou, S.: Exemplar-based face recognition from video. In: IEEE Intl. on Automatic Face and Gesture Recognition, pp. 175–180 (2002)
17. Hadid, A., Pietikainen, M.: From still image to video-based face recognition: An experimental analysis. In: IEEE Intl. Conf. on Automatic Face and Gesture Recognition, pp. 813–818 (2004)
18. Lloyd, S.P.: Least squares quantization in pcm. IEEE Trans. on Information Theory 28, 129–137 (1982)
19. Ahonen, T., Hadid, A., Pietikäinen, M.: Face Recognition with Local Binary Patterns. In: Pajdla, T., Matas, J(G.) (eds.) ECCV 2004. LNCS, vol. 3021, pp. 469–481. Springer, Heidelberg (2004)
20. Ahonen, T., Hadid, A., Pietikainen, M.: Face description with local binary patterns: Application to face recognition. IEEE Trans. on Pattern Analysis and Machine Intelligence 28, 2037–2041 (2006)
21. Hamm, J., Lee, D.D.: Grassmann discriminant analysis: A unifying view on subspace-based learning. In: Proc. Int. Conf. Machine Learning (ICML), pp. 376–383 (2008)
22. Hamm, J., Lee, D.D.: Extended grassmann kernels for subspace-based learning. In: Neural Information Processing Systems, pp. 601–608 (2009)
23. Wolf, L., Shashua, A.: Learning over sets using kernel principal angles. J. Mach. Learn. Res. 4, 913–931 (2003)
24. Belkin, M., Niyogi, P.: Laplacian eigenmaps and spectral techniques for embedding and clustering. Advances in Neural information Processing Systems 16 (2004)
25. Mika, S., Ratsch, G., Weston, J., Scholkoph, B., Mullers, K.R.: Fisher discriminant analysis with kernels. Neural Networks for Signal Processing (1999)
26. Viola, P., Jones, M.J.: Robust real-time face detection. International Journal of Computer Vision 57, 137–154 (2004)
27. Lee, K., Ho, J., Yang, M., Kriegman, D.: Visual tracking and recognition using probabilistic appearance manifolds. Computer Vision and Image Understanding 99, 303–331 (2005)
28. Wong, Y., Chen, S., Mau, S., Sanderson, C., Lovell, B.C.: Patch-based probabilistic image quality assessment for face selection and improved video-based face recognition. In: Computer Vision and Pattern Recognition Workshops (CVPRW), pp. 74–81 (2011)
29. Gross, R., Shi, J.: The cmu motion of body (mobo) database. Technical Report CMU-RI-TR-01-18, Robotics Institute, Pittsburgh, PA (2001)
30. Gorodnichy, D.O.: Video-based framework for face recognition in video. In: Second Workshop on Face Processing in Video in Proceedings of Second Canadian Conference on Computer and Robot Vision, pp. 330–338.
31. McCool, C., Marcel, S., Hadid, A., Pietikainen, M., Matejka, P., Cernocky, J., Poh, N., Kittler, J., Larcher, A., Levy, C., Matrouf, D., Bonastre, J.F., Tresadern, P., Cootes, T.: Bi-modal person recognition on a mobile phone using mobile phone data. In: IEEE ICME Workshop on Hot Topics in Mobile Multimedia (2012)

# Learning Hierarchical Bag of Words Using Naive Bayes Clustering

Siddhartha Chandra[1], Shailesh Kumar[2], and C.V. Jawahar[1]

[1] CVIT, IIIT Hyderabad
[2] Google, Hyderabad
siddhartha_c@students.iiit.ac.in,
shkumar@google.com, jawahar@iiit.ac.in

**Abstract.** Image analysis tasks such as classification, clustering, detection, and retrieval are only as good as the feature representation of the images they use. Much research in computer vision is focused on finding *better* or *semantically richer* image representations. Bag of visual Words (BoW) is a representation that has emerged as an effective one for a variety of computer vision tasks. BoW methods traditionally use low level features. We have devised a strategy to use these low level features to create "higher level" features by making use of the spatial context in images. In this paper, we propose a novel *hierarchical feature learning framework* that uses a *Naive Bayes Clustering* algorithm to convert a 2-D symbolic image at one level to a 2-D symbolic image at the next level with richer features. On two popular datasets, Pascal VOC 2007 and Caltech 101, we empirically show that classification accuracy obtained from the hierarchical features computed using our approach is significantly higher than the traditional SIFT based BoW representation of images even though our image representations are more compact.

## 1 Introduction

Over the years, research in computer vision has tried to narrow down the gap between raw image pixels and what humans see when they look at the image. The efforts to do so can be very broadly categorized into two classes. The first class of methods uses a robust representation based on relatively low level features (e.g. SIFT based Bag of Words (BoW) representations [1, 2]). BoW representations have received widespread success in a variety of computer vision tasks such as image classification and object detection [1–3] owing to their invariance to scale, spatial and rotational distortions. These methods also use domain knowledge. Over the years, much research has gone into improving the performance of models that employ BoW representations. Non-linear SVMs, specialized kernels of different kinds [4–7], and spatial pyramids [8] have all contributed to the success of these representations. Most of these approaches tend to increase the overall image representation size. While these methods have been successful in capturing diversity in image patches at low levels, it is hard to incorporate them into a hierarchical feature learning frameworks naturally as there is no systematic way to create higher level symbols from combinations of lower level discrete symbols.

K.M. Lee et al. (Eds.): ACCV 2012, Part I, LNCS 7724, pp. 382–395, 2013.
© Springer-Verlag Berlin Heidelberg 2013

The second class of methods continues to *enrich* low level features by using *hierarchical feature learning paradigms*. Most hierarchical feature learning approaches such as Deep Belief Networks [9], Convolutional Neural Networks [10], Convolutional Deep Belief Networks [11] and other hierarchical models [12] use simple building blocks such as a logistic function to learn complex overall models with many parameters to tune. Ideas like layered incremental training have made the training of these models practical. Further they can model translation invariance well using max pooling. The limitation in these models is that they need real-valued inputs at each layer in the hierarchy and hence the traditional BoW approaches that generate a large number of discrete symbols at lower levels cannot be naturally incorporated into such hierarchical feature learning frameworks. While the deep learning methods have been known to work well for a variety of simpler datasets such as ILSVRC 2010, ImageNet and Hollywood 2, they haven't enjoyed much success on more challenging datasets such as PASCAL [13].

Research into bridging the gap between these two directions exists. Hyperfeatures [14] exploit the spatial co-occurrence statistics at scales larger than their local input patches by aggregating local descriptors using methods such as GMM and LDA. This paper is a step forward in this direction and tries to combine the strengths of hierarchical feature learning and BoW learning paradigms. We propose a generic framework for building *discrete feature hierarchies* in an unsupervised fashion starting from any first level symbol image (e.g. dense SIFT visual words). The framework has two parts: (a) a novel *Naive Bayes Clustering* algorithm that clusters symbolic image patches using EM like updates to maximize the log likelihood of the data in terms of a mixture of naive Bayes discrete multi-variate distributions, and (b) a maximum pooling on neighboring patches using the posterior probabilities of clusters in data points to reduce the image size at the next level. Evaluations on Caltech 101 and Pascal VOC 2007 indicate our compact, meaningful representations outperform the traditional BoW and deep learnt representations.

## 2   Background

In this section we briefly summarize the two prominent directions in computer vision which endeavour to represent the visual world through features which are invariant to various external parameters. However, while the BoW approaches can improve by further exploiting the information content in the spatial layout of images, the deep learning methods can enhance their utility by overcoming the training and architectural complexity for learning large scale computer vision systems. We intend to learn from these two directions and take an approach that combines their powers to achieve superior representation.

### 2.1   Beyond Bag of Words

Visual BoW draws its inspiration from the analogous BoW models for document representation that ignore the order of words. Traditional image classification involves computing local features at interest points in an image and pooling these local features to give a global image representation. BoW essentially quantizes each local feature into one of the visual words using a codebook and then represents each image as a histogram of visual words. Computing the codebook involves identifying interesting local patches in an image, extracting features or keypoints such as SIFT from these local patches and finally clustering (usually using K-means) to group key points from the training images into clusters; the center of each cluster corresponds to a different visual word. Finally each SIFT vector is quantized by assigning it the label of the nearest cluster center. We represent each image as a histogram of the visual words, called the BoW representation.

BoW represents an image using the distribution of visual word occurrences. In doing so, it converts images of different sizes into fixed length representations. This is especially convenient for the classification task that need fixed dimensional inputs. However, BoW relies only on the appearance of the visual words and ignores their spatial layout. This characteristic imparts invariance to scale, translation and deformation, at the cost of discriminative power especially when the spatial layout is important.

There have been many recent attempts to overcome the limitations of BoW [15]. These include part generative models like [16] and frameworks that use geometric correspondence search [17]. These work well but are computationally expensive. BoW can be enhanced [18] by extending the codebook to include *doublets* which are pair-wise relations between features that lie in the same local neighbourhood. Spatial pyramids [8] was a major breakthrough in this direction; it incorporates spatial information by computing BoW representations for different image regions at different scales and concatenating these representations and finally uses a pyramid matching kernel [19] for classification. Almost everything in the book - from kernels [4–7] to sparsity [20] to local codes [6] has been attempted to enhance the power of these low level representations [21].

All these indicate the need of raising the semantic depth of the low level features discovered through the BoW process. Bringing context of neighboring features to define "higher level" features is clearly recognized as the next natural step here. As described in section 1, hyperfeatures [14] were devised especially to fulfil this need. In this paper, we continue to explore this middle ground.

## 2.2   Deep Learning

Deep learning networks [9, 11] and convolutional networks [10] represent an orthogonal school of thought. These are driven by the idea that good internal representations are hierarchical and can be learned directly from the data. These networks have hierarchical layers (also called *feature maps*) stacked together; each feature map learns artifacts in the image by assembling smaller artifacts learnt by the preceding feature maps. Pixels are assembled into edges, edges into object parts, object parts into objects, and objects into a scene; deep learning thus exploits the spatial information in the images. These levels represent the feature hierarchy.

Convolutional networks typically work on *overlapping* patches at each level (the overlap takes care of small translations) and summarize the features learnt in a neighbourhood by a pooling method. Popular pooling methods are (a) average pooling where the features computed over a region (called a cell) are averaged to give the feature representation of the cell and (b) max-pooling where the feature representation of the cell is the maximum of the features in the cell. Convolutional networks usually alternate between feature maps and pooling layers to achieve invariance to small translations and distortions.

Deep learning gives robust image representations. However *insufficient depth can hurt*. Also, training deep networks involves making many design decisions, huge training set, is computationally challenging and most of the feasible training algorithms are mostly approximations of the actual objective. (In fact, attempts at training deep networks had failed before [9].)

There have been a few attempts to bridge the gap between the two schools by taking the middle ground and developing frameworks that exploit the advantages of both [22]. In this paper, we intend to take a leap forward in this direction. Our approach involves deep / hierarchical learning of higher level discrete symbols from lower level discrete symbols (for instance BoW visual words) that lie in the same spatial neighbourhood. Our approach is different from traditional deep learning in that we work with symbols / visual words and not real valued features. A novel Naive Bayes Clustering method allows us to cluster combinations of low level symbols.

## 3   Naive Bayes Clustering

In order to build hierarchy of discrete features to compose symbols at the next level using the right juxtapositions of symbols at the previous level, we need a systematic way of dealing with the combinatorial explosion. For example, if we use 1000 low level features obtained from BoW and create higher level symbols from just $2 \times 2$ patches of SIFT visual words, the potential combinatorial space of discrete symbols at next level is $O(10^{12})$, clearly too prohibitive to just do traditional $2 \times 2$-gram histogram counting. If this were real-valued data, we could use any clustering technique but since this is symbolic data in a large vocabulary we need to use a non traditional clustering technique.

In this section we present a novel Naive Bayes clustering algorithm to cluster multi-variate discrete data in general and discrete image patches in particular. Note that in our experiments, we start with SIFT-BoW visual words; a discrete image patch is thus a patch of such visual words. To define a clustering algorithm, we need to define a "cost function", a "cluster representation" and of "update rules" to learn the cluster centers and cluster associations with data. First some notation: Let $\mathbf{X} = \{\mathbf{x}^n = (x_1^n \ldots x_D^n)\}_{n=1}^N$ be the set of $N$ data points. Each feature $X_d \in \mathbf{V}_d$ comes from a *discrete* feature vocabulary $\mathbf{V}_d = \{v_1^d \ldots v_{M_d}^d\}$ of size $M_d = |\mathbf{V}_d|$. In image domain, each 2-D discrete image patch of size $P \times P$ is treated as a one-dimensional vector of size $D = P^2$ and each symbol comes from the same vocabulary, (i.e. $\mathbf{V}_d = \mathbf{V}$ of dense SIFT clusters.)

## 3.1   Mixture of Multi-variate Discrete Naive Bayes

Mixture models [23] are commonly used to partition the data into meaningful clusters. Our patches are in $P \times P$ discrete space. Typically a parametric mixture model is learnt by maximizing a (log) likelihood objective over the data:

$$J(\Theta) = \log \prod_{n=1}^{N} P(\mathbf{x}^n) = \sum_{n=1}^{N} \log \sum_{k=1}^{K} P(k)P(\mathbf{x}^n|k). \qquad (1)$$

Depending on the nature of the data, the mixture density function $P(\mathbf{x}|k)$ takes different forms. For example when $\mathbf{x} \in R^D$ any real-valued multi-variate density function such as a full Gaussian can be used. In our case $\mathbf{x} \in \mathbf{V}^D$ and therefore in this paper, we propose to use the simplest multi-variate discrete density function, i.e. *Naive Bayes* (NB):

$$P(\mathbf{x}^n|k) = \prod_{d=1}^{D} P(x_d^n|k) \qquad (2)$$

In NB clustering, therefore we learn a "mixture-of-Naive Bayes" parametric generative model (Eq. 1) over a multi-variate discrete data by conveniently assuming independence among the features (Eq. 2). In general there are two constraints that are also part of the objective. The priors must add up to one and the density functions over all possible values that each feature can take for any given mixture component must also add up to one, i.e.,

$$\sum_{k=1}^{K} P(k) = 1, \sum_{m=1}^{M_d} P\left(v_m^d|k\right) = 1, \forall d = 1 \dots D \qquad (3)$$

A total of $K \times \left(1 + \sum_{d=1}^{D} M_d\right)$ parameters $\Theta = \left\{P(k), \{P(v_m^d)\}_{m=1}^{M_d}\right\}_{k=1}^{K}$ are learnt using an EM-algorithm with the following update rules for the E-step (Eq. 4) and smoothed M-step (Eq. 5 and 6) from iteration $t - 1$ to iteration $t$.

$$P_t(k|\mathbf{x}_n) = \frac{P_{t-1}(\mathbf{x}_n|k)P_{t-1}(k)}{\sum_{k'}^{K} P_{t-1}(\mathbf{x}_n|k')P_{t-1}(k')} \qquad (4)$$

$$P_t(k) = \frac{\lambda + \sum_{n=1}^{N} P_t(k|\mathbf{x}_n)}{\lambda K + N} \qquad (5)$$

$$P_t(v_m^d|k) = \frac{\lambda' + \sum_{n=1}^{N} \delta(x_{n,d} = v_m^d)P_t(k|\mathbf{x}_n)}{\lambda' M_d + N P_t(k)} \qquad (6)$$

Equation 4 computes the posterior probability of assigning a data point to cluster $k$ in the next iteration $(t)$ given the parameters at the previous iteration $(t-1)$. Equations 5 and 6 are the parameter updates based on the assignment of data points to the clusters in this iteration. $\delta$ is the *kronecker delta*. Here we employ basic laplacian smoothing that takes affect mostly if the number of points in a cluster is small compared to the vocabulary size.

## 3.2 Soft vs. Hard Clustering

The EM algorithm described above represents a soft clustering algorithm where each data point is assigned to all clusters using the posterior probabilities i.e., $P_t(k|\mathbf{x}_n)$ in each iteration. This increases the computational complexity of the other update rules by a factor of $K$. In traditional (hard) clustering in each iteration, a data point is assigned to the cluster with the highest posterior probability. The hard clustering version of the above soft clustering algorithm alternates between the assign cluster E-step (Eq. 7) and the cluster parameters M-step (Eq. 8 and 9):

$$\kappa_{t-1}(\mathbf{x}^n) = \arg\max_{k=1...K} \{P_{t-1}(\mathbf{x}_n|k)P_{t-1}(k)\} \tag{7}$$

$$P_t(k) = \frac{1}{N} \sum_{n=1}^{N} \delta\left(\kappa_{t-1}(\mathbf{x}^n) = k\right) \tag{8}$$

$$P_t\left(v_m^d|k\right) = \frac{\sum_{n=1}^{N} \delta\left(x_d^n = v_m^d\right)\delta\left(\kappa_{t-1}(\mathbf{x}^n) = k\right)}{\sum_{n=1}^{N} \delta\left(\kappa_{t-1}(\mathbf{x}^n) = k\right)} \tag{9}$$

Hard clustering is faster since parameter updates take $K$ times less time per iteration. Combined with a smarter initialization strategy discussed below, we found this to be better than soft clustering in terms of convergence and quality.

## 3.3 Smart Initialization

Sensitivity to initialization is a well known problem with clustering. Bad random initializations typically result in slow convergence, poor clustering quality and require multiple runs with different random initializations to generate the right final clusters. This randomness and uncertainty in clustering initialization can be mitigated by a number of smart initialization strategies [24]. In this paper, we employ a *farthest first point* (FFP) initialization. The goal of this initialization is to pick the initial $K$ clusters such that they "cover" the entire data space well by spreading themselves as far away from each other as possible. Representation score of a point is defined as the similarity of a data point with the nearest cluster. The similarity between two data points $\mathbf{x}^n$ and $\mathbf{x}^{n'}$, $sim(\mathbf{x}^n, \mathbf{x}^{n'}) = \sum_k \delta(x_d^n = x_d^{n'})$ The FFP algorithm works as follows:

1. Initialize:
   - First cluster randomly: $k \leftarrow 1, \mu_1 = \mathbf{x}^r$ where $r =$random$(\{1...N\})$
   - *Representation scores*: $R(\mathbf{x}^n|\mu_1) = sim(\mathbf{x}^n, \mu_1), \forall n = 1...N$
2. Sample least represented point as the next cluster. If there are more than one equally representative points, pick one randomly.:

$$\mu_{k+1} = \arg\min_{n=1...N} R(\mathbf{x}^n|\mu_1 \ldots \mu_k) \tag{10}$$

3. Update the representation scores of all data points:

$$R(\mathbf{x}^n|\mu_1 \ldots \mu_{k+1}) = \max\{R(\mathbf{x}^n|\mu_1 \ldots \mu_k), sim(\mathbf{x}^n, \mu_{k+1})\}, \forall n = 1...N$$

4. $k \leftarrow k+1$, repeat steps 2 through 4 while $k < K$

FFP based smart initialization gives significantly better clusters and faster convergence than traditional random initializations.

# 4   Learning Hierarchical Bag of Words

Any form of vector quantization gives a symbolic representation to the keypoints. Kmeans as a vector quantization framework has the limitation that it can cluster real valued keypoints only, because it has no distance metric to compare symbols. This is the primary hurdle that has prevented the evolution of models that learn hierarchical bags of features. As described in section 3.2, the NB clustering algorithm is designed to cluster symbolic data and hence it can be used to quantize discrete symbolic vectors. With this useful tool, we are prepared to exploit the principles of deep learning to learn features in the BoW domain.

## 4.1   Approach

We start conventionally by employing K-means on features computed at local image patches to give us symbol representations for the low level keypoints. Given these representations, we compute BoW representations of the images: we refer to these as our first level image representations / features. However, we do not lose the symbolic image yet, for it has spatial context. Adhering to the conventional mode of feature extraction, we collect keypoints (vectors of symbols) from patches in a dense grid over the level 1 symbol image. We quantize these symbolic vectors using the naive bayes clustering approach to get another level of symbols and another symbol image in turn. The symbols at this level are aggregations of the symbols at the previous level that lie in the same local neighbourhood. We compute the BoW representation of these level 2 symbol images and call these the second level image representations. We have thus devised a hierarchical feature extraction scheme that is independent of the way we get the visual words at any level: this process can be repeated any number of times to get a desired level of image representation. Figure 1 describes our approach.

## 4.2   Maximum Pooling

Spatial pooling is an idea borrowed from the deep learning community that introduces compactness in the representation and imparts invariance to distortions by reducing the spatial resolution. Conventionally, spatial pooling is done over a grid of cells where the keypoints within each cell are summarized by a single keypoint. For a cell $c$ spanning $P \times P$ symbolic keypoints ($\mathbf{x}^n, n = 1, \ldots, P^2$), we define the cell representative $\alpha_c$ to be the symbol with the maximum posterior probability as given by

$$\alpha_c = \arg\max_n \{P(\mathbf{x}_n | \kappa(x^n)) P(\kappa(x^n))\} \tag{11}$$

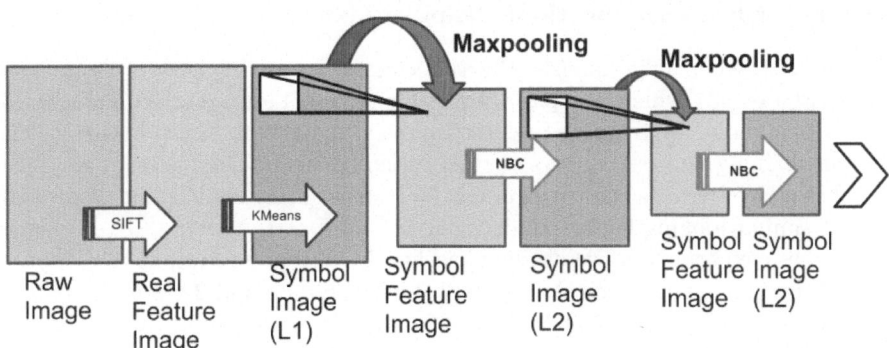

**Fig. 1.** Block diagram of our approach. SIFT features are computed on the raw image patches and quantized using K-means to get the first level symbol image. Henceforth, keypoints at any level of the hierarchy are collected from patches in a dense grid over the symbol image at the previous level. These keypoints are clustered using NB clustering and quantized to get the the symbol image at the current level. This process can be repeated any number of times. BoW representations can be computed using the symbol image at any level of the hierarchy and used for classification.

where $\kappa(x^n)$ is the cluster representative of $x^n$. In our experiments, we follow the usual convolutional network maxpooling protocol which uses non-overlapping patches of size $2 \times 2$ pixels.

## 5    Experiments, Results and Discussions

In this section, we use the NB clustering to learn hierarchical feature representations and use the learnt representations for the task of image classification. We first demonstrate our approach on a simple two class classification problem, and later show comprehensive results on two popular object classification datasets, namely Caltech 101 and Pascal VOC 2007. In this process, we gain insights into the learning by studying the effect of the parameters like the patch size $(p)$, the size of the symbol space at each level $(K)$ and the level of the hierarchy $(l)$. We argue that the method learns semantically meaningful concepts by assessing the objective we are trying to achieve. We also demonstrate that hierarchical representations learnt through the NB clustering of visual words are better representations and outperform the traditional BoW method of image classification.

**Experimental Setup:** In all the following experiments, we extract SIFT features over a dense grid using a scale of 12 and a shift of 6 pixels. Our baseline BoW representations are computed by clustering the SIFT vectors into 1000 visual words. For classification, we use a $\chi^2$ homogeneous kernel map [3] on the BoW histograms and use a linear pegasos SVM [25].

## 5.1   Two Class Classification: Okapi vs Llama

For the first set of experiments, the two classes we work with are llama and okapi (Figure 2a) which are part of the Caltech 101 dataset. We sample 15 images randomly for training and testing each from both these classes. This gives us training and testing sets of sizes 30 images each. These classes are hard to differentiate because the two animals look structurally similar and are found against similar looking backgrounds.

For these experiments, we use our baseline BoW representations to compute Level 2 features using patch sizes $p_2 = 2, 3$ with shifts 1 and 2 respectively and vocabulary size $K_2 = 50, 100, 150, 200, 250, 500$ (from this point on, we denote the patch size and the size of the symbol space at the $n^{th}$ level by $p_n$ and $K_n$ respectively). BoW on the level 2 features given by each combination of $p_2$ and $K_2$ gives us a different level 2 representation. We compute Level 3 features using the level 2 representation given by $p_2 = 2, K_2 = 200$. For level 3, we use $p_3 = 2$ with shift of 1 and $K_3 = 50, 100, 200$. We use classification accuracy as the performance metric in our evaluations in these experiments.

Figures 2b and 2c compare the classification performance of hierarchical representations with the baseline BoW. In 2b we fix the representation level ($l = 2$) and vary $K_2$ and $p_2$; in 2c we fix $p_2$ and vary the representation level ($l = 2, 3$) and $K_2$ and $K_3$. In 2b, level 2 features significantly outperform level 1 features. Also, a patch size of 3 works gives better accuracy. At the representation size of 200, the performance gap between level 1 and level 2 features is 30%. In 2c The plots demonstrate the improvement in classification accuracies as we build higher representations. For level 3, we hit the 100% accuracy bound at $K_3 = 100$ while for level 1, accuracy is merely 68% for $K_1 = 1000$. Hence we achieve 32% higher accuracies using $1/10^{th}$ representation size.

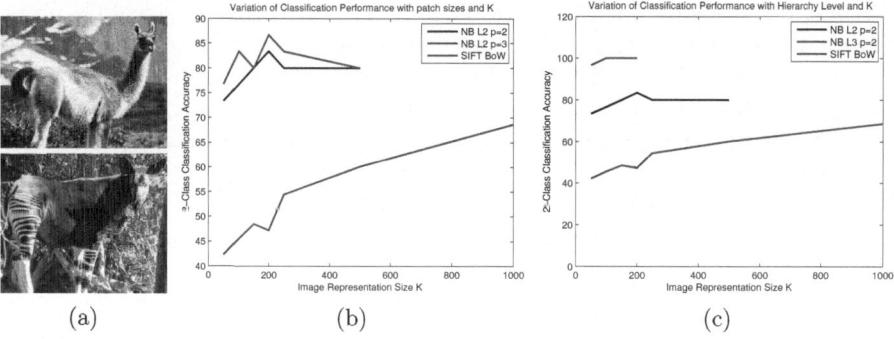

(a)                    (b)                              (c)

**Fig. 2.** Two-Class (Llama vs Okapi) Classification. (a) Llama (top) and Okapi (bottom) (b) Variation of accuracy with level 2 patch size and size of symbol space. (c) Classification accuracy based on Level 2,3 features; We chose p=2.

Figures 3a and 3b investigate what goes on at the core of the NB clustering algorithm during the vocabulary building procedure. We plot the average posterior probability per symbol per symbolic patch over the epochs of the training procedure. This is the average probability of a symbol to assume a particular position in a patch. This in turn determines the probability of a patch being part of a cluster of patches. In (c), we fix the level of representation ($l = 2$) while varying $p_2$ and $K_2$; in (d) we fix patch size and vary the representation level ($l = 2, 3$) and the number of clusters $K_2$ and $K_3$. It can be observed that bigger patches have lower average probabilities per symbol. This can be attributed to the fact that clustering a vector of 9 symbols is tougher than clustering a vector of 4 symbols because bigger patches are more complex in the number of ways the symbols are aligned in a patch. Another observation is that this probability increases as we increase the number of clusters. This can be explained by stating that increasing the number of clusters is allowing the arrangements of symbols in a patch more states to be in. Thus, each patch is more likely to find a state that it is most similar to. Finally, we comment on the increase in these probabilities across levels of the hierarchy. Figure 3b shows that the probabilities are higher for level 3 (for a fixed $K$). This shows that patches at this level are more likely (than patches at level 2) to find states / configuration of symbols that describe them. This has a direct bearing on the purity of the representations in terms of what they mean semantically.

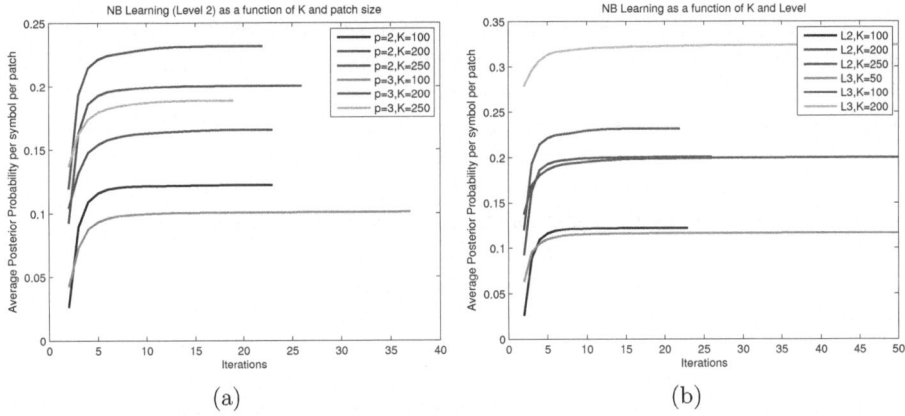

(a)                                    (b)

**Fig. 3.** (a) Plot of mean posterior probabilities per symbol per patch over epochs. Effect of the patch size (p) and size of symbol space (K) can be seen here. (b) NB Learning for different sizes of symbol space (K) across hierarchical levels 2 and 3. Higher probabilities for Level 3 show that the method is learning semantically meaningful concepts.

## 5.2   Caltech 101

Caltech 101 contains a total of 9146 images, split among 101 distinct object categories. In these experiments, we sampled 30 random images for training

Table 1: Classification accuracies on Caltech 101 for combinations of Spatial Pyramid and NB hierarchical features (and the baseline BoW). Table 2: Classification Accuracies on Caltech. BoW represents our baseline BoW results, BoW* represents the results quoted in [8]. Note that [8] uses pyramid kernel (and we use $\chi^2$) and different scale, shift for SIFT computation. NBC represents our best results corresponding to L2, $K_2 = 250$ with level 2 SPM.

**Table 1.** Caltech 101- NB + SP

| SPM | BoW | L2(250) | L3(200) |
|-----|-----|---------|---------|
| L 0 | $43.4 \pm 1.2\%$ | $60.4 \pm 0.7\%$ | $61.3 \pm 1.4\%$ |
| L 1 | $59.0 \pm 0.8\%$ | $68.2 \pm 0.8\%$ | $66.6 \pm 1.6\%$ |
| L 2 | $68.3 \pm 1.3\%$ | $72.4 \pm 0.6\%$ | $69.8 \pm 0.9\%$ |
| L 3 | $67.6 \pm 0.7\%$ | $67.8 \pm 1.1\%$ | $66.3 \pm 1.4\%$ |

**Table 2.** Classification on Caltech

| Method | Accuracy |
|--------|----------|
| BoW* [8] | $64.6 \pm 0.8\%$ |
| CDBN [11] | $65.4 \pm 0.5\%$ |
| BoW | $68.3 \pm 1.3\%$ |
| NBC | $72.4 \pm 1.8\%$ |

from each of the 101 categories, getting a total of 3030 training images; the rest of the images were treated as testing images; however, as in [8], we limited the number of testing images per category to 50. These experiments were repeated 5 times with random subsampling and the mean classification accuracies over the five experiments are reported. To compute the BoW codebook, we sampled 5 training images from each category (505 images in all). We trained a one-vs-rest SVM for each class and the test image was assigned the label of the classifier with the highest score and report the accuracy of the classification.

For level 2, we use patches of sizes $2 \times 2$ and $3 \times 3$ with shifts of 1 and 2 pixels respectively. To compute the level 2 vocabulary, we sample 5 images randomly from each class and further sample each of these images to collect 25% of the total keypoints per image; we use $K_2 = 100, 250$. For the third level, the patch size is $2 \times 2$ with a shift of 1 and $K_3 = 100, 200$, vocabulary is computed using 5 random training images per class and using 25% of the keypoints per image. The classification pipeline remains the same as in the baseline case.

The classification accuracies for these procedures can be seen in Tables 1 and 2. It can be seen that hierarchical features learnt using the NB clustering approach significantly outperform the baseline BoW representation. Table 1 compares the classification performance of the baseline BoW representation with features at levels 2 and 3 and also shows further improvement in classification performance by using spatial pyramids on top of the image representations derived through the various methods. Hence, the representative power of hierarchical features can be further enhanced by using spatial pyramids. Note that in these experiments, we use only the spatial pyramid representation and not the pyramid matching kernel. As mentioned earlier, we use a homogeneous $\chi^2$ kernel map; In Table 2, there are two rows devoted to BoW. BoW represents our baseline experiments (with $\chi^2$ kernel), BoW* reports the accuraries quoted in [8] (Note that [8] uses SIFT features computed at a scale of 16 and shift of 8, and a pyramid matching kernel).

Kindly note that while the spatial pyramid representation size increases many folds per level, our hierarchical representations typically become more compact. We achieve better classification performance despite this fact.

## 5.3  Pascal VOC 2007

Pascal VOC 2007 data set has a total of 9955 images, split into 5011 training and 4944 testing images, distributed across 20 object categories. We use the entire dataset for our experiments. In these experiments, the BoW codebook was computed by clustering the keypoints collected from 10 random training images from each category (200 images in all). The classification scheme here is different from our experiments on Caltech. Pascal dataset allows multiple object categories in the same image, hence computing classification accuracies by assigning the class label of the classifier that returns the highest score to the test image is not fair assessment. In this set of experiments, we train a classifier for each class and compute Average Precision (AP) over the ranked list of test images. We finally report the mean AP over all the classes. Note that for our final image representation, we use a $2^{nd}$ level spatial pyramid [8]. As mentioned in section 1, deep learning methods have not enjoyed much success on this challenging dataset. Unlike Caltech 101, where the images are aligned and centered, Pascal has significant variation in the scale, position and orientation of the object in the image; it also allows multiple objects in the image. Note that CDBN [11] results are not available on Pascal 2007.

For level 2 features, we experiment with patch sizes of $2 \times 2$, $3 \times 3$ with shifts of 1 and 2 respectively. To compute the level 2 vocabulary, we sample 10 images randomly from each class and further sample each of these images to collect 25% of the total keypoints per image; we use $K_2 = 100, 250$. For level 3, we use patches of size $2 \times 2$ with a shift of 1 and $K_2 = 100, 200$. We use the same classification pipeline to classify the features at level 2 and 3. Table 3 displays the classification results for the mentioned methods. Here again, we significantly outperform the baseline results. While the baseline representation achieves a mean AP of 52.8% using a representation size of 1000, our L3 representation achieves 57% at a smaller representation size of 200. Hence, our representation is both richer and more compact.

**Table 3.** Classification Results on the Pascal VOC 2007 dataset. The table shows mean classification APs over 20 classes.

| Method | SIFT BoW | L2 | L2 | L2 | L3 | L3 | L3 |
|--------|----------|-----|-----|-----|-----|-----|-----|
| p | - | 3 | 3 | 2 | 2 | 2 | 2 |
| K | 1000 | 100 | 250 | 100 | 250 | 100 | 200 |
| AP | 52.84 | 54.90 | 55.86 | 55.64 | 56.20 | 56.48 | 57.04 |

### 5.4  Discussion

Our results on two classes explore the semantic meaning of the learnt hierarchical representations. Empirical comparisions with spatial pyramids reveal that we can achieve better classification accuracies with a much smaller representation size. Both these methods endow BoW with means to use spatial context. However, while spatial pyramids intend to discover the same low level artifacts in different regions of the image, we learn aggregates of such low level artifacts in the hope that these artifacts are part of a larger context and repeating this process of aggregation over and over will eventually lead us to learning the objects we are trying to classify.

The complexity of our representation is dictated by the number of levels in the hierarchy, the size of the patches and the size of the symbol space at each level. Deciding the optimal complexity requires all these parameters to be taken into account. This is similar to determining the number of clusters in clustering or any other model complexity determination problem. We believe this is still an open issue that may be addressed by empirical parameter sweeps or regularization theory as research in this field continues. In this paper, we experiment with 2-3 levels of hierarchy.

By empirically outperforming both SPM and CDBN representations on the two datasets, we demonstrate that our representations are both richer and more *compact*. For example, in Table 3, our L3 representation of size 200 outperforms the baseline representation of size 1000 significantly. The performance of our approach can be further improved by allowing a larger representation size, i.e. by using multiple scales of SIFT features as in [21]. In these experiments, our primary focus was to demonstrate the superiority of our representation over traditional BoW.

## 6  Conclusions

In this paper we devised a clustering framework for symbolic data points which can be used to learn hierarchical features starting with discrete data (such as BoW symbols.) Our method attempts to bridge the gap between two directions of research by developing a framework that learns from both approaches. We produce experimental evidence to argue that our hierarchical representations are semantically meaningful. We back this claim by outperforming the traditional BoW and deep learning representations on popular image classification datasets. It is quite possible that there are better distance functions between discrete features that may improve the learning procedure and the representative power of such a framework.

## References

1. Sivic, J., Zisserman, A.: Video google: A text retrieval approach to object matching in videos. In: ICCV (2003)
2. Csurka, G., Dance, C.R., Fan, L., Willamowski, J., Bray, C.: Visual categorization with bags of keypoints. In: ECCV (2004)

3. Vedaldi, A., Zisserman, A.: Efficient additive kernels via explicit feature maps. In: CVPR (2010)
4. Perronnin, F., Sánchez, J., Mensink, T.: Improving the Fisher Kernel for Large-Scale Image Classification. In: Daniilidis, K., Maragos, P., Paragios, N. (eds.) ECCV 2010, Part IV. LNCS, vol. 6314, pp. 143–156. Springer, Heidelberg (2010)
5. van Gemert, J.C., Geusebroek, J.-M., Veenman, C.J., Smeulders, A.W.M.: Kernel Codebooks for Scene Categorization. In: Forsyth, D., Torr, P., Zisserman, A. (eds.) ECCV 2008, Part III. LNCS, vol. 5304, pp. 696–709. Springer, Heidelberg (2008)
6. Wang, J., Yang, J., Yu, K., Lv, F., Huang, T., Gong, Y.: Locality-constrained linear coding for image classification. In: CVPR (2010)
7. Zhou, X., Yu, K., Zhang, T., Huang, T.S.: Image Classification Using Super-Vector Coding of Local Image Descriptors. In: Daniilidis, K., Maragos, P., Paragios, N. (eds.) ECCV 2010, Part V. LNCS, vol. 6315, pp. 141–154. Springer, Heidelberg (2010)
8. Lazebnik, S., Schmid, C., Ponce, J.: Beyond bags of features: Spatial pyramid matching for recognizing natural scene categories. In: CVPR, pp. 2169–2178 (2006)
9. Hinton, G.E., Osindero, S., Whye Teh, Y.: A fast learning algorithm for deep belief nets. In: Neural Computation (2006)
10. Lecun, Y., Bottou, L., Bengio, Y., Haffner, P.: Gradient-based learning applied to document recognition. Proceedings of the IEEE, 2278–2324 (1998)
11. Lee, H., Grosse, R., Ranganath, R., Ng, A.Y.: Convolutional deep belief networks for scalable unsupervised learning of hierarchical representations. In: ICML (2009)
12. Riesenhuber, M., Poggio, T., Studies, E.: Hierarchical models of object recognition in cortex (1999)
13. Fergus, R., Yu, K., Ranzato, M.A., Lee, H., Salakhutdinov, R., Taylor, G.: Tutorial on deep learning methods for vision. In: CVPR 2012 Tutorial (2012), http://cs.nyu.edu/~fergus/tutorials/deep_learning_cvpr12/
14. Agarwal, A., Triggs, B.: Multilevel image coding with hyperfeatures. International Journal of Computer Vision (2008)
15. Quack, T., Ferrari, V., Leibe, B., Gool, L.V.: Efficient mining of frequent and distinctive feature configurations (2007)
16. Fei-Fei, L., Fergus, R., Perona, P.: Learning generative visual models from few training examples: An incremental bayesian approach tested on 101 object categories. In: WGMBV (2004)
17. Lazebnik, S., Schmid, C., Ponce, J.: A maximum entropy framework for part-based texture and object recognition. In: ICCV (2005)
18. Sivic, J., Russell, B., Efros, A., Zisserman, A., Freeman, W.: Discovering objects and their location in images. In: ICCV (2005)
19. Grauman, K., Darrell, T.: The pyramid match kernel: Discriminative classification with sets of image features. In: ICCV (2005)
20. Yang, J., Yu, K., Gong, Y., Huang, T.: Linear spatial pyramid matching using sparse coding for image classification. In: CVPR (2009)
21. Chatfield, K., Lempitsky, V., Vedaldi, A., Zisserman, A.: The devil is in the details: an evaluation of recent feature encoding methods. In: BMVC (2011)
22. lan Boreau, Y., Bach, F., Lecun, Y., Ponce, J.: Learning mid-level features for recognition (2010)
23. Bishop, C.M.: Pattern Recognition and Machine Learning. Information Science and Statistics (2007)
24. Arthur, D., Vassilvitskii, S.: K-means++: the advantages of careful seeding. In: SODA (2007)
25. Vedaldi, A., Fulkerson, B.: VLFeat: An open and portable library of computer vision algorithms (2008)

# Efficient Human Parsing
# Based on Sketch Representation

Meng Wang, Zhaoxiang Zhang, and Yunhong Wang

Laboratory of Intelligent Recognition and Image Processing,
Beijing Key Laboratory of Digital Media,
School of Computer Science and Engineering, Beihang University, Beijing, China

**Abstract.** In this paper, we present an efficient human parsing method which estimates human body poses from 2D images. Firstly we propose an edge sketch representation, which enhance critical information for pose estimation and prune the redundant. The sketch representation is generated by employing two sets of filters on extracted edges. Based on sketch representation, body part candidates can be located easily using parallel lines detection in Hough space. Then we use specifically trained linear SVM classifiers to detect each body part candidates based on parallel line feature. A dynamic programming algorithm is applied to calculate the MAP estimation based on standard pictorial structure model, which use a kinematic tree to describe human pose. To evaluate the representing ability of proposed sketch representation, as well as the accuracy and efficiency of our entire human pose estimation method, we run two sets of experiments on a sports image dataset respectively. Experimental results demonstrate that the human body parts in the images can be well described by our proposed sketch representation. Furthermore, our human pose estimation method is efficient and achieves comparable accuracy against the state-of-the-art.

## 1 Introduction

Image based human parsing method has great potential in many applications of computer vision, such as action recognition, crowd surveillance and human computer interaction. In these applications, human parsing method may be implemented as a preprocessing step which can provide more refined information of human body than raw image data. However, image data captured from real world is usually quite noisy, including various cloth color and texture, clutter background and intricate occlusions. Traditional human parsing method based on a kinematic tree model[1,2] may get in trouble on these non-ideal cases. Some researchers tried to augment traditional tree model using relations between unconnected nodes and proved these information was helpful to human pose estimation[3,4]. The efforts also include exploit priori knowledge of human body such as appearance symmetry[5], pairwise spatial relations[6] and balance of limb coordination[7].

K.M. Lee et al. (Eds.): ACCV 2012, Part I, LNCS 7724, pp. 396–407, 2013.
© Springer-Verlag Berlin Heidelberg 2013

When we trying to estimate human pose, some information is redundant. For example, the color and textures of a human body part will not make direct contributions on human pose estimation. Shape based features such as HOG[8] are widely used in object recognition, but HOG cannot describe the orientation of object. Common way using HOG feature to recognize rotated object is employing multiple HOG templates, which simultaneously cause computational cost increasing and accuracy decreasing. In this paper, we propose an edge sketch representation, which describes the image layout and contains most human pose information. To extract edge sketch, we employ two sets of filters on edge images. These two filter sets can prune small scale texture information and enhance large scale shape information respectively. Based on edge sketch representation, subsequent body part detection and pose estimation can be more efficient without lose critical information.

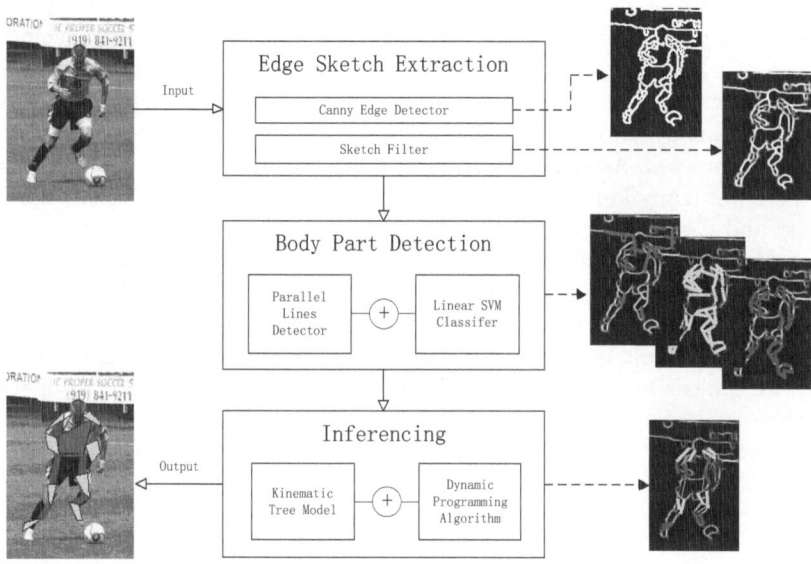

**Fig. 1.** Method Framework

Figure 1 illuminates the overall framework of our proposed human parsing method. As showing in the middle column, our human parsing method contains three main stages: The first stage is edge sketch extraction. In this stage a Canny edge detector is applied to find edges of the input image, and the edges are filtered to achieve the sketch representations. The second stage is body part detection. A parallel line detector and 9 linear SVM classifiers are applied to find all candidates of each human body part. The final stage is inferencing. As we use the standard kinematic tree model of human body, the optimal pose estimation given an input image is equivalent to the configurations of maximum posterior probability according to the kinematic tree model. We use an efficient dynamic programming algorithm to calculate the maximum posterior probability based on body part candidates detected in former stage and their spatial relations. The left two images in Figure 1 shows input image and output of our human parsing method, and the images on right side show some intermediate processing results of each stage. In the rest of this paper, we describe each stage of our human parsing method in Section 2, 3 and 4 respectively. The experimental results are showed and discussed in Section 5, and the conclusion and future plan are in Section 6.

## 2   Edge Sketch Extraction

As explained in section 1, critical information for image based human pose estimation includes shape, position, direction and scale of each body part. On the contrary, color and small scale texture information makes few contributions on human body pose estimation. We use edge image rather than original color image or gray scale image because edge image ignore these redundant information. Comparing with one or three channels, eight bits gray or RGB color image, using binary edge image heavily reduces both space and time computational cost for following processes. As edge detection is a well studied field in image processing, there are many kind of developed edge detection algorithms such as Sobel, Prewitt and Canny. In practice we choose Canny edge detector which achieves acceptable edge detection result on our test dataset. In our implementation we run Canny edge detection on each one of three channels of an RGB image respectively. Therefore we receive three edge detection results per image. As each edge detection result is a binary image(1 is an edge pixel and 0 is a non-edge pixel), we can easily merge these three edge detection results by an OR operator to get the final edge image. We find this trick brings better edge detection result than directly apply the edge detection algorithm on the gray scale image.

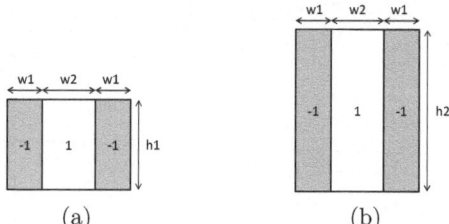

**Fig. 2.** Two filters

After edge extraction, we get a binary edge image from the original RGB image. The edge image contains no color information which is redundant for human pose estimation. However, the edge image still contains redundant information, such as patterns or textures on the clothes. Moreover, the critical information such as contours of body part may not complete and continuous. Small gaps may exist on a body part's contour, and clutter background edges may mix with the foreground objects. For the purpose of suppressing noise and enhancing critical information, two set of image filters are employed on edge image. Figure 2(a) shows one instance in the first set of filters. First set filters can suppress small scale textures such as crossings and circles, which usually are unrelated with human pose or even confuse the body part detectors. The second filter shown in Figure 2(b) gives high response for long straight edges and fills small gaps between segments, which often compose contours of body parts. In practise we set $w1 = 5$, $w2 = 10$, $h1 = 20$ and $h2 = 40$ pixels respectively, and rotate each filter constructing a filters set to adapt different edge orientations. Figure 3 shows the pipeline of edge Sketch extraction. The first column in Figure 3 are gray scale images, the second column are edge extraction result using Canny detector, the third and fourth columns are results applying filter 1 and filter 2 on edge image successively.

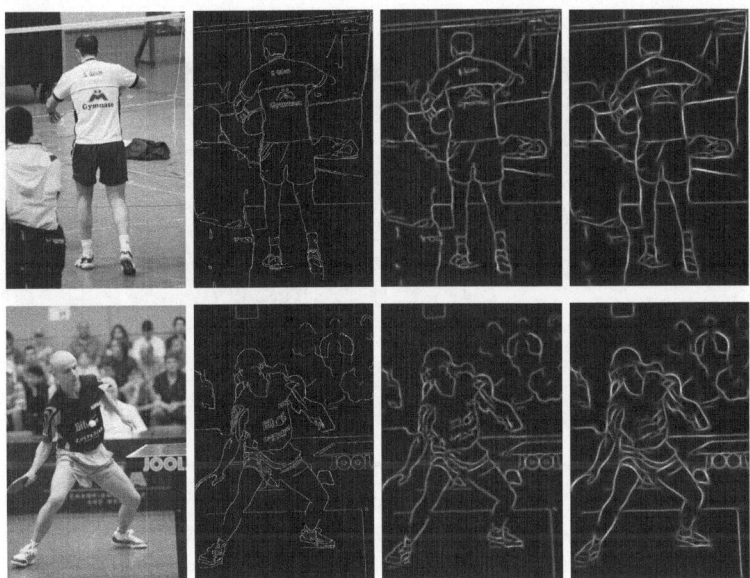

**Fig. 3.** Edge sketch representation

## 3 Body Part Detection

In most instances, projections of human body parts on image plane are close to rectangles, which can be depicted by its parallel edges. Head is an exception because its projection is quite inconstant, but head pose estimation can be assisted by some other methods such as face detection or head-shoulder $\Omega$ shape detection. Therefore, in this paper we focus on parsing remaining parts of human body except head, which is a chief difficult problem for recent human parsing methods.

### 3.1   Parallel Lines Detection

After edge sketch extraction stage, we have edge sketch representations which contain most long straight lines appeared in original RGB image. Because projections of human body parts are close to rectangles in most situations, we can find body part candidates by simply apply a rectangle detection. A rectangle contains two pairs of parallel lines, and these pairs of parallel lines can describe all important geometric characteristics $C = \{c, w, h, \theta\}$ of rectangle in a given coordinate system such as center position $c$, width $w$, height $h$, and orientation $\theta$. In fact, if one pair of parallel lines of a rectangle is located, the corresponding rectangle is determined. Therefore, a rectangle detection problem can be converted to a parallel lines detection problem by adding a simple constraint in order to control the length difference of two parallel lines. Thus we apply a parallel lines detection on the edge sketch image to generate possible body part candidates.

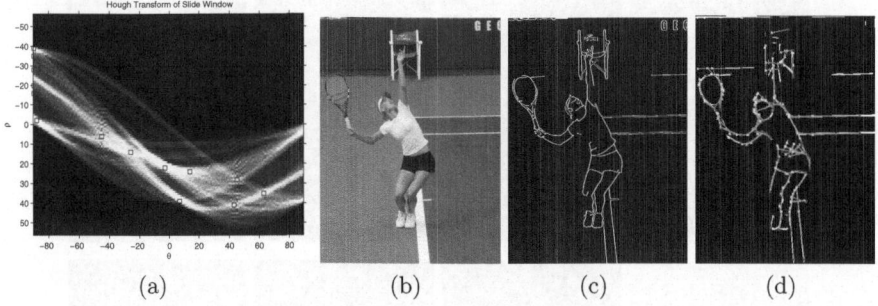

**Fig. 4.** Parallel lines detection

Hough transform are widely and successfully used in linear structure detection, because geometric characteristics of lines can be used directly in the Hough space. By search for parallel lines in hough space we can efficiently get all the rectangles in an image, namely all the candidates of human body parts. We apply a parallel detection algorithm which is a simpler version of [9], because actually we only need the principal pair (the pair which is longer) of parallel lines rather than both two. In practice we use a sliding window strategy to detect parallel lines in small image blocks, which brings more precise results. Figure 4 shows an example of parallel lines detection. Figure 4(a) shows a Hough transform result of a sliding window area, the horizon axis $\theta$ indicates orientation and the vertical axis $\rho$ indicates the distance from the origin. The small blue boxes indicate local maximums in the Hough space, typically means straight lines in the $xy$ plane. Therefore, in order to find parallel lines, we only need to find the local maximum (blue box) pairs which are close in $\theta$ axis. Figure 4(b) and 4(c) show original image, edge sketch representation respectively, and Figure 4(d) shows the parallel lines detection results, in which the green lines with yellow and red end points is the detected parallel line pairs.

## 3.2   Body Part Classification

This subsection describes our body part classification. As noted in parallel lines detection, each parallel line pair contains 4 attributes $C = \{c, w, h, \theta\}$. The likelihood of each body part then can be discriminatively determined based on these attributes, namely the features. 9 linear SVM classifiers are specifically trained for each body parts using particular labeled parallel line pair samples and random selected unlabeled samples, then these classifiers can determine whether a detected parallel line pair should belongs to a body part class (e.g. torso). By employing all body part classifiers, we can get all possible candidates of each body part class and reject those parallel line pairs as background which are not belong to any class. As a result of low feature dimension, the linear SVM classifiers perform quite efficient in practice. Figure 5 shows some results of body part classification on image sketch. Figure 5(a) shows all parallel lines detected in hough space, and following three images show candidates of torso, upper limbs and lower limbs respectively.

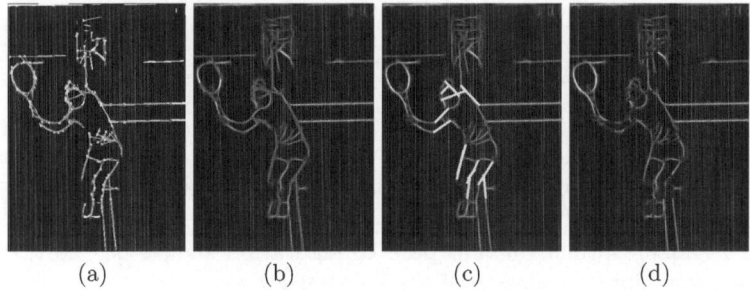

(a)            (b)            (c)            (d)

**Fig. 5.** Body part candidates

## 4   Kinematic Tree Model and Inference

As shown in Figure 6, most human parsing methods use a kinematic tree model $G = (V, E)$ to represent the pose of a human body appeared in an image. Each node $l_i \in V$ in this tree corresponding to a human body part, such as torso, head or left lower arm. The edges $(l_i, l_j) \in E$ in tree model indicate the connections between two body parts $l_i$ and $l_j$. So if we assign the torso node $l_1$ as root node, then head/upper limbs can be connected to torso node as child nodes, and lower limbs then connect to their corresponding parent nodes. After building tree model, we can compute configurations $Z$ of each human body part by estimate likelihood in each node $l_i$ and corresponding limb candidates

$$P(I|Z) \propto \prod_{i \in V} \phi_i(l_i) \propto \prod_{i \in V} \phi_i(c_i, w_i, h_i, \theta_i) \tag{1}$$

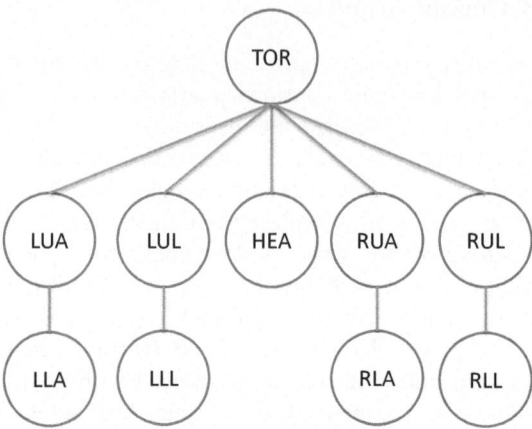

**Fig. 6.** Standard kinematic tree model

Considering spacial relations between connected nodes $l_i$, $l_j$, we have

$$P(Z) \propto \prod_{i,j \in E} \psi_{i,j}(l_i, l_j) \propto \prod_{i,j \in E} \psi_{i,j}((c_i, w_i, h_i, \theta_i), (c_j, w_j, h_j, \theta_j)) \qquad (2)$$

As we use parallel lines feature, we assume the spacial relations between connected nodes $l_i$, $l_j$ is Gaussian distribution. Thus we can easily train the $\psi_{i,j}(l_i, l_j)$ by a maximum likelihood estimation.

Then a global optimal human pose configuration should be the maximum posterior probability estimation of the kinematic tree model

$$P(Z|I) \propto P(I|Z)P(Z) \propto \prod_{i \in V} \phi_i(l_i) \prod_{i,j \in E} \psi_{i,j}(l_i, l_j) \qquad (3)$$

Standard kinematic tree model is based on an assumption that unconnected nodes are independent, but in some conditions this assumption maybe not valid.

Applying a dynamic programming algorithm [1], inference the maximum posterior probability pose estimation of kinematic tree model can be efficient with a computation complexity $O(cn)$, where $c$ is number of possible candidates and $n$ is the number of body parts in the model.

## 5    Experimental Results and Discussion

We test our human parsing method on Leeds Sports Pose Dataset [10]. This dataset is quite challenging because its images are captured from real-world sport scene and most human bodies in the images present strange poses and complex occlusions. To reduce complexity, the images in LSP dataset are cropped and scaled in order to normalize the length of the persons in images to about 150 pixels. For the purpose to compare with other methods, we following the evaluation criteria proposed in [11]: a body part estimation is accepted as a correct estimation only if the distance between each endpoint of estimation and ground-truth annotation are both less than half of the annotated limb length. For each experiments, we use first half (1000) images in the dataset to train our detectors and models, and the rest half are used for testing.

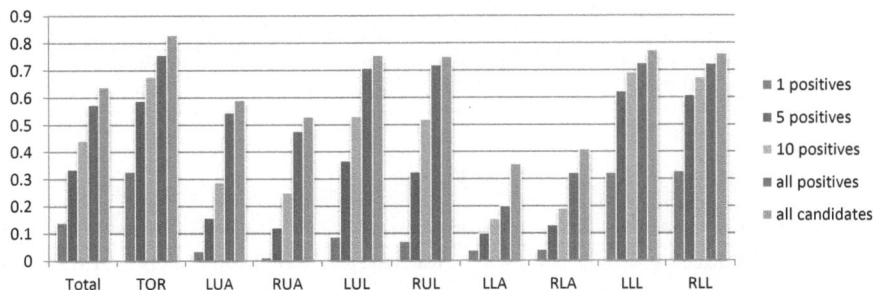

**Fig. 7.** Probability of correct estimation appears in different subsets of sorted candidates

## 5.1   Testing on Human Body Part Detection

In order to evaluate our proposed edge sketch representation and parallel line based part detector, our first experiment focus on body part detection. In this experiment, we apply our proposed edge sketch extraction and body part detection on each testing image, and record all the body part candidates which are found by the detectors. We sort candidates of each body part in descent order according to their SVM decision values, then we search for possible correct candidates which satisfy the evaluation criteria, and record which subset it appears. Figure 7 shows the probabilities of the correct candidates appear in different subsets of each sorted body part candidates list. In Figure 7, the first three bars of each body part indicate the probability of the correct estimation is ranked within the top 1, 5 and 10 positive candidates, and the fourth bar is the same probability of all positive candidates. The last bar of each body part is the probability of correct estimation appears in both positive and negative candidates (namely all candidates).

After survey Figure 7, we have following conclusions:

(1) The probability of correct estimation appears in all candidates is close to 75% in average. In other words, our parallel lines feature can cover nearly 75% human body parts in all images.

(2) In most human body parts (except LLA) the probability of correct estimation appears in all positives candidates and all candidates is close. This fact demonstrates that our linear SVM based body part detector can find most correct estimations.

(3) Body part likelihood is positive correlated with the decision values of SVM classifier, but such correlation is not strong enough.

**Table 1.** Comparison of correct estimation rates(in percentages) between different methods

| Method | Total | Torso | Upper Leg | Lower Leg | Upper Arm | Lower Arm |
|--------|-------|-------|-----------|-----------|-----------|-----------|
| Top 1 Pos | 14.0 | 32.7 | 7.9 | 32.4 | 2.4 | 3.9 |
| Our Method | 21.3 | 50.1 | 26.7 | 32.6 | 7.9 | 3.8 |
| Method a | 34.8 | 64.1 | 42.8 | 41.0 | 25.0 | 16.1 |
| Method b | 54.2 | 78.1 | 65.8 | 58.8 | 47.4 | 32.9 |
| All Pos | 57.4 | 75.6 | 71.3 | 72.4 | 51.0 | 26.1 |
| All Cad | 74.1 | 87.1 | 83.7 | 83.6 | 64.5 | 46.0 |

### 5.2 Comparison with Other Methods

We also test our complete human parsing method in the LSP dataset, Table 1 shows the comparison of correct estimation rates between our proposed method and two state-of-the-art methods. For comparison, we also place the probability of top 1 positive candidates, all positive candidates and all (both positive and negative) candidates in Table 1, which have same definition in Figure 7.

Method a and Method b in Table 1 are proposed in [12] and [10] respectively. Method a based on same linear SVM classifiers and standard pictorial structure models with our method, and the difference is that Method a uses HOG feature. Thus Method a is a good contrast method with our proposed method. By comparing the correct estimation rates of our method and Method a, we can conclude that our parallel line feature is not perform strictly as well as HOG feature on accuracy. However, the accuracy gap between these two methods is not very large. Method b also based on HOG feature, and by applying a heuristical mixture pictorial structure model strategy, this method achieve a great accuracy increase. As our parallel line feature also can be applied in such improved model, our method should still have a space for accuracy increasing.

Figure 8 shows some experimental results. Images in first row are original inputs, and the second row shows image sketches after two times filtering. Pose estimation results are showed in third and forth rows, which are based on kinematic tree model. In the third row, red, yellow and blue parallel lines indicate torso, upper limbs and lower limbs, and the thin green lines connecting each two body parts are soft connections between corresponding endpoints, which make the pose estimation results more reasonable. In the forth row, torsos and limbs are located by red and yellow quadrangles respectively.

### 5.3 Efficiency

We implement our algorithms using Matlab, and all experiments are executed on a 2.6GHz dual-core computer. The average running duration of 1000 test images is 4.26 seconds. To the best of our knowledge, our image sketch representation based human parsing method is more quickly than most other published

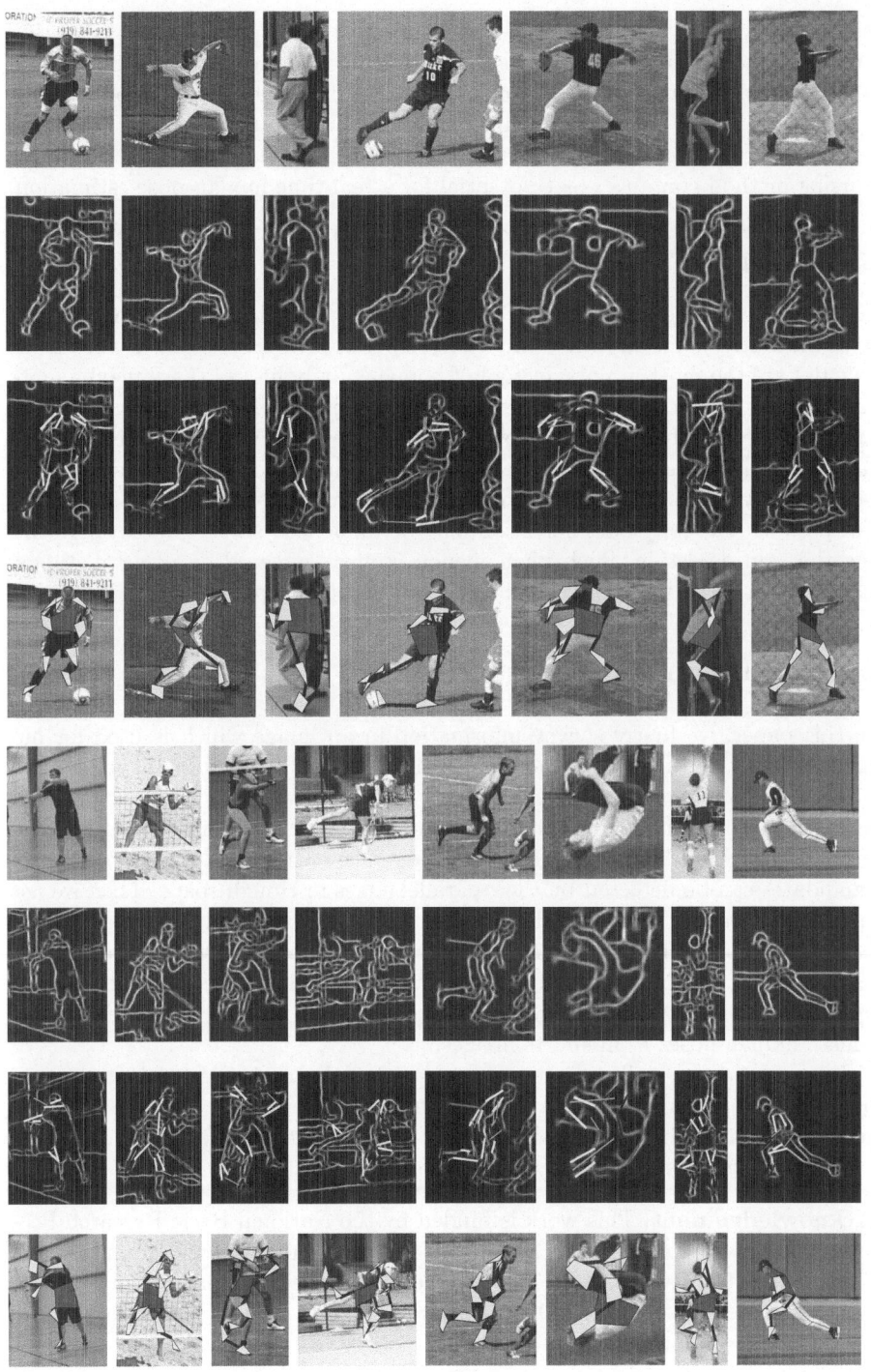

**Fig. 8.** Experiment results

methods, especially the methods based on gradient features. Since image filtering and parallel lines detection are the most time consuming parts of our method, a parallel optimization strategy may brings significant acceleration on running speed. Moreover, a native code implementation (e.g. a C/C++ version) may also execute more efficient. Therefore, our image sketch representation based human parsing method contains great potential for a real-time human pose estimation.

### 5.4    Discussion

As shown in the second row of Table 1, our proposed human parsing method is significantly weak on arm estimation. A possible interpretation is that arms (hands) are the most important tool of human's daily life, so there maybe more interactions between arms and external world objects. Moreover, arms are generally more close to human torsos and often present complicate occlusions in images. Considering our experiments are based on a sports image dataset, the occlusions and strange poses make accurate estimation even harder. Therefore our parallel line body part detection may be influenced severely when performing the arm detection. Such phenomenon is also appeared on other methods, namely arm detection is still a chief problem in human parsing field.

## 6    Conclusion and Future Plan

In this paper, we firstly survey information in an image which is used for human parsing. Because color and small scale textures are redundant for human pose estimation, we use edge images and employ two sets of filters to enhance long straight lines in edge sketch representation, which contain critical pose information of each body part. Based on edge sketch representation, body part candidates can be detected by their parallel edges in Hough space. Then we use specifically trained linear SVM classifiers to detect each body part candidates based on parallel line feature. A dynamic programming algorithm is applied to calculate the MAP estimation based on standard kinematic tree model. The experimental results demonstrate our human parsing method can efficiently estimate human poses from sports images.

In the future we will exploit improved pictorial structure models and apply our sketch representation and parallel line feature on them, and we will also survey the fusion of different features or cascade strategy for the purpose to achieve real-time high accuracy human parsing.

**Acknowledgement.** This work is funded by the National Basic Research Program of China (No.2010CB327902), the National Natural Science Foundation of China (No.61005016, No.61061130560), the Fundamental Research Funds for the Central Universities, and the Open Projects Program of National Laboratory of Pattern Recognition.

# References

1. Felzenszwalb, P.F., Huttenlocher, D.P.: Pictorial structures for object recognition. Int. J. Comput. Vision 61, 55–79 (2005)
2. Ramanan, D.: Learning to parse images of articulated bodies. In: Schölkopf, B., Platt, J., Hoffman, T. (eds.) Advances in Neural Information Processing Systems 19, pp. 1129–1136. MIT Press, Cambridge (2007)
3. Tian, T.P., Sclaroff, S.: Fast globally optimal 2d human detection with loopy graph models. In: 2010 IEEE Conference on Computer Vision and Pattern Recognition (CVPR), pp. 81–88 (2010)
4. Jiang, H., Martin, D.: Global pose estimation using non-tree models. In: IEEE Conference on Computer Vision and Pattern Recognition, CVPR 2008, pp. 1–8 (2008)
5. Ren, X., Berg, A., Malik, J.: Recovering human body configurations using pairwise constraints between parts. In: Tenth IEEE International Conference on Computer Vision, ICCV 2005, vol. 1, pp. 824–831 (2005)
6. Tran, D., Forsyth, D.: Improved Human Parsing with a Full Relational Model. In: Daniilidis, K., Maragos, P., Paragios, N. (eds.) ECCV 2010, Part IV. LNCS, vol. 6314, pp. 227–240. Springer, Heidelberg (2010)
7. Lan, X., Huttenlocher, D.: Beyond trees: common-factor models for 2d human pose recovery. In: Tenth IEEE International Conference on Computer Vision, vol. 1, pp. 470–477 (2005)
8. Dalal, N., Triggs, B.: Histograms of oriented gradients for human detection. In: IEEE Computer Society Conference on Computer Vision and Pattern Recognition, CVPR 2005, vol. 1, pp. 886–893 (2005)
9. Jung, C.R., Schramm, R.: Rectangle detection based on a windowed hough transform. In: Proceedings of the Computer Graphics and Image Processing, XVII Brazilian Symposium, SIBGRAPI 2004, pp. 113–120. IEEE Computer Society Press, Washington, DC (2004)
10. Johnson, S., Everingham, M.: Clustered pose and nonlinear appearance models for human pose estimation. In: Proceedings of the British Machine Vision Conference (2010), doi:10.5244/C.24.12
11. Ferrari, V., Marin-Jimenez, M., Zisserman, A.: Progressive search space reduction for human pose estimation. In: IEEE Conference on Computer Vision and Pattern Recognition, CVPR 2008, pp. 1–8 (2008)
12. Johnson, S., Everingham, M.: Combining discriminative appearance and segmentation cues for articulated human pose estimation. In: MLMotion 2009, pp. 405–412 (2009)

# Exclusive Visual Descriptor Quantization

Yu Zhang[1], Jianxin Wu[1], and Weiyao Lin[2]

[1] School of Computer Engineering, Nanyang Technological University, Singapore
[2] Department of Electronic Engineering, Shanghai Jiao Tong University, China

**Abstract.** Vector quantization (VQ) using exhaustive nearest neighbor (NN) search is the speed bottleneck in classic bag of visual words (BOV) models. Approximate NN (ANN) search methods still cost great time in VQ, since they check multiple regions in the search space to reduce VQ errors. In this paper, we propose ExVQ, an exclusive NN search method to speed up BOV models. Given a visual descriptor, a portion of search regions is excluded from the whole search space by a linear projection. We ensure that minimal VQ errors are introduced in the exclusion by learning an accurate classifier. Multiple exclusions are organized in a tree structure in ExVQ, whose VQ speed and VQ error rate can be reliably estimated. We show that ExVQ is much faster than state-of-the-art ANN methods in BOV models while maintaining almost the same classification accuracy. In addition, we empirically show that even with the VQ error rate as high as 30%, the classification accuracy of some ANN methods, including ExVQ, is similar to that of exhaustive search (which has zero VQ error). In some cases, ExVQ has even higher classification accuracy than the exhaustive search.

## 1 Introduction

Bag of visual words (BOV) has become a widely used practice in computer vision and related research, whose application include (but are not limited to) retrieval [1], scene recognition [2], and object categorization [3], etc. In spite of its simplicity, BOV achieves state-of-the-art performance in many problems.

In a classic BOV model, visual descriptors are first clustered to form a visual codebook, and the cluster centers are called visual codewords. A visual descriptor is then represented by the index of its nearest codeword. The procedure that maps a descriptor to its codeword index is called vector quantization (VQ). Finally, an image is represented by a histogram of the codeword indexes contained in this image. Classifiers are applied to these histograms to perform visual classification, e.g., in object or scene recognition. Recently, new BOV methods are also proposed, e.g., those based on the sparse coding [4][5].

In this paper, we limit our discussions to the classic BOV procedure, in which the vector quantization essentially performs a nearest neighbor (NN) search within all visual codewords, which is also the major speed bottleneck in applying BOV models. Two typical situations make this issue more prominent: large scale and real time. In large scale problems such as the TRECVID benchmark, weeks of time was needed even when computer clusters were used [6].

K.M. Lee et al. (Eds.): ACCV 2012, Part I, LNCS 7724, pp. 408–421, 2013.
© Springer-Verlag Berlin Heidelberg 2013

On the other hand, in real time applications where 30 or more images need to be processed per second, the VQ speed is again of paramount importance. We also observe that the VQ step occupies most of the processing time in BOV. Encoding an image in BOV is divided into three modules in [6]: point sampling, descriptor computation and VQ. Using the Caltech 101 [7] as an example, when we use densely sampled points and SIFT descriptors, the VQ time occupied from 87.53% to 96.56% of the total BOV processing time when the codebook size $K$ varies from 256 to 1024.

Approximate nearest neighbor (ANN) search is a natural choice to speed up the VQ process. In this paper, we propose ExVQ, an efficient ANN method, which greatly accelerates the VQ speed, without affecting the classification accuracy of BOV models.

ANN methods, e.g., FLANN [8], have shown great speedup effects in searching within large point sets. It has already been used in vector quantization in [9]. In this paper, our goal is to further improve the VQ speedup by maintaining the classification accuracy. First, we systematically evaluate the effect of ANN VQ errors to the subsequent visual classification stage. We show that some ANN methods, even with up to 30% VQ error rates, do not reduce the classification accuracy in object and scene recognition tasks.

Next, we propose a new ANN method to speed up the VQ process. Existing ANN methods follow a branch and bound strategy: split the search space into regions according to certain criterion, and assume that a point and its nearest neighbor will fall into the same region. Thus, the algorithm only needs to examine the few points in one region. We call this strategy the *inclusive* strategy. The inclusive assumption, however, rarely holds in reality. Thus, searching only one region leads to high VQ error rate. More regions (e.g., nearby ones) must also be examined, which increases the cost of ANN search. For example, FLANN has a parameter that specifies how many regions are to be checked.

In ExVQ, we use an *exclusive* strategy instead. For a BOV model, all clusters of visual descriptors, not only the codewords, are divided into three regions, $L$, $R$, and $I$. Instead of insisting that nearest neighbors of visual descriptors from $L$ must also reside inside $L$ (i.e., inclusive), we only assume that such neighbors will not appear in $R$ (and $I$ is a buffer region which is ignored in this process). ExVQ thus do not search through codewords from clusters in $R$. We will show that our exclusive assumption can be ensured to be correct (or almost correct) by learning a classifier that assigns all clusters into appropriate regions $L$, $R$, and $I$. In reality, we perform several exclusions in ExVQ, organized in a hierarchical tree structure.

Overall, the following contributions are presented in this paper:

- A systematic evaluation of the effects of VQ errors caused by ANN. We reveal that a high VQ error rate (e.g., 30%) does not necessarily reduce the classification accuracy of the BOV model.

- An exclusion strategy for ANN search. We ensure the correctness of the exclusion by learning classifiers, which also gives a reliable estimation of the VQ error.

- ExVQ, an ANN system for vector quantization in BOV. ExVQ requires only about 10–20% of the VQ time of the classic VQ, or half of that of FLANN. And, all three methods have indistinguishable classification accuracies.

## 2   Related Works

Vector quantization and its acceleration has long been studied in image and video coding. Tree-structure VQ methods such as TSVQ are popular because of its speed advantage [10]. Various branch-and-bound methods have also been used to find the exact or approximate NN with faster speed.

Tree structure is a useful tool to reduce search time. The hierarchical $k$-means tree can organize $O(n^m)$ items in a depth $m$ tree, in which every internal tree node has $n$ fan-out branches. A query then involves finding the path of the most similar nodes from the root of the tree toward a leaf node, which only requires $nm$ distance computations. It has been successfully used in object retrieval from large object databases with tens of thousands of objects [11][12]. Randomized trees and extremely randomized clustering forests have also shown excellent speed and accuracy in matching features and detecting objects [13][14].

The branch-and-bound strategy, which usually utilizes linear projections to split the search space, is also proven valuable in ANN search. $kd$-tree splits the search space into halves using a hyperplane (which is a special case of linear projection) on the dimension with the largest variance and continues to split iteratively until each node contains only one point. Randomized $kd$-trees and ensembles of them have shown acceleration up to the 30x with approximately 90% correct nearest neighbors [8], comparing to the exhaustive nearest neighbor search of SIFT descriptors.

Spill tree [15] is similar to the proposed ExVQ, in that they both adopt overlap (buffer) between the two split search sets. Spill tree splits the search set using a random projection. The overlap contains those search points within a small distance to the projection boundary. The difference is, ExVQ learns an accurate SVM classifier from the available visual descriptors and uses it to determine: which clusters, rather than data points, form the search sets or the overlap. Visual descriptors in the two split search sets, especially in the overlap, have zero (or almost zero) NN search error, which is not ensured in the spill tree. Similar strategy using a buffer to eliminate the decision error is also used in multi-class problem [16][17]. However, the method in [17] is very slow, which may take days to learn on the same dataset used in this paper.

Another family of methods use multiple linear projections to map the feature vector (or visual descriptor) into a short string with few binary bits, e.g., locality sensitive hashing (LSH) [18], Hamming embedding [19], and spectral hashing [20]. This strategy is particularly attractive for processing huge datasets. Their storage requirements are greatly reduced, although their NN search accuracy may be significantly lower than ANN methods such as FLANN.

In recent years, sparse coding [4][5] is popular in object recognition and classification, such as Locality-constrained Linear Coding (LLC) [4]. Multiple database points are assigned weights under the sparse constraint. In this paper, we will empirically compare ExVQ with LLC. Recently, product quantization [21] is also used for NN search. It can save search time and storage by quantizing the sub-vectors of the original high-dimension feature vector, which is, however, more suitable for retrieval applications rather than for visual recognition.

## 3   ExVQ: Exclusive Vector Quantization

In the BOV model, given a set of visual descriptors $X = \{x_0, x_1, ..., x_{N-1}\}$, by applying the $k$-means clustering, the cluster centers are used as a codebook $\{c_0, c_1, ..., c_{K-1}\}$, where $x_i, c_j \in \mathbb{R}^d, i = 0, 1, ..., N - 1, j = 0, 1, ..., K - 1$. A visual descriptor $x \in \mathbb{R}^d$ is quantized by the index of its nearest codeword as:

$$nn(x) = \underset{0 \leq i \leq K-1}{\arg\min}\ dist(x, c_i), \tag{1}$$

where $dist(\cdot, \cdot)$ can be any distance metric between two vectors. We consider the Euclidean distance in this paper, that is, $dist(x, c_i) = \|x - c_i\|_{\ell_2}$.

### 3.1   Effect of ANN VQ Errors to Classification

In an ANN method, we define the searched nearest neighbor index for a point $x$ as $ann(x)$. During an ANN based VQ process, a VQ error happens when $ann(x)$ is different from $nn(x)$. Intuitively, a high VQ error rate will lead to more classification errors in the subsequent visual classification stage. However, we find empirically that this is not the case. When certain ANN methods are used, a high VQ error rate (e.g., 30%) does not necessarily hurt the classification accuracy. Thus, we have the freedom to allow some VQ errors in order to accelerate the VQ process.

Fig. 1a shows one example of how the classification accuracy varies with the VQ error rate of FLANN. Although VQ errors vary from 5.70% to 32.44%, the classification accuracies are almost the same. This result seems counter intuitive. We conjecture that *it can be explained by the properties of the VQ errors*: some VQ errors are benign and will have minimal effect on the classification performance.

To validate this conjecture, we first define the error rank of $ann(x)$ using the following procedure. We calculate the distance of $x$ with each codeword $dist(c_i, x), i = 0, 1, ..., K - 1$, and store them in an array in the ascending order. The error rank of $ann(x)$ is defined as the index of $dist(c_{ann(x)}, x)$ in this sorted array. The error rank is 0 when $ann(x) = nn(x)$. Then we define the benign VQ error: a small portion of VQs ($< 30\%$ or around)[1] has error and the error ranks are small. This definition provides us with an empirical way to evaluate the property of VQ errors. In Fig. 1b, we show the histograms of ANN error ranks using FLANN with different check numbers, where the vertical axis is shown

---

[1] We find 30% is valid for most cases. More results will be shown in the experiment.

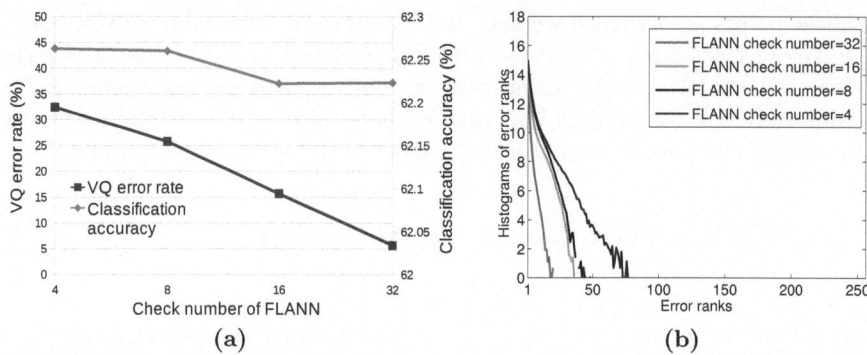

**Fig. 1.** (a) VQ error rate and classification accuracy (one round) using FLANN hierarchical $k$-means tree, on Caltech 101, when $K = 256$; (b) The histograms of ANN error ranks. The vertical axis is the frequency numbers shown *in natural logarithm*. We use FLANN hierarchical $k$-means tree with different check numbers on Caltech 101 when $K = 256$.

in natural logarithm. The error ranks of most VQ errors are close to 1, which supports our conjecture on benign VQ errors. More systematic results will be presented in Sec. 4.

### 3.2   ANN Search: Inclusion vs. Exclusion

When inclusive methods (e.g., LSH and FLANN) search the nearest neighbor of a visual descriptor in the codebook $\{c_0, c_1, ..., c_{K-1}\}$, they use linear projections to reduce the search range. With a linear projection $(\boldsymbol{w}, b), \boldsymbol{w} \in \mathbb{R}^d, b \in \mathbb{R}$, an inclusion strategy implicitly assumes that:

$$\forall \boldsymbol{x} \in \mathbb{R}^d, \mathrm{sgn}(\boldsymbol{w}^T \boldsymbol{c}_{nn(\boldsymbol{x})} + b) = \mathrm{sgn}(\boldsymbol{w}^T \boldsymbol{x} + b), \tag{2}$$

where $\mathrm{sgn}(\cdot)$ is the sign function.

However, in most cases, inclusive search methods fail to find the nearest neighbor in the reduced search range. Fig. 2 illustrates the inclusive NN search in the 2-D space. We use $k$-means to get 15 clusters from the randomly generated points. Each black star is the center of a cluster (i.e., codewords), which altogether form the codebook. Subject to the linear projection (the black line), 40% clusters (which are crossed by the line) violate the inclusive assumption. In reality, the inclusive assumption is violated even more seriously. Using a random linear projection on Caltech 101 ($K = 256, d = 128$), only about 10% clusters can guarantee Eq. 2. Thus the inclusive search methods usually need to check NN in multiple adjacent regions to maintain the search accuracy, which slows down the search speed.

We propose an exclusive NN search strategy to fulfill three goals: to reduce NN search time, to maintain a reasonable VQ error rate, and to ensure that the VQ errors are benign. In this strategy, the search range is reduced by excluding a portion of clusters (rather than data points) from the whole search space

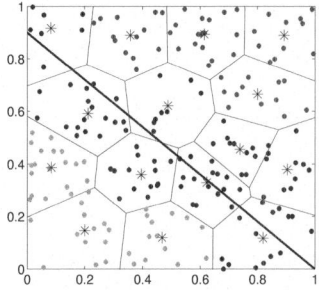

**Fig. 2.** Illustration of inclusive vs. exclusive NN search. The random projection violates the inclusive assumption. The exclusive strategy, however, can correctly excludes the red or the green clusters. This figure should be viewed in color.

subject to a linear projection. The exclusive NN search involves three index sets: the available search set $C$ containing the indexes of all clusters to be searched, the positive and negative exclusion sets $C_{+1}(L)$ and $C_{-1}(R)$, which are the index sets of clusters that can be excluded.

We illustrate the idea of exclusive NN search in Fig. 2. We first assign the indexes of red and green clusters to $C_{+1}$ and $C_{-1}$, respectively. Then, for a point above the linear projection, we search NN from the codewords within the red and blue clusters. Those green clusters $(C_{-1})$ can be safely excluded. In the inclusive strategy, for a point above the linear projection, its NN can be one of the blue-colored centers. Thus, regions in both sides of the black line are to be searched, that is, no cluster can be safely ignored.

In real-world NN search problems, a random linear projection may fail to produce high quality exclusion sets. Instead, we utilize existing examples to evaluate the irregular boundaries of exclusion clusters in $C_{+1}$ and $C_{-1}$. We use visual descriptors in all exclusion clusters to train an accurate linear classifier such that a high quality linear projection direction can be learned. This linear projection can accurately split the exclusion clusters on two sides.

Specifically, first, we calculate the inner product of the codeword in each cluster $c_i, i \in C = \{0, 1, ..., K-1\}$ with a random vector $r \in \mathbb{R}^d$ and sort the values in the ascending order. Then, we choose the desired exclusion portion $0 < p < 1/2$ and assign the indexes of clusters which codewords are of the $p \cdot |C|$ largest (smallest) values of $r^T c_i$ to $C_{+1}$ ($C_{-1}$). Next, we generate the positive training set $X_{+1} = \{x | x \in X, nn(x) \in C_{+1}\}$ and the negative training set $X_{-1} = \{x | x \in X, nn(x) \in C_{-1}\}$. Finally, we train a linear SVM classifier $(w, b)$ using $X_{+1}$ and $X_{-1}$:

$$\min_{w,b} \quad \frac{1}{2}\|w\|_2^2 + \alpha \sum_{x \in X_{+1}} \max(0, 1 - (w^T x + b))^2$$

$$+ \alpha \sum_{x \in X_{-1}} \max(0, 1 + (w^T x + b))^2, \tag{3}$$

where $\alpha$ is the trade off parameter.

After the linear SVM classifier is trained, we obtain $(\boldsymbol{w}, b)$, $C$, $C_{+1}$ and $C_{-1}$. For a visual descriptor $\boldsymbol{x} \in \mathbb{R}^d$, the exclusive NN search is defined as:

$$ann(\boldsymbol{x}) = \arg\min_i \|\boldsymbol{x} - \boldsymbol{c}_i\|_{\ell_2}, \tag{4}$$

$$\text{s.t. } i \in C - C_{-\text{sgn}(\boldsymbol{w}^T\boldsymbol{x}+b)}, \tag{5}$$

where $C - C_{-\text{sgn}(\boldsymbol{w}^T\boldsymbol{x}+b)}$ is the active search set of $\boldsymbol{x}$.

ExVQ and spill tree operates on different principles. ExVQ excludes one cluster entirely, which includes all points within the corresponding Voronoi cell. Thus, the nearest codewords of points in the rest search space never or rarely (depending on the training quality of the linear SVM classifier) exist in the exclusion set. In the spill tree, although a centroid may be far away from the exclusion region, its corresponding cluster (i.e., Voronoi cell) may have large overlap with it, that is, causing many VQ errors.

## 3.3   Tree-Structured ExVQ

One single exclusion is not enough in real-world applications. In ExVQ, we use multiple linear classifiers with a hierarchical tree structure. We implement ExVQ in an $L$-level complete binary tree, where each node is indexed level by level from 0 to $2^L - 2$. The $i$th node is related to three cluster index sets: $C^i, C^i_{+1}$ and $C^i_{-1}$, which are the available search set, and the positive and negative exclusion sets, respectively. First, in the root node, we set $C^0 = \{0, 1, ..., K-1\}$. Then, in the $i$th node, $C^i_{+1}$ and $C^i_{-1}$ are chosen from $C^i$ by a random vector $\boldsymbol{r}_i \in \mathbb{R}^d$ as described in Sec. 3.2, and to train a linear SVM classifier $(\boldsymbol{w}_i, b_i)$ according to Eq. 3. Next, we compute the available search sets for the the left and right children of the $i$th node as $C^{2i+1} = C^i - C^i_{-1}$ and $C^{2i+2} = C^i - C^i_{+1}$, respectively. Finally, the whole tree can be built recursively from the root. This process is detailed in Algorithm 1.

After the tree is built, we get $\{(\boldsymbol{w}_i, b_i), C^i, C^i_{+1}, C^i_{-1}\}$ in every node. For a query $\boldsymbol{x} \in \mathbb{R}^d$, the NN search is processed as follows: first, starting from the root node, we compute $\boldsymbol{w}_i^T\boldsymbol{x} + b_i$. If the value is positive, the exclusion process goes to process its left child, otherwise to the right. This process continues iteratively until a leaf node is reached. Then we output the active search set of the leaf node. Finally, the NN of $\boldsymbol{x}$ is acquired by exhaustively searching the active search set. We fully specify ANN search by ExVQ in Algorithm 2.

In ExVQ, the tree level $L$ and the exclusion portion $p$ can influence the search speed and the VQ error rate. Applying ExVQ to a visual descriptor, the number of distance computations in the NN search is: $\hat{K} = L + K(1-p)^L$.

If we assume that the VQ error rates caused by the exclusions from the same level nodes in the tree are the same, the whole VQ error rate of ExVQ can be estimated by:

$$e_{vq} = 1 - \prod_{l=1}^{L}(1 - pe_l), \tag{6}$$

---

**Algorithm 1.** Build tree-structure ExVQ

---

1: **Input**: Descriptors $\{\boldsymbol{x}_0, \boldsymbol{x}_1, ..., \boldsymbol{x}_{N-1}\} \subseteq \mathbb{R}^d$ and $K$ centers $\{\boldsymbol{c}_0, \boldsymbol{c}_1, ..., \boldsymbol{c}_{K-1}\}$, ExVQ tree level $L$ and an exclusion portion parameter $p$.
2: $C^0 \leftarrow \{0, 1, ..., K-1\}$
3: **for** $id = 0 \leftarrow 2^L - 2$ **do**
4:     $C_{+1}^{id} \leftarrow \emptyset, C_{-1}^{id} \leftarrow \emptyset$, $parent \leftarrow 0$
5:     **if** $id > 0$ **then**
6:         $parent = \lfloor \frac{id-1}{2} \rfloor$
7:     **end if**
8:     **if** $id$ is odd **then**
9:         $C^{id} \leftarrow C^{parent} - C_{-1}^{parent}$
10:     **else**
11:         $C^{id} \leftarrow C^{parent} - C_{+1}^{parent}$
12:     **end if**
13:     $a \leftarrow \emptyset, X_{+1} \leftarrow \emptyset, X_{-1} \leftarrow \emptyset$
14:     generate a random vector $\boldsymbol{r} \in \mathbb{R}^d$
15:     $a \leftarrow a \cup \boldsymbol{r}^T \boldsymbol{c}_i, \forall\, i \in C^{id}$
16:     **for** $i$ in $C^{id}$ **do**
17:         **if** $\boldsymbol{r}^T \boldsymbol{c}_i$ in the $p \cdot |C^{id}|$ biggest values of $a$ **then**
18:             $C_{+1}^{id} \leftarrow C_{+1}^{id} \cup i$
19:             $X_{+1} \leftarrow X_{+1} \cup \boldsymbol{x}_j, \forall\, j, nn(\boldsymbol{x}_j) == i$
20:         **end if**
21:         **if** $\boldsymbol{r}^T \boldsymbol{c}_i$ in the $p \cdot |C^{id}|$ smallest values of $a$ **then**
22:             $C_{-1}^{id} \leftarrow C_{-1}^{id} \cup i$
23:             $X_{-1} \leftarrow X_{-1} \cup \boldsymbol{x}_j, \forall\, j, nn(\boldsymbol{x}_j) == i$
24:         **end if**
25:     **end for**
26:     train a linear projection $(\boldsymbol{w}_{id}, b_{id})$ with positive set $X_{+1}$ and negative set $X_{-1}$
27: **end for**
28: **Output**: $\{(\boldsymbol{w}_i, b_i), C^i, C_{+1}^i, C_{-1}^i\}, i = 0, 1, ..., 2^L - 2$.

---

where $e_l$ is the VQ error rate caused by the exclusion in the $l$-th level. We note that $e_l$ is the generalization error of the linear classifiers in level $l$. Take Caltech 101 as an example, when $K = 256$, $L = 10$, $p = 1/5$, we get $\hat{K}/K = 14.64\%$. If we use the maximum training error of all linear SVM classifiers as an estimation for $e_l$, we estimate the VQ error as $e_{vq} = 14.45\%$ using Eq. 6, which provides a reasonable estimation of the actual VQ error rate (which is 11.13%).

## 4  Experiments

We use 4 datasets in our experiments: Caltech 101 (15 + 20) [7], scene 15 (100 + rest) [3], sports 8 (70 + 60) [22], and indoor 67 (80 + 20) [23]. X+Y for each dataset means the number of training and testing images used in every category, respectively. Following the suggestion from [24], we use SIFT ($d = 128$) for Caltech 101, and the CENTRIST ($d = 256$) descriptor for other datasets. We use the LIBLINEAR package [25] to train a linear SVM classifier in each node

---

**Algorithm 2.** NN search using ExVQ

---

1: **Input**: A visual descriptor $q \in \mathbb{R}^d$,
        $\{(w_i, b_i), C^i, C^i_{+1}, C^i_{-1}\}$, $i = 0, 1, ..., 2^L - 2$.
2: $id \leftarrow 0$
3: **while** $id < 2^L - 1$ **do**
4:    **if** $w_{id}^T q + b_{id} > 0$ **then**
5:        $id \leftarrow id \times 2 + 1$
6:    **else**
7:        $id \leftarrow id \times 2 + 2$
8:    **end if**
9: **end while**
10: **Output**:
11: $leaf = \lfloor \frac{id-1}{2} \rfloor$
12: **if** $id$ is odd **then**
13:    $ann(q) = \arg\min_{i \in (C^{leaf} - C^{leaf}_{-1})} \|q - c_i\|_{\ell_2}$.
14: **else**
15:    $ann(q) = \arg\min_{i \in (C^{leaf} - C^{leaf}_{+1})} \|q - c_i\|_{\ell_2}$.
16: **end if**

---

of the ExVQ tree. The trade off parameter in Eq. 3 is $\alpha = 0.01$. After the BOV representation of all images are created, we use a one-vs-all SVM classifier with the $\chi^2$ kernel $\kappa(x_1, x_2) = \sum_{i=1}^d \frac{2x_{1i}x_{2i}}{x_{1i}+x_{2i}}$ [26][27] for classification. For each dataset, five training / testing sets are randomly split and average accuracy and VQ time of these five rounds are reported, if not otherwise specified.

### 4.1   VQ Time vs. Classification Accuracy

First, we compare the VQ time and classification accuracy of ExVQ, FLANN and the exhaustive search, with different codebook size $K$. FLANN is a state-of-the-art ANN search method [8]. In all experiments, we use the hierarchical $k$-means tree (which leads to a higher classification accuracy than the randomized $kd$-trees) with default parameters in FLANN. For ExVQ, we fix the exclusion portion $p = 1/5$ and fix the tree level $L = 10$ for $K = 256$ and $L = 15$ for $K = 1024$. The results are shown in Table 1 ($K = 256$) and Table 2 ($K = 1024$).

ExVQ is much faster than FLANN while their classification accuracies are almost the same. In Table 1 and Table 2, the classification accuracy of ExVQ and FLANN on all four datasets have no statistically significant difference. However, ExVQ is about twice faster than FLANN no matter on the codebook with a small size ($K = 256$) or a large size ($K = 1024$). Both ExVQ and FLANN are much faster than the exhaustive search. ExVQ speed up NN search 5–10 times than the exhaustive search. Especially, in the indoor 67 dataset, when $K = 256$, ExVQ's classification accuracy is even significantly better than the exhaustive search.

When the codebook size is larger, the NN search speedup of ExVQ is more prominent. The search speedup of $K = 1024$ is about twice of that when $K = $

**Table 1.** VQ time $T_i$ (seconds) and classification accuracy (%) of various methods. $T_i/T_j$ is the speedup ratio between two methods. $i, j = 0, 1, 2$, $K = 256$.

| Dataset | ExVQ | | | | FLANN | | | Exhaustive | |
|---|---|---|---|---|---|---|---|---|---|
| | $T_0$ | $T_2/T_0$ | $T_1/T_0$ | Accuracy | $T_1$ | $T_2/T_1$ | Accuracy | $T_2$ | Accuracy |
| Caltech 101 | 129.2 | 4.86 | 2.83 | 61.87±0.25 | 365.0 | 1.72 | 62.22±0.72 | 627.8 | 62.63±0.55 |
| Scene 15 | 358.6 | 5.77 | 2.22 | 81.16±0.45 | 797.6 | 2.60 | 81.17±0.14 | 2070.8 | 81.36±0.42 |
| Sports 8 | 292.6 | 5.93 | 2.29 | 82.50±0.90 | 670.2 | 2.59 | 82.71±1.07 | 1736.2 | 82.33±1.28 |
| Indoor 67 | 471.6 | 5.78 | 2.53 | 35.75±1.09 | 1193.4 | 2.28 | 35.04±1.28 | 2724.6 | 34.76±1.39 |

**Table 2.** VQ time $T_i$ (seconds) and classification accuracy (%) of various methods. $T_i/T_j$ is the speedup ratio between two methods. $i, j = 0, 1, 2$, $K = 1024$.

| Dataset | ExVQ | | | | FLANN | | | Exhaustive | |
|---|---|---|---|---|---|---|---|---|---|
| | $T_0$ | $T_2/T_0$ | $T_1/T_0$ | Accuracy | $T_1$ | $T_2/T_1$ | Accuracy | $T_2$ | Accuracy |
| Caltech 101 | 277.0 | 8.92 | 1.90 | 65.08±0.50 | 526.6 | 4.69 | 65.53±0.62 | 2472.0 | 65.79±0.53 |
| Scene 15 | 660.2 | 12.36 | 2.41 | 83.17±0.32 | 1592.0 | 5.13 | 83.27±0.33 | 8162.4 | 83.53±0.20 |
| Sports 8 | 556.4 | 12.39 | 2.92 | 83.42±0.77 | 1622.2 | 4.25 | 83.67±1.22 | 6892.4 | 84.17±1.11 |
| Indoor 67 | 885.0 | 12.22 | 2.83 | 38.52±1.96 | 2503.2 | 4.32 | 38.91±1.30 | 10818.6 | 38.94±1.33 |

256, which is similar for FLANN. However, the larger the codebook size is, the more tree level ExVQ will need to achieve the speedup. This requirement usually costs more time in building the tree, mainly in training the linear SVM classifiers. When $K = 256$, building the 10-level tree costs 18.8–56.6 seconds on different datasets. The building time increases to 326–617 seconds using 15 levels when $K = 1024$. In the experiments, we keep the number of training descriptors from 40468 to 76219, to restrict the training time of linear SVM classifiers. Note that the classifiers are trained offline, and are trained for only once.

We also test a smaller check number for FLANN. When the check number is 4, FLANN is faster than default check number 32, but its VQ time is still at least 67% longer than ExVQ (or higher than 67% on different datasets). Furthermore, when $K = 1024$, the classification accuracy of FLANN with check number 4 is statistically significantly lower than that of ExVQ.

## 4.2  Properties of VQ Errors

For these datasets, the VQ error rates of ExVQ and FLANN are shown in Table 3. In some cases, the VQ error rates of ExVQ and FLANN are close. In many cases, the VQ error rate of ExVQ is higher than that of FLANN. However, as observed from Table 1 and Table 2, the difference in VQ error rates does not have impact on the classification performance. In fact, if we increase $L$ and reduce $p$, ExVQ can easily achieve both faster VQ speed and smaller VQ error rate than FLANN, with the cost of larger storage.

In practice, we don't need very large $L$, because ExVQ has benign VQ errors. We further evaluate the VQ errors generated by ExVQ in Fig. 3, which plots the histograms of error ranks for ExVQ. ExVQ error ranks are all within a small

**Table 3.** VQ error rates (%) of ExVQ and FLANN

|  | $K = 256$ | | $K = 1024$ | |
| --- | --- | --- | --- | --- |
| Dataset | ExVQ | FLANN | ExVQ | FLANN |
| Caltech 101 | 11.13 | 4.91 | 14.15 | 19.32 |
| Scene 15 | 4.99 | 3.20 | 18.64 | 7.14 |
| Sports 8 | 5.82 | 4.23 | 19.19 | 6.63 |
| Indoor 67 | 6.03 | 5.81 | 16.90 | 6.26 |

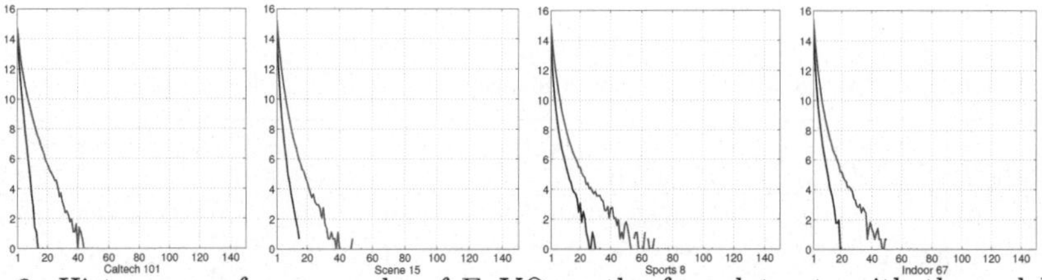

**Fig. 3.** Histograms of error ranks of ExVQ on the four datasets with the codebook size $K = 256$ (blue) and $K = 1024$ (red). The horizontal axis is the error rank and the vertical axis shows the frequency number plot in natural logarithm.

range (compared to the codebook size) close to 1, which we believe are benign to classification.

When the codebook size is larger, the maximum error rank is also lager. The maximum error rank for $K = 1024$ (red curve) is 2.57–3.15 times of that for $K = 256$ (blue curve). One may conjecture that the reduction in the number of training descriptors of each codeword makes the linear classifiers inaccurate when $K$ is larger. However, when we increase the training descriptors for $K = 1024$, we find that the maximum error rank is almost the same as that in Fig. 3. In fact, the VQ error rate is mostly dependent on the tree level $L$ and the exclusion portion $p$.

### 4.3 Effects of $L$ and $p$

$L$ and $p$ are the two parameters that can be tuned in ExVQ. In this section, we evaluate how $L$ and $p$ affect the trade off between the classification accuracy and the VQ time. First, we evaluate the classification accuracy and VQ time when we change $L$ with a fixed $p$. We change $L$ from 5 to 15 (with step size 2) and test on one round of Caltech 101 with $p = 1/5, K = 256$. The classification accuracy and the VQ time are shown in Fig. 4a. When $L$ is larger than 11, the VQ time is not reduced apparently. Besides, a larger $L$ can induce a higher VQ error. However, all classification accuracies are similar with different $L$. When $L$ is even larger, the VQ time cost will be bigger and the classification accuracy will drop.

Next, we evaluate ExVQ with different exclusion portion $p$ with a fixed $L$. We change $1/p$ from 3 to 11 (with step size 2) and fix $L = 10$ on one round of Caltech 101 with $K = 256$. The classification accuracy and the VQ time are shown in

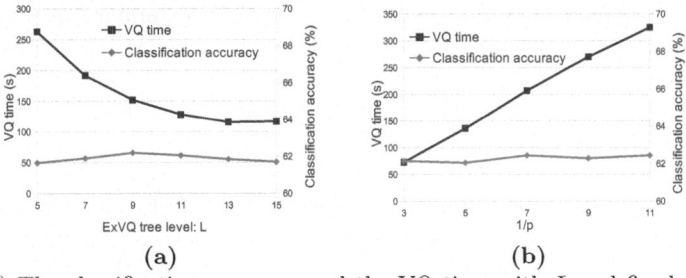

**Fig. 4.** (a) The classification accuracy and the VQ time with $L$ and fixed $p$; (b) The classification accuracy and the VQ time with $1/p$ and fixed $L$

**Table 4.** Comparison with other related methods on Caltech 101, $K = 1024$

| ANN methods | VQ time (s) | Accuracy (%) |
|-------------|-------------|--------------|
| ExVQ        | 280         | 65.17        |
| Spill tree  | 291         | 63.87        |
| LSH         | 3247        | 63.97        |
| LLC         | 4817        | 65.77        |

Fig. 4b. When $p$ is smaller, the training of linear classifiers in the tree will be more accurate. So the VQ error will be smaller. Meanwhile, in the leaf node of the ExVQ tree, the active search set will be larger, which leads to longer VQ time. However, the classification accuracies keep almost the same for different $p$. When $p$ is even smaller, the VQ time will cost more and the accuracy can be a little better (the linear projection is more accurate).

### 4.4   ExVQ and Other Related Methods

Finally, we compare ExVQ with more related methods including spill tree [15], LSH [18] and LLC [4]. We evaluate the VQ time and the classification accuracy of these methods on Caltech 101 with $K = 1024$. We use the same tree structure of ExVQ for spill tree: the same $L$ and $p$. So we can compare their classification accuracy under equivalent VQ time. We use the E$^2$LSH package[2] to implement LSH, which is to search all near neighbors within a radius $R$ of the query point. In order to use it in the BOV model, we search exhaustively from the returned results of LSH to get the nearest neighbor. In E$^2$LSH, we use multiple radius for near neighbor search to save the VQ time. For LLC, we use the published Matlab code[3] for testing. The results are shown in Table 4.

ExVQ has the shortest VQ time. Spill tree's VQ time is close, but its classification accuracy drops significantly. Meanwhile, the VQ error rate of spill tree (41% $\gg$ 30%, although the error ranks are small) is much more than that of ExVQ, which influences the classification accuracy. ExVQ has similar accuracy

---

[2] http://www.mit.edu/~andoni/LSH/

[3] http://www.ifp.illinois.edu/~jyang29/LLC.htm

with LLC, but is about 20 times faster. Note that this comparison is qualitative rather than quantitative, because different programming languages are used. We also want to point out that ExVQ uses only a single core, while LLC utilizes multiple cores of a six-core CPU. Since LLC also needs to search $k$NN, ExVQ can be used to accelerate it. LSH is effective in large scale NN search problems. However, it is not suitable to get the nearest neighbor from the codebook with $K = 1024$, which costs more time even than the exhaustive NN search. The VQ error of LSH is not benign: its histogram of error ranks has a long tail, and the maximum error rank is 997. LSH has a lower classification accuracy than ExVQ, which coincides with our conjecture about how VQ errors impact the classification.

## 5    Conclusions

We presented ExVQ, an approximate nearest neighbor (ANN) search method for vector quantization (VQ) in BOV models. ExVQ achieves 10x speedup than exhaustive search and 2x speedup than state-of-the-art ANN methods. The key insight in ExVQ is an exclusive strategy, which can safely reduce the search range. The exclusion's quality is guaranteed by learning an accurate classifier. Thus, it is more efficient than the commonly used inclusive strategy in ANN search. We also systematically evaluated how VQ errors affect the accuracy of BOV-based visual classification, and conclude that some VQ methods have benign VQ errors, which does not reduce the classification accuracy even with 30% VQ errors. On four benchmark datasets, ExVQ leads to indistinguishable accuracy rates with the exhaustive search method and the FLANN method.

Future works include the following issues. First, effective exclusive NN search on large databases (e.g., $K = 100,000$) will be investigated. Second, integration of multiple trees in ExVQ to further improve the NN search efficiency. Third, ExVQ can be extended to search NN using arbitrary distance metrics, e.g., histogram intersection kernel [28]. Finally, we want to work out a theoretical framework for analyzing the effect of VQ errors to classification.

**Acknowledgement.** This work was supported in part by the following grants: National Science Foundation of China grant (61001146) and Shanghai Pujiang Program (12PJ1404300).

## References

1. Sivic, J., Zisserman, A.: Video google: A text retrieval approach to object matching in videos. In: ICCV, pp. 1470–1477 (2003)
2. Fei-Fei, L., Perona, P.: A bayesian hierarchical model for learning natural scene categories. In: CVPR, vol. 2, pp. 524–531 (2005)
3. Lazebnik, S., Schmid, C., Ponce, J.: Beyond bags of features: Spatial pyramid matching for recognizing natural scene categories. In: CVPR, pp. 2169–2178 (2006)
4. Wang, J., Yang, J., Yu, K., Huang, T., Gong, Y.: Locality-constrained linear coding for image classification. In: CVPR, pp. 3360–3367 (2010)
5. Yang, J., Yu, K., Gong, Y., Huang, T.: Linear spatial pyramid matching using sparse coding for image classification. In: CVPR, pp. 1794–1801 (2009)

6. van de Sande, K.E.A., Gevers, T., Snoek, C.G.M.: Empowering visual categorization with the GPU. IEEE Transaction on Multimedia 13, 60–70 (2011)
7. Fei-Fei, L., Fergus, R., Perona, P.: Learning generative visual models from few training example: an incremental bayesian approach tested on 101 object categories. In: CVPR (2004)
8. Muja, M., Lowe, D.G.: Fast approximate nearest neighbors with automatic algorithm configuration. In: VISAPP, vol. 1, pp. 331–340 (2009)
9. Bhattacharya, S., Sukthankar, R., Jin, R., Shah, M.: A probabilistic representation for efficient large scale visual tasks. In: CVPR, vol. 2, pp. 2593–2600 (2011)
10. Gersho, A., Gray, R.M.: Vector quantization and signal compression. Springer (1991)
11. Nistér, D., Stewénius, H.: Scalable recognition with a vocabulary tree. In: CVPR, vol. 2, pp. 2161–2168 (2006)
12. Philbin, J., Chum, O., Isard, M., Sivic, J., Zisserman, A.: Lost in quantization: Improving particular object retrieval in large scale image databases. In: CVPR (2008)
13. Lepetit, V., Fua, P.: Keypoint recognition using randomized trees. IEEE TPAMI 28, 1465–1479 (2006)
14. Moosmann, F., Nowak, E., Jurie, F.: Randomized clustering forests for image classification. IEEE TPAMI 30, 1632–1646 (2008)
15. Liu, T., Moore, A.W., Gray, A., Yang, K.: An investigation of practical approximate nearest neighbor algorithms. In: NIPS (2004)
16. Marszałek, M., Schmid, C.: Constructing Category Hierarchies for Visual Recognition. In: Forsyth, D., Torr, P., Zisserman, A. (eds.) ECCV 2008, Part IV. LNCS, vol. 5305, pp. 479–491. Springer, Heidelberg (2008)
17. Gao, T., Koller, D.: Discriminative learning of relaxed hierarchy for large-scale visual recognition. In: ICCV (2011)
18. Datar, M., Immorlica, N., Indyk, P., Mirrokni, V.S.: Locality-sensitive hashing scheme based on p-stable distributions. In: Symposium on Computational Geometry, pp. 253–262 (2004)
19. Jegou, H., Douze, M., Schmid, C.: Improving bag-of-features for large scale image search. IJCV 87, 316–336 (2010)
20. Weiss, Y., Torralba, A., Fergus, R.: Spectral hashing. In: NIPS, vol. 21, pp. 1753–1760 (2009)
21. Jegou, H., Douze, M., Schmid, C.: Product quantization for nearest neighbor search. IEEE TPAMI 33, 117–128 (2011)
22. Li, L.J., Fei-Fei, L.: What, where and who? Classifying events by scene and object recognition. In: ICCV, pp. 261–268 (2007)
23. Quattoni, A., Torralba, A.: Recognizing indoor scenes. In: CVPR, pp. 413–420 (2009)
24. Wu, J., Rehg, J.M.: CENTRIST: A visual descriptor for scene categorization. IEEE TPAMI 33, 1489–1501 (2011)
25. Fan, R.E., Chang, K.W., Hsieh, C.J., Wang, X.R., Lin, C.J.: LIBLINEAR: A library for large linear classification. JMLR 9, 1871–1874 (2008)
26. Vedaldi, A., Zisserman, A.: Efficient additive kernels via explicit feature maps. IEEE TPAMI 34, 480–492 (2012)
27. Wu, J.: Power mean SVM for large scale visual classification. In: CVPR, pp. 2344–2351 (2012)
28. Wu, J., Rehg, J.M.: Beyond the Euclidean distance: Creating effective visual codebooks using the histogram intersection kernel. In: ICCV, pp. 630–637 (2009)

# Underwater Live Fish Recognition
# Using a Balance-Guaranteed Optimized Tree

Phoenix X. Huang, Bastiaan J. Boom, and Robert B. Fisher

School of Informatics, University of Edinburgh

**Abstract.** Live fish recognition in the open sea is a challenging multi-class classification task. We propose a novel method to recognize fish in an unrestricted natural environment recorded by underwater cameras. This method extracts 66 types of features, which are a combination of color, shape and texture properties from different parts of the fish and reduce the feature dimensions with forward sequential feature selection (FSFS) procedure. The selected features of the FSFS are used by an SVM. We present a Balance-Guaranteed Optimized Tree (BGOT) to control the error accumulation in hierarchical classification and, therefore, achieve better performance. A BGOT of 10 fish species is automatically constructed using the inter-class similarities and a heuristic method. The proposed BGOT-based hierarchical classification method achieves about 4% better accuracy compared to state-of-the-art techniques on a live fish image dataset.

## 1 Introduction

Live fish recognition in the open sea has been investigated by [1–4] for commercial and environmental applications like fish farming and a meteorologic monitoring. The detected fish are in 3D positions and against coral and sand as well as the open sea. Statistics about the specific oceanic fish species distribution besides an aggregate count of aquatic animals can assist biologists resolving issues ranging from food availability to predator-prey relationships [5, 6]. However, the recognition task is fundamentally challenging because fish can move freely and illumination levels change frequently in such environments [7, 8]. As a result, this task remains an outstanding research problem. Prior research is mainly restricted to constrained environments (*e.g.*, fish tanks [1], conveyor belts [9]). Strachan et al. [3] achieves the scores of 73%, 63% and 90%, respectively, on three types of fish. C. Spampinato et al. [10] classifies 360 images of ten different species and achieves an average accuracy of about 92%. R. Larsen et al. [11] classify three fish species and achieve a recognition rate of 76%. In contrast, this paper investigates novel techniques to perform effective live fish recognition in an unrestricted natural environment.

### 1.1 Related Work

**SVM Method.** The fish recognition task is seen as an application of multi-class classification, which has become an important and interesting research area

K.M. Lee et al. (Eds.): ACCV 2012, Part I, LNCS 7724, pp. 422–433, 2013.
© Springer-Verlag Berlin Heidelberg 2013

since the influence of machine learning theory. Over the last decade, SVM [12] has shown impressive accuracy on the multi-class classification task because of its maximum-margin advantages. However, SVM is originally designed for a binary classification task. Therefore, to enable multi-class classification, several mechanisms, such as one-vs-one and one-vs-rest, have been developed. This kind of multi-class classifier could be considered as a flat classifier because it classifies all classes at the same time [13] and omits the inter-class correlations. A shortcoming of the flat classifier is that it uses the same features to classify all classes without considering that some classes have certain similarities and can be better separated by some customized features.

**Hierarchical Classification Tree Method.** To overcome the problem of flat classifier, one possible solution is to integrate a domain knowledge database with the flat classifier and construct a tree to organize all classes hierarchically [14]. This strategy is called hierarchical classification which inherits from the divide and conquer tactic. Essentially, it uses a hierarchical classification procedure where a customized classifier is trained with specifical features at each level [15].

Hierarchical classification has several noticeable advantages. Firstly, it divides all classes into certain subsets and leaves similar classes for a later stage. This strategy balances the load of any single node. Secondly, unlike the flat classifier choosing a feature set based on the average accuracy over all classes, the hierarchical method applies a customized set of features to classify specific classes. As a result, it achieves better performance on similar classes. Thirdly, the hierarchical solution exploits the correlations between classes and finds the similar groupings. This is especially useful with a large number of categories [14]. Hierarchical structures are popular in document and image categorization. Mathis [16] organizes documents hierarchically by making use of the correlations between topical subjects. Deng *et.al.* [17] introduced a new dataset called ImageNet where a large scale hierarchical ontology of images are constructed based on the WordNet knowledge. However, these approaches use pre-defined hierarchical structures without considering how to construct a more accurate tree based on given classes.

Nonetheless, the hierarchical structure has a critical disadvantage called error accumulation. Each level of the hierarchical tree may have some classification errors. These errors are accumulated into deeper layers and reduce the average accuracy of the final result.

## 1.2   The Framework

In this paper, we propose a novel method to recognize fish in an unrestricted natural environment from underwater videos. We use the Balance-Guaranteed Optimized Tree (BGOT) to help resolve the error accumulation issue and make use of the inner-class similarities among fish species. The framework is illustrated in Fig 1.

In this paper we propose a hierarchical classification approach for live fish recognition. Furthermore, we use a heuristic method to construct an automatically

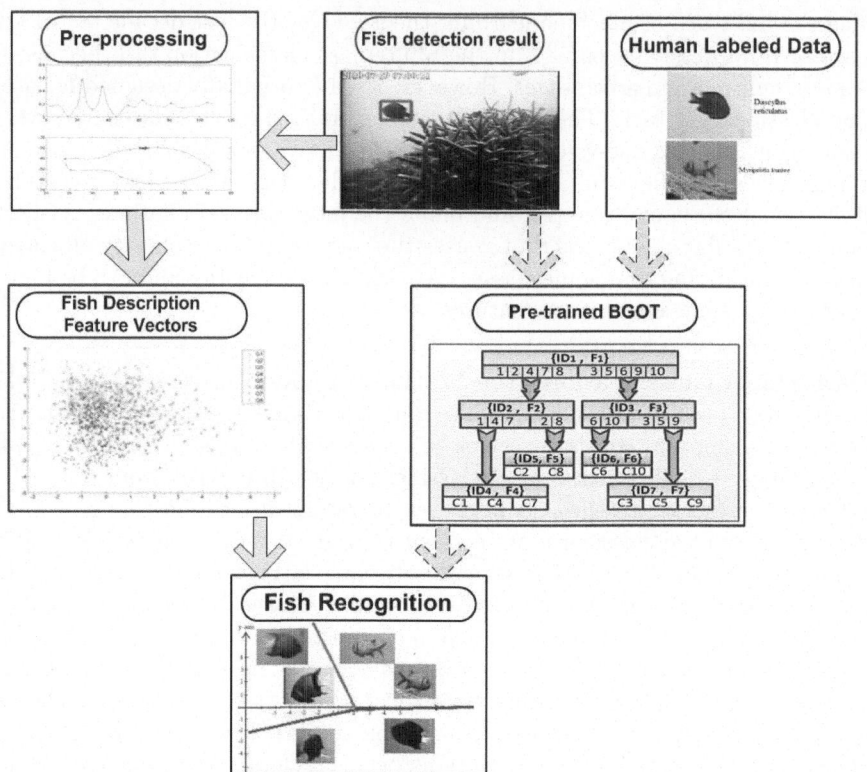

**Fig. 1.** The framework of our BGOT-based hierarchical classification system. The work flow of dotted arrows shows the training procedure and the solid arrows indicate the recognition procedure.

generated BGOT and the proposed method is evaluated on a live fish dataset. The algorithm itself is presented in section 2, including the mathematical explanation of hierarchical classification, a set of heuristics which help construct the hierarchical tree. In section 4, we compared the proposed BGOT tree to an Ada-boost [18] method and a flat SVM [12] (section 3) on a fish image set [19].

## 2    Hierarchical Classification Approach

Given a set of samples $\{x_i\}_{i=1}^n$, the feature vector $f_i = \{f_{i,1}, ..., f_{i,m}\}$ denotes the $m$ feature values for sample $x_i$. Let $\{y_i\}_{i=1}^n$ indicate the class label of $x_i$, and $y_i \in \{1, ..., c\}$ where $c$ is the number of classes. Our aim is to construct a classifier $h$ which uses the feature $f_i$ as input to predict the class label $\tilde{y}_i = h(f_i)$ that maximizes the classification accuracy.

A hierarchical classifier approach $h_{hier}$ is designed as a structured node set. Fundamentally, a node is defined as a triple: $\text{Node}_t = \{\text{ID}_t, \tilde{F}_t, \hat{C}_t\}$, where $\text{ID}_t$ is a unique node number, $\tilde{F}_t \subset \{f_1, ..., f_m\}$ is a feature subset chosen by a feature selection procedure that is found to be effective for classifying $\hat{C}_t$, which is a subset of classes and their groups. We only consider binary splits so each node has at most two groups. All samples that are classified as the same group will be transmitted into the same child node for later processing. An example with 10 classes is demonstrated in Figure 2, where the $ID_t$ and $\tilde{F}_t$ are illustrated in each node and $\hat{C}_t$ is described as local groups.

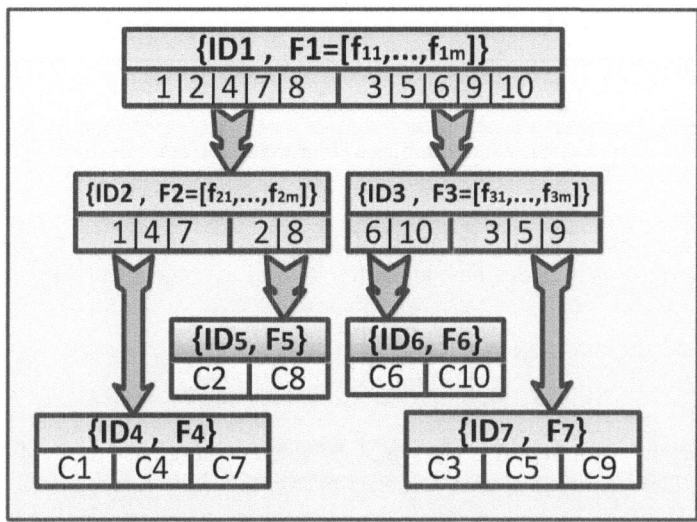

**Fig. 2.** Automatically generated tree (BGOT), the hierarchical example tree of 10 classes $(C1, ..., C_{10})$

## 2.1   Heuristic Method

In this paper, we propose two heuristics for how to organize a single classifier and construct a hierarchical tree with higher accuracy.

1. Arrange more accurate classifications at a higher level and leave similar classes to deeper layers.
2. Keep the hierarchical tree balanced to minimize the max-depth and control error accumulation.

Rule 1 recommends how to assign the single classifiers to a hierarchical tree. We consider the balanced tree $T_b$ in Figure 3(a) with sample number $n_i$. This tree has 4 classes $\{c_1, c_2, c_3, c_4\}$ and each single classifier has a different accuracy $\{p_1, p_2, p_3\}$. The average accuracy is calculated as $p_1 * \frac{1}{2}(p_2 + p_3)$ assuming all classes have equal magnitude. The best accuracy is achieved by assigning

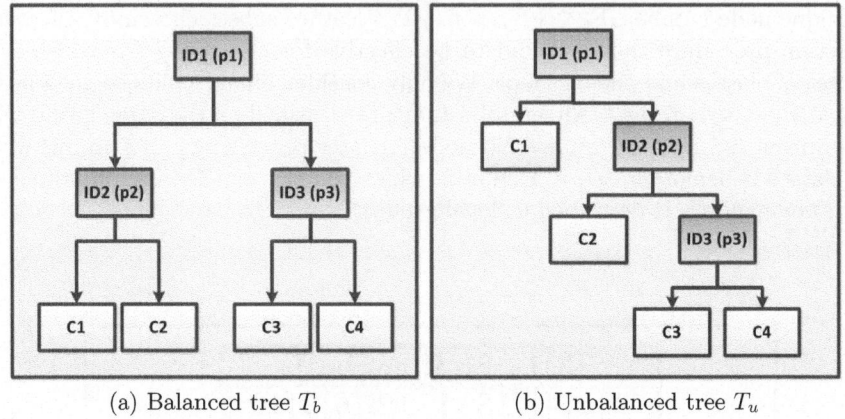

(a) Balanced tree $T_b$         (b) Unbalanced tree $T_u$

**Fig. 3.** Examples of hierarchical trees

the most accurate classifier to node $ID_1$. Generally, the result of a balanced hierarchical tree of N nodes has depth $log_2 N$ and average accuracy:

$$P_b = \prod_{i=1}^{log_2 N} \widetilde{P}_i = \prod_{i=1}^{log_2 N} \frac{1}{2^{(i-1)}} \sum_{s=2^{(i-1)}}^{2^i - 1} p_s \tag{1}$$

where $p_s$ is the accuracy of node $s$ and $\widetilde{P}_i$ is the average accuracy of all nodes in layer i. The hierarchical tree achieves better accuracy if we choose the more accurate classifiers at higher layers which equates to assigning these nodes a higher weight. In the future, we will think more about how to construct the hierarchical tree if classes are not at equal size.

Rule 2 is explained by comparing two sample trees: a balanced tree $T_b$ and an unbalanced tree $T_u$. These examples are shown in Figure 3. Let us assume each class has the same number of samples $n_i$ and each classifier has an equal accuracy p. In $T_b$, each class is classified with an accuracy $p^2$, while the average accuracy in $T_u$ is $\frac{1}{4}(p + p^2 + 2p^3)$. We can prove that $P_b > P_u$, for $0.5 < p < 1$. To generalize, a balanced tree of N nodes has average accuracy:

$$P_b = p^{log_2 N} \tag{2}$$

and unbalanced accuracy:

$$P_u = \frac{1}{N} (\sum_{i=1}^{N-1} p^i + p^{N-1}) \tag{3}$$

for $0.5 < p < 1$, $P_b > P_u$. Thus a more balanced hierarchical tree with $log_2 N$ depth suppresses error accumulation, and achieves better accuracy than an unbalanced tree.

## 2.2 Algorithm of Generating BGOT

The BGOT is based on the two heuristics of the last section: keep the hierarchical tree balanced and optimize the performance by putting more accurate nodes at the top layers. In the fish recognition task, some species of fish are more similar than others and the similarity is summarized from the confusion matrix. We illustrate the algorithm of generating BGOT below:

```
Input: class C1 to Cn
begin c := [C₁, ..., Cₙ]
    level := 0
    construct(c, level);
where
proc construct(c, n) ≡
    if n > MAXDEPTH then exit fi;
    comment: find the best binary split of given classes on whole feature set;
    [cLeft, cRight] := ChooseSplit(c);
    comment: The ChooseSplit function splits the class set into equal-size subsets;
    featureSet = FeatureSelection(cLeft, cRight);
    comment: the minimum splitting is set to 3 to limit the max depth;
    if size(cLeft) > 3 then
                        construct(cLeft, n + 1)
    fi;
    if size(cRight) > 3 then
                        construct(cRight, n + 1)
    fi;
end
```

An example BGOT is shown in Fig 2, where 10 classes are arranged into 3 layers. The first layer splits all classes into two groups: C1, C2, C4, C7, C8 and C3, C5, C6, C9, C10. Then it chooses the feature subset to maximize the average accuracy of these groups. This procedure keeps on until all groups have less than 4 classes.

## 3    Experiment with Fish Recognition

Our data is acquired from a live fish dataset with 3179 fish images of the 10 different species shown in Figure 4. This figure shows the fish species name and the numbers of images. As can be seen, the data is very imbalanced where the first two species account for 2564 images. The fish detection and tracking software described in [19] is used to obtain the fish images. The fish species are manually labeled by following instructions from marine biologists.

Figure 3 shows some hard fish examples: blurred, occlusion by other fish or background objects, which include coral, the sea flower and open sea.

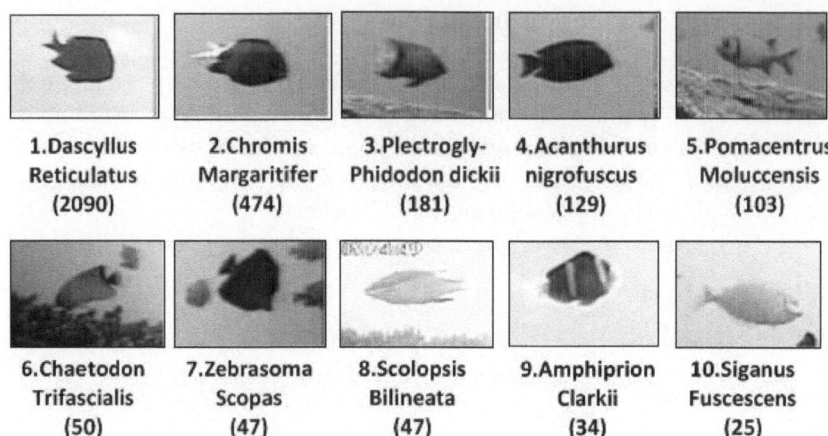

| 1.Dascyllus Reticulatus (2090) | 2.Chromis Margaritifer (474) | 3.Plectrogly- Phidodon dickii (181) | 4.Acanthurus nigrofuscus (129) | 5.Pomacentrus Moluccensis (103) |
| --- | --- | --- | --- | --- |
| 6.Chaetodon Trifascialis (50) | 7.Zebrasoma Scopas (47) | 8.Scolopsis Bilineata (47) | 9.Amphiprion Clarkii (34) | 10.Siganus Fuscescens (25) |

**Fig. 4.** Top 10 species of fish in underwater videos

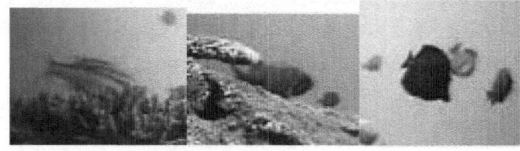

**Fig. 5.** Hard fish examples

### 3.1   Feature Extraction

After constructing the fish dataset, some pre-processing procedures are undertaken to improve the recognition rate. Firstly, the Grabcut algorithm [20] is employed to segment fish from the background. Secondly, we propose a streamline hypothesis, which uses the assumption that the head is smoother than the tail. We calculate the fish orientation by weighting each contour pixel with its local curvature scale, and we use this algorithm to align all fish horizontally where the head of the fish is located on the right. we align the fish images to the same direction before further processing. This procedure is carried out based on a streamline assumption, which assumes that most fish have a smoother head than tail because fish need a more frictional tail (caudal fin) to swim and help them keep balance. In order to find the tail side, we smooth the fish boundary with a Gaussian filter to eliminate some noise, and then calculate the curvature of each boundary pixel as following [21, 22]:

$$\kappa(u,\sigma) = \frac{X_u(u,\sigma)Y_{uu}(u,\sigma) - X_{uu}(u,\sigma)Y_u(u,\sigma)}{(X_u(u,\sigma)^2 + Y_u(u,\sigma)^2))^{\frac{3}{2}}} \tag{4}$$

where $X_u(u,\sigma)/X_{uu}(u,\sigma)$ and $Y_u(u,\sigma)/Y_{uu}(u,\sigma)$ are the first and the second derivative of $X(u,\sigma)$ and $Y(u,\sigma)$, respectively; $X(u,\sigma)$ and $Y(u,\sigma)$ are the convolution result of 1-D Gaussian kernel function $g(u, \sigma)$ with fish boundary coordinates $x(u)$ and $y(u)$. However, the pixel curvature is sensitive to local corners and we normalize it using the logarithm function:

$$\kappa_{normalize} = \begin{cases} log(\kappa) & \text{if } \kappa \geq 1 \\ -log(2 - \kappa) & \text{if } \kappa < 1 \end{cases} \tag{5}$$

The fish boundary coordinates are weighted by their local curvature and the vector from the center of mask to the curvature weighed center estimates the tail orientation. A typical fish orientation procedure is illustrated in Figure 6. The fish orientation method achieves 95% accuracy using 1000 manually labeled fish images. Finally, every fish image is divided into four parts (head/tail/top/bottom) according to the relative positions from the fish center.

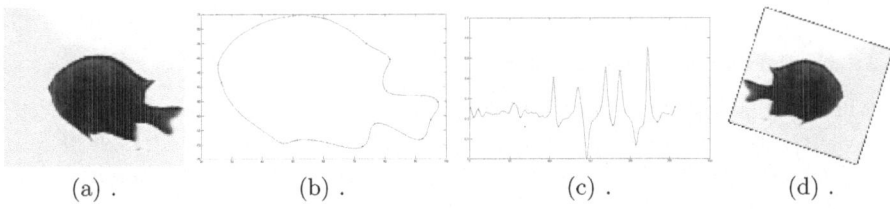

(a) .                (b) .                (c) .                (d) .

**Fig. 6.** Fish orientation demonstration: (a) original fish image; (b) fish boundary after gaussian filter; (c) curvature along fish boundary; (d) oriented fish image

After this, 66 types of feature are extracted. These features are a combination of color, shape and texture properties in different parts of the fish such as tail/head/top/bottom, as well as the whole fish. We use normalized color histogram in the Red&Green channel and the Hue component in HSV color space. These color features are normalized to minimize the effect of illumination changes. We recompute the range of every bin according to the average distribution over all samples and map them into a 11-bin histogram to take full advantage of all bins, as shown below:

$$\widetilde{B}_i = \sum_{j=a_i}^{a_{i+1}} B_j \qquad s.t. \qquad a_i = min\{X \in \mathbb{N}^+ \mid \Sigma_{j=1}^{X}\overline{B}_j \geq \frac{i}{11}\} \tag{6}$$

where $B_j, j \in \{1, ..., 50\}$ is the original color histogram bin, $\overline{B}_j, j \in \{1, ..., 50\}$ is the averaged histogram over all samples and $\widetilde{B}_i, i \in \{1, ..., 11\}$ is the recomputed bin.

In order to describe the fish texture, we calculate the co-occurrence matrix, Fourier descriptor and gabor filter. The grey level co-occurrence matrices describe the co-occurrence frequency of two grey scale pixels at a given distance $d$ [10]:

$$C_{\Delta u, \Delta v}(i,j) = \sum_{p=1}^{n} \sum_{q=1}^{m} \begin{cases} 1 & \text{if } I(p,q) = i \text{ and } I(p + \Delta u, q + \Delta v) = j \\ 0, & \text{otherwise} \end{cases} \quad (7)$$

The frequency is calculated for several orientations $\lambda$. We compute Contrast, Correlation, Energy, Entropy, Homogeneity, Variance, Inverse Difference Moment, Cluster Shade, Cluster Prominence, Max Probability, Auto correlation, Dissimilarity. These 12 features are useful as they are the first selected features by the feature selection procedure.

Histogram of oriented gradients and Moment Invariants, as well as Affine Moment Invariants, are employed as the shape features. Furthermore, some specific features like tail/head area ratio, tail/body area ratio, *etc.* are also included. All features are normalized by subtracting the mean and dividing by the standard deviation (z-score normalized).

### 3.2 Hierarchical Classification

As the SVM is firstly designed for binary classification problem, we introduce a one-vs-one strategy with a voting mechanism to convert the binary SVM into a multi-class classifier [12]. Based on the multi-class classifier, we designed two classifiers (see Figure 2):

1. A flat SVM classifier, which classifies all 10 classes simultaneously, is implemented as a baseline classifier.
2. An automatically generated tree (BGOT) is designed by recursively choosing a binary split which has the best accuracy in given classes. We choose binary splitting to keep the tree balanced.

An Ada-boost method [18], which boosts on individual features, is also implemented as a comparison method.

### 3.3 Results and Analysis

The experiment is based on 3179 fish images with a 6-fold cross validation procedure. The training and testing sets are isolated so fish images from the same trajectory sequence are not used during both training and testing. Sequential forward feature selection is applied at each node. We then train a customized classifier at each node for specific classes. Results are listed in Table 1 where the AP and AR results are averaged over all classes rather than over all fish. This is because of the greatly unbalanced class sizes.

The accuracy of a classification system is evaluated as Average Recall (AR), Average Precision (AP) and Accuracy over Count (AC). Generally, given True Positive / False Positive / False Negative, the AR is defined as:

$$AR = \frac{1}{c} \sum_{j=1}^{c} \left( \frac{TruePositive_j}{TruePositive_j + FalseNegative_j} \right) \quad (8)$$

where c is the number of classes. The second score is Average Precision (AP) over all species. It is the probability that the classification results are relevant to specified species, as shown below:

$$AP = \frac{1}{c} \sum_{j=1}^{c} \left( \frac{TruePositive_j}{TruePositive_j + FalsePositive_j} \right) \tag{9}$$

The third metric is the accuracy over all samples (Accuracy over Count, AC), which is defined as the proportion of correct classified samples among the whole dataset. The AC is calculated as following:

$$AC = \frac{\sum_{j=1}^{c} TruePositive_j}{\sum_{j=1}^{c} (TruePositive_j + FalsePositive_j)} \tag{10}$$

We compare the hierarchical classification against the Ada-boost method (75.3% AR) and flat SVM classifier (86.3% AR). The automatically generated hierarchical tree (BGOT), which chooses the best splitting by exhaustively searching all possible combinations while remaining balanced, achieves an AR of (90.0%). The search procedure takes several hours and a possible improvement is to integrate the hierarchical method with domain knowledge like taxonomy, which helps organize similar species for later processing, instead of exhaustive searching. In the average precision (AP) score, the proposed BGOT method is about 6% better than the baseline SVM method, which are 85.8% and 91.7%, respectively. The Ada-boost method is 76.9% in AP. The AC score of BGOT is tested in a t-test with 95% confidence of significant improvement than the SVM method and Ada-boost method. We calculate the average AC rates at each level in the hierarchy (BGOT): 0.977 (Level 1), 0.9725 (Level 2), 0.950 (Level 3).

**Table 1.** Fish recognition result. * means significant improvement with 95% confidence.

| Algorithm | AR | AP | AC |
|---|---|---|---|
| Ada-boost | 0.753 ± 0.091 | 0.769 ± 0.092 | 0.923 |
| Flat SVM | 0.863 ± 0.052 | 0.858 ± 0.061 | 0.934 |
| BGOT method | 0.900 ± 0.042 | 0.917 ± 0.045 | 0.950* |

The individual class recall/precision is shown in Figure 7 and 8. The hierarchical approaches achieve a better accuracy than the flat SVM classifier because they arrange the similar species (1,4,7) into the same group and add fish-tail features to distinguish these species. The flat SVM method misclassified some fish from species 4 to species 8, which achieves a better precision in species 4.

## 4   Conclusion

In this paper we propose a hierarchical classification approach for live fish recognition. Furthermore, we propose a set of heuristics which are helpful to construct

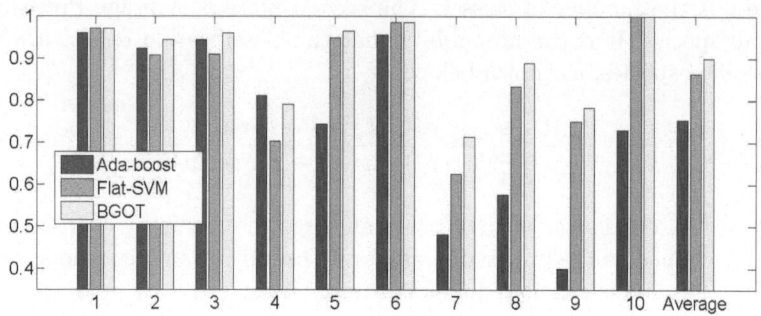

**Fig. 7.** Recall of 10 species. The BGOT method is better than the baseline method.

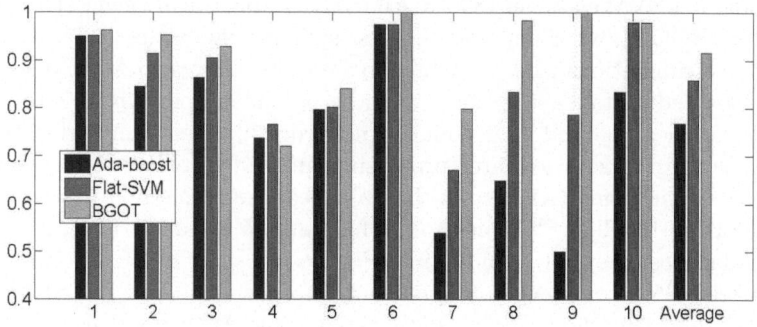

**Fig. 8.** Precision of 10 species. The BGOT method is better than the baseline method (class 4 is an exception, and is discussed in the result section).

a hierarchical tree. The proposed method is evaluated on a live fish dataset and the automatically generated hierarchical tree (BGOT) achieves c. 4% improvement of the average recall (AR) compared to the flat SVM classifier.

**Acknowledgements.** This work is supported by the Fish4Knowledge project, which is funded by the European Union Seventh Framework Programme [FP7/2007-2013].

# References

1. Lee, D., Schoenberger, R.B., Shiozawa, D., Xu, X., Zhan, P.: Contour matching for a fish recognition and migration-monitoring system. In: Proc. of SPIE, vol. 5606, pp. 37–48 (2004)
2. Ruff, B.P., Marchant, J.A., Frost, A.R.: Fish sizing and monitoring using a stereo image analysis system applied to fish farming. Aquacultural Engineering 14, 155–173 (1995)

3. Strachan, N.J.C., Nesvadba, P., Allen, A.R.: Fish species recognition by shape analysis of images. Pattern Recognition 23, 539–544 (1990)
4. Okamoto, M., Morita, S., Sato, T.: Fundamental study to estimate fish biomass around coral reef using 3-dimensional underwater video system. In: OCEANS 2000 MTS/IEEE Conference and Exhibition, vol. 2, pp. 1389–1392 (2000)
5. Rova, A., Mori, G., Dill, L.M.: One fish, two fish, butterfish, trumpeter: Recognizing fish in underwater video. In: IAPR Conference on Machine Vision Applications, pp. 404–407 (2007)
6. Zion, B., Shklyar, A., Karplus, I.: In-vivo fish sorting by computer vision. Aquacultural Engineering 22, 165–179 (2000)
7. Strachan, N.J.C.: Length measurement of fish by computer vision. Computers and Electronics in Agriculture 8, 93–104 (1993)
8. Toh, Y.H., Ng, T.M., Liew, B.K.: Automated fish counting using image processing. In: International Conference on Computational Intelligence and Software Engineering, pp. 1–5 (2009)
9. Strachan, N.J.C.: Recognition of fish species by colour and shape. Image and Vision Computing 11, 2–10 (1993)
10. Spampinato, C., Giordano, D., Salvo, R.D., Chen-Burger, Y.H., Fisher, R.B., Nadarajan, G.: Automatic fish classification for underwater species behavior understanding. In: Proceedings of the First ACM International Workshop on Analysis and Retrieval of Tracked Events and Motion in Imagery Streams, pp. 45–50 (2010)
11. Larsen, R., Ólafsdóttir, H., Ersbøll, B.: Shape and texture based classification of fish species. In: Proceedings of SCIA, pp. 745–749 (2009)
12. Chih-Chung, C., Chih-Jen, L.: LIBSVM: a library for support vector machines. ACM Trans. Intell. Syst. Technol. 2, 1–27 (2011)
13. Carlos, S., Alex, F.: A survey of hierarchical classification across different application domains. Data Mining and Knowledge Discovery 22, 31–72 (2010)
14. Deng, J., Berg, A.C., Li, K., Fei-Fei, L.: What Does Classifying More Than 10,000 Image Categories Tell Us? In: Daniilidis, K., Maragos, P., Paragios, N. (eds.) ECCV 2010, Part V. LNCS, vol. 6315, pp. 71–84. Springer, Heidelberg (2010)
15. Gordon, A.D.: A review of hierarchical classification. J. Royal Stat. Soc. 150, 119–137 (1987)
16. Mathis, C.: Classification using a hierarchical bayesian approach. In: Proc. of ICPR, vol. 4, pp. 103–106 (2002)
17. Deng, J., Dong, W., Socher, R., Li, L., Li, K., Fei-Fei, L.: ImageNet: a large-scale hierarchical image database. In: CVPR, pp. 248–255 (2009)
18. Freund, Y., Schapire, R.E.: A Decision-Theoretic generalization of on-Line learning and an application to boosting. Computational Learning Theory 904, 23–37 (1995)
19. Nadarajan, G., Chen-Burger, Y., Fisher, R., Spampinato, C.: A flexible system for automated composition of intelligent video analysis. In: Proc. of ISPA, pp. 259–264 (2011)
20. Rother, C., Kolmogorov, V., Blake, A.: GrabCut: interactive foreground extraction using iterated graph cuts. ACM Trans. on Graphics (TOG), 309–314 (2004)
21. He, X.C., Yung, N.H.C.: Curvature scale space corner detector with adaptive threshold and dynamic region of support. In: International Conference on Pattern Recognition, vol. 2, pp. 791–794. IEEE Computer Society (2004)
22. Mokhtarian, F., Suomela, R.: Robust image corner detection through curvature scale space. IEEE Transactions on PAMI 20, 1376–1381 (1998)

# Local 3D Symmetry
# for Visual Saliency in 2.5D Point Clouds

Ekaterina Potapova, Michael Zillich, and Markus Vincze

Automation and Control Institute, Vienna University of Technology

**Abstract.** Many models of visual attention have been proposed in the past, and proved to be very useful, e.g. in robotic applications. Recently it has been shown in the literature that not only single visual features, such as color, orientation, curvature, etc., attract attention, but complete objects do. Symmetry is a feature of many man-made and also natural objects and has thus been identified as a candidate for attentional operators. However, not many techniques exist to date that exploit symmetry-based saliency. So far these techniques work mainly on 2D data. Furthermore, methods, which work on 3D data, assume complete object models. This limits their use as bottom-up attentional operators working on RGBD images, which only provide partial views of objects. In this paper, we present a novel local symmetry-based operator that works on 3D data and does not assume any object model. The estimation of symmetry saliency maps is done on different scales to detect objects of various sizes. For evaluation a Winner-Take-All neural network is used to calculate attention points. We evaluate the proposed approach on two datasets and compare to state-of-the-art methods. Experimental results show that the proposed algorithm outperforms current state-of-the-art in terms of quality of fixation points[1].

## 1 Introduction

Attention has been studied extensively for many years [1–4]. The value of attention, e.g. for robotic applications, has been demonstrated by Aloimonos *et al.* [5]. Many attentional systems concentrate on pre-attentive features, such as color contrast, orientation, curvature, etc. It has been shown, however, that not only single popping out features attract bottom-up attention, but also complete objects do [6, 7].

Symmetry is one of the characteristics of human-made and natural objects, and thus can be seen as an objectness measure. Kootstra *et al.* [8] showed that human eye fixations can be predicted well by symmetry. Many symmetry operators exist [9–13], which can be divided into two major groups: operators working on 2D data, and operators working on 3D data. Among the 2D operators one well-known operator was developed by Reisfeld *et al.* [9] which detects context-free generalized symmetry based on magnitude orientations of image gradients.

---

[1] The research leading to these results has received funding from the Austrian Science Fund (FWF) under project TRP 139-N23 InSitu.

K.M. Lee et al. (Eds.): ACCV 2012, Part I, LNCS 7724, pp. 434–445, 2013.
© Springer-Verlag Berlin Heidelberg 2013

This symmetry operator was extended by Heidemann *et al.* [10] to a local color symmetry operator. Loy and Zelinsky [11] proposed to detect local radial symmetries in an image using a special transform. Kootstra *et al.* [14] proposed a 2D symmetry saliency operator based on the symmetry operator by Reisfeld *et al.* [9]. This saliency operator is able to detect symmetrical regions at different scales. The basic idea is that symmetries are computed over multiple scales and then summed in across-scale addition manner to obtain a master saliency map. Kootstra *et al.* [14] showed that this approach works better than classical contrast model saliency [15]. Mitra *et al.* [16] gave an extensive overview of the existing methods to detect different types of symmetries in 3D geometries. Methods based on search in oriented histograms [17], spectral analysis [12], feature-graph matching [13] and many others were indicated. The majority of 3D algorithms work on a complete 3D model of an object to detect symmetries. This property limits their use as bottom-up attentional operators working on RGBD images, i.e. partial views of objects.

In this paper, we propose a new 3D symmetry-based saliency operator, calculating a measure of context-free local symmetry from a 3D point cloud. The proposed symmetry operator is used to predict fixation points for further attention-driven segmentation or detailed exploration of the scene. We show that a 3D symmetry-based saliency operator reflects the notion of objectness better than the currently existing 2D symmetry-based saliency operator by Kootstra *et al.* [14] and the classical saliency operator by Itti *et al.* [15]. We extensively evaluated both methods on two databases. The first database consists of images showing table scene, and the second one of scenes of complete rooms. Both in quantity and quality of fixations, the proposed algorithm outperforms previous work.

The paper is structured as follows: In Section 2, we describe our proposed 3D symmetry-based saliency operator. Section 3 presents the evaluation results to demonstrate our approach. We compare our methods to Kootstra *et al.* [14] and Itti *et al.* [15]. Section 4 concludes the paper.

## 2   Method

In this section, we describe the method for calculating local symmetries in 3D. The algorithm is based on detecting reflective symmetries using principal axes of Extended Gaussian Images built from patches' normals.

### 2.1   3D Symmetry Model

The 3D reflective symmetry is calculated from a depth image $D$ (Fig. 1). Based on the depth image $D$, we create a point cloud $P$, so that $\forall p\,(r,c) \in P$:

$$p\,(r,c) = (x,y,z) \tag{1}$$

where $(r,c)$ are row-column coordinates in the depth image, $(x,y,z)$ are 3D point coordinates. For each point $p$ a normal $\boldsymbol{n}_p$ is estimated. The normal to a point in the point cloud is estimated as the normal of a plane tangent to the neighboring surface [18].

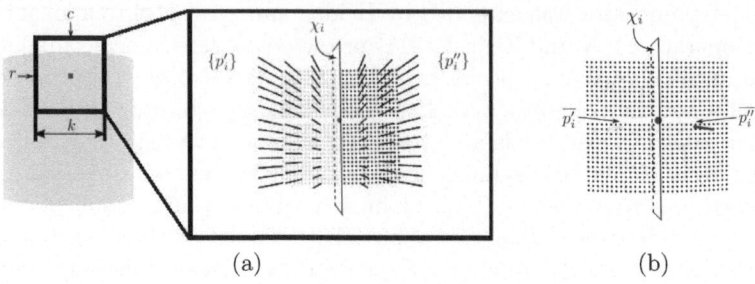

(a) (b)

**Fig. 1.** The depth image of a cylinder (artificial data) is shown on Figure 1(a), with the point $p(r, c)$ for which the symmetry is calculated (highlighted in red), and the kernel $\Phi(p)$ shown as a black square. The subset of points $\{p\} = \Phi(p) \bigcap P$ is shown in 3D on the right side. Subsets $\{p'_i\}$ and $\{p''_i\}$ are shown in yellow and blue respectively, with the reflective plane $\chi_i$ between the two point subsets. Normals $n_p$ are shown as black lines. In Figure 1(b) examples of $\overline{p'_i}, \overline{\mathbf{n'_i}}$ and $\overline{p''_i}, \overline{\mathbf{n''_i}}$ are shown in yellow and blue respectively.

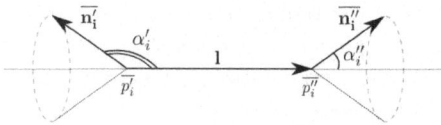

**Fig. 2.** Visual illustration for the calculation of angles $\alpha'_i$ and $\alpha''_i$. l is the line connecting the two mean points $\overline{p'_i}$ and $\overline{p''_i}$. $\alpha'$ is the angle between mean normal $\overline{\mathbf{n'_i}}$ and l, and $\alpha''$ is the angle between mean normal $\overline{\mathbf{n''_i}}$ and l.

$\Phi(p)$ defines the symmetry kernel as a squared patch, centered around $p$ (Fig. 1) with side length $k$. The amount of 3D symmetry at the given location $p(r, c)$ is estimated on the subset of points $\{p\} = \Phi(p) \bigcap P$.

Sun et al. [17] proposed to use an Extended Gaussian Image built from point normals to detect symmetries of a model. Minovic et al. [19] proved that planes of reflective symmetries are perpendicular to the directions of the principal axes. Thus, to detect planes of reflective symmetries from the patch we build an Extended Gaussian Image from the patch's point normals, and calculate the principal axes $\gamma = \{\gamma_1, \gamma_2. \gamma_3\}$ of the Extended Gaussian Image using Principal Component Analysis (PCA). The corresponding symmetry reflective planes $\chi_i$ $(i = 1, 2, 3)$ are defined as planes going through the point $p(r, c)$ with the plane normal equal to the corresponding principal axis $\gamma_i$.

For a given reflective plane $\chi_i$ the point set $\{p\}$ is divided into two subsets $\{p'_i\}$ and $\{p''_i\}$, so that $\forall p \in \{p\}$:

$$p \in \begin{cases} \{p'_i\} & \text{if } d_H(p, \chi_i) > 0 \\ \{p''_i\} & \text{if } d_H(p, \chi_i) < 0 \end{cases} \tag{2}$$

where $d_H(p, \chi_i)$ is the signed Euclidean distance from point $p$ to the plane $\chi_i$ (Fig. 1). The signed Euclidean distance is the distance from the plane according to the Hessian normal form.

The amount of 3D reflective symmetry is relative to a given plane $\chi_i$ for a given subset of points $\{p\}$ and defined as:

$$\Omega_i(\Phi(p)) = \exp(-\triangle D_i) \cdot \exp(-\triangle d_i) \cdot \omega_1 \cdot \omega_2 \tag{3}$$

The multiplication of all four components reflects the fact, that we are searching for patches that are symmetrical in all four aspects (see below).

$\triangle D_i$ represents the difference in depth values between mean points:

$$\triangle D_i = \left| D\left(\overline{p_i'}\right) - D\left(\overline{p_i''}\right) \right| \tag{4}$$

$$\overline{p_i'} = \frac{1}{N'} \sum_{p_j \in \{p_i'\}} p_j \tag{5}$$

$$\overline{p_i''} = \frac{1}{N''} \sum_{p_j \in \{p_i''\}} p_j \tag{6}$$

where $N'$ and $N''$ are numbers of points in the subsets $\{p'\}$ and $\{p''\}$ respectively, and $\overline{p'}$ and $\overline{p''}$ are mean points of the respective subsets. $\triangle D_i$ reflects the fact, that we are only interested in symmetries, that are facing our view point.

$\triangle d_i$ represents the difference in distances from mean points $\overline{p'}$ and $\overline{p''}$ to the reflective plane $\chi_i$:

$$\triangle d_i = \left| d\left(\overline{p_i'}, \chi_i\right) - d\left(\overline{p_i''}, \chi_i\right) \right| \tag{7}$$

where $d(p, \chi_i)$ is the unsigned Euclidean distance from the point $p$ to the plane $\chi_i$. $\triangle d_i$ reflects the fact that we are not only searching for patches with symmetrical orientations, but also for patches that can be divided into two subpatches, which are equally sized and symmetrically positioned in 3D space.

$\omega_1$ is a coefficient measuring the co-planarity between the line $\mathbf{l}$ connecting $\overline{p_i'}$ and $\overline{p_i''}$ and the two mean normals $\overline{\mathbf{n_i'}}$ and $\overline{\mathbf{n_i''}}$ (Fig. 2):

$$\omega_1 = |[\overline{\mathbf{n_i'}} \times \overline{\mathbf{n_i''}}] \times \mathbf{l}| \tag{8}$$

$$\mathbf{l} = \frac{\overline{p_i'} - \overline{p_i''}}{\|\overline{p_i'} - \overline{p_i''}\|} \tag{9}$$

$$\overline{\mathbf{n_i'}} = \frac{\sum_{p_i \in \{p_i'\}} \mathbf{n_{p_i}}}{\|\sum_{p_i \in \{p_i'\}} \mathbf{n_{p_i}}\|} \tag{10}$$

$$\overline{\mathbf{n_i''}} = \frac{\sum_{p_i \in \{p_i''\}} \mathbf{n_{p_i}}}{\|\sum_{p_i \in \{p_i''\}} \mathbf{n_{p_i}}\|} \tag{11}$$

where $\overline{p'_i}$ and $\overline{p''_i}$ are mean points of the subsets $\{p'_i\}$ and $\{p''_i\}$ respectively, and $\overline{\mathbf{n}'}$ and $\overline{\mathbf{n}''}$ are mean normals.

$\omega_2$ shows the similarity between mean normal directions based on the symmetry operator from Reisfeld *et al.* [9] and is calculated as following (Fig. 2):

$$\omega_2 = (1 - \cos(\alpha' + \alpha'')) \cdot (1 - \cos(\alpha' - \alpha'')) \tag{12}$$

where $\alpha'$ is the angle between mean normal $\overline{\mathbf{n}'_i}$ and $\mathbf{l}$, and $\alpha''$ is the angle between mean normal $\overline{\mathbf{n}''_i}$ and $\mathbf{l}$. Basically this operator gives the largest value to regions, where normals are oriented completely opposite and the smallest value to regions, where normals have the same orientation (i.e. flat surfaces).

Ideally the factors $\triangle D_i$, $\omega_2$ and $\omega_2$ should be calculated on each pair of opposite points and then summed up after multiplication. Due to small errors in the calculation of normals this approach is not very robust. Moreover, it is computationally expensive. Using only the mean points and normals to represent subpatches is a common approximation which proved to be accurate enough for our computations.

The amount of 3D symmetry $s(x, y)$ at a given pixel $p(r, c)$ is equal to:

$$s(r, c) = \begin{cases} 0 & \text{if } D(r, c) = 0 \\ \max_{i=1,2,3}\{\Omega_i\left(\Phi\left(p\left(r, c\right)\right)\right)\} & \text{if } D(r, c) > 0 \end{cases} \tag{13}$$

where $D(r, c) = 0$ means that no depth information is available at this point.

Due to the nature of the 3D symmetry operator convex and concave regions will obtain the same symmetry values. While in everyday scenarios the majority of objects, that are claimed to be symmetric by humans, are rarely concave. To eliminate concave regions the following equation is applied:

$$s(r, c) = \begin{cases} 0 & \text{if } (\alpha' > \pi/2 \text{ and } \alpha'' < \pi/2) \text{ or } (\alpha' < \pi/2 \text{ and } \alpha'' > \pi/2) \\ s(r, c) & \text{otherwise} \end{cases} \tag{14}$$

## 2.2   Multi-scale Symmetry-Based Saliency Map

To calculate a multi-scale symmetry-based saliency map a Gaussian pyramid of depth images is created. For each depth map the respective point cloud is calculated. 3D based symmetry maps $s_l$ are calculated on every scale $l$ of the pyramid. This results in a pyramid of symmetry maps. A master saliency map $S$ is obtained by across scale addition [15] of the symmetry pyramid:

$$S(r, c) = \bigoplus_{l=L_1}^{L_2} s_l(r, c) \tag{15}$$

where $L_1$ is the finest scale and $L_2$ is the coarsest scale. The calculation on different scales allows to detect symmetries of different sizes in a computationally effective manner.

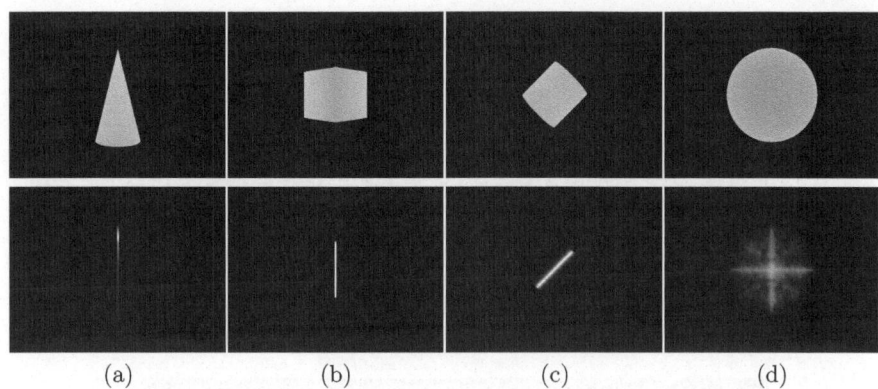

(a)                    (b)                    (c)                    (d)

**Fig. 3.** Examples of symmetry maps calculated on artificial data. In the first row artificially created depth images of a cone, a rotated cube, a rotated cylinder and a sphere are shown in columns (a), (b), (c), (d) respectively. The second row shows the corresponding 3D symmetry-based maps calculated using only one scale $l = 0$ and kernel size $k = 30$.

### 2.3 Attention Points

The multi-scale symmetry-based saliency map $S$ is used as input to the Winner-Take-All (WTA) neural network [20] to calculate attention points. Attention points can be used as seed points for attention-driven segmentation [21] or as fixations for further investigation of the region like zooming in or foveation. This approach for scene investigation is highly useful in such applications as robot navigation, robot localization and object detection. It can significantly reduce the search space and automatically point to interesting objects or areas, without exhaustive and computationally expensive exploration of the whole scene.

## 3 Evaluation

The quality of symmetry-based saliency maps was evaluated on artificial data, as well as on real data. Usually saliency operators are evaluated by comparing saliency results with eye-tracking data. This approach is useful when the task on hand is to build a system that tries to explain the human visual attention system. Since our task is to build an attention system that can be useful in robotic tasks, we chose a different approach for evaluation.

Our evaluation consists of several parts. At first, we evaluated the quality of attention points by detecting how many different objects were covered by the attention system with a given number of fixations, the so-called Hit Ratio (HR). Secondly, because our algorithm depends on the size of the kernel, we evaluate the variance of the fixation results under different kernel sizes.

Our experiments were done against the 2D symmetry saliency operator proposed by Kootstra et al. [14] and against the orientation-contrast saliency operator proposed by Itti et al. [15].

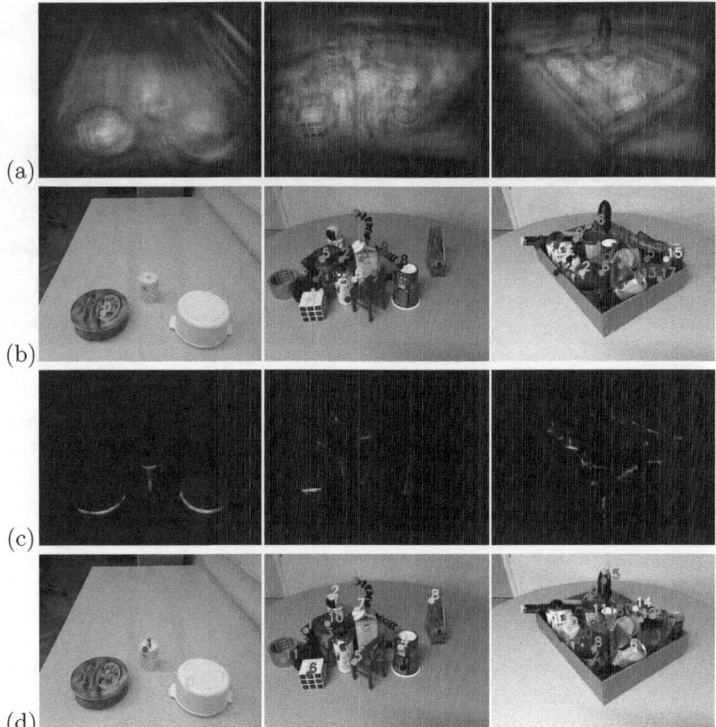

**Fig. 4.** Examples of images from the Table Objects Scene Database (TOSD) from Vienna University of Technology. Row (a) shows examples of 2D symmetry-based maps [14] overlaid with original images. Respective attention points calculated from 2D symmetry-based maps using WTA are shown in row (b). 2D symmetry-based maps were calculated on scales $l = 1..5$ using an external kernel $k_1 = 11$ and an internal kernel $k_2 = 5$ (for detailed parameters explanation see [14]). Row (c) shows 3D symmetry-based maps calculated using the proposed method and overlaid with original images. Respective attention points are shown in row (d). 3D symmetry-based maps were calculated on scales $l = 0..4$ using kernel $k = 15$.

## 3.1   Evaluation on Artificial Data

To prove that our 3D symmetry operator is performing as expected, we have tested it on artificially created data. Artificially created data was produced from rendering mathematical models of different objects with known shape (i.e. cylinders, cubes, spheres, cones). Results of symmetry operators are shown in Fig. 3.

From the presented results it is clearly visible that the proposed method works perfectly for synthetic examples. However, the result for the sphere (Fig. 3, (d)) visually does not look perfect, due to artifacts of the visualization process. Symmetry values for the sphere are quite small (note that, as explained in Section 2.1, surface patches, that are rather flat locally, result in small values of $\omega_2$). For visualization in Fig. 3 values were normalized to a visible range, which in this case led to an amplification of small errors from the normal calculation step.

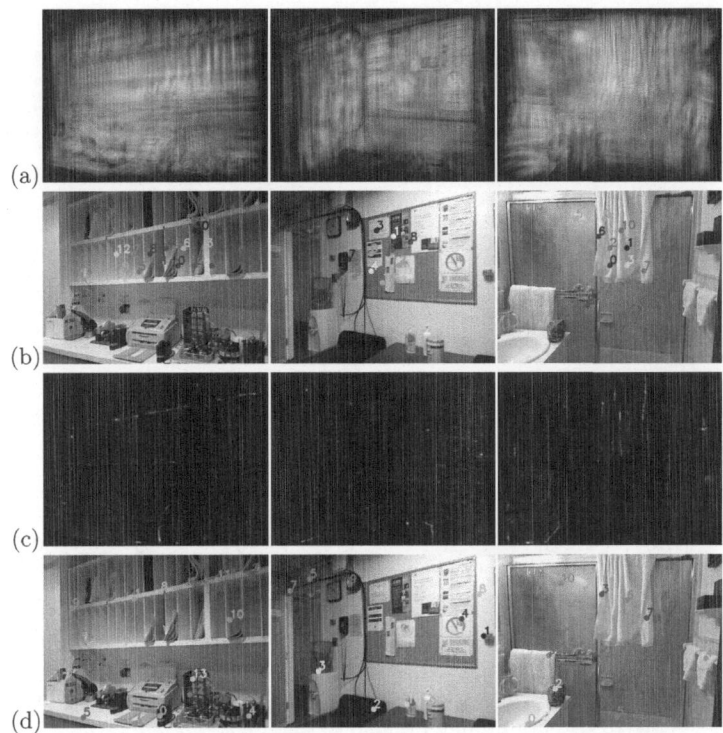

**Fig. 5.** Examples of images from the New York University Depth Database (NYUDD). Row (a) shows 2D symmetry-based maps [14] overlaid with original images. Respective attention points calculated from 2D symmetry-based maps using WTA are shown in row (b). 2D symmetry-based maps were calculated on scales $l = 1..5$ using an external kernel $k_1 = 11$ and an internal kernel $k_2 = 5$ (for detailed parameters explanation see [14]). Row (c) shows 3D symmetry-based maps calculated using the proposed method and overlaid with original images. Respective attention points are shown in row (d). 3D symmetry-based maps were calculated on scales $l = 0..4$ using kernel $k = 15$.

## 3.2 Evaluation on Real Data

Symmetry-based saliency maps were evaluated on two RGB-D databases. The first database is the Table Object Scene Database (TOSD) from Vienna University of Technology[2]. The database consists of 244 different table scenes including free-standing objects, multiple occluded objects and piles of objects. All objects in the TOSD were hand-labeled with outlining polygons. Examples of images from the database and respective saliency maps are shown in Fig. 4.

The second database on which we evaluated our results was the New York University Depth Dataset (NYUDD)[3] which consists of more than 1000 densely labeled images of more that 400 different indoor scenes (Fig. 5).

---

[2] https://repo.acin.tuwien.ac.at/tmp/permanent/TOSD.zip

[3] http://cs.nyu.edu/ silberman/datasets/nyu_depth_v2.html

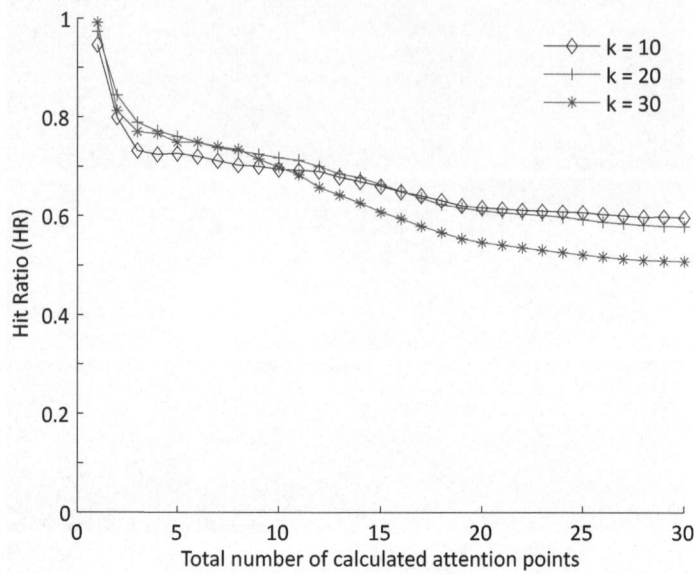

**Fig. 6.** Hit Ratio (HR) against the total number of calculated attention points for kernel sizes $k = 10$, $k = 20$, $k = 30$. As can be seen from the plot the kernel size does not have a big influence on the performance of the proposed algorithm when the total number of calculated attention points is smaller than 30.

From symmetry-based saliency maps attention points were calculated using the Winner-Take-All neural network. Attention points are evaluated with respect to the Hit Ratio (HR).

The Hit Ratio (HR) shows the percentage of unique attention points being situated inside different objects:

$$HR = \frac{n}{N} \tag{16}$$

where $N$ is the total number of calculated attention points and $n$ is the number of different attended objects. A perfect attention mechanism will hit every object exactly once, resulting in a HR equal to one.

### 3.3 Choosing the Size of the Kernel

Our algorithm depends on exactly one settable parameter - the kernel size $k$. We have evaluated the performance of the proposed method with different kernel sizes ($k = 10$, $k = 20$ and $k = 30$) on the TOSD. Results are shown on Fig. 6. As can be seen from the plot the size of the kernel does not influence the performance much, when the number of calculated attention points is smaller than 10. This result is expected, because symmetry maps are calculated on different scales. This allows to detect symmetrical objects of different sizes regardless of the kernel size. However, with the kernel size $k = 30$ the performance drops significantly

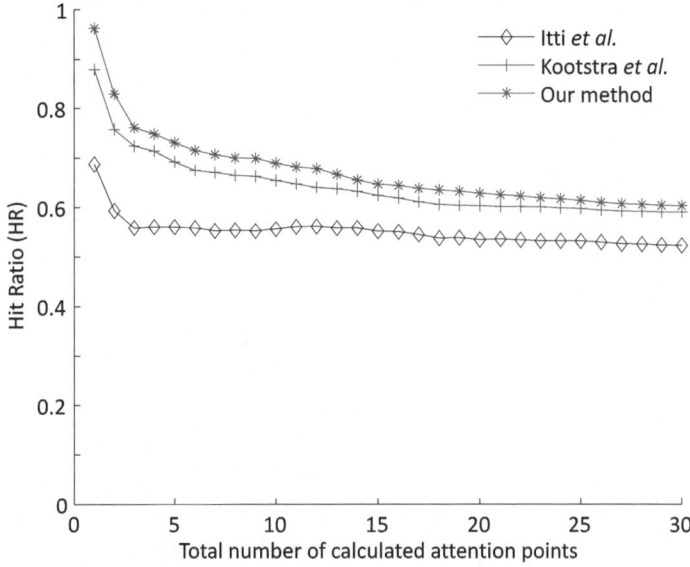

**Fig. 7.** Comparison plot of the Hit Ratio (HR) against the total number of calculated attention points for the Table Objects Scene Database (TOSD) for different types of saliency maps: the orientation-contrast model [15], the 2D symmetry-based model [14] and our proposed 3D symmetry-based model

after around 10 attention points. This is easily explained, due to the fact that typical sizes of objects in the TOSD are smaller than 50 pixels. It means that after all relatively big objects were detected in cluttered scenes, smaller objects were ignored. These results suggests that smaller kernels are to be preferred (a value of 15 was chosen in subsequent experiments). And the detection of larger objects can then be done on coarser scales.

### 3.4   Evaluation on the Databases

Fig. 7 and Fig. 8 show comparison plots of the HR against the total number of calculated attention points for the TOSD and for the NYUDD respectively. As can be seen from the plot the use of 3D symmetry-based saliency maps improves the quality of attention points up to 10% starting from the first fixation. An interesting observation can be made from the plots. An improvement for the NYUDD is more noticeable than for the TOSD. While for the TOSD the average HR is higher. Explanations to these effects lie in the types of scenes. The TOSD consists of crowded table scenes, while the NYUDD presents room scenes. The probability to hit any object in the TOSD just by selecting a random point is much higher than in the NYUDD. It also means that a perfect saliency operator for TOSD should take much more complicated information into account, than only early vision processes, e.g. early segmentation.

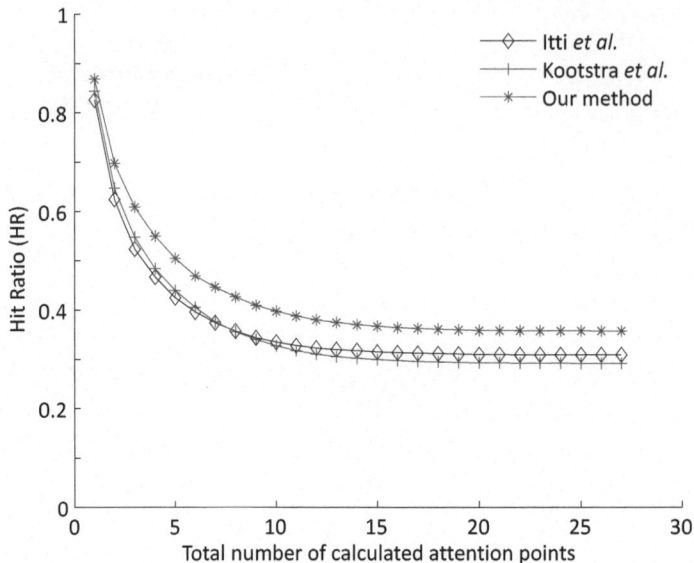

**Fig. 8.** Comparison plot of the Hit Ratio (HR) against the total number of calculated attention points for the New York University Depth Dataset (NYUDD) for different types of saliency maps: the orientation-contrast model [15], the 2D based symmetry map [14] and our proposed method

## 4   Conclusion

In the presented paper, we discussed a new algorithm for calculating a 3D symmetry-based saliency map. The proposed algorithm is based on finding local reflective symmetries using Extended Gaussian Images and normal direction dissimilarities. From these saliency maps attention points using a Winner-Take-All neural network were extracted. The quality of attention points was evaluated on two databases (the TOSD and the NYUDD) against the Hit Ratio. Result were compared to two saliency methods: the orientation-contrast method [15] and the 2D symmetry-based method [14]. We showed that the proposed algorithm works better in terms of Hit Ratio (HR). Future work will concentrate on finding a way to combine both 2D and 3D symmetry models to gain better results on a variety of different types of scenes.

## References

1. Treisman, A.M., Gelade, G.: A feature-integration theory of attention. Cognitive Psychology 12, 97–136 (1980)
2. Koch, C., Ullman, S.: Shifts in selective visual attention: Towards the underlying neural circuitry. Human Neurobiology 4, 219–227 (1985)
3. Wolfe, J.M., Cave, K.R., Franzel, S.L.: Guided search: An alternative to the feature integration model for visual search. Journal of Experimental Psychology: Human Perception & Performance 15, 419–433 (1989)

4. Tsotsos, J.: Analyzing vision at the complexity level. Behavioral and Brain Sciences 13, 423–469 (1990)
5. Aloimonos, J., Weiss, I., Bandyopadhyay, A.: Active vision. International Journal of Computer Vision 1, 333–356 (1988)
6. Einhauser, W., Spain, M., Perona, P.: Objects predict fixations better than early saliency. Journal of Vision 8, 1–26 (2008)
7. Scholl, B.J.: Objects and attention: the state of the art. Cognition 80, 1–46 (2001)
8. Kootstra, G., Nederveen, A., Boer, B.d.: Paying attention to symmetry. In: Proc. of the British Machine Vision Conference, pp. 1115–1125. BMVA Press (2008)
9. Reisfeld, D., Wolfson, H., Yeshurun, Y.: Context free attentional operators: the generalized symmetry transform. International Journal of Computer Vision 14, 119–130 (1995)
10. Heidemann, G.: Focus-of-attention from local color symmetries. IEEE Trans. on Pattern Analysis and Machine Intelligence (2004)
11. Loy, G., Zelinsky, A.: Fast radial symmetry for detecting points of interest. IEEE Trans. on Pattern Analysis and Machine Intelligence 25, 959–973 (2003)
12. Chertok, M., Keller, Y.: Spectral symmetry analysis. IEEE Trans. on Pattern Analysis and Machine Intelligence 32, 1227–1238 (2010)
13. Berner, A., Wand, M., Mitra, N.J., Mewes, D., Seidel, H.P.: Shape analysis with subspace symmetries. Computer Graphics Forum 30, 277–286 (2011)
14. Kootstra, G., Bergstroem, N., Kragic, D.: Using symmetry to select fixation points for segmentation. In: Proc. of 20th International Conference on Pattern Recognition, pp. 3894–3897 (2010)
15. Itti, L., Koch, C., Niebur, E.: A model of saliency-based visual attention for rapid scene analysis. IEEE Trans. on Pattern Analysis and Machine Intelligence 20, 1254–1259 (1998)
16. Mitra, N.J., Pauly, M., Wand, M., Ceylan, D.: Symmetry in 3d geometry: Extraction and applications. In: Eurographics State-of-the-art Report (2012)
17. Sun, C., Sherrah, J.: 3d symmetry detection using the extended gaussian image. IEEE Trans. on Pattern Analysis and Machine Intelligence 19, 164–168 (1997)
18. Rusu, R.B.: Semantic 3D Object Maps for Everyday Manipulation in Human Living Environments. PhD thesis, Computer Science department, Technische Universitaet Muenchen, Germany (2009)
19. Minovic, P., Ishikawa, S., Kato, K.: Symmetry identification of a 3-d object represented by octree. IEEE Trans. on Pattern Analysis and Machine Intelligence 15, 507–514 (1993)
20. Lee, D.K., Itti, L., Koch, C., Braun, J.: Attention activates winner-take-all competition among visual filters. Nature Neuroscience 2, 375–381 (1999)
21. Mishra, A.K., Aloimonos, Y.: Visual segmentation of simple objects for robots. In: Robotics: Science and Systems (2011)

# Exploiting Features – Locally Interleaved Sequential Alignment for Object Detection

Karel Zimmermann, David Hurych, and Tomáš Svoboda

Czech Technical University, Faculty of Electrical Engineering,
Department of Cybernetics, Center for Machine Perception, Karlovo Náměstí 13,
Prague, 121-35, Czech Republic

**Abstract.** We exploit image features multiple times in order to make
sequential decision process faster and better performing. In the decision process features providing knowledge about the object presence
or absence in a given detection window are successively evaluated. We
show that these features also provide information about object position
within the evaluated window. The classification process is sequentially
interleaved with estimating the correct position. The position estimate
is used for steering the features yet to be evaluated. This locally interleaved sequential alignment (LISA) allows to run an object detector
on sparser grid which speeds up the process. The position alignment
is jointly learned with the detector. We achieve a better detection rate
since the method allows for training the detector on perfectly aligned
image samples. For estimation of the alignment we propose a learnable
regressor that approximates a non-linear regression function and runs in
negligible time.

## 1 Introduction

Image features coupled with an appropriate learning and classification scheme
have proved to be widely applicable [1, 2]. Richer features and SVM based classifiers have reached impressive results in object recognition [3–7]. However,
richer features and classifiers are more costly. Applying them in a sliding window scheme can be prohibive in realtime applications. The problem is addressed
in [8] where a branch and bound approach is proposed finding the correct position of the search window. The search starts from a larger window is branched in
one dimension and bounded by a quality function learned on rich features, typically bag of visual words. Kokkinos [9] combines branch and bound technique [8]
with deformable part models [3]. He adapts the dual trees data structure for the
branch and bound, which prioritizes the search of promising image area and ignores the rest. Thanks to that he achieves exactly the same results as with [3],
but on average 10 times faster. Still, the combined approach needs few seconds
for decent images.

We propose an alternative approach. Our motivation is a real-time detection
of relatively small objects in large images. Very simple features are employed. We
show that features which are used for the object detection contain also knowledge

K.M. Lee et al. (Eds.): ACCV 2012, Part I, LNCS 7724, pp. 446–459, 2013.
© Springer-Verlag Berlin Heidelberg 2013

about the accurate object position in its local neighbourhood – *alignment*. We embody the alignment estimation into the object detection process in the way which does not increase the computational complexity. The detector and alignment are learned jointly. Experiments show a significant improvement, especially when detection time is constrained. As far as we know, no previous work shows that alignment can be estimated completely free of charge during the detection process.

We demonstrate this idea on a Sequential Decision Process (SDP) similar to Waldboost [10]. In a SDP, features are successively evaluated and a classifier cumulatively estimates *confidence* about the object presence in a given detection window. After each feature, the confidence is updated by a value from a hash table indexed by feature values. Once the confidence is sufficiently low the window is rejected and the process continues on the following window. We extend a SDP by exploiting the same features used for the confidence estimation to estimate local object *alignment* (e.g. position or scale) within the evaluated window. Whenever the accumulated knowledge about the alignment is sufficiently accurate the alignment is applied and the process continues on aligned coordinates. From now on, both the confidence and the alignment are estimated more efficiently, since it is easier to distinguish well aligned positive samples from the background or to estimate the alignment from a closer neighborhood. This process continues until the rejection or acceptance is reached as in the classical SDP. Note that since the alignment is estimated from the same features as the SDP, the per feature running time is preserved, because alignment updates are obtained from the same hash table (and the same column) as the confidence updates. We call this extension Sequential Decision Process with *Local Interleaved Sequential Alignment* (SDP with *LISA*).

Despite their tremendous efficiency of simple features the whole detection process does not allow exhaustive search when applied on large images and small objects. The detector is applied on a subset of possible positions and scales and trained on artificially perturbed positive data. This widens the visual classes even more. One approach is to break the positive class into small visually compact sub-classes which are easy to distinguish. If each sub-class is detected by an independently trained detector, then the running time also grows exponentially with the dimension of the detection grid. To decrease the running time, decision trees have been introduced. Since decision trees eventually break the training set into small subsets, large training sets are often needed. We may consider the alignment, computed by a regression function from a single feature in the SDP, to be an embranchment, which influences positions of the successively evaluated features. In this sense it corresponds to a special type of a huge but finite decision tree[1] for a discrete regression function or even infinite tree for a continuous regression function, the learning of which is intractable. In contrast to decision trees, we eventually do not break the training set into small subsets, therefore the learning is well-posed even for reasonably small training sets. Space does not allow for a full review; we refer the reader to Huang et al. [2] for a more detailed discussion.

---

[1] For example if a quantized regression function assigns 20 possible values to each feature, then after evaluating 200 features the decision tree has $1.6^{260}$ leaves.

Recently, Ali et al. [11] propose to estimate rotations of some features (as the dominant gradient direction) before the detection takes place. Here the rotation of the feature corresponds to the one dimensional alignment space. In their approach the alignment space for each feature is exhaustively searched. Hence, the running time also grows almost exponentially with the alignment space dimensionality.

In contrast to this, we interleave object detection and alignment regression. Since the regression functions successively estimate alignment of the currently evaluated window, the detector runs on increasingly good aligned features. Since we re-use detection features for the regression, almost no additional computations are needed and the running time does not grow with the dimension of the alignment space.

The use of sequence of linear predictors (regressors) for alignment estimation was proposed in [12]. They proposed a method for learning of the optimal sequence of predictors for particular object. The learning process is explicitly minimizing the computational complexity of alignment estimation for user defined alignment precision. In comparison we propose to learn multiple sequences of piecewise linear regressors, which approximate a non-linear regression functions.

The paper [13] proposes a similar idea to [12]. They propose to learn a fixed sequence of weak regressors, where each regressor is a random fern. Sequence of random ferns forms a non-linear estimator, which requires a large amount of data for training (depending on the depth of each fern). Similarly to us, the authors in [13] generate artificially perturbed image samples to obtain the necessary amount of training data.

## 2   SDP with LISA Classification

We divide the classification process into $K$ stages where both the confidence and the alignment are cumulatively estimated from individual features. In each stage $k$, we have a detection function $d_k : \mathbb{R} \to \mathbb{R}$ which assigns a real-valued contribution to the confidence coming from the feature value, and a regression function $r_k : \mathbb{R} \to \mathbb{R}^2$ which assigns a two dimensional contribution to the alignment coming from the same feature value. Then there is a threshold $\theta_k \in \mathbb{R}$ (estimated during the learning), which allows to reject windows with the so far accumulated confidence lower than $\theta_k$. It is not desirable to apply accumulated alignment after each feature because not every single feature has the discriminative power for good quality displacement estimation in both the training and validation data. Yet the same feature in combination with other features is useful.

Therefore, we also introduce a binary value: $z_k = \mathtt{TRUE}$ means that the accumulated alignment is applied on feature $k+1$, while $z_k = \mathtt{FALSE}$, means that the alignment is accumulated, but not immediately applied on the following feature. Since we need to apply the alignment on some features, we define a feature function $f_k : \mathbb{R}^n \times \mathbb{R}^2 \to \mathbb{R}$ as a mapping which assigns a feature value to a window with image data $I \in \mathbb{R}^n$, with $n$ pixels and an alignment $\mathbf{a} \in \mathbb{R}^2$. For the sake of

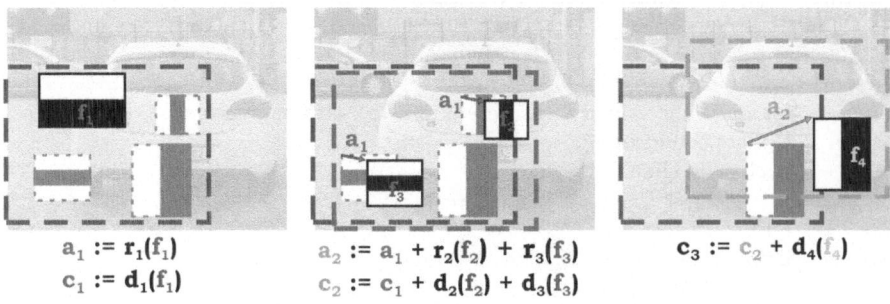

$$\mathbf{a}_1 := \mathbf{r}_1(f_1)$$
$$c_1 := \mathbf{d}_1(f_1)$$

$$\mathbf{a}_2 := \mathbf{a}_1 + \mathbf{r}_2(f_2) + \mathbf{r}_3(f_3)$$
$$c_2 := c_1 + \mathbf{d}_2(f_2) + \mathbf{d}_3(f_3)$$

$$c_3 := c_2 + \mathbf{d}_4(f_4)$$

**Fig. 1. Classification:** Three steps of SDP with LISA are depicted. Left image shows initial position of the sliding window with all features. In the initial position, only the feature 1 is evaluated and from its value the first alignment $\mathbf{a}_1$ and confidence $c_1$ are computed. In the middle image the alignment $\mathbf{a}_1$ is applied on features 2 and 3. Note, that the applied alignment $\mathbf{a}_2$ is updated by contribution of two regressors, not just one. Also note, that the alignment $\mathbf{a}_1$ was not applied on feature 4. In the right image the last feature is moved from its initial position by accumulated alignment $\mathbf{a}_2$.

simplicity, we refer to the feature function as to the *feature* and to image data in the window as to the *window*. Each feature is selected from a feature pool $\mathcal{F}$. Based on the above introduced notation, we define the strong classifier as a sequence:

$$H = [f_1, d_1, \theta_1, r_1, z_1, \ldots, f_k, d_k, \theta_k, r_k, z_k, \ldots, f_K, d_K, \theta_K]. \tag{1}$$

Algorithm 1 summarizes how the SDP with LISA decides about object presence or absence in a given window $I$ with the given strong classifier $H$. See also Figure 1 In the algorithm, we denote $c_k$ as the confidence and $\mathbf{a}_k$ as the alignment, both accumulated up to the stage $k$. Especially, $\mathbf{a}$ refers to the alignment which is applied on currently evaluated features. Note, that there are two alignments: (i) accumulated up to stage $k$ denoted by $\mathbf{a}_k$ and (ii) applied $\mathbf{a}$, which is not up-to-date by purpose.

## 3   SDP with LISA Joint Learning

The expected output from the learning is the strong classifier $H$, Eq. (1). Inputs to the learning process are *training* and *validation* sets. In the beginning of each training stage, the training set with the following structure is available:

$$\mathcal{T} = \{I^1, \mathbf{t}^1, \ldots, I^p, \mathbf{t}^p, I^{p+1} \ldots I^N, y^1 \ldots y^N\},$$

where $I^1, \ldots, I^p$ are positive image data, $I^{p+1}, \ldots, I^N$ are negative image data, $y^1 \ldots y^N$ are labels and $\mathbf{t}^1 \ldots \mathbf{t}^p$ are correct alignments of artificially perturbed positive data. The validation set $\mathcal{V}$ has a similar structure.

For the sake of simplicity, we introduce $[[\Psi]]$ to be a binary function equal to 1 if a statement $\Psi$ is TRUE and 0 otherwise, and $[h_1\ h_2\ \ldots\ h_k]$ to be the

---

**Algorithm 1.** Classification of a single window by SDP with LISA

---
1: Initialize $\mathbf{a} = \mathbf{0}, \mathbf{a}_0 = \mathbf{0}, c_0 = 0, k = 1$.
2: **while** $k \leq K$ **do**
3:       Estimate the value of feature $v = f_k(I, \mathbf{a})$ with alignment $\mathbf{a}$.
4:       Update confidence $c_k \leftarrow c_{k-1} + d_k(v)$.
5:       **if** $c_k < \theta_k$ **then**
6:             reject the window and break,
7:       **end if**
8:       Estimate alignment $\mathbf{a}_k = \mathbf{a}_{k-1} + r_k(v)$.
9:       **if** $z_k = \text{TRUE}$ **then**
10:             update the applied alignment $\mathbf{a} \leftarrow \mathbf{a}_k$
11:       **end if**
12:       $k \leftarrow k + 1$
13: **end while**

---

concatenation of sequences $h_1, \ldots, h_k$. We also introduce the error $E(H, \mathcal{V}) = \sum_i [[H(I_i) \neq y_i]]$ of the strong classifier $H$ on validation data $\mathcal{V}$. For the sake of completeness we define: $E(\emptyset, \mathcal{V}) = \infty$.

The joint SDP and LISA learning, see Algorithm 2, successively builds a strong classifier $H$. Current stage is denoted by lower index $k$, training samples are indexed by upper index $i$. Since we do not know in advance whether to use the *accumulated alignment* or the *applied alignment* in the current stage, we keep two strong classifiers which differ only by the used alignment in the last stage. We denote $H_k$ the strong classifier which applies the *applied alignment* $\mathbf{a}^i$ in the beginning of stage $k$, and $\widehat{H}_k$ as the strong classifier which applies the *accumulated alignment* $\mathbf{a}^i_{k-1}$ in the beginning of stage $k$. In the beginning, the strong classifier is empty and both accumulated $\mathbf{a}^i_0$ and applied $\mathbf{a}^i$ alignments are zero. Then features $f_k, \widehat{f}_k$ and corresponding weak classifiers $d_k, \widehat{d}_k$, minimizing weighted training error are found. The learning of the weak classifiers will be explained later in section 5. Symbols $f_k, d_k$ denote the feature and the weak classifier estimated for the case where the used alignment is $\mathbf{a}^i$. Similarly $\widehat{f}_k, \widehat{d}_k$ denote feature and weak classifier found for the case where used alignment is the $\mathbf{a}^i_{k-1}$. Rejection thresholds $\theta_k$ and $\widehat{\theta}_k$ are set in order to preserve the required maximum number of false negatives FN per learning stage. The FN limit is defined by user to achieve the required running time similarly to [14]. In lines 8-12, validation errors of both strong classifiers are compared, and the one with the lower error is selected (denoted $H_k$). Training weights are updated in line 15. Finally the training data $\mathcal{T}$ are updated (line: 16) by the new negative samples which are collected as false positives (FP) of the current strong classifier $H_k$. The algorithm continues until the validation error starts to increase.

## 4    Regression Functions for Alignment

As already noted in section 2, the use of a regressor which was learned on just one feature over the training samples may not be profitable and may increase

**Algorithm 2.** Learning of SDP with LISA

1: input: $\mathcal{T}, \mathcal{V}, \mathcal{F}$

2: $r_{\emptyset} = \emptyset, k = 1, g = 1, \gamma = 1, \mathbf{a}^i = \mathbf{0}, \mathbf{a}_0^i = \mathbf{0}, w^i = 1/N, i = 1, \ldots, N.$

3: **while** $E(H_k, \mathcal{V}) \leq E(H_{k-1}, \mathcal{V})$ **do**

    *//Find features, weak classifiers and thresholds with different alignments*

4:    $[f_k d_k \theta_k] \leftarrow$ *learn_weak_cls*$(\mathcal{T}, \mathcal{V}, \mathcal{F}, \mathbf{a}^i)$

5:    $[\widehat{f}_k \widehat{d}_k \widehat{\theta}_k] \leftarrow$ *learn_weak_cls*$(\mathcal{T}, \mathcal{V}, \mathcal{F}, \mathbf{a}_{k-1}^i)$

    *//Create strong classifiers $H_k, \widehat{H}_k$*

6:    $H_k = \Big[ H_{\gamma-1} \, [z_\gamma \ f_\gamma \ d_\gamma \ \theta_\gamma \ r_\gamma] \ldots$
    $\ldots [z_{k-1} \ f_{k-1} \ d_{k-1} \ \theta_{k-1} \ r_{k-1}] [\text{FALSE} \ f_k \ d_k \ \theta_k] \Big]$

7:    $\widehat{H}_k = \Big[ H_{\gamma-1} \, [z_\gamma \ f_\gamma \ d_\gamma \ \theta_\gamma \ r_\gamma] \ldots$
    $\ldots [z_{k-1} \ f_{k-1} \ d_{k-1} \ \theta_{k-1} \ r_{k-1}] [\text{TRUE} \ \widehat{f}_k \ \widehat{d}_k \ \widehat{\theta}_k] \Big]$

    *//Comparison of validation errors decides, whether the applied alignment*
    *//will be updated in learning and as well as during the classification*

8:    **if** $E(H_k, \mathcal{V}) \geq E(\widehat{H}_k, \mathcal{V})$ **then**

    *//Replace $H_k$ by $\widehat{H}_k$*

9:    $H_k \leftarrow \widehat{H}_k$

10:   $\gamma \leftarrow k$

    *//Update the applied alignment*

11:   $\mathbf{a}^i \leftarrow \mathbf{a}_{k-1}^i, i = 1 \ldots p$

12:   **end if**

    *//Jointly learn a group of regressors on last few features*

13:   $\{r_\gamma, \ldots, r_k\} \leftarrow$ *learn_regressors*$(f_\gamma, \ldots, f_k)$

    *//Update accumulated alignment*

14:   $\mathbf{a}_k^i = \mathbf{a}^i + r_\gamma(f_\gamma(I^i, \mathbf{a}^i)) + \ldots + r_k(f_k(I^i, \mathbf{a}^i)),$
    $i = 1, \ldots, N$

    *//Update weights of training samples*

15:   $w^i = \exp(-y^i \cdot H_k(I^i)), i = 1, \ldots, N$

    *//Collect new negative samples as FPs of H and update $\mathcal{T}$*

16:   **update:** $\mathcal{T}$

17:   $k \leftarrow k + 1$

18: **end while**

Split the current classifier into two classifiers $H_k$ $\widehat{H}_k$

Select features and weak classifiers for:

$H_k$ which will keep on using the old alignment

$\widehat{H}_k$ which will apply up-to-date alignment

Compare validation errors of both classifiers and choose the better one

Train regressors which minimize residual alignment error

Update data and classifier

the validation error. The learning waits for the right number of features, gathered from the stage of last applied alignment update (line 11 of Algorithm 2), for which the jointly learned regressors yield better alignment and lower the validation error of the detector.

Hence the regressors $r_k$ are not learned separately for each feature $k$, but jointly over more features (line 13 of Algorithm 2). We denote the set of successive features for which we will jointly learn the group of regressors by $S \subset \mathcal{F}$, and a set of indexes $J = \{k|f_k \in S\}$. Regressors are learned to lower the alignment error $(\mathbf{t}^i - \mathbf{a}^i)$ of preceding regressors. Formally,

$$\arg\min_{r_j, \forall j \in J} \sum_{i=1}^{p} \left\| \sum_{\forall j \in J} \left( r_j(f_j(I^i, \mathbf{a}^i)) \right) - (\mathbf{t}^i - \mathbf{a}^i) \right\|_F^2, \tag{2}$$

where $\mathbf{t}^i$ is the correct alignment and $\mathbf{a}^i$ is the accumulated alignment estimated by preceding regressors.

A non-linear regression usually yields higher precision than a linear one. Yet we need to keep the low computational complexity. We propose to approximate a non-linear regression function by partitioning of each feature's space (dividing the feature space into $U$ bins), where into each bin of each feature we fit a linear function. Each regressor $r_j$ is in fact a set of coefficients of several linear functions – one function for each feature bin. We test three types of linear functions, where each feature's $f_j$ contribution to estimation of the displacement parameter $t_j^i$ in one bin $u$ is computed as follows

$$t_j^i = \lambda_{ju} f_j \left( I^i, \mathbf{a}^i \right), \tag{3}$$

$$t_j^i = \lambda_{ju} f_j \left( I^i, \mathbf{a}^i \right) + \omega_{ju}, \tag{4}$$

$$t_j^i = \omega_{ju}. \tag{5}$$

Two types of feature space partitionings were tested. Non-proportional one divides the space into bins of equal sizes and the proportional one divides the space into bins of sizes proportional to the training data density. Each bin contains the same number of training samples. See Figure 2 for example of partitioning into 7 bins with all three tested functions fitted into the training data of one feature.

The optimal coefficients of group of regressors solving (2) are estimated by a least squares method. Let us denote $\mathrm{L} = \left[ \mathbf{l}^1 \mathbf{l}^2 \ldots \mathbf{l}^p \right]$ as the matrix of training samples, where each vector $\mathbf{l}^i$ contains values of features $f_j, \forall j \in J$ of training sample $i$ and columnwise matrix $\mathrm{T} = \left[ \mathbf{t}^1 - \mathbf{a}^1 \ \mathbf{t}^2 - \mathbf{a}^2 \ \ldots \ \mathbf{t}^p - \mathbf{a}^p \right]$ with the ground truth displacement parameters. Than the least squares solution of (2) may be written in a compact form $\mathrm{TL}^+$, where $^+$ denotes the Moore-Penrose pseudo-inverse [15] of a matrix. The same equation is used for learning of all three types of tested piecewise linear functions with any number of bins. The only difference is in the composition of vectors of training samples $\mathbf{l}^i$ in the training matrix $\mathrm{L}$. Normally each row of matrix $\mathrm{L}$ corresponds to values of a single feature over all training examples. We extend the number of rows corresponding

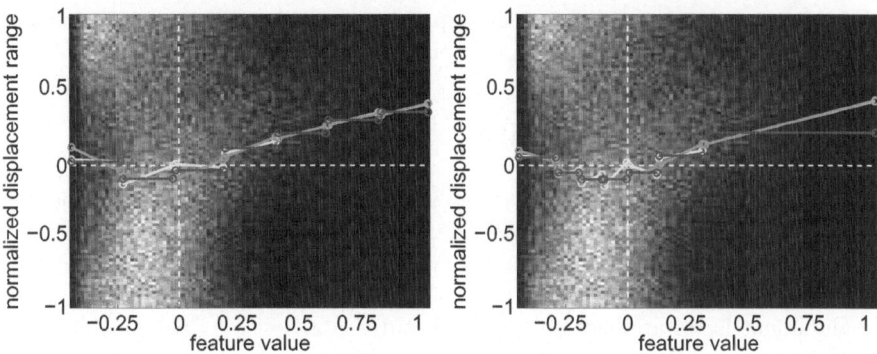

**Fig. 2. Examples of tested piecewise linear regression functions:** The density of the training data for one feature (samples depicted as white dots) with fitted regression functions. The left image corresponds to *non-proportional partitioning* and the right image to the *proportional partitioning*. Yellow color corresponds to fitted function (3), green color function (4) and red color function (5).

to each feature to $U$ (the number of bins), where the feature's value fills only the position of the corresponding bin in each training example. Lets suppose, for example, that we want to partition the feature space into three bins. Than the row of L corresponding to one feature $f_j$ over all training examples expands into $3 \times p$ matrix $\Lambda_j = \begin{bmatrix} 0 & f_j(I^2, \mathbf{a}^2) & 0 \\ f_j(I^1, \mathbf{a}^1) & 0 & \dots & 0 \\ 0 & 0 & f_j(I^p, \mathbf{a}^p) \end{bmatrix}$. When we want to use the intercept parameter $\omega_{ju}$ in the regression functions (4) and (5), we also need the expansion $\Omega_j = \begin{bmatrix} 0 & 1 & 0 \\ 1 & 0 \dots 0 \\ 0 & 0 & 1 \end{bmatrix}$. The training matrices used for learning of the regression functions (3), (4) and (5) are extended as follows

$$L_{(3)} = \begin{bmatrix} \Lambda_{j_1} \\ \Lambda_{j_2} \\ \vdots \end{bmatrix}, L_{(4)} = \begin{bmatrix} \Lambda_{j_1} \\ \Omega_{j_1} \\ \Lambda_{j_2} \\ \Omega_{j_2} \\ \vdots \end{bmatrix}, L_{(5)} = \begin{bmatrix} \Omega_{j_1} \\ \Omega_{j_2} \\ \vdots \end{bmatrix}. \tag{6}$$

We evaluate the alignment error and speed of the three linear functions for different numbers of bins on the validation data. The piecewise constant function (5) is significantly less time consuming than the other two. In order to estimate the displacement contribution from one feature value, we just need to read a constant value from particular bin. For a reasonable number of bins ($U \geq 9$) the function (5) quickly reaches the alignment precision of functions (3) and (4). Also the partitioning proportional to the training data density yields lower validation error than the one with equally sized bins. In our implementation we proportionally partition each feature space into 20 bins, where each contains a constant regression function (5). The approximation allows for computation free evaluation during classification phase, see the next section.

## 5  Implementation Details

Both the weak classifier $d_k$ and the weak regressor $r_k$ in stage $k$ are implemented as a single hash table (see Table 1 for example). Therefore getting the regression contribution from one feature means to read it from the same row of the same hash-table. Hence the only additional cost we pay during the classification for the alignment is its application on the features positions. As we consider only translation the application means only two additions per feature point. In our

**Table 1.** A part of one hash-table encoding the confidence and 2D displacement for one feature in stage $k$

| feature bin | $(-\infty, -0.015)$ | $\langle -0.015, 1.44 \rangle$ | $\langle 1.44, 2.76 \rangle$ | $\langle 2.76, 3.87 \rangle$ | $\langle 3.87, 5.24 \rangle$ | ... |
|---|---|---|---|---|---|---|
| confidence | $-1$ | 0 | $-0.25$ | 0.85 | 0.74 | ... |
| rows alignment | 0 | 0.01 | 0.25 | $-0.09$ | $-0.08$ | ... |
| cols alignment | 0 | $-0.47$ | $-0.49$ | $-0.01$ | 0.14 | ... |

implementation, for each feature $f_k \in \mathcal{F}$ from the feature-pool $\mathcal{F}$, we divide feature space into $U$ bins $B_u$, $u = 1 \ldots U$ of sizes proportional to the training data density[2]. In the $k$-th hash table we denote the classifier data corresponding to $u$-th bin as $D_k(u)$. Let us denote $J_u = \{i | f(I^i, \mathbf{a}^i) \in B_u\}$, i.e. the set of indexes of training examples which fall into bin $B_u$. Then the value $D_k(u)$ in the hash table by which the weak classifier contributes to the overall confidence (when the feature falls into bin $B_u$) is computed as follows:

$$D_k(u) = \arg\min_{d_k} \sum_{i \in J_u} w^i \cdot (d_k(f_k(I^i, \mathbf{a}^i)) - y^i)^2 = \frac{\sum_{i \in J_u} w^i \cdot y^i}{\sum_{i \in I_h} w^i}. \quad (7)$$

In the weak classifier learning process the same procedure is performed for each bin and each feature from the feature pool. Finally, we use the feature (and corresponding hash table) which yields the lowest error. Such approach is coincident with Gentleboost technique [16].

## 6  Experiments

We conduct our experiments on two datasets: (i) rear-view cars dataset (RVC) and (ii) labeled faces in the wild dataset (LFW) [17]. In the rest of this section, we describe datasets in details and introduce different detection grids used in the following experiments. In section 6.1 we experimentally verify that, under

---

[2] Except the size of border bins which are $[-\infty, \texttt{min\_value}]$ and $[\texttt{max\_value}, +\infty]$.

a computational time constraint, LISA yields a significant improvement in the detection rate. In section 6.2 we show that on the fixed density of the detection grid, we achieve both the better detection rate and lower number of features, which need to be evaluated. In addition to that, we show what we lose by re-using the detection feature for the regression instead of selecting special features for regression.

*Datasets Description:* In the RVC dataset, we have collected 1500 of positive samples in different scales, each $10\times$ randomly perturbed within the range of corresponding translations, see Figure 3. To train LISA we manually labeled very accurate ground truth data. We have also collected 6000 background images, which contains approximately 15Gpxl of negative data. The LFW is free of charge widely used dataset containing approximately 13000 positive images. The same amount of negative data consisting of 6000 background images ($\approx$ 15Gpxl of negative data) is used.

*Running Time:* We enforce the time constraint by requiring the same average number of features evaluated in 1 Mpxl of image data. More formally, let us denote the number of detection windows per 1Mpxl of image data as NoW (Number of Windows). In the sparse grid NoW $= 0.84\cdot10^6/$1Mpxl, in the medium grid NoW $= 1.90\cdot10^6/$1Mpxl ($\approx 4\times$ more windows must be evaluated), in the dense grid NoW $= 7.6 \cdot 10^6/$1Mpxl, ($\approx 9\times$ more windows must be evaluated). Let us denote the average number of features evaluated per 1 detection window as FpW (Features per Window). Then the average *per image detection time* is proportional to the Total number of Features TnF evaluated in 1Mpxl of image data TnF $=$ FpW$\cdot$NoW. Note, that it is not easy to achieve exactly the same TnF, especially on different detection grids. In order to assure a fair comparison, we use such a setting in which TnF of SDP with LISA is smaller or equal to TnF of SDP, see for example Figure 4(b).

*Detection Grids:* In the following experiments SDP and SDP with LISA running on sparse, medium, and dense detection grid are compared. For detectors running in the sparse-grid (with detection step equal to 20% of the object size), positive data were perturbed in the range of $\pm10\%$ of the object size. Similarly for detection in medium-grid, positive data were perturbed in the range of $\pm5\%$

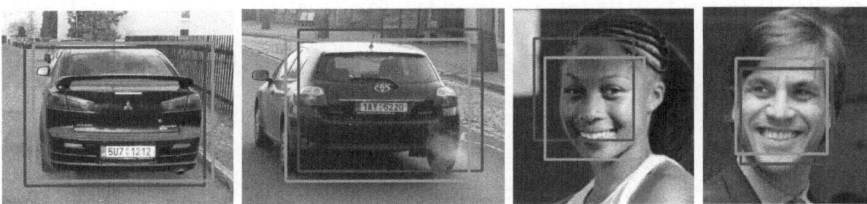

**Fig. 3. Positive Data:** Four randomly perturbed samples. Perturbed training window shown in red, correct object position in green. Two left images are taken from RCV dataset and two right images from LFW dataset.

of the object size. Note that in our training resolution (60pxl) the alignment error of 1% is under the size of 1 pixel, therefore it cannot be compensated. Grids differ only by sparsity of positions, the scale step remains the same throughout all the experiments.

## 6.1 SDP vs. SDP with LISA on the CRV Dataset

We experimentally verify, that under a computational time constraint, LISA yields a significant improvement in the detection rate. For the sake of simplicity, we summarize the comparison in Table 2. It shows, FN rate for the setting in which the detectors have approximately 1 FP per 100 Mpxl of image data, i.e. $FP = 10^{-2}$. SDP and SDP with LISA are compared on the same level of TnF. All detectors were learned for different grid densities. Only those detectors, which achieved the best results on a given TnF level are shown. More detailed analysis, including ROC curves for all grids follows in the rest of this section.

**Table 2.** Comparison of FN rates for fixed number of FP per 1Mpxl equal to $10^{-2}$ for SDP and SDP with LISA. Results corresponds to ROC curves in Figure 4.

| TnF | 3.6M | 5M | 10M | 25M |
|---|---|---|---|---|
| **SDP with LISA** | 0.173 | 0.153 | 0.112 | − |
| **SDP** | | 0.73 | 0.247 | 0.181 | 0.170 |

When the running time is limited, the detector trained on perfectly aligned data must decide about the object presence/absence after the evaluation of only a small number of features to reach the TnF limit, which significantly deteriorates its detection rate. The detection rate on the same TnF-level is always improved, when the LISA is used, see for example red curves in Figure 4(a). Naturally, the higher the TnF level, the smaller advantage comes from using the LISA, see results for TnF ≈ 5M in Figure 4(b) and for TnF ≈ 10M in Figure 4(c). Eventually, improvement in the detection rate for TnF = 10M is apparent only from $FP \leq 10^{-1}$ , compare black and red curves in Figure 4(c).

We push the comparison to the limit by relaxing the time constraint and allowing to run the SDP on a dense grid using as many features as needed, see 4(d). Then the best is to train the SDP on perfectly aligned data, which makes application of LISA redundant. It essentially makes no sense to align already aligned data. Detection rate of such SDP is shown by blue dashed line in Figure 4(d). Such SDP has 6× higher TnF, than SDP with LISA on sparse-grid (red solid line), and 3× higher TnF (red dashed line), than SDP with LISA on medium-grid. Figure also shows, that SDP with LISA with TnF=5.3M has the same detection rate as SDP with TnF=16M. We can see that, for lower FPs the SDP with LISA on the medium-grid (red dashed line) achieves even better detection rate than the SDP on the dense-grid (blue dashed line). We explain this behaviour, by remaining ground-truth inaccuracy, which is compensated by LISA generalization.

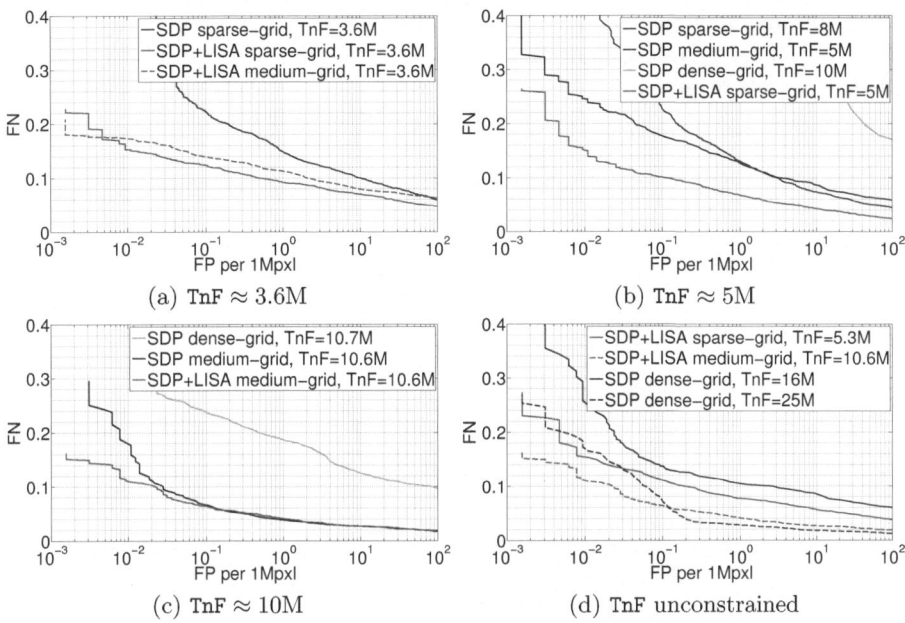

**Fig. 4. ROC curves (FP per 1 Mpxl) for CRV dataset:** SDP with a sparse (blue), medium (black) and dense (green) detection grid vs. the SDP with LISA (red). False positives are measured per 1 Mpxl of the background data, false negatives per dataset.

## 6.2 SDP vs. SDP with LISA Comparison on LFW Dataset

In this experiment, we show that on a fixed density of the detection grid, we achieve both the better detection rate and lower TnF. We demonstrate these results on the same detection grids as were used in the previous experiment. In addition to that, we show what we lose by re-using the detection feature for regression, instead of selecting special features for regression, by performing the experiment in which regression features are also selected by boosting during the training process.

Figure 5(a,b,c) shows ROC curves of SDP (blue) and SDP with LISA (red) detector on LFW dataset for the detection in different detection grids. Especially for the dense detection detection grid, we also show ROC curve for SDP with LISA with Special regression Feature (SDP+LISA+SF in green). This experiment shows, what one can achieve when a special regression feature is used to estimate the alignment in each detection stage. Figure 5(d) shows corresponding Mean Regression Error (MRE) as a function of the number of evaluated features. In SDP no alignment is performed, therefore the MRE is constant (here we normalize MRE to make this value equal to one). SDP with LISA exhibits slower descent than SDP+LISA+SF, because detection features are not that suitable for the regression. Nevertheless the asymptotic value of the MRE on the testing data (dashed line) is similar. Hence, the SDP+LISA+SF achieves accurate alignment faster and rejects background window earlier. As a consequence of that, only 15M features is used for detection, however additional 30M of special features are needed for the regression. Totally TnF = 45M features are used, which is almost twice as many than for SDP with LISA.

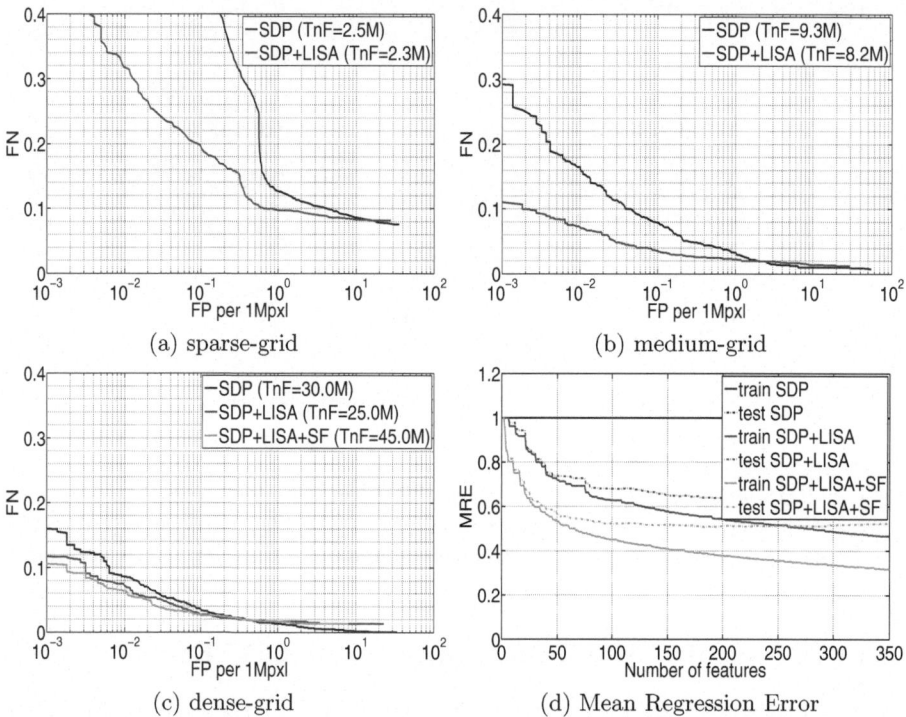

(a) sparse-grid

(b) medium-grid

(c) dense-grid

(d) Mean Regression Error

**Fig. 5. ROC curves (FP per 1 Mpxl) for LFW dataset:** SDP (blue) vs. SDP with LISA (red) with a sparse, medium and dense detection grids. False positives are measured per 1 Mpxl of background data, false negatives per dataset.

## 7   Conclusion

We have proposed an efficient approach for exploiting features for both classification/detection and alignment. The alignment interleaves with sequential decision process. It allow the detector to run on a sparser grid and compute fewer features. The alignment is computed by a regressor which is learned jointly with the classifier. The regressor approximates a non-linear function and allows a hash table implementation and is thus tremendously efficient.

We have experimentally verified, that using the Locally Interleaved Sequential Alignment (LISA) in a Sequential Detection Process (SDP) significantly improves the detection rate if the detection time is limited. We have also shown that the same detection rate is achievable with approximately 3× lower detection time in average. In addition to that it was shown that on the same detection grid SDP with LISA exhibits both better detection rate and better detection time.

**Acknowledgement.** The first and second authors were supported by the Czech Science Foundation Projects P103/11/P700 and P103/10/1585 respectively. The third author was supported by EC project FP7-ICT-247870 NIFTi. Any opinions expressed in this paper do not necessarily reflect the views of the European Community. The Community is not liable for any use that may be made of the information contained herein.

# References

1. Viola, P., Jones, M.J.: Robust real-time face detection. International Journal of Computer Vision 57, 137–154 (2004)
2. Huang, C., Ai, H., Li, Y., Lao, S.: Vector boosting for rotation invariant multi-view face detection. In: ICCV, pp. 446–453 (2005)
3. Felzenszwalb, P., Girshick, R., McAllester, D., Ramanan, D.: Object detection with discriminatively trained part-based models. IEEE Transactions on Pattern Analysis and Machine Intelligence 32, 1627–1645 (2010)
4. Dalal, N., Triggs, B.: Histograms of oriented gradients for human detection. In: CVPR, pp. 1–8 (2005)
5. Vedaldi, A., Gulshan, V., Varma, M., Zisserman, A.: Multiple kernels for object detection. In: ICCV, pp. 606–613 (2009)
6. Harzallah, H., Jurie, F., Schmid, C.: Combining efficient object localization and image classification. In: ICCV, pp. 237–244 (2009)
7. Zhu, Q., Yeh, M.C., Cheng, K.T., Avidan, S.: Fast human detection using a cascade of histograms of oriented gradients. In: CVPR, vol. 2, pp. 1491–1498 (2006)
8. Lampert, C.H., Blaschko, M.B., Hoffmann, T.: Efficient subwindow search: A branch and bound framework for object localization. IEEE Transactions on Pattern Analysis and Machine Intelligence 31, 2129–2142 (2009)
9. Kokkinos, I.: Rapid deformable object detection using dual-tree branch-and-bound. In: Advances in Neural Information Processing Systems (NIPS), pp. 2681–2689 (2011)
10. Šochman, J., Matas, J.: Waldboost - learning for time constrained sequential detection. In: CVPR, pp. 150–157 (2005)
11. Ali, K., Fleuret, F., Hasler, D., Fua, P.: A real-time deformable detector. IEEE Transactions on Pattern Analysis and Machine Intelligence 34, 225–239 (2012)
12. Zimmermann, K., Matas, J., Svoboda, T.: Tracking by an optimal sequence of linear predictors. IEEE Transactions on Pattern Analysis and Machine Intelligence 31, 677–692 (2009)
13. Dollar, P., Welinder, P., Perona, P.: Cascaded pose regression. In: 2010 IEEE Conference on Computer Vision and Pattern Recognition (CVPR), pp. 1078–1085 (2010)
14. Bourdev, L., Brandt, J.: Robust object detection via soft cascade. In: CVPR, vol. 2, pp. 236–243 (2005)
15. Penrose, R.: A generalized inverse for matrices. Mathematical Proceedings of the Cambridge Philosophical Society 51, 406–413 (1955)
16. Friedman, J., Hastie, T., Tibshirani, R.: Additive logistic regression: a statistical view of boosting. Annals of Statistics 28, 2000 (1998)
17. Huang, G.B., Ramesh, M., Berg, T., Learned-Miller, E.: Labeled faces in the wild: A database for studying face recognition in unconstrained environments. Technical Report 07-49, University of Massachusetts, Amherst (2007)

# Efficient and Scalable
# 4th-Order Match Propagation

David Ok, Renaud Marlet, and Jean-Yves Audibert

Université Paris-Est, LIGM (UMR CNRS), Center for Visual Computing
École des Ponts ParisTech, 6-8 av. Blaise Pascal, 77455 Marne-la-Vallée, France

**Abstract.** We propose a robust method to match image feature points taking into account geometric consistency. It is a careful adaptation of the match propagation principle to 4th-order geometric constraints (match quadruple consistency). With our method, a set of matches is explained by a network of locally-similar affinities. This approach is useful when simple descriptor-based matching strategies fail, in particular for highly ambiguous data, e.g., with repetitive patterns or where texture is lacking. As it scales easily to hundreds of thousands of matches, it is also useful when denser point distributions are sought, e.g., for high-precision rigid model estimation. Experiments show that our method is competitive (efficient, scalable, accurate, robust) against state-of-the-art methods in deformable object matching, camera calibration and pattern detection.

## 1 Introduction

Establishing correspondences between sets of features detected in images arises in many vision tasks, e.g., object matching, camera calibration and pattern detection. In many cases, distinctive feature descriptors and simple matching strategies [1, 2] successfully produce a reasonably good set of matches w.r.t. the task requirements: large enough to carry meaningful information and with a large enough proportion of true positives (little contamination by false positives). But in ambiguous settings, e.g., when similar objects occur several times (e.g., windows on a facade, rocks in a landscape) or when distinctive textures are lacking, these matching strategies may fail and jeopardize the whole task. Yet, more robust correspondences can be found using the geometric consistency of feature location. Methods that try to address this issue fall into three main categories.

The first category includes RANSAC-based methods [3, 4], possibly in conjunction with Hough-based clustering [5]. They are fast and robust if the noise in the data can be estimated and if the percentage of inliers (i.e., true correspondences) among the set of candidate correspondences is of order 10% or greater. But this is hardly the case for pattern detection and ambiguous feature matching, where true correspondences can be less than 5%. Besides, the correspondences are explained by a number of independent homographies, i.e., disjoint planar facets [4, 5]. There is no relation among homographies other than looking for a totally new homography at the periphery of a previous one, which is inappropriate for curved surfaces and deformations.

K.M. Lee et al. (Eds.): ACCV 2012, Part I, LNCS 7724, pp. 460–473, 2013.
© Springer-Verlag Berlin Heidelberg 2013

In constrast, the second kind of approaches explicitly handles such cases. Correspondence selection is formulated there as a hypergraph matching problem that exploits geometric cues [6–11]. However, the algorithmic complexity can be prohibitive in practice: given $n$ points, time $O(n^d \log n)$ has been reported for $d$-order potentials and after a number of approximations [9]. Such methods hardly scale to thousands of interest points, which would correspond to huge (gigabytes) affinity tensors, even after sparsification. Moreover, not all of them define how to discriminate inliers from outliers. Many hypergraph matchers only look for a bijection: a match is always found for any point, although dummy points can be added to attract outliers [12]. Some authors also use a threshold on the computed match confidence [12], but the confidence value is relative and cannot be easily associated to a geometric, understandable measure, leaving the user clueless for setting a sensible threshold value. Besides, looking for a single explanation of all correspondences may be an issue for scenes with moving objects.

Methods in the third category solve many local correspondence problems through simultaneous match propagation [13–15]: different seeds are grown and adapt to different transformations. However, these approaches basically exploit 2nd-order constraints and heavily depend on affine shape adaptation. They are thus not or poorly applicable to features that are not affine-covariant, such as DoG-SIFT [1]. Moreover, as shown by our experiments, affine shape determination is not very precise and shape adaptation can thus be significantly noisy. Even if optimized during propagation [14], affine shapes lack robustness. Some approaches also require the images to be available [13, 14], as opposed to only working on the set of abstract feature points. In addition, these methods cope with a reasonable amount of matching ambiguity, but fail to limit detection when the set of possible correspondences is strongly contaminated by outliers.

Our method tries to overcome the above drawbacks. It is a careful adaptation of the match propagation principle to 4th-order geometric constraints (macth quadruple consistency). Our framework explains a set of matches by a continuous network of locally-similar affinities which are determined from neighboring matches rather than by the affine shape of a single match. Our approach enjoys many good properties. It works on any kind of feature point (not only affine-covariant) and different types of features can even be freely mixed, for denser, more uniform or more precise correspondences. Besides, it does not require the image pixels after detection, contrary to most propagation based methods. Although it has no global view of all correspondences (contrary to non-approximating hypergraph matchers), it produces very reliable matches. It can tell inliers from outliers and it is robust to high outlier contamination rates. It adapts to scenes that have to be explained by different, separate models or by continuous model deformation. Last, it scales to hundreds of thousands of matches, both in time and space.

The rest of the paper is organized as follows. Section 2 states the optimization problem we try to solve. Section 3 and 4 present our algorithm and our pattern matcher. Section 5 evaluates our method for deformable object matching, camera calibration and pattern detection (accurate localization). Section 6 concludes.

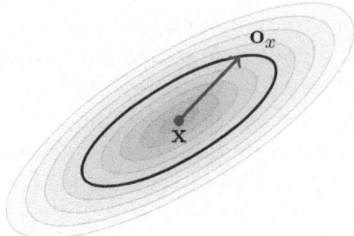

(1) the position $\mathbf{x} \in \mathbb{R}^2$ of the feature in the image, which we note by a font change only for readability,

(2) a shape $\mathcal{S}_x$ representing the (possibly anisotropic) scale of the feature, encoded by a scale matrix $\mathbf{\Sigma}_x \in \mathbb{R}^{2 \times 2}$,

(3) an orientation $\mathbf{o}_x$,

(4) a feature descriptor $\mathbf{v}_x$.

**Fig. 1.** Geometric information of a feature

## 2    Problem Statement

Before formulating the problem, we lay down a few definitions and notations. Let $\mathcal{X}$ and $\mathcal{Y}$ be two sets of features extracted respectively from two images, and let $\mathcal{M} \subseteq \mathcal{X} \times \mathcal{Y}$ be a given set of possible matches. In the following, we denote a match by $m = (x, y)$. It is typically a pair of features whose descriptors are close, or close enough compared to other close descriptors. Note that $\mathcal{M}$ may include numerous ambiguities, i.e., any number of matches with the same feature $x$ or $y$. ($\mathcal{M}$ can even be $\mathcal{X} \times \mathcal{Y}$.) A set of matches $R \subset \mathcal{M}$ is called a *region*.

### 2.1    Feature Information

The sets of features and matches can freely mix detectors and descriptors of different kinds, e.g., Harris-affine or Hessian-affine interest points [16], DoG-SIFT blobs and descriptors [1], MSER regions [17]. But a meaningful match can only involve a detector-descriptor pair of the same kind.

For each kind $f$ of feature (a detector-descriptor pair), and each feature $x$ of kind $f$, we assume that the information illustrated in Fig. 1 is available. Note that, while affine-covariant keypoint scales are elliptic, e.g., with a Harris-affine detector, others such as DoG-SIFT scales are isotropic, i.e., circular. The orientation is typically given by the dominant gradient direction around $x$ at some appropriate scale. The feature descriptor abstracts the image around $x$, also at some appropriate scale, for comparison with other detected features.

### 2.2    Match Consistency Under Affinity Constraint

Feature information, besides descriptors, provides the ground for assessing the geometric consistency of a set of features. If $x$ and $y$ match, and if $\phi$ is a local affinity relating image 1 around $x$ to image 2 then: the position $\phi(\mathbf{x})$ should be close to $\mathbf{y}$, taking scale into account; shape $\phi(\mathcal{S}_x)$ should be close to shape $\mathcal{S}_y$; and orientation $\phi(\mathbf{o}_x)$ should be close to orientation $\mathbf{o}_y$. Symmetrically, this should also be true of $(y, x)$ for the inverse affinity $\phi^{-1}$. We elaborate these notions.

"Being close" hinges on the specific characteristics of the kind of feature. We assume that each detector for a feature kind $f$ comes with its *associated repeatability expectations*, that depend, e.g., on the detector precision and parameters

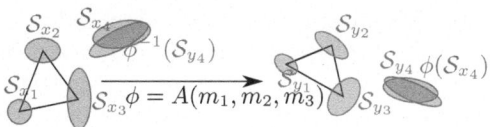

**Fig. 2.** Affine consistency of match $m_4$ w.r.t. $\phi = A(m_1, m_2, m_3)$

or on the maximum expected change in images (viewpoint, illumination, etc.). Based on this knowledge, we can test position, shape and orientation consistency between two features $\phi(x)$ and $y$. Standard definitions include a threshold on the distance between the positions, possibly taking scale into account based on $\phi(\mathcal{S}_x)$ and/or $\mathcal{S}_y$. The *scale-sensitive distance* to $x$ (resp. to $y$) is defined as:

$$d_x(\mathbf{x}') = (\mathbf{x}' - \mathbf{x})^T \boldsymbol{\Sigma}_x (\mathbf{x}' - \mathbf{x}) \tag{1}$$

Joint with a threshold on the Jaccard distance (overlap) between co-centered $\phi(\mathcal{S}_x)$ and $\mathcal{S}_y$, it is used to estimate detector repeatability [16].

It can be combined with an orientation angle threshold. Note that a typical threshold value for the Jaccard distance is 0.4 [18]. However, because we use a local affine approximation (see below), this threshold can be loosened, e.g., to 0.6. This prevents the unwanted, premature rejection of possible matches.

Assuming we know the expected precision of position $\delta_p$, the expected precision of shape $\delta_s$ and the expected precision of orientation angle $\delta_o$, we define predicate a $\mathbb{P}_f$ to test simultaneously position, shape and orientation consistency:

$$\mathbb{P}_f(x_1, x_2) = (d_{x_1}(\mathbf{x}_2) < \delta_p) \wedge \left(1 - \frac{\text{area}(\mathcal{S}_{x_1} \cap \mathcal{S}_{x_2})}{\text{area}(\mathcal{S}_{x_1} \cup \mathcal{S}_{x_2})} < \delta_s\right) \wedge (\mathbf{o}_{x_1}.\mathbf{o}_{x_2} > \cos(\delta_o)) \tag{2}$$

Predicate $\mathbb{P}_\phi$ assesses the consistency of a match under an affinity constraint $\phi$:

$$\mathbb{P}_\phi(x, y) \stackrel{\text{def}}{=} \mathbb{P}_f(\phi(x), y)) \wedge \mathbb{P}_f(x, \phi^{-1}(y)) \tag{3}$$

Namely, an $f$-match $m = (x, y)$ is *position-, shape- and orientation consistent w.r.t. affinity* $\phi$ iff $\mathbb{P}_f$ holds both for $(\phi(x), y)$ and $(x, \phi^{-1}(y))$.

Finally, we define a predicate $\mathbb{P}_d$ (used for match propagation) that tests relative, scaled distance consistency: two $f$-matches $m = (x, y)$ and $m' = (x', y')$ are *(scaled-)distance-consistent* iff the distance of $x'$ to $x$, relative to the scale of $x$, is close enough to the distance of $y'$ to $y$, relative to the scale of $y$:

$$\mathbb{P}_d(m, m') \stackrel{\text{def}}{=} \frac{\min(d_x(\mathbf{x}'), d_y(\mathbf{y}'))}{\max(d_x(\mathbf{x}'), d_y(\mathbf{y}'))} > 1/2 \tag{4}$$

### 2.3   Region Consistency

The feature correspondence problem relies on two kinds of assumptions. First, if $(x, y)$ is a good match, the image around $x$ should be similar to the image around $y$. This photometric criterion translates into features having "close enough" descriptors. Second, given a set of matches $(x_i, y_i)_{1 \leq i \leq n}$, the relative position of feature $x_i$ w.r.t. others features $(x_j)_{j \neq i}$ is expected to be similar to the relative position of $y_i$ w.r.t. other features $(y_j)_{j \neq i}$. This criterion is mainly geometric, i.e., based on the relative coordinates of the features. But it also has an indirect, photometric flavor as the feature shapes and orientations also have to agree when relating $x_i$ and $y_i$ in the context of $(x_j, y_j)_{j \neq i}$.

The geometric assumption only holds locally. Geometric consistency is thus only expected in independent image regions, i.e., separate sets of features. Accordingly, we define the consistency of a given single region as well as the region-wise consistency of a set of separate regions. We will actually be looking for a subpartition $\mathcal{R} = (R_i)_{1 \leq i \leq n}$ of $\mathcal{M}$ such that each region $R_i$ is affine-consistent. (A set of regions $\mathcal{R}$ is a *subpartition* of $\mathcal{M}$ iff it is a partition of a subset of $\mathcal{M}$.)

*Local Affinity.* A consistent region can be defined as a set of matches locally related by an affine homography [16]. We actually do not define a consistent region by a single affinity but by many. This particular setting provides a valuable flexibility allowing a region to adapt to substantial non-affine transformations (cf. §5.1). Given a triple of matches $(m_i)_{1 \leq i \leq 3} = (x_i, y_i)_{1 \leq i \leq 3}$, one can construct a unique affine transformation $\phi = A((m_i)_{1 \leq i \leq 3})$ between images 1 and 2 that maps $\mathbf{x}_i$ to $\mathbf{y}_i$ for all $1 \leq i \leq 3$. This only makes sense if the positions are not *degenerate*, i.e., if the points are not aligned, and more generally if the triangles corresponding to the feature triples in both images do not have too sharp angles. Now the affine-consistency of a given match $m$ can be defined as the conjunction of the position, shape and orientation consistency of $m$ w.r.t. affinity $\phi$. Specifically, we say that $m$ is *affine-consistent* with matches $(m_i)_{1 \leq i \leq 3}$ iff $(m_i)_{1 \leq i \leq 3}$ is not degenerate and $\mathbb{P}_\phi(m)$ holds for $\phi = A((m_i)_{1 \leq i \leq 3})$. Fig. 2 illustrates this concept.

*Region Affine-Consistency.* As 3 matches can always be related by an affinity, region affine-consistency makes sense for at least 4 matches. It is our 4th-order constraint. A quadruple of matches $(m_i)_{1 \leq i \leq 4}$ is *affine-consistent* iff for all $1 \leq i \leq 4$, $m_i$ is affine-consistent with $(m_j)_{1 \leq j \leq 4, j \neq i}$. This is extended to a region using chains of affine-consistent quadruples. First, given a region $R \subset \mathcal{M}$, a pair of matches $m, m' \in R$ are said *affine-consistent in $R$* iff there exists a sequence $(m_{1,i}, m_{2,i}, m_{3,i}, m_{4,i})_{1 \leq i \leq n}$ of affine-consistent quadruples in $R$ from $m$ to $m'$, i.e., s.t. $m = m_{1,1}$, $m_{4,i} = m_{1,i+1}$ for $1 \leq i < n$, and $m_{4,n} = m'$. Then, a region $R$ is said *affine-consistent* iff any different matches $m, m' \in R$ are affine-consistent. By extension, a subpartition $\mathcal{R} = (R_i)_{1 \leq i \leq r}$ of $\mathcal{M}$ is said affine-consistent iff each region $R_i$ is affine-consistent. An important property is that, given two affine-consistent regions $R, R'$ such that $R \cap R' \neq \varnothing$, $R \cup R'$ is affine-consistent.

*Maximal Consistency.* Finally, we are interested in finding a maximum number of meaningful matches; the actual number of underlying regions does not matter.

Given a set of regions $\mathcal{R}$, we thus define the *size of $\mathcal{R}$*, noted $\|\mathcal{R}\|$, as the number of matches occurring in $\mathcal{R}$, i.e., $\|\mathcal{R}\| = |\bigcup_{R \in \mathcal{R}} R|$. If $\mathcal{R}$ is a subpartition of $\mathcal{M}$, this reduces to $\|\mathcal{R}\| = \sum_{R \in \mathcal{R}} |R|$. If we can additionally impose that

---

**Algorithm 1.** Region growing from a seed match $m_1$.

---

**Notations:**
- $\mathcal{N}_K(m)$: $K$ nearest matches of $m$ that are scaled-distance consistent.
- $C$: matches that are scaled-distance consistent w.r.t. at least 1 match in $R$. When $C$ is modified, it is always kept sorted by increasing distrust score.

1: **procedure** GROWREGION($m_1, K$)
2:     Pick matches $m_2, m_3 \in \mathcal{N}_K(m_1)$
3:     $R \leftarrow \{m_i\}_{1 \leq i \leq 3}$                ▷ *Initialize R with seed*
4:     $C \leftarrow \bigcup\limits_{1 \leq i \leq 3} \mathcal{N}_K(m_i) \setminus R$          ▷ *Initialize C*
5:     **while** $\exists\, (m, m', m'', m''') \in C \times R^3$ affine-consistent **do** ▷ LOCALSEARCH *(algo 2.)*
6:         $R \leftarrow R \cup \{m\}$                      ▷ *Grow R*
7:         $C \leftarrow C \cup (\mathcal{N}_K(m) \setminus R)$     ▷ *Ensure that matches in R are excluded*
8:     **end while**
9:     Return $R$
10: **end procedure**

---

the number $|\mathcal{R}|$ of underlying regions be minimal, the subpartition of $\mathcal{M}$ into affine-consistent regions with maximum size is actually unique (if any).

Our feature matching problem can now be stated: *Find the affine-consistent subpartition $\mathcal{R}$ of $\mathcal{M}$ of maximum size, then minimum cardinality.*

*Ambiguity Freedom.* Different tasks have different requirements regarding match ambiguity. For instance, whereas repeated pattern detection overtly calls for ambiguous matches, scene tracks used for estimating camera calibration parameters require unambiguous matches. A variant of our feature matching problem additionally require ambiguity-freedom, at the region or subpartition level. Note that uniqueness is not guaranteed in this case. More formally, a match $(x, y)$ is *unambiguous in M* iff for all $(x', y') \in M \setminus \{(x, y)\}$, $x \neq x'$ and $y \neq y'$; a region $R$ is *ambiguity-free* iff for any match $m \in R$, $m$ is unambiguous in $R$; and a set of regions $\mathcal{R}$ is *ambiguity-free* iff $R$ is ambiguity-free for all $R \in \mathcal{R}$.

## 3 Match Propagation Procedure

Due to the highly combinatorial nature of this optimization problem, we propose an algorithm and a set of heuristics that efficiently determine an affine-consistent subpartition of $\mathcal{M}$ of large size, and small cardinality, possibly ambiguity-free. Although we do not satisfy the global extremality constraints, our experiments show that our local maxima yield very good sets of matches (cf. §5).

The algorithm follows a region growing scheme. Given an initial region consisting of a triple of potential matches, we iteratively add more matches into the region provided they are geometrically consistent with some triple of matches already in the region. When no more match can be added, the region is considered as valid iff it is large enough. More regions can be grown by re-running the algorithm on the remaining potential matches. See Algorithm 1. for details.

Besides, if unambiguity is required, any match $(x, y)$ is checked for ambiguity before being added to a growing region $R$. If there already is a match $(x, y')$ or $(x', y)$ in $R$, then $(x, y)$ is removed from the remaining potential matches and associated to $R$, but without contributing to $|R|$.

The key ingredients of the algorithm are additional heuristics for growing the regions, that prevent a combinatorial explosion and only explore a limited number of pertinent cases, most likely matches being tried first. They enable a selective evaluation of concistency checks, in particular the shape consistency which can be computationally intensive. They are presented in the following.

*Ordering and Limiting Potential Matches.* Matches $(x, y)$ are ordered by increasing distrust score, defined as follows. Let $D$ be a distance in the descriptor space, e.g., Euclidean distance for SIFT. For a descriptor $\mathbf{v}_x \in \mathcal{V}_{\mathcal{X}}$, let $\mathbf{v}_y^1, \mathbf{v}_y^2 \in \mathcal{V}_{\mathcal{Y}}$ be respectively its nearest neighbor (1-NN) and its second nearest neighbor (2-NN). The distrust score (or Lowe score [1]) of match $m = (x, y)$ is defined as

$$L_{\mathcal{X} \to \mathcal{Y}}(x, y) = \frac{D(\mathbf{v}_x, \mathbf{v}_y^1)}{D(\mathbf{v}_x, \mathbf{v}_y^2)} \leq 1 \tag{5}$$

The smaller the score $L_{\mathcal{X} \to \mathcal{Y}}(m)$ is, the less ambiguous match $m$ is. Usually, a set of reliable matches is obtained with matches $m$ such that $L_{\mathcal{X} \to \mathcal{Y}}(m) \leq \ell$. Typically, $\ell$ ranges in $[0.6; 0.8]$. However, doing so discards ambiguous matches. To avoid it, the distrust score is extended as follows:

$$L_{\mathcal{X} \to \mathcal{Y}}(x, y) = \begin{cases} \frac{D(\mathbf{v}_x, \mathbf{v}_y)}{D(\mathbf{v}_x, \mathbf{v}_y^2)} & \text{if } \mathbf{v}_y = \mathbf{v}_y^1 \quad \leq 1 \\ \frac{D(\mathbf{v}_x, \mathbf{v}_y)}{D(\mathbf{v}_x, \mathbf{v}_y^1)} & \text{if } \mathbf{v}_y \neq \mathbf{v}_y^1 \quad \geq 1 \end{cases} \tag{6}$$

$$L(m) = \min\left(L_{\mathcal{X} \to \mathcal{Y}}(m), L_{\mathcal{Y} \to \mathcal{X}}(m)\right). \tag{7}$$

$L_{\mathcal{X} \to \mathcal{Y}}(x, y)$ quantifies an ambiguous match $(x, y)$ by the relative proximity of $\mathbf{v}_y$ with respect to its 1-NN. $L(m)$ makes the distrust score symmetric. Note that using max rather than min would delay too much the analysis of 1-to-many ambiguities. In our work, $\mathcal{M}$ is the set of matches $m$ such that $L(m) \leq \ell$, where $\ell$ can be greater than 1. Consequently, $\mathcal{M}$ is much more ubiquitous than with the usual Lowe criterion, for a better support of repetitive patterns.

*Local Search for Region Growing.* When trying to grow a region $R$ with a match $m = (x, y) \in C$ (line 5 of Algorithm 1.), we prune the search of a triple of matches $(m', m'', m''')$ by considering only close matches, i.e., matches $(x', y') \in R$ such that $x'$ is among the $k$ nearest neighbors of $x$, or $y'$ is among the $k$ nearest neighbors of $y$. Specifically, line 5 of Algorithm 1. actually calls Algorithm 2. to find a triple of matches that provides affine consistency to candidate match $m$.

*Sidedness Constraint.* We also introduce a sidedness constraint that, experimentally, is very efficient in pruning the search and more efficient than the one in [14].

**Algorithm 2.** Local search for region growing.

---

**Notation:** $\mathcal{W}_k(m)$: neighborhood of $m$ containing $k$ nearest matches in $R$.

```
 1: procedure LOCALSEARCH(R, C)
 2:     for m = (x, y) ∈ C do
 3:         find its nearest match m' ∈ R
 4:         for (m'', m''') ∈ Wₖ(m') × Wₖ(m') do
 5:             return (m, m', m'', m''') if affine-consistent
 6:         end for
 7:     end for
 8:     return ∅
 9: end procedure
```

---

The general idea is that if $m_1 = (x_1, y_1)$ and $m_2 = (x_2, y_2)$ are good matches, then the directed lines $\overrightarrow{x_1 x_2}$ and $\overrightarrow{y_1 y_2}$ should define corresponding half spaces. More formally, given two points $\mathbf{u}, \mathbf{v} \in \mathbb{R}^2$, the half space on the left of $\overrightarrow{\mathbf{uv}}$ is $E(\mathbf{u}, \mathbf{v}) = \{\mathbf{w} \in \mathbb{R}^2 \mid \det(\mathbf{v} - \mathbf{u}, \mathbf{w} - \mathbf{u}) > 0\}$. A match $(x, y)$ is *side-consistent* w.r.t. matches $(x_1, y_1), (x_2, y_2)$ iff $\mathbf{x} \in E(\mathbf{x}_1, \mathbf{x}_2) \Leftrightarrow \mathbf{y} \in E(\mathbf{y}_1, \mathbf{y}_2)$. When evaluating a match candidate $m$ for growing a region $R$, $m$ can be excluded if there are $m_1, m_2 \in R$ such that $m$ is not side-consistent w.r.t. matches $m_1, m_2$.

For robustness, the sidedness consistency applies only to matches $(x, y)$ such that $\mathbf{x}$ (resp. $\mathbf{y}$) is not to close to line $\overrightarrow{x_1 x_2}$ (resp. $\overrightarrow{y_1 y_2}$). This prevents spurious match rejections caused by non-affine transformations or due to the imprecision of feature localization. For efficiency, we limit consistency checks for a region $R = (x_i, y_i)_{1 \leq i \leq n}$ to the contour edges of the convex hulls associated respectively to $(\mathbf{x}_i)_{1 \leq i \leq n}$ and $(\mathbf{y}_i)_{1 \leq i \leq n}$. We also impose that at any step of the region growing, the contour vertices of the convex hull of the points already matched in $\mathcal{X}$ should correspond to the contour vertices of the convex hull of the points already matched in $\mathcal{Y}$. The sidedness-checking procedure in [14] operates over all pairs of matches in a given region $R$, and thus performs $O(|R|^2)$ line checks. Our sidedness check operates only on the perimeter of $R$, rather than the whole area. The number of line checks is thus linear in the number of vertices on the contour of the convex hull, which is in practice $O(\sqrt{|R|})$.

## 4    Repetitive Pattern Search

Our feature matching algorithm can easily be turned into a pattern matcher. Given a object model $M_0$ defined by a geometric region $I_0$ in some input image $I$, the goal is to retrieve all objects that are similar to $M_0$ in some image $J$ (possibly equal to $I$), i.e., to find image regions in $J$ that are similar to $I_0$. We consider the case where $I_0$ is defined as the interior of a polygon $P_0$.

For this, we define $\mathcal{X}_0$ as the set of features inside polygon $P_0$ in $I$ and $\mathcal{Y}$ as the set of features in $J$ not in $\mathcal{X}_0$. We then grow regions of $\mathcal{M} \subset \mathcal{X}_0 \times \mathcal{Y}$ as described above, allowing ambiguity on $\mathcal{X}_0$. The resulting set of regions $\mathcal{R} = (R_i)_{1 \leq i \leq n}$ corresponds to discovered pattern instances. The image region in $J$ corresponding to a set of matches $R_i$ can be retrieved by assuming local affinity transformations from $I$ to $J$. More formally, given a vertex $\mathbf{u} \in \mathbb{R}^2$ of polygon $P_0$ in $I$, let $x_1, x_2, x_3$ be the geometrically closest 3 features in $I$ such that there are matches $(m_j)_{1 \leq j \leq 3} = (x_j, y_j)_{1 \leq j \leq 3} \in R_i$. Then the corresponding polygon vertex in image $J$ is $A(m_1, m_2, m_3)(\mathbf{u})$. The polygon $P_i$ formed by such vertices defines an image region $J_i$ of $J$ that delineates the matched object $M_i$.

More pattern instances can be found by removing features in $\mathcal{R}$ from $\mathcal{Y}$ and reusing recursively image regions $(J_i)_{1 \leq i \leq n}$ as new input patterns, until no new pattern instance is found. To reduce the risk of pattern drifting, the patterns have to be explored in breadth-first search.

## 5   Results

We used the same parameters for *all* our experiments, which indicates the stability of our method. The region growing parameters defined in §3 are defined as $K = 80$ and $k = 10$. A region $R$ is deemed valid iff $|R| \geq 7$. In the reported experiments, we processed on average $N = 5000$ points per image (sometimes tens of thousands) and 15 matches per point, i.e., $|\mathcal{M}| = 75,000$ on average. The number of matches per point, up to 650 in our examples, depends on the ambiguity of the descriptor value. A complete region-growing trial can take up to 4 seconds, for a very large and dense region. For deformable object matching and calibration, we performed 1000 attempts to grow regions; for pattern detection, all possible seeds were explored.

### 5.1   Deformable Object Matching

We evaluated our method on deformable object matching using the ETHZ Toys dataset (40 images of 9 models, and 23 test images), testing each model image against each test image. We compared with Ferrari et al. [14], Kannala et al. [13] and Cho et al. [15], as reported in their papers. For a fair comparison, we used MSER and Harris-affine features with SIFT descriptors, like [15]. Methods [13, 14] additionally use color information and dense photometric information.

Performance is reported in the ROC curve on the left part of Fig. 3, which depicts the detection rate versus false positive rate, letting a detection threshold vary. (An object is considered as detected if the number of produced matches,

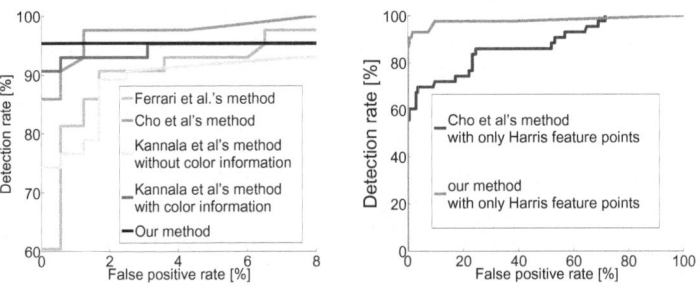

**Fig. 3.** ROC curves on the ETHZ Toys dataset

**Table 1.** Some images of the *Books* dataset and calibration results

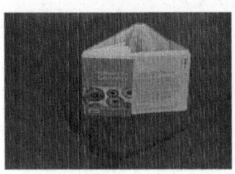 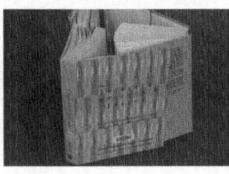

| Methods | Cameras | Match Time |
|---------|---------|------------|
| Ours | **20/31** | 60 mn |
| [1] + [3] | 5/31 | **5 mn** |
| [15] | 7/31 | 2880 mn |
| [14] | 2/31 | 540 mn |

**Table 2.** Some images of the *Mars* dataset and calibration results

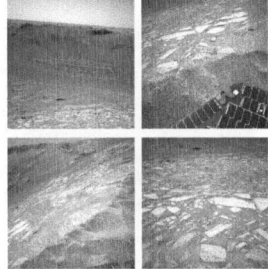

| Methods | # Cams | MSRE | # Tracks |
|---------|--------|------|----------|
| Ours | **60/60** | $5.00 \times 10^{-2}$ | **75, 966** |
| [1] $(\ell = 0.3)$ + [3] | 22/60 | $\mathbf{2.00 \times 10^{-2}}$ | 3, 266 |
| [1] $(\ell = 0.4)$ + [3] | 30/60 | $3.13 \times 10^{-2}$ | 5, 598 |
| [1] $(\ell = 0.5)$ + [3] | **33/60** | $47.50 \times 10^{-2}$ | 1, 131 |
| [1] $(\ell = 0.6)$ + [3] | 28/60 | $5.68 \times 10^{-2}$ | 6, 378 |
| [1] $(\ell = 0.7)$ + [3] | 28/60 | $6.47 \times 10^{-2}$ | 6, 533 |
| [1] $(\ell = 0.8)$ + [3] | 28/60 | $8.27 \times 10^{-2}$ | **6, 667** |
| [1] $(\ell = 0.9)$ + [3] | 28/60 | $8.84 \times 10^{-2}$ | 6, 564 |

summed over all its model views, exceeds this threshold.) Our method outperforms others, except for high false positive rate. This makes our method attractive for object matching tasks that tolerate only few wrong detections.

We performed a second experiment with the same dataset and the same parameters as Cho et al. [15], but only considering Harris affine features, which are reported to be among the most ambiguous affine-covariant features [18]. The right part of Fig. 3 confirms that our method is less prone to false detection, as it outperforms Cho et al.'s method both for low and high false positive rates.

## 5.2 Accurate and Scalable Matching for Camera Calibration

We tested a calibration task using Bundler [19] as a black-box taking as input a set of matches. We used two pathological datasets, which are hard to calibrate: *Books* (31 images) and *Mars* (60 images)[1]. In *Books* (cf. Table 1), matching ambiguities arises from the uniform background and the chair, as well as the repeated letters on the covers. We calibrate (here with Harris-affine features) many more cameras than Ferrari et al.'s [14], Cho et al.'s [15], and a baseline consisting in a Lowe criterion [1] followed by a RANSAC filter [3] estimating the fundamental matrix. In *Mars* (cf. Table 2), the landscape is very flat and the numerous rocks create ambiguous matches. Yet all 60 cameras are calibrated successfully with our method (with DoG features), contrary to RANSAC, which only calibrates half of the cameras. The mean squared reprojection error (MSRE, in pixels) and the number of consistent scene tracks also compare favorably. Our implementation has actually been used in the 3D-reconstruction chain of the winners of the *PRoVisG Mars 3D Challenge 2011*, from which this dataset is extracted. For this dataset, all 1770

---

[1] PRoVisG Mars 3D Challenge, http://cmp.felk.cvut.cz/mars/

**Table 3.** For a given number $|\mathcal{M}|$ of potential matches, number $N$ of corresponding features and average running time, on all image pairs of [18]'s dataset

| $\|\mathcal{M}\|$ | 3,000 | 10,000 | 30,000 | 100,000 |
|---|---|---|---|---|
| DoG | 2,676  0.21 s | 5,342  0.42 s | 7,027  0.70 s | 7,027  1.36 s |
| MSER | 1,585  0.84 s | 2,283  1.11 s | 2,283  1.46 s | 2,283  1.83 s |
| Hessian | 2,190  1.71 s | 5,054  3.02 s | 5,922  3.35 s | 5,922  3.99 s |
| Harris | 2,178  1.59 s | 6,250  3.62 s | 10,273  3.58 s | 10,623  4.01 s |

possible image pairs are considered in 3.5 hours using parallelization on a 8-core CPU Xeon 2.8GHz machine.

We also compared with a method for tensor-based, 3rd-order hypergraph matching [9], with image 1 and 4 of the *graffiti* dataset used in [18], where the ground truth homography $\mathbf{H}$ is known. DoG features were detected and described with the SIFT descriptor. We evaluated the accuracy $a$, i.e., the proportion of actually correct matches among produced ones, as a function of the number $N_f$ of features to match. To enable comparison, we experimented with various feature sets such that $|\mathcal{X}| = |\mathcal{Y}| = N_f$ and there is a bijection between $\mathcal{X}$ and $\mathcal{Y}$ such that for each $x \in \mathcal{X}$, there is a unique $y \in \mathcal{Y}$ satisfying $\|\mathbf{H}x - y\| \leq 5$ pixels, and likewise when permuting $\mathcal{X}$ and $\mathcal{Y}$. For bare TM (3rd-order affinities only), performance is poor: $a \leq 0.80$ for $N_f \leq 20$ and $a \leq 0.05$ for $N_f \geq 30$. Adding 1st-order SIFT descriptors to 3rd-order affinities improves it: $0.75 \leq a \leq 0.85$ for $N_f \leq 200$. But our method achieves better results: $0.95 \leq a$ for $N_f \leq 200$.

Although our theoretical complexity is $O(BN^2 \log N + \log |\mathcal{M}|)$, where $N$ is the number of features and $B$ the maximum degree of ambiguity of matches in $\mathcal{M}$, it is less than quadratic in $N$ in practice, as illustrated in Table 3 on [18]'s dataset. (DoG is faster as it requires no ellipse intersection computation.) It is better, e.g., than tensor-based matching [9], which would be here $O(N^3 \log N)$ or $O(N^4 \log N)$, or agglomerative clustering [15], which is at least $O(|\mathcal{M}|^2)$.

### 5.3   Accurate Pattern Localization: Window Detection

We experimented with pattern detection, looking for windows in building facades. Although this problem has already been attacked [20–23], *accurate* localization has been treated very little for unrectified images. Window localization is challenging because of the wide range of appearance variety, the lack of texture, and the illumination variations. Unrectified images adds up to these challenges. Windows are then related by homographies or affinities: they may vary in size and shape, and it is difficult to detect small windows with almost no texture.

We used *eTRIMS* [24] for evaluation, which displays many different architectural and building styles, with annotations for windows. We selected the 45 images having at least 6 windows. For each image, we indicated seed windows manually and we generated rectified images for comparison purposes. In the case where images are rectified, they are indicated either manually or by a trained cascade classifier (CC) [25]. Then our pattern search retrieves missing windows.

To apply our repetitive pattern search, DoG, Harris-Affine and MSER features are extracted in each image and described by the SIFT descriptor. We only keep

**Table 4.** Example image and results on the *eTRIMS* dataset. (CC) is the cascade classifier run solely to detect windows. (Manual+ours) and (CC+ours) are methods where input window quadrilaterals are respectively provided manually and by the classifier (CC) combined with our method to retrieves missing windows.

|  |  | Rectified images | | Unrectified Images |  |
|---|---|---|---|---|---|
| Methods | | TPR | TNR | TPR | TNR |
| Manual+ours | | 75% | 96% | 71% | 98% |
| CC+ours | | 60% | 93% | N/A | N/A |
| CC | | 46% | 96% | N/A | N/A |

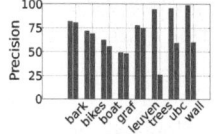 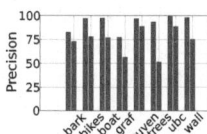 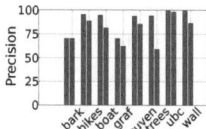 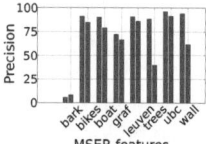

**Fig. 4.** Precision (%) of region growing on Mikolajczyk et al's. dataset (images 1-3). Affinities are computed from match triples (green) or single matches (red).

matches whose distrust score is less than 1.2, i.e., matches within 20% of the best match (description-wise). The bounding box of the pattern windows is dilated by 15% before search, to include some surrounding information, and shrunk back when instances are found to estimate the window region accurately.

The methods are compared in terms of mean true positive rate ($\overline{\text{TPR}}$) and mean true negative rate ($\overline{\text{TNR}}$), which should ideally be close to 1. Results are reported in Table 4. In case the image is not rectified, the $\overline{\text{TPR}}$, loses 4 points w.r.t. the rectified case. This slight degradation is chiefly due to estimation errors of the geometric transformation between the matched patterns. Shift and size errors between the geometric region of the detected pattern and the estimated image region also accumulates. Still, our method achieves a very low $\overline{\text{FPR}}$ of 2%.

## 5.4   Affinity Estimation: Triple vs Single Match

Finally, as discussed in the introduction, we evaluate the interest of match triples $(m, m', m'')$ to construct accurate and robust affinities vs resorting to single matches $m = (x, y)$, using the shapes $(\mathcal{S}_x, \mathcal{S}_y)$ and orientation $(\mathbf{o}_x, \mathbf{o}_y)$. Experiments with Mikolajczyk et al.'s dataset [18] demonstrate that our region growing process performs consistently and significantly better when affinities $\phi$ are estimated with match triples. Each dataset consists of 6 images. For each dataset and for a given kind of feature $f$, we extract all feature points of type $f$. We match image 1 to images 2–5. Initial $f$-matches are obtained and ranked with Lowe's criterion. The distrust threshold is set to $\ell = 1$. On average, our region growing deals with $7,000$ to $28,000$ $f$-matches with an outlier proportion of at least 75%. We compare the performance of our region growing in terms of precision for both variants: triples and single matches (see Fig. 4).

Precision rates for triples are consistently better. We give two explanations. First, orientation estimation is often unstable; it remains sensitive to illuminations changes, blurring and compression. Second, local affinities estimated from the shape of DoG features are unsurprisingly inaccurate and consequently produces worse precision rates in general. Even when elliptic features are used, affinities estimated from triples still produce much better results in many cases.

## 6    Conclusion

We have proposed a feature matching method that enforces photometric and geometric consistency. As illustrated by our experiments, it is efficient, scalable, accurate and robust, even in the presence of high ambiguity, improving over other existing methods. This allows applications in repetitive pattern detection.

Our approach belongs to the region-growing/match-propagation family [26]. Although it uses known ideas for matching under affinity constraint [18], it includes original ingredients and, as a whole, provides a unique blend. Our propagation is based on local affinities like [13–15], not pixel adjacency [26, 27], flow [26] or similitudes [28]. Our affinities are computed from match triples (any kind of feature points, possibly in combination), not necessarily affine correspondences [14, 15], 2nd moment matrix plus gradient orientation [13], or patch transformations [26, 28]. Our affinity constraint is 4th-order and sensitive to feature scale, not 2nd-order [6, 8, 15], 3rd-order [10] and photometric [9], or 4th-order reduced to points [7, 10]. For precision and robustness, each match of our growing regions selects nearby scale-consistent candidates; each candidate (best first) then looks for a nearby consistent triple in the region. It is simpler that the expansion-contraction phases of [14]. In [13], a region point only defines a single affinity to select admissible candidates, while in [15], growing is via agglomerative clustering. Our propagation is isotropic, image-order insensitive, scale-invariant and adapts to varying detection density like [15], contrary to fixed-size grid in model image [14], fixed-size pixel neighborhood [13, 26, 27] or reference image [28]. We are purely based on features, like [15], rather than photometric similarity. We do not require images (pixels) after feature detection, unlike [13, 14, 26–28], nor a regular flow of images [27] or epipolarly rectified image pairs [27]. All these characteristics are crucial for robustness and precision in difficult settings.

**Acknowledgements.** This work is part of IMAGINE, a joint research project between Ecole des Ponts ParisTech (ENPC) and CSTB.

## References

1. Lowe, D.G.: Distinctive image features from scale-invariant keypoints. International Journal of Computer Vision 60, 91–110 (2004)
2. Tola, E., Lepetit, V., Fua, P.: Daisy: An efficient dense descriptor applied to wide-baseline stereo. IEEE Trans. Pattern Anal. Mach. Intell. 32, 815–830 (2010)
3. Fischler, M.A., Bolles, R.C.: Random sample consensus: A paradigm for model fitting with applications to image analysis and automated cartography. Commun. ACM 24, 381–395 (1981)
4. Pritchett, P., Zisserman, A., Zisserman, A.: Wide baseline stereo matching. In: ICCV, pp. 754–760 (1998)

5. Brown, M., Lowe, D.: Invariant features from interest point groups. In: BMVC, pp. 656–665 (2002)
6. Leordeanu, M., Hebert, M.: A spectral technique for correspondence problems using pairwise constraints. In: ICCV, pp. 1482–1489 (2005)
7. Zass, R., Shashua, A.: Probabilistic graph and hypergraph matching. In: CVPR (2008)
8. Choi, O., Kweon, I.S.: Robust feature point matching by preserving local geometric consistency. Comput. Vis. Image Underst. 113, 726–742 (2009)
9. Duchenne, O., Bach, F., Kweon, I.S., Ponce, J.: A tensor-based algorithm for high-order graph matching. IEEE Trans. PAMI 33, 2383–2395 (2011)
10. Chertok, M., Keller, Y.: Efficient high order matching. IEEE Transactions on Pattern Analysis and Machine Intelligence 32, 2205–2215 (2010)
11. Cho, M., Lee, J., Lee, K.M.: Reweighted Random Walks for Graph Matching. In: Daniilidis, K., Maragos, P., Paragios, N. (eds.) ECCV 2010, Part V. LNCS, vol. 6315, pp. 492–505. Springer, Heidelberg (2010)
12. Zheng, Y., Doermann, D.: Robust point matching for nonrigid shapes by preserving local neighborhood structures. Tr. PAMI 28 (2006)
13. Kannala, J., Rahtu, E., Brandt, S., Heikkila, J.: Object recognition and segmentation by non-rigid quasi-dense matching. In: CVPR, pp. 1–8 (2008)
14. Ferrari, V., Tuytelaars, T., Van Gool, L.: Simultaneous Object Recognition and Segmentation by Image Exploration. In: Pajdla, T., Matas, J(G.) (eds.) ECCV 2004. LNCS, vol. 3021, pp. 40–54. Springer, Heidelberg (2004)
15. Cho, M., Lee, J., Lee, K.M.: Feature correspondence and deformable object matching via agglomerative correspondence clustering. In: ICCV (2009)
16. Mikolajczyk, K., Schmid, C.: An Affine Invariant Interest Point Detector. In: Heyden, A., Sparr, G., Nielsen, M., Johansen, P. (eds.) ECCV 2002, Part I. LNCS, vol. 2350, pp. 128–142. Springer, Heidelberg (2002)
17. Matas, J., Chum, O., Urban, M., Pajdla, T.: Robust wide baseline stereo from maximally stable extremal regions. In: BMVC, pp. 384–393 (2002)
18. Mikolajczyk, K., Tuytelaars, T., Schmid, C., Zisserman, A., Matas, J., Schaffalitzky, F., Kadir, T., Gool, L.V.: A comparison of affine region detectors. IJCV 65, 43–72 (2005), http://www.robots.ox.ac.uk/~vgg/research/affine/
19. Snavely, N., Seitz, S.M., Szeliski, R.: Modeling the world from internet photo collections. Int. J. Comput. Vision 80, 189–210 (2008)
20. Lee, S.C., Nevatia, R.: Extraction and integration of window in a 3D building model from ground view image. In: CVPR (2), pp. 113–120 (2004)
21. Ali, H., Seifert, C., Jindal, N., Paletta, L., Paar, G.: Window detection in facades. In: ICIAP, pp. 837–842 (2007)
22. Haugeard, J.E., Philipp-Foliguet, S., Precioso, F.: Windows and facades retrieval using similarity on graph of contours. In: ICIP, pp. 269–272 (2009)
23. Recky, M., Leberl, F.: Windows detection using k-means in cie-lab color space. In: ICPR, pp. 356–359 (2010)
24. Korč, F., Förstner, W.: eTRIMS Image Database for interpreting images of man-made scenes. Technical Report TR-IGG-P-2009-01, University of Bonn (2009)
25. Viola, P.A., Jones, M.J.: Robust real-time face detection. IJCV 57, 137–154 (2004)
26. Lhuillier, M., Quan, L.: Match propagation for image-based modeling and rendering. Tr. PAMI 24, 1140–1146 (2002)
27. Cech, J., Sanchez-Riera, J., Horaud, R.: Scene flow estimation by growing correspondence seeds. In: CVPR, pp. 3129–3136 (2011)
28. HaCohen, Y., Shechtman, E., Goldman, D.B., Lischinski, D.: Non-rigid dense correspondence with applications for image enhancement. SIGGRAPH 30 (2011)

# Hierarchical Object Representations for Visual Recognition via Weakly Supervised Learning

Tianzhu Zhang[1], Rui Cai[2], Zhiwei Li[2], Lei Zhang[2], and Hanqing Lu[1]

[1] Institute of Automation, Chinese Academy of Sciences, Beijing 100190, P.R. China
[2] Microsoft Research Asia, Beijing 100080, P.R. China
{tzzhang,luhq}@nlpr.ia.ac.cn, {ruicai,zli,leizhang}@microsoft.com

**Abstract.** In this paper, we propose a weakly supervised approach to learn hierarchical object representations for visual recognition. The learning process is carried out in a bottom-up manner to discover latent visual patterns in multiple scales. To relieve the disturbance of complex backgrounds in natural images, bounding boxes of foreground objects are adopted as weak knowledge in the learning stage to promote those visual patterns which are more related to the target objects. The difference between the patterns of foreground objects and backgrounds is relatively vague at low-levels, but becomes more distinct along with the feature transformations to high-levels. In the test stage, an input image is verified against the learnt patterns level-by-level, and the responses at each level construct a hierarchy of representations which indicates the occurring possibilities of the target object at various scales. Experiments on two PASCAL datasets showed encouraging results for visual recognition.

## 1 Introduction

Recent research efforts have indicated that adopting hierarchical representations is a very promising way to improve visual recognition and classification [1–7]. Multiple levels of features organized in a hierarchical structure can summarize images from various scales, and can incorporate spatial information to increase distinguishability.

The most straightforward yet successful way to construct hierarchical features is to extract a series of statistics (e.g.averaging histogram [3] or max-pooling [5]) at multiple scales based on the bottom-level local appearance descriptors (e.g.gray-scale or SIFT [8]). To better characterize spatial information, a more sophisticated manner is to learn new descriptors for each level of the hierarchical structure. Specifically, descriptors of an upper-level are usually generated through some kind of (especially, nonlinear) transformation of the features of the underneath level. In this way, high-level descriptors are capable of characterizing more complex and discriminative visual patterns (e.g.contours, corners, and angles, beyond low-level oriented edges [4]). This multi-level learning strategy has been proved to be quite successful. Well-known methods following such a strategy include the hyper-features [1], convolutional restricted Boltzmann machines [4], and hierarchical sparse coding [2, 6, 7].

K.M. Lee et al. (Eds.): ACCV 2012, Part I, LNCS 7724, pp. 474–485, 2013.
© Springer-Verlag Berlin Heidelberg 2013

Almost all the aforementioned approaches are unsupervised and do not distinguish foreground objects and context backgrounds in feature learning . An unavoidable drawback here is that the learnt features are prone to be disturbed by background noise. This is especially serious for methods which learn descriptors level-by-level, where noise is likely to be magnified in the process of feature transformations. This is because the signal-to-noise-ratio drops at high-levels, as a patch of larger-scale may include more background noise. Therefore, these methods mainly work on datasets like face, handwriting, and those in the Caltech-101 dataset [9]. Such object images are usually with relatively clean background, and the foreground objects dominate the pictures.

By contrast, it is more challenge to do visual recognition of natural images, such as those in the PASCAL VOC dataset [10]. In a natural image, the object to be classified may be small, located at an unnoticeable corner, and mixed with complex background and other objects. Empirical studies show that, in this situation, it is still possible to achieve good performance if both the feature learning and recognition are restricted to only working on foreground objects [11]. However, such an assumption is impractical as the locations of foreground objects are typically unknown in the recognition stage.

In this paper, we propose a weakly supervised approach to learn hierarchical object representations for visual recognition of natural images, where the locations of foreground objects are only required in the training stage. The proposed approach basically follows the existing hierarchical structures, to learn features (visual patterns) level-by-level. The main difference is that, in this paper, the foreground object locations are employed to vote which learnt visual patterns are more related to objects. In low-levels, foreground objects and backgrounds are still very likely to share similar visual patterns; however, the non-linear transformations (e.g.convolution or max-pooling) that combine low-level patterns can make the high-level patterns more distinguishable. Especially, the voting from foreground objects is involved in the feature transformations, to highlight foreground object patterns and suppress background patterns. In this way, patterns at high-levels tend to describe foreground objects, and are considered as "detectors" in recognition to verify whether an image contains such objects. This also explains why our approach does not need information of foreground locations in recognition. Some examples are shown in Fig. 2 to provide a concrete illustration to the proposed idea.

## 2    Related Work

Visual object recognition has attracted considerable research efforts over the last few years. A noticeable trend is to learn hierarchical features which can provide more comprehensive representations to objects. The most well-known hierarchical feature representation is the spatial pyramid matching (SPM) kernel [3], which divides an images into multi-scale pathes and computes the bag-of-feature histogram for each path. These patch-based histograms are finally concatenated to form a vector representation of the image. To extend SPM, Yang et al. [5] proposed the ScSPM model which introduces sparse coding [12] and max-pooling into the feature extraction. In [5], sparse coding replaces the traditional K-means vector quantization to construct bag-of-feature dictionary; and max-pooling replaces the averaging histogram in SPM. Both sparse coding and max-pooling have been frequently adopted by existing research work for visual recognition.

Beyond the simple multi-scale statistics in the SPM and ScSPM models, another popular trend to learn hierarchical feature representations is to construct a series of new "dictionaries" or "codebooks" for each level (scale), to enable those high-level features to describe more complicated spatial patterns. Representative work in this direction includes the "deep learning" framework [13] which build multi-level Restricted Boltzmann Machines (RBM) (also called "deep belief network" (DBN)) to encode latent visual patterns [4], and the hierarchical sparse coding methods [6, 7] which believe sparse representation is more biological plausible. In this paper, we follow the multi-level sparse coding framework, and use the learnt sparse code bases to characterize latent visual patterns.

The hierarchical features can also be learnt in a supervised fashion. With the category labels of visual objects, back-propagation like strategies have been leveraged to make the features more discriminative over different categories. For hierarchical sparse coding, a back-projection based dictionary learning was proposed in [6]; and for deep belief network, a common practice is to add a supervised layer as the top level of the network [13]. There are also other hierarchical representation methods [14, 15]. However, most of existing hierarchical representation methods [4, 6, 13, 14] work on clean object images (e.g., face, digits), and suffer from background noises when working on natural images. By contrast, the proposed approach is working on natural images. It is interesting in distinguishing foreground objects from backgrounds with weakly supervised information (e.g.bounding box of a foreground object), and can gradually remove noises and promote object-related patterns.

## 3    Algorithms

Given an image collection, which consists of multiple classes of objects and objects appear in complex backgrounds, e.g.the PASCAL VOC 2007 dataset [10], our goal is to learn hierarchical representations for each class of objects. In the training process, we assume that each image has bounding boxes to specify where the objects are.

**Learning Representations in Layer-1:** To simplify the notations, we assume that all images are $N \times N$, even though there is no limitation that the inputs must be square and equally sized images. Moreover, we use one image to present the algorithm. It is easy to generalize equations to multiple images by a simple sum operation. An illustration architecture of the proposed algorithm is shown in Fig. 1.

We first divide a whole image into $m \times m$ overlapping patches, and the spacing between two adjacent patches is $n$ pixels, e.g.$m$ is 8 and $n$ is 4 in our experiments. This schema leads to a very dense sampling to the image, and can effectively

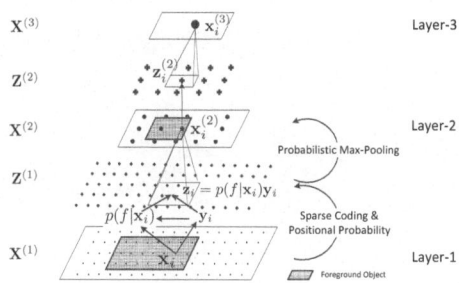

**Fig. 1.** The illustration architecture of the proposed algorithm to learn hierarchical representations. At the level $\ell$, a descriptor $\mathbf{x}_i^{(\ell)}$ is first translated into sparse codes $\mathbf{y}_i^{(\ell)}$, which is further weighed by the smoothed conditional probability $p(f|\mathbf{x}_i^{(\ell)})$ to highlight components related to foreground objects (shown in the area of red rectangle). In this way, a new descriptor $\mathbf{z}_i^{(\ell)}$ is generated for the $i$-th patch, based on which a probabilistic max-pooling is carried out to produce the descriptor of next level, i.e., $\mathbf{x}_i^{(\ell+l)}$.

prevent splitting of visual patterns. To represent a patch, we extract a 128-dimensional SIFT descriptor [8]. In this way, the image is represented by a $128 \times M$ matrix, where $M = ((N - m)/n + 1) \times ((N - m)/n + 1)$ is the number of patches. As proposed in [5], we adopt a simultaneous sparse coding technique to learn a basis set [16]. The problem is defined as

$$\min_{\mathbf{y},\mathbf{B}} \sum_{i=1}^{M} \|\mathbf{x}_i - \mathbf{B}\mathbf{y}_i\| + \gamma |\mathbf{y}_i| \\ s.t. \ \|\mathbf{b}_k\| \leq c, \forall k = 1, 2, ..., K \tag{1}$$

where $\mathbf{x}_i$ is the SIFT descriptor for the $i$-th patch, $\mathbf{B} = \{\mathbf{b}_k, 1 \leq k \leq K\}$ is a basis set with $K$ column vectors, $\mathbf{y}_i$ are coefficients, $\gamma$ and $c$ are constants. Eq. (1) can be efficiently solved by an iterative algorithm, in which the variables, $\{\mathbf{y}_i, \ 1 \leq i \leq M\}$ and $\mathbf{B}$, are optimized alternatively [16]. Once we have learned a basis set, we run a standard sparse coding solver to compute the coefficients $\mathbf{y}_i$ for each patch. $\mathbf{y}_i = \{y_{ik}, 1 \leq k \leq K\}$ is a $K$-dimensional column vector, while most of its elements are zero. $\{\mathbf{b}_k, 1 \leq k \leq K\}$ can be considered as $K$ latent visual patterns, and $y_{ik}$ denotes the correlation between the $i$-th patch and the $k$-th pattern.

We simply notate the object area in an image as "foreground", $f$, which is often specified by a bounding box, and the other part of the image as "background". Given a patch $\mathbf{x}_i$ , we define the *positional probability* that it belongs to the foreground as

$$p_{pos}(f|\mathbf{x}_i) = \frac{area(\mathbf{x}_i \cap f)}{area(\mathbf{x}_i)} \tag{2}$$

where $area(.)$ means the area of a region, and $\mathbf{x}_i \cap f$ means the common part of the $i$-th patch and the foreground. Thus, if a patch completely appears in background, its positional probability will be zero, otherwise it will be non zero.

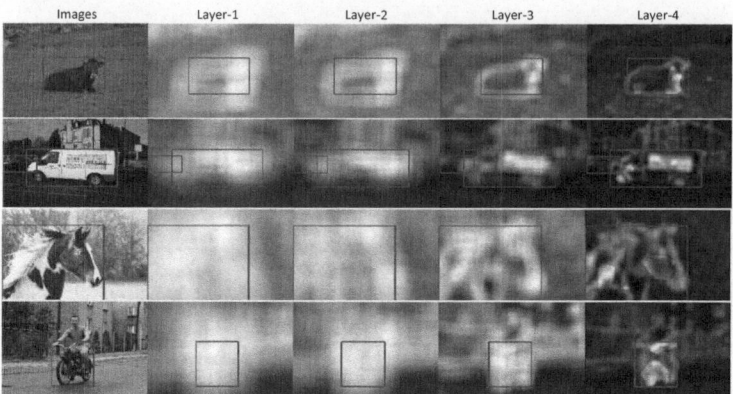

**Fig. 2.** The probability maps of $p(f|\mathbf{x}_i)$ for Layer-1 to Layer 4, on several object categories from VOC 2006 dataset [17]. Locations of foreground objects are shown with red rectangles (bounding boxes). The bright parts of a probability map indicate high probability of the related regions being associated with foreground objects. It's clear that with the increasing of layers, the foreground objects become more distinguishable on the probability maps.

Consequently, we can compute the probability that a basis $\mathbf{b}_k$ belongs to the foreground by a voting strategy

$$p(f|\mathbf{b}_k) = [y_{1k}, ..., y_{Mk}][p_{pos}(f|\mathbf{x}_1), ..., p_{pos}(f|\mathbf{x}_M)]^T \qquad (3)$$

Here, $y_{ik}$ can be deemed as an indicator of whether $\mathbf{b}_k$ is correlated with the patch $\mathbf{x}_i$, and $p(f|\mathbf{b}_k)$ averages over patches to estimate the probability score that the basis $\mathbf{b}_k$ being associated with the foregrounds. After obtaining these scores, they can be normalized to get the corresponding probabilities. Consequently, the smoothed conditional probability that a patch $\mathbf{x}_i$ (with respect to its sparse code $\mathbf{y}_i$) belongs to the foregrounds is defined as in Eq.(4).

$$p(f|\mathbf{x}_i) = \sum_{k=1}^{K} p(f|\mathbf{b}_k)y_{ik} \qquad (4)$$

This probability contains two kinds of information, i.e. whether the patch appears in the foreground, and whether its sparse code is similar to codes often appearing in the foreground. The second column of Fig. 2 shows some example images. The probability map contains some high probability points in the background, and have a few low probability points in the foreground (Note, our approach is neither to generate saliency maps nor locate objects. Its goal is to learn object-specific representations which are robust to noises. The probability map-like illustrations are just used to show effectiveness of the models). This fact indicates that only from a descriptor of a local patch, we cannot confidently know whether it belongs to the foreground or the background.

Finally, we multiply the sparse code $\mathbf{y}_i$ with the smoothed probability $p(f|\mathbf{x}_i)$ to generate a new descriptor for the patch $\mathbf{x}_i$, as

$$\mathbf{z}_i = p(f|\mathbf{x}_i)\mathbf{y}_i \tag{5}$$

For those patches which do not belong to the foreground, or whose codes $\mathbf{y}_i$ are not similar to codes of patches appearing in the foreground, their new codes $\mathbf{z}_i$ are likely to be zero. In this way, we represent an image as an $M \times K$ matrix $\mathbf{Z}$. As shown in Fig. 1, this representation will be the input of the second layer.

**Learning Representations in Layer-2:** The second layer is constructed by merging adjacent patches in the first layer, to describe spatial information in a larger scale. The new patch size is $(2 \times m) \times (2 \times m)$, and the spacing between two adjacent patches is still $n$ pixels . A spatial max-pooling technique similar to [5] is adopted here to generate the input descriptors $\mathbf{x}_i^{(2)}$ for the second layer, as

$$\begin{aligned}
\mathbf{x}_i^{(2)} &= \phi\left(\mathbf{z}_j^{(1)}, j \in A_i^{(2)}\right) \\
&= \max_{j \in A_i^{(2)}}\left(\left.\left|p(f|\mathbf{x}_j^{(1)})\mathbf{y}_j^{(1)}\right|\right._{abs}\right)
\end{aligned} \tag{6}$$

where $\phi(.)$ is the max-pooling function defined on the collection of patches $A_i^{(2)}$ in Layer-1, and $|.|_{abs}$ is the element-wise absolute value of a vector. In Fig. 1, to distinguish from the max-pooling work in [5], we termed $\phi(.)$ as *probabilistic max-pooling*, as the foreground probabilities $p(f|\mathbf{x}_i^{(1)})$ participate in the pooling. From now on, we will add a superscript $^{(1)}$ for the variables in Layer-1, e.g.$\mathbf{z}_j^{(1)}$ is the $\mathbf{z}_j$ in the last section.

Once we have obtained the new descriptors $\mathbf{x}_i^{(2)}$, we re-run a simultaneous sparse coding to estimate a basis set, and then re-compute those probabilities for bases and patches as in Eq. (2)–(4). The only difference between Layer-1 and Layer-2 is their inputs. In Layer-1, the inputs are SIFT descriptors of patches, while in Layer-2 the inputs are sparse codes obtained by probabilistic max-pooling. The third column of Fig. 2 illustrates the probabilities of patches obtained in Layer-2. The number of noisy points are much smaller than in Layer-1. This fact indicates that high level structures are helpful to resolve confusion in low layers.

From Layer-2, it is easy to generalize the algorithm to Layer-3 and higher layers. The fourth and fifth columns of Fig. 2 show the probability map in Layer-3 and Layer-4. With the increasing of layers, only complex and intrinsic visual patterns of objects are preserved, while other patterns are almost vanishing. The obtained hierarchical model is represented as $< \mathbf{B}^{(\ell)}, p(f|\mathbf{b}_k^{(\ell)}) >$, where $k \in [1, K^{(\ell)}]$, $\ell \in [1, L]$, and $L$ is the maximum level of the model.

**Discussion:** To explain why the noisy points are vanishing, let's see the objective function of simultaneous sparse coding in Layer-2, as

$$\begin{aligned}
&\min_{\mathbf{y}^{(2)}, \mathbf{B}^{(2)}} \sum_{i=1}^{M^{(2)}} \left\|\mathbf{x}_i^{(2)} - \mathbf{B}^{(2)}\mathbf{y}_i^{(2)}\right\| + \gamma\left|\mathbf{y}_i^{(2)}\right| \\
&= \min_{\mathbf{y}^{(2)}, \mathbf{B}^{(2)}} \sum_{i=1}^{M^{(2)}} \left\|\phi(\mathbf{z}_j^{(1)}, j \in A_i^{(2)}) - \mathbf{B}^{(2)}\mathbf{y}_i^{(2)}\right\| + \gamma\left|\mathbf{y}_i^{(2)}\right|
\end{aligned} \tag{7}$$

If a patch $\mathbf{x}_j^{(1)}$ is neither in the foreground nor similar to patches in the foreground, its descriptor $\mathbf{z}_j^{(1)} = p(f|\mathbf{x}_j^{(1)})\mathbf{y}_j^{(1)}$ is close to zero, and consequently $\mathbf{x}_i^{(2)}$ is more likely to be zero. A zero variable will have no impact to the basis set learned by the objective function in Eq. (7). Thus, the newly learned bases $\mathbf{B}^{(2)}$ focuses its energy on explaining those patches which are in the foreground themselves or similar to patches in foreground in Layer-1. The elimination to noise is a key insight of this paper, which differentiates our approach from existing hierarchical representation learning works, e.g.hierarchical sparse coding [6] and convolutional restricted Boltzmann machines [4].

A more straightforward approach to learning object representations is to just use patches in the bounding box. By considering a fact that some patches appearing in a bounding box may be meaningless patches (e.g., grass around a horse), we designed the learning approach as in this paper. For such a noisy patch in the foreground, although its positional probability $p_{pos}(f|\mathbf{x}_i^{(\ell)})$ is 1, its foreground probability $p(f|\mathbf{x}_i^{(\ell)})$ is almost zero because most of its similar patches appear in the background. In brief, patches in backgrounds will help remove meaningless patches in foreground bounding boxes, and consequently remove meaningless combinations in higher layers.

# 4 Object Category Recognition

The learned hierarchical models can be applied in many applications, e.g.object recognition and detection. In this paper, we use object category recognition to demonstrate their usages. Assuming we have an image collection with $C$ classes of objects, and consequently we can train $C$ hierarchical models.

## 4.1 Feature Extraction

Given an image, we extract its hierarchical representations at each level of a given learned model $\{< \mathbf{B}^{(\ell)}, p(f|\mathbf{b}_k^{(\ell)}) >, 1 \leq \ell \leq L\}$. Essentially, the model tells us the latent visual patterns ($\mathbf{B}^{(\ell)}$) at each level, as well as the correlation of each pattern to the target object class ($p(f|\mathbf{b}_k^{(\ell)})$). In this way, we do not need bounding box of objects anymore in this process. The extracting approaches are very similar in all layers.

In Layer-1, the process consists of the following steps:
1-1) Dividing the image into $m \times m$ overlapping cells, in which the spacing is $n$ pixels, and then extracting SIFT descriptors for all the patches.
1-2) Solving a standard sparse coding problem to compute sparse code $\mathbf{y}_i^{(1)}$ for each patch, where the basis set is $\mathbf{B}^{(1)}$.
1-3) Computing foreground probability $p(f|\mathbf{x}_i^{(1)})$, and then sparse code $\mathbf{z}_i^{(1)}$ for each patch, in which the probability of basis is $p(f|\mathbf{b}_k^{(1)})$.

In Layer-2 and higher layers, the process consists of the following steps:
2-1) Running max-polling with respect to $\mathbf{Z}^{(\ell-1)}$ to obtain initial representations $\mathbf{x}_i^{(\ell)}$ for each patch.

2-2) Solving a standard sparse coding problem to compute sparse code $\mathbf{y}_i^{(\ell)}$ for each patch, where the basis set is $\mathbf{B}^{(\ell)}$.

2-3) Computing foreground probability $p(f|\mathbf{x}_i^{(\ell)})$, and then sparse code $\mathbf{z}_i^{(\ell)}$ for each patch, in which the probability of basis is $p(f|\mathbf{b}_k^{(\ell)})$.

If we apply a model of the $i$-th category to images not containing the $i$-th class object, the responses $\mathbf{y}_i^{(\ell)}$ and $\mathbf{z}_i^{(\ell)}$ are likely to be zeros. However, for images which contain the $i$-th class objects, they are likely to have some non-zero responses, which will be the key discriminative features.

Considering the numbers of patches are different due to various image sizes, the patch-based sparse codes $\mathbf{z}_i^{(\ell)}$ are aggregated via applying a $3 \times 3$ grid at each level. Histogram of the sparse codes are computed over patches in the same grid, to form a $(9 \times K^{(\ell)})$-dimensional vector for the $\ell$-th level. In total, the feature length is $9 \times \sum_{\ell=1}^{L} K^{(\ell)}$.

### 4.2  Classifier Training

We have trained hierarchical models for each object class, and extracted features with respect to each model for each image in the whole image collection. Thus, for each image, it has $C + 1$ kinds of features, i.e.$[F_0, F_1, ..., F_C]$, where $F_0$ is an object independent feature and $F_{i>0}$ is hierarchical features for $i$-th category. To obtain $F_0$, we run spatial max-pooling with respect to the outputs of step (1-1)~(1-2) to encode spatial information in a SPM manner, as proposed in [3, 5], which has been demonstrated as one of the state-of-the-art representations for object recognition.

We train an one-vs-others SVM classifier for each category, in which linear kernel is adopted [5]. We use a concatenation of $F_0$ and $F_i$ as features to train the $i$-th classifier. For example, to train a binary classifier for the 2-nd class, the feature is $[F_0, F_2]$. The output of each classifier is a probability score. Thus, we can decide the predication result of a test image by ranking its probabilities belonging to various categories.

## 5  Experiments

In this section, we present experimental results that validate the effectiveness of our proposed method on two PASCAL benchmark datasets. We also conduct a thorough comparison with the most related methods.

### 5.1  Experiment Setup

We conducted experiments on two publicly available and popular PASCAL VOC Challenges databases, i.e.2006 [17] and 2007 [10]. The VOC 2006 dataset contains 10 classes in 5,304 images, on which a total of 9,507 annotated objects can be found. The VOC 2007 dataset contains 20 classes in 9,963 images with 24,640 annotated objects. These datasets are split into a fixed training, validation, and

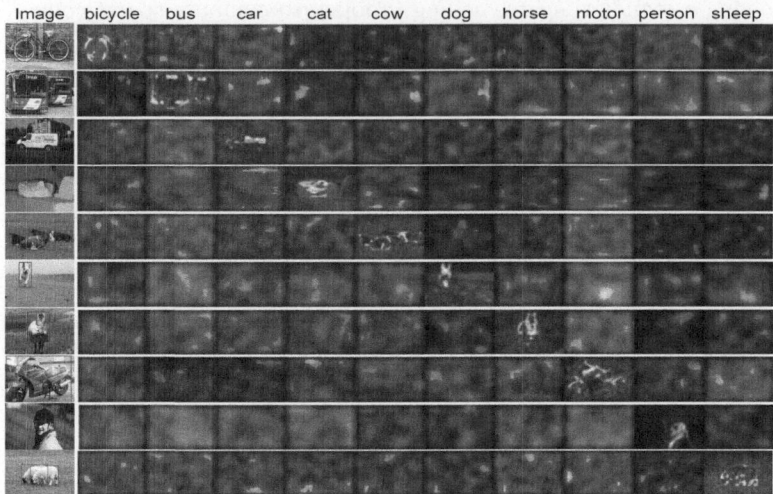

**Fig. 3.** Visualization of model responses. Each row shows an example image from one object class. Each column shows a hierarchical model learned for an object class. A cell [i, j] shows the responses of the $i$-th image with respect to the $j$-th model. Only the responses to the Level 3 models ($p(f|\mathbf{x}_i^{(3)})$) are shown in this table.

test set. In the VOC 2006 database the training set contains 1277 images. The validation set has 1341 images and the test set 2686 images. The VOC 2007 database has 2501 training images, 2510 validation images, and 4952 test images.

In all experiments, we fix the patch size $m = 8$, spacing $n = 4$, $K^{(\cdot)} = 200$ in all layers. We trained a four-layer model for each object class. The codebook size for the $F_0$ feature is set to 4000. The total dimensionality of an $F_{i>1}$ feature for all the four layers is 7200. SVM classifiers are trained by the LIBLINEAR tool. Due to the linear kernel, we only have one SVM parameter, i.e.the $C$ of $C$-$SVM$. We merged the train and validation set to a new training set. 10-fold cross validation is adopted to find an optimal $C$. Due to the goal of this paper, we mainly want to evaluate the performance of the learned hierarchical models. Therefore unlike competitors of the VOC Challenges, we only sample one kind size of patches, generate one kind of descriptor, and do not do any post processing to improve performance. The simple settings make this work easy to repeat. To facilitate the comparison with existing literatures, we adopt Area Under ROC curve (AUC) to measure performances on VOC 2006 dataset [17], and mean Average Precision (mAP) to measure performances on VOC 2007 [10].

### 5.2    Visualization of Model Response

Given a dataset with $C$ classes of objects, we learn a hierarchical model for each class of objects. In the prediction stage, given an input image without bounding box to objects, we apply the $C$ models to extract $C$ kinds of features. In terms

**Table 1.** Performance on VOC 2006. Evaluated by Area Under ROC curve (AUC).

| | bicycle | bus | car | cat | cow | dog | horse | motorbike | person | sheep | **average** |
|---|---|---|---|---|---|---|---|---|---|---|---|
| ScSPM | 0.862 | 0.926 | 0.915 | 0.865 | 0.857 | 0.763 | 0.814 | 0.893 | 0.748 | 0.925 | 0.857 |
| Visual Bits[18] | 0.842 | 0.930 | 0.759 | 0.782 | 0.875 | 0.790 | 0.761 | 0.671 | 0.782 | 0.722 | 0.791 |
| 2006 winner[17] | 0.948 | 0.981 | 0.975 | 0.937 | 0.938 | 0.876 | 0.926 | 0.969 | 0.855 | 0.956 | 0.936 |
| Ours | 0.923 | 0.974 | 0.956 | 0.918 | 0.904 | 0.820 | 0.884 | 0.943 | 0.794 | 0.942 | 0.906 |

**Table 2.** Performance on VOC 2007. Evaluated by mean Average Precision (mAP).

| | BOF[11] | Object[11] | ScSPM | Ours |
|---|---|---|---|---|
| bottle | 0.192 | 0.197 | 0.196 | 0.237 |
| chair | 0.449 | 0.454 | 0.502 | 0.525 |
| diningtable | 0.276 | 0.580 | 0.443 | 0.509 |
| pottedplant | 0.156 | 0.263 | 0.239 | 0.255 |
| sofa | 0.369 | 0.519 | 0.459 | 0.518 |
| tv | 0.409 | 0.516 | 0.475 | 0.496 |
| bird | 0.378 | 0.387 | 0.405 | 0.449 |
| cat | 0.437 | 0.508 | 0.534 | 0.543 |
| cow | 0.274 | 0.376 | 0.349 | 0.364 |
| dog | 0.367 | 0.374 | 0.391 | 0.412 |
| horse | 0.692 | 0.568 | 0.753 | 0.761 |
| sheep | 0.284 | 0.427 | 0.417 | 0.441 |
| bicycle | 0.462 | 0.621 | 0.567 | 0.616 |
| bus | 0.496 | 0.624 | 0.538 | 0.585 |
| car | 0.690 | 0.813 | 0.714 | 0.751 |
| motorbike | 0.491 | 0.592 | 0.568 | 0.587 |
| train | 0.686 | 0.742 | 0.693 | 0.738 |
| aeroplane | 0.702 | 0.752 | 0.688 | 0.727 |
| boat | 0.623 | 0.574 | 0.656 | 0.684 |
| person | 0.792 | 0.836 | 0.794 | 0.818 |
| mean AP | 0.461 | 0.536 | 0.519 | 0.551 |

of facilitating category recognition, we expect that an image containing the $i$-th class object only generates non-zero responses to the $i$-th model, while generates zero responses to the other models. Fig. 3 illustrates the cross model probabilities $p(f|x_i^{(3)})$ for some example images from the VOC 2006 dataset. From these figures, we can see only the responses along the diagonal are significant, other responses are not significant.

## 5.3   Object Category Recognition

Table 1 and Table 2 show the categorization performance of different approaches on VOC 2006 and 2007 dataset respectively. For VOC 2006 dataset, two baseline approaches are selected, *ScSPM* and *Visual Bits* [18]. ScSPM is implemented by ourselves with the feature $F_0$. Visual Bits is a supervised dictionary learning

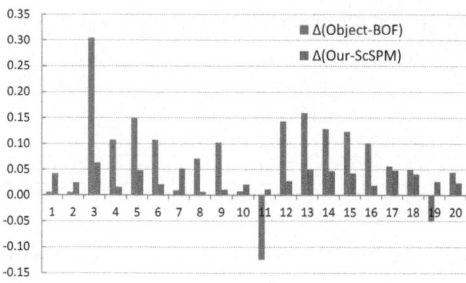

**Fig. 4.** Relative improvements of performance for the 20 categories of the VOC 2007 dataset due to considering of object areas

approach [18]. We also list the results of 2006 winners, which utilizes a bunch of features and mixes classification methods. Our performance is close to the winners'. The results indicate the effectiveness of the learned hierarchical models, which improves the feature extraction.

For VOC 2007 dataset, three approaches are compared with ours: *BOF* (a bag-of-features based classifier implemented by [11]), *Object* (both training and testing are conducted within bounding boxes to objects, and the area is represented by BOF models [11]), and *ScSPM* with feature $F_0$ [5]. Due to different implementations, performance of these approaches may be a little different from the reports of their authors. Results of our implementation are comparable with many easy to repeat works, e.g. [5]. Our approach significantly outperformed the *Object* approach, which is an ideal setting for object category recognition. This result indicates i) The hierarchical features are good complementary to the whole image features; ii) the learned visual patterns are better representations for objects than the common BOF models.

Fig. 4 shows the relative improvements due to taking the object areas into considering on VOC 2007 dataset. The relative improvement of BOF model is defined as $\Delta(Object - BOF)$ (Element-wise differences of the second and third columns of Table 2), which shows the effectiveness of information containing in the object area. The relative improvement of our approach is defined as $\Delta(Ours - ScSPM)$, which shows the effectiveness of the proposed hierarchical representations to objects. From this figure, we can see that the trends of the two improvements are coherent, that is, if the *Object* method can significantly improve the performance, our approach can improve too, and vice versa. This result indicates that our approach is able to capture useful visual patterns only in object areas, as well suppress the influence of complex background.

## 6    Conclusion

In this paper, we presented a weakly supervised approach to learning hierarchical representations for visual recognition. The experimental results are quite promising. First, it is observed that the learning process can filter background noise and highlight patterns of foreground objects. Second, based on the learnt object models, the extracted hierarchical features can help increase the recognition accuracy remarkably.

**Acknowledgment.** This work was supported by 973 Program (2010CB327905) and National Natural Science Foundation of China (61070104, 60835002).

# References

1. Agarwal, A., Triggs, B.: Hyperfeatures – Multilevel Local Coding for Visual Recognition. In: Leonardis, A., Bischof, H., Pinz, A. (eds.) ECCV 2006. LNCS, vol. 3951, pp. 30–43. Springer, Heidelberg (2006)
2. Kavukcuoglu, K., Sermanet, P., Boureau, Y.L., Gregor, K., Mathieu, M., LeCun, Y.: Learning convolutional feature hierarchies for visual recognition. In: NIPS (2010)
3. Lazebnik, S., Schmid, C., Ponce, J.: Beyond bags of features: Spatial pyramid matching for recognizing natural scene categories. In: CVPR (2) (2006)
4. Lee, H., Grosse, R., Ranganath, R., Ng, A.Y.: Convolutional deep belief networks for scalable unsupervised learning of hierarchical representations. In: ICML (2009)
5. Yang, J., Yu, K., Gong, Y., Huang, T.S.: Linear spatial pyramid matching using sparse coding for image classification. In: CVPR, pp. 1794–1801 (2009)
6. Yang, J., Yu, K., Huang, T.S.: Supervised translation-invariant sparse coding. In: CVPR (2010)
7. Zeiler, M.D., Krishnan, D., Taylor, G.W., Fergus, R.: Deconvolutional networks. In: CVPR (2010)
8. Lowe, D.G.: Distinctive image features from scale-invariant keypoints. Int. J. Comput. Vis. 60, 91–110 (2004)
9. Li, F.F., Fergus, R., Perona, P.: Learning generative visual models from few training examples: An incremental Bayesian approach tested on 101 object categories. Computer Vision and Image Understanding 106, 59–70 (2007)
10. Everingham, M., Van Gool, L., Williams, C.K.I., Winn, J., Zisserman, A.: The PASCAL Visual Object Classes Challenge 2007 (VOC2007) Results (2007)
11. Uijlings, J.R.R., Smeulders, A.W.M., Scha, R.J.H.: What is the spatial extent of an object? In: CVPR (2009)
12. Zhang, T., Ghanem, B., Liu, S., Ahuja, N.: Robust visual tracking via multi-task sparse learning. In: CVPR, pp. 2042–2049 (2012)
13. Bengio, Y.: Learning deep architectures for AI. Foundations and Trends in Machine Learning 2, 1–127 (2009)
14. Fidler, S., Boben, M., Leonardis, A.: A Coarse-to-Fine Taxonomy of Constellations for Fast Multi-class Object Detection. In: Daniilidis, K., Maragos, P., Paragios, N. (eds.) ECCV 2010, Part V. LNCS, vol. 6315, pp. 687–700. Springer, Heidelberg (2010)
15. Serre, T., Wolf, L., Bileschi, S., Riesenhuber, M., Poggio, T.: Robust object recognition with cortex-like mechanisms. IEEE TPAMI 29, 411–426 (2007)
16. Lee, H., Battle, A., Raina, R., Ng, A.Y.: Efficient sparse coding algorithms. In: NIPS, pp. 801–808 (2006)
17. Everingham, M., Zisserman, A., Williams, C.K.I., Van Gool, L.: The PASCAL Visual Object Classes Challenge 2006 (VOC2006) Results (2006)
18. Yang, L., Jin, R., Sukthankar, R., Jurie, F.: Unifying discriminative visual codebook generation with classifier training for object category recognition. In: CVPR (2008)

# Invariant Surface-Based Shape Descriptor for Dynamic Surface Encoding

Tony Tung and Takashi Matsuyama

Kyoto University, Graduate School of Informatics, Japan
tung@vision.kuee.kyoto-u.ac.jp, tm@i.kyoto-u.ac.jp

**Abstract.** This paper presents a novel approach to represent spatio-temporal visual information. We introduce a surface-based shape model whose structure is invariant to surface variations over time to describe 3D dynamic surfaces (e.g., obtained from multiview video capture). The descriptor is defined as a graph lying on object surfaces and anchored to invariant local features (e.g., extremal points). Geodesic-consistency-based priors are used as cues within a probabilistic framework to maintain the graph invariant, even though the surfaces undergo non-rigid deformations. Our contribution brings to 3D geometric data a temporally invariant structure that relies only on intrinsic surface properties, and is independent of surface parameterization (i.e., surface mesh connectivity). The proposed descriptor can therefore be used for efficient dynamic surface encoding, through transformation into 2D (geometry) images, as its structure can provide an invariant representation for 3D mesh models. Various experiments on challenging publicly available datasets are performed to assess invariant property and performance of the descriptor.

## 1 Introduction

It is one of the major goals of natural sciences to find invariant properties. In the 90s, computer vision scientists found several projectively invariant properties (e.g., viewpoint, illumination and curvature invariants) to characterize 3D object shape for recognition tasks [1, 2]. As it is difficult to find invariants on general 3D shapes that are not planar (or simple), local descriptors are used as well to model invariants and represent 3D object surface as a collection of small patches [3].

In this paper, we propose a new invariant surface-based shape descriptor for dynamic geometric objects, that is invariant to surface parameterization (e.g., surface mesh complexity or connectivity) and visual features (e.g., texture) as it relies only on intrinsic surface properties and geodesic paths. The descriptor is defined as a graph lying on object surface and anchored to invariant local features (e.g., extremal points). Positions of graph edges and nodes are optimized using a Bayesian probabilistic framework driven by two *geodesic consistency* cues: when surfaces undergo non-rigid deformations over time, the overall graph structure remains invariant to surface variations. We show that the descriptor can be applied for efficient encoding of 3D video data (or free-viewpoint video), which are becoming a popular media [4–7]. Particularly, when each 3D video

K.M. Lee et al. (Eds.): ACCV 2012, Part I, LNCS 7724, pp. 486–499, 2013.
© Springer-Verlag Berlin Heidelberg 2013

frame is reconstructed individually using multiview stereo techniques, the produced 3D surface models have no geometric consistency between each other: vertex number and mesh connectivity are different. It is then not trivial to find an optimal encoding scheme for the data structure. Moreover, as no adaptive resolution streaming mechanism exists for 3D video, communication and telepresence applications are still tedious on low-bandwidth networks. Although 3D video data can be post-processed to obtain meshes with consistent topology and connectivity [8–11], how to cope with geometry variations is still unclear (e.g., when the mesh resolution has to dynamically change). Here, inspired by [12], we propose to use the new invariant surface-based shape descriptor as cut graphs that cut open surface meshes for parameterization into a square domain. As the cut graphs are invariant regardless of mesh resolution, 3D video data can be transformed into sequences of 2D (geometry) images that are suitable for any 2D video encoding technology (e.g., MPEG-4). Related work is discussed in Sect. 2. The invariant surface-based shape descriptor is presented in Sect. 3. Section 4 introduces 3D video data encoding using the proposed model. Section 5 describes various experiments on challenging datasets. Section 6 concludes the paper with discussions.

## 2  Related Work

Several multi-view video capture systems were developed in the recent years [4–7] to provide a new media that gives users free-viewpoint visualization of 3D objects in motion (namely 3D video). Unlike depth maps (2.5D data) which are unclosed surface, 3D video data represent objects in full 3D as a sequence of reconstructed closed surfaces (3D meshes). This technology has potentially several applications in medicine, culture, communication, entertainment, etc. In practice, 3D video data are reconstructed frame-by-frame using multi-view stereo techniques [13].

To encode a sequence of 3D meshes, the state-of-the-art consists mainly of: (1) methods to compress every frame independently [14]; since redundant information between frames is not managed, encoding cannot be optimal. (2) techniques designed for 3D animation sequences [15–18]; as they are dedicated to meshes sharing the same connectivity, they cannot be applied directly to 3D video data (without post-processing with a surface alignment method [8–11]) and for adaptive bitrate streaming purpose.

On the other hand, the literature has provided numerous 3D shape models based on volume, surface, global or local properties (e.g., medial axis [19], skeleton-curve [20], Reeb graphs [21]). Although most of descriptors can capture intrinsic shape property, they are not suited for dynamic representation as their structure is usually too noisy. Similarly, skeleton fitting approaches can capture intrinsic information of shape based on surface or volume [22–24], but are not particularly invariant in time and often need prior knowledge on the shape to be described (e.g., a human skeleton). Moreover, once the structure (e.g., topology) is found, its relationship to surface variations is usually lost [25].

We propose a new surface-based shape descriptor that has invariant property to surface variations, and can be used as a cut graph [16, 26] to encode 3D video data using a transformation into 2D video, by cutting and parameterizing 3D surface meshes on image planes (see Sect. 4 and [12, 27]). To our knowledge, no similar model has been designed [1, 2, 28].

## 3   Invariant Surface-Based Shape Representation

### 3.1   Local Feature Extraction

Let us assume that dynamic surfaces representing real-world objects in motion can be approximated by compact 2-manifold meshes. We consider geodesic distances to characterize surface intrinsic properties, as geodesic distances are invariant to pose, and robust to shape variations when normalized [9, 21]. Let $\mu : \mathcal{S} \to \mathbb{R}$ denote the continuous function defined on the object surface $\mathcal{S}$:

$$\mu(v) = \int_{\mathcal{S}} g(v, s) dS, \tag{1}$$

where $g : \mathcal{S}^2 \to \mathbb{R}$ is the geodesic distance between two points on $\mathcal{S}$. Eq. 1 is the geodesic integral function whose critical points can be used to characterize shape (see Morse theory [29, 30]). For example, local maxima usually correspond to limb extremities of humans or animals while the global minimum corresponds to the body center. We use a Reeb graph to robustly identify and match critical points over time using geometry and topology information [21, 31–33] (see Fig. 1).

### 3.2   Temporal Geodesic Consistency

**Definition 1.** Assuming a set of $N$ points $\mathcal{B} = \{b_1, ..., b_N\}$ defined on a 2-manifold $\mathcal{S}$, the points $v_1$ and $v_2$ on $\mathcal{S}$ are said geodesically consistent with respect to $\mathcal{B}$ if and only if:

$$\forall i \in [1, N], \quad |g(v_1, b_i) - g(v_2, b_i)| \le \epsilon, \tag{2}$$

where $\epsilon \to 0$. If the points in $\mathcal{B}$ do not have any particular configuration of alignment or symmetry, the geodesic consistency property can be used to uniquely locate points on $\mathcal{S}$ when $N > 2$. In practice, the unicity is verified by checking the number of intersections of isovalue lines from $\mathcal{B}$, and ambiguities are solved by increasing $N$ or adding geometric constraints (e.g., Euclidean distance).

**Definition 2.** Assuming a set of $N$ points $\mathcal{B}^t = \{b_1^t, ..., b_N^t\}$ defined on a deformable 2-manifold $\mathcal{S}^t$ at time $t \in [t_b, t_e]$, the points $v_1^t$ and $v_2^t$ on $\mathcal{S}^t$ are said temporally geodesically consistent with respect to $\mathcal{B}^t$ in $[t_b, t_e]$ if and only if:

$$\forall t \in [t_b, t_e], \forall i \in [1, N], \quad |g(v_1^t, b_i^t) - g(v_2^{t+\delta}, b_i^{t+\delta})| \le \epsilon, \tag{3}$$

where $t_b < t_e$, $t + \delta \in [t_b, t_e]$ and $\epsilon \to 0$. $g$ is normalized using the maximum geodesic distance over all pairs of points on $\mathcal{S}^t$ to preserve geodesic consistency when surfaces undergo non-rigid deformations (e.g., scale changes). Figure 1 illustrates temporal geodesic consistency with respect to critical points (top: 8, bottom: 5) extracted automatically using local geometry and topology properties (see [33]). Ambiguity maps are obtained by counting the number of candidate pairs $(v_1^t, v_2^{t+\delta})$ when $\epsilon > 0$. We observe that the regions located around object centers have very low ambiguity (i.e., numerical approximation is not an issue). In practice, we can search for $v_2^{t+\delta} = \arg\min_{v \in \mathcal{S}^t} \sum_{i=1}^{N} |g(v_1^t, b_i^t) - g(v, b_i^{t+\delta})|$.

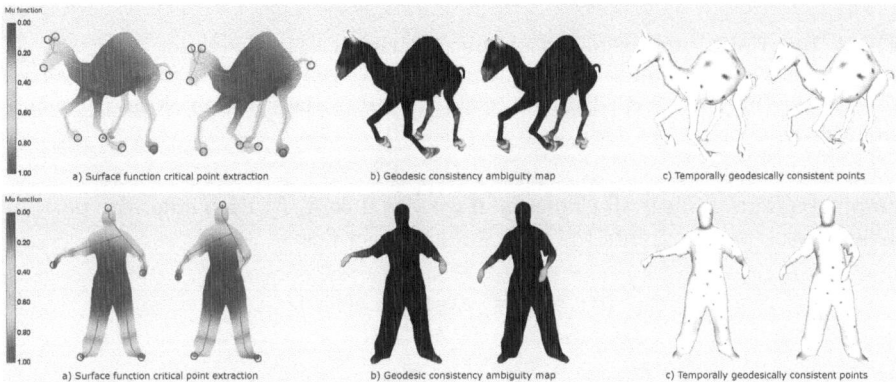

**Fig. 1. Temporal Geodesic Consistency.** a) Critical points extracted on surface mesh using Reeb graphs [33]. b) Geodesic consistency ambiguity map (darker means less position ambiguity). c) 50 temporally consistent points chosen randomly.

### 3.3 Invariant Surface-Based Graph Construction

**Definition 3.** Let $\mathcal{C}^t = \{c_1^t, ..., c_N^t\}$ denote a set of invariant local features (e.g., local extrema) on $\mathcal{S}^t$ that are tracked over time in $[t_b, t_e]$. The surface-based shape descriptor $\mathcal{T}(\mathcal{V}^t, \mathcal{P}^t)$ is a graph on $\mathcal{S}^t$ whose nodes $\mathcal{V}^t$ are temporally geodesically consistent with respect to $\mathcal{C}^t$ in $[t_b, t_e]$. Every edge in $\mathcal{P}^t$ of $\mathcal{T}$ is linked to a feature in $\mathcal{C}^t$, and nodes of $\mathcal{T}$ represent edge junctions. Here, an edge consists of a path[1] on $\mathcal{S}^t$. To maintain the graph structure invariant over time independently from the parameterization of $\mathcal{S}^t$, we develop a probabilistic framework where edge positions are optimized using two geodesic consistency cues (see Fig. 2), while being located in regions of low ambiguity (see Def. 2).

**Construction.** First, we define an initial graph structure $\rho_0$ on $\mathcal{S}^{t_b}$ at $t_b$ as either the global minimum (i.e., one point) given by Eq. 1 if $\mathcal{S}^{t_b}$ is genus-0, or as a graph cutting handles if the genus is higher (see [34], [35] and Sect. 4). Second, we initialize the graph: $\rho \leftarrow \rho_0$. The graph $\mathcal{T}$ is then built by iteratively adding the shortest edge linking a local feature (e.g., local maxima) in $\mathcal{C}^{t_b}$ to the current

---

[1] A path on a surface is a set of points linked two-by-two by a line.

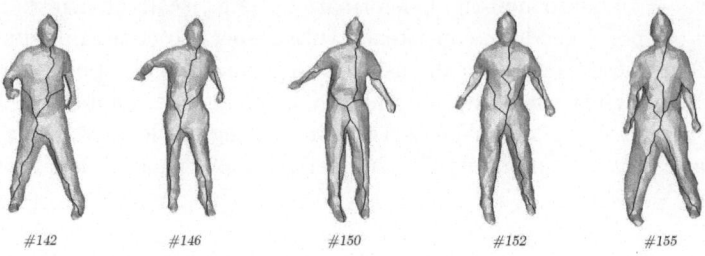

**Fig. 2. Invariant surface-based shape descriptor.** The descriptor is a graph (in blue) defined on the object surfaces. Graph nodes are maintained geodesically consistent over time, whereas edges vary adaptively to surface deformations. (Bouncing sequence.)

graph structure $\rho$ until all elements in $\mathcal{C}^{t_b}$ are linked. At each step, the path $\rho_j$ given by the pair of points $(c_j^{t_b}, v_j^{t_b}) \in \mathcal{C}^{t_b} \times \rho$ verifies:

$$(c_j^{t_b}, v_j^{t_b}) = \underset{(c,v) \in \mathcal{C}^{t_b} \times \rho}{\arg\min} \; g(c, v). \qquad (4)$$

$\rho_j$ is linked to $\rho$: $\rho \leftarrow \rho \cup \rho_j$, and $v_j^{t_b}$ is inserted into the set $\mathcal{V}^{t_b}$ (initially empty). When every feature in $\mathcal{C}^{t_b}$ is linked to $\rho$, we obtain $\rho = (\bigcup \rho_j) \cup \rho_0$ and we finally set: $\mathcal{T} \leftarrow \rho$ at $t_b$.

For all $t > t_b$, the invariant model is obtained by building a graph whose nodes have temporal geodesic consistency with the prior graph nodes and are located at local maxima or in non-ambiguous regions.. The problem is formulated as an MRF to find the optimal paths linking the graph nodes using intrinsic surface properties, so that graph constructions across time are independent from surface parameterization. The algorithm to construct a graph at $t$ is the following:

1. Extract local features $\mathcal{C}^t = \{c_1^t, ..., c_N^t\}$ on $\mathcal{S}^t$ using Eq. 1 and match them to prior ones in $\mathcal{C}^{t-1}$ (e.g., using geometry and topology information [33]).
2. Derive an initial structure $\rho_0^t$ on $\mathcal{S}^t$ geodesically consistent to the prior one. Note that for genus-0 surface, $\rho_0^t$ is usually a point located around the object center. Set the graph at $t$: $\rho^t \leftarrow \rho_0^t$.
3. Edges that link the features $\mathcal{C}^t$ to the current graph structure $\rho^t$ are added iteratively, and in the same order as the prior steps. Let $\mathcal{P}^t = \{p_i^t\}$ denote the set of points forming a path (a graph edge) linking a feature $c^t$ to a node $v^t$ at $t$, and $\mathcal{D}^t = \{d_i^t\}$ denote the set of points forming the shortest path linking $c^t$ to $v^t$ (e.g., using Dijkstra's algorithm). To obtain the optimal path $\mathcal{P}^t = \{p_i^t\}$, the problem is expressed as a MAP-MRF where the surface mesh vertices at $t$

serve as sites. Probabilities of $p_i^t$ to be at some positions at $t$ are computed given known priors $\mathcal{P}^{t-1}$ and $\mathcal{D}^t$. The posterior probability to maximize is:

$$\Pr(\mathcal{P}^t|\mathcal{D}^t,\mathcal{P}^{t-1}) \propto \prod_i E_d(p_i^t,d_i^t)E_p(p_i^t,p_i^{t-1}) \prod_i \prod_{j\in\mathcal{N}(i)} V(p_i^t,p_j^t), \qquad (5)$$

where $E_d$ and $E_p$ are the local evidence terms for a point $p_i^t$ to be at positions inferred from $d_i^t$ and $p_i^{t-1}$ respectively, $\mathcal{N}(i)$ is the neighborhood of $i$, and V is a pair-wise smoothness assumption (so that $\mathcal{P}^t$ forms a path on $\mathcal{S}^t$). $E_d$ and $E_p$ are defined as what follows:

$$E_d(p_i^t,d_i^t) = f_d(\sum_{k\in[1,N]} ||g(p_i^t,c_k^t) - g(d_i^t,c_k^t)||), \qquad (6)$$

$$E_p(p_i^t,p_i^{t-1}) = f_p(\sum_{k\in[1,N]} ||g(p_i^t,c_k^t) - g(p_i^{t-1},c_k^{t-1})||), \qquad (7)$$

where $f_d$ and $f_p$ are Gaussian distributions centered on $d_i^t$ and $p_i^{t-1}$ respectively, $g$ is the normalized geodesic distance, $c_k^t \in \mathcal{C}^t$ and $c_k^{t-1} \in \mathcal{C}^{t-1}$. Note that indices were simplified for clarity: $\mathcal{P}^{t-1}$, $\mathcal{P}^t$ and $\mathcal{D}^t$ may not have the same number of elements, and $d_i^t$ and $p_i^{t-1}$ are the closest point to $p_i^t$ on $\mathcal{D}^t$ and $\mathcal{P}^{t-1}$. Hence, Eq. 5 estimates the probability of $\mathcal{P}^t$ to be geodesically consistent to the previous edge $\mathcal{P}^{t-1}$, while being influenced by the shortest path $\mathcal{D}^t$. Let $\mathcal{P}^\star$ denote the optimal path linking the feature $c^t$ to the node $v^t$. Thus, we have to estimate:

$$\mathcal{P}^\star = \arg\max_{\{\mathcal{P}^t\}} \Pr(\mathcal{P}^t|\mathcal{D}^t,\mathcal{P}^{t-1}), \qquad (8)$$

where $\{\mathcal{P}^t\}$ denotes all the possible paths linking $c^t$ to $v^t$. Shortest paths are added one-by-one to avoid edge overlapping when linking local features. $E_d$ acts as a force that attracts the path to a state where the stress is lower (see Fig. 2) when an elastic deformation occurs or in case of surface noise (e.g., 3D reconstruction artifact). As well, $E_d$ prevents the model to be subject to error accumulation over time, causing drift effects. On the other hand, $E_p$ maintains the graph structure consistent over time, which can be crucial for some applications (see Sect. 4).

$\rho^t$ is obtained by iteratively adding paths $\mathcal{P}_j^\star$ linking $c_j^t \in \mathcal{C}^t$ to the current graph at node $v_j^t$. $v_j^t$ is the closest point on the current graph to:

$$\bar{v}_j^t = \arg\min_{v\in\rho_t}[\lambda.g(\hat{v}_j^t,v) + (1-\lambda).g(\check{v}_j^t,v)], \qquad (9)$$

where $\hat{v}_j^t$ is the point in $\mathcal{S}^t$ geodesically consistent to $v_j^{t-1}$ in $\mathcal{S}^{t-1}$ with respect to $\mathcal{C}^t$, $\check{v}_j^t$ is the intersection point given by the shortest path from $c_j^t$ to $\rho^t$, and $\lambda = 0.5$ is a weight. (Temporal priors are discarded if $\lambda = 0$.) In addition, $v_j^t$ is constrained to belong to the edge derived from the edge containing $v_j^{t-1}$. The structure of $\mathcal{T}$ is therefore maintained invariant over time. Note that priors can be extended to $\{\mathcal{P}^{t-k}\}_{t_b<k<t}$.

4. Repeat Step 3. until every feature in $\mathcal{C}^t$ is linked to $\rho^t$. Finally, the graph $\mathcal{T}$ at $t$ is given by $\rho^t \leftarrow (\bigcup \mathcal{P}_j^{\star,t}) \cup \rho_0^t$.

5. Set $t \leftarrow t + 1$ and repeat Step 1. to 4. for all $t < t_e$.

Note that the optimization problem in Step 3. can be effectively solved by dynamic programming. Finally, as illustrated in Fig. 3 we obtain a graph that is invariant over time regardless of the surface parameterization (i.e., mesh complexity and connectivity).

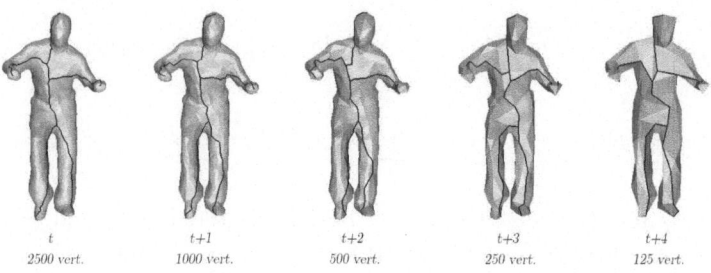

| $t$ | $t+1$ | $t+2$ | $t+3$ | $t+4$ |
| 2500 vert. | 1000 vert. | 500 vert. | 250 vert. | 125 vert. |

**Fig. 3. Invariant property against surface parameterization.** The graph structure is maintained invariant even though the surface mesh complexity and connectivity change. Here, the number of vertices varies from 2500 to 125 vertices. (Lock sequence.)

## 4    3D Video Data Encoding

The surface-based shape descriptor $\mathcal{T}$ introduced in the previous section can provide an invariant structure to 3D data obtained independently, such as a sequence of 3D meshes obtained from multiple view stereo [4, 6, 13]. Hence, we propose to apply the descriptor for 3D video data encoding using a strategy inspired by the geometry images [12].

For each frame, the graph structure of $\mathcal{T}$ is used as a cut graph $\rho$ that cuts and opens the 3D surface mesh $M$ into a disk (a genus-0 chart). $M$ is then mapped onto a flat parameter domain, which will be used as an image plane. Finally, $M$ is resampled on a regular grid, where the 3D coordinates XYZ are scaled and stored as RGB pixel components to form a 2D (geometry) image $\mathcal{I}$. To retrieve $M$ from $\mathcal{I}$, RGB values are simply reconverted to 3D coordinates. When applying the transformation on a sequence of 3D meshes, the process returns a sequence of images (i.e., a video). As the graph structure is invariant over the sequence, consecutive frames vary smoothly and can therefore be efficiently encoded using any popular codec for 2D video. Note that if a lossy compression method is used for encoding and alters the border of $\mathcal{I}$, cracks may be observed on the reconstructed surface around the cut $\rho$. In that case, a post-processing step (e.g., mesh joining or hole filling) may be necessary to preserve the topology of the initial mesh. The advantage of the proposed invariant surface-based shape descriptor for 3D video encoding is at least twofold:

1. The shape descriptor can be used as cut graphs to produce smoothly varying geometry images from real-world 3D video data independently from the
   surface parameterization, i.e., even though the mesh resolution or connectivity is inconsistent between consecutive frames. Hence the model allows
   for adaptive bitrate streaming application, whereas state-of-the-art methods
   cannot be applied [16, 27].
2. In standard parameterization approaches [12, 27, 36], the computation of
   the cut graph $\rho$ is obtained iteratively and requires several parameterization
   steps to detect all the local extrema one-by-one (e.g., using triangle geometric stretch). On the other hand, the proposed strategy is one-shot, and still
   guarantees that the generated cut path passes through all local extrema of
   $M$ (i.e., surface protrusions), which is a crucial condition to preserve the geometry accuracy after transformation. When the cut graphs are well defined,
   the transformation can be used for lossless compression of 3D meshes.

**Topology Change.** As the cut graph passes through all extrema, critical points
usually lie at the boundaries of the parameter domain. When surface topology
changes, the number of critical points may vary, and the graph structure can
locally change. This results in a discontinuity between consecutive geometry images that cannot be avoided. On the other hand, it guarantees that the original
surface topology is preserved and can be reconstructed from a single chart. Otherwise a surface alignment method could be applied as preprocessing [9–11], but
large resolution variations as shown in Fig. 3 would not be handled and original
topology would be lost. Methods that estimate global geodesic distortions for
shape matching are usually robust to local surface deformation [9, 37]. However,
the measures can be strongly affected by surface topology changes, as opposed to
the proposed descriptor which is only locally affected. Figure 4 shows geometry
image discontinuities when altering geodesic consistency of nodes and adding an
arbitrary critical point. As critical points are matched across time, image regions
with no perturbation remain aligned (see left part of images).

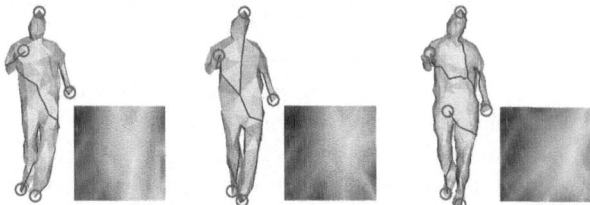

**Fig. 4.** (Left and Center) Geometry images show discontinuities when graph nodes are
not geodesically consistent. (Right) Adding an arbitrary critical point alters locally the
image boundaries. (Bouncing sequence.)

## 5    Experimental Results

**Datasets.** For experimental validations, we have tested the algorithm on publicly available datasets of 3D video reconstructed from multi-view images [6, 10].
They consist of real subjects wearing loose clothing and performing various actions, such as dancing or jumping. Surfaces can therefore vary a lot between two
consecutive frames when the motion is fast. Our experiments aim to assess the
invariant property of the proposed descriptor regardless of surface parameterization, and its performance (e.g., reconstruction accuracy) when applied for 3D
video adaptive bitrate streaming. We use 3D mesh sequences processed by [11]
as the surface genus is theoretically consistent over the sequences. (In practice,
3D video data can be post-processed using a surface alignment method to prevent surface topology changes [8–11].) In addition, we remeshed the sequences
to cancel all mesh connectivity consistency, and produced mixed resolution 3D
video data containing alternatively 3D meshes of 1000, 500, 250 and 125 vertices.

We perform comparisons to a state-of-the-art parameterization technique [27],
where cut graphs are obtained by iterative parameterizations. The approach, here
named Geometry Image Sequence (GIS), is known to optimally encode closed 3D
surface meshes. Results obtained with our proposed technique on mesh sequences
having same resolution are denoted 'fixed', whereas results obtained on sequences
with meshes having various resolutions are denoted 'mixed'. Computation time
for a 1000 vertex mesh is in the order of seconds on dual-core PC.

**Invariant Property Evaluation.** To assess the invariant property of the descriptor to surface variations and its ability to produce consistent geometry images that varies smoothly, the mean square error of pixel values (MSE) between
consecutive geometry images is computed (smaller MSE is better). It allows us
to estimate how much the geometry images vary over a sequence. In our experiments, the size of geometry images has been fixed to $128 \times 128$ pixels (encoded
in RGB with 8bit per pixel component) for the sake of consistent comparison.
(To achieve optimal streaming, the geometry images should indeed be resized
with respect to the mesh resolution.) Table. 1 shows average MSE obtained on
various sequences. The proposed descriptor shows remarkable invariant property
between consecutive frames: average MSE(fixed) values are very low. Moreover,
the resolution changes do not affect the performance: MSE(mixed) are low as
well. Note that as GIS does not contain any stabilization mechanism: average
MSE(GIS) values are high and are given for comparison.

Fig. 5 shows MSE for the Lock sequence. The other sequences return similar
results. Figure 6 illustrates invariant graphs obtained with our approach with
fixed and mixed mesh resolution.

**Reconstruction Accuracy.** To assess the reconstruction accuracy of geometry images obtained from the invariant surface-based shape descriptor used as
cut graphs, Hausdorff distances are computed between original meshes and reconstructed meshes [38]. Average Hausdorff distances $\Delta$ between ground truth
sequences and reconstructed surfaces by GIS and our proposed method (with

**Table 1.** Average MSE of pixel values between consecutive geometry images

|           | MSE(GIS) | MSE(fixed) | MSE(mixed) |
|-----------|----------|------------|------------|
| Bouncing  | 35302    | 2886       | 3224       |
| Crane     | 28485    | 1670       | 2025       |
| Handstand | 30671    | 1261       | 3125       |
| Kickup    | 27700    | 1938       | 3753       |
| Lock      | 22466    | 1700       | 3037       |
| Samba     | 35302    | 2886       | 3282       |

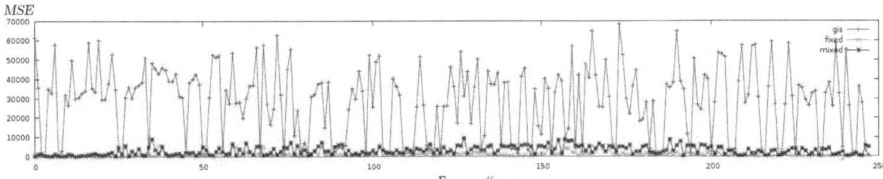

**Fig. 5. MSE of Lock sequence.** Our approach produces geometry images that vary very smoothly regardless of surface mesh complexity and connectivity.

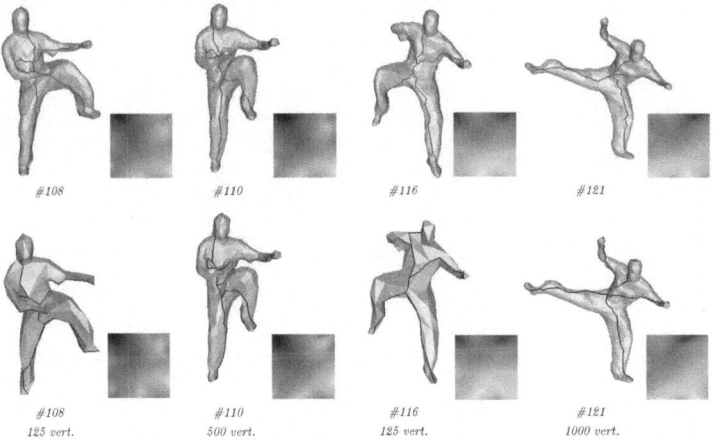

**Fig. 6. Graph invariant property regardless of surface mesh complexity and connectivity.** (top) shows a mesh sequence with 1000 vertices. (bottom) shows the same sequence with meshes at different resolutions. Although surface parameterizations are different, the proposed surface-based shape descriptor computed on the Lock sequence shows invariant property and adaptivity: graphs and geometry images remain similar.

fixed resolution) are reported in Table. 2. We can observe similar performances between the proposed approach and GIS as $\Delta$ is very low for both methods. Results between original data and simplified meshes (125 vertices) are given for comparison (see $\Delta$(ref)).

As shown in Figure 7, our method can achieve accurate reconstruction (comparable to GIS) while using an original one-shot processing, as opposed to standard iterative parameterizations employed by GIS. Additional examples are given in

**Table 2.** Average Hausdorff distances $\Delta$ to ground truth

|          | $\Delta$(GIS) | $\Delta$(proposed) | $\Delta$(ref) |
|----------|---------------|--------------------|---------------|
| Bouncing | 0.0122        | 0.0126             | 0.0885        |
| Crane    | 0.0126        | 0.0132             | 0.0729        |
| Handstand| 0.0119        | 0.0122             | 0.0920        |
| Kickup   | 0.0118        | 0.0120             | 0.0862        |
| Lock     | 0.0079        | 0.088              | 0.0783        |
| Samba    | 0.0223        | 0.0237             | 0.0913        |

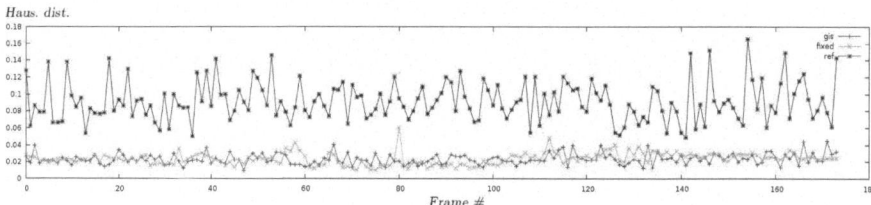

**Fig. 7. Hausdorff distances $\Delta$ for Samba sequence.** Our approach allows accurate reconstruction of mesh sequences comparable to state-of-the-art implementation [27]).

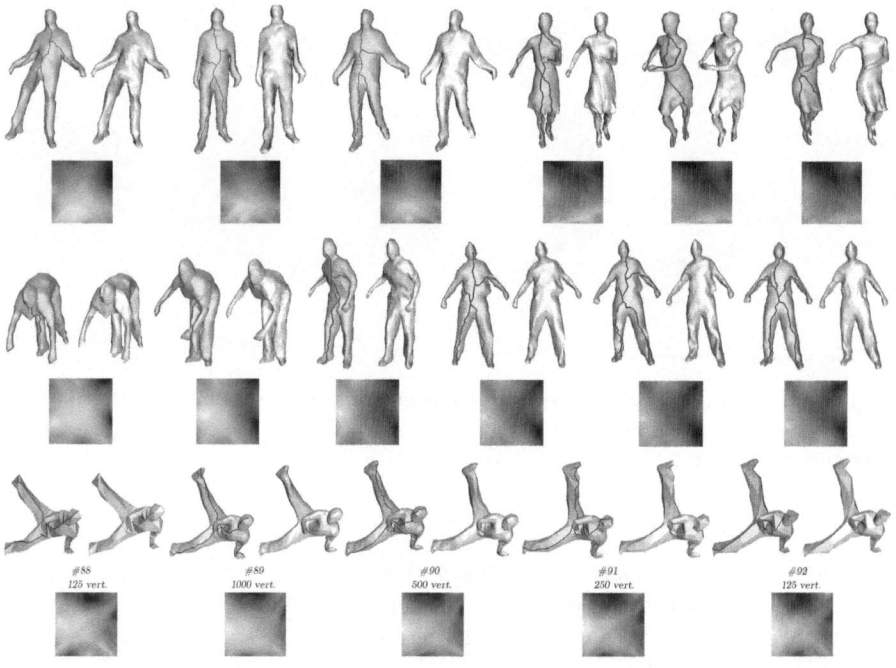

**Fig. 8. Encoding and reconstruction.** Surface-based graphs are shown in red and blue (for mixed resolutions), reconstructions are shown in grey. Although surfaces undergo strong variations, the invariant surface-based shape descriptor produces smoothly varying geometry images and accurate surface reconstruction. Sequences are: (Top) Crane and Samba, (Middle) Handstand, (Bottom) Kickup.

**Table 3.** 3D video encoding. For each format, the size of each sequence is given in KB. Standard H.264/MPEG-4 is used for compression of geometry images (128 × 128p).

|           | #fr. | OFF(zip) | GIS   | Proposed |
|-----------|------|----------|-------|----------|
| Bouncing  | 174  | 16,300   | 304.4 | 169.9    |
| Crane     | 173  | 14,100   | 283.7 | 162.7    |
| Handstand | 173  | 24,700   | 283.4 | 154.7    |
| Kickup    | 219  | 29,900   | 365.1 | 197.0    |
| Lock      | 249  | 32,400   | 388.2 | 204.0    |
| Samba     | 174  | 22,200   | 304.0 | 173.2    |

Fig. 8 showing the descriptor invariant property to surface undergoing large deformations.

**Encoding Performance.** Table. 3 shows 3D video encoding performance with respect to different strategies. Our method clearly performs better.

# 6   Conclusion

We present a novel invariant shape descriptor to represent spatio-temporal visual information that varies over time, such as 3D dynamic surfaces. The proposed descriptor consists in a surface-based graph that lies on object surfaces, and is anchored to local features. The overall graph structure is made invariant to surface variations using surface intrinsic geometric properties while surfaces undergo non-rigid deformation. In particular, the graph is defined within a probabilistic framework using temporal geodesic consistency cues as priors, and is independent to surface parameterization. Hence, the descriptor can be used to bring an invariant structure to 3D geometric data that are produced independently, such as 3D video obtained from multiple view stereo.

We show that the proposed shape descriptor can be employed as surface cut graphs, which enables 3D surface models to be transformed into 2D (geometry) images using a one-shot strategy while geometry is accurately preserved. Moreover, the invariant property of the representation allows the production of smoothly varying images, regardless of the 3D surface mesh complexity and connectivity. Therefore, the approach is suitable for adaptive bitrate streaming of 3D video data, which was a challenging issue as state-of-the-art techniques are only designed to optimally encode 3D animated mesh sequences sharing a same mesh connectivity. For further research, additional surface features such as color (when available) may be exploited.

**Acknowledgments.** This work was supported in part by the JST-CREST project "Creation of Human-Harmonized Information Technology for Convivial Society", and the JSPS (Wakate-B No. 23700170).

# References

1. Forsyth, D.A., Mundy, J.L., Zisserman, A., Coelho, C., Heller, A., Rothwell, C.: Invariant descriptors for 3d object recognition and pose. IEEE PAMI 13 (1991)
2. Mundy, J., Zisserman, A.: Geometric invariance in computer vision. MIT Press (1992)
3. Rothganger, F., Lazebnik, S., Schmid, C., Ponce, J.: 3d object modeling and recognition using local affine-invariant image descriptors and multi-view spatial constraints. IJCV 66, 231–259 (2006)
4. Matsuyama, T., Wu, X., Takai, T., Nobuhara, S.: Real-time 3d shape reconstruction, dynamic 3d mesh deformation, and high fidelity visualization for 3d video. CVIU 96, 393–434 (2004)
5. Allard, J., Ménier, C., Raffin, B., Boyer, E., Faure, F.: Grimage: Markerless 3d interactions. ACM SIGGRAPH - Emerging Technologies (2007)
6. Starck, J., Hilton, A.: Surface capture for performance-based animation. IEEE CGA (2007)
7. de Aguiar, E., Stoll, C., Theobalt, C., Ahmed, N., Seidel, H.P., Thrun, S.: Performance capture from sparse multi-view video. ACM Trans. Graphics 27 (2008)
8. Starck, J., Hilton, A.: Spherical matching for temporal correspondence of non-rigid surfaces. In: IEEE ICCV (2005)
9. Bronstein, A.M., Bronstein, M.M., Kimmel, R.: Calculus of non-rigid surfaces for geometry and texture manipulation. IEEE Trans. VCG, 902–913 (2007)
10. Vlasic, D., Baran, I., Matusik, W., Popovic, J.: Articulated mesh animation from multi-view silhouettes. ACM Trans. Graphics 27 (2008)
11. Cagniart, C., Boyer, E., Ilic, S.: Probabilistic Deformable Surface Tracking from Multiple Videos. In: Daniilidis, K., Maragos, P., Paragios, N. (eds.) ECCV 2010, Part IV. LNCS, vol. 6314, pp. 326–339. Springer, Heidelberg (2010)
12. Gu, X., Gortler, S., Hoppe, H.: Geometry images. ACM SIGGRAPH (2002)
13. Seitz, S., Curless, B., Diebel, J., Scharstein, D., Szeliski, R.: A comparison and evaluation of multi-view stereo reconstruction algorithms. In: IEEE CVPR (2006)
14. Alliez, P., Gotsman, C.: Recent advances in compression of 3d meshes. In: Advances in Multiresolution for Geometric Modelling. Springer (2005)
15. Alexa, M., Müllen, W.: Representing animations by principal components. Computer Graphics Forum 19 (2000)
16. Briceno, H., Sandler, P., McMillian, L., Gortler, S., Hoppe, H.: Geometry videos: A new representation for 3d animations. In: Eurographics/SIGGRAPH Symp. Computer Animation, pp. 136–146 (2003)
17. Karni, Z., Gotsman, C.: Compression of soft-body animation sequence. Computers & Graphics 28, 25–34 (2004)
18. Mamou, K., Zaharia, T., Preteux, F., Stefanoski, N., Ostermann, J.: Frame-based compression of animated meshes in mpeg-4. In: IEEE ICME (2008)
19. Blum, H.: A transformation for extracting new descriptors of shape. Models for the Perception of Speech and Visual Form (1967)
20. Cornea, N., Silver, D., Yuan, X., Balasubramanian, R.: Computing hierarchical curve skeletons of 3d objects. The Visual Computer 21, 945–955 (2005)
21. Hilaga, M., Shinagawa, Y., Kohmura, T., Kunii, T.L.: Topology matching for fully automatic similarity estimation of 3d shapes. ACM SIGGRAPH, 203–212 (2001)
22. Carranza, J., Theobalt, C., Magnor, M., Seidel, H.-P.: Free-viewpoint video of human actors. ACM Trans. Graphics 22, 569–577 (2003)

23. Palagyi, K., Kuba, A.: A parallel 3d 12-subiteration thinning algorithm. Graph. Models and Image Proc. 61, 199–221 (1999)

24. Baran, I., Popovic, J.: Automatic rigging and animation of 3d characters. ACM Trans. Graphics 26, 27 (2007)

25. Tung, T., Matsuyama, T.: Topology dictionary for 3d video understanding. IEEE Trans. PAMI 34, 1645–1657 (2012)

26. Habe, H., Katsura, Y., Matsuyama, T.: Skin-off: Representation and compression scheme for 3d video. In: Picture Coding Symposium (2004)

27. Saboret, L., Alliez, P., Lévy, B.: Planar parameterization of triangulated surface meshes. In: CGAL Reference Manual. CGAL Editorial Board, 4.0 edition (2012)

28. Mortara, M., Patanè, G.: Affine-invariant skeleton of 3d shapes. Shape Modeling International (2002)

29. Morse, M.: The calculus of variations in the large. American Mathematical Society, Colloquium Publication 18, New York (1934)

30. Pascucci, V., Scorzelli, G., Bremer, P.T., Mascarenhas, A.: Robust on-line computation of reeb graphs: Simplicity and speed. ACM Trans. Graphics 26 (2007)

31. Edelsbrunner, H., Harer, J., Mascarenhas, A., Pascucci, V.: Time-varying reeb graphs for continuous space-time data. In: Symp. Computational Geometry (2004)

32. Klein, T., Ertl, T.: Scale-space tracking of critical points in 3d vector fields. In: Proc. Topology-Based Methods in Visualization (2005)

33. Tung, T., Schmitt, F.: The augmented multiresolution reeb graph approach for content-based retrieval of 3d shapes (code on webpage). Int'l J. Shape Modeling 11, 91–120 (2005)

34. Taubin, G., Rossignac, J.: Geometric compression through topological surgery. ACM Trans. Graphics 17, 84–115 (1998)

35. Erickson, J., Har-Peled, S.: Optimally cutting a surface into a disk. Discrete & Computational Geometry 31, 37–59 (2004)

36. Floater, M.: Parametrization and smooth approximation of surface triangulations. CADG 14, 231–250 (1997)

37. Mémoli, F., Sapiro, G.: A theoretical and computational framework for isometry invariant recognition of point cloud data. Found. Comput. Math. 5, 313–347 (2005)

38. Cignoni, P., Rocchini, C., Scopigno, R.: Metro: measuring error on simplified surfaces. Computer Graphics Forum 17, 167–174 (1998)

# Linear Discriminant Analysis
# with Maximum Correntropy Criterion

Wei Zhou and Sei-ichiro Kamata

Waseda University, Japan

**Abstract.** Linear Discriminant Analysis (LDA) is a famous supervised feature extraction method for subspace learning in computer vision and pattern recognition. In this paper, a novel method of LDA based on a new Maximum Correntropy Criterion optimization technique is proposed. The conventional LDA, which is based on L2-norm, is sensitivity to the presence of outliers. The proposed method has several advantages: first, it is robust to large outliers. Second, it is invariant to rotations. Third, it can be effectively solved by half-quadratic optimization algorithm. And in each iteration step, the complex optimization problem can be reduced to a quadratic problem that can be efficiently solved by a weighted eigenvalue optimization method. The proposed method is capable of analyzing non-Gaussian noise to reduce the influence of large outliers substantially, resulting in a robust classification. Performance assessment in several datasets shows that the proposed approach is more effectiveness to address outlier issue than traditional ones.

## 1 Introduction

In many data measurement problems, observation data often lies in a lower dimensional subspace which can be obtained from the original high dimensional data space. Such a lower dimensional subspace, especially the linear subspace, has many important applications in computer vision or pattern recognition, such as object recognition [1], motion estimation [2]. Among these subspace methods, linear discriminant analysis (LDA) [3] is one of the most popular methods. LDA tries to find a set of projections that maximize the ratio of the between-class distance to the within-class distance. These projections constitute a low-dimensional linear subspace by which the data structure in the original input space can be effectively captured.

In general, LDA approaches [3] [4] utilize the Frobenius norm (L2-Norm) (we call it LDA-L2 in the following) to measure the between-class and within-class distances. Thus, the process of training may be dominated by outliers since the between-class or within-class distances is determined by the sum of squared distances. Recently, in order to solve the outlier problem, Li [5] proposed rotation invariant L1-norm (notated as R1-norm) based linear discriminant analysis (we call it LDA-R1 in the following). The R1-norm is determined by the sum of elements without being squared. Thus, the R1 norm is less sensitive to outliers than L2-norm. However, in the spatial dimension, squared data is still used.

K.M. Lee et al. (Eds.): ACCV 2012, Part I, LNCS 7724, pp. 500–511, 2013.
© Springer-Verlag Berlin Heidelberg 2013

Moreover, LDA-R1 takes a lot of time to achieve convergence for a large dimensional input space and it can not effectively handle large outlier problem. In this paper, instead of maximizing variance which is based on L2-norm, maximum correntropy criterion (MCC) [6] based linear discriminant analysis (we denote it as LDA-MCC) is proposed, which is a useful measurement to handle non-Gaussian noise with large outliers. From the viewpoint of Information Theoretic Learning (ITL), LDA-MCC is a natural extension of LDA by replacing MSE criterion by MCC and has several appealing advantages: 1) It is robust to outliers as well as rotationally invariant. 2) Optimal solutions of the proposed method are the principal eigenvectors of a robust covariance matrix corresponding to the largest eigenvalues.

The remainder of this paper is organized as follows: Problem formulation will be described in section 2. In section 3, the solution of the proposed method will be introduced and experiments are presented in section 4. Finally, conclusions and future work are discussed in section 5.

## 2   Problem Formulation

Assume we have a set of samples $X = \{\{x_i^l\}_{i=1}^{N_l}\}_{l=1}^{C} \in \mathbb{R}^{d \times n}$, $N_l$ of which belong to class $\omega_l$ $(l = 1, 2, ..., C)$, where $n$ and $d$ denote the number of samples and the dimension of the original input space, respectively. And $n = \sum_{l=1}^{C} N_l$. In LDA-L2, the objective is to seek $t$ projections $Y = \{\{y_i^l\}_{i=1}^{N_l}\}_{l=1}^{C} \in \mathbb{R}^{t \times n}$ by means of $t$ linear transformation vectors $W \in \mathbb{R}^{d \times t}$, which embeds the original $d$ dimension into $t$ dimension vector space such that $t < d$. Let $\text{Tr}(.)$ be the trace of its matrix argument, $S_b$ be the between-class scatter matrix, and $S_w$ be the within-class scatter matrix, which are formulated as: $S_b = \sum_{l=1}^{C}(m_l - m)(m_l - m)^T$ and $S_w = \sum_{l=1}^{C} \sum_{i=1}^{N_l}(x_i^l - m_l)(x_i^l - m_l)^T$. Here $m_l = (1/N_l) \sum_{i=1}^{N_l} x_i^l$ is the mean of the samples belonging to class $\omega_l$, and $m = (1/n) \sum_{l=1}^{C} N_l m_l$ is the global mean of the samples. LDA-L2 aims to find an optimal transformation $W$ by maximizing the ratio of $\text{Tr}(S_b)$ and $\text{Tr}(S_w)$ as following problem

$$\max_{W} J_{L2} = \max_{W} \frac{\text{Tr}(S_b)}{\text{Tr}(S_w)} \\ = \frac{W^T S_b W}{W^T S_w W} \tag{1}$$

The denominator of the objective function $J_{L2}$ can be simply to $W^T S_w W = I$, since it is invariant with respect to rescaling of the vectors $W \rightarrow \beta W$ ($\beta$ is some coefficient). Thus, the problem of maximizing $J_{L2}$ can be converted into the following constrained optimization problem:

$$\max_{W} \quad W^T S_b W \\ s.t. \quad W^T S_w W = I \tag{2}$$

It is known that the L2-norm is sensitive to outliers and recently, R1-norm approach [5] was presented to solve this problem. In this case, the problem becomes finding $W$ that maximizes the following objective function:

$$\max_{W} J_{R_1} = (1 - \alpha) \sum_{l=1}^{C} \sqrt{||W^T(m_l - m)||^2} - \\ \alpha \sum_{l=1}^{C} \sum_{i=1}^{N_l} \sqrt{||W^T(x_i^l - m_l)||^2} \tag{3}$$

However, for a large dimensional input space, it takes a lot of time to achieve convergence, and in the spatial dimension, squared data is still used. Thus, R1-norm approach is not effective and efficient for larger outlier problems. In this paper, we try to use Maximum Correntropy Criterion (MCC) to measure the between-class scatter instead of Mean Square Error (MSE). In practice, the correntropy is defined as a generalized similarity measure between two arbitrary random variables $A$ and $B$:

$$V_{n,\sigma}(A, B) = \frac{1}{n} \sum_{l=1}^{n} k_\sigma(a_l - b_l) \tag{4}$$

When kernel function $k_\sigma(.)$ is Gaussian kernel $g(x) = exp(-x^2/2\sigma^2)$, then

$$V_{n,\sigma}(A, B) = \frac{1}{n} \sum_{l=1}^{n} g(a_l - b_l) \tag{5}$$

In order to measure the similarity of two random variables $A$ and $B$, MSE uses all the samples in the input space while correntropy is just determined by kernel function along the line $a_l = b_l$. This important property intuitively explains the reason that the correntropy is superior to MSE if the residual of $A - B$ is non-symmetric or with nonzero mean.

In ITL, it has been pointed out that MSE is a global measurement while MCC is a local measurement [6]. By global, that means all the data points in the joint space will contribute equally to the value of the measurement and the locality of MCC means that the value is mainly determined by the kernel function. Since an outlier is far away from the data cluster, then its contribution to estimating correntropy will be smaller so that it always receives a low value in the matrix. Therefore, the outliers will have weaker influence on the estimation as correntropy increases. As a result, LDA-MCC is robust against outliers even large outliers occur.

Substituting $a_l = (m_l - m)$ and $b_l = WV_l$ into Eq.(5), here, $V_l = W^T(m_l - m)$ is a projected vector, and we can obtain a novel maximum correntropy criterion based LDA as follows:

$$\begin{aligned} \max_{W} \quad & J_{MCC} = \sum_{l=1}^{C} g((m_l - m) - WV_l) \\ s.t. \quad & W^T S_w W = I \end{aligned} \tag{6}$$

Since $W$ is orthonormal and then

$$g((m_l - m) - WV_l) = g(\sqrt{||(m_l - m) - WW^T(m_l - m)||^2}) \\ = g(\sqrt{(m_l - m)^T(m_l - m) - (m_l - m)^T WW^T(m_l - m)}) \tag{7}$$

let $M_l = (m_l - m)$ then the Eq.(6) can be converted into following objective function:

$$\max_{W} \quad J_{MCC} = \sum_{l=1}^{C} g(\sqrt{M_l^T M_l - M_l^T W W^T M_l})$$
$$s.t. \quad W^T S_w W = I \tag{8}$$

## 3   Linear Discriminant Analysis with Maximum Correntropy Criterion

Recently, Information theoretic learning (ITL) has been proved more efficient to data analysis problems. ITL utilizes probability density function of the data, estimated by Parzen kernel estimator [7], as the cost function.

### 3.1   Optimization

In ITL, the half-quadratic technique [8] [9] is often used to solve nonlinear ITL optimization problem. And in our study, half quadratic based algorithm is also applied to solve Eq.(8). According to the theory of convex conjugated functions [8], we can get the following proposition.

Proposition: There exists a convex conjugated function $\varphi$ of $g(x)$ such that

$$g(x) = \max_{p'}(p'\frac{||x||^2}{\sigma^2} - \varphi(p')) \tag{9}$$

where $p' \in R$ is a scalar variable, and for a fixed $x$, the maximum is reached at $p' = -g(x)$ [9]. Substituting Eq.(9) into Eq.(8), we can get an augmented objective function in the enlarged parameter space then the Eq.(6) can be converted into

$$\max_{W,P} \quad J_{MCC} = \sum_{l=1}^{C}(p_l(M_l^T M_l - M_l^T W W^T M_l) - \varphi(p_l))$$
$$s.t. \quad W^T S_w W = I \tag{10}$$

where $P = [p_1, p_2, ..., p_C]$ is storing the auxiliary variables introduced in the Half-Quadratic optimization. Consequently, we can optimize $(W, P)$ by iterations as:

$$\max_{W,P} \mathcal{L} = J_{MCC} - \lambda(W^T S_w W - I) \tag{11}$$

Then, according to Lagrangian method, a weighted traditional LDA problem can be obtained as follows

$$(S_w)^{-1} S_b P W = \lambda W \tag{12}$$

where $P$ is a diagonal matrix whose diagonal entity $p(l,l) = -p_l$ and $p_l = -g(\sqrt{M_l^T M_l - M_l^T W W^T M_l})$. Thus, the final algorithm of LDA-MCC is listed in Algorithm 1.

---

**Algorithm 1. LDA-MCC**

---

**Require:** $X = \{\{x_i^l\}_{i=1}^{N_l}\}_{l=1}^C \in \mathbb{R}^{d \times n}, t \leq d$
  Initialization: $W = [w_1, w_2, ..., w_t] \in \mathbb{R}^{d \times t}, W^T W = I$
  **while** not converge **do**
    1. Calculate $p_l = -g(\sqrt{M_l^T M_l - M_l^T W W^T M_l})$
    2. Update $W$ according to $(S_w)^{-1} S_b P W = \lambda W$
  **end while**
  **return** $W \in \mathbb{R}^{d \times t}$

---

### 3.2   Convergence of LDA-MCC

Let $r$ be the iteration number of Algorithm 1. then

$$\begin{aligned}
J_{MCC}^{r+1} - J_{MCC}^r &= J_{MCC}(W^{r+1}, P^{r+1}) - J_{MCC}(W^r, P^r) \\
&= [J_{MCC}(W^{r+1}, P^{r+1}) - J_{MCC}(W^r, P^{r+1})] \\
&\quad + [J_{MCC}(W^r, P^{r+1}) - J_{MCC}(W^r, P^r)]
\end{aligned} \tag{13}$$

Based on the Proposition and Eq.(12), $W^{r+1}$ and $P^{r+1}$ is the optimization value for $J_{MCC}^{r+1}$ and $J_{MCC}^r$, respectively. Then $J_{MCC}(W^{r+1}, P^{r+1}) - J_{MCC}(W^r, P^{r+1})$ $\geq 0$ and $J_{MCC}(W^r, P^{r+1}) - J_{MCC}(W^r, P^r) \geq 0$. So $J_{MCC}^{r+1} - J_{MCC}^r \geq 0$. That is, the objective function $J_{MCC}^r|_{r=1,2,...}$ increases monotonically. In the other side, apparently, $J_{MCC}^r|_{r=1,2,...}$ function has an upper bound Thus, we can get that $J_{MCC}^r|_{r=1,2,...}$ converges.

## 4   Experiments

In this section, the proposed approach is applied to some pattern recognition problems and the performance is compared with those of LDA-L2 and LDA-R1. This work follows the lines of correntropy [6] and estimates the bandwidth $\sigma$ by Silvermans rule [10].

### 4.1   Toy Set

The first experiment is based on a toy set composed of ten samples clustered into two category with an additional large outlier as shown in Fig.1(a).

To evaluate the effectiveness of LDA-MCC which is less sensitivity to outlies, the outlier sample (plotted as triangle at the top-right corner of Fig.1(a)) is intentionally added into the training samples of Class 1 before classification. For this kind of data, LDA-L2, LDA-R1 and LDA-MCC are applied and the projection vectors are $w_{L2} = [-0.7071, 0.7071]^T$, $w_{R1} = [-0.76431, 0.6448]^T$ and $w_{MCC} = [-0.8784, 0.4779]^T$. The final learning results are plotted as 1-dimensional signals in Fig.1(b) , Fig.1(c) and Fig.1(d) corresponding to LDA-L2, LDA-R1 and LDA-MCC, respectively. After the step of dimension reduction. Clearly, the between-class scatter of the two-class samples except for the outlier sample in Fig.1(d) is much larger than that in Fig.1(b) and Fig.1(c). In this

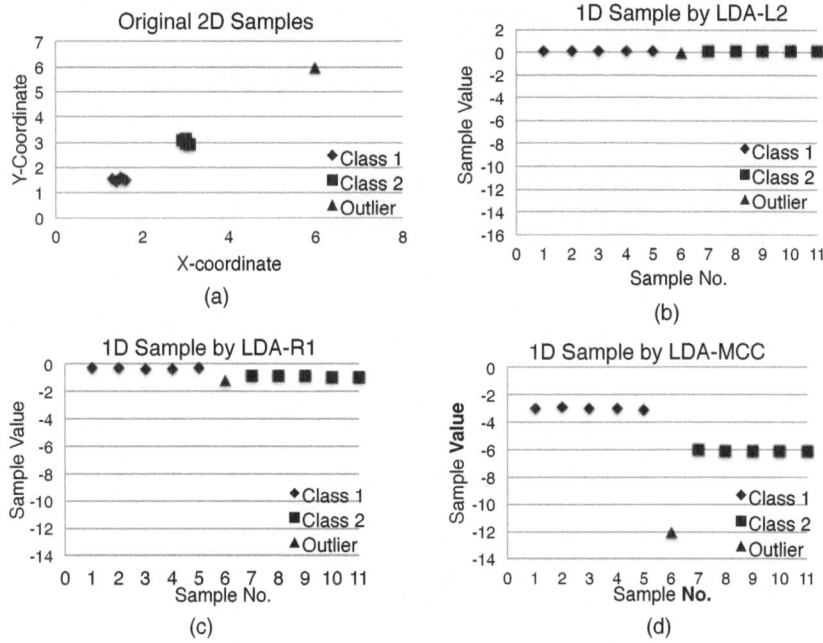

**Fig. 1.** (a) Samples in toy set (b) Results of LDA-L2 (c) Results of LDA-R1 (d) Results of LDA-MCC

experiment, LDA-MCC is randomly initialized and only two iterations are taken for convergence, while LDA-R1 converges in four iterations. Thus, the proposed method is more powerful to address the outlier problem.

## 4.2   Brodatz Texture Dataset

The second experiment is to evaluate the classification performance over the subset of Brodatz Texture Dataset [11]. In this dataset, 20 images are selected as category("real" images) and one image is selected as outlier image(shown in Fig.2).

At first, each image is normalized into $128 \times 128$ size, and then is non-overlapping divided into 16 regions. 5 regions per category and 1 region in outlier image are used as gallery and others per category are treated as probe. The final classification results are shown in Fig.3, where x-axis corresponds to the reduced dimension and y-axis is associated with the accuracy. From this figure, we can see the proposed method is less sensitive to outlier than the other two traditional approaches. In average, the proposed method can achieve about 6 percent higher than LDA-R1 and 11 percent higher than LDA-L2 approach. Moreover, form Dim. 30 to Dim. 40, the accuracy of LDA-R1 drops significantly, that means the projection weights from Dim. 30 to Dim. 40 obtained by LDA-R1 are very sensitivity to the outlier while LDA-MCC is much stable.

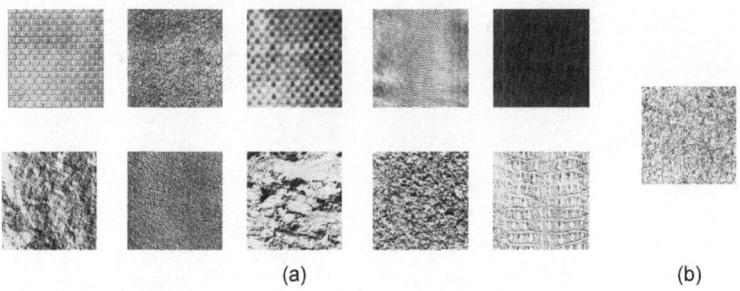

Fig. 2. Samples in Brodatz Texture Dataset (a) "real" images (b)outlier image

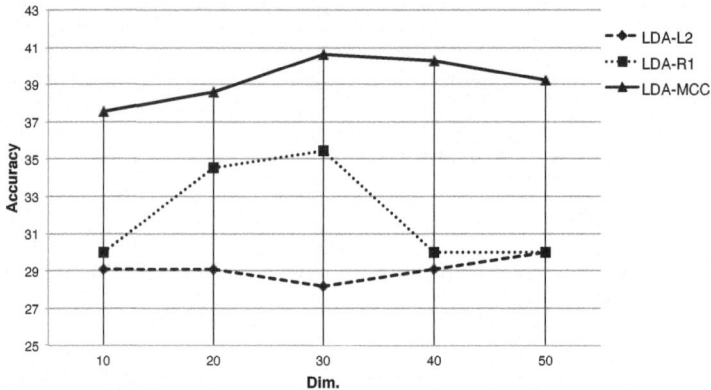

Fig. 3. Accuracy in Brodatz Texture Dataset

## 4.3 ORL Dataset

The third experiment is evaluated over the ORL dataset [12]. All images are gray scale and normalized to a resolution of $32 \times 32$ pixels. Among these 400 images, 30 percent were randomly selected and occluded with a rectangular noise consisting of random black and white dots whose size was $10 \times 10$, located at a random position. For a better illustration, some training samples are shown in Fig.4. 3 images per person are used for training and others are for testing. Simple 1-nearest-neighbor(1NN) classifier is used for the final classification. The performance is shown in Fig.5. The average number of iterations for LDA-MCC is 6.25 while 9.7 for LDA-R1. From this figure, we can see that the proposed method is the outstanding one and can obtain about 10 percent or 35 percent than LDA-R1 and LDA-L2, respectively.

Moreover, in this figure, when the reduced dimension is very small, the proposed method can get significant performance. In order to see how the accuracy changes in small dimension, another experiment is carried out and the result is

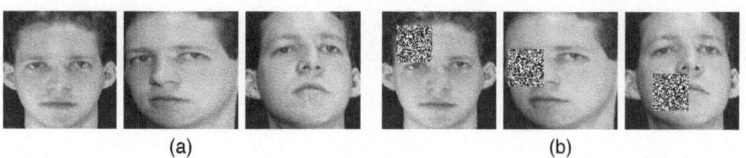

**Fig. 4.** ORL dataset (a) Original Images (b) Corresponding Images with occlusion

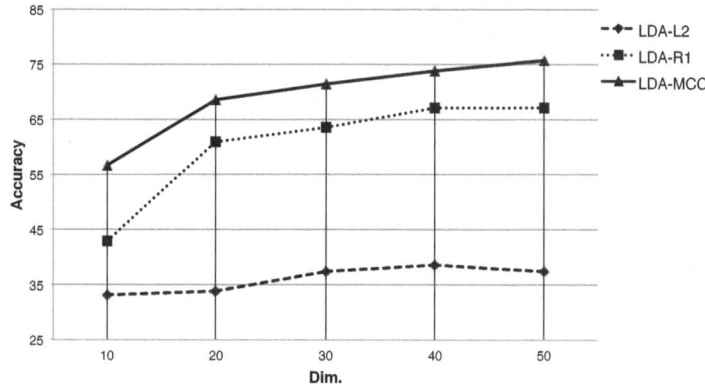

**Fig. 5.** Accuracy in ORL Dataset

shown in Fig.6. From this figure, we can see more clear about the effectiveness of the proposed method.

Finally, the accuracy on ORL dataset and the average training time are concluded in Table 1, here, PCA-L2 [13] means L2 norm based PCA while PCA-L1 [14] is L1 norm based PCA. From this table, we can see that our proposed method has higher performance than traditional ones.

**Table 1.** Recognition rate and computation cost on ORL dataset

| method | Recognition Rate | Average number of iterations | Average time (s) |
|---|---|---|---|
| LDA-L2 | 38.6 | / | / |
| LDA-R1 | 67.1 | 9.7 | 21.8 |
| PCA-L2 [13] | 49.5 | / | / |
| PCA-L1 [14] | 68.1 | / | / |
| LDA-MCC | 75.7 | 6.25 | 10.9 |

In next experiment, the proposed method is applied to face reconstruction problem and the performance is compared with those of other methods. We applied LDA-L2, LDA-R1, LDA-MCC and extracted various numbers of features.

By using only a fraction of features, we could compute the average reconstruction error with respect to the original unoccluded images as Eq.(14).

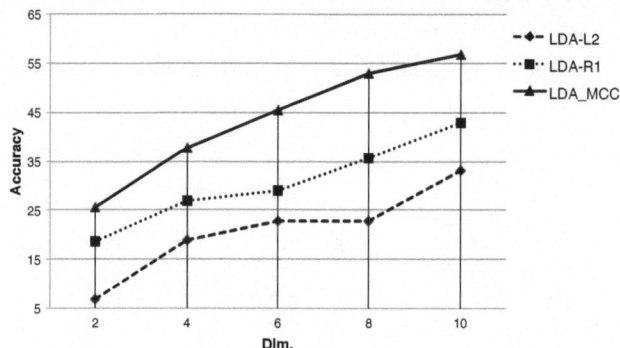

**Fig. 6.** Classification results for small dimension in ORL Dataset

$$e(m) = \frac{1}{n} \sum_{i=1}^{n} ||X^{org} - WW^T X||_2 \tag{14}$$

Here, $n$ is the number of samples, which is 400 in this case, $X^{org}$ and $X$ are the original unoccluded image and the image used in the training, respectively. Fig.7 shows the average reconstruction errors for various numbers of extracted features. In this figure, even when the number of extracted features is small, the average reconstruction error of the proposed method is smaller than LDA-L2 and LDA-R1 approaches.

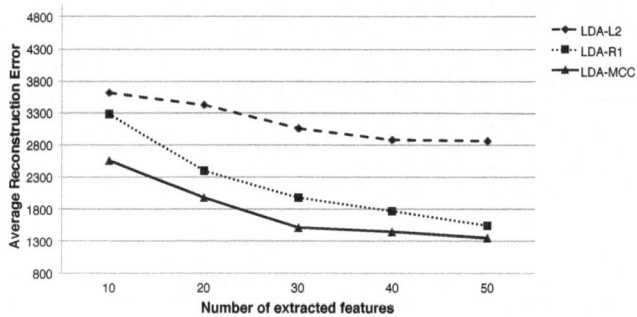

**Fig. 7.** Average reconstruction errors for ORL dataset

## 4.4   AR Dataset

The AR [15] dataset consists of over 3,200 color images of the frontal images of faces of 126 subjects. Each subject has 26 different images, including frontal views of with different facial expressions, lighting conditions and occlusions. For each subject, these images were recorded in two different sessions which are separated by two weeks, each session consisting of 13 images. For the experiments reported in this section, 60 different individuals were randomly selected from this database. Then there are 1560 images in our experiments. All images were manually cropped and resized to 80 by 60. Some example images of one person are shown in Fig.8.

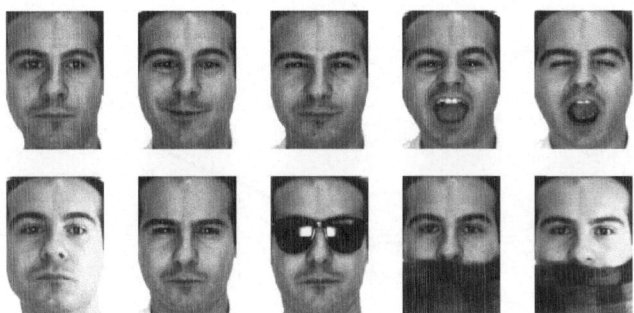

**Fig. 8.** Some samples from AR dataset

In this evaluation, the recognition performances of the different algorithms on AR database are compared. Six samples of each individual are randomly selected as gallery (training images), and the remaining ones are used for probe (testing images). In our study, we perform 5 times to randomly choose the training set and calculate the average recognition rates. Some classification results are listed in Fig.9, where we can see that the proposed method has higher performance than LDA-L2 and LDA-R1. In general, LDA-MCC can obtain about 10 percent or 20 percent than LDA-R1 and LDA-L2, respectively. And the average number of iterations for LDA-MCC is 10.1 while 25.3 for LDA-R1. Thus, we can see clearly that LDA-R1 takes much more computation cost to achieve convergence in larger dimensional input space, such as face recognition application, than LDA-MCC. Base on this evaluation, our proposed method is more effective and efficient than the traditional approaches to solve facial expression, illumination or occlusions issues.

In Fig.10, only low-dimensional space is focused on since we want to make a comparison of the most discriminant features for the proposed method and some related algorithms. Same as Fig.9, the proposed methods can extract more discriminant features.

Finally, the average accuracy and time cost for training on AR dataset is concluded in Table 2, and our proposed methods are superior to the traditional approaches.

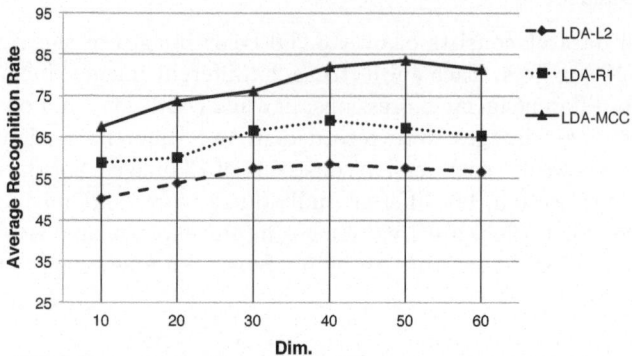

**Fig. 9.** Classification results in AR Dataset

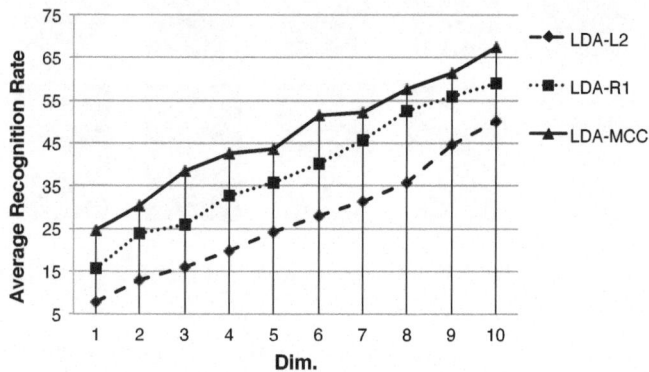

**Fig. 10.** Classification results for small dimension in AR Dataset

**Table 2.** Recognition rate and computation cost on AR dataset

| method | Recognition Rate | Average number of iterations | Average time (s) |
|---|---|---|---|
| LDA-L2 | 58.6 | / | / |
| LDA-R1 | 69.1 | 25.3 | 87.8 |
| PCA-L2 [13] | 55.2 | / | / |
| PCA-L1 [14] | 73.2 | / | / |
| LDA-MCC | 83.7 | 10.1 | 30.5 |

## 5    Conclusions and Future Work

In this paper, we proposed a novel method of LDA with MCC, which better characterizes the between-class separability. The proposed objective function is robust to outliers and can be efficiently optimized by the half-quadratic optimization technique. For each iteration step, the complex correntropy objective can be reduced to a weighted traditional LDA optimization problem. The proposed subspace method not only successfully suppresses the negative effects of outliers but also it is invariant to rotations. Experimental results have demonstrated the effectiveness of the proposed method compared to the existing approaches.

In out future work, first, how to apply MCC to with-class distance and how to extend MCC to matrix or tensor based LDA will be studied. Second, some specific applications, such as facial expression recognition, using the proposed method will be evaluated.

# References

1. Geng, Y., Shan, C., Hao, P.: Square loss based regularized lda for face recognition using image sets. In: CVPRW, pp. 99–106 (2009)
2. Landon, J., Jeffs, B., Warnick, K.: Model-based subspace projection beamforming for deep interference nulling. IEEE Transactions on Signal Processing 60, 1215–1228 (2012)
3. McLachlan, G.J.: Discriminant analysis and statistical pattern recognition. Wiley (1992)
4. Zhao, W., Chellappa, R., Krishnaswamy, A.: Discriminant analysis of principal components for face recognition. In: 3rd International Conference on Automatic Face and Gesture Recognition (1998)
5. Li, X., Hu, W., Wang, H., Zhang, Z.: Linear discriminant analysis using rotational invariant l1 norm. Neurocomputing, 2571–2579 (2010)
6. Liu, W., Pokharel, P.P., Principe, J.C.: Correntropy: Properties and applications in non-gaussian signal processing. IEEE Trans. Signal Process 55, 5286–5298 (2007)
7. Parzen, E.: On estimation of a probability density function and mode. The Annals of Mathematical Statistics 33, 1065–1076 (1962)
8. Rockfellar, R.: Convex analysis. Princeton Univ., Princeton (1970)
9. Yuan, X., Hu, B.: Robust feature extraction via information theoretic learning. In: Proceedings of the 26th Annual International Conference on Machine Learning, pp. 1193–1200 (2009)
10. Silverman, B.W.: Density estimation for statistics and data analysis. Chapman and Hall, London (1986)
11. http://www.ux.uis.no/tranden/brodatz.html
12. http://www.cl.cam.ac.uk/research/dtg/attarchive/facedatabase.html
13. Turk, M.A., Pentland, A.P.: Face recognition using eigenfaces. In: IEEE Conference on Computer Vision and Pattern Recognition (1991)
14. Kwak, N.: Principal component analysis based on L1-norm maximization. IEEE Trans. Pattern Anal. Mach. Intell. 30, 1672–1680 (2008)
15. Martnez, A., Benavente, R.: The ar-face database. CVC Technical Report 24 (1998)

# AfNet: The Affordance Network

Karthik Mahesh Varadarajan and Markus Vincze

Vienna, Austria

**Abstract.** There has been a growing need to build an object recognition system that can successfully characterize object constancy, irrespective of lighting, shading, occlusions, viewpoint variations and most importantly, deal with the multitude of shapes, colors and sizes in which objects are found. Affordances on the other hand, provide symbolic grounding mechanisms that enable linking features obtained from visual perception with the functionality of the objects, which provides the most consistent and holistic characterization of an object. Recognition by Component Affordances (RBCA) is a recent theory that builds affordance features for recognition. As an extension of the psychophysical theory of Recognition by Components (RBC) to generic visual perception, RBCA is well suited for cognitive visual processing systems which are required to perform implicit cognitive tasks. A common task is to substitute a cup for a mug, bottle, jug, pitcher, pilsner, beaker, chalice, goblet or any other unlabeled object, but with a physical part affording the ability to hold liquid and a part affording grasping by a human hand, given the goal of 'finding an empty cup' and no cups are available in the work environment of interest. In this paper, we present affordance features for recognition of objects. Using a set of 25 structural and 10 material affordances we define a database of over 250 common household objects. This database called the Affordance Network or AfNet is available as community development framework and is well suited for deployment on domestic robots. Sample object recognition results using AfNet and the associated inference engine that grounds the affordances through visual perception features demonstrate the effectiveness of the approach.

## 1 Introduction

Affordances for cognitive object recognition have received close attention in recent years. Recent major contributions in the field have been from [1, 18], which use explicit modeling of the interacting agent for affordance and hence object recognition. However such approaches are neither scalable nor comprehensive, since they suffer from a representation deadlock resulting from the fact that modeling of the agent and its actions are necessary to model the object and the former task is a challenge in itself. For example, in order to model a 'sittable' object, it is necessary to model the 'human' or 'child' or 'dog' in the first place, which is not just superfluous, but also non-trivial. It becomes necessary to model only attributes of the 'human' that relate to the object being detected. This in turn is entirely defined by the 'sittable object' in this case. A more holistic approach would be characterize objects without modeling agents but in terms of

K.M. Lee et al. (Eds.): ACCV 2012, Part I, LNCS 7724, pp. 512–523, 2013.
© Springer-Verlag Berlin Heidelberg 2013

attributes such as scales, position, pose that would enable a human agent to interact with it. For the purpose of visual perception systems, it is possible to take for granted the agent of action to be human and build affordance definitions as intrinsic properties of the object (at scales/pose ascertained for an average human). There have also been recent advances towards the use of object attributes towards recognition [16, 17] in the framework of Zero-shot learning. However, the choice, types and suitability of attributes is rather arbitrary. On the other hand, in this domain, a related paradigm of conceptual equivalence classes for cognitive representation of object categories has been recently introduced [3]. These classes are defined as sets of objects that are functionally equivalent. For most cognitive visual processing applications such as robotic manipulation tasks in domestic environments, these classes represent the optimally sufficient and necessary representation for object recognition. These classes are defined based on the theory of Recognition by Component Affordances (RBCA). These affordances are not just an arbitrary set of features for object representation. Instead affordances present an evolutionary and psychophysical model to visual perception grounded in the evolutionary psychophysical theory of '$k$-TR' [6]. Affordances [7] have been used as a feature for object recognition in the past. However, there has been a lack of an exhaustive affordance theory that is capable of handling the wide variety of object types in man-made physical world. Current affordance theories are too disparate and incomprehensive to support practical object recognition. There have been some recent attempts at using affordances for robotics [10, 11, 12]. The MACS project [11] is the most significant of these efforts. The major contribution of the MACS project is affordance cueing, which has been implemented using machine learning and is limited to perceptibility of traversability and a few other forms relevant to the robot at hand, but not as a holistic tool for object feature representation. Various ontologies have also been used recently for semantic object retrieval. Semantic Web, OWL (Web Ontology Language) based systems are being increasingly used. The most significant of semantic knowledge acquisition and representational systems is the ConceptNet. In the domain of robotic vision systems, the most popular system is the KnowRob (Knowledge Processing for Robots), which uses reasoners and machine learning tools such as Prolog, Mallet and Weka, operating on ontology databases such as researchCyc and OMICS (indoor common-sense knowledge database). However, these systems use explicit 3D models for object representation hence curtailing scalability of the system. Furthermore, they lack suitable representations for implicit cognitive processing. The theory of RBCA and Equivalence Classes help overcome these issues. Recognition by component parts and semantic definitions based on parts is a well explored area. Furthemore, recognition using functional parts and their linkages has been studied earlier [19, 20, 21]. However, none of these approaches have defined an ontology that goes beyond recognizing the very basic 2-part objects such as hammers or deal with affordances beyond the very basic 'sittability' and 'containability'. There is a definite lack of an affordance based ontology that can deal with the wide variety of objects in the world.

## 2   Algorithm

The main contribution of this paper is in defining a concise set of affordance features for cognitive object recognition leading to AfNet - The Affordance Network database that represents objects in terms of affordance features. These features are scalable, representative of conceptual equivalence classes and provide for cognitive visual perception and scene understanding systems. The resulting framework, called the Visual Cognitive Engine (VCE) is discussed in the paper with demonstration of its efficiency in recognizing generic everyday objects together with task related implicit cognitive processing.

These functionally related object types form an equivalence class and detection of the equivalence category is an optimally sufficient and necessary condition for task related visual perception and object manipulation. RBCA in the human visual perception system is supported by the '$k$-TR' theory. Our Visual Cognitive Engine (VCE) is composed of a Range Processing Module and an Inference Engine which uses multiple ontologies, along with abstract features which we define in this paper- affordance features leading to the Affordance Network (AfNet) database. Symbol binding schemes permit task based recognition of affordances from RGB-D data. AfNet is successful in describing over 250 everyday objects (Fig 1) through RBCA using 35 (Fig 2) affordance types. Thus, we present a novel schema that goes beyond the very basic of affordances such as sittability and containability and objects such as hammers and beds that form the limit of current state-of-the-art algorithms that use affordances or semantics based object definitions.

### 2.1   $k$-TR Theory of Affordances

The '$k$-TR' theory [6] presents the first holistic and scalable attempt to explaining the modeling and recognition of objects in the human visual perception using affordances going beyond [19, 20, 21] in providing concise, yet highly expressive affordance features. '$k$-TR' hypothesizes a two-step process to visual perception and recognition of objects. The first level is based on an evolutionary cognitive algorithmic process (k) - that learns abstract functional visual primitives such as flatness, concavities etc. The second level depends on repeated learning of correlated local features in the object space (TR) - instances such as 'small cylinders' etc. A first attempt at modeling '$k$-TR' features or '$k$-TRONs' for object recognition was presented in [2]. Saliency models using the '$k$-TR' model have been presented in [22] and '$k$-TR' and affordance based language for cognitive robot task description in [23].

### 2.2   Recognition by Component Affordances (RBCA) and $k$-TRONs

Biederman's Recognition by Components (RBC) [8] theory puts forward a schema for visual object recognition based on geons. Though concise, this theory suffers from several serious drawbacks. Most importantly, it does not provide models for cognitive, semantic or intuitive processes that form the basis of object categorization. Of several computer vision theories based on extension of geon-like paradigms, the theory of RBCA addresses this issue successfully. RBCA states that recognition occurs primarily (at the holistic $k$ level) through the detection of part affordances. $k$-TRON features (a combination of '$k$' and 'TR') are essentially part based. 'TR' features are (a) global features such as simple 2D shapes such as squares, circles or 3D shapes such as cylinders, cubes, (b) local features such as color or texture On the other hand, '$k$' features are essentially affordance features- (a) Structural affordances- functions rendered by an object as a result of its geometric structure (such as flatness or concavity), (b) Material affordances- rendered by the material properties of the object. Humans are capable of categorizing previously unseen objects with uncharacteristic color, texture, size and shape into its right class, without apriori knowledge about the exact instance name of the object. $k$-TR hypothesizes that this ability of humans is due to the inference of abstract knowledge about the object based on the paradigm of 'Conceptual Equivalence Classes' [3]. This mechanism also forms the highest level of abstraction or minimal essential subset of the '$k$' processes that are key to object constancy. In other words, the Structural Affordance schema forms core and primal mechanism for object constancy and recognition.

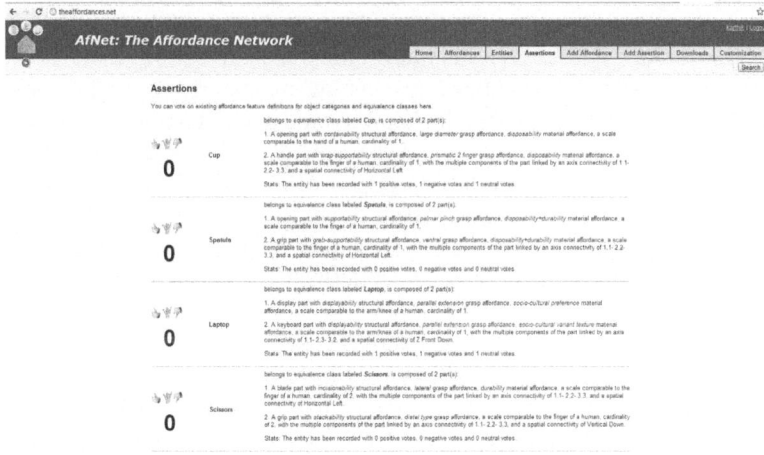

**Fig. 1.** Affordance based definitions for a slice of the AfNet Ontology

## 2.3   Affordance Features and AfNet – The Affordance Network

The Structural Part Affordance Schema first presented in [3] and supported by [5] has been extended leading to the creation of the Affordance Network database (AfNet), (available for download, see Fig 1. for samples from the database), while providing an interactive user interface to update affordance definitions. This database represents each conceptual equivalence class in terms of various structural affordance definitions, grasp affordances and topological relationships between the various components which constitute the object in question, while providing symbol binding mechanisms for these affordances. For eg. the definition for a pen is stated as belonging to Equivalence Class labeled Pen, composed of 1 part(s): 1. A Generic part with Engraveability structural affordance, Writing Tripod grasp affordance, a scale comparable to the Finger of a human, cardinality of 1. The definition for a Knife is: belongs to Equivalence Class labeled Knife, composed of 2 part(s): 1. A Blade part with Incisionability structural affordance, Lateral grasp affordance, Durability material affordance, a scale comparable to the Finger of a human, cardinality of 1, 2. A Handle part with Grab-supportability structural affordance, Ventral grasp affordance, a scale comparable to the Finger of a human, cardinality of 1, with the multiple components of the object linked by an axis connectivity of 1,1- 2,2- 3,3, and a spatial connectivity of Horizontal Left. AfNet is structured similar to ConceptNet, ImageNet, WordNet etc. and is built to complement these databases in providing a holistic object recognition system. AfNet also defines the scale of the object parts (in abstract measures with respect to the human arm: labels 'f' through 'a' denoting sizes comparable to finger upto arm). In addition, abstract topological relationships (axial and spatial connectivity) between the object parts each of which provides an affordance is also defined. These are defined with respect to the Part Connectivity Calculus (PCC) [15]. Since Gibson's fundamental work on affordances [7], there have been various disparate and arbitrary definitions of affordance features in use for computer vision. AfNet provides the first holistic and concise set of affordances. This affordance feature set as demonstrated by the AfNet database of object affordance definitions describe over 250 most common objects using just 25 (+10) affordance primitives. These are classified as (a) Structural affordances that corresponds to inferred knowledge about the 2D/3D shape of the object. For example, detection of a cylindrical or circular shape corresponding to a part of the object or as a whole, indicates a Roll-ability affordance. Example of an object affording roll-ability is the vehicle tire. Similarly, a flat or slightly convex part indicates a structural and hence function affordance of Support-ability, indicating that the part/object is capable of supporting other objects over it. The seat of a chair is an example of an object part that provides the support-ability affordance. A 3D structure with a high degree of convexity supports an affordance of Contain-ability. Cups, mugs and beakers provide this affordance. Detection of a sharp tip indicates an affordance of Engrave-ability. Pens, styluses, pencils exhibit this affordance. It should be noted that structural affordance definitions are key to equivalence class recognition, while the secondary affordances are required for fine grained categorization of conceptual equivalence classes or instance based object recognition that might be essential for certain robot applications.

## 3    Symbol Grounding – Range Processing Module of the VCE

We employ the algorithms of [13, 14] combined with a Semantic Part Segmentor for building our Range Processing Module for the VCE. The symbol grounding from range (and color images) uses the following pipeline.

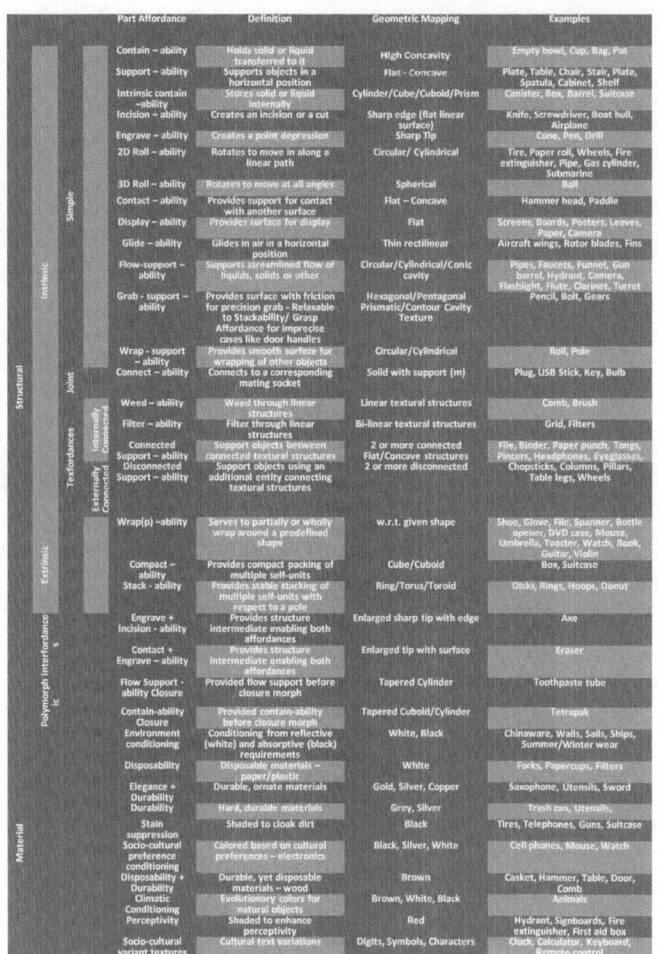

**Fig. 2.** Partial list of affordance features

Range Data Pre-Processing: Range pre-processing (Fig 3) is carried out using a combination of Depth Diffusion for sparsity reduction [13, 14] and Bilateral Filtering for surface normalization. The diffusion is carried out using a PDE heat solver based on the Iterative Back Substitution (IBS) algorithm. An MRF based region classifier is used to guide the diffusion, through determination of neighborhood similarity (of texture). The core equation for diffusion that represents the change in pixel values $u$ with time $t$ are given by

$$\frac{\partial u(r,t)}{\partial t} = c\left(\frac{\partial^2 u(r,t)}{\partial x^2} + \frac{\partial^2 u(r,t)}{\partial y^2}\right) \qquad (1)$$

Part Detection from Range Images: We employ a novel part segmentor to detect parts in range images. This segmentor [4] is based on semantic scene information and depth and curvature edges and regions, followed semantic edge selection

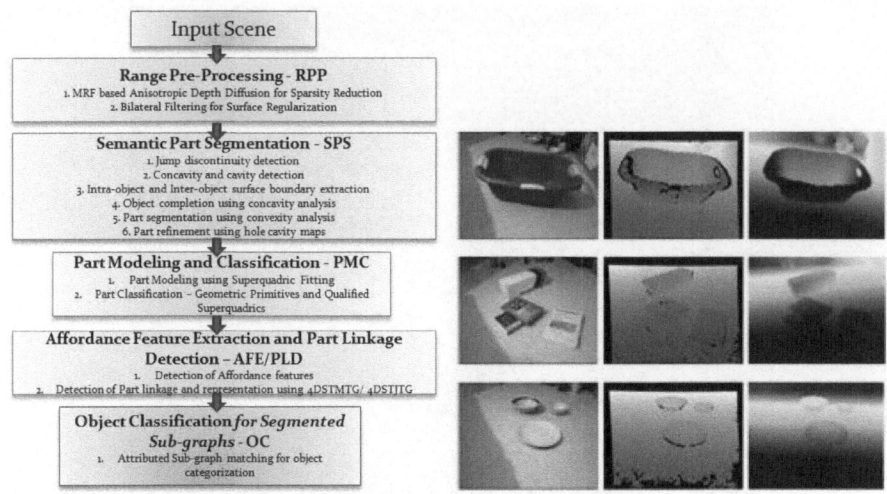

**Fig. 3.** Left: Range Processing Pipeline of the Visual Cognitive Engine (VCE). Right: Input depth maps and depth maps after diffusion.

```
FringeTriDiagSolver := {InitializeSolution,
InitializeMatrixComputation,      i_iter -> 0,
        While[{CurrEps > EpsTol && i_iter < MaxItr && AbsErr > AbsErrTol},{

                            i_iter -> i_iter + 1,


StorePreviousResult,
ForwardSubstitution,BackwardSubstitution,
ComputeMaximumResidual}]      }
```

**Fig. 4.** Iterative Back Substitution (IBS) Algorithm for solving tridiagonal linear systems with fringes

and region merging to identify the most consistent object regions. Based on a number of processes, including detection of cavities, concavities (Fig 5) and other semantic cues, part segmentation is carried out.

Part Recognition using Superquadric Fitting: The detected parts are then fit (using Levelberg Marquardt Algorithm -LMA optimized using Particle Swarms -PSO) to geometric primitives using Superquadrics that are defined using a 15 parameter feature space (6 DOF pose, 2 model parameters, 4 deformation parameters - bending and tapering, 3 scale parameters). The fitting function is given by

$$F^{\epsilon_1}(x, y, z) = \left( \left( \left( \frac{x}{a_1} \right)^{\frac{2}{\epsilon_2}} + \left( \frac{y}{a_2} \right)^{\frac{2}{\epsilon_2}} \right)^{\frac{\epsilon_2}{\epsilon_1}} + \left( \frac{z}{a_3} \right)^{\frac{2}{\epsilon_1}} \right)^{\epsilon_1} \tag{2}$$

The geometric primitive labels (such as cuboid, cylinder, cone etc.) are then identified by classification of the Superquadric parameters. Based on abstract

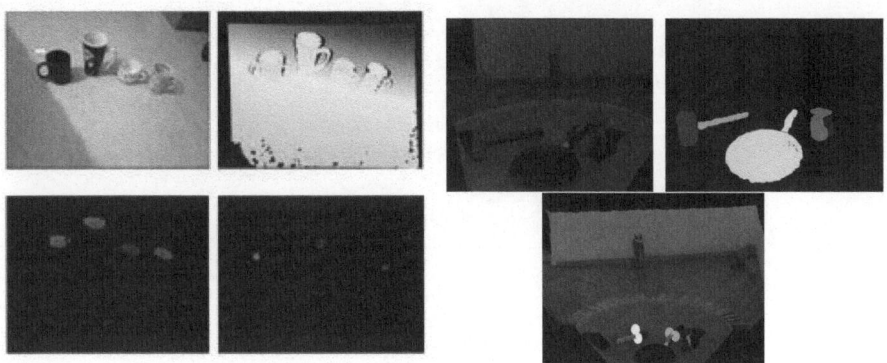

**Fig. 5.** Left: (Top to bottom, left to right) Color image, input depth map, detected concavities and cavity map. Right: (Left to Right) Input 3D scene, detected parts, detected graspable handle affordances.

geometric information obtained from the part segments (such as flat, convex, concave etc) as well as based on the type of SQ fit, the part affordance is detected (Fig 5).

### 3.1   Symbol Grounding – Inference Engine

The Inference Engine of the VCE is responsible for the selection of the right object (object providing the right affordance) given an input query. The Inference Engine uses the AfNet database to find a match corresponding to the query of interest. If a direct match amongst the equivalence class members is found, this definition is used for pattern matching with a high confidence score. In case of a no match, the engine uses WordNet and ConceptNet to find the most relevant object in the scene (Fig 6). Each object in the scene is represented as a graph with its parts defining nodes along with vector attributes that may be symbolic (such as affordances) or metric (scales). In the given scene of interest, the queried object for the given task is found using attributed graph matching of the concept node built for the query with all geometrical objects found in the scene. Given the limited number of objects in a given scene, the matching process is fast and accurate. Refer to Figure 11 for sample graph definitions.

## 4   Results and Evaluation

As seen from figure 2, each affordance presents a unique symbol grounding/ binding mechanism, that is detected using the processing pipeline demonstrated in figure 3. However, it can be seen that some of the structural geometries corresponding to the affordances partially overlap, resulting in affordance ambiguities. Furthermore, some structural geometries are difficult to detect, especially in cluttered scenes. Figure 7 shows the true positive vs false positive rates obtained in the identification of various affordances in an office environment across

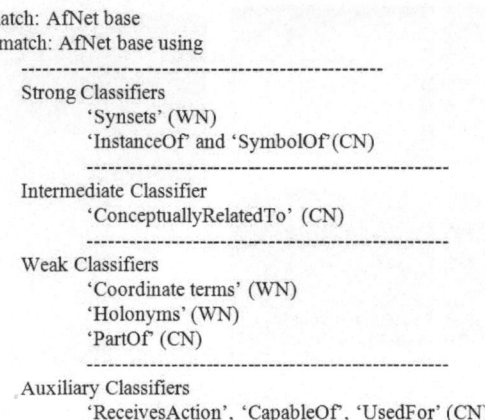

Fig. 6. Partial inference mechanism for Visual Query Match - Levels of matching

20 scenes each with 25 objects posssessing different affordances. It can be seen that while certain affordances such as supportability are easily detected, others such as connectability are poorly discerned. Additional results for classification of objects with different affordance features can be found in the supplementary materials.

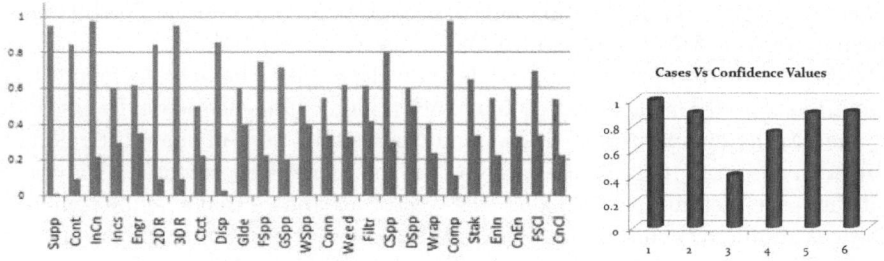

Fig. 7. Left: True (blue) and false positive (red) detection rate for affordance features (Ref Fig 2) Right: Confidence levels returned by VCE for the 6 test cases in Fig 10

The system can also be evaluated on a case by case basis through a set of queries associated with perception tasks. The query tasks and corresponding scenes are shown in Figure 8. The graphs generated for each test case are also shown in figure 8. Further detailed examples are presented in supplementary materials. Intermediate results from the Range Processing modules of the Visual Cognitive Engine are also shown in the figure. It should be noted that the current version of the Inference Engine of the VCE primarily depends on the AfNet for object feature definitions, as opposed to using ConceptNet and WordNet for object representation. These ontologies are used as auxiliary knowledge bases to aid in the parsing of query terms that AfNet does not provide explicit definitions for.

The input RGB and depth images of the scene are shown in rows A and B. Results of range image pre-processing are presented in rows C and D. Depth diffusion results are shown in C, while the depth normals after surface regularization are shown in D. Row E depicts results of concavity detection. Intermediate object candidates are shown in F. Final object detection results after semantic processing using concavity and cavity information are shown in G, followed by part detection results in row H. Each part is shaded in a different color in row H. The regularized scene is shown in row I. Row J shows selective results of superquadric fitting for each scene with respect to the object of interest, as chosen by the Inference Engine in response to the user query. Each setting required the robot to scan the given scene for an object of interest in response to a task query. (a) For the first scene, a search query of box was presented. AfNet maps the equivalence class corresponding to boxes with the intrinsic containability affordance, which is grounded through cylinder/cuboid/prism geometric mappings. Hence, other surfaces corresponding to books are discarded, while the box is chosen for further processing. In this case the weighted confidence score returned is 0.9 corresponding to the classification confidence from the Superquadric parameters. The book in the scene is not returned due to its thin structure (b) In the second scene, the system is presented with a search query for 'plate'. Using the supportability affordance returned by AfNet, the VCE rejects the bowls in the scene, with an output confidence of 1.0. (c) For the third scene, a search query for 'jug' was presented. It should be noted that the query 'jug' is not available in the equivalence class database, hence causing the search to be non-trivial. Using WordNet based parsing, renders the part affordance of 'containability' with a weight measure of 2 (out of 10), based on frequency scores for primary (from definition text) and secondary characteristics (from other attributes). ConceptNet also renders the 'containability' affordance along with a 'HasA' attribute of 'handle' which provides the grasp affordance for the given case. The attributed graph for the given query is simple and is composed of nodes for 'containability' part affordance and a 'handle' - small diameter grasp affordance with an overall weighted confidence score of 0.415 (1.66/4) (using concept and textual unit definitions of 1 and 3 respectively). The range image processing algorithms yield both the mugs in scene as results (prioritized by the closest object), since these objects contain concavities (affordance: containability) and handles (grasp affordance) that match the query graph attributes exactly (normalized HEOM score of 1). (d) The fourth scene contains considerable clutter and a query of mug was presented to the system. Using an affordance mapping of Containability from AfNet, the disposable container in the scene is returned with confidence level of 0.75 (since part functional affordance is matched while, grasp affordance is not - missing handle from definition of mug). Nevertheless, it is the best cognitive result for the given test case. (e) In the fifth case, a search query for bench is requested. Using an AfNet match corresponding to supportability affordances with respect to two staggered orthogonal parts - the seat and the back, the chair in the scene is returned as the result with a confidence level of 0.9 (since the legs are missing in the viewpoint) . (f) In the sixth case, a search query - 'basket' is presented. The range processing module of the VCE returns the handles and the concave bodies of the bag which afford Containability. The confidence score on the resulting affordance description is 0.91 (3.64/4) (WordNet returns a high frequency score of 8). The overall confidence levels for each test scenario is listed in Fig. 7, with the confidence levels returned by VCE for the 6 test cases based on both strong classifiers (AfNet) and weak classifiers (ConceptNet, WordNet).

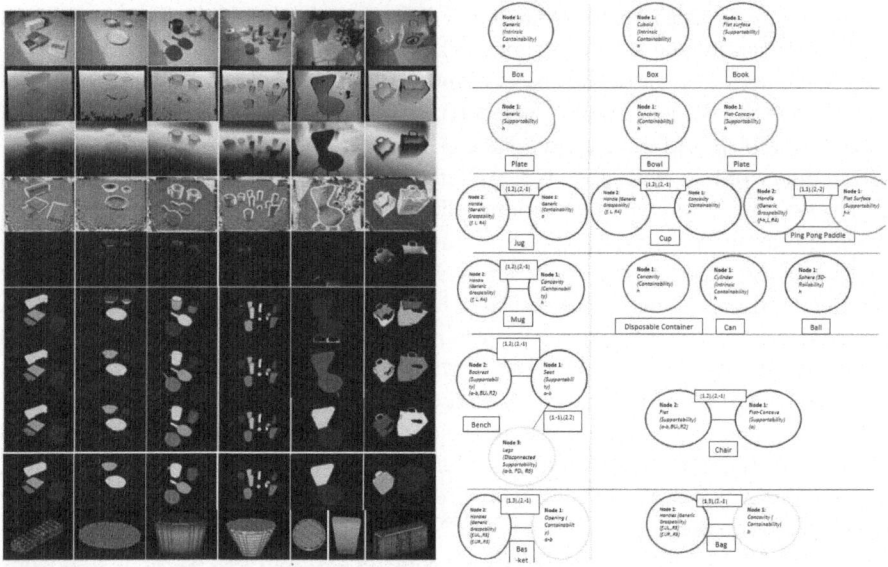

**Fig. 8.** Left: Rows (A) Sample scenes (B) Input depth map (C) Diffused depth map (D) Depth normals after surface regularization (E) Concavity map (F) Object candidates (G) Object map (H) Part map (I) Regularized scene (J) Superquadric fitting of parts based on cognitive query processing. Right: Query Attributed Graphs (Left panel - query label shown in box) and Object Attributed Graphs (Right panel) to be matched for each scene on the left.

### 4.1   Conclusion

In this work, we have presented details about our affordance feature set for generic and scalable object detection and the structure of a novel Visual Cognitive Engine that uses affordance features, representation, storage and implicit task based cognitive processing. The various components of the framework and modules that the VCE interacts with are also presented. A detailed evaluation of the Range Processing and the Inference Engine modules of the VCE are also presented. The recognition process in the VCE is abstracted through the representation of Conceptual Equivalence Classes. These form the Structural Affordance Schema Layer of the 'k-TR' theory. This also forms the minimal complete or holistic component of the theory within the scope of object recognition. Use of AfNet enables support for processing over 250 commonly found object types. Extension of this database as well as enhancement of the VCE form current scope of work.

# References

1. Grabner, H., Gall, J., van Gool, L.: What Makes a Chair a Chair? In: CVPR, pp. 1529–1536 (2011)
2. Varadarajan, K.M., Vincze, M.: Holistic Visual Cognitive Recognizer using Part based Local, Global, Semantic and Affordance Features. In: CVPR W (2011)
3. Varadarajan, K.M., Vincze, M.: Affordance based Part Recognition for Grasping and Manipulation. In: ICRA W (2011)
4. Varadarajan, K.M., Vincze, M.: Object Part Segmentation and Classification in Range Images for Grasping. In: ICAR (2011)
5. Varadarajan, K.M., Vincze, M.: Knowledge Representation and Inference for Grasp Affordances. In: Crowley, J.L., Draper, B.A., Thonnat, M. (eds.) ICVS 2011. LNCS, vol. 6962, pp. 173–182. Springer, Heidelberg (2011)
6. Varadarajan, K.M.: Karmic Tabula Rasa k-TR - A Theory of Visual Perception. In: ISP (2011)
7. Gibson, J.J.: The Theory of Affordances. In: Shaw, R., Bransford, J. (eds.) (1977) ISBN 0-470-99014-7
8. Biederman I.: Recognition - by - components: a theory of human image understanding. Psych. Rev. (1994)
9. MacDorman, K.F.: Responding to affordances: Learning and projecting a sensorimotor mapping. In: ICRA (2000)
10. Fitzpatrick, P., et. al: Learning about objects through action. In: ICRA (2003)
11. Stoytchev, A.: Toward learning the binding affordances of objects. In: AAAI Symposium on Dev. Robotics (2005)
12. Sahin, E., et al.: To afford or not to afford. Adaptive Behavior 15(4), 447–472 (2007)
13. Varadarajan, K.M., Vincze, M.: Real-Time Depth Diffusion for 3D Surface Reconstruction. In: ICIP (2010)
14. Varadarajan, K.M., Vincze, M.: Surface Reconstruction for RGB-D Data using Real-Time Depth Propagation. In: ICCV W (2011)
15. Varadarajan, K.M., Vincze, M.: 4D Space-Time Mereotopogeometry. In: PCC ICRA (2013)
16. Lampert, C.H., Nickisch, H., Harmeling, S.: Learning to detect unseen object classes by between class attribute transfer. In: CVPR (2009)
17. Parikh D., Grauman K.: Relative Attributes. In: ICCV (2011)
18. Gupta, A., Satkin, E., Efros, I., Hebert, M.: From 3D Scene Geometry to Human Workspace. In: CVPR (2011)
19. Winston, P.H., Binford, T.O., Katz, B., Lowry, M.: Learning physical description from functional definitions, examples, and precedents. MIT Press (1984)
20. Stark, L., Bowyer, K.: Achieving generalized object recognition through reasoning about association of function to structure. PAMI (1991)
21. Rivlin, E., Dickinson, S.J., Rosenfeld, A.: Recognition by functional parts. In: CVIU (1995)
22. Varadarajan, K.M., Vincze, M.: K-TR Theory of Semantic Saliency. In: ICPR (2012)
23. Varadarajan, K.M., Vincze, M.: AfkTRAANS: The language of Cognitive Robots. In: AAAI Robotics and Multimedia Satellite Event (2012)

# A Directed Graphical Model
# for Linear Barcode Scanning
# from Blurred Images

Ling Chen *

Department of Computer Science
Southwestern University of Finance and Economics, China
lchen@swufe.edu.cn

**Abstract.** Image blur is one of the major issues deteriorating the capability of a linear barcode scanning system. In this work, linear barcode scanning is treated under the perspective of stochastic modeling and inference. A directed graphical model is proposed to characterize the relationship between barcode value and its out-of-focused waveforms, based on which highly effective inference process can be implemented, allowing decoding barcode in real-time on mobile devices, directly from blurred images. The value of the proposed model is its potential to enlarge the operating range of current linear barcode scanning systems with no need for dedicated hardware components and making linear barcode scanning at close-up distance on fixed-focus lens a reality.

## 1 Introduction

Out-of-focus blur is one of the most prominent issues which often undermines the performance of or even totally invalidates a barcode scanning system. This is especially the case for linear barcode (also called 1D barcode, refer Fig. 1 for an example), in which information is normally encoded into bars and spaces of varying predefined dimensions. Features for locating these bars and spaces, such as boundary of bars and spaces or peaks of barcode waveform, are usually searched and utilized as the basis of many current barcode scanning systems [1, 2], leading to their dependency on the capability of recovering this type of features, which usually diminish or even totally disappear when the barcode is located outside the *depth of field* (DOF) of the optical system.

There exists research efforts of reading barcodes under severe image blur at the signal processing and analysis level . A main school of thought is to treat this problem in the image restoration/deblurring domain [3–6]. But the iterative nature of this categories of methods makes the computation very time consuming, not feasible for real-time barcode scanning in real world situations.

In this paper we present a directed graphical model for linear barcode reading which is robust to severe out-of-focus blur. For an EAN-13 or UPC-A barcode

* This work is supported in part by SWUFE under Grant 211QN10055 and by WuXi AiDingGe Info. Tech. Co., Ltd.

K.M. Lee et al. (Eds.): ACCV 2012, Part I, LNCS 7724, pp. 524–535, 2013.
© Springer-Verlag Berlin Heidelberg 2013

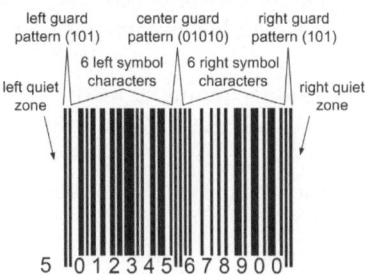

**Fig. 1.** Example of a 1D barcode. It is an EAN-13 barcode and the encoded value is 5012345678900. EAN-13 barcode is composed of 95 modules (narrow elements), the width of each module is called the X-dimension or simply the module width.

(refer [7]), the maximum out-of-focus blur can be handled by the current implementation of the proposed directed graphical model is up to the width of one symbol character, which is 7 times the module width of a EAN/UPC barcode. Unlike barcode image restoration methods, which usually try to reconstruct the original barcode image or scanline and then use traditional barcode scanning methods to get the code value, the proposed new system tries to classify the observed barcode signal directly through stochastic modeling and inference, without image deblurring, which is usually a mathematically ill-defined problem, computationally difficult to be dealt with.

## 2    Motivations of Stochastic Modeling for Linear Barcode Scanning

The *point spread function* (PSF) $h(x, y)$ of the linear shift invariant out-of-focus blurring process can be modeled as a uniform circular disk [8]:

$$h(x, y) = \begin{cases} 0, \sqrt{x^2 + y^2} > r \\ 1/(\pi r^2), \sqrt{x^2 + y^2} \leq r \end{cases} \tag{1}$$

where the blur radius $r$ represents the out-of-focus level. The *line spread function* (LSF) corresponding to Eq. (1) is

$$h(x) = \frac{2}{\pi r^2} \sqrt{r^2 - x^2}, \quad -r \leq x \leq r \tag{2}$$

As linear barcode is a composition of line segments of various widths, if a scanline is extracted from the out-of-focus blurred barcode image, the extracted scanline is actually the standard barcode symbol scanline convoluted with the LSF of out-of-focus blur, plus the additive noise, i.e.,

$$g(x) = h(x) \otimes f(x) + n(x),$$

where $f(x)$ is the standard barcode symbol scanline, $g(x)$ is the observed scan-line, $\otimes$ represents the 1-dimensional linear convolution operator, and $n(x)$ is the additive noise.

In the context of linear barcode scanning, if we denote the traditional scanning system (e.g., [9, 2]) as $S_{\text{traditional}}$ and the code value as $\mathbf{c}$, image restoration based methods normally try to get an estimation $\hat{f}(x, y)$ of the original image $f(x, y)$, then use $S_{\text{traditional}}$ to map the estimation to the barcode value, i.e.,

$$S_{\text{traditional}} : \hat{f}(x, y) \mapsto \mathbf{c}.$$

We claim that it is possible to directly cope with the degraded barcode signal, such as a scanline $g(x)$ extracted from the out-of-focus blurred barcode image, and design a linear barcode scanning system $S$, which directly maps the degraded barcode signal to the barcode value, i.e.,

$$S : g(x) \mapsto \mathbf{c}.$$

This claim is based on the observation that a linear barcode symbol has finite number of code values; and each code value relates to a specific barcode wave-form differentiable from all other barcode waveforms of different code value. If background noise is ignored, then at any out-of-focus level, the degraded barcode waveforms are still differentiable from each other. More formally, suppose $f_1(t)$ and $f_2(t)$ are waveforms of two different linear barcode symbols. After out-of-focus blurring, we get degraded waveforms $g_1(t) = f_1(t) \otimes h(t)$ and $g_2(t) = f_2(t) \otimes h(t)$. As $f_1(t) \neq f_2(t)$, by noticing the non-zero property of out-of-focus LSF and the linearity of the out-of-focus blurring system, it can be easily seen that $g_1(t) \neq g_2(t)$. Based on this observation, if creating a bank of reference waveforms of all possible barcode values according to a specific out-of-focus blur level, then linear barcode scanning can be accomplished by comparing the degraded waveform extracted from the blurred image with the reference wave-forms to find one reference waveform most similar to the degraded waveform. And if the similarity surpasses certain predefined threshold, the barcode value corresponding to the selected reference waveform can be treated as the output of the scanning system; otherwise, the scanning process failed.

It should be noticed that a brute force comparison of the degraded bar-code waveform with all reference waveforms can be computationally prohibitive. Therefore efficient methods which can give real-time performance on carrying out the comparison process is needed. And stochastic modeling can fulfill this task, as presented below.

## 3    Linear Barcode Symbol Decomposition and State Variable Sequence Modeling

As each linear barcode symbol is composed of a series of concatenated symbol characters, and each character is discrete valued, we can always find a scheme to decompose a linear barcode symbol into a sequence of information units. Each information unit is discrete valued and is composed of one or more neighboring symbol characters. For example, an EAN-13 barcode (refer Fig. 1) is composed of 12 symbol characters. If each information unit is chosen to be composed of only one symbol character, then an EAN-13 barcode is composed of 12 information units; If each information unit is chosen to be composed of two symbol characters, then an EAN-13 barcode is composed of 6 information units. In the context of linear barcode scanning, we treat each information unit as a state variable; and each linear barcode can be represented by a state variable sequence of length $T$. All state variables are 1D discrete random variables. The value of each state variable is determined by the value of corresponding symbol character or characters. The value of any state variable is not observable (hidden) and can only be estimated from the observed barcode waveform. All state variables are independent from each other. We denote each state variable as $s_t$, where $t = 1, 2, ..., T$ represents the location of a specific state variable in the state variable sequence. We denote the state space of a state variable $s_t$ as $\{1, 2, ..., N_t\}$. It means at time $t$ the number of states is $N_t$ and all these states are represented by number 1 to $N_t$. We denote state variable sequence as $\mathbf{s} = (s_1, s_2, ..., s_T)$.

Then it can be easily seen that the prior of each state variable follows a uniform distribution, i.e., $P[s_t = i] = 1/N_t, 1 \leq i \leq N_t$. It will be clear in next section that in any linear barcode symbol decomposition scheme, the number of symbol characters associated with a state variable is determined by out-of-focus blur level. For example, if the out-of-focus blur level is less or equal to the width of one symbol character, there should be only one symbol character associated with a state variable; if the out-of-focus blur level is greater than the width of one symbol character but is less or equal to the width of two symbol characters, there should be two symbol character associated with one state variable.

It should be noticed that in the context of linear barcode scanning, the value of state variable at different location $t$ may have different meanings as symbol characters at different location may come from different symbol character encodings. Number set $\{1, 2, ..., N_t\}$ is only used to index all possible states which are corresponding to all valid symbol characters at a specific location $t$, the same state value at different locations may mean different symbol characters. Use EAN-13 barcode as an example (refer [7]), the symbol character at location $t = 1$ can only be selected from symbol character set A. Whereas at location $t = 2$ to $t = 6$, the symbol character can be selected from either symbol character set A or symbol character set B. And at location $t = 7$ to $t = 12$, the symbol character can only be selected from symbol character set C. Therefore when $s_1 = 1$, it means the symbol character selected at location 1 is the first character of character set A; and when $s_7 = 1$, it means the symbol character selected at location 7 is the first character of character set C. That is, although in this case $s_1 = s_7$, these two state variables are actually representing different symbol characters.

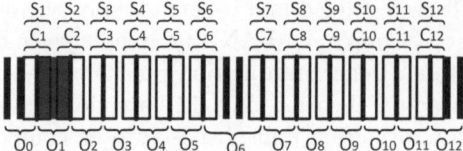

**Fig. 2.** A scanline segmentation scheme of EAN-13 barcode under the condition that the out-of-focus blur level is less or equal to the width of one symbol character. In this figure each symbol character is represented by $c_t$, $t = 1, 2, ..., 12$. Each rectangle beneath $c_t$ represents space occupied by each symbol character (For the convenience of differentiating neighbouring symbol characters, neighbouring rectangles are artificially separated). A bold line segment is drawn in each rectangle in order to delineate the middle point of each rectangle. Given that the out-of-focus level is less or equal to the width of one symbol character, the symbol decomposition scheme can be that each state variable is associated with one symbol character, as illustrated in this figure, where each state variable is represented by $s_t$. If scanline is segmented by the middle point of each rectangle (one segment is illustrated by the gray area in the figure), it can be easily noticed the waveform of each segmentation is only dependent on neighbouring state variables on its immediate left and right and is independent of all other state variables. Each observation variable corresponding to each waveform segment is represented by $\mathbf{o}_t$, $t = 0, 1, ..., 12$.

## 4    Linear Barcode Scanline Segmentation and Observation Sequence Modeling

Based on state variable sequence modeling of linear barcode, when out-of-focus blur level is less than one half of the total length of a barcode symbol, given a scanline of a barcode symbol and the out-of-focus blur level, we can always determine a linear barcode scanline segmentation scheme, to make that each waveform segment in the scanline segmentation scheme is jointly determined by only two neighbouring state variables and is independent of any other state variables in the state variable sequence (The waveform segment located at the boundary area of the scanline is solely determined by the first state variable or the last state variable). An example scanline segmentation scheme of EAN-13 barcode is given in Figure 2 in which the out-of-focus blur level is less or equal to the width of one symbol character. In this figure, each state variable contains one symbol character. Similarly, if the out-of-focus blur is greater than the width of one symbol character and is less or equal to the width of two symbol characters, each state variable can be made to contain two consecutive symbol characters, etc.

After scanline segmentation, each waveform segment can be treated as an observation variable; and the scanline can be represented by an observation variable sequence. All observation variables are multi-dimensional random variables. The value of each observation variable is observable and is jointly determined by two consecutive state variables (The two boundary observation variables located on the two sides of the scanline are individually determined by the first state variable and the last state variable). We denote each observation variable as $\mathbf{o}_t$ with dimension $D_t$, where $t = 0, 1, ..., T$. We denote observation variable sequence as $\mathbf{O} = (\mathbf{o}_0, \mathbf{o}_1, ..., \mathbf{o}_T)$. Denote multi-dimensional constant $\boldsymbol{\mu}_t(i, j) = [\mu_1, \mu_2, ..., \mu_{D_t}]'$, where $t = 1, 2, ..., T - 1$, as the standard reference waveform segment at the detected out-of-focus level when the values of two consecutive state variables $s_t$ and $s_{t+1}$ are $i$ and $j$, respectively. Denote multi-dimensional constant $\boldsymbol{\mu}_t(i) = [\mu_1, \mu_2, ..., \mu_{D_t}]'$, where $t = 0$ or $t = T$, as the standard reference waveform segment at the detected out-of-focus level when the value of the first or the last state variable is $i$.

The standard reference waveform segments can be calculated offline. The procedure of determining the value of the standard reference waveform segment is:

- For $t = 0$, choose state variable value $s_0 = i$, the out-of-focus kernel corresponding to the detected blur level is convoluted with the standard waveform of the first symbol character corresponding to state variable value $i$. After convolution, the part on the right side of the middle point of the resulting waveform is cut off and the remaining waveform segment is $\boldsymbol{\mu}_0(i)$. Repeat this procedure for $i = 1, 2, ..., N_0$ to get $\boldsymbol{\mu}_0(i)$, $i = 1, 2, ..., N_0$.

- Similarly, we can get $\boldsymbol{\mu}_T(i)$, $i = 1, 2, ..., N_T$, except the cut-off part after convolution is on the left side of the middle point of the resulting waveform.

- For $t = 1, 2, ..., T - 1$, choose state variable values $s_t = i$ and $s_{t+1} = j$, the out-of-focus kernel corresponding to the detected blur level is convoluted with the standard waveform of two consecutive symbol characters corresponding to state variable value $i$ and $j$. After convolution, the part located in between the original middle points of the two consecutive symbol characters are kept as $\boldsymbol{\mu}_t(i, j)$, $i = 1, 2, ..., N_t$ and $j = 1, 2, ..., N_{t+1}$.

It should be noticed that if guard patterns are defined (such as EAN-13/UPC-A barcode) for a specific symbology type, they should be integrated into the standard reference waveform segmentation scheme described above.

Then if we assume the background noise is Gaussian, i.e., $\mathcal{N}(0, \sigma^2)$, it can be easily seen that the conditional distribution of observation variable $p(\mathbf{o}_t | s_t = i, s_{t+1} = j)$ follows multi-dimensional Gaussian $\mathcal{N}(\boldsymbol{\mu}_t(i, j), \Sigma)$ where $t = 1, 2, ..., T - 1$ and $\Sigma$ is an unit matrix scaled by $\sigma^2$, i.e.,

$$\Sigma = \sigma^2 I_{D_t} = \sigma^2 \times \begin{bmatrix} 1 & 0 & ... & 0 \\ 0 & 1 & ... & 0 \\ \vdots & \vdots & \ddots & \vdots \\ 0 & 0 & ... & 1 \end{bmatrix}_{D_t \times D_t}$$

When $t = 0$ or $t = T$, the conditional distribution of observation variable $p(\mathbf{o}_0 | s_1 = i)$ or $p(\mathbf{o}_T | s_T = i)$ follows multi-dimensional Gaussian $\mathcal{N}(\boldsymbol{\mu}_0(i), \Sigma)$ or $\mathcal{N}(\boldsymbol{\mu}_T(i), \Sigma)$.

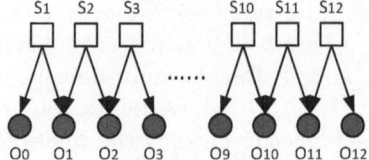

**Fig. 3.** An example of the joint modeling of state variable sequence **s** and observation sequence **O** for EAN-13 barcode, under the condition that the out-of-focus blur level is less or equal to the width of one symbol character. In the figure discrete distributed random variables are represented as squares; continuous distributed random variables are represented as circles. Shaded means observable, clear means non-observable (hidden). The conditional dependence relationships among random variables are denoted as directed edges.

## 5    Joint Modeling of State Variable Sequence and Observation Sequence

Based on above discussion, the stochastic relationship between linear barcode symbol value (represented by state variable sequence) and the observed scanline (represented by observation variable sequence) can be depicted as a directed graphical model. Fig. 3 illustrates an example of such model where the symbology type is EAN-13 and the out-of-focus level is less or equal to the width of one symbol character. To summarize, the directed graphical model is characterized by the following:

1. $T$, the length of state variable sequence. And $T+1$ is the length of observation variable sequence.
2. $N_t$, $t = 1, ..., T$, the state variable $s_t$'s state space.
3. $\mathbf{s} = (s_1, s_2, ..., s_T)$, the state variable sequence.
4. $P[s_t = i] = 1/N_t, 1 \leq i \leq N_t$, the state variable $s_t$'s distribution, which is the discrete uniform distribution.
5. Depending on the location $t$, the standard reference waveform segment at the detected out-of-focus level has two different cases:
   - $\boldsymbol{\mu}_t(i) = [\mu_1, \mu_2, ..., \mu_{D_t}]'$, where $i = 1, ..., N_t$, $t = 0$ or $t = T$.
   - $\boldsymbol{\mu}_t(i, j) = [\mu_1, \mu_2, ..., \mu_{D_t}]'$, where $i = 1, ..., N_t$, $j = 1, ..., N_{t+1}$, and $t = 1, 2, ..., T - 1$.
6. Depending on the location $t$, the conditional distribution of observation variables has two different cases:
   - When $t = 0$ or $t = T$, the observation variable is only dependent on the first state variable or the last state variable, therefore the conditional distributions are:

$$b_0^i(\mathbf{o}_0) = p(\mathbf{o}_0|s_1 = i) = \mathcal{N}(\boldsymbol{\mu}_0(i), \Sigma)$$

where $i = 1, 2, ..., N_0$ and

$$b_T^i(\mathbf{o}_T) = p(\mathbf{o}_T|s_T = i) = \mathcal{N}(\boldsymbol{\mu}_T(i), \Sigma)$$

where $i = 1, 2, ..., N_T$.

- In other cases, the observation variable is dependent on state variable $s_t$ and $s_{t+1}$, the conditional distributions are:

$$b_t^{i,j}(\mathbf{o}_t) = p(\mathbf{o}_t|s_t = i, s_{t+1} = j) = \mathcal{N}(\boldsymbol{\mu}_t(i,j), \Sigma)$$

where $i = 1, 2, ..., N_t$ and $j = 1, 2, ..., N_{t+1}$.

From now on, we use $\lambda$ to represent the complete parameter set of this directed graphical model. Given the directed graphical model $\lambda$, the value of a linear barcode can be inferred by finding an "optimal" state variable sequence. The symbol characters' values corresponding to the optimal state variable values will be treated as the inferred barcode value. The process is detailed in the section below.

## 6    Barcode Value Determination Based on Optimal State Sequence Finding

Given the observation sequence $\mathbf{O} = (\mathbf{o}_0, \mathbf{o}_1, ..., \mathbf{o}_T)$ and the directed graphical model $\lambda$, we define the optimal state variable sequence $\mathbf{s}^* = (s_1^*, s_2^*, ..., s_T^*)$ as the sequence which maximize the posterior probability $p(\mathbf{s}|\mathbf{O}, \lambda)$, i.e.,

$$\mathbf{s}^* = \arg\max_{\mathbf{s}} p(\mathbf{s}|\mathbf{O}, \lambda) \tag{3}$$

Eq. (3) is equivalent to find $\mathbf{s}^*$ which maximize the joint probability $p(\mathbf{s}, \mathbf{O}|\lambda)$, i.e.,

$$\mathbf{s}^* = \arg\max_{\mathbf{s}} p(\mathbf{s}, \mathbf{O}|\lambda) \tag{4}$$

In order to calculate Eq. (4), we define the quantity

$$\delta_t(i) = \max_{s_1 s_2 ... s_{t-1}} p(s_1 s_2 ... s_{t-1}, s_t = i, \mathbf{o}_0 \mathbf{o}_1 ... \mathbf{o}_{t-1}|\lambda) \tag{5}$$

that is, $\delta_t(j)$ is the maximum joint probability of $(s_1 s_2 ... s_t)$ and $(\mathbf{o}_0 \mathbf{o}_1 ... \mathbf{o}_{t-1})$ when $s_t = i$. By induction, we have

$$\delta_{t+1}(j) = \max_i [\delta_t(i) \cdot b_t^{i,j}(\mathbf{o}_t)] \cdot P[s_{t+1} = j] \tag{6}$$

In order to retrieve the best state variable sequence, the arguments that maximized Eq. (6) at each $t$ and $j$ need to be recorded. Array $\psi_t(j)$ is used for this purpose. The complete procedure for finding the optimal state variable sequence is a variation of Viterbi algorithm [10] and can be stated as follows:

1. Initialization:

$$\delta_1(i) = b_0^i(\mathbf{o}_0) \cdot P[s_1 = i], \tag{7}$$

$$\psi_1(i) = 0, \tag{8}$$

where    $1 \leq i \leq N_0$.

(a)                                              (b)

**Fig. 4.** Examples of images captured by HTC Desire device. (a) is better focused whereas in (b) the out-of-focus blur is easily perceivable.

2. Recursion:

$$\delta_t(j) = \max_{1 \leq i \leq N_{t-1}} [\delta_{t-1}(i) \cdot b_{t-1}^{i,j}(\mathbf{o}_{t-1})] \cdot P[s_t = j], \tag{9}$$

$$\psi_t(j) = \arg \max_{1 \leq i \leq N_{t-1}} [\delta_{t-1}(i) \cdot b_{t-1}^{i,j}(\mathbf{o}_{t-1})], \tag{10}$$

where $2 \leq t \leq T$ and $1 \leq j \leq N_t$.

3. Termination:

$$P^* = \max_{1 \leq i \leq N_T} [\delta_T(i) \cdot b_T^i(\mathbf{o}_T)], \tag{11}$$

$$s_T^* = \arg \max_{1 \leq i \leq N_T} [\delta_T(i) \cdot b_T^i(\mathbf{o}_T)]. \tag{12}$$

4. Optimal state variable sequence backtracking:

$$s_t^* = \psi_{t+1}(s_{t+1}^*), \quad t = T - 1, T - 2, ..., 1. \tag{13}$$

If $P^* = p(\mathbf{s}^*, \mathbf{O}|\lambda)$ is greater than a predefined threshold value, the barcode value corresponding to $\mathbf{s}^*$ is treated as the output of linear barcode scanning system.

## 7    Results

A linear barcode scanning system is built based on the proposed directed graphical model. To compare the proposed system with other linear barcode scanning systems, we tried some online barcode decoding services by checking the decodability of images prepared by us when these services are used. One service is from DataSymbol.[1]. The other is from ZXing.[2] To our awareness, the work in [11] gives ZXing, the popular open source barcode image processing library the

---

[1]  http://www.datasymbol.com/barcode-recognition-sdk/barcode-reader/
online-barcode-decoder.html

[2]  http://zxing.org/w/decode.jspx

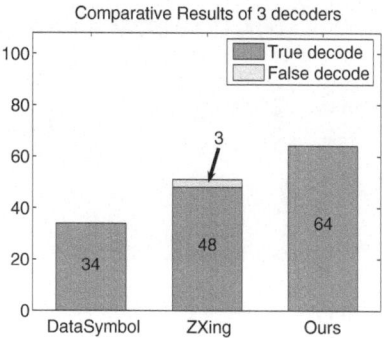

**Fig. 5.** Comparative results of DataSymbol, ZXing, and our system on 108 images captured by HTC Desire

capability of handling out-of-focus blurs. We prepared 108 images captured by a HTC Desire device, an Android smart phone carrying an auto-focus camera module. These 108 images were captured by pointing the phone at one single barcode when its images were continuously taken. During the image capturing process, the auto-focus functionality is continuously called on the device with a period around 4 seconds. Therefore some of these 108 images are in focus, others contain various level of out-of-focus blur. Fig. 4 gives two example images captured for testing. One of the image is in-focus whereas the other is out-of-focus. Fig. 5 illustrates the testing results. It is observed that DataSymbol's barcode scanning system can only handle well focused barcode images. While ZXing's system is able to decode more images, it starts to have false decodes among the testing images. Our proposed system achieves a 59% decode ratio and no false decode is observed among the testing images.

To test the effectiveness of the proposed system on mobile phones embedded with fixed-focus lens, a barcode image database is created, containing more than 1000 barcode images captured by various camera phones with fixed-focus lenses. Images are all taken from real product packaging, bearing lots of variations such as foreground/background color, symbol size, lighting conditions, etc. Fig. 6 gives some examples. The out-of-focus level of these images is mainly around 0.2-0.9 of the width of 1 symbol character. It's found that when the decoding rate is around 30%, the false positive rate is less than 3%. And 240 images captured by Nokia E50 and Motorola XT502 in our barcode image database are tested against the two online barcode scanning systems, as images of these two devices lead to the best and worst performance in our system. Its found that none of these images are decodable by the two online barcode scanning systems.

Our proposed system is implemented in C and tests are performed on a PC with an Intel Core 2 Duo CPU @ 2.33GHz and 0.99GB of RAM. Without counting opening and loading image data and procedures not directly related to decoding, such as printing information on the command window, the average processing time for a QVGA ($320 \times 240$ pixels) sized image is 15.57 milliseconds.

**Fig. 6.** Examples of barcode images in our database

The system is also implemented and tested on phone devices of multiple smart phone platforms such as Symbian (s60v3, s60v5, Symbian^3, Symbian Anna, Symbian Belle) and Android (2.1 and above). Real-time processing is achieved as the system even works well on Nokia E50 which uses an ARM 9 processor at 235MHz of clock rate. The scanning system is integrated with a mobile application called iDigMobi, a mobile internet based product searching and sharing service. [3]

## 8    Conclusion

This paper presented a directed graphical model for linear barcode scanning. The model specifically considered the relationship between out-of-focus blur and linear barcode waveforms, enabled a systematic approach in handling excessive out-of-focus blur in digital image based linear barcode scanning systems. The idea is generic and can be extended to handle other image blurs such as motion blur by incorporating other type of image blurs into the line spread function.

## References

1. Wachenfeld, S., Terlunen, S., Jiang, X.: Robust recognition of 1-d barcodes using camera phones. In: 19th International Conference on Pattern Recognition, ICPR 2008, pp. 1–4. IEEE (2008)
2. Joseph, E., Pavlidis, T.: Bar code waveform recognition using peak locations. IEEE Trans. Pattern Anal. Machine Intell. 16, 630–640 (1994)
3. Esedoglu, S.: Blind deconvolution of bar code signals. Inverse Problems 20, 121–135 (2004)
4. Dridi, N., Delignon, Y., Sawaya, W., Septier, F.: Blind detection of severely blurred 1d barcode. In: GLOBECOM, pp. 1–5. IEEE (2010)
5. Qu, L., Tu, Y.: Change point estimation of bilevel functions. Journal of Modern Applied Statistical Methods 5, 347–355 (2006)
6. Choksi, R., van Gennip, Y.: Deblurring of one dimensional bar codes via total variation energy minimization. SIAM J. Imaging Sci. 3, 735–764 (2010)

---

[3] http://www.idigmobi.com

7. ISO: ISO/IEC 15420:2000 Information technology — Automatic identification and data capture techniques — Bar code symbology specification — EAN/UPC. International Organization for Standardization (2000)
8. Kundur, D., Hatzinakos, D.: Blind image deconvolutions. IEEE Signal Process. Mag. 13, 43–63 (1996)
9. Pavlidis, T., Swartz, J., Wang, Y.: Fundamentals of bar code information theory. Computer 23, 74–86 (1990)
10. Forney, G.D.: The viterbi algorithm. Proc. IEEE 61, 268–278 (1973)
11. Zamberletti, A., Gallo, I., Carullo, M., Binaghi, E.: Neural image restoration for decoding 1-d barcodes using common camera phones. In: Proceedings of 5th International Conference on Computer Vision Theory and Applications, VISAPP 2010, pp. 5–11 (2010)

# A Probabilistic 3D Model Retrieval System Using Sphere Image

Ke Ding and Yunhui Liu

Department of Mechanical and Automation Engineering,
The Chinese University of Hong Kong

**Abstract.** The view-based 3D model retrieval systems represent a 3D model using its projected views, and retrieve 3D models by comparing the projected views. Most of the existing view-based 3D model retrieval systems only analyze the features of the projected views, while the spatial arrangements of the viewpoints are not well considered. In this paper, we propose a new 3D model descriptor called sphere image, which is defined as a sphere with a large number of viewpoints distributed on it. Each viewpoint is regarded as a "pixel", associated with a projected view. The feature of the projected view is quantized into a vector, regarded as the "intensity". We also propose a probabilistic graphical model for 3D model matching, and develop a 3D model retrieval system to test our approach. The proposed approach was evaluated on the Princeton shape benchmark. Experimental results indicate that our approach outperforms most of the existing 3D model retrieval systems in respect of retrieval precision and computation cost.

## 1    Introduction

As the number of 3D models on the Internet is growing rapidly, 3D model retrieval system has become a necessity. To develop a 3D model retrieval system, researchers address the challenge on two aspects: (1) 3D model representation, which means extracting and analyzing appropriated features to describe 3D models. (2) 3D model comparison, which means matching the 3D model descriptors.

[1] [2] [3] proposed detailed surveys on 3D model retrieval systems. Numerous methods are proposed for 3D model representation. Kazhdan et al. [4] proposed the Spherical Harmonic descriptor for 3D model representation. Ohbuchi et al. [5] used the projected views to describe 3D models, and applied the SIFT [6] features to quantize the projected views. Chen et al. [7] represented the 3D model using the Light Field descriptor, which is composed of 10 projected views. Vranić et al. [8] used the continuous Karhunen-Loeve transform and the fast Fourier Transform to build a ray-based 3D model descriptor. Mademlis et al. [9] decomposed a 3D model into several parts, and represented the 3D model by an attributed graph, which is constructed based on the connectivity of the parts.

According to different types of the features, 3D model descriptors can be divided into view-based descriptors, graph-based descriptors, geometry-based

K.M. Lee et al. (Eds.): ACCV 2012, Part I, LNCS 7724, pp. 536–547, 2013.
© Springer-Verlag Berlin Heidelberg 2013

descriptors, etc. We focus our research on the view-based 3D model descriptor. As Shilane [10] showed, the view-based 3D model descriptor, such as the Light Field descriptor, presented promising performance on retrieval precision. However, most of the view-based 3D model descriptors have limitations on computation cost. For example, the Light Field descriptor [7] matches 3D models by pairwise comparing the projected views. The Light Field descriptor needs a 3D model alignment process, because it is not invariant to the rotation of the 3D model. To reduce the computation cost, researchers proposed several methods, such as Ansary et al. [11], Ohbuchi et al. [12] and Gao et al. [13] [14] [15]. The other limitation for the view-based 3D model descriptors is that the spatial arrangements of the viewpoints are not well considered. Most of the current view-based 3D model descriptors focus on quantizing the projected views into different descriptors, the positions of the viewpoints are not well considered.

In this paper we present a new 3D model descriptor, called sphere image. The sphere image is actually a sphere with a large number of viewpoints distributed on it. Each viewpoint is regarded as a "pixel", which is associated with a projected view of the 3D model. Each projected view is described by a Fourier descriptor, which is regarded as the "intensity" of the "pixel". Our approach do not match the 3D models by pairwise comparing the projected views. We treat all the projected views as an entity. The viewpoints and the rendered projected views constitute a sphere image, which preserves the information of the positions of viewpoints ("pixels") and the features of projected views ("intensities"). Using the sphere image, we can easily introduce some image processing techniques to the field of 3D model retrieval.

For the 3D model matching process, we first divide the sphere image into several regions, then form a "star graph" by connecting the regions and the center of the sphere. Inspired by Boiman [16], we propose a probabilistic model for 3D model retrieval. The similarity between the 3D query model and the 3D models in database can be measured by the joint likelihood. We also present a statistical inference process for 3D model comparison.

The main contributions of this paper are: (1) We present a new view-based 3D model descriptor, called the sphere image. The spatial arrangements of the viewpoints and the features of the projected views are both considered. (2) We propose a new probabilistic model, and an efficient matching algorithm for 3D model retrieval. (3) We develop a 3D model retrieval system to test our approach.

This paper is organized as follows. Section 2 discusses the details of the sphere image, section 3 presents the new probabilistic model for 3D model retrieval. Section 4 presents the experimental results. Finally, a brief conclusion appears in section 5.

## 2   Sphere Image

Vision is the most intuitive way for human to represent an object. For most of the existing view-based 3D model retrieval systems, people usually use one or several projected views to describe a 3D model, and then retrieve the 3D model

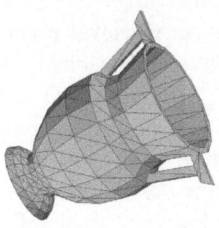

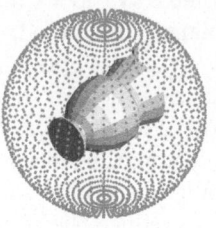

(a) The 3D model of
vase.

(b) The sphere image of the 3D
model of vase.

**Fig. 1.** An example of the sphere image. Each blue dot denotes a viewpoint, which is associated with a projected view.

by pairwise matching the projected views. However, the projected views can be very different from various viewpoints. Although we can increase the number of projected views to represent the 3D model more precise, it can result in expensive computation cost and storage space. Also, most of the existing view-based 3D model descriptors only analyze the features of the projected views, the spatial arrangements of the viewpoints are not well considered.

Unlike the existing view-based 3D model descriptors, we simply use one sphere image to describe a 3D model. The sphere image is defined as a sphere, which is composed of thousands of viewpoints. The viewpoints are regarded as "pixels", and the projected views associated with the viewpoints are regarded as the "intensities". In our implementation, the number of projected views is 2475. Figure 1b shows a sphere image of the 3D model of vase. Each blue dot denotes a viewpoint, which is associated with a projected view. One advantage of the sphere image is that all the viewpoints and the projected views are considered as an image, therefore, some image processing techniques can be easily introduced into the field of 3D model retrieval. The other advantage is that the spatial arrangements of the viewpoints are considered.

The process for constructing a sphere image is illustrated below:

1. Build a sphere with the number of $N$ viewpoints.
2. Translate and scale the 3D model to ensure sure that it is contained in the sphere. Since the viewpoints are distributed on the sphere, the position of each viewpoint is denoted by a three dimensional vector. The origin point of the coordinate system is the center of the sphere.
3. Render the projected views of the 3D model.
4. Quantize the projected views into the Fourier descriptors.

The feature descriptor of the projected view is regarded as the "intensity" of the pixel (viewpoint). Numerous features and feature descriptors can be applied to represent the projected view, such as the SIFT [6], the Zernike moment. To reduce the retrieval time, we only analyze the contour of the projected view, without considering its inside details. The contour is extracted by the Canny edge detection algorithm [17], and is quantized into a set of Fourier coefficients using the Fourier descriptor. A Fourier descriptor is composed of a set of Fourier coefficients, which are obtained by applying the Fourier transform on shape features. The Fourier descriptor has the advantage of being invariant to translation, rotation and scaling. The fine details of the contour only affect the high frequency parts of the coefficients.

The contour is described by the centroid distance, which is defined as:

$$r(t) = ([x(t) - x_c]^2 + [y(t) - y_c]^2)^{1/2}, \quad t = 0, 1, ..., N - 1 .\tag{1}$$

where $(x_c, y_c)$ is the center of the contour, $(x(t), y(t))$ denotes a boundary point.

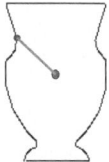

**Fig. 2.** The contour of the 3D model of vase

Figure 2 shows a contour of the 3D model of vase. The red point denotes the center of the contour. The blue point denotes a point on the contour, and the green straight line denotes the centroid distance.

The Fourier transform of $r(t)$ is given by:

$$a_n = \frac{1}{n} \sum_{t=0}^{N-1} r(t) exp(\frac{-j2\pi nt}{N}), \quad n = 0, 1, ..., N - 1 .\tag{2}$$

The coefficients $a_n$, $n = 0, 1, ..., N - 1$, are consisted of the Fourier descriptor of the contour. The importance of the Fourier coefficients are not the same. For a Fourier descriptor $FD[a_0, a_1, a_2, a_3..., a_n]$, the coefficients on the left (low frequency) are more important, because they describe the general shape of the contour. And the right side (high frequency) of the coefficients are less important, because they represent the fine details of the shape feature. Given this fact, we cannot simply use the Euclidean distance to compare Fourier descriptors. In our implementation, we compare the Fourier descriptors by attaching weight $w_i$ (empirically defined) for every coefficient. For instance, we have two Fourier descriptor: $FD_1 [a_0, a_1, a_2..., a_n]$ and $FD_2 [b_0, b_1, b_2..., b_n]$, the similarity of these two descriptors is:

$$Similarity = \sqrt{\sum_{i=1}^{n} w_i(a_i - b_i)^2} .\tag{3}$$

Consider we extract the number of $N$ views $\{V_1, V_2, ..., V_N\}$ to describe a 3D model, then the sphere image is composed of $N$ "pixels". And if we represent each projected view using a Fourier descriptors with $M$ coefficients, then it means the "intensity" of each "pixel" is described by a vector with the length of $M$.

## 3   3D Model Matching

After the previous steps, each 3D model is represented by a sphere image. The position of the "pixel" is represented by the spatial arrangements of the viewpoints, and the "intensity" of the "pixel" is denoted by the Fourier descriptor of the projected view. We introduce a pictorial structure to the 3D model retrieval problem. This idea is inspired by Felzenszwalb and Huttenlocher [18], they proposed an algorithm for matching pictorial structures to images. A pictorial structure is a collection of parts arranged in a deformable configuration. In our method, a sphere image is divided into several regions. Each region is represented by a projected view from the center of the region, and the spatial arrangements of the viewpoints are represented by the connections between the regions' centers and the sphere's center.

We use the clustering method to segment the sphere image. Since the number of regions of a sphere image cannot be determined beforehand, we cannot simply use the K-means clustering. In out mehtod, we apply the Gaussian means (G-means) [19] clustering algorithm, which adapts the number of clusters.

A 3D model is represented by a collection of regions $R = \{r_1, ..., r_n\}$, $r_i$ denotes the $i$th region of the sphere image. Each region is consisted of a number of viewpoints. The locations of the regions are denoted by $l = \{l_1, ..., l_n\}$. Figure 3 shows an example of the pictorial structure of a 3D model. Each region is represented by a characteristic view, which is extracted from the viewpoint at the center of the region. We connect the center of the region to the center of the sphere, and obtain a "star graph", as the Figure 3b shows. Each region is associated with two attributes: (1) The region descriptor, which is the Fourier descriptor extracted from the viewpoint at the center of the region. (2) The location, which is the connection between the region and the center of the sphere.

Inspired by Boiman [16], we propose a probabilistic model for 3D model retrieval. A statistical formulation process and an inference process are provided.

### 3.1   Statistical Formulation

Consider a 3D model query $\mathcal{Q}$, and a 3D model denoted by $\mathcal{T}$ in database, $\mathcal{T} \in \mathcal{DB}$, where $\mathcal{DB}$ denotes the database. The similarity between these two 3D models can be measured by the joint likelihood:

$$P(\mathcal{Q}, \mathcal{T}) = P(\mathcal{T}|\mathcal{Q})P(\mathcal{Q}) . \tag{4}$$

The regions of the sphere image are represented by Fourier descriptors, denoted by $\{d_1, ..., d_n\}$, where $n$ is the number of the regions of a sphere image. $n$ is obtained by G-means clustering, it is not a constant, it changes with respect to different 3D models. The location of a region is represented by a three dimensional vector, which is denoted by $l$. We search for a similar geometric configuration of

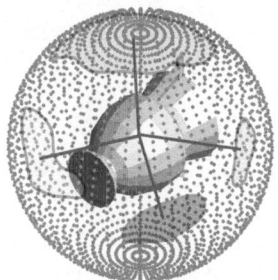

(a) The surface of the view sphere is classified into several regions.

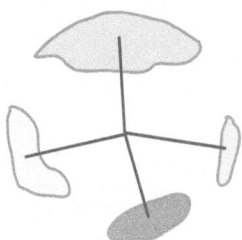

(b) The star graph constructed by the regions.

**Fig. 3.** Ensembles of regions in sphere image

regions with similar properties. The similarity between the 3D model query $\mathcal{T}$ and the 3D model $\mathcal{Q}$ from the database is measured by:

$$P(\mathcal{Q}, \mathcal{T}) = P(c_{\mathcal{Q}},\ d_{\mathcal{Q}}^1, ..l_{\mathcal{Q}}^1, ..,\ c_{\mathcal{T}},\ d_{\mathcal{T}}^1, ..l_{\mathcal{T}}^1, ..) \ . \tag{5}$$

Where $c_{\mathcal{Q}}$ and $c_{\mathcal{T}}$ are the centers of the 3D models $\mathcal{Q}$ and $\mathcal{T}$. $d_{\mathcal{Q}}^i$ denotes the Fourier descriptor of the $i$th region of the 3D model query $\mathcal{Q}$, and $l_{\mathcal{Q}}^i$ denotes the location of the $i$th region of the 3D model query $\mathcal{Q}$.

To simplify the computation process, we make a standard Markovian assumption to compute the joint likelihood $P(\mathcal{Q}, \mathcal{T})$. Given a descriptor $d_{\mathcal{T}}^i$, the corresponding query's region descriptor $d_{\mathcal{Q}}^i$ is assumed to be independent of the other regions' descriptors. The similarity between the query region $d_{\mathcal{Q}}^i$ and the region $d_{\mathcal{T}}^i$ in database is measured using the Gaussian distribution:

$$P(d_{\mathcal{Q}}^i | d_{\mathcal{T}}^i) = \alpha_{\mathcal{D}} \exp(-(d_{\mathcal{Q}}^i - d_{\mathcal{T}}^i)^T \Sigma_{\mathcal{D}}^{-1} (d_{\mathcal{Q}}^i - d_{\mathcal{T}}^i)) \ . \tag{6}$$

Where $\alpha_{\mathcal{D}}$ is an empirically determined constant, and $\Sigma_{\mathcal{D}}$ is a constant covariance matrix, which captures the allowable deviation of the descriptors.

Similarly, we model the similarity between the positions of the regions by:

$$P(l_{\mathcal{Q}}^i | l_{\mathcal{T}}^i,\ c_{\mathcal{T}},\ c_{\mathcal{Q}}) = \alpha_{\mathcal{L}} \exp(-((l_{\mathcal{Q}}^i - c_{\mathcal{Q}}) - (l_{\mathcal{T}}^i - c_{\mathcal{T}}))^T \Sigma_{\mathcal{L}}^{-1} ((l_{\mathcal{Q}}^i - c_{\mathcal{Q}}) - (l_{\mathcal{T}}^i - c_{\mathcal{T}}))) \ . \tag{7}$$

Where $\alpha_{\mathcal{L}}$ is an empirically determined constant, and $\Sigma_{\mathcal{L}}$ is a constant covariance matrix, which captures the allowed deviations of the locations of the regions.

In the database $\mathcal{DB}$, the relations of the region descriptor $d_{\mathcal{T}}^i$ and the corresponding location $l_{\mathcal{T}}^i$ is measured as:

$$P(d_{\mathcal{T}} | l_{\mathcal{T}}) = \begin{cases} 1, & (d_{\mathcal{T}}, l_{\mathcal{T}}) \ \epsilon \ \mathcal{DB} \\ 0, & \text{otherwise} \ . \end{cases} \tag{8}$$

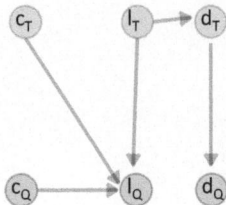

**Fig. 4.** The probabilistic graphical model for 3D model retrieval. The blue circles denote the variables in database, and the orange circles denote the query variables. (The figure is best viewed in color.)

As the Figure 4 shows, we can factor the joint likelihood $P(\mathcal{Q}, \mathcal{T})$ as follows:

$$P(c_{\mathcal{T}},\ d_{\mathcal{T}}^1, ..l_{\mathcal{T}}^1, .., \ c_{\mathcal{Q}},\ d_{\mathcal{Q}}^1, ..l_{\mathcal{Q}}^1, ..) = \alpha \Pi P(l_{\mathcal{Q}}^i | l_{\mathcal{T}}^i,\ c_{\mathcal{T}},\ c_{\mathcal{Q}}) P(d_{\mathcal{Q}}^i | d_{\mathcal{T}}^i) P(d_{\mathcal{T}} | l_{\mathcal{T}}) \ . \tag{9}$$

### 3.2 Inference Process

For the inference process of 3D model retrieval, the objective is seeking a 3D model which maximizes its MAP (maximum a-posterior probability) assignment:

$$\begin{aligned} \underset{X}{max} P(c_{\mathcal{T}},\ d_{\mathcal{T}}^1, ..l_{\mathcal{T}}^1, .., \ c_{\mathcal{Q}},\ d_{\mathcal{Q}}^1, ..l_{\mathcal{Q}}^1, ..) \\ = \alpha \underset{i}{\Pi} \ \underset{l_{\mathcal{T}}^i}{max} P(l_{\mathcal{Q}}^i | l_{\mathcal{T}}^i,\ c_{\mathcal{T}},\ c_{\mathcal{Q}}) \underset{d_{\mathcal{T}}^i}{max} P(d_{\mathcal{Q}}^i | d_{\mathcal{T}}^i) P(d_{\mathcal{T}}^i | l_{\mathcal{T}}^i) \ . \end{aligned} \tag{10}$$

To reduce the computation cost for the MAP assignment, we apply the Belief Propagation algorithm. First, we choose a region from the query's sphere image, denoted by $(d_{\mathcal{Q}}^i,\ l_{\mathcal{Q}}^i)$. Then we compare the region $d_{\mathcal{Q}}^i$ with the regions' descriptors $d_{\mathcal{T}}^i$ in database, with respect to the location $l_{\mathcal{T}}^i$. The process can be considered as passing a message $m_{dl}^i$ from the node $d_{\mathcal{T}}^i$ to the node $l_{\mathcal{T}}^i$, regarding its belief in the location $l_{\mathcal{T}}^i$:

$$m_{dl}^i(l_{\mathcal{T}}^i) = \underset{d_{\mathcal{T}}^i}{max} P(d_{\mathcal{Q}}^i | d_{\mathcal{T}}^i) P(d_{\mathcal{T}}^i | l_{\mathcal{T}}^i) \ . \tag{11}$$

Second, for the locations $l_{\mathcal{T}}^i$ in the database, we pass a message about the induced possible origin locations $c_{\mathcal{T}}$:

$$m_{lc}^i(c_{\mathcal{T}}) = \underset{l_{\mathcal{T}}^i}{max} P(l_{\mathcal{Q}}^i | l_{\mathcal{T}}^i,\ c_{\mathcal{T}},\ c_{\mathcal{Q}}) m_{dl}(l_{\mathcal{T}}^i) \ . \tag{12}$$

## 4    Experiments

In this section, we conduct experiments based on the Princeton shape benchmark [10] data sets, and compare our method with some existing 3D model retrieval systems. We first present the experimental setup, and then the experimental results as compared to the other methods.

## 4.1   Experimental Setup

To test our proposed method, we have developed a 3D model retrieval system, which runs on an Intel Xeon computer (CPU 2.83GHz). Figure 5 shows the appearance of our 3D model retrieval system. There are three buttons on the left of the figure, named "Refresh", "Query" and "Recognition". The window on the right of the figure shows the retrieval results, ranking from the most similar to the least similar.

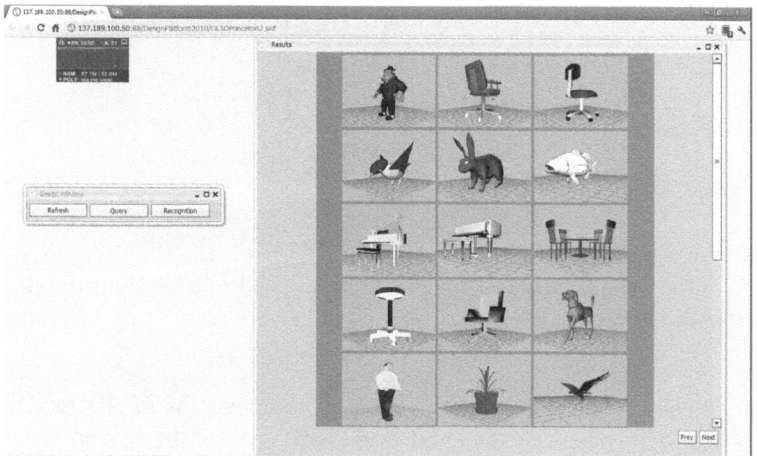

**Fig. 5.** The appearance of our 3D model retrieval system

The Princeton shape benchmark data sets contain 1814 3D models collected from the Internet. All the 3D models are manually classified according to their functions and forms. The Princeton shape benchmark data sets are consisted of two data sets. One is the training set, which contains 907 3D models with 90 classes; the other is the test set, which contains 907 3D models with 92 classes. Figure 6 shows a few examples of 3D models from the Princeton shape benchmark data sets.

We evaluated our proposed 3D model descriptor using some evaluation methods proposed by [10], including the nearest neighbor, the first tier, the second tier, the E-measure, the Discounted Cumulative Gain (DCG) and the precision-recall curve. The details of these evaluation methods are illustrated as following:

1. **precision-recall curve**: The *Precision* is the ratio of the retrieved 3D models that are relevant to the query. The *Recall* is the ratio of the successfully retrieved 3D models that are relevant to the query.
2. **Nearest Neighbor**: Measure the percentage of the correctly retrieved 3D models. Higher score indicates better performance on retrieval precision.
3. **First Tier and Second Tier**: Measure the percentage of correctly retrieved 3D models within the top $K$ matches, where $K$ is related to the size of the

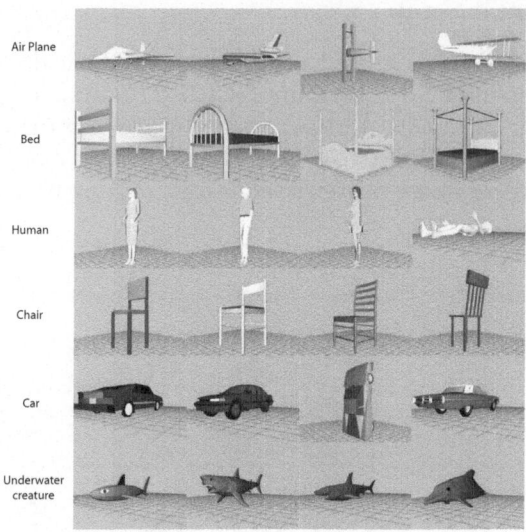

**Fig. 6.** The thumbnail images of six classes of 3D models from the Princeton shape benchmark data sets.

query's class. Consider a query's class is composed of $M$ 3D models, then $K = M$ - 1 for the first tier, and $K = 2(M$ - 1) for the second tier. Higher score indicates better performance on retrieval precision.

4. **E-measure**: Measure the precision and recall for a fixed number of retrieved 3D models. The idea is that people are more interested in the top $C$ of the retrieved 3D models. We choose $C = 32$ in our implementation. The E-measure is defined as $2/(\frac{1}{Precision} + \frac{1}{Recall})$.

5. **Discounted Cumulative Gain (DCG)**: Measure the ranking list of the retrieved 3D models, where the correct results in front of the ranking list weight heavier than the correct results in the end of the ranking list.

## 4.2    Experimental Results

We used the precision-recall curve to evaluate the performance between our method and several existing 3D model retrieval methods, including the Spherical Harmonics Descriptor (SHD) [4], the D2 descriptor [20], the Absolute Angle Distance (AAD) descriptor [21], the linearly Parameterized Statistics (PS) descriptor [21], the Surflet-Pair Relations Histogram (SPRH) descriptor [22] and the Light Field Descriptor (LFD) [7]. The experiment was conducted by pairwise comparing all the 3D models in database, resulting in a $907 \times 907$ distance matrix for every 3D model retrieval method. The Princeton shape benchmark utilities were applied to analyze the distance matrix. Figure 7 shows the precision-recall curve based on the Princeton shape benchmark test set. Each curve represents the average result over all classified 3D models in the database. The Light Field

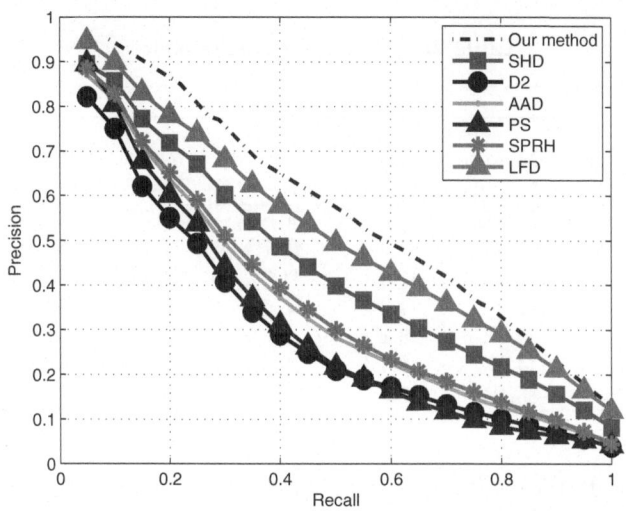

**Fig. 7.** Precision-recall curve of our proposed method versus the other 3D model retrieval methods. This plot was generated using the Princeton evaluation utilities. (The figure is best viewed in color.)

descriptor outperforms most of the 3D model retrieval methods, which is the same as showed by Shilane et al. [10]. Our approach outperforms all of these methods on average. This is because we apply more projected views to describe a 3D model, and also consider the positions of the viewpoints.

Table 2 shows the evaluation results on the nearest neighbor, the first tier, the second tier, the E-measure and the DCG. The LFD presents the second best performance as compared to other 3D model retrieval methods. On average, the nearest neighbor score of our method is 6% higher than the LFD, the first tier and the second titer scores of our method are 9%, 4% higher than the LFD, the E-measure score of our method is 10% higher than the LFD, and the DCG score of our method is 6% higher than the LFD.

**Table 1.** Average Matching time for different 3D model retrieval methods

| Descriptors | Average Matching Time (s) |
| --- | --- |
| SHD | 0.004846 |
| Our method | 0.006764 |
| AAD | 0.009619 |
| D2 | 0.016352 |
| PS | 0.016575 |
| SPRH | 0.016839 |
| LFD | 0.062311 |

**Table 2.** The Retrieval Performance

| Shape Descriptor | Discrimination | | | | |
|---|---|---|---|---|---|
| | Nearest Neighbor | First Tier | Second Tier | E-Measure | DCG |
| Our method | 69.8% | 41.2% | 50.8% | 30.7% | 68.1% |
| LFD | 65.8% | 37.9% | 48.7% | 27.9% | 64.3% |
| SHD | 55.3% | 31.0% | 41.3% | 24.0% | 58.5% |
| SPRH | 47.2% | 24.2% | 33.6% | 19.9% | 52.1% |
| AAD | 45.6% | 23.1% | 32.7% | 19.4% | 51.3% |
| PS | 44.0% | 19.4% | 26.0% | 15.6% | 47.6% |
| D2 | 35.1% | 17.9% | 26.1% | 15.4% | 45.2% |

The computation time for 3D model matching is also analyzed. In our experiment, each 3D model was compared with all the 3D models from the Princeton shape benchmark test set. Since the Princeton shape benchmark test set contains 907 3D models, then each 3D model was compared with 907 3D models, and the total comparing times is $907 \times 907$. The average time for each matching is illustrated Table 1. Compared with the Light Field Descriptor (LFD) [7], the Spherical Harmonics descriptor (SHD) [4], the D2 descriptor [20], the Absolute Angle Distance (AAD) descriptor [21], the linearly Parameterized Statistics (PS) descriptor [21], the Surflet-Pair Relations Histogram (SPRH) descriptor [22], our method presents the second best performance. The SHD is the most fast 3D model retrieval method in this experiment. The first reason is that the dimension of the SHD is smaller than the other methods. The Second reason is that the SHD is rotationally invariant, and thus it needs not to align 3D models.

## 5    Conclusion

In this paper, we proposed a new view-based 3D model descriptor, called the sphere image. Both the spatial arrangements of the viewpoints and the features of the projected views are considered in the sphere image. Using the sphere image, we can easily introduce some image processing techniques to the field of 3D model retrieval. We proposed a new probabilistic method for 3D model retrieval, and developed a 3D model retrieval system to test our approach. Experimental result shows that our method outperforms most of the existing 3D model retrieval methods.

## References

1. Tangelder, J., Veltkamp, R.: A survey of content based 3d shape retrieval methods. In: Proceedings of the Shape Modeling International (SMI), pp. 145–156 (2004)
2. Bustos, B., Keim, D.A., Saupe, D., Schreck, T., Vranić, D.V.: Feature-based similarity search in 3d object databases. ACM Computing Surveys 37, 345–387 (2005)

3. Bimbo, A.D., Pala, P.: Content-based retrieval of 3d models. ACM Trans. on Multimedia Computing, Communications and Applications 2, 20–43 (2006)
4. Kazhdan, M., Funkhouser, T., Rusinkiewicz, S.: Rotation invariant spherical harmonic representation of 3d shape descriptors. In: Proceedings of the Eurographics/ACM SIGGRAPH Symposium on Geometry Processing, pp. 156–164. Eurographics Association (2003)
5. Ohbuchi, R., Osada, K., Furuya, T., Banno, T.: Salient local visual features for shape-based 3d model retrieval. In: IEEE Int. Conf. on Shape Modeling and Applications, pp. 93–102 (2008)
6. Lowe, D.G.: Object recognition from local scale-invariant features. In: Proceedings of the 7th IEEE Int. Conf. on Computer Vision, vol. 2, pp. 1150–1157 (1999)
7. Chen, D., Tian, X., Shen, Y., Ouhyoung, M.: On visual similarity based on 3d model retrieval. Computer Graphics Forum, 223–232 (2003)
8. Vranić, D., Saupe, D., Richter, J.: Tools for 3d-object retrieval: Karhunen-loeve transform and spherical harmonics. In: IEEE 4th Workshop on Multimedia Signal Processing, pp. 293–298 (2001)
9. Mademlis, A., Daras, P., Axenopoulos, A., Tzovaras, D., Strintzis, M.G.: Combining topological and geometrical features for global and partial 3-d shape retrieval. IEEE Trans. on Multimedia 10, 819–831 (2008)
10. Shilane, P., Min, P., Kazhdan, M., Funkhouser, T.: The princeton shape benchmark. In: Proceedings of the Shape Modeling Applications, pp. 167–178 (2004)
11. Ansary, T.F., Daoudi, M., Vandeborre, J.P.: A bayesian 3d search engine using adaptive views clustering. IEEE Trans. on Multimedia 9, 78–88 (2007)
12. Ohbuchi, R., Furuya, T.: Accelerating bag-of-features sift algorithm for 3d model retrieval. In: SAMTWorkshop Semantic 3-D Media, pp. 22–30 (2008)
13. Gao, Y., Wang, M., Zha, Z.J., Tian, Q., Dai, Q., Zhang, N.: Less is more: Efficient 3d object retrieval with query view selection. IEEE Trans. on Multimedia 13, 1007–1018 (2011)
14. Gao, Y., Wang, M., Tao, D., Ji, R., Dai, Q.: 3-d object retrieval and recognition with hypergraph analysis. IEEE Transactions on Image Processing 21, 4290–4303 (2012)
15. Gao, Y., Dai, Q., Zhang, N.Y.: 3d model comparison using spatial structure circular descriptor. Pattern Recognition 43, 1142–1151 (2010)
16. Boiman, O., Irani, M.: Detecting irregularities in images and in video. In: IEEE International Conference on Computer Vision (ICCV), vol. 1, pp. 462–469 (2005)
17. Canny, J.: A computational approach to edge detection. IEEE Trans. on Pattern Analysis and Machine Intelligence 8, 679–698 (1986)
18. Felzenszwalb, P.F., Huttenlocher, D.P.: Efficient matching of pictorial structures. In: Proceedings of the IEEE Conference on Computer Vision and Pattern Recognition, vol. 2, pp. 66–73 (2000)
19. Hamerly, G., Elkan, C.: Learning the $k$ in $k$-means. In: Neural Information Processing Systems, pp. 281–288. MIT Press (2003)
20. Osada, R., Funkhouser, T., Chazelle, B., Dobkin, D.: Matching 3d models with shape distributions (2001)
21. Ohbuchi, R., Otagiri, T., Ibato, M., Takei, T.: Shape-similarity search of three-dimensional models using parameterized statistics. In: Proceedings of the Pacific Graphics, pp. 265–274 (2002)
22. Wahl, E., Hillenbrand, U., Hirzinger, G.: Surflet-pair-relation histograms: A statistical 3d-shape representation for rapid classification. In: 3DIM 2003, pp. 474–482 (2003)

# Model Based Training, Detection and Pose Estimation of Texture-Less 3D Objects in Heavily Cluttered Scenes

Stefan Hinterstoisser[1], Vincent Lepetit[3], Slobodan Ilic[1], Stefan Holzer[1], Gary Bradski[2], Kurt Konolige[2], and Nassir Navab[1]

[1] CAMP, Technische Universität München (TUM), Germany
[2] Industrial Perception, Palo Alto, CA, USA
[3] CV-Lab, École Polytechnique Fédérale de Lausanne (EPFL), Switzerland

**Abstract.** We propose a framework for automatic modeling, detection, and tracking of 3D objects with a Kinect. The detection part is mainly based on the recent template-based LINEMOD approach [1] for object detection. We show how to build the templates automatically from 3D models, and how to estimate the 6 degrees-of-freedom pose accurately and in real-time. The pose estimation and the color information allow us to check the detection hypotheses and improves the correct detection rate by 13% with respect to the original LINEMOD. These many improvements make our framework suitable for object manipulation in Robotics applications. Moreover we propose a new dataset made of 15 registered, 1100+ frame video sequences of 15 various objects for the evaluation of future competing methods.

## 1 Introduction

Many current vision applications, such as pedestrian tracking, dense SLAM [2], or object detection [1], can be made more robust through the addition of depth information. In this work, we focus on object detection for Robotics and Machine Vision, where it is important to efficiently and robustly detect objects and estimate their 3D poses, for manipulation or inspection tasks. Our approach is based on LINEMOD [1], an efficient method that exploits both depth and color images to capture the appearance and 3D shape of the object in a set of templates covering different views of an object. Because the viewpoint of each template is known, it provides a coarse estimate of the pose of the object when it is detected.

However, the initial version of LINEMOD [1] has some disadvantages. First, templates are learned online, which is difficult to control and results in spotty coverage of viewpoints. Second, the pose output by LINEMOD is only approximately correct, since a template covers a range of views around its viewpoint. And finally, the performance of LINEMOD, while extremely good, still suffers from the presence of false positives.

In this paper, we show how to overcome these disadvantages, and create a system based on LINEMOD for the automatic modeling, detection, and tracking

K.M. Lee et al. (Eds.): ACCV 2012, Part I, LNCS 7724, pp. 548–562, 2013.
© Springer-Verlag Berlin Heidelberg 2013

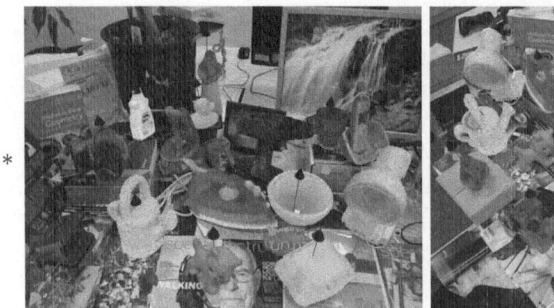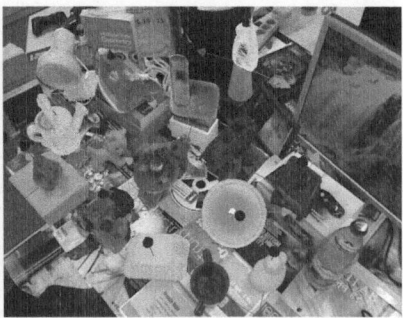

**Fig. 1.** 15 different texture-less 3D objects are simultaneously detected with our approach under different poses on heavy cluttered background with partial occlusion. Each detected object is augmented with its 3D model. We also show the corresponding coordinate systems.

of 3D objects with RGBD sensors. Our main insight is that a 3D model of the object can be exploited to remedy these deficiencies. Note that accurate 3D models can now be created very quickly [2–5], and requiring a 3D model beforehand is not a disadvantage anymore. For industrial applications, a detailed 3D model often exists before the real object is even created.

Given a 3D model of an object, we show how to generate templates that cover a full view hemisphere by regularly sampling viewpoints of the 3D model. We also show how the 3D model can be used to obtain a fine estimate of the object pose, starting from the one provided by the templates. Together with a simple test based on color, this allows us to remove false positives, by checking if the object under the recovered pose aligns well with the depth map. Moreover, we show how to define the templates only with the most useful appearance and depth information, which allows us to speed up the template detection stage. The end result is a system that significantly improves the original LINEMOD implementation in performance, while providing accurate pose for applications.

In short, we propose a framework that is easy to deploy, reliable, and fast enough to run in real-time. We also provide a dataset made of 15 registered, 1100+ frame video sequences of 15 various objects for the evaluation of future competing methods. In the remainder of this paper we first discuss related work, briefly describe the approach of LINEMOD, introduce our method, represent our dataset and present an exhaustive evaluation.

## 2   Related Work

3D object detection and localization is a difficult but important problem with a long research history. Methods have been developed for detection in photometric images and range images, and more recently, in registered color/depth images. We discuss these below.

**Camera Images.** We can divide image-based object detection into two broad categories: learning-based and template approaches. Learning-based systems generalize well to the objects of particular class like human faces [6], cars [7, 8], or other objects [9]. Their main limitations are the limited set of object poses they accept, and the large training database and time. In general, they also do not return an accurate estimate of the object 3D pose.

To overcome these limitations, researchers tried to learn the object appearance from 3D models [7, 8, 10]. The approach of Stark *et al.* [7] relies only on 3D CAD models of cars and Liebelt and Schmid [8] combine geometric shape and pose priors with natural images. Both of these approaches work well and also generalize to object classes, but they are not real-time capable, require expensive training and cannot handle clutter and occlusions well. In [10] authors use a number of viewpoint-specific shape representations to model the object category. They rely on contours and introduce a novel feature called BOB (bag of boundaries), which at a given point in the image is a histogram of boundaries from image contours in training images. This feature is later used in the shape context descriptor for template matching. While it generalizes well, it is far from real-time and cannot find a precise 3D pose. In contrast, our method is real-time capable, can learn new objects online from 3D models, can handle large amount of clutter and moderate occlusions and can detect multiple objects simultaneously.

As discussed in [1], template-based approaches [11–14] typically do not require large training sets or time, as the templates are acquired quickly from views of the object. However, all these approaches are either susceptible to background clutter or too slow for real-time performance.

**Range Images.** Detection of 3D objects in range data has a long history; a review can be found in [15]. One of the standard approaches for object pose estimation is ICP [16]; however this approach requires an initial estimate and is not suited for object detection. Approaches based on 3D features are more suitable and are usually followed by ICP for the pose refinement. Some of these methods (which assume that a full 3D model is available) include spin-images [17], point pairs [18, 19], and point-pair histograms [20, 21]. These methods are usually computationally expensive, and have difficulty in scenes with clutter. The method of Drost *et. al* [18] can deal with clutter; however, its efficiency and performance depend directly on the complexity of the 3D scene, which makes it difficult to use in real-time applications.

**RGBD Images.** In recent years, a number of methods that rely on RGBD sensors have been introduced—among them [22] which is subject to object classification, pose estimation and reconstruction. Similar to us the training data set is composed of depth and image intensity cues and the object classes are detected using a modified Hough transform. While being quite effective in real applications these approaches still require exhaustive training on large data sets. In [23] Lei *et al.* study the recognition problem at both the category and the instance level. In addition they provide a large data set of 3D objects. However, they have neither demonstrated that their approach work on heavily cluttered scenes in real time nor that it returns 3D pose as our method does.

# 3   Approach

Our approach to object detection is based on LINEMOD [1]. LINEMOD is an efficient method to detect multi-modal templates in the Kinect output, a depth map registered to a color image. The LINEMOD templates sample the possible appearances of the objects to detect, and are built from densely sampled image gradients and depth map normals. When a template is found, it provides not only the object's 2D location in the image, but also a coarse estimate of its pose, as the templates can easily be labeled with this information.

In the reminder of the paper, we will show how we generate the templates automatically from a 3D model with a regular sampling. We also show how we speed up detection time by keeping only the most useful information in the templates, how we compute a fine estimate of the object 3D pose, and how we exploit this pose and the object color to detect outliers.

## 3.1   Exploiting a 3D Model to Create the Templates

In contrast to online learning approaches [1, 14, 24–26], we build a set of templates automatically from CAD 3D models. This has several advantages. First, online learning requires physical interaction of a human operator or a robot with their environment, and therefore takes time and effort. Furthermore, it usually takes an educated user and careful manual interaction to collect a well sampled training set of the object that covers the whole pose range. Online methods usually follow a greedy approach and they are not guaranteed to lead to optimal results in terms of trade-off between efficiency and robustness.

### 3.1.1 Viewpoint Sampling
Viewpoint sampling is crucial in LINEMOD. We have to balance the trade-off between the coverage of the object for reliability and the number of template for efficiency. As in [27], we solve this problem by recursively dividing an icosahedron, the largest convex regular polyhedron. We substitute each triangle into four almost equilateral triangles, and iterate several times. As illustrated in Fig. 2, the vertices of the resulting polyhedron give us then the two out-of-plane rotation angles for the sampled pose with respect to the coordinate center. In practice we stop at 162 vertices on the upper hemisphere for a good trade-off. Two adjacent vertices are then approximately 15 degrees apart. In addition to the these two out of plane rotations, we also created templates for different in-plane rotations. Furthermore, we generate templates at different scales by using different sized polyhedrons, using a step size of 10 cm.

### 3.1.2 Reducing Feature Redundancy
LINEMOD relies on two different features: color gradients, computed from the color image, and surface normals, computed from the object 3D model. Both are discretized to a few values by the algorithm. The color gradients are taken at each image location as the gradient of largest magnitude over the 3 color channels. The LINEMOD templates are made from these two features computed

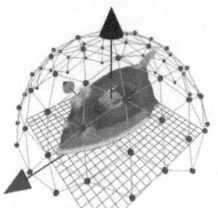 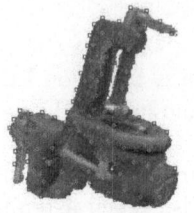 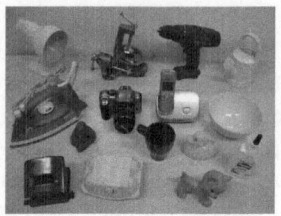

**Fig. 2. Left:** Sampling the viewpoints of the upper hemisphere for template generation: Red vertices represent the virtual camera centers used to generate templates. Note, that the camera centers are uniformly sampled. **Middle:** The selected features: Color gradient features are displayed in red, surface normal features in green. The features are quasi uniformly spread over the areas where they represent the object best. **Right:** 15 different texture-less 3D objects used in our experiments.

densely. We show here that we can consider only a subset of the features used in LINEMOD. This speeds up the detection with no loss of accuracy.

**Color Gradient Features:** We keep only the main color gradient features located on the contour of the object silhouette, because we focus on texture-less objects which exhibit no or only little texture on the interior of the object silhouette, and because the texture of a given CAD 3D model is not always available.

For each sampled pose generated by the method described above, we first compute the object silhouette by projecting the 3D model under this pose. By subtracting the eroded silhouette from its original version we quickly obtain the silhouette contour. We then compute all the color gradients that lie on the silhouette contour and sort them with respect to their magnitudes. This is important since our silhouette edge is not guaranteed to be only one pixel broad. We then use a greedy approach where we iterate through this sorted list, starting from the gradient with the strongest magnitude, and take the first feature that appears in this list. We then remove from the list the features whose image locations are close—according to some distance threshold—to the picked feature location, and we iterate.

If we have finished iterating through the list of features before a desired number of features is selected, we decrease the distance threshold by one and start the process again. The threshold is initially set to the ratio of the area covered by the silhouette and the number of features that are supposed to be selected. This heuristic is reasonable since the silhouette contour is usually a one pixel broad edge such that the initial threshold is simply the maximal possible distance between two features if these are spread uniformly on an ideal one pixel broad silhouette. As a result, our efficient method ensures that the selected features are both robust and, at the same time, almost uniformly spread on the silhouette (see Fig. 2).

**Surface Normal Features:** In contrast to color gradient features, we chose the surface normal features to be selected on the interior of the object silhouette.

This is because the surface normals on the borders of the projected object are often not estimated reliably, or not recovered at all.

As in LINEMOD we discretize the normals computed from the depth map by considering their orientations. The first difference is that in the case of the template generation, the depth map is computed from the object 3D model, not acquired by the Kinect.

We first remark that normals surrounded by normals of similar orientation are recovered more reliably. We therefore want to keep these normals during the creation of the template, and discard the less stable ones. To do so, we first create a mask for each of the 8 possible values of discretized orientations from the depth map generated for the object under the considered pose.

For each of the 8 masks, we then weight each normal with the distance to the mask boundary. Large distances indicate normals surrounded with normals of similar orientation. Small distances indicate normals surrounded by different normals, or normals close to the object silhouette boundaries, and we first directly reject the normals with a weight smaller than a specific distance—we use 2 in practice.

However, we can not rely on the weights only to select the normals we want to keep among the remaining ones. This is because large areas with similar normals would have a too great influence on the resulting template, and therefore, we normalize the weights by the size of the mask they belong to.

We then proceed as for the selection of the color gradients. We first create a list of the surface normals, ranked according to their normalized weights, and iteratively select the normals we keep in the final template. It ensures an quasi uniform spreading of the selected normals (see Fig. 2). Here, the threshold is set to the square root of the ratio of the area covered by the rendered object and the number of features we want to keep.

## 3.2   Postprocessing Detections

For each template detected by LINEMOD—starting with the one with the highest similarity score, we first check the consistency of this detection by comparing the object color with the content of the color image at its location. If it passes the test, we estimate the 3D pose of the corresponding object. We reject all detections whose 3D pose estimates have not converged properly. Taking the first $n$ detections that passed all checks, we do a final pose estimate for the best of them. We use this final estimate in an ultimate depth test for the validity of the detection. As shown in the results section, these additional tests make our approach much more reliable than LINEMOD.

### 3.2.1 Coarse Outlier Removal by Color

Each detected template provides a coarse estimate of the object pose that is good enough for an efficient check based on color information. We consider the pixels that lie on the object projection according to the pose estimate, and count how many of them have the expected color. We decide a pixel has the expected color if the difference between its hue and the object hue (modulo $2\pi$) is smaller than a threshold—considering the hue makes the test robust to light changes. If the percentage of pixels that have their expected color is not large enough (at least 70% in our implementation), we reject the detection as false positive.

In practice we do not take into account the pixels that are too close to the object projection boundaries, to be tolerant to the inaccuracy of the current pose estimate. This can be done efficiently by eroding the object projection beforehand.

We still have to handle black and white objects. Since black and white are not covered by the hue component, we map them to the hue values of similar colors: black to blue and white to yellow. This is done by checking the corresponding saturation and value component before we compute the absolute difference. In case the value component is below a threshold $t_v$, we set the hue value to blue. If the value component is larger than $t_v$ and the saturation component below a threshold $t_s$, we set the hue component to yellow. In our case $t_s = t_v = 0.12$.

### 3.2.2 Fast Pose Estimation and Outlier Rejection Based on Depth

For the detections that passed the previous color check, we refine the pose estimate provided by the template detection. This is performed with the Iterative Closest Point algorithm to align the 3D model surface with the depth map. The initial translation is estimated from the depth values covered by the initial model projection.

For efficiency, we first subsample the 3D points from the depth map that lie on the object projection or close to it. To speed up point-to-point matching, we use the efficient voxel-based ICP method of [28], which relies on a grid that can be pre-computed for each object. For robustness, at each iteration $i$, we compute the alignment using only the inlier 3D points. The inlier points are the ones that fall within a distance to the 3D model smaller than an adaptive threshold $t_i$.

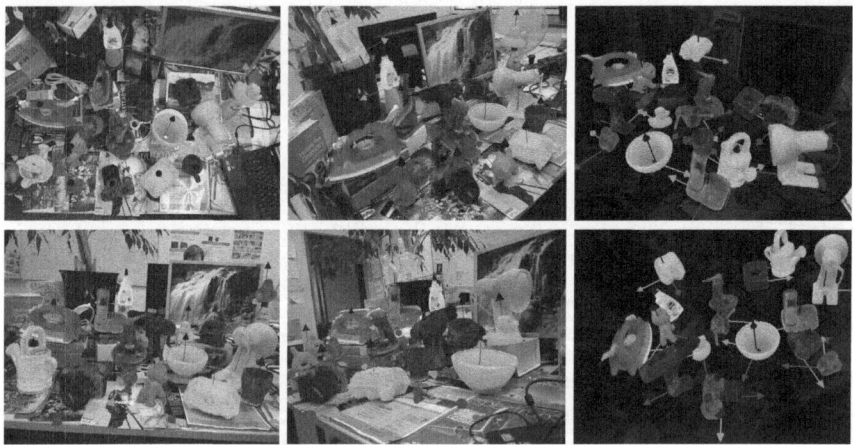

**Fig. 3.** 15 different texture-less 3D objects are simultaneously detected under different poses on heavy cluttered background with partial occlusion and illumination changes. Each detected object is augmented with its 3D model and its coordinate systems.

$t_0$ is initialized to the size of the object, $t_{i+1}$ is set to three times the average distance of the inliers to the 3D model at time $i$. After convergence, if the average distance of the inliers to the 3D model is too large, we reject the detection as false positive.

We repeat this until $n = 3$ detections passed this check or no detections are left. Then we perform a slower but finer ICP for the best of these $n$ detections by considering all the points from the depth map that lie on the object projection or close to it. The best detection is found by comparing the number of inliers and their average distance to the 3D model. The final ICP is followed by a final depth test. For that, we consider the pixels that lie on the object projection according to the final pose estimate, and count how many of them have the expected depth. We decide a pixel has the expected depth if the difference between its depth value and the projected object depth is smaller than a threshold. If the percentage of pixels that have their expected depth is not large enough (at least 70% in our implementation), we finally reject the detection as false positive. Otherwise, we we say that the object was found with the final pose.

## 4    Experiments

For comparison, we created a large dataset of 15 registered video sequences of 15 texture-less 3D objects. Each object was sticked to the center of a planar board with markers attached to it, for model and image acquisition. The markers on the board provided the corresponding ground truth poses. Each object was reconstructed first using a set of images and the corresponding poses using a simple voxel based approach. After reconstruction, we added close range and far range 2D and 3D clutter to the scene and took the evaluation sequences. Each sequence contains more than 1,100 real images from different view points. In order to guarantee a well distributed pose space sampling of the dataset pictures, we uniformly divided the upper hemisphere of the objects into equally distant pieces and took at most one image per piece. As a result, our sequences provide uniformly distributed views from 0-360 degree around the object, 0-90 degree tilt rotation, 65 cm-115 cm scaling and ±45 degree in-plane rotation. For each object, we visualized the cameras color coded with respect to their distance to the object center in the second column of Figs. 5 and 6.

Since it was already shown in [29] that LINEMOD outperforms DOT [14], HOG [30], TLD [26] and the method of Steger *et al.* [13], we compare our method only to the one of Drost *et al.* [18]. For [18], we use the binaries kindly provided by the authors that run on Intel Xeon E5345 processor with 2.33 GHz and 32 GB RAM. All the other experiments were performed on a standard notebook with an Intel i7-2820QM processor with 2.3 GHz and 8 GB of RAM. For obtaining the image and the depth data we used the Primesense$^{(tm)}$ PSDK 5.0 device.

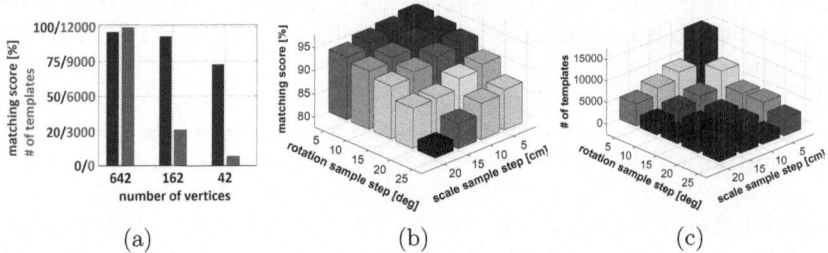

(a)                    (b)                    (c)

**Fig. 4.** Quality of the detections for drilling machine data set with respect to the viewpoint sampling steps. **(a)** The matching scores for different numbers of vertices (see Sec. 3.1). A good trade-off between speed and robustness are 162 vertices for the upper hemisphere. **(b),(c)**: the matching score decreases if the sample steps increase. We also display the number of templates with respect to the sampling steps: we made sure that all necessary poses were covered. A good trade-off between speed and robustness is a rotation sampling step of 15 degree and a scale sampling step of 10 cm.

**Table 1.** Recognition rates for $k_m = 0.1$. The first column gives the results of our method using automatically generated templates (see Sec. 3.1). The second and third columns give recognition numbers if no postprocessing is performed. For the second column, we use the best (with respect to the ground truth) out of the first $n = 3$ detections with the highest similarity score. For the third column, we only evaluate the detection with the highest similarity score. In the fourth and fifth column, we give the average runtime of our method and the one of Drost *et al.* [18] per frame.

| Approach | Our Appr. | Drost[18] | LINEMOD3 | LINEMOD1 | Our Appr. | Drost[18] |
|---|---|---|---|---|---|---|
| Sequence (#pics) | Matching Score | | | | Speed | |
| Ape (1235) | **95.8%** | 86.5% | 86.3% | 69.4% | **127ms** | 22.7s |
| Bench Vise (1214) | **98.7%** | 70.7% | 98.0% | 94.0% | **115ms** | 2.94s |
| Driller (1187) | **93.6%** | 87.3% | 91.8% | 81.3% | **121ms** | 2.65s |
| Cam (1200) | **97.5%** | 78.6% | 93.4% | 79.5% | **148ms** | 2.81s |
| Can (1195) | **95.4%** | 80.2% | 91.3% | 79.5% | **122ms** | 1.60s |
| Iron (1151) | **97.5%** | 84.9% | 95.9% | 88.8% | **116ms** | 3.18s |
| Lamp (1226) | **97.7%** | 93.3% | 97.5% | 89.8% | **125ms** | 2.29s |
| Phone (1224) | **93.3%** | 80.7% | 88.3% | 77.8% | **157ms** | 4.70s |
| Cat (1178) | **99.3%** | 85.4% | 97.9% | 88.2% | **111ms** | 7.52s |
| Hole punch (1236) | **95.9%** | 77.4% | 90.5% | 78.4% | **110ms** | 8.30s |
| Duck (1253) | **95.9%** | 46.0% | 91.4% | 75.9% | **104ms** | 6.97s |
| Cup (1239) | **97.1%** | 68.4% | 87.9% | 80.7% | **105ms** | 16.7s |
| Bowl (1232) | **99.9%** | 95.7% | 99.7% | 99.5% | **97ms** | 5.18s |
| Box (1252) | **99.8%** | 97.0% | 99.8% | 99.1% | **101ms** | 2.94s |
| Glue (1219) | **91.8%** | 57.2% | 80.9% | 64.3% | **135ms** | 4.03s |
| Average (18241) | **96.6%** | 79.3% | 92.7% | 83.0% | **119ms** | 6.3s |

## 4.1  Robustness

In order to evaluate our approach, we first have to define an appropriate matching score for a 3D model $\mathcal{M}$: having the ground truth rotation $\mathbf{R}$ and translation $\mathbf{T}$ and the estimated rotation $\tilde{\mathbf{R}}$ and translation $\tilde{\mathbf{T}}$, we compute the average distance of all model points $\mathbf{x}$ from their transformed versions:

$$m = \operatorname*{avg}_{\mathbf{x} \in \mathcal{M}} \| (\mathbf{R}\mathbf{x} + \mathbf{T}) - (\tilde{\mathbf{R}}\mathbf{x} + \tilde{\mathbf{T}}) \| . \tag{1}$$

We say that the model was correctly detected and the pose correctly estimated if $k_m d \geq m$ where $k_m$ is a chosen coefficient and $d$ is the diameter of $\mathcal{M}$. We still have to define a matching score measure for objects that are ambiguous or have a subset of views under which they appear to be ambiguous. Such objects ("cup","bowl","box" and "glue") are shown in Fig. 6. We define the corresponding matching score as:

$$m = \operatorname*{avg}_{\mathbf{x}_1 \in \mathcal{M}} \operatorname*{min}_{\mathbf{x}_2 \in \mathcal{M}} \| (\mathbf{R}\mathbf{x}_1 + \mathbf{T}) - (\tilde{\mathbf{R}}\mathbf{x}_2 + \tilde{\mathbf{T}}) \| . \tag{2}$$

Since it was already shown in [29] that LINEMOD outperforms DOT [14], HOG [30], TLD [26] and the method of Steger et al. [13], we evaluate our new pipeline with the approach of Drost et al. [18]. This approach – contrary to the before mentioned ones – does not only perform detection but also pose estimation of general 3D objects. For our experiments, we set $n = 3$ and used the optimal training parameters as described in Sec. 4.3. As one can see in the graphs shown in Fig. 5 and 6, our new approach outperforms Drost et al. [18].

In addition, we compared the output of our new pipeline to the detection results of LINEMOD. For the latter, we simply used the pose composed by the rotation under which the detected template was created and the translation coming from the depth map. Here, we evaluated two strategies: for the first one, we only took the pose of the detected template whose similarity score was largest (LINEMOD1). Since our new pipeline evaluates several hypotheses, we also added curves where we took the best pose with respect to the ground truth one out of the three best detected templates (LINEMOD3). For both cases, we can see that our new pipeline drastically increases the recognition performance.

We also show the matching results for $k_m = 0.1$ in Table 1. Matches with $k_m = 0.1$ are also found visually correct. In this table, we see that our new pipeline outperforms the approach of Drost et al. [18] by average 17.3% and improves the recognition results by average 13% w.r.t. the original LINEMOD.

Furthermore, we also evaluated our new approach on the ape, duck and cup dataset of [1] where we compared our automatically trained LINEMOD against the manually learned LINEMOD.Our new pipeline obtains almost no false positves and a superior true positive rate of 98.7% for the cup sequence (compared to [1]: 96.8%), 98.2% for the ape sequence (compared to [1]: 97.9%) and 99.5% for the duck sequence (compared to [1]: 97.9).

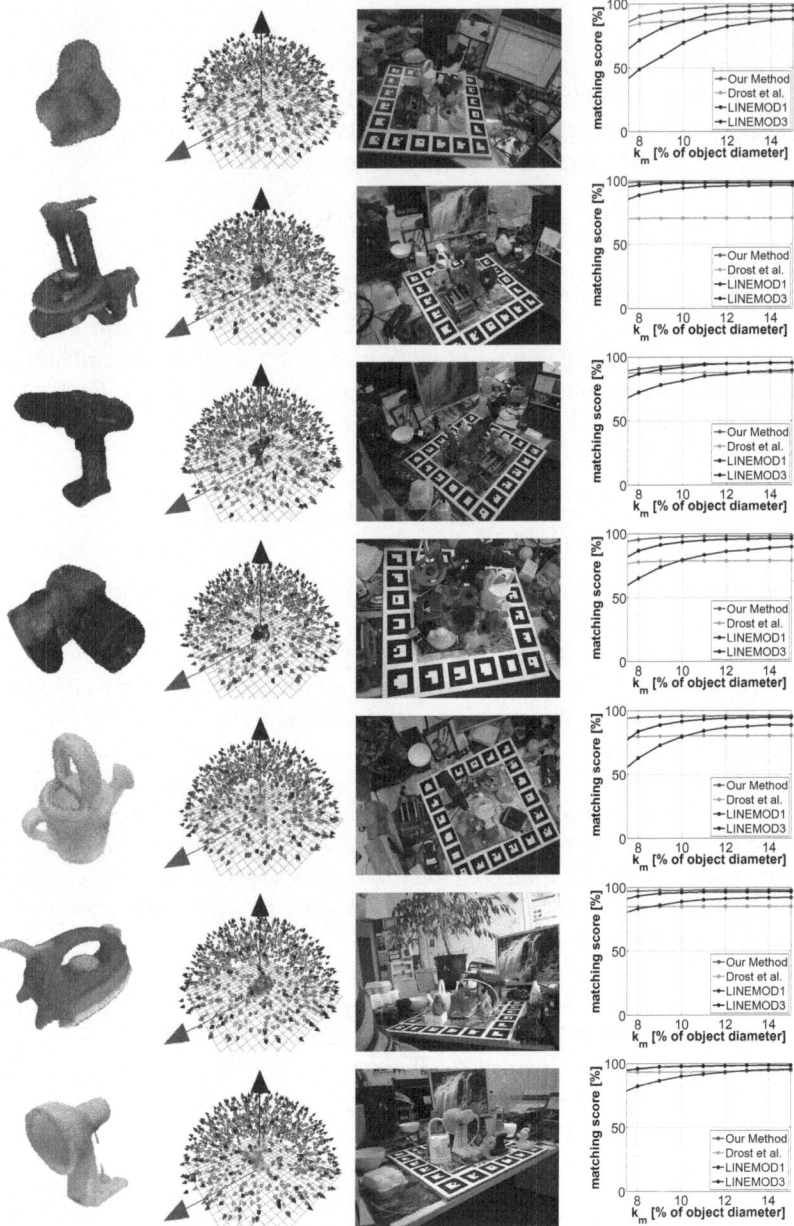

**Fig. 5.** In our experiments, different texture-less 3D objects are detected in real-time under different poses on heavy cluttered background. **Left:** Some 3D reconstructed models. **Middle Left:** The pose space of the dataset images. The distance of the cameras to the object is color coded. **Middle Right:** One test image with the correctly recognized object. The 3D model of the object is augmented. **Right:** The matching scores with respect to different $k_m$. **The datasets is public available at http://campar.in.tum.de/twiki/pub/Main/StefanHinterstoisser**.

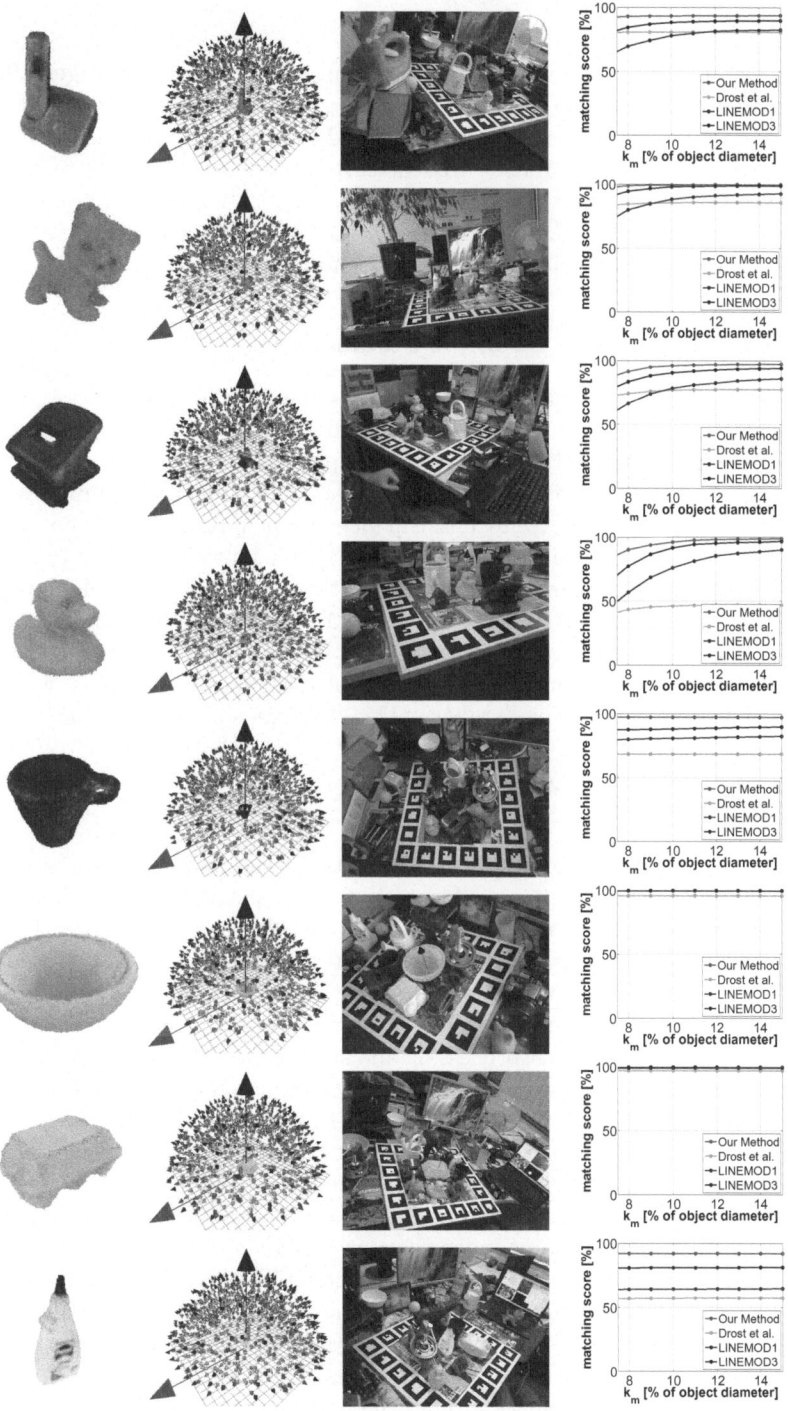

**Fig. 6.** Another set of 3D objects we used in our extensive experiments. **The datasets is public available at** http://campar.in.tum.de/twiki/pub/Main/StefanHinterstoisser.

## 4.2   Speed

As we see in Tab. 1, our whole recognition pipeline needs in average 119ms to detect an object in the pose range of 0-360 degree around the object, 0-90 degree tilt rotation, 65 cm-115 cm scaling and ±45degree in-plane rotation. This is 53 times faster than the approach of Drost *et al.* and allows real-time recognition. To cover this pose range we need 3,115 templates. Unoptimized training lasts from 17 seconds for the "ape" object to 50 seconds for the "bench vise" object and is dependent on the number of vertices to render.

## 4.3   Choosing Training Sample Parameters

In order to choose the right parameters for training, we initially took the drill sequence and evaluated our method with respect to the training parameters. As we can see in the first graph of Fig. 4, sampling the viewpoints with 162 vertices is a good trade-off between robustness and the number of templates which have to be matched. The speed performance of our approach is proportional to this number and thus, using less templates implies shorter runtime. In addition we made experiments, how the sampling of the scale and the in-plane rotation influences the robustness and the runtime. As we can see in middle and right graphs of Fig. 4, a good trade-off is a scale step of 10 cm and a rotation step of 15 degrees. As we found out, the choice of these parameters gave very good results for all objects in our database. Therefore, we set them once and for all.

## 5   Conclusion

We have presented a framework for automatic learning, detection and pose estimation of 3D objects using a Kinect. As a first contribution, we showed how we automatically reduce feature redundancy for color gradients and surface normals and how we automatically learn templates from a 3D model. For the latter, we provide a solution of pose space sampling which guarantees a good trade-off between detection speed and robustness. As a second contribution, we provided novel means for efficient postprocessing and showed that the pose estimation and the color information allow us to check the detection hypotheses and to improve the correct detection rate by 13% with respect to the original LINEMOD. Furthermore, we showed that we significantly outperform the approach of Drost *et al.* [18]—a commercial state-of-the-art detection approach that is able to estimate the object pose. Our final contribution is the proposal of a new dataset made of 15 registered, 1100+ frame video sequences of 15 various texture-less objects for the evaluation of future competing methods. The novelty of our sequences with respect to state-of-the-art datasets is the combination of the following features: First, for each sequence and each image, we provide the corresponding 3D model of the object and its ground truth poses. Second, each sequence uniformly covers the complete pose space around the registered object. Third, each image contains heavy close range and far range 2D and 3D clutter.

# References

1. Hinterstoisser, S., Cagniart, C., Holzer, S., Ilic, S., Konolige, K., Navab, N., Lepetit, V.: Multimodal Templates for Real-Time Detection of Texture-Less Objects in Heavily Cluttered Scenes. In: ICCV (2011)
2. Newcombe, R.A., Izadi, S., Hilliges, O., Molyneaux, D., Kim, D., Davison, A.J., Kohli, P., Shotton, J., Hodges, S., Fitzgibbon, A.: KinectFusion: Real-Time Dense Surface Mapping and Tracking. In: ISMAR (2011)
3. Pan, Q., Reitmayr, G., Drummond, T.: ProFORMA: Probabilistic Feature-based On-line Rapid Model Acquisition. In: BMVC (2009)
4. Weise, T., Wismer, T., Leibe, B., Gool, L.V.: In-hand Scanning with Online Loop Closure. In: International Workshop on 3-D Digital Imaging and Modeling (2009)
5. Newcombe, R.A., Lovegrove, S.J., Davison, A.J.: DTAM: Dense Tracking and Mapping in Real-Time. In: ICCV (2011)
6. Viola, P., Jones, M.: Fast Multi-View Face Detection. In: CVPR (2003)
7. Stark, M., Goesele, M., Schiele, B.: Back to the Future: Learning Shape Models from 3D Cad Data. In: BMVC (2010)
8. Liebelt, J., Schmid, C.: Multi-View Object Class Detection With a 3D Geometric Model. In: CVPR (2010)
9. Ferrari, V., Jurie, F., Schmid, C.: From Images to Shape Models for Object Detection. In: IJCV (2009)
10. Payet, N., Todorovic, S.: From contours to 3d object detection and pose estimation. In: ICCV, pp. 983–990 (2011)
11. Gavrila, D., Philomin, V.: Real-Time Object Detection for "smart" Vehicles. In: ICCV (1999)
12. Huttenlocher, D., Klanderman, G., Rucklidge, W.: Comparing Images Using the Hausdorff Distance. TPAMI (1993)
13. Steger, C.: Similarity Measures for Occlusion, Clutter, and Illumination Invariant Object Recognition. In: Radig, B., Florczyk, S. (eds.) DAGM 2001. LNCS, vol. 2191, pp. 148–154. Springer, Heidelberg (2001)
14. Hinterstoisser, S., Lepetit, V., Ilic, S., Fua, P., Navab, N.: Dominant Orientation Templates for Real-Time Detection of Texture-Less Objects. In: CVPR (2010)
15. Mian, A.S., Bennamoun, M., Owens, R.A.: Automatic Correspondence for 3D Modeling: an Extensive Review. International Journal of Shape Modeling (2005)
16. Zhang, Z.: Iterative Point Matching for Registration of Free-Form Curves. In: IJCV (1994)
17. Johnson, A.E., Hebert, M.: Using Spin Images for Efficient Object Recognition in Cluttered 3 D Scenes. TPAMI (1999)
18. Drost, B., Ulrich, M., Navab, N., Ilic, S.: Model Globally, Match Locally: Efficient and Robust 3D Object Recognition. In: CVPR (2010)
19. Mian, A.S., Bennamoun, M., Owens, R.: Three-Dimensional Model-Based Object Recognition and Segmentation in Cluttered Scenes. TPAMI (2006)
20. Rusu, R.B., Blodow, N., Beetz, M.: Fast Point Feature Histograms (FPFH) for 3D Registration. In: International Conference on Robotics and Automation (2009)
21. Tombari, F., Salti, S., Di Stefano, L.: Unique Signatures of Histograms for Local Surface Description. In: Daniilidis, K., Maragos, P., Paragios, N. (eds.) ECCV 2010, Part III. LNCS, vol. 6313, pp. 356–369. Springer, Heidelberg (2010)
22. Sun, M., Bradski, G., Xu, B.-X., Savarese, S.: Depth-Encoded Hough Voting for Joint Object Detection and Shape Recovery. In: Daniilidis, K., Maragos, P., Paragios, N. (eds.) ECCV 2010, Part V. LNCS, vol. 6315, pp. 658–671. Springer, Heidelberg (2010)

23. Lai, K., Bo, L., Ren, X., Fox, D.: Sparse distance learning for object recognition combining rgb and depth information. In: ICRA, pp. 4007–4013 (2011)
24. Grabner, M., Grabner, H., Bischof, H.: Learning Features for Tracking. In: CVPR (2007)
25. Ozuysal, M., Calonder, M., Lepetit, V., Fua, P.: Fast Keypoint Online Learning and Recognition. TPAMI (2010)
26. Kalal, Z., Matas, J., Mikolajczyk, K.: P-N Learning: Bootstrapping Binary Classifiers by Structural Constraints. In: CVPR (2010)
27. Hinterstoisser, S., Benhimane, S., Lepetit, V., Fua, P., Navab, N.: Simultaneous Recognition and Homography Extraction of Local Patches With a Simple Linear Classifier. In: BMVC (2008)
28. Fitzgibbon, A.: Robust Registration fo 2D and 3D Point Sets. In: BMVC (2001)
29. Hinterstoisser, S., Ilic, S., Sturm, P., Navab, N., Fua, P., Lepetit, V.: Gradient Response Maps for Real-Time Detection of Texture-Less Objects. TPAMI (2012)
30. Dalal, N., Triggs, B.: Histograms of Oriented Gradients for Human Detection. In: CVPR (2005)

# Boosting with Side Information

Jixu Chen[1], Xiaoming Liu[2], and Siwei Lyu[3]

[1] GE Global Research, Niskayuna, NY
chenji@ge.com
[2] Michigan State University, East lansing, MI
liuxm@cse.msu.edu
[3] University at Albany, SUNY, Albany, NY
slyu@albany.edu

**Abstract.** In many problems of machine learning and computer vision, there exists side information, i.e., information contained in the training data and not available in the testing phase. This motivates the recent development of a new learning approach known as *learning with side information* that aims to incorporate side information for improved learning algorithms. In this work, we describe a new training method of boosting classifiers that uses side information, which we term as *AdaBoost+*. In particular, AdaBoost+ employs a novel classification label imputation method to construct extra weak classifiers from the available information that simulate the performance of better weak classifiers obtained from the features in side information. We apply our method to two problems, namely handwritten digit recognition and facial expression recognition from low resolution images, where it demonstrates its effectiveness in classification performance.

## 1 Introduction

Classification plays a central role in the solutions of many computer vision problems. A classifier is a parametric function that takes input $\mathbf{x} \in \mathcal{R}^d$ and predicts its class label $y \in \{0, 1, \cdots, C\}$. The conventional approach to obtain a classifier is with supervised learning that uses a training set of data $(\mathbf{x}_1, \cdots, \mathbf{x}_N)$ and their corresponding class labels $(y_1, \cdots, y_N)$. The semi-supervised learning approach [6] relaxes on the requirement of a fully labelled training set, and can be used to learn a classifier with a mixture of labelled and unlabelled training data.

However, in many practical applications, there may be extra sources of information other than the training data and class labels, and to which we only have access when training the classifier. For instance, in face recognition, besides images of faces and their corresponding subjects' identities, we can have other information in training, such as the age, gender, skin color, etc. In this work, we call such features as *side information*, and correspondingly, we call features that are present in both training and testing as *available information*.

Side information arises because some aspects of a classification problem cannot be specified via the class labels and the training data[1]. Therefore, it should be

---

[1] In the most general sense, labels of the training set can also be regarded as side information.

K.M. Lee et al. (Eds.): ACCV 2012, Part I, LNCS 7724, pp. 563–577, 2013.
© Springer-Verlag Berlin Heidelberg 2013

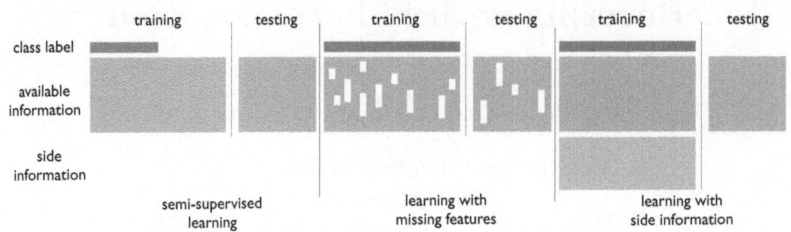

**Fig. 1.** Graphical illustrations of settings of different learning paradigms

differentiated from missing features, which are subsets of composing categories of data that are unavailable in the testing and/or training sets [24,1,14,27,10]. More importantly, typical techniques addressing missing features such as *data imputation*, where the missing features are replaced with their predictions from the available information, may not be used to handle side information. Predicting side information could be a more difficult task than directly learning the classifier from available information, as in the cases when side information corresponds to more complex and higher dimensional features. On the other hand, predicting side information may not be of particular relevance to the classification task, which could be regarded as unnecessary and wasteful in practical applications.

Incorporating side information into the construction of the classifier may be beneficial because it provides alternative means for the system designer to input more prior knowledge into the learned classifier. Yet, because side information is not present when the classifier is deployed to classify a previously unseen datum, it has been largely ignored in the current practice of automatic learning of classifiers. This motivates the recent development of a new learning approach known as *learning with side information* (also known as learning with privileged information) [33,32,25]. The general idea of learning with side information is to use a hypothetical classifier built with available and side information together as an oracle of performance upper-bound to guild the training of the classifier using only available information. Recent results in learning theory [21,25] have suggested that using side information can improve the learning rate in the training of the classifier, and may be particularly useful when the training data set is relatively small. In practice, learning with side information has shown promising performance gain when it is incorporated in the training of the SVM classifiers (an algorithm known as SVM+) and applied to handwritten digit recognition, time series prediction, and protein classification [33,32]. Learning with side information can also find abundant applications in computer vision. For instance, to obtain an effective classifier that can recognize faces in low resolution still images from surveillance cameras, we can use high resolution images (e.g., mug-shots) or video clips as side information.

Here, we explore the potential of combining side information to improve boosting classifiers, which we call *AdaBoost+*. Boosting has been widely used in many computer vision problems (such as face or expression recognition), because it is constructed from simple base classifiers, e.g. decision stumps or linear cuts, which facilitates extracting interpretable rules from the decision boundary.

In particular, AdaBoost+ does not attempt to impute the side information with available information, which as we have mentioned, could lead to a more difficult problem. Instead, it uses *classification label imputation* to construct extra weak classifiers from the available information that simulate the performance of better weak classifiers obtained from features in side information. We apply AdaBoost+ to two problems, namely handwritten digit recognition and facial expression recognition from low resolution images, where it demonstrates its effectiveness in classification performance.

## 2   Related Works

In machine learning, side information has been employed in the context of unsupervised learning, in particular, in distance metric learning [34], constrained clustering [4] and similarity kernel learning [17]. In the unsupervised learning context, the side information is usually cast in the form of pairwise constraints, while few work discusses using side information in the form of extra features.

In comparison, there are fewer works discussing the use of side information for supervised learning. The recent work of Vapnik [33,25] has shown that a learning algorithm trained with the help of both side information (SVM+), as well as the available information, provides improved performance over a machine trained only on the available information (SVM). In the SVM+ algorithm, side information is used to predict the optimal slack variables in the SVM objective function. In statistical analysis, missing features usually cause biased estimation of statistics or model parameters. To improve the estimation, we can either delete the examples with missing features (list-wise deletion, pairwise deletion) or impute the missing features [24,13,27] (regression imputation, hot deck imputation, multiple imputation and EM). A few works focusing on the problem of missing features only in testing data set [14,10,27]. In particular, if the missing feature indices are known, it shows that simply imputing the missing features will give an even worse result than using only the observed features [27]. Our work demonstrates that an improved performance can be achieved by using the missing feature in testing as side-information in the training phase.

In computer vision, the attribute-based object recognition [11,18] uses discrete attribute as side information. These attributes are semantic visual qualities of objects, such as 'red', 'striped', 'wood', etc. Most of the attribute-based methods are similar to imputation, i.e., the missing attributes in the testing data is imputed by attribute classifiers. These methods are different from our work in two significant ways. First, they only focus on low-dimensional discrete attribute labels, while our work is applicable to more general types of side information including discrete labels (Sec. 5.1), high-dimensional continuous data (Sec. 5.2), time series data or 3D structure of proteins [33]. Second, they use the attributes as mid-level features and have to learn attribute classifiers, which may or may not be relevant to the actual classification task. In contrast, we use side-information as extra relevant information with an explicit goal of improving the final classification performance.

There are some prior works on boosting with side information [36] for medical applications where the side information is the actual domain knowledge of a particular application, rather than the data in our work. Side information is also different from the prior work using 'side' data [29,7], which performs unsupervised learning using a data set with relative information and an auxiliary 'side' data set with irrelevant information. The irrelative information in the 'side' data is minimized in learning.

## 3   Side Information and Classification Performance

We start with a simple analysis on the relationship between side information and classification performance. For simplicity, we consider binary classification, and a classifier is defined as $f(\tilde{\mathbf{x}}) : \mathcal{X} \mapsto \{-1, +1\}$, which maps data to the binary class $\tilde{\mathbf{x}} \in \mathcal{X}$ to the corresponding binary class labels. The optimal performance of a binary classification problem is lower bounded by the Bayesian error, $P(y \neq f(\tilde{\mathbf{x}})|\tilde{\mathbf{x}})$ [5], which itself is lower bounded by the conditional entropy $H(y|\tilde{\mathbf{x}})$, a direct corollary of applying the Fano's inequality [9]. In other words, the probability of incorrectly predicting $y$ based on information from $\tilde{\mathbf{x}}$ is constrained by the remaining uncertainty of $H(y|\tilde{\mathbf{x}})$ about $y$ when $\tilde{\mathbf{x}}$ is known. In this sense, $H(y|\tilde{\mathbf{x}})$ provides a general metric of classification performance independent of the particular choice of $f$.

Next, we consider data as a composite of the available information $\mathbf{x}$ and the side information $\mathbf{z}$, $\tilde{\mathbf{x}} = (\mathbf{x}, \mathbf{z})$. Then, we have $H(y|\mathbf{x}, \mathbf{z}) \leq H(y|\mathbf{x})$, since $H(y|\mathbf{x}) - H(y|\mathbf{x}, \mathbf{z}) = I(y, \mathbf{z}|\mathbf{x})$, where the conditional mutual information $I(y, \mathbf{z}|\mathbf{x})$ is always non-negative [9]. Therefore, including side information may lead to the reduction of the conditional uncertainty about the class label $y$ given input data, which could correspond to a lower Bayesian error. Furthermore, the optimal classification performance when the side information is available in training but withheld in testing is expected to be sandwiched between of the optimal performances of the two other ideal classifiers, one constructed with only available information and the other constructed with both available and side information. In particular, when the performance gap between the two ideal classifiers is significant, the latter can be used as an oracle to guide the training for more effective use of the side information.

So far, our analysis only pertains to the ideal case when we have access to the joint distribution of data and class labels, corresponding to an infinitely large labelled training data set. When finite training data sets are used, recent results in learning theory [21,25] show that under some fairly general conditions, learning with side information can lead to provably faster learning rate (in some cases, it gives rise to exponential improvement in the learning rates [21]), i.e., more reduction in classification error per additional training example. This makes learning with side information particularly useful in classification problems with high dimensional data and limited training data sets.

---

**Algorithm 1.** Boosting with Side Information (Adaboost+)

---

**input:** $N$ training samples of $\tilde{\mathbf{x}}_i = (\mathbf{x}_i, \mathbf{z}_i) \in \mathcal{R}^{D+E}$, with available information $\{\mathbf{x}_i\}_{i=1..N}$ and side information $\{\mathbf{z}_i\}_{i=1..N}$ and class labels $\{y_i\}_{i=1..N}$.
**output:** Boosted classifier $f^T(\mathbf{x}) = \sum_{t=1}^{T} \alpha^t h^t(\mathbf{x})$
**Initialization:** Set initial classifier : $f^0(\mathbf{x}) = 0$.
**for** $t = 1$ to $T$ **do**
  Using $\{\tilde{\mathbf{x}}_i\}_{i=1..N}$ as training data, build a *Type-I* classifier for each feature.
  Select top K weak classifiers $h_I^t(\tilde{\mathbf{x}})$ and the corresponding $\alpha^t$ that minimize the training error, Eq.(1).
  **for** $k = 1$ to $K$ **do**
    **if** $h_I^t(\tilde{\mathbf{x}})$ is built with a feature from side information **then**
      Train a regressor $\mathcal{R}^t$ from available information to this weak classifier.
      Build a *Type-II* weak classifier $h_{II}^t(\mathbf{x})$ on this regressor (Eq. 4).
      Replace the original *Type-I* classifier with $h_{II}^t(\mathbf{x})$.
      Update the corresponding $\alpha^t$ (Eq. 3).
      Update the corresponding training error.
    **else**
      Keep the original *Type-I* weak classifier $h_I^t(\mathbf{x})$ and its corresponding error.
    **end if**
  **end for**
  Add the updated top one weak classifier into the final boosting classifier $f^t(\mathbf{x}) = f^{t-1}(\mathbf{x}) + \alpha^t h^t(\mathbf{x})$.
**end for**

---

# 4    Boosting with Side Information

In this section, we will describe our algorithm to incorporates side information into an AdaBoost classifier, named *AdaBoost+*. The basic idea of boosting is to produce a strong classifier by linearly combining a set of weak classifiers, each may be learned from one single feature, in an iterative learning procedure. During each iteration, one optimal weak classifier will be selected based on the strong classifier up to the previous iteration, from one feature in the feature pool. In particular, for our scenario of learning with side information, the feature pool includes features from both available information and side information. In this paper, we assume that during the iterative process, there is at least one weak classifier learned from side information will be considered as optimal for a certain iteration, comparing to all weak classifiers from available information.

If this assumption cannot be satisfied, i.e., the weak classifier from available information always leads to a lower error rate on the training data than that of the side information while combining with the existing strong classifier, our method will be degenerated into the conventional AdaBoost. When this assumption can be satisfied, we assert that there is a possibility for a boosted classifier constructed with features from both available and side information to achieve better classification performance than a classifier built with available information alone. One simple reason for this assertion is that the particular feature of side information chosen during the iteration may serve as an oracle to guide the boosting on how to use the available information more effectively. In our paper such guidance is achieved by classification label imputation, which uses an auxiliary regressor from available information to simulate the binary classification outputs of the weak classifier from side information.

### 4.1   Algorithm

Let us first introduce the basic notations in the subsequent description. The training data set of the boosting classifier includes corresponding examples of available information $\{\mathbf{x}_i\}_{i=1..N}$ and side information $\{\mathbf{z}_i\}_{i=1..N}$, with binary class labels $\{y_i\}_{i=1..N}$. Note that for $i$th training sample, its available information, $\mathbf{x}_i \in \mathcal{R}^D$, and side information, $\mathbf{z}_i \in \mathcal{R}^E$ can be from different feature spaces. We also denote the complete training data by combining available information and side information as: $\tilde{\mathbf{x}}_i = (\mathbf{x}_i, \mathbf{z}_i) \in \mathcal{R}^{D+E}$, where $\mathbf{x}_i = (x_i^1, ..., x_i^D)$ and $\mathbf{z}_i = (z_i^1, ..., z_i^E)$, respectively. From the training data, our goal is to learn a boosted strong classifier $f^T(\mathbf{x}) = \sum_{t=1}^{T} \alpha^t h^t(\mathbf{x})$.

This algorithm is summarized in Algorithm 1 and the algorithm diagram is shown in Figure 2. As in the general framework of boosting, our algorithm starts with an initial classifier $f^0(\mathbf{x}) = 0$. Then from the whole set of training data, $\{\tilde{\mathbf{x}}_i\}_{i=1..N}$, we learn a *Type-I* classifier, $h_I(\mathbf{x}) = p \cdot (sign)(x^d - \theta)$, for each feature corresponding to available information and side information. Specifically, $h_I(\mathbf{x})$ is a decision stump, where $d$ is the index of the selected feature, $\theta$ is the threshold, and $p \in \{+1, -1\}$ is the polarity of the weak classifier. We then select the top $K$ weak classifiers $h_I^t(\tilde{\mathbf{x}})$ and their corresponding $\alpha^t$ that minimize the training error in Eq. 1.

$$E = \sum_{i=1}^{N} e\left(y_i, f^{t-1}(\mathbf{x}_i) + \alpha^t h_I^t(\tilde{\mathbf{x}}_i)\right), \tag{1}$$

where $e(\cdot, \cdot)$ is the error function in comparing the class label with the classifier output. The choice of function $e(\cdot)$ differs among different boosting algorithms, and we adopt the one for Adaboost [12], which is given by:

$$e\left(y_i, f(\mathbf{x}_i)\right) = \exp(-y_i f(\mathbf{x}_i)). \tag{2}$$

Given a weak classifier $h^t(\mathbf{x})$, its corresponding $\alpha^t$ to minimize Eq. 1 is computed as:

$$\alpha^t = 0.5 \log\left((1 - \epsilon^t)/\epsilon^t\right), \tag{3}$$

where $\epsilon^t = \frac{\sum_{i=1}^{N} w_i \cdot [y_i \neq h^t(\mathbf{x}_i)]}{\sum_{i=1}^{N} w_i}$ is the weighted error of this classifier, and the weight $w_i = \exp(-y_i f^{t-1}(\mathbf{x}_i))$ depends on the previous strong classifier.

In the second step of the training, if any one of the top $K$ *Type-I* classifiers is from side information, we replace it with a regressor from available information that optimally match the binary outputs of that *Type-I* weak classifier. In actual testing when side information is not available, such regressor can mimic the effect of side information since the outputs of the *Type-I* weak classifier have been approximated from this regressor. Specifically, for each one of top $K$ *Type-I* weak classifier that is from side information, we train an auxiliary regressor,

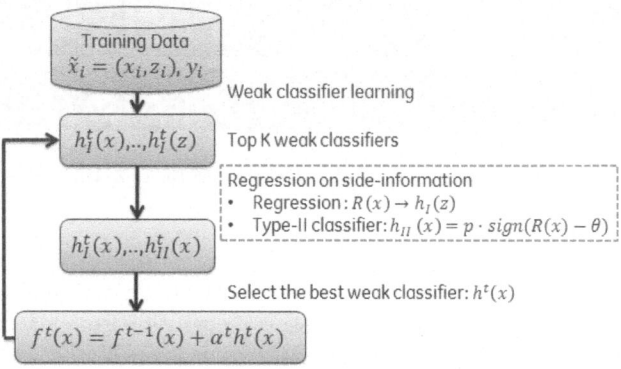

**Fig. 2.** The algorithm diagram of boosting with side information (Adaboost+)

$R^t(\mathbf{x}) \to h_I^t(\mathbf{z})$, that uses available information to predict the binary output of this weak classifier. Note that our method is different from using a regression to predict all the features in side information from available information, which is the typical practice of data imputation. In contract, we call our method as classification label imputation, which is applicable to side information with much higher dimensions than the available information (see the experiment in Sec. 5.2). Based on the regressor's output, we construct a *Type-II weak classifier*, which is defined as:

$$h_{II}(\mathbf{x}) = p \cdot (sign)[R(\mathbf{x}) - \theta]. \tag{4}$$

In principle, any regression method can be used in our algorithm. Considering the efficiency and effectiveness, we use the Gaussian Process Regression (GPR) [26] in our experiment. GPR is a non-parametric regression which assumes the regression function following gaussian process. Given the training data of input/output pairs $\{\mathbf{x}_i, y_i\}_{i=1..N}$, the regression output of a new input $\mathbf{x}^*$ can be derived as a Gaussian distribution, and we use its mean as the regression output:

$$y* = R(\mathbf{x}_*) = \mathbf{K}_*^T (\mathbf{K})^{-1} \mathbf{Y}, \tag{5}$$

where $\mathbf{K}$ is a $N \times N$ matrix whose entries are the kernel functions (RBF kernel [26] in our experiment) of the training data: $k(\mathbf{x}_i, \mathbf{x}_j)$. $\mathbf{K}_*$ and $\mathbf{Y}$ are $N$ dimensional vectors whose entries are $k(\mathbf{x}_i, \mathbf{x}^*)$ and $y_i$ respectively. To train a GPR, we only need to estimate the covariance matrix $\mathbf{K}$ on the training data.

After the top $K$ classifiers are updated, we select the top one weak classifier into the final classifier for the current iteration. Notice that if all the top classifiers are selected from available information, they do not need to update and our algorithm degenerates to conventional Adaboost. We choose $K > 1$, because the imperfection of the regression may change the ranking of the top $K$ weak classifiers. Since very low ranked classifiers has little chance to be top ranked, we set $K = 5$ in our experiments, which seems working well in practices.

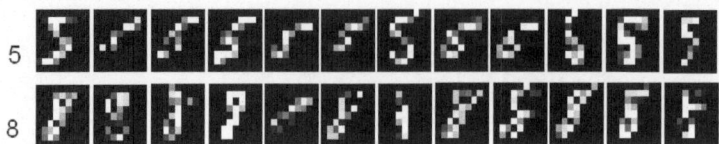

**Fig. 3.** Examples of handwritten digits in $10 \times 10$image

# 5  Experiments

We now demonstrate the effectiveness of our algorithm on two applications, hand-written digit recognition and facial expression recognition from low resolution images, each of which uses different types of side information. Note that in both cases, rather than developing methods of performance better than the state-of-the-art, our emphasis here is to showcase that the boosting with side information can lead to better performance in comparison to the conventional boosting algorithm.

## 5.1  Handwritten Digits Recognition

In the first set of experiments, we consider the problem of handwritten digit recognition from images. As shown in Fig. 3, we use the data set provided by [33], which consists of low-resolution images ($10 \times 10$ pixels) of handwritten digits 5 and 8. As in [33], we use 100 images (maximally available to the public) as training set and 1866 images as the test set. Furthermore, for every training image, 21 holistic (poetic) descriptions are provided by an independent expert. Each description can be translated to a discrete value. Some of these descriptions (with range of possible values) are: two-part-ness (0-5); tilting to the right (0-3); uniformity (0-3), etc. Note that these descriptions are not available for the test images and thus are treated as side information in our method.

Our goal is to learn a boosted classifier using the available information (100 dimensional vectors of the vectorized pixel values) and the side information (21 dimensional vectors from the quantized textual descriptions). The classification errors using different training data sizes are shown in Fig. 4(a). For each training data size smaller than 100, 12 different subsets are randomly selected from the training data. Thus, we perform train and test 12 times and report the average and standard deviation of these 12 testing errors. We also compare with the regression imputation [24], i.e., the missing side information in the testing data is recovered by the predicted value from a regression, and the augmented features with both side information and available information are used for classification. Here, we learn a Gaussian process regression to predict the side information from the available information. When the training data size is 100 (only test once), the classification error is 13.23%, 11.47% and 10.08% for imputation, Adaboost and Adaboost+ respectively. We can see that the imputation result is even worse than Adaboost. This is consistent with the previous imputation result [24] and the attribute-based methods [30,11] which show that using side information/attributes in an unselective manner does not necessarily improve the classification. In [11], the classification performance can be improved only when good discriminative attributes are carefully selected.

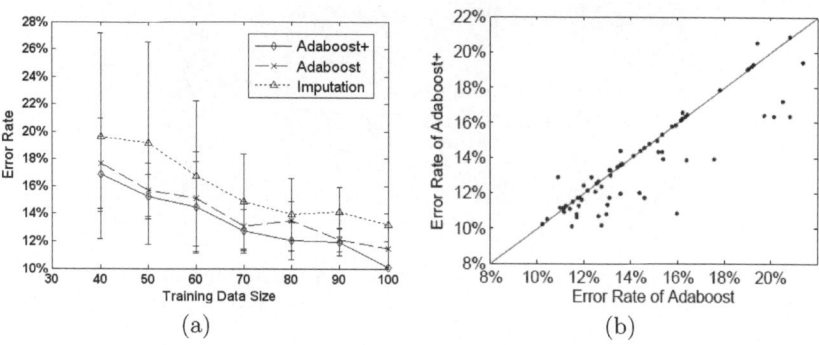

**Fig. 4.** (a) Performance comparison with various training data sizes. (b) Scatter plot of error rates of 73 tests. Adaboost+ is equal or better than Adaboost in 63 tests.

Using the side information, Adaboost+ outperforms Adaboost in general. The scatter plot in the top panel of Fig. 4 compares the Adaboost and Adaboost+ testing performances of the classifiers trained using each randomly selected training subset. We can see that Adaboost+ outperforms Adaboost in most tests.

A direct comparison with SVM+ [33] is difficult. On one hand, SVM and boosting are two very different classification techniques. On the other hand, [33] used 4000 images as an extra validation set for tuning the parameters in SVM and SVM+. This validation set does not have accompanying textual descriptions as side information. In order to have a fair comparison with SVM+, we also use this validation set in our boosted classifier. Specifically, after applying Algorithm 1 on the training set, we obtain a set of selected features (some features are from regression). We then extract these features for the validation data, from which we build a Adaboost classifier. Given the same training, validation and testing data as [33], the classification results of Adaboost+ and SVM+ are shown in Fig. 5.

These results suggest that it is easy to incorporate the validation data without side information into the Adaboost+ algorithm, and compared to Fig. 4(a) the variance of the results reduces significantly due to the large amount of validation data. More importantly, note that the side information improves the classification performances of both SVM and Adaboost. For instance, using 90 training samples, the average error rate of SVM is reduced from 8.2% to 6.7% (SVM+), and the average error rate of Adaboost is reduced from 6.5% to 5.3% (Adaboost+). Lastly, we notice that the errors of Adaboost and Adaboost+ decrease given larger training data size, but this decrease is not as fast

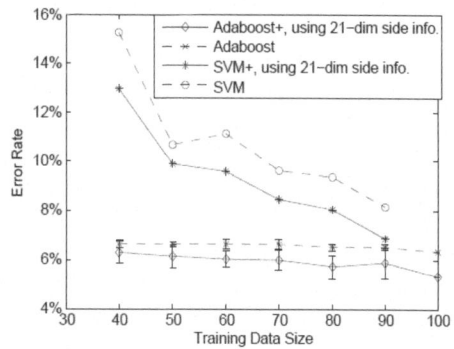

**Fig. 5.** Digit recognition with validation data. SVM and SVM+ results are from [32].

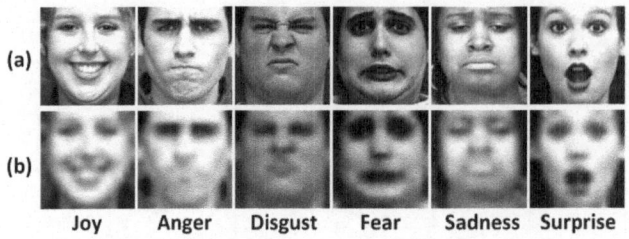

Joy    Anger    Disgust    Fear    Sadness    Surprise

**Fig. 6.** HR (a) and LR (b) images of six prototype emotions in the Cohn-Kanade database (©Jeffrey Cohn) . LR is re-scaled to the same size ($128 \times 128$) as HR.

as those of SVM-based classifiers. The reason is that Adaboost directly combines a large amount of validation data (4000 samples) with training data (100 samples) in training, while SVM uses training data to learn support vectors and uses validation data to tune the hyper-parameter. Therefore, the training data size plays a more important role in SVM. It is difficult to directly compare SVM+ and Adaboost+ because the ways of using validation data are different. However, we can see Adaboost+ is achieving better performance than SVM+ with the same training and validation data, and the gap between Adaboost and Adaboost+ is significant.

### 5.2   Facial Expression Recognition

Facial expression provides critical cues for the internal emotions of a human subject, and expression recognition is an important problem in computer vision. Most of the current works [35,3,8] assumes high resolution face images. However, many practical scenarios call for expression recognition based on low-resolution images, for instance when the images are captured with low resolution web-cams or surveillance cameras. In this section, we consider a system of facial expression recognition that uses low-resolution images, but is trained with high resolution images as side information.

We used the Cohn-Kanade (CK) Facial Expression database [20], which is considered today's de-facto standard for comparative studies in facial expression analysis. This database consists of 100 subjects who are instructed to perform a series of 23 facial displays, six of which are prototype emotions, i.e., anger, disgust, fear, joy, sadness and surprise. For our experiment, we select 300 image sequences from the database. The length of the sequences varies between 9 and 60 frames. Each of the sequences consists of expressions from neutral to one of the six prototype emotions. In the original CK database, only the peak expression of each sequence is labeled. Here, we perform recognition on every frame based on the frame-by-frame expression label in [31]. We randomly separate the subjects into two folds, and perform two-fold cross-validation to make sure the training and testing images are from different subjects.

Given the original image resolution of $640 \times 490$, we simulate the low-resolution (LR) image recognition by normalizing the face region to a $16 \times 16$ small image (Fig. 6). Previous experiment [22] on CK database has shown that the recognition

**Table 1.** Area under ROC for six expressions

| Expression | LR (Adaboost) | HR | LR interpolation | LR+ (Adaboost+) |
|---|---|---|---|---|
| Anger | 0.786 | 0.910 | 0.705 | 0.815 |
| Disgust | 0.855 | 0.919 | 0.833 | 0.897 |
| Fear | 0.688 | 0.732 | 0.634 | 0.721 |
| Joy | 0.954 | 0.959 | 0.521 | 0.944 |
| Sadness | 0.832 | 0.886 | 0.802 | 0.875 |
| Surprise | 0.976 | 0.992 | 0.773 | 0.980 |
| Average | 0.849 | 0.899 | 0.711 | 0.872 |

rate decreases significantly in low-resolution images. To address this problem, previous work focus on extracting robust features from LR images [23,28]. Here, we suppose the corresponding high-resolution (HR) face images are available as training data, and we propose to use these HR images as side information to learn a better classifier. This application is related to the popular super-resolution approaches [16,15,19] in face recognition, which uses HR images in training data to learn a mapping from LR image to HR images. The test LR image is mapped to a HR image for recognition. However, our approach is fundamentally different from those methods because we extract complimentary and discriminative side information from HR images rather than reconstructing the HR images themselves. Specifically, we extract $128 \times 128$ HR face images from the training image sequences (Fig. 6). Local binary pattern (LBP) feature [2] is extracted from the HR and LR images respectively. We chose LBP due to its demonstrated effectiveness for expression recognition in low-resolution image [28]. Similar to [28], we divide the HR image into 64 regions of $16 \times 16$ pixels [2] and apply the $LBP_{8,2}^{u2}$ operator to extract a 59-bin histogram from each region. Original LBP combines these histograms to form a long feature vector ($59 \times 64$) for the face image. For efficiency, we map the 59 dimension vector to a two-dimensional LDA space. Thus, the final feature vector has $2 \times 64 = 128$ dimensions. Similarly, the feature from the side information (one HR image) also has 128 dimensions.

Using Adaboost or Adaboost+ classifier, we compare the result of different settings as follows:

- LR recognition: Adaboost is trained on LR and tested on LR. This is the baseline in LR-based expression recognition.
- HR recognition: Adaboost is trained on HR and tested on HR. This ideal case provides an upper bound for LR-based recognition.
- LR-interpolate recognition: Adaboost is trained on HR and tested on re-scaled LR though interpolation. This is an naive approach to test on LR by using HR as training data.
- LR+ recognition: Adaboost+ is trained on LR with HR as side information and tested on LR.

---

[2] Before feature extraction, LR image is firstly re-scaled to $128 \times 128$ through cubic interpolation.

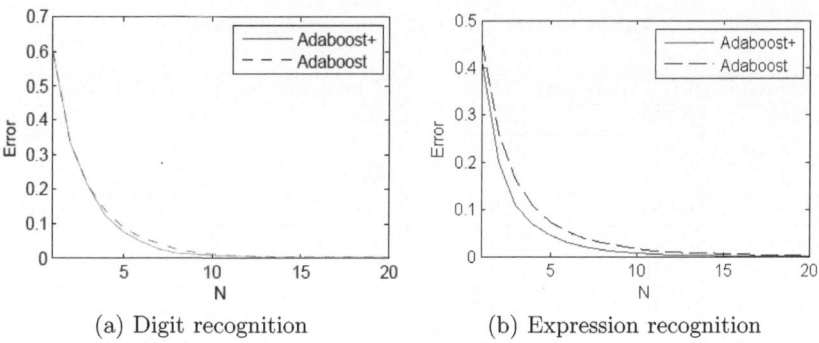

(a) Digit recognition          (b) Expression recognition

**Fig. 7.** Comparison of training error for the top $N$ features

In [28,22], only the average recognition rates are reported without false alarm. To provide a comprehensive evaluation, the area under ROC (AUC) for six expressions are shown in Table 1. As expected, the performance of HR recognition is the upper-bound (average AUC=0.899). Using HR as side information, the LR recognition rate can be improved towards the upper-bound (average AUC is improved from 0.849 to 0.872). We observe that this improvement is more significant for subtle expressions, i.e., anger, disgust, fear and sadness. But for expressions such as surprise and joy, the improvement is marginal. We also notice that the naive approach of interpolating the LR image does not work well. One possible reason is that the classifier trained on HR relies more on high frequency features, which are not presented in interpolated LR images.

## 5.3    Side Information in Different Applications

In different applications, side information are extracted from different sources, have different meanings and have difference influences on the final classifier. Here, we compare the side information in the above two applications.

In AdaBoost+, a feature from side information is selected only when it can further decrease the error function in Eq. 2. We show the average error function of the top $N$ features in Fig. 7. As expected, the error of Adaboost+ decreases faster than Adaboost indicating a more economic use of weak classifiers based on effective side information. We also observe that the side information (HR image) in expression recognition is more effective. Compared to the poetic descriptions in digit recognition, HR image provides more information to the available feature (LR image). This can also be observed in the number of features selected from side information. In the top 20 features, average 5.5 features are selected from side information in expression recognition, while only 0.71 features are selected in digit recognition. These results are consistent with the theoretical analysis [21,25], which suggests that using side information can accelerate the convergence of learning errors.

# 6    Conclusions

Side information that is contained in the training data but not available in testing exists in many problems in machine learning and computer vision. This motivates the recent development of a new learning approach known as *learning with side information* that aims to incorporate side information for improved training of learning algorithms. In this work, we describe a new training method of boosting classifiers that uses side information, known as AdaBoost+. In particular, we propose a novel *classification label imputation* method to construct extra weak classifiers from the available information that simulate the performance of better weak classifiers obtained from features in side information. The experiments on two vision problems demonstrate the effectiveness of our method in improving classification performance compared to AdaBoost classifier trained without using side information.

There are several important extensions of the current work that we would like to further pursue. First, note that in the most general sense, learning with side information is similar to semi-supervised learning and learning with missing features, where a classifier is obtained with partially missing information. In semi-supervised learning, this corresponds to missing labels, and in learning with side information, this corresponds to the absence of side information in the testing phase. Therefore, we are interested in extending the current work to a more general setting that combines missing label, feature and side information. This would provide a unification of all these different learning algorithms, and can also find many applications in machine learning and computer vision. Second, we believe that many problems in computer vision can benefit from the incorporation of side information, and we like to extend the boosting with side information framework to other computer vision problems.

# References

1. Ahmad, S., Tresp, V.: Some solutions to the missing feature problem in vision. In: NIPS (1998)
2. Ahonen, T., Hadid, A., Pietikainen, M.: Face description with local binary patterns: Application to face recognition. IEEE T-PAMI 28(12), 2037–2041 (2006)
3. Bartlett, M.S., Littlewort, G., Frank, M., Lainscsek, C., Fasel, I., Movellan, J.: Recognizing facial expression: machine learning and application to spontaneous behavior. In: CVPR (2005)
4. Basu, S., Bilenko, M., Mooney, R.J.: A probabilistic framework for semisupervised clustering. In: KDD (2004)
5. Bishop, C.M.: Pattern Recognition and Machine Learning, 1st edn. Information Science and Statistics. Springer (2007)
6. Chapelle, O., Schölkopf, B., Zien, A.: Semi-Supervised Learning. MIT Press, Cambridge (2006)
7. Chechik, G., Tishby, N.: Extracting relevant structures with side information. In: NIPS (2002)
8. Cohen, I., Sebe, N., Garg, A., Chen, L.S., Huang, T.S.: Facial expression recognition from video sequences: temporal and static modeling. CVIU 91(1-2), 160–187 (2003)

9. Cover, T., Thomas, J.: Elements of Information Theory, 2nd edn. Wiley-Interscience (2006)
10. Dekel, O., Shamir, O., Xiao, L.: Learning to classify with missing and corrupted features. Machine learning (2010)
11. Farhadi, A., Endres, I., Hoiem, D., Forsyth, D.: Describing objects by their attributes. In: CVPR (2009)
12. Friedman, J., Hastie, T., Tibshirani, R.: Additive logistic regression: a statistical view of boosting. Annals of Statistics 28(2), 337–407 (2000)
13. Garcia-Laencina, P.J., Sancho-Gomez, J.-L., Figueiras-Vidal, A.R.: Pattern classification with missing data: a review. Neural Comput. Appl. 19(2), 263–282 (2010)
14. Globerson, A., Roweis, S.: Nightmare at test time: robust learning by feature deletion. In: ICML (2006)
15. Gunturk, B.K., Batur, A.U., Altunbasak, Y., Hayes III, M.H., Mersereau, R.M.: Eigenface-domain super-resolution for face recognition. IEEE T-IP 12(5), 597–606 (2003)
16. Hennings-Yeomans, P.H., Baker, S., Kumar, B.V.K.V.: Simultaneous super-resolution and feature extraction for recognition of low-resolution faces. In: CVPR (2008)
17. Hoi, S.C.H., Jin, R., Lyu, M.R.: Learning nonparametric kernel matrices from pairwise constraints. In: ICML (2007)
18. Hwang, S.J., Sha, F., Grauman, K.: Sharing features between objects and their attributes. In: CVPR (2011)
19. Jia, K., Gong, S.: Multi-modal tensor face for simultaneous super-resolution and recognition. In: ICCV (2005)
20. Kanade, T., Cohn, J.F., Tian, Y.: Comprehensive database for facial expression analysis. In: FG (2000)
21. Kuusela, P., Ocone, D.: Learning with side information: PAC learning bounds. J. Comput. Syst. Sci. 68(3), 521–545 (2004)
22. Tian, Y.-l.: Evaluation of face resolution for expression analysis. In: CVPRW (2004)
23. Liao, S., Fan, W., Chung, A.C.S., Yeung, D.-Y.: Facial expression recognition using advanced local binary patterns, tsallis entropies and global appearance features. In: ICIP (2006)
24. Little, R.J.A., Rubin., D.B.: Statistical Analysis with Missing Data. John Wiley and Sons, Inc. (1987)
25. Pechyony, D., Vapnik, V.: On the theory of learning with privileged information. In: NIPS (2010)
26. Rasmussen, C.E., Williams, C.K.I.: Gaussian Processes for Machine Learning. MIT Press (2005)
27. Saar-Tsechansky, M., Provost, F.: Handling missing values when applying classification model. Journal of Machine Learning Research 8, 1623–1657 (2007)
28. Shan, C., Gong, S., McOwan, P.W.: Robust facial expression recognition using local binary patterns. In: ICIP (2005)
29. Shashua, A., Wolf, L.: Kernel Feature Selection with Side Data Using a Spectral Approach. In: Pajdla, T., Matas, J(G.) (eds.) ECCV 2004. LNCS, vol. 3023, pp. 39–53. Springer, Heidelberg (2004)
30. Su, Y., Allen, M., Jurie, F.: Improving object classification using semantic attributes. In: BMVC (2010)
31. Tong, Y., Liao, W., Ji, Q.: Facial action unit recognition by exploiting their dynamic and semantic relationships. IEEE T-PAMI 29(10), 1683–1699 (2007)
32. Vapnik, V., Vashist, A.: A new learning paradigm: Learning using privileged information. Neural Networks 22(5-6), 544–557 (2009)

33. Vapnik, V., Vashist, A., Pavlovitch, N.: Learning using hidden information (learning with teacher). In: IJCNN (2009)
34. Xing, E.P., Ng, A.Y., Jordan, M.I., Russell, S.: Distance metric learning, with application to clustering with side-information. In: NIPS (2003)
35. Zeng, Z., Pantic, M., Roisman, G.I., Huang, T.S.: A survey of affect recognition methods: Audio, visual, and spontaneous expressions. IEEE T-PAMI 31(1), 39–58 (2009)
36. Zhang, L., Samaras, D., Tomasi, D., Volkow, N., Goldstein, R.: Machine learning for clinical diagnosis from functional magnetic resonance imaging. In: CVPR (2005)

# Generalized Mutual Subspace Based Methods for Image Set Classification

Takumi Kobayashi

National Institute of Advanced Industrial Science and Technology, Japan
takumi.kobayashi@aist.go.jp

**Abstract.** The subspace-based methods are effectively applied to classify *sets* of feature vectors by modeling them as subspaces. It is, however, difficult to appropriately determine the subspace dimensionality in advance for better performance. For alleviating such issue, we present a generalized mutual subspace method by introducing *soft weighting* across the basis vectors of the subspace. The bases are effectively combined via the soft weights to measure the subspace similarities (angles) without definitely setting the subspace dimensionality. By using the soft weighting, we consequently propose a novel mutual subspace-based method to construct the discriminative space which renders more discriminative subspace similarities. In the experiments on 3D object recognition using image sets, the proposed methods exhibit stably favorable performances compared to the other subspace-based methods.

## 1 Introduction

In recent visual recognition tasks, *sets* of images (feature vectors) are effectively employed; *e.g.*, image frames in a video sequence for face recognition [1–4] and multiple still images captured from various angles for 3D object recognition [5, 6]. Those image sets capture various appearance changes of objects, providing more discriminative clues for classification than a single-shot image alone. Thus, the recognition systems utilizing those sets exhibit superior performances [1, 7].

The subspace models are successfully applied to classify the sets of vectors [5–13]. The vector set is represented by its underlying subspace spanned by a small number of the principal basis vectors. The angle between a vector and a subspace [14] is mathematically extended to the canonical angle between subspaces [7, 15, 16] which is a fundamental measurement for classifying the sets. The canonical angles measured in the original vector space, however, are not necessarily favorable from the viewpoint of discriminating classes, and for improving classification performances, apart from kernelization [6, 13], it is important to discriminatively measure those canonical angles. For that purpose, much research effort has been made for constructing the discriminative space [5, 8–11]. Those methods render the space such that the embedded subspaces are discriminatively separated in terms of the canonical angles, as in Fisher discriminant analysis [17] which makes the pair-wise vector distance more discriminative.

K.M. Lee et al. (Eds.): ACCV 2012, Part I, LNCS 7724, pp. 578–592, 2013.
© Springer-Verlag Berlin Heidelberg 2013

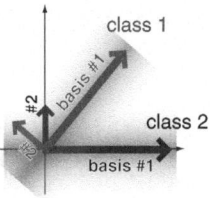

**Fig. 1.** The arrows indicate the directions of the bases with the variances (arrow length) in two classes. The one-dimensional subspaces (longer arrows) discriminate the two class, but they coincide when employing two-dimensional subspace. The proposed method can properly distinguish them with soft weighting based on the variances.

The subspace-based methods, however, involve the crucial issue regarding the dimensionality of the subspace. Users are required in advance to appropriately determine the subspace dimensionality for better performance. Each of the basis vectors in the set, given by an eigen-decomposition (PCA), is subject to the decision whether it is employed to support the subspace or not, based on the eigenvalues (variances). Such *binary* decision may significantly affect the performance as shown in Fig. 1, and the proper number of the bases, *i.e.*, the subspace dimensionality, is not known a priori depending on the overlap among the classes. The importance of the bases should be defined smoothly according to the eigenvalues (variances) rather than in such a binary form.

We propose generalized mutual subspace based methods for alleviating the issue regarding the subspace dimensionality. The proposed methods introduce *soft weighting* on the basis vectors composing the subspace, without definitely picking up a small number of the principal bases. We generalize the mutual subspace method (MSM) [7] by using the soft weighting to effectively combine the bases for computing subspace angles. In addition, we reformulate the constrained mutual subspace method (CMSM) [8, 9] constructing the discriminative space and give it theoretical justification. The reformulation also enables us to generalize the method by incorporating the soft weighting. The proposed methods effectively exploit all the bases, some of which are even less contributive to support the subspace, via the soft weighting. In summary, our contributions are 1) to introduce the soft weighting across the bases for effectively computing the subspace angles in MSM, 2) to reformulate CMSM with theoretical justification and 3) to propose a novel method for constructing the discriminative space based on the reformulation with the soft weighting.

This paper is organized as follows: in the next section, we briefly review the methods of MSM and CMSM and describe the novel reformulation of CMSM. In Sec.3, the details of the proposed methods are described and Sec.4 shows the experimental results on 3D object recognition. We conclude this paper in Sec.5.

## 2   Subspace Based Methods

The subspace model is effectively applied to classify not only a feature vector [14] but also a set of feature vectors [7] that is our main concern in this paper. The set of feature vectors is represented by the subspace and thereby samples are those subspaces, not vectors.

## 2.1 Mutual Subspace Method (MSM)

Let the $i$-th set of feature vectors be denoted by $X_i = [x_{i1}, \cdots, x_{in_i}] \in \Re^{d \times n_i}$ where $x_{ij} \in \Re^d$ is the $j$-th $d$-dimensional feature vector in the $i$-th set. The set of vectors is modeled by the subspace spanned by the principal basis vectors: we first apply an eigen-decomposition to $X_i X_i^\top = V_i \Lambda_i V_i^\top$ where $V_i, \Lambda_i = \mathtt{diag}(\{\lambda_{il}\}_{l=1}^d) \in \Re^{d \times d}$ are the eigenvectors and the eigenvalue diagonal matrix, respectively, and then exploit the eigenvectors of the $m_i$ larger eigenvalues as the orthonormal principal vectors $\hat{V}_i \in \Re^{d \times m_i}$.

To classify the set of vectors, $i.e.$, the subspace, the similarity measure is defined by the canonical angles [15, 16] between the subspaces, called mutual subspace method (MSM) [7]:

$$\cos \theta_{ij}^{(k)} = \max_{q_{ik} \in \Re^{m_i}, q_{jk} \in \Re^{m_j}} q_{ik}^\top \hat{V}_i^\top \hat{V}_j q_{jk}, \quad k = 1, \cdots, \min[m_i, m_j] \qquad (1)$$

$$s.t., \|q_{ik}\| = \|q_{jk}\| = 1, \ q_{ik}^\top q_{ik'} = q_{jk}^\top q_{jk'} = 0, \ k \neq k'.$$

This is computed by applying singular value decomposition (SVD) to $\hat{V}_i^\top \hat{V}_j$:

$$\hat{V}_i^\top \hat{V}_j = Q_i \Theta_{ij} Q_j^\top, \qquad (2)$$

where $Q_i, Q_j$ are the singular vectors composed of $q_{ik}, q_{jk}$ and $\Theta_{ij}$ is the singular-value diagonal matrix whose diagonal elements are the singular values $\{\cos \theta_{ij}^{(k)}\}_k$. The $k$-th canonical vectors $\hat{V}_i q_{ik}$ and $\hat{V}_j q_{jk}$ provide the $k$-th canonical angle $\cos \theta_{ij}^{(k)}$. In this paper, we define the similarity measure by $s_{ij} = \mathtt{tr}(\Theta_{ij}^2)$. The measure $s_{ij}$ becomes high for the similar subspaces and low for the distinct ones, and they are fed to $k$-NN classifications.

It should be noted that in MSM the subspace dimensionality $m_i$ is crucial for better classification performances, since the larger $m_i$ causes the measure $s_{ij}$ to be uniformly high for any pairs of subspaces; $s_{ij} = d, \forall i, j$ in case of $m_i = d$. There is no theoretical way to appropriately determine the dimensionality, and thus users are required in advance to carefully tune the dimensionality, which is an exhaustive procedure from the practical viewpoint.

## 2.2 Constrained Mutual Subspace Method (CMSM)

In the above section, we have described how MSM works on classifying sets of feature vectors in the original vector space. The original space, however, is not necessarily favorable in terms of discriminating the subspaces, and it is desirable to embed those subspaces into the more discriminative space as in Fisher discriminant analysis (FDA) [17]. For that purpose, some methods have been proposed for constructing the discriminative space to make the subspace angles measured in that space more discriminative [5, 8–11]. In this paper, we focus on the constrained mutual subspace method (CMSM) [8, 9] due to its simple formulation and promising performances.

Each class is represented by the subspace $\hat{V}^{[c]} \in \Re^{d \times m_c}$, $c = 1, \cdots, C$, and let the collection of those subspace bases be denoted by $\bar{V} = [\hat{V}^{[1]}, \cdots, \hat{V}^{[C]}]$. CMSM produces the projection vectors $D$ by the eigenvectors of the smaller eigenvalues in the following eigenvalue problem:

$$\bar{V}\bar{V}^{\top}D = D\Sigma, \ s.t., D^{\top}D = I, \tag{3}$$

where $\Sigma = \texttt{diag}(\{\sigma_l\}_l)$ is the eigenvalue diagonal matrix. In [8], it is shown that those projection vectors of the smaller eigenvalues are based on the differential vectors between the canonical vectors, which discriminatively separate the subspaces.

In a more practical case that multiple subspaces $\{\hat{V}_i^{[c]}\}_{i=1}^{n_c}$ are given in each class, a heuristic approach is presented in [9]: CMSM is repeatedly applied to *within-class* subspaces and *between-class* ones as follows.

1. **Within-Class:** In the $c$-th class, the representative subspace $P^{[c]}$ is obtained by applying CMSM to $\bar{V}^{[c]} = [\hat{V}_1^{[c]}, \cdots, \hat{V}_{n_c}^{[c]}]$ as $\bar{V}^{[c]}\bar{V}^{[c]\top} = P^{[c]}\Sigma^{[c]}P^{[c]\top}$.
2. **Between-Class:** CMSM is applied to $\bar{V} = [P^{[c]}, \cdots, P^{[c]}]$ in (3) to get the projection vectors $D$.

## 2.3   Reformulation of CMSM

In this paper, we give justification to CMSM in a different way from [8, 9] by reformulating (3); the proposed method is founded on the reformulation (see Sec.3). We consider the following dual eigenvalue problem of (3):

$$\bar{V}^{\top}\bar{V}Q = Q\Sigma, \ s.t., Q^{\top}Q = I, \tag{4}$$

and the projection matrix $D$ is retrieved by

$$D = \bar{V}Q\Sigma^{-\frac{1}{2}}, \tag{5}$$

since $\bar{V} = D\Sigma^{\frac{1}{2}}Q^{\top}$ (SVD). The novel formulation (4) provides the coefficients $Q$ on the basis vectors, like coefficients on support vectors in SVM [18], to construct discriminative space. We can give two interpretations (justifications) to (4) as follows.

1) **Differential Canonical Vectors.** The reformulation (4) simply shows that the projection vectors are based on the differential vectors between canonical vectors. Suppose the two class subspaces $\hat{V}_1, \hat{V}_2$ and $\bar{V} = [\hat{V}_1, \hat{V}_2]$. The dual eigenvalue problem (4) is described by

$$\bar{V}^{\top}\bar{V}\frac{1}{\sqrt{2}}\begin{bmatrix} Q_1 & Q_1 \\ Q_2 & -Q_2 \end{bmatrix} = \begin{bmatrix} I & \hat{V}_1^{\top}\hat{V}_2 \\ \hat{V}_2^{\top}\hat{V}_1 & I \end{bmatrix}\frac{1}{\sqrt{2}}\begin{bmatrix} Q_1 & Q_1 \\ Q_2 & -Q_2 \end{bmatrix}$$

$$= \frac{1}{\sqrt{2}}\begin{bmatrix} Q_1+Q_1\Theta_{12} & Q_1-Q_1\Theta_{12} \\ Q_2\Theta_{12}+Q_2 & Q_2\Theta_{12}-Q_2 \end{bmatrix} = \frac{1}{\sqrt{2}}\begin{bmatrix} Q_1 & Q_1 \\ Q_2 & -Q_2 \end{bmatrix}\begin{bmatrix} I+\Theta_{12} & 0 \\ 0 & I-\Theta_{12} \end{bmatrix}.$$

where $Q_1, Q_2, \Theta_{12}$ are the singular vectors and the singular values in (2). Thus, the projection vectors of the smaller eigenvalues are $D = \frac{1}{\sqrt{2}}(\hat{V}_1 Q_1 - \hat{V}_2 Q_2)(I - \Theta_{12})^{-\frac{1}{2}}$, which are (normalized) differential vectors between the canonical vectors, $\hat{V}_1 Q_1$ and $\hat{V}_2 Q_2$, of those two classes. This shows that the eigenvalues less than 1 exhibit the discriminative power, rendering the differential canonical vectors for the projections.

**2) Minimization of Pair-Wise Canonical Angles.** The eigenvalue problem (4) is also derived from the following optimization:

$$\min_{\|\boldsymbol{q} \triangleq [\boldsymbol{q}^{[1]^\top}, \cdots, \boldsymbol{q}^{[C]^\top}]^\top\|=1} \sum_{c,c'|c \neq c'}^{C} \boldsymbol{q}^{[c]^\top} \hat{\boldsymbol{V}}^{[c]^\top} \hat{\boldsymbol{V}}^{[c']} \boldsymbol{q}^{[c']} + \boldsymbol{q}^\top \boldsymbol{q} = \boldsymbol{q}^\top \bar{\boldsymbol{V}}^\top \bar{\boldsymbol{V}} \boldsymbol{q}, \quad (6)$$

where we use $\hat{\boldsymbol{V}}^{[c]^\top} \hat{\boldsymbol{V}}^{[c]} = \boldsymbol{I}$, $\forall c$. The second term $\boldsymbol{q}^\top \boldsymbol{q}$ $(= 1)$ is the same as the constraint, which thus makes no effect on the optimization. Roughly speaking, the first term $J \triangleq \sum_{c \neq c'} \boldsymbol{q}^{[c]^\top} \hat{\boldsymbol{V}}^{[c]^\top} \hat{\boldsymbol{V}}^{[c']} \boldsymbol{q}^{[c']}$ amounts to sum of canonical angles between different classes $c$ and $c'$ as in (1). The eigenvalue less than 1 indicates $J < 0$ in which the discriminative coefficients $\boldsymbol{q}$ are extracted.

The another merit of the reformulation (4) is that we can give theoretical justification to the heuristic procedure [9] described in Sec.2.2 for dealing with multiple subspaces in each class. Based on the above-mentioned second interpretation, we consider the optimization problem to minimize the canonical angles between classes while maximizing those within classes, which is formulated as in FDA [17] by

$$J = \min_{\boldsymbol{q}} \frac{\sum_{c,c'|c \neq c'}^{C} \sum_{i}^{n_c} \sum_{j}^{n_{c'}} \boldsymbol{q}_i^{[c]^\top} \hat{\boldsymbol{V}}_i^{[c]^\top} \hat{\boldsymbol{V}}_j^{[c']} \boldsymbol{q}_j^{[c']}}{\sum_{c}^{C} \sum_{i,j|i \neq j}^{n_c} \boldsymbol{q}_i^{[c]^\top} \hat{\boldsymbol{V}}_i^{[c]^\top} \hat{\boldsymbol{V}}_j^{[c]} \boldsymbol{q}_j^{[c]} + \boldsymbol{q}^\top \boldsymbol{q}} = \min_{\boldsymbol{q}} \frac{\boldsymbol{q}^\top \boldsymbol{R}_B \boldsymbol{q}}{\boldsymbol{q}^\top \boldsymbol{R}_W \boldsymbol{q}} \quad (7)$$

$$\Rightarrow \boldsymbol{R}_B \boldsymbol{Q} = \boldsymbol{R}_W \boldsymbol{Q} \tilde{\boldsymbol{\Sigma}} \Leftrightarrow \boldsymbol{R}_T \boldsymbol{Q} = \boldsymbol{R}_W \boldsymbol{Q} \boldsymbol{\Sigma}, \ s.t., \boldsymbol{Q}^\top \boldsymbol{Q} = \boldsymbol{I}, \quad (8)$$

where $\boldsymbol{\Sigma} = \tilde{\boldsymbol{\Sigma}} + \boldsymbol{I}$ and

$$\boldsymbol{R}_W = \begin{bmatrix} \bar{\boldsymbol{V}}^{[1]^\top} \bar{\boldsymbol{V}}^{[1]} & & \\ & \ddots & \\ & & \bar{\boldsymbol{V}}^{[C]^\top} \bar{\boldsymbol{V}}^{[C]} \end{bmatrix} = \texttt{blkdiag}(\{\bar{\boldsymbol{V}}^{[c]^\top} \bar{\boldsymbol{V}}^{[c]}\}_{c=1}^C) \succcurlyeq 0,$$

$$\boldsymbol{R}_T = [\bar{\boldsymbol{V}}^{[1]}, \cdots, \bar{\boldsymbol{V}}^{[C]}]^\top [\bar{\boldsymbol{V}}^{[1]}, \cdots, \bar{\boldsymbol{V}}^{[C]}] \succcurlyeq 0, \quad \boldsymbol{R}_B = \boldsymbol{R}_T - \boldsymbol{R}_W,$$

where `blkdiag` constructs a block-diagonal matrix. The projection matrix is given in a manner similar to (5) by

$$\boldsymbol{D} = [\bar{\boldsymbol{V}}^{[1]}, \cdots, \bar{\boldsymbol{V}}^{[C]}] \boldsymbol{Q} \boldsymbol{\Sigma}^{-\frac{1}{2}}. \quad (9)$$

As in (6), $\boldsymbol{q}^\top \boldsymbol{R}_B \boldsymbol{q}$ and $\boldsymbol{q}^\top \boldsymbol{R}_W \boldsymbol{q}$ measure *between-class* and *within-class* canonical angles, respectively. This proposed formulation has the following properties with respect to the projection vectors $\boldsymbol{D}$ and the eigenvalues $\boldsymbol{\Sigma} = \texttt{diag}(\{\sigma_l\}_l)$.

**Theorem 1.** *The projection vectors (9) produced via (8) are the same as the projections by the heuristic procedure [9] described in Sec.2.2.*

*Proof.* We apply SVD to $\bar{\boldsymbol{V}}^{[c]} = \boldsymbol{P}^{[c]} \boldsymbol{\Sigma}^{[c]} \boldsymbol{Q}^{[c]^\top}$, and define a block-diagonal matrix $\boldsymbol{R}_W^{-\frac{1}{2}} = \texttt{blkdiag}(\{\boldsymbol{Q}^{[c]} \boldsymbol{\Sigma}^{[c]^{-1}}\}_{c=1}^C)$ such that $\boldsymbol{R}_W^{-\frac{1}{2}^\top} \boldsymbol{R}_W \boldsymbol{R}_W^{-\frac{1}{2}} = \boldsymbol{I}$. By using these, (8) is transformed into

$$\boldsymbol{R}_W^{-\frac{1}{2}^\top} \boldsymbol{R}_T \boldsymbol{R}_W^{-\frac{1}{2}} \boldsymbol{Q}' = \boldsymbol{Q}' \boldsymbol{\Sigma}, \ s.t., \boldsymbol{Q}'^\top \boldsymbol{Q}' = \boldsymbol{I}, \ \text{where } \boldsymbol{Q} = \boldsymbol{R}_W^{-\frac{1}{2}} \boldsymbol{Q}'. \quad (10)$$

The left-hand-side matrix results in

$$\boldsymbol{R}_W^{-\frac{1}{2}^\top}\boldsymbol{R}_T\boldsymbol{R}_W^{-\frac{1}{2}} = \boldsymbol{R}_W^{-\frac{1}{2}^\top}[\bar{\boldsymbol{V}}^{[1]},\cdots,\bar{\boldsymbol{V}}^{[C]}]^\top[\bar{\boldsymbol{V}}^{[1]},\cdots,\bar{\boldsymbol{V}}^{[C]}]\boldsymbol{R}_W^{-\frac{1}{2}}$$
$$= [\boldsymbol{P}^{[1]},\cdots,\boldsymbol{P}^{[C]}]^\top[\boldsymbol{P}^{[1]},\cdots,\boldsymbol{P}^{[C]}]. \tag{11}$$

This is the same procedure as within-class CMSM to obtain the class representative subspaces $\boldsymbol{P}^{[c]}$ in [9]. $\bar{\boldsymbol{V}} = [\boldsymbol{P}^{[1]},\cdots,\boldsymbol{P}^{[C]}]$ is decomposed via SVD by

$$\bar{\boldsymbol{V}} = \boldsymbol{D}\boldsymbol{\Sigma}^{\frac{1}{2}}\boldsymbol{Q}'^\top,$$

where $\boldsymbol{D}$ corresponds to the projection vectors heuristically given in [9] and $\boldsymbol{Q}'$ is the eigenvectors in (10). The projection vectors (9) are finally described by

$$\boldsymbol{D}^{dual} = [\bar{\boldsymbol{V}}^{[1]},\cdots,\bar{\boldsymbol{V}}^{[C]}]\boldsymbol{Q}\boldsymbol{\Sigma}^{-\frac{1}{2}} = [\bar{\boldsymbol{V}}^{[1]},\cdots,\bar{\boldsymbol{V}}^{[C]}]\boldsymbol{R}_W^{-\frac{1}{2}}\boldsymbol{Q}'\boldsymbol{\Sigma}^{-\frac{1}{2}}$$
$$= [\boldsymbol{P}^{[1]},\cdots,\boldsymbol{P}^{[C]}]\boldsymbol{Q}'\boldsymbol{\Sigma}^{-\frac{1}{2}} = \bar{\boldsymbol{V}}\boldsymbol{Q}'\boldsymbol{\Sigma}^{-\frac{1}{2}} = \boldsymbol{D}. \quad \square$$

**Theorem 2.** *The eigenvalues in (8) are bounded in* $0 \le \sigma_l \le C$, $\forall l$.

*Proof.* $\boldsymbol{R}_T \succcurlyeq 0$ and $\boldsymbol{R}_W \succcurlyeq 0$ lead to $\sigma_l \ge 0$, $\forall l$. By (10) and (11), the maximum eigenvalue is obtained by

$$\max_l \sigma_l = \max_{\|\boldsymbol{q}\|=1} \boldsymbol{q}^\top[\boldsymbol{P}^{[1]},\cdots,\boldsymbol{P}^{[C]}]^\top[\boldsymbol{P}^{[1]},\cdots,\boldsymbol{P}^{[C]}]\boldsymbol{q}, \tag{12}$$

where $\boldsymbol{P}^{[c]}$ is the orthonormal vectors since $\bar{\boldsymbol{V}}^{[c]} = \boldsymbol{P}^{[c]}\boldsymbol{\Lambda}^{[c]}\boldsymbol{Q}^{[c]^\top}$ (SVD). Here, we consider $\boldsymbol{P}^{[c]}\boldsymbol{q}^{[c]} = \bar{q}^{[c]}\bar{\boldsymbol{p}}^{[c]}$ where $\|\bar{\boldsymbol{p}}^{[c]}\| = 1$ and $\bar{q}^{[c]} = \sqrt{\boldsymbol{q}^{[c]^\top}\boldsymbol{q}^{[c]}}$, and $[\boldsymbol{P}^{[1]},\cdots,\boldsymbol{P}^{[C]}]\boldsymbol{q} = [\bar{\boldsymbol{p}}^{[1]},\cdots,\bar{\boldsymbol{p}}^{[C]}]\bar{\boldsymbol{q}}$ where $\bar{\boldsymbol{q}} = [\bar{q}^{[1]},\cdots,\bar{q}^{[C]}]^\top \in \Re^C$. Thus, the right-hand side in (12) is bounded in

$$\bar{\boldsymbol{q}}^\top[\bar{\boldsymbol{p}}^{[1]},\cdots,\bar{\boldsymbol{p}}^{[C]}]^\top[\bar{\boldsymbol{p}}^{[1]},\cdots,\bar{\boldsymbol{p}}^{[C]}]\bar{\boldsymbol{q}} \le \bar{\boldsymbol{q}}^\top\boldsymbol{1}\boldsymbol{1}^\top\bar{\boldsymbol{q}} \le C, \; s.t. \; \|\bar{\boldsymbol{q}}\| = 1,$$

where we use $\|\bar{\boldsymbol{q}}\| = \|\boldsymbol{q}\| = 1$ and $\bar{\boldsymbol{p}}^{[c']^\top}\bar{\boldsymbol{p}}^{[c]} \le 1$, $\forall c, c'$. $\square$

## 3   Proposed Methods

As mentioned in Sec.2.1, the crucial issue in the subspace-based methods is how to determine the dimensionality of the subspace. For alleviating it, the main idea in this paper is to introduce *soft weighting* across the basis vectors of the subspace instead of definitely selecting a small number of the principal bases.

### 3.1   Generalized Mutual Subspace Method (gMSM)

The determination of the subspace dimensionality is regarded as picking up the principal basis vectors, which further corresponds to designing the binary weights on all the bases as shown in Fig. 2; 1/0 indicates whether the basis is picked up or not. We relax the binary (hard) weighting to *soft weighting*. Let $\boldsymbol{\omega} \in [0,1]^d$ be the soft weights on the bases and $\boldsymbol{\Omega} = \text{diag}(\boldsymbol{\omega}) \in \Re^{d \times d}$. The soft weight is illustrated in Fig. 2 compared to the binary one. By incorporating the weights into MSM in (1), the generalized MSM (gMSM) is defined by

$$\max_{\boldsymbol{q}_i^\top\boldsymbol{\Omega}_i^{-2}\boldsymbol{q}_i=1,\boldsymbol{q}_j^\top\boldsymbol{\Omega}_j^{-2}\boldsymbol{q}_j=1} \boldsymbol{q}_i^\top\boldsymbol{V}_i^\top\boldsymbol{V}_j\boldsymbol{q}_j \Leftrightarrow \max_{\boldsymbol{q}_i'^\top\boldsymbol{q}_i'=1,\boldsymbol{q}_j'^\top\boldsymbol{q}_j'=1} \boldsymbol{q}_i'^\top\boldsymbol{\Omega}_i\boldsymbol{V}_i^\top\boldsymbol{V}_j\boldsymbol{\Omega}_j\boldsymbol{q}_j', \tag{13}$$

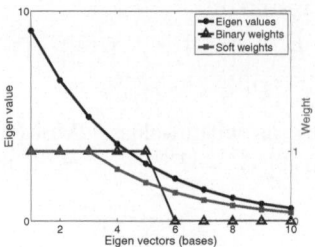

**Fig. 2.** Weights on basis vectors. The binary weight indicates five dimensions of the subspace and the soft weight is created by $w_3$ in (15).

where $\boldsymbol{q}_i = \boldsymbol{\Omega}_i \boldsymbol{q}_i'$ and $\boldsymbol{V}_i$ indicates the orthonormal bases given by an eigendecomposition of $\boldsymbol{X}_i \boldsymbol{X}_i^\top = \boldsymbol{V}_i \boldsymbol{\Lambda}_i \boldsymbol{V}_i^\top$. As in (2), the generalized canonical angles are computed by

$$\boldsymbol{\Omega}_i \boldsymbol{V}_i^\top \boldsymbol{V}_j \boldsymbol{\Omega}_j = \boldsymbol{Q}_i' \boldsymbol{\Theta}_{ij} \boldsymbol{Q}_j'^\top, \ s_{ij} = \mathrm{tr}(\boldsymbol{\Theta}_{ij}^2), \tag{14}$$

and the $k$-th canonical vectors are described by $\boldsymbol{V}_i \boldsymbol{q}_i = \boldsymbol{V}_i \boldsymbol{\Omega}_i \boldsymbol{q}_i'$ and $\boldsymbol{V}_j \boldsymbol{\Omega}_j \boldsymbol{q}_j'$. In this formulation for measuring the generalized canonical angle, the soft weights on the bases work in the constraint $\boldsymbol{q}^\top \boldsymbol{\Omega}^{-2} \boldsymbol{q} = 1$; the smaller weight $\omega_l$ decreases the coefficient $q_l$, and especially $\omega_l \to 0$ enforces $q_l \to 0$. The gMSM in (13) obviously reduces to the ordinary MSM in (1) by $\boldsymbol{\omega} \in \{0,1\}^d$ (binary weights) since $[\hat{\boldsymbol{V}}_i, \boldsymbol{0}] = \boldsymbol{V}_i \boldsymbol{\Omega}_i$. While in MSM the classification performance is, like quantization errors, sensitive to the dimensionality indicated by the binary weights, the soft weights in gMSM effectively combine the bases to compute the subspace angles.

The only issue is how to design the soft weights. Since the dimensionality is usually determined based on the variances corresponding to the eigenvalues in $\boldsymbol{X}\boldsymbol{X}^\top = \boldsymbol{V}\boldsymbol{\Lambda}\boldsymbol{V}^\top$, the soft weights are also set according to the eigenvalues by

$$\boldsymbol{\omega} = \mathrm{w}_m(\boldsymbol{\lambda}), \ \text{where } \boldsymbol{\Lambda} = \mathrm{diag}(\boldsymbol{\lambda}) \ \text{and } \mathrm{w}_m(\boldsymbol{\lambda}) = \min\left[\frac{\lambda}{\lambda_m}, 1\right], \tag{15}$$

where $\lambda_m$ is the $m$-th eigenvalue in $\boldsymbol{\lambda} \in \Re^d$ in descending order and min operates on each component of the vector in comparison to 1, enforcing $\omega \le 1$. This weighting evaluates the importance of the basis vector by the variance relative to $\lambda_m$; the basis of the larger variance is more important. In most cases, the first principal basis vector indicate the direction of the subspace, which results in significantly large $\lambda_1$, and the second or later ones capture the spread of the distribution around that direction. Thus, we suggest to use $m > 1$; the soft weights with $m = 3$ are illustrated in Fig. 2.

## 3.2   Generalized Constrained Mutual Subspace Method (gCMSM)

Along with gMSM, CMSM is also generalized by incorporating the soft weights into the optimization problem (6) of the reformulated CMSM:

$$\min_{\boldsymbol{q}^\top \bar{\boldsymbol{\Omega}}^{-2} \boldsymbol{q} = 1} \sum_{c,c' | c \ne c'}^{C} \boldsymbol{q}^{[c]^\top} \boldsymbol{V}^{[c]^\top} \boldsymbol{V}^{[c']} \boldsymbol{q}^{[c']} + \boldsymbol{q}^\top \bar{\boldsymbol{\Omega}}^{-2} \boldsymbol{q} \tag{16}$$

$$\Leftrightarrow \min_{q^\top \bar{\Omega}^{-2}q=1} q^\top (R_T - I + \bar{\Omega}^{-2})q \Leftrightarrow \min_{q'^\top q'=1} q'^\top (\bar{\Omega}R_T\bar{\Omega} - \bar{\Omega}^2 + I)q', \quad (17)$$

where $q \triangleq [q^{[1]^\top}, \cdots, q^{[C]^\top}]^\top = \bar{\Omega}q'$, $\bar{\Omega} = \texttt{blkdiag}(\{\Omega^{[c]}\}_{c=1}^C)$ and $R_T = \bar{V}^\top\bar{V}$, $\bar{V} = [V^{[1]}, \cdots, V^{[C]}]$. This results in the following eigenvalue problem:

$$(\bar{\Omega}R_T\bar{\Omega} - \bar{\Omega}^2 + I)Q' = Q'\Sigma, \ s.t., Q'^\top Q' = I, \quad (18)$$

and by using the eigenvectors of the smaller eigenvalues, the projection vectors are obtained by

$$D = \bar{V}Q\Sigma^{-\frac{1}{2}} = \bar{V}\bar{\Omega}Q'\Sigma^{-\frac{1}{2}}. \quad (19)$$

As in the ordinary CMSM, the gCMSM also implies the differential vectors between the canonical vectors as follows. Suppose two class bases $V_1, V_2$ and $\bar{V} = [V_1, V_2]$, $\bar{\Omega} = \texttt{blkdiag}(\Omega_1, \Omega_2)$. The eigenvalue problem (18) is described by

$$(\bar{\Omega}R_T\bar{\Omega} - \bar{\Omega}^2 + I)\frac{1}{\sqrt{2}}\begin{bmatrix} Q_1' & Q_1' \\ Q_2' & -Q_2' \end{bmatrix} = \begin{bmatrix} I & \Omega_1 V_1^\top V_2 \Omega_2 \\ \Omega_2 V_2^\top V_1 \Omega_1 & I \end{bmatrix} \frac{1}{\sqrt{2}}\begin{bmatrix} Q_1' & Q_1' \\ Q_2' & -Q_2' \end{bmatrix}$$

$$= \frac{1}{\sqrt{2}}\begin{bmatrix} Q_1'+Q_1'\Theta_{12} & Q_1'-Q_1'\Theta_{12} \\ Q_2'\Theta_{12}+Q_2' & Q_2'\Theta_{12}-Q_2' \end{bmatrix} = \frac{1}{\sqrt{2}}\begin{bmatrix} Q_1' & Q_1' \\ Q_2' & -Q_2' \end{bmatrix}\begin{bmatrix} I+\Theta_{12} & 0 \\ 0 & I-\Theta_{12} \end{bmatrix},$$

where we use $\Omega_1 V_1^\top V_2 \Omega_2 = Q_1'\Theta_{12}Q_2'^\top$ (SVD) in gMSM (14). The projection vectors are described by using the eigenvectors of the smaller eigenvalues as $D = (V_1\Omega_1 Q_1' - V_2\Omega_2 Q_2')(I - \Theta_{12})^{-\frac{1}{2}}$, which are differential vectors between the canonical vectors of the two classes in gMSM.

The proposed gCMSM has the following property for the projection vectors.

**Theorem 3.** *The projection vectors in* (19) *have the norms less than* 1.

*Proof.* The squared norm of the projection vector is

$$p^\top p = \sigma^{-\frac{1}{2}}q^\top \bar{V}^\top \bar{V}q\sigma^{-\frac{1}{2}} = \sigma^{-\frac{1}{2}}q'^\top \bar{\Omega}R_T\bar{\Omega}q'\sigma^{-\frac{1}{2}}$$

$$= \sigma^{-\frac{1}{2}}q'^\top (\bar{\Omega}R_T\bar{\Omega} - \bar{\Omega}^2 + I)q'\sigma^{-\frac{1}{2}} - \sigma^{-\frac{1}{2}}q'^\top (I - \bar{\Omega}^2)q'\sigma^{-\frac{1}{2}} \quad (20)$$

$$\leq \sigma^{-\frac{1}{2}}q'^\top \sigma q'\sigma^{-\frac{1}{2}} = q'^\top q' = 1, \quad (21)$$

where we use $I - \bar{\Omega}^2 \succcurlyeq 0$ since the weights are $\omega_l \leq 1, \forall l$, and the eigenvalue problem (18) for transforming (20) to (21), and $\|q'\| = 1$ to get the last equality. $\square$

### 3.3  gCMSM for Multiple Subspaces

The gCMSM is also extended so as to cope with multiple subspaces in each class. According to (7) and (16), the optimization problem is formulated by

$$J = \min_q \frac{\sum_{c,c'|c\neq c'}^C \sum_i^{n_c} \sum_j^{n_{c'}} q_i^{[c]^\top} V_i^{[c]^\top} V_j^{[c']} q_j^{[c']}}{\sum_c^C \sum_{i,j|i\neq j}^{n_c} q_i^{[c]^\top} V_i^{[c]^\top} V_j^{[c]} q_j^{[c]} + q^\top \bar{\Omega}^{-2}q} \quad (22)$$

$$= \min_q \frac{q^\top R_B q}{q^\top (R_W - I + \bar{\Omega}^{-2})q} \Rightarrow R_B Q = (R_W - I + \bar{\Omega}^{-2})Q\tilde{\Sigma}$$

$$\Leftrightarrow (R_T - I + \bar{\Omega}^{-2})Q = (R_W - I + \bar{\Omega}^{-2})Q\Sigma \quad (23)$$

$$\Leftrightarrow (\bar{\Omega}R_T\bar{\Omega} - \bar{\Omega}^2 + I)Q' = (\bar{\Omega}R_W\bar{\Omega} - \bar{\Omega}^2 + I)Q'\Sigma, \tag{24}$$

where $\Sigma = \tilde{\Sigma} + I$, $Q = \bar{\Omega}Q'$ and

$$\bar{V}^{[c]} = [V_1^{[c]}, \cdots, V_{n_c}^{[c]}], \quad \bar{V} = [\bar{V}^{[1]}, \cdots, \bar{V}^{[C]}],$$

$$\bar{\Omega}^{[c]} = \texttt{blkdiag}(\{\Omega_i^{[c]}\}_{i=1}^{n_c}), \quad \bar{\Omega} = \texttt{blkdiag}(\{\bar{\Omega}^{[c]}\}_{c=1}^{C}),$$

$$R_W = \texttt{blkdiag}(\{\bar{V}^{[c]^\top}\bar{V}^{[c]}\}_{c=1}^{C}) \succcurlyeq 0, \quad R_T = \bar{V}^\top\bar{V} \succcurlyeq 0, \quad R_B = R_T - R_W.$$

The projection vectors are given by using the eigenvectors of the smaller eigenvalues as

$$D = \bar{V}Q\Sigma^{-\frac{1}{2}} = \bar{V}\bar{\Omega}Q'\Sigma^{-\frac{1}{2}}. \tag{25}$$

The generalized eigenvalue problem (24) is transformed to a standard eigenvalue problem as follows. We apply an eigen-decomposition to $\bar{\Omega}^{[c]}\bar{V}^{[c]^\top}\bar{V}^{[c]}\bar{\Omega}^{[c]} - \bar{\Omega}^{[c]^2} + I = Q'^{[c]}\Sigma^{[c]}Q'^{[c]^\top}$, which is *within-class* gCMSM, and define $R_W'^{-\frac{1}{2}} = \texttt{blkdiag}(\{Q'^{[c]}\Sigma^{[c]^{-\frac{1}{2}}}\}_{c=1}^{C})$ such that $R_W'^{-\frac{1}{2}^\top}(\bar{\Omega}R_W\bar{\Omega} - \bar{\Omega}^2 + I)R_W'^{-\frac{1}{2}} = I$. Therefore, (24) is transformed into

$$R_W'^{-\frac{1}{2}^\top}(\bar{\Omega}R_T\bar{\Omega} - \bar{\Omega}^2 + I)R_W'^{-\frac{1}{2}}Q'' = Q''\Sigma, \ s.t., Q''^\top Q'' = I, \ \text{where } Q' = R_W'^{-\frac{1}{2}}Q''. \tag{26}$$

The left-hand-side matrix is

$$R_W^{-\frac{1}{2}^\top}(\bar{\Omega}R_T\bar{\Omega} - \bar{\Omega}^2 + I)R_W^{-\frac{1}{2}}$$
$$= [P^{[1]}, \cdots, P^{[C]}]^\top[P^{[1]}, \cdots, P^{[C]}] - \texttt{blkdiag}(\{P^{[c]^\top}P^{[c]}\}_{c=1}^{C}) + I,$$

where $P^{[c]} = \bar{V}^{[c]}\bar{\Omega}^{[c]}Q'^{[c]}\Sigma^{[c]^{-\frac{1}{2}}}$ indicates the projection vectors in the $c$-th within-class gCMSM in (19), and the final projection vectors (25) are described by $D = \bar{V}\bar{\Omega}R_W^{-\frac{1}{2}}Q''\Sigma^{-\frac{1}{2}} = [P^{[1]}, \cdots, P^{[C]}]Q''\Sigma^{-\frac{1}{2}}$. Therefore, (26) is regarded as *between-class* gCMSM using the vectors produced by *within-class* gCMSM. The procedure for this method is shown in Algorithm 1 and the practical details are described in the next section.

This proposed method has the following properties regarding the projection vectors $D$ and the eigenvalues $\Sigma = \texttt{diag}(\{\sigma_l\}_l)$.

**Theorem 4.** *The projection vectors in* (25) *have the norms less than 1.*

*Proof.* The squared norm of the projection vector is

$$d^\top d = \sigma^{-\frac{1}{2}}q'^\top\bar{\Omega}\bar{V}^\top\bar{V}\bar{\Omega}q'\sigma^{-\frac{1}{2}}$$
$$= \sigma^{-\frac{1}{2}}q'^\top(\bar{\Omega}R_T\bar{\Omega} - \bar{\Omega}^2 + I)q'\sigma^{-\frac{1}{2}} - \sigma^{-\frac{1}{2}}q'^\top(I - \bar{\Omega}^2)q'\sigma^{-\frac{1}{2}}$$
$$\leq \sigma^{-\frac{1}{2}}q'^\top\sigma(\bar{\Omega}R_W\bar{\Omega} - \bar{\Omega}^2 + I)q'\sigma^{-\frac{1}{2}} = q''^\top q'' = 1,$$

where we use $I - \bar{\Omega}^2 \succcurlyeq 0$ and the eigenvalue problems (24) and (26). $\square$

**Theorem 5.** *The eigenvalues in* (24) *are bounded in* $0 \leq \sigma_l \leq C$, $\forall l$.

*Proof.* The weights $\omega \leq 1$ result in $\bar{\Omega}^{-2} - I \succcurlyeq 0$. Thus, since $R_T - I + \bar{\Omega}^{-2} \succcurlyeq 0$ and $R_W - I + \bar{\Omega}^{-2} \succcurlyeq 0$, we get $\sigma_l \geq 0$, $\forall l$ in (23). By using $R_W - I + \bar{\Omega}^{-2} \succcurlyeq R_W$, the eigenvalues are upper-bounded by

$$\max_l \sigma_l = \max_q \frac{q^\top R_B q}{q^\top(R_W - I + \Omega^{-2})q} + 1 \leq \max_q \frac{q^\top R_B q}{q^\top R_W q} + 1 = \max_q \frac{q^\top R_T q}{q^\top R_W q} \leq C,$$

---

**Algorithm 1.** gCMSM training

---

**Input:** $\boldsymbol{X}_i^{[c]} \in \Re^{d \times n_{ci}}$: $d$-dimensional feature vectors of the $i$-th set in the $c$-th class.

1: **for** $c = 1$ to $C$ **do**

2:　　Subspace: $\boldsymbol{X}_i^{[c]} \boldsymbol{X}_i^{[c]\top} = \boldsymbol{V}_i^{[c]} \mathtt{diag}(\lambda_i^{[c]}) \boldsymbol{V}_i^{[c]\top}$, $i = 1, \cdots, n_c$.

3:　　$\bar{\boldsymbol{V}}^{[c]} = [\boldsymbol{V}_1^{[c]}, \cdots, \boldsymbol{V}_{n_c}^{[c]}]$, $\bar{\boldsymbol{\Omega}}^{[c]} = \mathtt{diag}([\mathsf{w}_m(\lambda_1^{[c]})^\top, \cdots, \mathsf{w}_m(\lambda_{n_c}^{[c]})^\top]^\top)$.

4:　　*Within-class* gCMSM: $\bar{\boldsymbol{\Omega}}^{[c]} \bar{\boldsymbol{V}}^{[c]\top} \bar{\boldsymbol{V}}^{[c]} \bar{\boldsymbol{\Omega}}^{[c]} - \bar{\boldsymbol{\Omega}}^{[c]2} + \boldsymbol{I} = \boldsymbol{Q}^{[c]} \boldsymbol{\Sigma}^{[c]} \boldsymbol{Q}^{[c]\top}$,
$$\boldsymbol{P}^{[c]} = \bar{\boldsymbol{V}}^{[c]} \bar{\boldsymbol{\Omega}}^{[c]} \boldsymbol{Q}^{[c]} \boldsymbol{\Sigma}^{[c]-\frac{1}{2}}.$$

5:　　Cut-off the vectors: $\boldsymbol{P}^{[c]} \leftarrow \{\boldsymbol{p}_l^{[c]} | \|\boldsymbol{p}_l^{[c]}\|^2 > \epsilon\}$, $\boldsymbol{p}_l^{[c]}$: the $l$-th column vector in $\boldsymbol{P}^{[c]}$.

6: **end for**

7: $\bar{\boldsymbol{P}} = [\boldsymbol{P}^{[1]}, \cdots, \boldsymbol{P}^{[C]}]$, 　$\boldsymbol{O} = \mathtt{blkdiag}(\{\boldsymbol{P}^{[c]\top} \boldsymbol{P}^{[c]}\}_{c=1}^C)$: block-diagonal matrix.

8: *Between-class* gCMSM: $(\bar{\boldsymbol{P}}^\top \bar{\boldsymbol{P}} - \boldsymbol{O} + \boldsymbol{I})\boldsymbol{Q} = \boldsymbol{Q}\boldsymbol{\Sigma}$, $\boldsymbol{D} = \bar{\boldsymbol{P}}\boldsymbol{Q}\boldsymbol{\Sigma}^{-\frac{1}{2}}$.

9: Cut-off the projections: $\boldsymbol{D} \leftarrow \{\boldsymbol{d}_l | \sigma_l < \tau\}$, $\boldsymbol{d}_l$: the $l$-th column vector in $\boldsymbol{D}$.

**Output:** Projection vectors: $\boldsymbol{D} \in \Re^{d \times L}$.

---

**Algorithm 2.** gMSM classification

---

**Input:** $\{\boldsymbol{X}_i, y_i\}_{i=1}^n$: pairs of $d$-dimensional feature vectors $\boldsymbol{X}_i \in \Re^{d \times n_i}$ and a class label
　　$y_i \in \{1, \cdots, C\}$ of the $i$-th set for training,
　　$\boldsymbol{X}_t$: feature vectors of a set for test.

1: Subspace in gCMSM space: $\boldsymbol{D}^\top \boldsymbol{X}_t = \boldsymbol{V}_t \mathtt{diag}(\lambda_t) \boldsymbol{U}_t^\top$, $\boldsymbol{\Omega}_t = \mathtt{diag}(\mathsf{w}_m(\lambda_t))$.

2: **for** $i = 1$ to $n$ **do**

3:　　Subspace in gCMSM space: $\boldsymbol{D}^\top \boldsymbol{X}_i = \boldsymbol{V}_i \mathtt{diag}(\lambda_i) \boldsymbol{U}_i^\top$, $\boldsymbol{\Omega}_i = \mathtt{diag}(\mathsf{w}_m(\lambda_i))$.

4:　　Similarity: $s_{ti} = \mathtt{tr}(\boldsymbol{\Theta}_{ti}^2)$, where $\boldsymbol{\Omega}_t \boldsymbol{V}_t^\top \boldsymbol{V}_i \boldsymbol{\Omega}_i = \boldsymbol{Q}_t \boldsymbol{\Theta}_{ti} \boldsymbol{Q}_i^\top$ (SVD).

5: **end for**

6: $k$-NN: $y = k\mathrm{NN}(\{s_{ti}, y_i\}_{i=1}^n)$.

**Output:** Estimated class label of the test set $\boldsymbol{X}_t$: $y$.

---

where the last inequality is obtained from Theorem 2. And, as in CMSM (Sec.2.3), $\sigma_l < 1$ indicates $J < 0$ in (22), producing the discriminative coefficients $\boldsymbol{q}$. 　□

## 3.4 Procedure for Classification

For classifying sets of feature vectors, we first train by gCMSM the discriminative space in which the gMSM is subsequently performed to compute the subspace angles. The training procedure by gCMSM is shown in Algorithm 1. In the line 5, we cut off the class representative vectors $\boldsymbol{P}^{[c]}$ which are fed into *between-class* gCMSM in the line 8. By Theorem 3, the vectors $\boldsymbol{P}^{[c]}$ have the norms less than 1, and there are negligible vectors whose norms are close to 0. By eliminating those vectors, the eigenvalue problem in the line 8 is sufficiently speeded up without changing the result; in this paper, we set $\epsilon = 0.1$. In the line 9, we extract the discriminative projection vectors of the smaller eigenvalues based on Theorem 5; note that the projection vectors of the eigenvalues less than 1 are discriminative, and we set $\tau = 0.9999$.

The procedure to classify sets is shown in Algorithm 2. We apply gMSM in the discriminative space produced by Algorithm 1 and then $k$-NN, say $k = 1$.

## 4    Experimental Results

We conducted the experiments on 3D object classification by using ETH-80 [19] and RGB-D [20] datasets.

### 4.1    ETH-80 Dataset

ETH-80 dataset [19] consists of eight categories, each of which contains 10 objects with 41 images of different views. The images were transformed into gray-scale and resized to $32 \times 32$ pixels after subtracting background as shown in Fig. 3, resulting in 1024-dimensional image vectors. For evaluation, we applied two-fold cross validation; the 10 objects in each category are partitioned into two folds of five objects for training and test. We randomly repeated the validation 10 times and reported the averaged classification performance. Two types of experimental protocol were employed; 'experiment 1' is to use all of 41 views and 'experiment 2' is to randomly pick up 15 views for test while using all views in training.

First, we validated the theorems that the proposed method (Algorithm 1) is based on. For Theorem 3 used in the line 5 of Algorithm 1, the norms of the class representative vectors $\boldsymbol{p}_l^{[c]}$ produced by within-class gCMSM are shown in Fig. 4a where those vectors are sorted in descending order of the eigenvalues $\sigma_l^{[c]}$. Some of those vectors have tiny norms and by eliminating those tiny vectors, the computational cost in the subsequent between-class gCMSM is significantly reduced; actually the computation time for gCMSM is reduced to 0.19 sec from 2.13 sec on Xeon 3.33GHz. For Theorem 5 in the line 9 of Algorithm 1, the eigenvalues $\sigma_l$ of gCMSM are shown in Fig. 4b along with the norms of the projection vectors $\boldsymbol{d}_l$ to validate Theorem 4. We can see that around $\sigma_l = 1$ the projection vectors have smaller norms and are less contributive to the projections; we exploit the projections of $\sigma_l < \tau = 0.9999$.

We then analyzed the performances of the proposed methods; gMSM in (13) measures canonical angles in the original vector space while the methods of gCMSM in (18, 24) perform in the discriminative space. Note that there are two types of gCMSM; gCMSM in (18), denoted by gCMSM-mono, groups all the vectors of each class into a single set which is further represented by a mono-subspace, while gCMSM in (24) deals with each object's image set individually. Fig. 5 shows the performances on various $m$ used in the weighting function $\mathsf{w}_m$ in (15). The gCMSM produces the best performance, demonstrating that 1) the discriminative space contributes to improve the performances in comparison to gMSM and 2) the optimization considering *within-class* measures as well as *between-class* ones is effective compared to gCMSM-mono. The proposed methods are also compared to the other subspace-based methods, MSM [7], OSM [10], DCC [5], CMSM [8], as shown in Fig. 5 and Table 1. For fair comparison, the subspace dimensionality is set by the number $m$ in the weighting function for gCMSM. As is the case with gCMSM, CMSM is superior to CMSM-mono. The proposed gCMSM produces stably high performances on various $m$ due to soft weighting, which are superior to the others. In the experiment 2, we used only a

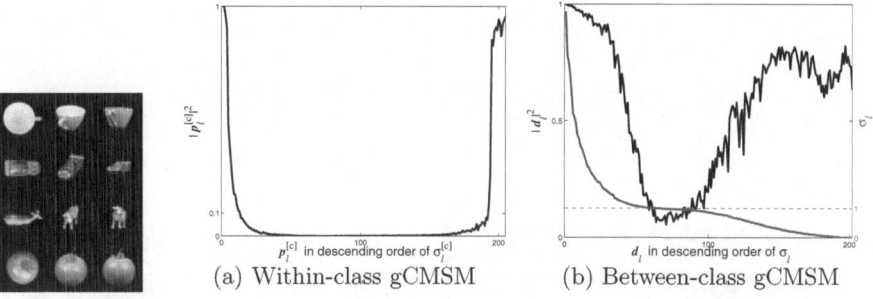

(a) Within-class gCMSM    (b) Between-class gCMSM

**Fig. 3.** ETH80        **Fig. 4.** Norms of projection vectors with eigenvalues

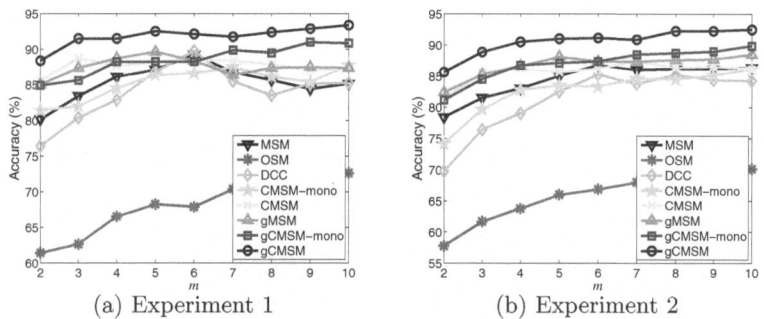

(a) Experiment 1                (b) Experiment 2

**Fig. 5.** ETH-80 dataset

subset of images of objects in test, making the test set different from the training ones. Even though the principal directions of the image sets are highly sensitive to the variations in pose, the proposed gCMSM exhibits superior performance which is almost the same as in the experiment 1, while the others are degraded.

## 4.2   RGB-D **Dataset**

RGB-D dataset [20] contains color and depth images of 300 physically distinct objects in 51 categories. This dataset is composed of video sequences for each object as it is spun around on a turntable at constant speed. The video data is recorded by the camera mounted at three different views of approximately 30, 45 and 60 degrees from the horizon with 20 Hz providing about 250 RGB+depth frames in a sequence. For this experiment, we subsampled the video sequences at every fifth frame to obtain about 40,000 RGB-depth image pairs. The object regions were extracted by background subtraction based on the depth and then resized into $32 \times 32$ pixels both for RGB and depth images, as shown in Fig. 6. Thus, we obtain the depth features of 1024 dimensionality as well as the gray-scale features transformed from RGB.

The proposed methods are compared to the other methods by using each of gray-scale and depth features. The results are shown in Fig. 7 and Table 2,

**Table 1.** Best accuracies (%) on **ETH-80** dataset

| Method | MSM | OSM | DCC | CMSM | gMSM | gCMSM |
|--------|-----|-----|-----|------|------|-------|
| Exp.1 | 89.25 | 72.63 | 89.75 | 88.75 | 89.63 | **93.38** |
| Exp.2 | 86.75 | 70.13 | 85.25 | 87.50 | 88.50 | **92.50** |

RGB 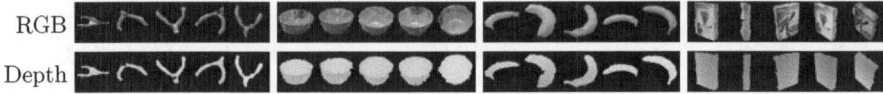 Depth

**Fig. 6.** RGB-D dataset

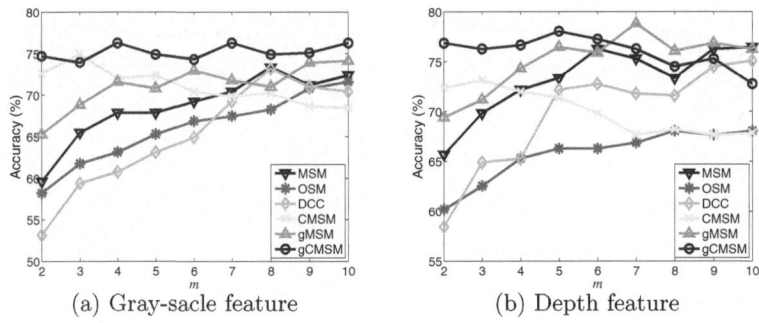

(a) Gray-sacle feature　　　　　(b) Depth feature

**Fig. 7.** RGB-D dataset

**Table 2.** Best accuracies (%) on **RGB-D** dataset

| Method | MSM | CMSM | OSM | DCC | gMSM | gCMSM | [20] | [21] |
|--------|-----|------|-----|-----|------|-------|------|------|
| Gray-scale | 73.33 | 74.90 | 71.57 | 73.14 | 74.12 | **76.27** | 74.7 | 76.1 |
| Depth | 76.47 | 73.14 | 68.04 | 75.10 | **78.82** | 78.04 | 66.8 | 75.7 |

demonstrating the proposed gCMSM produces stably high performances compared to the others; the best accuracies are competitive even with the state-of-the-art results [20, 21]. The proposed methods are more effectively applied to the depth features than to the image features, which is contrast to [20, 21] using sophisticated local features such as SIFT. The depth values depending on the object's distance give less effective clues for classification in the local features, while the global structure (distribution) of the depth values is effectively extracted by the subspace. effective for classification. On the other hand, the appearance (gray-scale) features are affected by the textures and slightly degrade the performance.

# 5    Conclusion

We have proposed generalized mutual subspace based methods. A *soft weighting* is introduced across the bases of the subspace instead of definitely picking up only principal basis vectors. The soft weights are constructed according to the variances, *i.e.*, eigenvalues, associated with the bases. The generalized MSM is proposed to effectively combine the bases via the soft weights for measuring the subspace angles. In addition, CMSM is reformulated with theoretical justification, and the reformulation also enables us to generalize the CMSM by incorporating the soft weighting for providing the discriminative space. In the experiments on 3D object recognition using ETH-80 and RGB-D datasets, the proposed methods exhibited stably favorable performances compared to the other subspace-based methods.

# References

1. Wang, R., Shan, S., Chen, X., Gao, W.: Manifold-manifold distance with application to face recognition based on image set. In: CVPR (2008)
2. Wang, T., Shi, P.: Kernel grassmannian distances and discriminant analysis for face recognition from image sets. Pattern Recognition Letters 30, 1161–1165 (2009)
3. Shakhnarovich, G., Fisher III, J.W., Darrell, T.: Face Recognition from Long-Term Observations. In: Heyden, A., Sparr, G., Nielsen, M., Johansen, P. (eds.) ECCV 2002, Part III. LNCS, vol. 2352, pp. 851–865. Springer, Heidelberg (2002)
4. Arandjelović, O., Shakhnarovich, G., Fisher, J., Cipolla, R., Darrell, T.: Face recognition with image sets using manifold density divergence. In: CVPR, pp. 581–588 (2005)
5. Kim, T.K., Kittler, J.V., Cipolla, R.: Discriminative learning and recognition of image set classes using canonical correlations. IEEE Transaction on Pattern Analysis and Machine Intelligence 29, 1005–1018 (2007)
6. Wu, J., Fukui, K.: Multiple view based 3d object classification using ensemble learning of local subspaces. In: ICPR (2008)
7. Yamaguchi, O., Fukui, K., Maeda, K.: Face recognition using temporal image sequence. In: FG, pp. 318–323 (1998)
8. Fukui, K., Yamaguchi, O.: Face recognition using multi-viewpoint patterns for robot vision. In: International Symposium of Robotics Research, pp. 192–201 (2003)
9. Fukui, K., Yamaguchi, O.: Constrained mutual subspace method using a generalized difference subspace. IEICE Trans. on Info. & Syst. 87D, 1622–1631 (2004)
10. Oja, E.: Subspace Methods for Pattern Recognition. Research Studies Press (1983)
11. Kim, T.K., Kittler, J.V., Cipolla, R.: On-line learning of mutually orthogonal subspaces for face recognition by image sets. IEEE Transaction on Image Processing 19, 1067–1074 (2010)
12. Kim, T.K., Arandjelović, O., Cipolla, R.: Learning over sets using boosted manifold principal angles (bompa). In: BMVC, pp. 779–788 (2005)
13. Wolf, L., Shashua, A.: Learning over sets using kernel principal angles. Journal of Machine Learning Research 4, 913–931 (2003)
14. Watanabe, S., Pakvasa, N.: Subspace method of pattern recognition. In: ICPR, pp. 25–32 (1973)

15. Björck, Å., Golub, G.H.: Numerical methods for computing angles between linear subspaces. Mathematics of Computation 27, 579–594 (1973)
16. Hotelling, H.: Relations between two sets of variates. Biometrika 28, 321–372 (1936)
17. Duda, R.O., Hart, P.E., Stork, D.G.: Pattern Classification, 2nd edn. Wiley-Interscience (2001)
18. Vapnik, V.: Statistical Learning Theory. Wiley (1998)
19. Leibe, B., Schiele, B.: Analyzing appearance and contour based methods for object categorization. In: CVPR, pp. 409–415 (2003)
20. Lai, K., Bo, L., Ren, X., Fox, D.: A large-scale hierarchical multi-view rgb-d object dataset. In: ICRA, pp. 1817–1824 (2011)
21. Bo, L., Lai, K., Ren, X., Fox, D.: Object recognition with hierarchical kernel descriptors. In: CVPR, pp. 1729–1736 (2011)

# Simultaneous Monocular 2D Segmentation, 3D Pose Recovery and 3D Reconstruction

Victor Adrian Prisacariu, Aleksandr V. Segal, and Ian Reid

University of Oxford

**Abstract.** We propose a novel framework for joint 2D segmentation and 3D pose and 3D shape recovery, for images coming from a single monocular source. In the past, integration of all three has proven difficult, largely because of the high degree of ambiguity in the 2D - 3D mapping. Our solution is to learn nonlinear and probabilistic low dimensional latent spaces, using the Gaussian Process Latent Variable Models dimensionality reduction technique. These act as class or activity constraints to a simultaneous and variational segmentation – recovery – reconstruction process. We define an image and level set based energy function, which we minimise with respect to 3D pose and shape, 2D segmentation resulting automatically as the projection of the recovered shape under the recovered pose. We represent 3D shapes as zero levels of 3D level set embedding functions, which we project down directly to probabilistic 2D occupancy maps, without the requirement of an intermediary explicit contour stage. Finally, we detail a fast, open-source, GPU-based implementation of our algorithm, which we use to produce results on both real and artificial video sequences.

## 1 Introduction

The three tasks of 2D segmentation, 3D pose tracking and 3D shape recovery are fundamental to computer vision so there exists a large amount of research for each of them. Their interdependence is however often ignored and they are treated either separately or in pairs. For example, some systems recover 2D segmentation and 3D pose jointly, but require a fixed, known 3D model. Others jointly optimise 3D shape and 3D pose but require high quality segmentations.

In this paper we develop a method for simultaneous 2D segmentation, 3D pose recovery and 3D shape recovery, from one or multiple images coming from a monocular camera. The main issue with this aim has always been the very high ambiguity in the mapping from 2D silhouette to 3D pose and 3D shape. To deal with this we learn nonlinear and probabilistic low dimensional latent shape spaces. We represent shapes implicitly, as 3D level set functions, which we project (using known camera calibration) directly to 2D occupancy maps. Such an occupancy map is represented probabilistically with the $p = 0.5$ level giving the implicit representation of the contour. Both pose and shape recovery problems are cast as a single, joint minimisation of an image based energy function, searching inside an n-dimensional space jointly comprising 6 pose DoFs

K.M. Lee et al. (Eds.): ACCV 2012, Part I, LNCS 7724, pp. 593–606, 2013.
© Springer-Verlag Berlin Heidelberg 2013

and n-6 shape DoFs. Segmentation results automatically from the projection of the recovered 3D shape with the recovered 3D pose.

Our work is based on ideas from monocular 3D pose recovery. Assuming a *fixed* 3D shape, there are works such as [1–4] which propose methods for level-set based, monocular, simultaneous 3D pose recovery and 2D segmentation. A first such attempt was made in [1], where a level set-based Chan-Vese like energy function [5], with an added 2D shape term, is minimised alternately, first in an unconstrained manner, then as a function of the 6 DoF 3D pose of the known 3D model. The unconstrained part of the minimisation is removed in [2], where the energy function is evolved approximately, only as a function of 3D pose. A first variational approach to this problem was introduced in [3]. Here a region based (but not level set) energy function, summing an integral over the foreground with one over the background, is differentiated wrt. the pose parameters, using the Leibniz-Reynolds transport theorem. This results in an integral along the 2D contour and two surface integrals on the inside and outside regions of the contour. As in [5], the authors measure image statistics using the region's mean color and variance. This simple formulation allows their two surface integrals to collapse, which would not happen with a more complex energy function. A similar joint optimisation is used in [4], but the contour of the projection is represented implicitly (instead of explicitly as in [3]) as the zero-level of a level set embedding function. This allows for simpler math and more complex region statistics, which results in a larger convergence basin with fewer local minima.

Recovering 3D shape (along with 3D pose and 2D segmentation) is an extremely underconstrained problem, especially in the monocular case we are looking at in this paper. That is to say that the mapping from a 3D shape – pose pair is hugely multimodal. It is therefore unlikely that a full unconstrained 3D shape recovery could be performed successfully with no prior knowledge of pose or segmentation. There exist various methods for adding shape information to the segmentation and tracking process. For example, [6] represent shape knowledge probabilistically, using level set embedding functions and probabilistic confidence maps. This is added to the segmentation process in a maximum a posteriori fashion. Alternatively, instead of learning a model from multiple shapes, [7] use a single shape, but model 2D deformations using a homography. Perhaps the most common solution to our problem comes in the form of low dimensional latent shape spaces. In [8] for example, principal component analysis (PCA) is used to capture the variance in the space of shapes. Segmentation is then cast as a minimisation of an image-based error function in space. The similar method if [9] introduces nonlinearity by using Kernel PCA instead of PCA, followed by [10], where nonlinear and probabilistic spaces are used, by replacing Kernel PCA with GP-LVM. Nonlinearity is essential because most shape spaces tend to be nonlinear and modelling nonlinearity will decrease the number of dimensions needed to capture the shape variance. For example, in [10], a 2 dimensional GP-LVM space captures as much variance as a 10 dimensional PCA space.

The work most similar to ours is [11]. Here the authors look at improving image segmentation by use of spaces of 3D shapes. They use Kernel PCA to learn these spaces and represent shapes implicitly using 3D level set embedding functions. The pose optimisation is the same as [3] i.e. using the Leibniz-Reynolds transport theorem and the simple image statistics of [5]. While their system does indeed produce both pose and shape, the authors only look at its segmentation ability. 3D poses and 3D shapes are never shown, quantified or examined.

Similar to this work, we use nonlinear dimensionality reduction to capture shape variance. Unlike [11] however, we use a method that is also probabilistic, in the form of Gaussian Process Latent Variable Models (GP-LVM). Our solution is better suited to capturing shape variance, compared to either PCA or Kernel PCA, as shown in [10, 12]. The GP-LVM generative process is closed form without making any assumptions on the type of energy function, as is done in [11]. This makes it faster and less prone to local minima. Finally, [11] needs manual tuning for the parameters of the kernel embedding functions, which makes it prone to overfitting. GP-LVM learn these parameters automatically. Our method is also similar to [12]. Here GP-LVM is used to learn joint spaces between 2D shapes and other various types of sets of parameters, ranging from 3D pose, to eye gaze and to 3D shape. One of the applications the authors explore is 3D reconstruction. While their system is able to generate 3D shapes, these are not used directly in the optimisation. They learn a shared 2D silhouette – 3D shape space and optimise for the 2D side view by finding the low dimensional latent space that generates the 2D contour that best segments the given image. This latent point is then back-projected to the set of parameters space. 3D shape is recovered when the sets of parameters describes a 3D shape. The obvious flaw of this system is that it will only recover 3D shape when the object is in a predefined (and pretrained) pose. Our method does not have this limitation.

From a fixed model 3D tracker point of view, our system is similar to [4], in that we minimise a level set based energy function wrt. the pose of known 3D model. Unlike [4] though, we represent shapes with 3D distance transforms which we project directly into 2D contour embedding functions. We do not render a vertex-based 3D model and then compute a 2D distance transform, as it is done in [4]. Our method therefore is, to our knowledge, the only *true* level set based 3D tracker, as other works always represent either the 3D shape or its 2D projection contour explicitly at some stage of the algorithm. One advantage of this formulation is that it naturally allows all points on the 3D shape to be considered in the optimisation, not just the ones that are visible from a given pose. As shown in [4], these are important to consider because, often, it is the invisible 3D points (under the current pose) that lead to changes in the shape of the projection. Another advantage is that it makes the energy function minimisation suitable for high level, GPU based, parallelisation.

When working with rigid objects, as they are being tracked throughout a sequence of frames, their shape does not change. Previous works ignored this fact. Here we impose shape consistency by alternating between optimising pose individually for each frame and shape jointly over multiple frames.

Consequently, our method has the following advantages over previous work: (i) we can generate more accurate models from our latent spaces (compared to

PCA or Kernel PCA based methods); (ii) the generated shapes are stable across multiple frames; (iii) the formulation for the rigid object tracking part of our system is more principled and parallelisable.

The remainder of this paper is structured as follows: we begin by describing our energy function in Section 2. We continue in Sections 3 and 4 with details about the minimisation wrt. pose and wrt. shape, respectively. The way we maintain shape consistency is presented in Section 5. Implementation details are explained in Section 6. We show results obtained by applying our method to several images and videos in Section 7 and conclude in Section 8.

## 2   Energy Function

Standard level-set based segmentation aims to minimise an integral over the entire image with the following form:

$$E(\phi) = \int_{\Omega} H_e(\phi)r_f(x) + (1 - H_e(\phi))r_b(x)d\Omega \tag{1}$$

where $\Omega$ is the image domain, $x$ is a pixel in this domain, $\phi$ is the 2D level set embedding function, $H_e$ is the smoothed Heaviside function and $r_f$ and $r_b$ are two monotonically decreasing functions, measuring per pixel foreground and, respectively, background model matching scores.

Our energy function is similar:

$$E(\Phi) = \sum_{x \in \Omega} \left( \pi(\Phi)r_f(x) + (1 - \pi(\Phi))r_b(x) \right) \tag{2}$$

where $\Phi$ is a 3D level set embedding function (instead of the usual 2D one denoted by $\phi$) (discretised as an $256 \times 256 \times 256$ voxel cube). $\pi(\Phi)$ projects $\Phi$ to the equivalent of a smoothed Heaviside i.e. a function of value 1 inside the projection and 0 outside, with a smooth transition between the two regions.

To obtain $r_f$ and $r_b$ we first manually segment a few frames from the video to be analysed (between 5 and 7 frames from videos with lengths of 100 to 300 frames). Next, we extract $3 \times 3$ patches for each pixel in a band around the edge of each manual segmentation, combining RGB colour value and gradient orientation at that pixel. We then use these patches to train a two class random forest classifier, in a manner similar to [13]. We used 32 trees of depth 6. This method leads to considerably better image statistics when compared to either [4] or [11]. This step is not to be confused with a full image segmentation: here we are simply replacing the *per pixel* probability of foreground and background that is more usually obtained from a colour model with the probability obtained from a random forest classifier; this is *not* the segmentation step but analogous to the unary term in an MRF framework.

To define $\pi(\Phi)$ we interpret $\Phi$ as the log odds transform of a probability field:

$$\Phi(l) = \log \frac{p_{inside}}{1 - p_{inside}} \tag{3}$$

where $l = (x, y, z)$ represents a 3D voxel location inside the level set function and $p_{inside}$ quantifies the probability of $l$ being inside the closed 3D shape embedded by the level set function. $p_{inside}$ is then extracted using the sigmoid function as:

$$p_{inside}(l) = sigmoid(\Phi(l)) = \frac{\exp(\Phi(l))}{1 + \exp(\Phi(l))} \tag{4}$$

It then follows that, for any image pixel $(u, v)$, we can define a $p_{fg}$ as the probability of $(u, v)$ being the projection of a voxel from inside the 3D level set:

$$p_{fg}(u, v) = 1 - \prod_{l \text{ on ray}} \left(1 - p_{inside}(l)\right) \tag{5}$$

with the product being computed for all 3D points that project to $(u, v)$.

For numerical stability we use the log space to compute this probability. We also introduce a parameter $\zeta$ which controls the smoothness of the transition between the inside and outside regions. Therefore, our final energy function is:

$$\pi(\Phi) = 1 - \exp\left(\sum_{l \text{ on ray}} \log\left(1 - \frac{e^{\Phi(l)\zeta}}{e^{\Phi(l)\zeta} + 1}\right)\right) \tag{6}$$

The smoothness parameter $\zeta$ is constant throughout our tests, with a value of 0.75. An example 3D model and corresponding projection is shown in Figure 1.

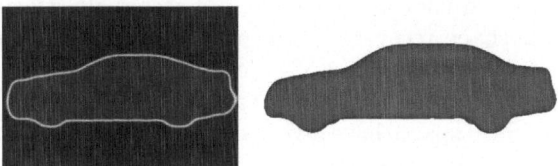

**Fig. 1.** Example 3D model and projection: left – projection, blue represents $p_{fg} = 0$, red represents $p_{fg} = 1$; right – the 3D model that generated the projection

## 3   Pose Optimisation

We optimise pose in a manner similar to [4], by differentiating the energy function wrt. the 6 pose parameters $\lambda_i$, $i \in \{1, \ldots, 6\}$, three for transform and three for rotation. We use the Rodrigues notation to parametrise rotation.

The derivative follows as:

$$\frac{\partial E}{\partial \lambda_i} = -\sum_{x \in \Omega} \left((r_f(x) - r_b(x)) \exp(\ldots) \sum_{l \text{ on ray}} \frac{e^{\Phi(l)\zeta}}{e^{\Phi(l)\zeta} + 1} \frac{\partial l}{\partial \lambda_i}\right) \tag{7}$$

where $\exp(\ldots)$ is as defined in Equation 6 and:

$$\frac{\partial l}{\partial \lambda_i} = \left(\frac{\partial l}{\partial x} \frac{\partial x}{\partial \lambda_i} + \frac{\partial l}{\partial y} \frac{\partial y}{\partial \lambda_i} + \frac{\partial l}{\partial z} \frac{\partial z}{\partial \lambda_i}\right) \tag{8}$$

with $[x, y, z]$ being OpenGL-style 3D normalised device coordinates. This representation allows $\pi(\Phi)$ to be responsible only for an orthogonal projection, making the selection of the points on the projection ray much easier.

Therefore, we can write:

$$\frac{\partial x}{\partial \lambda_i} = -f_u \frac{1}{Z^2} \left( Z \frac{\partial X}{\partial \lambda_i} - X \frac{\partial Z}{\partial \lambda_i} \right) \quad \frac{\partial y}{\partial \lambda_i} = -f_v \frac{1}{Z^2} \left( Z \frac{\partial Y}{\partial \lambda_i} - Y \frac{\partial Z}{\partial \lambda_i} \right)$$

$$\frac{\partial z}{\partial \lambda_i} = -\frac{1}{Z^2} \frac{\partial Z}{\partial \lambda_i} \tag{9}$$

where $(f_u, f_v)$ represent the focal distance expressed in horizontal and vertical pixels and $[X, Y, Z]$ are 3D points in camera coordinates and functions of the pose (i.e. $R$ and $T$) and their respective coordinates in the object frame (i.e. inside the level set voxel cube), $[X_0, Y_0, Z_0]$.

Finally, $\frac{\partial X}{\partial \lambda_i}$, $\frac{\partial Y}{\partial \lambda_i}$ and $\frac{\partial Z}{\partial \lambda_i}$ are computed analytically in a straightforward manner and $\frac{\partial l}{\partial x}$, $\frac{\partial l}{\partial y}$ and $\frac{\partial l}{\partial z}$ are computed numerically.

## 4   Shape Optimisation

As mentioned in the introduction, the mapping from a single silhouette to a 3D pose – 3D shape pair is hugely multimodal and ambiguous. There is less ambiguity when multiple frames are available, but, especially when those frames are consecutive, 3D shape recovery is still underconstrained. If however an assumption can be made on the class of object or on the activity the object is performing, a space for that class/activity can be learned and used to constrain the shape recovery. Such spaces have a very high dimensionality ($256 \times 256 \times 256$ dimensions in our case), but often actually lie on much lower dimensional manifolds. We find these manifolds using a nonlinear and probabilistic dimensionality reduction technique, called Gaussian Process Latent Variable Models [14].

Given a set of $n$ variables $\mathbf{Y} = [\mathbf{y}_1, \ldots, \mathbf{y}_n]$ of dimensionality $d$, GP-LVM learns a set of variables $\mathbf{X} = [\mathbf{x}_1, \ldots, \mathbf{x}_n]$, of dimensionality $q$, with $q \ll d$, and the hyperparameters of a Gaussian Process (GP) mapping $\mathbf{X}$ to $\mathbf{Y}$. This is done by applying standard nonlinear optimisation techniques to maximise the probability of the data $\mathbf{Y}$, jointly wrt. the latent variables $\mathbf{X}$ and the hyperparameters of the GP. This probability is written as:

$$P(\mathbf{Y}|\mathbf{X}) = \prod_{i=1}^{n} \mathcal{N}(\mathbf{y}_i|0, \mathbf{K}) \tag{10}$$

where $\mathbf{K}_{ij} = \kappa(\mathbf{x}_i, \mathbf{x}_j)$ is GP covariance matrix and $\kappa(\cdot, \cdot)$ is the GP kernel:

$$\kappa(\mathbf{x}_i, \mathbf{x}_j) = \theta_1 \exp\left( -\frac{\theta_2}{2} ||\mathbf{x}_i - \mathbf{x}_j||^2 \right) + \theta_3 + \theta_4 \delta_{ij} \tag{11}$$

with $\delta_{ij}$ being Kronecker's delta function and $\theta_{1-4}$ the GP hyperparameters.

The remainder of the GP-LVM learning process is beyond the scope of this paper and the interested reader is referred to [14].

To improve the likelihood of a good convergence, and to precondition the descriptors, in a manner similar to [12], we do not learn the space of level sets directly, but rather compute discrete cosine transforms (DCTs) for each level set and learn the space of DCT harmonic coefficients. We use 25 DCT harmonics for each 3D dimensions, for a total of $25 \times 25 \times 25$ harmonics. This is essential and a very important difference from [11]. Holding in memory a small dataset of just 100 exemplars of $256 \times 256 \times 256$ voxels requires 6.4GB of RAM memory available. This makes it very difficult to extend to larger datasets. The DCT compression allows is to work with the same dataset using just 5.96MB of RAM.

Given a $25 \times 25 \times 25$ descriptor $\mathbf{y}_p$, our level set function $\Phi$ is therefore the inverse DCT of $\mathbf{y}_p$, so $\Phi = IDCT(\mathbf{y}_p)$. $\mathbf{y}_p$ is also the high dimensional counterpart of a low dimensional latent point $\mathbf{x}_p$, so $\mathbf{y}|\mathbf{X} \sim N(\mu_p, \sigma_p^2)$, with:

$$\mu_p = \kappa(\mathbf{x}_p, \mathbf{X})\mathbf{K}^{-1}\mathbf{Y} \qquad \sigma_p^2 = \kappa(\mathbf{x}_p, \mathbf{x}_p) - \kappa(\mathbf{x}_p, \mathbf{X})\mathbf{K}^{-1}\kappa(\mathbf{x}_p, \mathbf{X})^T \qquad (12)$$

As with the pose optimisation, to optimise shape, we differentiate our energy function, now wrt. each dimension of $\mathbf{x}$, which we denote by $\mathbf{x}_q$ :

$$\frac{\partial E}{\partial \mathbf{x}_q} = -\sum_{x \in \Omega}\left((r_f(x) - r_b(x))\exp(...)\sum_{l \text{ on ray}}\frac{e^{\Phi(l)}}{e^{\Phi(l)} + 1}\frac{\partial l}{\partial \mathbf{x}_q}\right) \qquad (13)$$

It can be shown that the derivative of the inverse DCT is the inverse DCT of the derivative. It follows that $\frac{\partial l}{\partial \mathbf{x}_q} = IDCT\left(\frac{\partial \mu}{\partial \mathbf{x}_q}\right)$, with:

$$\frac{\partial \mu}{\partial \mathbf{x}_q} = \frac{\partial \kappa(\mathbf{x}_q, \mathbf{X})}{\partial \mathbf{x}_i}\mathbf{K}^{-1}\mathbf{Y} \qquad (14)$$

with $\mu$ defined in Equation 12.

The derivative of $\kappa(\cdot, \cdot)$ follows in a straightforward manner.

In [10, 12], where a 2D version of this GP-LVM based shape optimisation is proposed, the authors also use the variance $\sigma^2$ to drive the optimisation only along areas of the latent space with high likelihood. Throughout our testing, we did not find this to be necessary in the 3D case.

## 5    Shape Consistency

When multiple frames are available, the shape of a rigid object should be consistent among all the frames. The naive, adhoc solution to this problem is to choose a single informative frame, find the shape in this frame and use this shape to recover the pose (and implicitly the segmentation) in all the other frames. This is not often a good strategy, as we are unlikely to find a single frame that completely disambiguates the 3D shape, even when using a latent space shape prior.

A common solution to this problem, used throughout the 3D reconstruction literature, is to alternately iterate between shape and pose optimisations. We take a similar approach, by alternating between shape iterations (over all the frames) and pose iterations (for each frame separately). We can perform optimisation in joint space (and indeed have done so), but our experiments suggest that separating these into alternation between pose and shape has no penalty in terms of accuracy, and confers the convenience that we can impose fixed shape over over many frames rather more conveniently.

Since our energy function is a sum of per pixel values, it extends naturally to multiple frames:

$$E(\Phi) = -\sum_{f=1}^{F} \sum_{x \in \Omega_v} \Big( \pi_{\lambda_v}(\Phi) r_f(x) + (1 - \pi_{\lambda_v}(\Phi)) r_b(x) \Big) \qquad (15)$$

where $f$ is the frame, $F$ is the total number of frames and $\pi_{\lambda_v}(\Phi)$ is the projection of $\Phi$ according to the pose parameters $\lambda_v$. The derivative of this energy function wrt. shape is just the sum of the derivatives wrt. shape for each individual frame.

When a new frame is available, we proceed as follows:

– Iterate pose for the new frame using the approximation from the previous frame.
– Repeat until convergence:
  • Iterate the $q$ shape parameters, over all frames (using Equation 15).
  • Iterate the $6 \times f$ pose parameters over all frames, using the new shape.

Note that the same formulation also extends to multiple views coming from different cameras, but this is beyond the scope of this paper.

## 6   Implementation

To start the tracking process, the user must provide at least one manually segmented image and initial values for the latent point and pose. Potentially, these values could be obtained automatically using a classifier, while the manually segmented image could be obtained automatically using an unconstrained segmenter. Given these initial assumptions, the remaining operations are automatic.

Our algorithm is well suited for large scale parallelism, most operations being either per pixel or per voxel. To take advantage of this we have used the NVIDIA CUDA framework [15] to implement the complete inference algorithm (except for the random forest classification) on the GPU. The complete source code for our implementation is available online at http://www.robots.ox.ac.uk/$\sim$lav.

A standard joint shape pose iteration of our algorithm proceeds as follows:

– Compute the GP-LVM posterior mean using Equation 12.
– Create the level set voxel cube by decompressing the GP-LVM posterior mean with the inverse DCT transform.
– Compute the GP-LVM posterior mean gradient using Equation 14.
– Compute $\frac{\partial l}{\partial x_q}$ using the inverse DCT transform.
– Project the voxel cube using our projection function (Equation 6).
– Compute and sum per voxel derivatives w.r.t. pose and shape.

**Table 1.** Per iteration processing times

| Processing Stage | Time |
|---|---|
| GP-LVM posterior mean computation | 0.51 ms |
| Compute level set voxel cube with the inverse DCT on the GP-LVM mean | 31.17 ms |
| GP-LVM posterior mean gradient | 0.21 ms |
| $\frac{\partial l}{\partial \mathbf{x}_q}$ for a two dimensional space (using the inverse DCT) | 58.15 ms |
| Voxel cube projection | 2.69 ms |
| Per voxel shape/pose derivative | 7.12 ms |

A detailed summary of the processing times required for each of these steps is shown in Table 1. We used $640 \times 480$ images and an NVIDIA GTX 480 video card. The average processing time per pose iteration is $\sim 10ms$ and per shape iteration is $\sim 100ms$. Our algorithm usually converges within 25-50 iteration, so our average per image processing time is between 2.5 and 5 seconds. Note however that (i) in the pose optimisation case, around half the processing time is spent doing the final summation and (ii) in the shape optimisation case, $\sim 90\%$ processing time is spent doing the inverse DCT. Furthermore, since, potentially, the shape does not need to be iterated for every frame, with some further optimisations, our algorithm would be suitable for real time applications.

## 7   Results

We tested our algorithm using a two dimensional latent space learned from a 100 car dataset built from Google SketchUp models. For this we show several qualitative examples, a quantitative comparison between the 2D segmentation and 3D reconstruction accuracy obtained by our algorithm and the one of [12] and a quantitative comparison between the 3D poses generated by our method and those of the PTAM system of [16]. We also compare our random forest classifier (RF) with the pixel wise posteriors formulation of [4, 10, 12, 17] (PWP) and provide evidence maintaining shape consistency constraints improves results.

Figure 2 shows our car shape latent space. Blue indicates low variance (i.e. a trusted region of the space) while red indicates high variance (a region with low probability of generating valid shapes). A sample run of our system using this space is shown in Figure 3. Here we intentionally started far from the correct value to show that our algorithm is able to converge despite gross shape and pose errors. We adapted both shape and pose simultaneously and the algorithm converged in $\sim 300$ gradient descent iterations. More powerful optimisation methods could potentially be used, as there are no mathematical impediments to computing a second derivative of our energy function (unlike standard level set formulations that often require the derivative of the Dirac delta).

Two tracking results using the car latent space, for two different types of car (sedan and hatchback), are shown in Figure 6. Both cars are being tracked successfully throughout their respective sequences.

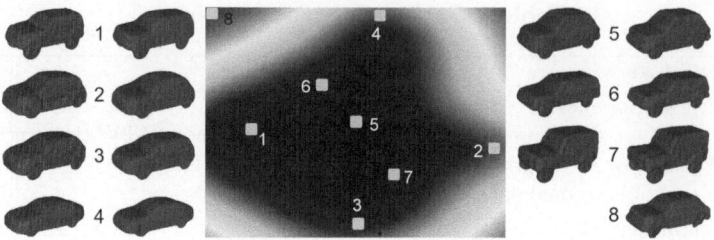

**Fig. 2.** Example 2D latent space, capturing car inter-class variance. From each shape pair, left represents the ground truth and right the generated one. Shapes 1-7 are points inside the low variance region of the space (in blue), while shape 8 is from the high variance area (in red). The sample from the high variance area does not have a corresponding ground truth because it was not part of the original training data.

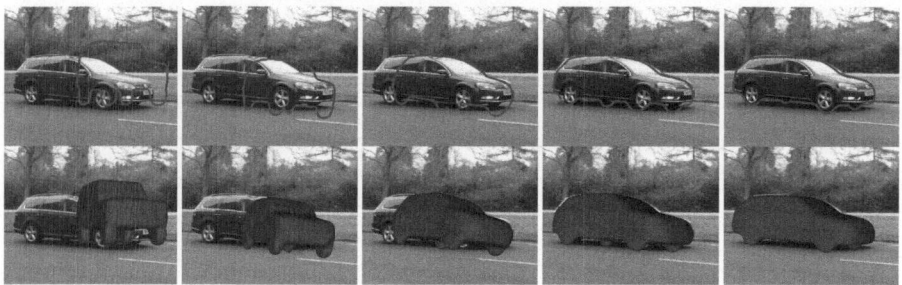

**Fig. 3.** Example shape and pose convergence for our algorithm

In Figure 4 we compare the 2D segmentation and 3D reconstruction accuracies of our system and the one from [12], where shared shape spaces are learned between 2D car side views and 3D car models. When the system from [12] is shown a car side view the results are good. In all other poses however, the system from [12] fails, whereas ours does not.

Figure 5 shows a comparison between our method and the simultaneous location and mapping PTAM method of [16]. Here, on the same video sequence, we tracked the pose of the camera using PTAM and the pose of the car using our system. The two system produce very similar poses, in spite of the fact that PTAM uses features from the whole image, while our method uses just features from the contour of the car.

In Figure 7 we compare the pixel wise fg/bg separation obtained by using RFs and the PWP formulation of [4, 10, 12, 17]. For each pixel, a fg probability $P_f$ and a bg probability $P_b$ are computed using both methods. Figure 7 shows the difference between the two probabilities, where $P_f - P_b > 0$. The RF classifier achieves better separation, which in turn leads to more reliable tracking.

Enforcing shape consistency is essential. Figure 8 shows two charts, test 1 corresponding to the video sequence from Figure 9 and test 2 for the one in Figure 9. We ran each sequence twice, once with and once without shape consistency

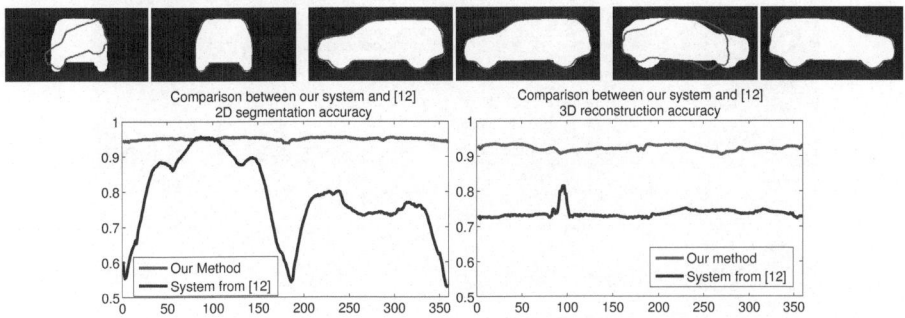

**Fig. 4.** 2D Segmentation and 3D reconstruction comparison with the system from [12]. We used a known 3D model which we rotated 360 degrees around the Z axis. Example frames are shown above, with results from [12] on the left and our results on the right. On the charts, the X axis shows rotation angle and the Y axis shows accuracy.

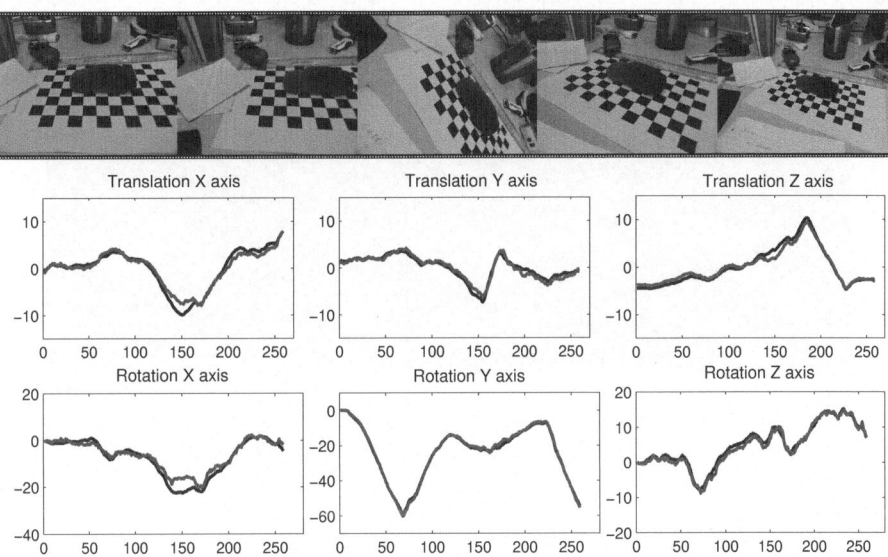

**Fig. 5.** 3D pose tracking comparison between our method (red) and the system from [16] (blue). The video sequence used is shown above. The X axis shows the frame number while the Y axis shows centimetres for transition and degrees for rotation.

constraints. Both times the result was smoother when shape consistency was used. Furthermore, in the second example the lack of shape consistency leads to a complete failure of tracking. As shown in Figure 9, when the cyclist occludes the car, not using shape consistency causes the algorithm to incorrectly adapt shape, ultimately leading to failure. When shape consistency is kept the algorithm can use information from unoccluded frames, which insures stable tracking.

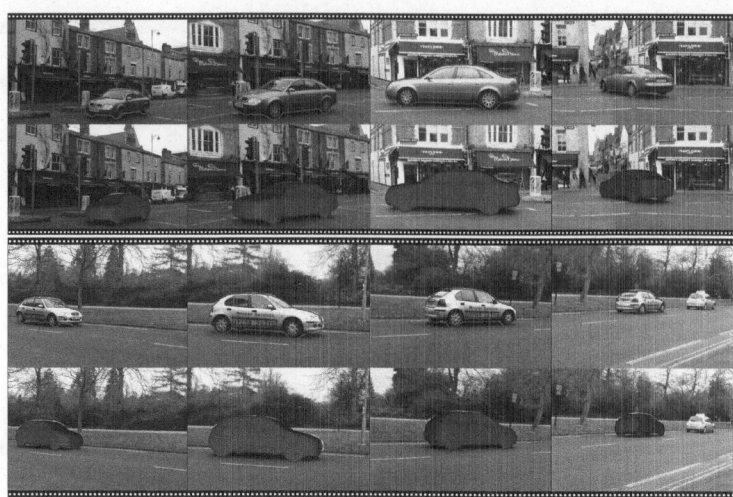

**Fig. 6.** Film strips showing our algorithm successfully tracking different types of cars in different environments

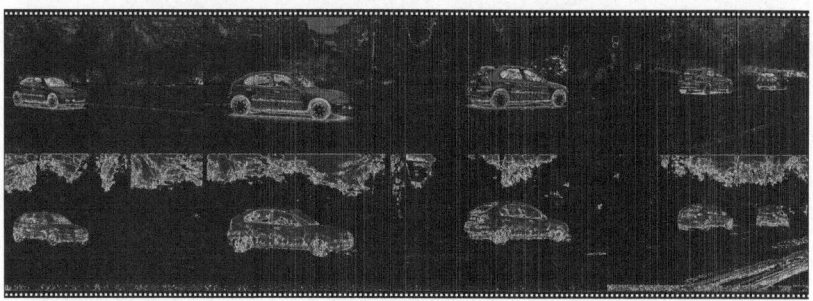

**Fig. 7.** Comparison between the foreground / background separation provided by the PWP method used of [4, 10, 12, 17] and our RF classifier. Warm colours indicate high probability and cold ones low probability.

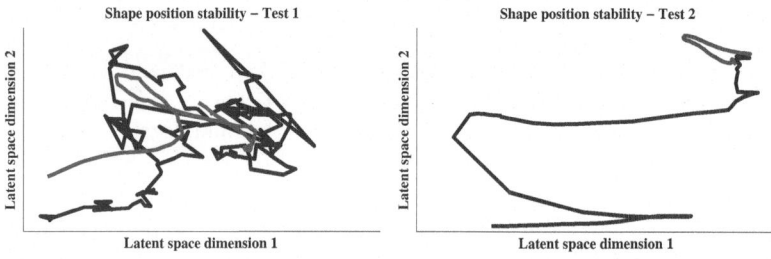

**Fig. 8.** Charts showing recovered latent space positions, with (in red) and without (in blue) shape consistency. When shape consistency is used the trajectories in the recovered latent space is smoother and tighter.

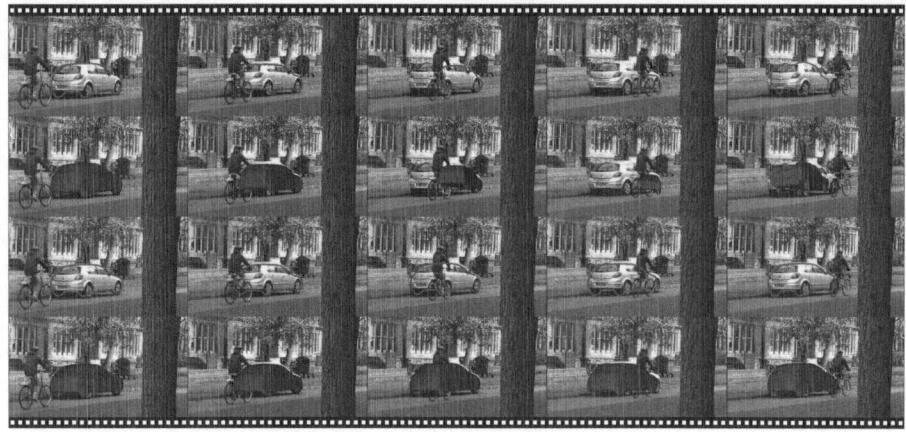

**Fig. 9.** Failure due to occlusion, combined with lack of shape consistency. When the cyclist passes in front of the camera and shape consistency is not kept the system fails (top two rows). When information from multiple frames is integrated the system successfully tracks through the occlusions (bottom two rows).

## 8   Conclusions

In this article we proposed a method for simultaneous 2D segmentation, 3D pose recovery and 3D shape reconstruction. We have shown that constraining the shape search space with Gaussian Process Latent Variable Models latent spaces is effective and leads to high quality reconstructions. The rigid body part of our formulation is, to our knowledge, the first true level set based tracker, since we don't switch from implicit shape representations to explicit ones at any point during the algorithm. Shapes are represented via 3D level set embedding functions (discretised as voxel cubes) and are projected down directly to 2D occupancy maps, avoiding the need for an explicit contour representation. We also propose a fast, potentially real time, GPU based implementation, which we make available online as an open source package.

One possible extension to this work is the processing of MRI or Ultrasound data. Shared spaces, as used [12], between 3D shapes and sets of parameters could also be learned. This could, for example, enable articulated poses to be recovered as part of our current framework.

**Acknowledgement.** This work was supported by the REWIRE FP7 project and by EPSRC through a doctoral prize award.

# References

1. Rosenhahn, B., Brox, T., Weickert, J.: Three-dimensional shape knowledge for joint image segmentation and pose tracking. IJCV 73, 243–262 (2007)
2. Schmaltz, C., Rosenhahn, B., Brox, T., Cremers, D., Weickert, J., Wietzke, L., Sommer, G.: Region-Based Pose Tracking. In: Martí, J., Benedí, J.M., Mendonça, A.M., Serrat, J. (eds.) IbPRIA 2007. LNCS, vol. 4478, pp. 56–63. Springer, Heidelberg (2007)
3. Dambreville, S., Sandhu, R., Yezzi, A., Tannenbaum, A.: Robust 3D Pose Estimation and Efficient 2D Region-Based Segmentation from a 3D Shape Prior. In: Forsyth, D., Torr, P., Zisserman, A. (eds.) ECCV 2008, Part II. LNCS, vol. 5303, pp. 169–182. Springer, Heidelberg (2008)
4. Prisacariu, V.A., Reid, I.: PWP3D: Real-Time Segmentation and Tracking of 3D Objects. IJCV, 1–20
5. Vese, L.A., Chan, T.F.: A multiphase level set framework for image segmentation using the mumford and shah model. IJCV 50, 271–293 (2002)
6. Rousson, M., Paragios, N.: Prior Knowledge, Level Set Representations & Visual Grouping. IJCV 76, 231–243 (2008)
7. Riklin-raviv, T., Kiryati, N., Sochen, N.: Prior-based segmentation and shape registration in the presence of projective distortion. IJCV 72, 309–328 (2007)
8. Tsai, A., Yezzi, A., Wells, W., Tempany, C., Tucker, D., Fan, A., Grimson, E., Willsky, A.: A shape-based approach to the segmentation of medical imagery using level sets. T-MI 22, 137–154 (2003)
9. Dambreville, S., Rathi, Y., Tannenbaum, A.: A framework for image segmentation using shape models and kernel space shape priors. T-PAMI 30, 1385–1399 (2008)
10. Prisacariu, V., Reid, I.: Nonlinear shape manifolds as shape priors in level set segmentation and tracking. In: CVPR 2011, pp. 2185–2192 (2011)
11. Sandhu, R., Dambreville, S., Yezzi, A., Tannenbaum, A.: A Nonrigid Kernel-Based Framework for 2D-3D Pose Estimation and 2D Image Segmentation. T-PAMI 33, 1098–1115 (2011)
12. Prisacariu, V., Reid, I.: Shared shape spaces. In: ICCV 2011 (2011)
13. Santner, J., Unger, M., Pock, T., Leistner, C., Saffari, A., Bischof, H.: Interactive Texture Segmentation using Random Forests and Total Variation. In: BMVC 2009 (2009)
14. Lawrence, N.: Probabilistic non-linear principal component analysis with gaussian process latent variable models. JMLR 6, 1783–1816 (2005)
15. NVIDIA: NVIDIA CUDA Programming Guide 4.1 (2012)
16. Klein, G., Murray, D.: Parallel tracking and mapping for small AR workspaces. In: ISMAR 2007, pp. 1–10 (2007)
17. Bibby, C., Reid, I.: Robust Real-Time Visual Tracking Using Pixel-Wise Posteriors. In: Forsyth, D., Torr, P., Zisserman, A. (eds.) ECCV 2008, Part II. LNCS, vol. 5303, pp. 831–844. Springer, Heidelberg (2008)

# Joint Kernel Learning
# for Supervised Image Segmentation

Jongmin Kim, Youngjoo Seo, Sanghyuk Park,
Sungrack Yun, and Chang D. Yoo

Department of EE, KAIST, Daejeon, Korea
{waterboy0309,minerrba,shine0624,yunsungrack}@kaist.ac.kr,
cdyoo@ee.kaist.ac.kr

**Abstract.** This paper considers a supervised image segmentation algorithm based on joint-kernelized structured prediction. In the proposed algorithm, correlation clustering over a superpixel graph is conducted using a non-linear discriminant function, where the parameters are learned by a kernelized-structured support vector machine (SSVM). For an input superpixel image, correlation clustering is used to predict the superpixel-graph edge labels that determine whether adjacent superpixel pairs should be merged or not. In previous works, the discriminant functions for structured prediction were generally chosen to be linear with the model parameter and joint feature map. However, the linear model has two limitations: complex correlations between two input-output pairs are ignored, and the joint feature map should be explicitly designed. To cope with these limitations, a nonlinear discriminant function based on a joint kernel, which eliminates the need for explicit design of the joint feature map, is considered. The proposed joint kernel is defined as a combination of an *image similarity kernel* and an *edge-label similarity kernel*, which measure the resemblance of two input images and the similarity between two edge-label pairs, respectively. Each kernel function is designed for fast computation and efficient inference. The proposed algorithm is evaluated using two segmentation benchmark datasets: the Berkeley segmentation dataset (BSDS) and Microsoft Research Cambridge dataset (MSRC). It is observed that the joint feature map implicitly embedded in the proposed joint kernel performs comparably or even better than the explicitly designed joint feature map for a linear model.

## 1 Introduction

Image segmentation is a task of splitting an image into disjoint regions such that each region is homogeneous. It is a crucial preprocessing step for many high-level computer vision tasks including image/scene understanding and annotation. The resulting segmented image improves the performance and speed of the subsequent labeling task for the following reasons. *First*, the assumption that each region contains only a single class label serves as a good prior for many labeling tasks. *Second*, each homogeneous region allows consistent feature extraction to incorporate contextual information over the region with preserved

K.M. Lee et al. (Eds.): ACCV 2012, Part I, LNCS 7724, pp. 607–621, 2013.
© Springer-Verlag Berlin Heidelberg 2013

object boundaries. *Third*, the region-based processing significantly reduces the computational complexity of the successive labeling task: the number of large homogeneous regions is much smaller than the number of pixels.

Recently, structured learning and prediction frameworks have been successfully adopted for various computer vision tasks [1–6], by mitigating local prediction errors using a global discriminant function. As a method of structured prediction for image segmentation, correlation clustering over a superpixel graph has shown much promise [6]: given an oversegmented superpixel image in Figure 1 as input, the correlation clustering outputs a superpixel graph in which the edge labels determine whether adjacent superpixel pairs should be merged or not based on their similarity.

For structured prediction, a discriminant function that is linear to the model parameter and the joint-feature function of input and output, referred to as a *joint feature map*, is often used; however, the linear discriminant function is associated with the following two limitations. *First*, the function only considers the given input-output pair, while ignoring information incorporated in the correlations with other input-output pairs. *Second*, explicit design of the joint feature map is required; this is not desirable since the information pertaining to optimal high-dimensional feature space is ambiguous.

To overcome these limitations, this paper proposes an image segmentation algorithm using a non-linear discriminant function based on a joint-kernel function, which is learned with a kernelized-SSVM. The joint kernel is a function that measures the similarity between two input-output pairs. By properly designing the joint-kernel function, complex high-level relationships between couples of input-output pairs can be incorporated into the embedded Reproducing Kernel Hilbert Spaces (RKHS). Moreover, compared to the explicitly defined joint feature map, the joint-kernel function can be more intuitively designed as long as it represents the similarity between two input-output pairs. The proposed joint-kernel combines two component kernels, such as the *image similarity kernel* and *edge-label similarity kernel*, which measure the resemblance of two input images and the correlations between two edge-label pairs, respectively. The key idea is that the joint feature map implicitly embedded in the proposed joint kernel performs comparably or even better than the explicitly designed joint feature map for linear discriminant function.

Recently, non-linear structured learning approaches based on a joint-kernel and kernelized-SSVM have been proposed for several computer vision tasks, such as object localization [1, 2] and object segmentation [7]. The main bottlenecks of using a joint-kernel are the high computational complexity at test-time prediction and intractable inference of the non-linear discriminant function. For instance, in object localization, the inference problem was solved with an elaborately developed branch-and-bound algorithm [1], while in [7] the joint-kernel was designed such that efficient graph-cut inference can be used for object segmentation. In this paper, each component kernel is designed for fast computation at test time using pre-trained binary classifiers. Also, the kernel function is designed to be linear to the output variable, which allows efficient inference by linear programming (LP) relaxation.

The rest of the paper is organized as follows. Section 2 describes correlation clustering for image segmentation. Section 3 describes large-margin training using kernelized-SSVM. In Section 4, the proposed joint-kernel functions are presented, which is the main contribution of this paper. In Section 5, a number of experiments and comparative results are presented and discussed, and Section 6 concludes the paper.

## 2   Correlation Clustering over Superpixel Graph

The proposed segmentation algorithm is based on correlation clustering over superpixel image as shown in Figure 1. For a given undirected graph $\mathcal{G} = (\mathcal{V}, \mathcal{E})$ which consists of superpixels as nodes and the boundary between two adjacent superpixels as edges, the correlation clustering predicts a binary label $y_{jk}$ for an edge $(j, k) \in \mathcal{E}$ to be either 1 if nodes $j$ and $k$ should be *clustered*, or 0 otherwise. As a result, the correlation clustering produces a validly-partitioned image as shown on the right side of Figure 1, where the edges colored with green and red represent label 0 and 1, respectively. The correlation clustering requires a similarity function that measures the correlation between two adjacent superpixels. For example in [6], a linear discriminant function is defined by a sum of similarities between all adjacent superpixel pairs in an image $\mathbf{x}$ multiplied by the edge label $\mathbf{y}$ such as

$$
\begin{aligned}
F(\mathbf{x}, \mathbf{y}; \mathbf{w}) &= \sum_{(j,k)\in\mathcal{E}} \mathrm{Sim}(\mathbf{x}, j, k; \mathbf{w}) y_{jk} \\
&= \sum_{(j,k)\in\mathcal{E}} \langle \mathbf{w}, \phi_{jk}(\mathbf{x}) \rangle y_{jk} = \langle \mathbf{w}, \Phi(\mathbf{x}, \mathbf{y}) \rangle
\end{aligned}
\tag{1}
$$

Here, $\mathrm{Sim}(\mathbf{x}, j, k; \mathbf{w})$ measures the similarity between the two adjacent superpixels $j$ and $k$ by inner product of parameter vector $\mathbf{w}$ and the joint feature map

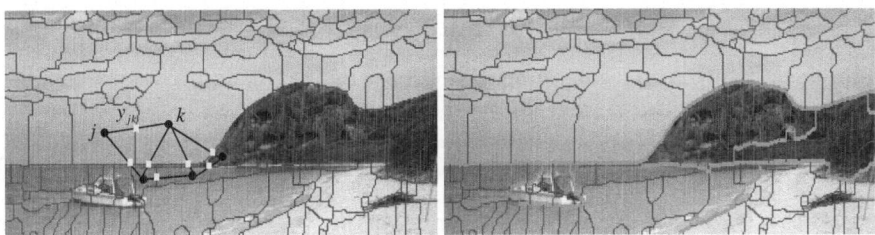

**Fig. 1.** Left: superpixel image and superpixel graph for correlation clustering. Right: an example of valid partitioning.

$\Phi(\mathbf{x}, \mathbf{y})$. The $\Phi$ is a function that maps the input-output pair into the high-dimensional joint-feature space, and $\Phi(\mathbf{x}, \mathbf{y})$ is the joint-feature vector which is a combined-feature representation of input and output [8]. Then, the edge label $\hat{\mathbf{y}}$ is inferred by maximizing the discriminant function $F$ such that

$$\hat{\mathbf{y}} = \arg \max_{\mathbf{y} \in \mathcal{Y}} F(\mathbf{x}, \mathbf{y}; \mathbf{w}) \tag{2}$$

Although predicting a valid partitioning is generally an NP-hard problem, the Eq.(2) is efficiently solved by approximation using multicut LP relaxation [5, 9]. Also, the linearity of the function $F$ allows large-margin training of the parameter using linear-SSVM which will be described in Section.3.1. However, the linear discriminant function cannot take into account correlations between the input sample and the training samples, and it needs fairly high-demensional joint feature map to sufficiently model the input-output relationship. Therefore, the linear model relies on manually designed joint feature map: for example, in Eq.(1), the joint feature map is defined as $\Phi(\mathbf{x}, \mathbf{y}) = \sum_{(j,k) \in \mathcal{E}} \phi_{jk}(\mathbf{x}) y_{jk}$, which does not guarantee a good high-dimensional feature representation. The main contribution of this paper is considering a non-linear discriminant function using joint kernels, to find better joint feature space embedded in the kernel function for enhanced segmentation performance. In Section.3.2, the kernelized-SSVM for learning the non-linear discriminant function is presented.

## 3    Image Segmentation via Structured-SVM Learning

### 3.1    Linear-SSVM: Structured Learning in Primal Domain

In this section, a large-margin training based on structured-SVM is described. To find the parameter vector $\mathbf{w}$ of the linear discriminant function $F(\mathbf{x}, \mathbf{y}; \mathbf{w})$, the following constrained-optimization problem referred to as margin scaling [10–12] is solved.

$$
\begin{aligned}
\min_{\mathbf{w}, \boldsymbol{\xi}} \quad & \frac{1}{2} \|\mathbf{w}\|^2 + \frac{C}{N} \sum_{n=1}^{N} \xi_n \\
\text{s.t.} \quad & d(\mathbf{x}_n, \mathbf{y}; \mathbf{w}) \geq \Delta(\mathbf{y}_n, \mathbf{y}) - \xi_n, \quad \mathbf{y} \in \mathcal{Y} \setminus \mathbf{y}_n, \ \forall n, \\
& \xi_n \geq 0, \ \forall n
\end{aligned}
\tag{3}
$$

Here, $d(\mathbf{x}_n, \mathbf{y}; \mathbf{w})$ is the difference of the discriminant function values between the ground-truth label $\mathbf{y}_n$ and the predicted label $\mathbf{y}$ such as

$$d(\mathbf{x}_n, \mathbf{y}; \mathbf{w}) = F(\mathbf{x}_n, \mathbf{y}_n; \mathbf{w}) - F(\mathbf{x}_n, \mathbf{y}; \mathbf{w}), \tag{4}$$

and $\xi_n$ is a slack variable to allow training error for $\mathbf{x}_n$ and $C$ is the balance coefficient to control the trade-off between the training error minimization and the margin maximization. The loss function $\Delta(\mathbf{y}_n, \mathbf{y})$ is an error measurement of predicting a label $\mathbf{y}$ given the correct label $\mathbf{y}_n$. In this paper, a modified hamming loss [6] is used to overcome the unbalance problem.

The optimization problem of Eq.(3) has exponential number of constraints with respect to the dimensionality of $\mathbf{y}$. Thus, the cutting-plane algorithm [8, 13] is used to reduce the number of constraints. In the algorithm, the most violated label for $n$th training data is inferred as

$$\bar{\mathbf{y}}_n = \arg\max_{\mathbf{y}\in\mathcal{Y}/\mathbf{y}_n} [\Delta(\mathbf{y}_n, \mathbf{y}) - d(\mathbf{x}_n, \mathbf{y}; \mathbf{w})] \tag{5}$$

and then added to the constraint set. Note that the considered loss function is decomposable over the test edges for efficient inference of $\bar{\mathbf{y}}_n$ in Eq.(5). Given the constraint set, the optimization problem can be solved using quadratic programming(QP).

## 3.2 Kernelized-SSVM: Structured Learning in Dual Domain

This section describes kernelized-SSVM that is used to learn the non-linear discriminant function proposed in this paper. Using standard Lagrangian duality techniques, the optimization problem in Eq.(3) is replaced with the following dual QP [8].

$$\max_{\alpha} -\frac{1}{2} \sum_{i,\bar{\mathbf{y}}_i\neq\mathbf{y}_i} \sum_{j,\bar{\mathbf{y}}_j\neq\mathbf{y}_j} \alpha_{i\bar{\mathbf{y}}_i}\alpha_{j\bar{\mathbf{y}}_j} J_{(i\bar{\mathbf{y}}_i)(j\bar{\mathbf{y}}_j)} + \sum_{i,\bar{\mathbf{y}}_i\neq\mathbf{y}_i} \alpha_{i\bar{\mathbf{y}}_i}\Delta(\mathbf{y}_i, \bar{\mathbf{y}}_i) \tag{6}$$

$$s.t. \quad \alpha \geq 0, \quad \sum_{i,\bar{\mathbf{y}}_i\neq\mathbf{y}_i} \alpha_{i\bar{\mathbf{y}}_i} \leq \frac{C}{N}, \quad \forall i = 1,...,N$$

Here, the coefficient matrix $J$ for quadratic term is defined as

$$\begin{aligned} J_{(i\bar{\mathbf{y}}_i)(j\bar{\mathbf{y}}_j)} &= \left\{ (\Phi(\mathbf{x}_i, \mathbf{y}_i) - \Phi(\mathbf{x}_i, \bar{\mathbf{y}}_i)) \cdot (\Phi(\mathbf{x}_j, \mathbf{y}_j) - \Phi(\mathbf{x}_j, \bar{\mathbf{y}}_j)) \right\} \\ &= K((\mathbf{x}_i, \mathbf{y}_i), (\mathbf{x}_j, \mathbf{y}_j)) - K((\mathbf{x}_i, \mathbf{y}_i), (\mathbf{x}_j, \bar{\mathbf{y}}_j)) \\ &\quad - K((\mathbf{x}_i, \bar{\mathbf{y}}_i), (\mathbf{x}_j, \mathbf{y}_j)) + K((\mathbf{x}_i, \bar{\mathbf{y}}_i), (\mathbf{x}_j, \bar{\mathbf{y}}_j)) \end{aligned} \tag{7}$$

where $K((\mathbf{x}_i, \mathbf{y}_i), (\mathbf{x}_j, \mathbf{y}_j))$ is the joint-kernel function of two input-output pairs $(\mathbf{x}_i, \mathbf{y}_i)$ and $(\mathbf{x}_j, \mathbf{y}_j)$, and is defined as the inner product of two embedded joint feature maps such as

$$K((\mathbf{x}_i, \mathbf{y}_i), (\mathbf{x}_j, \mathbf{y}_j)) = \langle \Phi(\mathbf{x}_i, \mathbf{y}_i), \Phi(\mathbf{x}_j, \mathbf{y}_j) \rangle \tag{8}$$

The solution of the dual problem gives a set of weights $\alpha$ for the support vectors. Then, the discriminant function $F(\mathbf{x}, \mathbf{y}; \alpha)$ is written as,

$$F(\mathbf{x}, \mathbf{y}; \alpha) = \sum_{i=1}^{N} \sum_{\bar{\mathbf{y}}_i\in\mathcal{Y}/\mathbf{y}_i} \alpha_{i\bar{\mathbf{y}}_i}\{K((\mathbf{x}_i, \mathbf{y}_i), (\mathbf{x}, \mathbf{y})) - K((\mathbf{x}_i, \bar{\mathbf{y}}_i), (\mathbf{x}, \mathbf{y}))\} \tag{9}$$

and a loss-augmented inference for cutting-plane learning is formulated as follows:

$$\mathbf{y}^* = \arg\max_{\mathbf{y}}[F(\mathbf{x}, \mathbf{y}; \alpha) + \Delta(\mathbf{y}_i, \mathbf{y})] \tag{10}$$

In this paper, for efficient inference of Eq.(9) and Eq.(10) using LP, the joint-kernel is designed to be decomposable over the edges of test sample $(\mathbf{x}, \mathbf{y})$ such as,

$$K((\mathbf{x}_i, \mathbf{y}_i), (\mathbf{x}, \mathbf{y})) = \sum_{e \in \mathcal{E}} K_e((\mathbf{x}_i, \mathbf{y}_i), (x_e, y_e)) \tag{11}$$

Here, $x_e$ and $y_e$ are the feature vector and label of $e$th edge of $(\mathbf{x}, \mathbf{y})$, respectively. Then, $K_e$ is the atomic kernel which measures the correspondence between the $i$th training sample $(\mathbf{x}_i, \mathbf{y}_i)$ and the $e$th edge of test sample $(\mathbf{x}, \mathbf{y})$.

## 4    A Joint Kernel Function for Image Segmentation

One of the main contributions of this paper is the design of joint kernel functions in Eq.(8). The proposed kernel functions evaluate the quality of the mutual match between two image-edge label pairs; If two images are similar, the kernel response is high in case the edge labels are similar as well. In contrast, if the edge labels are not matched for two similar images, the kernel response should be low. Compared to the conventional linear SSVMs based on explicitly modeled joint feature map $\Phi(\mathbf{x}, \mathbf{y})$, the proposed algorithm has two main advantages: *First*, by using the joint-kernel function, the explicit knowledge of non-linear mapping to higher dimensional space is not required. *Second*, non-linear discriminant functions based on joint kernels allow to encode complex relationships between two training image-edge label pairs. The proposed joint-kernel is defined as follows:

$$K((\mathbf{x}^l, \mathbf{y}^l), (\mathbf{x}^r, \mathbf{y}^r)) = \sum_{t \in \mathcal{F}} \beta_t \Lambda_t(\mathbf{x}^l, \mathbf{x}^r) \Theta_t((\mathbf{x}^l, \mathbf{y}^l), (\mathbf{x}^r, \mathbf{y}^r)) \tag{12}$$

Here, $(\mathbf{x}^l, \mathbf{y}^l)$ and $(\mathbf{x}^r, \mathbf{y}^r)$ are the training sample and test sample, respectively. And, $\mathcal{F}$ is the set of low-level features, e.g. $\mathcal{F} = \{\text{color, texture, shape}\}$. Therefore, as shown in Eq.(12), the complete joint-kernel is composed of the weighted sum of several component kernels, each of which is built using one type of low-level feature. Image similarity kernel $\Lambda_t$ measures the similarity between two input images, and edge-label similarity kernel $\Theta_t$ measures the correlation of the two input-output pairs. Although the proposed kernel function is multiplicative form, note that $\Theta_t((\mathbf{x}^l, \mathbf{y}^l), (\mathbf{x}^r, \mathbf{y}^r))$ is not in the most prominent factor form such as $K((\mathbf{x}^l, \mathbf{y}^l), (\mathbf{x}^r, \mathbf{y}^r)) = K_\mathcal{X}(\mathbf{x}^l, \mathbf{x}^r) \cdot K_\mathcal{Y}(\mathbf{y}^l, \mathbf{y}^r)$ which does not consider the correlation between input and output. In the following subsections, each component kernels in Eq.(12) is described in detail.

### 4.1    Edge-Label Similarity Kernel

The edge-label similarity kernel $\Theta_t((\mathbf{x}^l, \mathbf{y}^l), (\mathbf{x}^r, \mathbf{y}^r))$ is designed to be a linear combination of two different kernel functions, such as

$$\Theta_t((\mathbf{x}^l, \mathbf{y}^l), (\mathbf{x}^r, \mathbf{y}^r))$$
$$= \gamma_t \Theta_t^{local}((\mathbf{x}^l, \mathbf{y}^l), (\mathbf{x}^r, \mathbf{y}^r)) + (1 - \gamma_t) \Theta_t^{global}((\mathbf{x}^l, \mathbf{y}^l), (\mathbf{x}^r, \mathbf{y}^r)) \tag{13}$$

**Local Binary Model Kernel.** The local binary model kernel tries to measure how good a label $\mathbf{y}^r$ is to the input image $\mathbf{x}^r$ using a merge/split prediction model learned from $\mathbf{x}^l$ and label $\mathbf{y}^l$. In other words, if the input-output relationship of $(\mathbf{x}^r, \mathbf{y}^r)$ is similar to the input-output relationship of $(\mathbf{x}^l, \mathbf{y}^l)$, the kernel value is high. If the two relationships are not similar, the kernel value is low. To achieve this property, we model the input-output relationship of $(\mathbf{x}^l, \mathbf{y}^l)$ as binary SVM classifier trained with the data $D = \{(\mathbf{f}_e^l, y_e^l)\}_{e=1,...,|E^l|}$, where $\mathbf{f}_e^l$ and $y_e^l$ are the low-level feature and the binary label of $e$th edge of $(\mathbf{x}^l, \mathbf{y}^l)$, respectively. Then, the kernel function measures how well the edges of $(\mathbf{x}^r, \mathbf{y}^r)$ are classified by the trained binary classifier trained from $(\mathbf{x}^l, \mathbf{y}^l)$. We can then write the kernel expression as:

$$
\Theta^{local}((\mathbf{x}^l, \mathbf{y}^l), (\mathbf{x}^r, \mathbf{y}^r))
$$
$$
= \frac{1}{|E^{(r)}|} \sum_{e \in E^{(r)}} \sigma(\mathbf{v}^l \cdot \mathbf{f}_e^r + b^l) y_e^r + \{1 - \sigma(\mathbf{v}^l \cdot \mathbf{f}_e^r + b^l)\}(1 - y_e^r) \quad (14)
$$

Here, $\mathbf{v}^l$ is the weight vector of the binary classifier trained from $(\mathbf{x}^l, \mathbf{y}^l)$, and $b^l$ is a bias. $\mathbf{f}_e^r$ and $y_e^r$ are the low-level feature and the binary label of $e$th edge of $(\mathbf{x}^r, \mathbf{y}^r)$, respectively. $\sigma(\cdot)$ is a sigmoid function, with the following definition:

$$
\sigma(\mathbf{v}^l \cdot \mathbf{f}_e^r + b^l) = \frac{\exp(\mathbf{v}^l \cdot \mathbf{f}_e^r + b^l)}{1 + \exp(\mathbf{v}^l \cdot \mathbf{f}_e^r + b^l)} \quad (15)
$$

where $\sigma(\mathbf{v}^l \cdot \mathbf{f}_e^r + b^l)$ represents the probability that the feature $\mathbf{f}_e^r$ to be labeled as $y_e^r = 1$ by the classifier $\mathbf{v}^l$. Note that $\mathbf{v}^l$ is trained using the edge label-feature pairs in $(\mathbf{x}^l, \mathbf{y}^l)$ only, and can be considered as *local* binary model of feature-edge label pairs in $(\mathbf{x}^l, \mathbf{y}^l)$. Therefore, we define $\sigma(\mathbf{v}^l \cdot \mathbf{f}_e^r + b^l)$ as *the local classifier response* of the $\mathbf{f}_e^r$ to $(\mathbf{x}^l, \mathbf{y}^l)$. Figure 2 shows how the local binary model kernel works. In the first column, the ground-truth label $\mathbf{y}^l$ and the most violated constraint $\bar{\mathbf{y}}^l$ are presented. The histograms given in the first and the second row represents the distribution of the local classifier responses of the edges of $(\mathbf{x}^l, \mathbf{y}^l)$, with respect to the binary classifiers trained with $(\mathbf{x}^l, \mathbf{y}^l)$ and $(\mathbf{x}^l, \bar{\mathbf{y}}^l)$, respectively. In the first row, the classifier responses are high because $(\mathbf{x}^l, \mathbf{y}^l)$ fits to the classifier trained with $(\mathbf{x}^l, \mathbf{y}^l)$. In contrast, in the second row, the classifier responses are low because $(\mathbf{x}^l, \mathbf{y}^l)$ does not fit to the classifier trained with $(\mathbf{x}^l, \bar{\mathbf{y}}^l)$. Thus, $\Theta^{local}((\mathbf{x}^l, \mathbf{y}^l), (\mathbf{x}^l, \mathbf{y}^l))$ has high value while $\Theta^{local}((\mathbf{x}^l, \bar{\mathbf{y}}^l), (\mathbf{x}^l, \mathbf{y}^l))$ has low value. The kernel has three properties: *First*, the kernel is asymmetric. However, previous studies on asymmetric kernel show that learning via asymmetric kernels can be treated in the same way as symmetric kernels, provided that the kernel is positive definite [14, 15]. *Second*, the kernel is linear to $\mathbf{y}^r$, which enables efficient inference using LP. *Third*, at prediction time, the kernel can be evaluated fast by using pre-trained local binary classifiers.

**Global Binary Model Kernel.** The global binary model kernel $\Theta^{global}$ is constructed in similar fashion to $\Theta^{local}$, but measures how well each edge-label

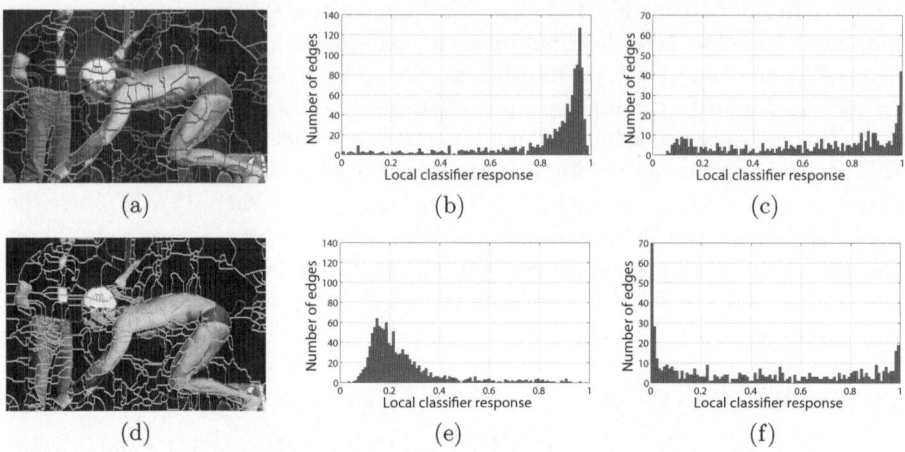

**Fig. 2.** Row 1: The ground-truth label $\mathbf{y}^l$ (a), the histogram of local classifier responses of the edges with ground-truth $y = 1$ (b) and $y = 0$ (c). Row 2: The violated constraint $\bar{\mathbf{y}}^l$ (d) and the histogram of local classifier responses of the edges with ground-truth $y = 1$ (e) and $y = 0$ (f).

pair follows a global merge/split prediction model built using all training samples. The kernel is defined as the product of global classifier responses of two input-output pairs, such as

$$\Theta^{global}((\mathbf{x}^l, \mathbf{y}^l), (\mathbf{x}^r, \mathbf{y}^r))$$

$$= \left[ \frac{1}{|E^{(l)}|} \sum_{e \in E^{(l)}} \sigma(\mathbf{v}^G \cdot \mathbf{f}_e^l + b^G) y_e^l + \left\{ 1 - \sigma(\mathbf{v}^G \cdot \mathbf{f}_e^l + b^G) \right\} (1 - y_e^l) \right]$$

$$\cdot \left[ \frac{1}{|E^{(r)}|} \sum_{e \in E^{(r)}} \sigma(\mathbf{v}^G \cdot \mathbf{f}_e^r + b^G) y_e^r + \left\{ 1 - \sigma(\mathbf{v}^G \cdot \mathbf{f}_e^r + b^G) \right\} (1 - y_e^r) \right] \quad (16)$$

Here, the $\mathbf{v}^G$ is the weight of the global classifier trained with *all* edges existing in the entire training image-label pairs. In contrast to the local binary model kernel in Section 4.1, the global binary model kernel is symmetric. Also, the kernel is linear to $\mathbf{y}^r$, which enables efficient inference using LP.

### 4.2   Image Similarity Kernel

The image similarity kernel $\Lambda(\mathbf{x}^l, \mathbf{x}^r)$ is used to regulate the edge-label similarity kernels presented in Section 4.1. The motivation of this kernel is that for a given test image, the edge prediction should rely more on the training images which are *similar* to the test image, rather than the training images significantly different from the test image. To achieve this property, the image similarity kernel is designed to measure the degree of overlap between the two feature distributions.

By using the image similarity kernel, the given test image reliably refers to the classifiers of training images for which the value of image similarity kernel is high enough. Figure 3 shows the idea of image similarity kernel. On the left side, the two images are quite similar and there is a large overlap between the two feature distributions (orange and green). In this case, the binary model kernels are reliable because the corresponding binary classifier performs well on the edges of the given test image. On the other hand, the two images on the right side are not similar, and the two feature distributions are apart from each other. In this case, the binary model kernels are unreliable, because the corresponding binary classifier does not fit the edges on the given test image. The designed image similarity kernel is similar to the Pyramid Match Kernel(PMK) [16], and formulated as follows:

$$\Lambda(\mathbf{x}^l, \mathbf{x}^r) = \frac{1}{Z} \sum_{d=1}^{D} \sum_{i=0}^{L-1} w_i \mathcal{I}_i(H_d(\mathbf{x}^l), H_d(\mathbf{x}^r)) \tag{17}$$

Here, $Z$ is the normalization constant to make the range of $\Lambda$ to be $[0, 1]$, where $Z = D \times \sum_{i=0}^{L-1} w_i$. $H_d(\mathbf{x})$ is the histogram of $d$th elements of the D-dimensional feature vectors in image $\mathbf{x}$. $\mathcal{I}$ is the histogram intersection function [16] which measures the overlap between the two histogram's bins such as

$$\mathcal{I}(A, B) = \sum_{j=1}^{r} min(A^{(j)}, B^{(j)}), \tag{18}$$

where $A$ and $B$ are histograms with $r$ bins, and $A^{(j)}$ denotes the count of the $j$th bin of $A$. In Eq.(17), $i, L$ and $w_i$ are the index of pyramid level, the total number of levels and the level weights, respectively [16]. In this work, we set $r = 256, L = 5, w_i = 2^{-i}$.

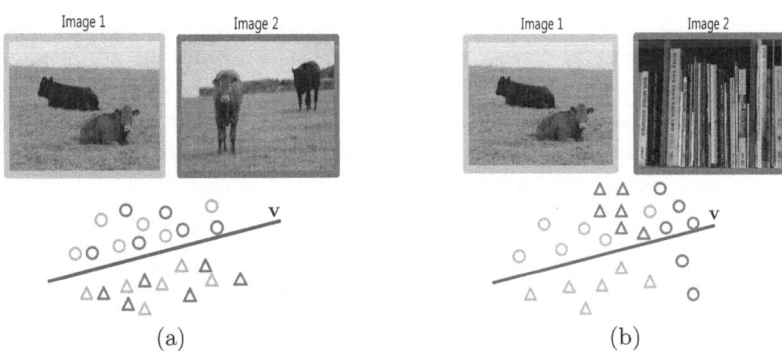

**Fig. 3.** The feature distributions of (a) similar image pair, and (b) dissimilar image pair. In (a), the overlap between the two distributions are large($\Lambda$ is high), while in (b) the two distributions are apart from each other($\Lambda$ is low).

### 4.3   Learning the Relative Weights between Kernels

Because of the additive structure of the proposed joint kernel, the relative weights $\beta_t$ in Eq.(12) and $\gamma_t$ can be learned using Multiple Kernel Learning(MKL) algorithm [17, 18]. In [18], the kernel weights $\{\beta, \gamma\}$ and the support vector weights $\alpha$ are optimized in an alternating way.

## 5   Experiments

To evaluate the effectiveness of the proposed algorithm, three different kinds of experiments are presented:

1. *Segmentation performance with various feature kernels*: To show that the additive structure of the proposed kernel corresponds to the combination of several low-level features, we compare the performance of using each single low-level feature kernel with the performance of using multiple kernels.
2. *Segmentation performance with different kernel combinations*: To show the effectiveness of the three types of proposed kernels ($\Theta^{local}$, $\Theta^{global}$ and $\Lambda$), we evaluate the segmentation performances with different kernel combinations.
3. *Comparison with other algorithms*: To show the effectiveness of the proposed joint-kernel framework, we compare qualitative and quantitative results with other state-of-the art image segmantation algorithms.

### 5.1   Experimental Setup

**Datasets.** Two benchmark datasets are used for evaluation: Berkeley segmentation dataset (BSDS) [19] and Microsoft Research Cambridge dataset (MSRC) [20]. The BSDS contains 300 natural images that explicitly divided into disjoint 200 training image subsets and 100 test images subsets. Since each image of the dataset is segmented by five different human subjects on average, we defined a single probabilistic (real-valued) ground-truth segmentation of each for training. The MSRC dataset contains 591 natural images and 23 object classes with pixelwise labeling. We seperate the whole dataset into 45% training, 10% validation, and 45% test subsets, following [20]. The performance was evaluated using the clean ground-truth object instance labeling of [21]. On average, all algorithms used in the experiment are set to produce 30 disjoint regions on BSDS dataset and 15 disjoint regions on MSRC dataset.

**Data Preparation.** The input superpixel images are obtained by gPb contour detector and the oriented watershed transform [22]. We initially obtained the edge labels from the boundaries of the baseline superpixels (374 superpixels per image in BSDS, 732 superpixels per image in MSRC ) and then use these boundary edge information to conduct experiments. The average number of edges in each image are 2072 for BSDS dataset and 1035 for MSRC dataset, respectively.

**Feature Vector.** For the low-level feature, the following pairwise feature vectors that reflect the correspondence between adjacent superpixels are used.

1. Color difference (26-dim): The RGB/HSV color distances(absolute differences, $\chi^2$-distances, earth mover's distances) between two adjacent superpixels.
2. Texture difference (29-dim) : The texture distances(absolute differences, $\chi^2$-distances, earth mover's distances) between two adjacent superpixels.
3. Shape/localtion difference (5-dim): The 5-dimensional shape/location feature proposed in [23].

**Performance Metric.** Four performance metrics are used to evaluate the proposed algorithm as follows: probabilistic Rand index (PRI) [24], variation of information (VOI) [25], segmentation covering (SCO) [22], and boundary displacement error (BDE) [26]. As the predicted segmentation is close to the ground-truth segmentation, the PRI and SCO are increased while the VOI and BDE are decreased.

## 5.2 Experimental Results

**Segmentation Performance with Various Feature Kernels.** The goal of this experiment is to validate the additive structure of the proposed kernel in Eq.(12), where the total kernel is defined as a multiple kernel which is a linear combination of several single kernels constructed with single low-level feature. For this, we compare the segmentation performance of the multiple kernel with the performances when only single kernel is used. The results are shown in Table 1. On both datasets, the performance of the multiple kernel at the last line is better than each single kernel in the first three rows. This observation draws a straightforward but important conclusion: adding more kernels has the same effect as increasing the feature dimension, which leads to performance improvement.

**Table 1.** Segmentation performance with different feature combinations

| Dataset | BSDS | | | | MSRC | | | |
|---|---|---|---|---|---|---|---|---|
| Feature type | PRI | VOI | SCO | BDE | PRI | VOI | SCO | BDE |
| Color(26dim) | 0.782 | 1.915 | 0.566 | 12.640 | 0.765 | 1.766 | 0.612 | 11.092 |
| Texture(29dim) | 0.752 | 2.172 | 0.502 | 13.860 | 0.755 | 2.010 | 0.572 | 10.295 |
| shpae/location(5dim) | 0.765 | 2.468 | 0.483 | 15.537 | 0.743 | 2.201 | 0.549 | 11.571 |
| Multiple(60dim) | **0.792** | **1.905** | **0.567** | **11.710** | **0.780** | **1.621** | **0.632** | **9.588** |

**Segmentation Performance with different Kernel Combinations.** The goal of this experiment is to demonstrate the effectiveness of three component kernels proposed in this paper: The local binary model kernel ($\Theta^{local}$), global binary model kernel ($\Theta^{global}$) and image similarity kernel ($\Lambda$). For this, we compared the segmentation performances using three different kernel combinations,

**Table 2.** Segmentation performance with different kernel combinations

| Dataset | BSDS | | | | MSRC | | | |
|---|---|---|---|---|---|---|---|---|
| Kernel type | PRI | VOI | SCO | BDE | PRI | VOI | SCO | BDE |
| $\Theta^{local}$ | 0.788 | 1.980 | 0.552 | 11.776 | 0.772 | 1.648 | 0.621 | 10.686 |
| $\Theta^{local} + \Theta^{global}$ | 0.790 | **1.903** | 0.566 | **11.686** | 0.773 | 1.645 | 0.626 | 10.348 |
| $\Lambda(\Theta^{local} + \Theta^{global})$ | **0.792** | 1.905 | **0.567** | 11.710 | **0.780** | **1.621** | **0.632** | **9.588** |

and the results are shown in Table 2. For both datasets, the combination of local and global kernel (middle) improves the performances compared to using local kernel only (top). The result shows that the errors caused by ambiguities of local classifiers can be compensated by the global classifier to some degree. In the bottom line, performances with image similarity kernel are presented. For MSRC dataset, the usage of $\Lambda$ clearly improves the performance, while for BSDS dataset it does not. One reasonable explanation about this phenomenon is as follows. In the MSRC dataset, the images of the same class are quite similar to each other, and the effect of image similarity kernel is clear in this case since for a given test image, the kernel gives more weight to the similar training images for prediction. In contrast, in the BSDS dataset, all images look much different from each other, and the image similarity kernel is not effective in this case.

**Comparison with Other Algorithms.** In this experiment, the proposed algorithm is compared to the following state-of-the-art image segmentation algorithms: gPb-owt-ucm [22], gPb-Hoiem [23] and pairwise correlation clustering [6]. The result is presented in Table 3. For MSRC dataset, the proposed joint-kernel algorithm achieves the best performances on all segmentation metrics. Remarkably, the proposed algorithm outperforms the pairwise correlation clustering [6] which uses linear discriminant function with explicit joint feature map

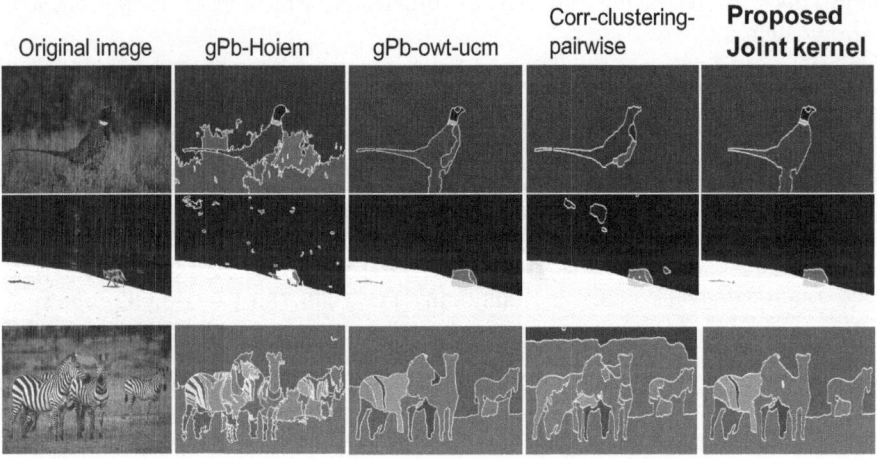

**Fig. 4.** Qualitative segmentation results on BSDS dataset

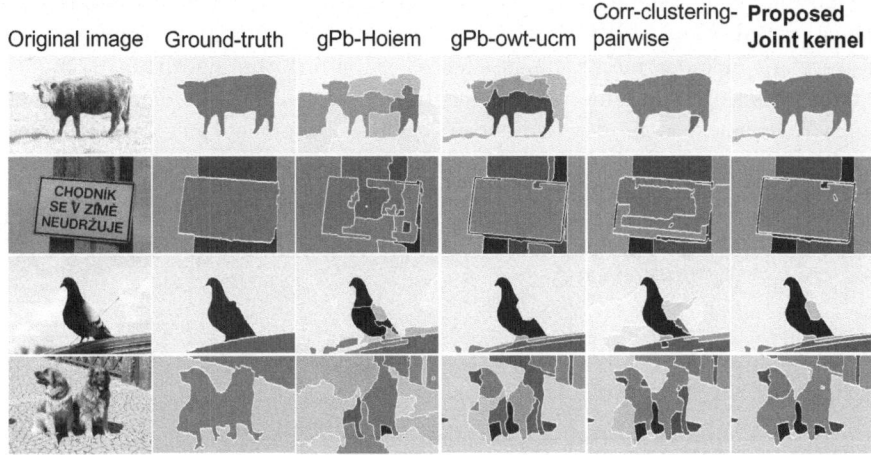

**Fig. 5.** Qualitative segmentation results on MSRC dataset

**Table 3.** Quantitative results of image segmentation

| Dataset | BSDS | | | | MSRC | | | |
|---|---|---|---|---|---|---|---|---|
| Algorithm | PRI | VOI | SCO | BDE | PRI | VOI | SCO | BDE |
| gPb-Hoiem [23] | 0.776 | 2.268 | 0.507 | 13.266 | 0.615 | 2.915 | 0.341 | 14.367 |
| gPb-owt-ucm [22] | **0.794** | 1.909 | **0.571** | **11.461** | 0.779 | 1.675 | 0.628 | 9.800 |
| Corr-Cluster-Pairwise [6] | 0.792 | 1.960 | 0.558 | 11.598 | 0.761 | 1.722 | 0.605 | 9.686 |
| **Proposed Joint-kernel** | 0.792 | **1.905** | 0.567 | 11.710 | **0.780** | **1.621** | **0.632** | **9.588** |

as in Eq.(1). For BSDS dataset, the state-of-the art gPb-owt-ucm shows the best performance. However, the performance of the proposed algorithm is not only comparable, but still outperforms the pairwise correlation clustering. Figure 4 and Figure 5 show some example segmentations on BSDS and MSRC datasets, respectively.

## 6   Conclusion

In this paper, an image segmentation algorithm based on correlation clustering using non-linear discriminant function has been presented to solve the limitations of linear model. The main contribution is the design of joint-kernel function, which incorporates the correlation between two input-output pairs. Instead of using explicit joint feature function, the proposed algorithm tries to find a better joint feature that is embedded in a properly-designed joint-kernel function. The experimental results showed that the joint feature map implicitly embedded in the proposed joint-kernel function works comparable or even better than the explicitly defined high-dimensional joint feature function used in the predominant linear structured prediction model. The proposed algorithm showed comparable image segmentation performance with several state-of-the-art algorithms on BSDS and MSRC datasets, both quantitatively and qualitatively. Our future work includes many things such as extending the algorithm to higher-order correlation clustering, improving binary model kernels using non-linear binary classifier, designing kernel which considers output-output correlation and developing more promising image similarity kernel.

**Acknowledgement.** This work was supported by the National Research Foundation of Korea(NRF) grant funded by the Korea government(MEST) (No.2012-0005378 and No.2012-0000985).

# References

1. Blaschko, M.B., Lampert, C.H.: Learning to Localize Objects with Structured Output Regression. In: Forsyth, D., Torr, P., Zisserman, A. (eds.) ECCV 2008, Part I. LNCS, vol. 5302, pp. 2–15. Springer, Heidelberg (2008)
2. Blaschko, M., Lampert, C.: Object localization with global and local context kernels. In: BMVC (2009)
3. Ladicky, L., Russell, C., Kohli, P., Torr, P.H.S.: Associative hierarchical crfs for object class image segmentation. In: ICCV, pp. 739–746 (2009)
4. Lempitsky, V., Vedaldi, A., Zisserman, A.: A Pylon Model for Semantic Segmentation. In: NIPS (2011)
5. Nowozin, S., Jegelka, S.: Solution stability in linear programming relaxations: Graph partitioning and unsupervised learning. In: ICML (2009)
6. Kim, S., Nowozin, S., Kohli, P., Yoo, C.D.: Higher-Order Correlation Clustering for Image Segmentation. In: NIPS (2011)
7. Bertelli, L., Yu, T., Vu, D., Gokturk, B.: Kernelized structural SVM learning for supervised object segmentation. In: CVPR, pp. 2153–2160 (2011)
8. Joachims, T., Finley, T., Yu, C.N.J.: Cutting-plane training of structural SVMs. Machine Learning 77, 27–59 (2009)
9. Chopra, S., Rao, M.R.: The partition problem. Mathematical Programming 59, 87–115 (1993)
10. Tsochantaridis, I., Joachims, T., Hofmann, T.: Large Margin Methods for Structured and Interdependent Output Variables. JMLR 6, 1453–1484 (2005)
11. Vapnik, V.: Statistical Learning Theory. Wiley and Sons Inc., New York (1998)
12. Taskar, B., Guestrin, C., Koller, D.: Max-margin Markov networks. In: NIPS (2003)
13. Kelley, J.E.: The cutting-plane method for solving convex programs. Journal of the Society for Industrial Applied Mathematics 8, 703–712 (1960)
14. Tsuda, K.: Support vector classifier with asymmetric kernel functions. In: European Symposium on Artificial Neural Networks (1999)
15. Wu, W., Xu, J., Li, H., Oyama, S.: Asymmetric Kernel Learning. Microsoft Technical Report (2010)
16. Grauman, K., Darrell, T.: The pyramid match kernel: Discriminative classification with sets of image features. In: ICCV, pp. 1458–1465 (2005)
17. Lanckriet, G.R.G., Cristianini, N., Bartlett, P., Ghaoui, L.E., Jordan, M.I.: Learning the kernel matrix with semidefinite programming. JMLR 5, 27–72 (2004)
18. Rakotomamonjy, A., Bach, F., Canu, S., Grandvalet, Y.: SimpleMKL. JMLR 9, 2491–2521 (2008)

19. Martin, D., Fowlkes, C., Tal, D., Malik, J.: A Database of Human Segmented Natural Images and its Application to Evaluating Segmentation Algorithms and Measuring Ecological Statistics. In: ICCV, pp. 416–423 (2001)
20. Shotton, J., Winn, J., Rother, C., Criminisi, A.: *TextonBoost*: Joint Appearance, Shape and Context Modeling for Multi-class Object Recognition and Segmentation. In: Leonardis, A., Bischof, H., Pinz, A. (eds.) ECCV 2006. LNCS, vol. 3951, pp. 1–15. Springer, Heidelberg (2006)
21. Malisiewicz, T., Efros, A.A.: Improving spatial support for objects via multiple segmentations. In: BVMC (2007)
22. Arbelaez, P., Maire, M., Fowlkes, C., Malik, J.: Contour detection and hierarchical image segmentation. IEEE TPAMI 33, 898–916 (2011)
23. Hoiem, D., Efros, A.A., Hebert, M.: Recovering surface layout from an image. IJCV 75, 151–172 (2007)
24. Rand, W.M.: Objective criteria for the evaluation of clustering methods. Journal of the American Statistical Association, 846–850 (1971)
25. Meila, M.: Comparing clusterings: an axiomatic view. In: ICML, pp. 577–584 (2005)
26. Freixenet, J., Muñoz, X., Raba, D., Martí, J., Cufí, X.: Yet Another Survey on Image Segmentation: Region and Boundary Information Integration. In: Heyden, A., Sparr, G., Nielsen, M., Johansen, P. (eds.) ECCV 2002, Part III. LNCS, vol. 2352, pp. 408–422. Springer, Heidelberg (2002)

# Application of Heterogenous Motion Models towards Structure Recovery from Motion

Rohith M.V. and Chandra Kambhamettu

Video/Image Modeling and Synthesis (VIMS) Lab,
Dept. of Computer and Information Sciences, University of Delaware,
Delaware, USA
{rohithmv,chandrak}@udel.edu

**Abstract.** Non-rigid structure estimates are often performed under the assumption that linear combination of a few rigid basis shapes can describe the deformation. However, the quality of reconstruction suffers as the number of basis shapes increase. When a natural video (which may contain rigid, articulated and non-rigid objects together with camera motion) is to be processed, the complexity of motion precludes use of rigid SFM methods. We propose that this problem may be approached using the notions of heterogeneity, articulation and stationarity. In this paper, we present a scheme for structure recovery based on motion classification and automatic selection of reconstruction algorithms for each scene object. Rigid, low-rank non-rigid and articulated structures are reconstructed separately. Using sub-sequence stationarity graphs, these are stitched together to form a coherent structure. We tested our method on data from human motion capture for objective analysis and provide results on natural videos.

## 1 Introduction

Non-rigid structure from motion algorithms are being explored for a variety of applications such as 2D to 3D conversion of existing video sequences, human motion analysis and human computer interaction. It is often achieved by analyzing the trajectories of a sparse set of feature points over the length of the given sequence. Movement of feature points in monocular imagery depends on camera motion as well as deformation of objects in the scene. Separating these components is especially difficult when the deformation in the scene is complex. To render the problem tractable, several assumptions have been proposed - the non-rigid structure can be composed from linear combinations of basis structures [1–3], the non-rigid component is small or the scene is made of piecewise rigid structures [4]. There have also been different models of non-rigid deformations such as multiple rigid motions [5], surface deformation [6] and articulated motion [7]. These works attempt to recover the geometry of the entire scene using a single model of deformation. However, schemes that use motion segmentation [8, 9] to handle regions of scene differently are also being explored [10–12]. These schemes are motivated from observations in natural videos which contain purely

K.M. Lee et al. (Eds.): ACCV 2012, Part I, LNCS 7724, pp. 622–635, 2013.
© Springer-Verlag Berlin Heidelberg 2013

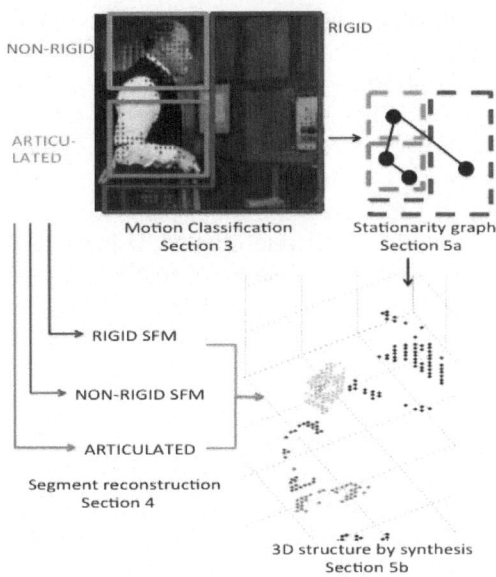

**Fig. 1.** Our scheme for estimating 3D structure from videos. Multiple reconstructions are obtained from appropriate SFM algorithms automatically selected using motion classification. Using a sub-sequence stationarity graphs, these reconstructions are synthesized into a coherent structure.

articulated objects or a combination of rigid and non-rigid objects. In this paper, we attempt to improve structure estimation by exploiting the following features often found in natural videos :

- Heterogeneity - Not all the features in the scene undergo non-rigid motion.
- Articulation - Groups of features may have rigidity constraints.
- Stationarity - Non-rigid motion of features may be intermittent.

The above characteristics are especially true in cases of sequences where the camera is in motion while capturing a static background scene and deforming foreground objects (often referred to as tracking or dolly shots). Del Bue *et al.*[10] have explored partially rigid scenes in the context of face modeling. Fayad *et al.*[11] and MV *et al.*[12] use motion segmentation to identify articulated objects in the scene. The main contributions of our method are: (i) an automatic method for reconstructing a heterogeneous non-rigid scene using motion segmentation and deformation analysis (ii) a novel method of synthesis of reconstructions from independent models using sub-sequence stationarity. Though works such as [10–12] have used motion segmentation towards registration, they each have relatively simple models of non-rigid motion and cannot respond to the heterogeneities in the scene. Our algorithm uses characteristics of feature trajectories to apply a suitable combination of rigid and non-rigid SFM algorithms.

As outlined in Figure 1, the feature tracks are first segmented and classified into rigid, low-rank non-rigid and articulated motions. Depending on the nature of deformation found in each segment, a suitable algorithm for reconstruction is automatically selected. When sections of the scene are independently reconstructed, the spatial relation between them cannot be estimated as the various reconstructions may have different global scales and orientations. For this, we introduce the notion of sub-sequence stationarity - that is intervals of similar motion among feature tracks of different objects. Using such intervals of relative rigidity among the segments, the ambiguity of spatial relations may be removed. Note that this does not require all parts of the scene to be rigid at the same interval. Based on the relative motion between the various segments at various intervals in the sequence, a graph is built that decides propagation of global motion estimates. This enables synthesis of structures estimated in the previous step to create a coherent reconstruction of the scene.

As the initial segmentation is carried out based on characteristics of feature tracks, our method does not require prior information about the number of objects, geometry of the articulated links or surface templates. The proposed method is applicable even when a scene contains a mixture of motions, as the automatic selection of motion models ensures that a suitable algorithm is applied for each of them. The alignment issues faced in [11] do not affect our method as we exploit the sub-sequence stationarity to obtain the spatial relations. Though this assumes relative rigidity between segments during the scene, we observe that this is often satisfied in natural videos. If information about the camera motion or calibration is available, it can be easily incorporated into the reconstruction of rigid segments and the method automatically carries it over to other segments.

We apply our method to datasets generated with real 3D structures and synthetic camera motion in order to provide insight into the working of the method and provide objective analysis of performance. We also test our method on a variety of real datasets to demonstrate its efficacy. Comparisons with other motion segmentation methods demonstrate that our method is more generic in terms of the feature point distribution and complexity of motion. We describe our approach to segmentation and classification of motion in section 3. In section 4, we present the methods we use for structure estimation of segments and in section 5 we present the synthesis using sub-sequence stationarity. We present results on human motion and natural videos in section 6 and conclude in section 7.

## 2   Background

### 2.1   Motion Segmentation

Successfully segmenting regions of a video based on their motion is often dependent on the nature of the deformations present. Vidal *et al.* [8] use GPCA based framework to identify multiple rigid motions. Del Bue *et al.* [10] employ deformability index [13] to segment the scene into rigid and non-rigid parts. The method is based on motion trajectories lying in different subspaces. However, these methods cannot be applied to articulated motion as there is a considerable overlap in the subspaces of trajectories which are connected. To segment articulated motions, Yan and Pollefeys [9] propose a method based on spectral clustering of affinity derived from principal angles between the subspaces to segment subspaces. They also provide a graph algorithm which constructs a kinematic chain based on shared subspaces. This method cannot be extended to complex objects due to the restriction of minimum number of samples required (which grows exponentially with number of subspaces [11]). Ross et al. [7] use probabilistic graphical models to estimate the evolution of joint angles and classification of features to links. There have also been other methods which use link length constraints to estimate joint angles [14]. However, since they use sample consensus as their underlying mechanism for grouping trajectories, they perform poorly on limited tracks available in most video sequences. Fayad et al. [11] pose segmentation of articulated motion as a labeling problem. Pairwise costs are assigned depending on the reprojection errors and graph-cut based optimization is used to solve for labels. Since this approach depends heavily on the spatial proximity of points of the same segment, it may not be feasible in cases where the points are unevenly distributed across segments of articulated objects. We use a segmentation approach close to [12], which performs motion segmentation using subspace clustering as in [9], but employs a different affinity function that is insensitive to distance of feature point from the axis of articulation. In addition, we also analyze the resultant subspaces using deformability index [13] to obtain the nature of non-rigid motion present in the segment.

## 2.2 Non-rigid Structure from Motion

As noted earlier, a number of non-rigid structure from motion algorithms have been proposed [1, 2, 4] which perform structure recovery for all the scene points in a uniform manner. Akhter et al.[15] use DCT basis for trajectory bases to obtain a dual representation of SFM problem. In this paper however, as we concentrate on heterogenous treatment of scene points based on segmentation, we restrict our discussion of related works to those that handle articulated motion and combinations of multiple motion types. Tresadern and Reid [14] use factorization to solve purely articulated motion based on segmentation using RANSAC. Paladini et al. [3] present a method based on iterative factorization. The estimates are projected onto a manifold of metric constraints to preserve the relation between points of the same sub-model (or link in the case of articulated structures). This method provides alternate methods of handling articulated and general non-rigid deformation. It does not include a method to automatically select the appropriate algorithm for a given scene. Gotardo and Martinez [16] use complementary rank 3 subspaces to reconstruct complex motion using single factorization. Tresadern and Reid [17] utilize a rank constraint based factorization algorithm to align video sequences based on deformation. Fayad et al. [11] solve the problem of articulated structure from motion using the factorization with constraints on rotation matrices. This method independently reconstructs each segment in a different frame of reference and hence needs a post-processing

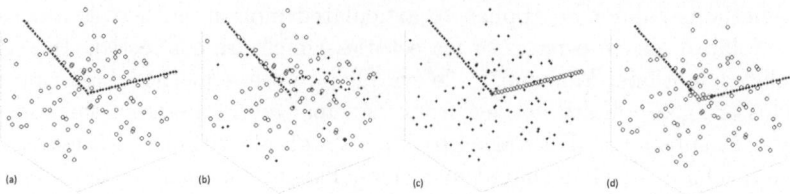

**Fig. 2.** Comparison of motion segmentation algorithms. The data was generated by adding an articulated object with a single link within a rigidly moving random point cloud. In each figure, the hollow and filled markers indicate points identified as rigid points and non-rigid respectively. (a) Ground Truth (b) Method of principal angles [9] (c) Method using deformability index [10] (d) Our method.

step of stitching the segments to provide a coherent reconstruction. They use 3D Euclidean distances between pairs of corresponding points as a measure of alignment. Though the method performs well on purely articulated objects, it cannot be easily extended to scenes that involve rigid and non-rigid parts. The method assumes that the stitched components are all physically connected. This assumption may not be true in cases where an object is disjoint from the scene. The method by Del Bue *et al.* [10], which handles rigid and non-rigid components, assumes that these two components can still be described together using a small number of basis shapes. This assumption holds for scenes with single objects such as faces, but is violated in scenes such as Figure 1 where the non-rigid object is separate from the rigid background. This also affects the method of hierarchical non-rigid SFM [12] which separates the low-rank non-rigid and articulated motion. Our method does not suffer from these disadvantages as we exploit sub-sequence stationarity to merge various segments.

## 3    Motion Segmentation and Classification

Since our scheme aims at reconstructing objects in the scene based on their rigidity, we start with dividing the feature trajectories in a video sequence into different segments. The segmentation is performed using a variant of the algorithm proposed in [12] which is sensitive to proximity of features. This algorithm is designed to identify articulated motions and disjoint motion segments. We use it to classify the segments into articulated and non-articulated segments. The non-articulated segments may actually be either rigid or non-rigid segments. These are identified using deformability index [13] subsequently. We now discuss the details of segmentation and classification steps.

### 3.1    Motion Segmentation

Given the observation matrix $W$ constructed from the coordinates of the feature trajectories, we estimate a preliminary motion and shape estimate using factorization in the form $W = CMAS$[12]. Though this does not represent the actual motion and structure matrices, the subspace properties shown in [9, 12] ensure that trajectories of feature points that move rigidly with respect to each other lie in the same subspace. Equation 1 shows the affinity measure suggested in [12]. $H_{ij}$ represents the affinity between the features $i$ and $j$, where $S_i$ is the $i^{th}$ column of shape matrix $S$ and $^+$ represents the pseudo-inverse.

$$H_{ij} = \exp(- \sum_{1 \leq k \leq K} | [S_i \ S_j] ([S_i \ S_j]^+ S_k) - S_k|^2) \tag{1}$$

We define a modified affinity measure $H'_{ij}$ which includes the average Euclidean distance between the feature points $(u_{ij})$, as $H'_{ij} = H_{ij} + \alpha \exp(-u_{ij})$. Here $\alpha$ controls the weight of proximity over trajectory similarity and $K$ is the number of feature points. We then use the normalized cuts [18] algorithm to segment the various segments. We will refer to these groups of trajectories as motion segments.

An example of this segmentation scheme is shown in Figure 2 which compares our method with a method that performs articulated motion segmentation [9] and a method for separating rigid and non-rigid motion based on deformability index [10]. We see that our method performs better than both the compared methods. In case the background feature points of a scene is spread over the image in different locations (such as in Figure 1), this method may identify them as different motion segments due to the proximity term in the affinity function. This is handled in the next step of motion classification. However, this implies that we cannot build the kinematic chain based on the results of segmentation algorithm alone as there may be rigid points in the scene that may be close to the articulated motion segments and using a proximity based linking may result in erroneous kinematic chains. Hence, we build kinematic chains only after the multiple rigid segments are grouped and separated. We tested our motion segmentation algorithm on the Hopkins 155 Motion segmentation dataset [19] and achieved an overall segmentation accuracy of 90.02% (cases in which the number of motion segments were correctly identified). More details are available in the supplementary material.

### 3.2 Motion Classification

Once segments are identified, we need to distinguish between rigid segments and those containing low-rank non-rigid motion. Any separated rigid components which are part of the same object (or which share common global rotation and translation) are then joined. To perform the classification of segments, we employ a measure of deformation called deformability index [13] which has proven effective in human gait studies and other non-rigid motion problems. The deformability index is a measure of the number of basis shape components needed to model the deformation observed in the scene. Hence, if the scene is completely rigid, the deformation index is one and it increases with the complexity of the deformation. For each non-articulated motion segment, we classify it as a rigid segment if its deformability index is less than or equal to 1.5. Though the index is ideally 1 for rigid segments, additional basis shapes are sometimes needed to handle tracking noise which does not fit the distribution assumed in estimating the index. Other non-articulated motion segments with higher index are classified as non-rigid. The motion segmentation accuracy depends on the complexity of the scene and feature tracking errors. We have simulated such errors by artificially changing the segmentation results and the results are presented in section 6.

Since there may be feature trajectories in a video that may be physically distant but share the same motion model (for example feature points belonging to background of the scene separated in the image due to a foreground object), we must combine such rigid components together. Motion segments that are classified as either non-rigid or articulated are excluded from this test. The remaining rigid objects are combined pairwise to check if they can be described using the same model. If $W_1$ and $W_2$ contain the columns of the observation matrix $W$ that belong to two motion segments, we estimate the rank of the matrix $W'_{12}$ given by equation 2, where $\tilde{W}_1$ and $\tilde{W}_2$ are columns of $W_1$ and $W_2$ modified so that each row of $W'_{12}$ has a zero mean. Although a scene may have many feature tracks, they will be grouped into a few motion segments. Hence, the check for shared motion model may be performed by checking pairs of segments.

$$W'_{12} = [\tilde{W}_1, \tilde{W}_2] \tag{2}$$

Since the absolute rank of $W'_{12}$ may be large, we check for approximate rank using the method in [8]. If the rank is close to three [10], the segments are combined into the same rigid segment. Once all the rigid segments are identified, the remainder of the segments classified as articulated in the previous step are processed to build kinematic chains. As the global rigid components are now removed, the articulated segments can now be linked together based on proximity between their extremal points in the subspace (as in [12]). The results of motion classification can be seen in Figure 4 middle column. Using the classification performed in this stage, we can choose the appropriate structure estimation algorithm for each segment (Section 4).

## 4   Structure Estimation

Non-rigid structure estimates are often performed under the assumption that a few rigid basis shapes may be linearly combined to describe the deformation. As shown in [3, 11, 12], the quality of reconstruction suffers as the number of basis shapes increase. When a natural video (which may contain rigid, articulated and non-rigid objects together with camera motion) is to be processed, the complexity of motion precludes use of methods such as [1, 2]. Instead, if a method handles the various objects separately, suitable algorithms may be applied to each segment based on the motion observed (Section 3). In this section, we describe the algorithms we use for each type of segment.

$$
W_r = \begin{bmatrix} R_1 \\ R_2 \\ \vdots \\ R_N \end{bmatrix} \begin{bmatrix} s_1 & s_2 & \cdots & s_K \end{bmatrix} \tag{3}
$$

**Rigid Segments:** The rigid segments contain trajectories which do not deform during the entire video sequence. Common rigid segments include the static background in a given scene (e.g., the book case and the chair in the Marple2 sequence shown in Figure 1). The rigid feature trajectories are dependent only on their fixed geometry in the scene and camera motion. Hence the observation matrix of rigid scene trajectories $W_r$ can be written as in Equation 3, which describes an observation matrix of $N$ frames of video with $K$ rigid points. Each $R_i$ is a $2 \times 3$ matrix and each $s_j$ is a 3x1 vector. The observation of a point $i$ during frame $j$, which is a 2x1 vector of image coordinates is given by $R_j s_i$.

We note that the $W_r$ matrix is preprocessed to center the points in each frame to remove the translational component of the camera/scene motion. There are a variety of algorithms available for rigid structure estimation, however we use the method by Oliensis and Hartley [20] which is provided as part of SFM toolbox [21]. We also use bundle adjustment to refine the estimated structure and motion parameters.

**Non-rigid Segments:** Some objects in the scene such as human faces, clothes and other objects undergo deformation which may be effectively modeled (in isolation) by a linear combination of basis shapes. To clarify the point further, the linear combination model holds only when feature trajectories of a single object are considered. In this case, we use the model in Equation 4. It represents the observation matrix $W_{nr}$ of $K$ feature points over $N$ frames factorized into $M$ basis shapes. $l_{ij}$ represents the contribution of $j$th model to the $i$th frame whereas $s_{uv}$ represents the coordinate of $u$th point in the basis shape $v$.

$$
W_{nr} = \begin{bmatrix} l_{11}R_1 & \cdots & l_{1M}R_1 \\ \vdots & \ddots & \vdots \\ l_{N1}R_N & \cdots & l_{NM}R_N \end{bmatrix} \begin{bmatrix} s_{11} & \cdots & s_{K1} \\ \vdots & \ddots & \vdots \\ s_{1M} & \cdots & s_{KM} \end{bmatrix} \tag{4}
$$

After experimenting with a number of algorithms, we found two algorithms that seem to perform well for these segments. The first is the method of hierarchical priors proposed by Torresani et al.[2] and the other is method of metric reproductions by Paladini et al. [3]. We present results with both the algorithms.

**Articulated Segments:** Articulated objects in natural videos commonly consist of human limbs, although they may include robotic arms and other appliances when an industrial setting is encountered. Such objects are often characterized by rigid segments which rotate relative to each other on a joint or pivot. The trajectories of all the points that belong to one link or section of the object lie on a linear subspace [9]. This allows the trajectories to be ordered or sorted, enabling us to identify the extreme or pivotal points of each link. Since no prior information is available about the nature of objects present in the scene, we assume that each joint is a universal joint, allowing the link connected to undergo motion with two degrees of freedom. Intuitively, the degrees of freedom represent rotation within and out of the image plane. Using each pair of points on a given link, we can obtain an estimate of these angles. Due to tracking error and movement of feature points parallel to the axis of rotation (e.g., sliding of shirt along the arm), some of these estimates may be inaccurate. These are handled using sample consensus to eliminate outliers. Note that the sign of the out of plane angle cannot be resolved by this method, however this is handled in the synthesis section. We reconstruct the articulated segments using the method presented in [12].

## 5   Synthesis of Multiple Structures

Since the reconstructions are performed independently in Section 4, they exist in different frames of reference. These have to be synthesized into a single reconstruction to get a coherent structure estimate. Fayad *et al.* [11] perform this using 3D Euclidean distance between corresponding points of different structures. However, to guarantee a valid reconstruction, their method requires that all the structures be physically connected. That is, all the structures must be part of a single object. This poses great restriction when applied to scenes containing multiple objects. Hence, we propose an alternate method of synthesis which does not depend on physical connectivity between scene elements.

Our method is based on the observation that, in natural videos, parts of different objects may become stationary with respect to each other during a small interval during the video sequence. Note that, if an object in a scene is never stationary with respect to any other object in the scene, its relative position cannot be determined with certainty using feature trajectories alone (occlusions and other cues may be used to obtain depth ordering). Though, at first, this appears as a severe restriction on the videos that can be analyzed, we observed that most natural videos satisfy stationarity. This is because, in case of deforming objects, it is sufficient if part of the object becomes stationary with respect to another object. For example, if we consider a video of a human running, it is sufficient that only the arm or the leg become stationary with respect to a background object. Since videos are often captured at a suitably high enough frame rate, we can extract several frames where the motion of an arm, leg or torso is quite small. We use tests of rigidity on feature trajectories to identify such regions of sub-sequence stationarity. A graph is built by identifying the pairwise rigid relations at different intervals in the sequence. The pairs of segments are reconstructed together in their stationary intervals to obtain their relative spatial relations. Corresponding complete reconstructions of segments are warped to match this arrangement.

## 5.1   Sub-sequence Stationarity

Whenever the feature tracks of two motions segments move together in the video as if they are part of one rigid object, we refer to them as being stationary with respect to each other. Segments may be stationary with respect to each other for the whole duration of the video sequence (different objects in a static background) or only during a short interval within the sequence. Let $W_1$ and $W_2$ be the columns of observation matrix containing the feature tracks of two motions segments. If these segments are relatively stationary in frames $i$ to $j$, then they satisfy Equation 5.

$$\text{rank}(\widehat{W_1}) = \text{rank}(\widehat{W_2}) = \text{rank}([\widehat{W_1}, \widehat{W_2}]) \qquad (5)$$

Here $\widehat{W_1}$ and $\widehat{W_2}$ contain the rows of $W_1$ and $W_2$ corresponding to the frames $i$ through $j$. This relation may be shown to hold based on the rank property of observation matrices containing rigidly moving feature points. By checking the validity of the above relation, we can identify pairwise stationary intervals of segments. To make the problem computationally tractable, we use fixed windows of 8 frames with an overlap of 4 frames. For set of 8 frames, the column subspace of the corresponding rows of the observation matrices is computed using SVD factorization. The column eigenvectors corresponding to the three largest singular values are retained. If the tracks of $W_2$ can be reconstructed using the column basis vectors extracted from $W_1$, then they can be treated as rigid segments. Though limiting the window size may be considered somewhat restrictive, it is necessary to reduce the computational complexity. Using preset windows as mentioned above, the subspace basis for each of the column vectors will only need to be identified once and the rigidity of several segments can be verified in parallel. We choose a threshold of reconstruction error based on the estimate of feature tracking error to decide whether a pair of segments can be classified as stationary. An alternate algorithm may be devised using the technique of Generalized SVD, but it would require a new decomposition for each pair of segments.

After all the pairwise stationary segments are identified, we construct a graph with the motion segments as nodes. An edge is introduced between two segments if they are relatively stationary during some interval. Note that, multiple edges may be introduced between nodes if there is more than one interval of stationarity and multiple paths may exist between pairs of nodes in the graph. To obtain a single path for propagation, we extract the minimum spanning tree of the graph using corresponding subspace reconstruction errors as weights. Sample graphs may be seen in Figure 4. The root of spanning tree is identified as the motion segment that undergoes least deformation (usually the segment which covers the static background features).

## 5.2   Alignment of Structures from Combined and Individual Estimates

Consider the structure estimates from two rigid motion segments $W_1$ and $W_2$ as $S_1$ and $S_2$, respectively (individual reconstructions containing all frames). There

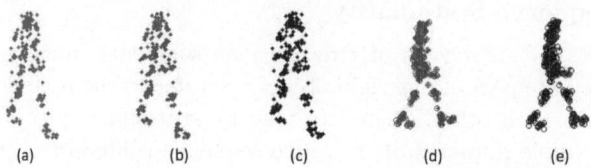

**Fig. 3.** Reconstruction of human motion data. (a) Ground truth 3D points for frame 300. (b) 3D Reconstruction from our method using [3] (c) 3D Reconstruction from our method using [2] (d) Overlay of reconstruction (b) with ground truth (e) Overlay of reconstruction in (c) with ground truth.

are no feature points common between the two segments, as motion segments are disjoint. However, using the stationary sub-sequences identified in the previous subsection, we can obtain new reconstructions containing feature points from pairs of stationary segments. Following the notation of the previous subsection, the observation matrices $[\widehat{W_1}, \widehat{W_2}]$ is reconstructed using the rigid SFM methods discussed in the earlier section. We refer to the resultant set of 3D points as $\hat{S_{12}}$. This result may be improved by using the camera motion estimate from the SFM results of $W_1$ or $W_2$ (individual reconstructions containing all frames) as an initialization for the factorization process. The choice is resolved by picking the segment with the lowest deformability index.

The reconstructions of stationary frames provide us with a frame of reference which describes the spatial relation between the points belonging to different motion segments. We are now able to perform alignment of different motion segments using the sub-sequence reconstruction as an intermediate reference. This is illustrated in Equation 6 where the transformations $T_1$ and $T_2$ aligns the points from $S_1$ and $S_2$ to $\widehat{S_{12}}$ respectively.

$$S_1 \xrightarrow{T_1} \widehat{S_{12}} \underset{T_2}{\overset{T_2^{-1}}{\rightleftharpoons}} S_2. \tag{6}$$

The points in $S_1$ can now be transformed into the reference frame of $S_2$ using the transformation $T_1 T_2^{-1}$. The reconstructions of uncalibrated algorithms are in general related by a bijective mapping between projective spaces (*collineation*) and hence this must be the nature of $T_1$ and $T_2$. This is estimated using by minimizing the distance between the two point sets in the projective sense using the least squares method [22]. If the structures $S_1$ and $S_2$ are not rigid, then the transformations are estimated based on the average structure observed during the interval of stationarity.

Using the tree generated in the previous subsection, we can now align the point sets incrementally along the paths of the tree till all the point sets are aligned with the root node. To reiterate, unlike [11], we do not need the feature points from the motion segments to be physically connected to estimate their spatial relation.

# 6    Results

## 6.1    Human Motion Data

For quantitative results on human motion, we used the MOCAP data from Motion capture lab at CMU Graphics Lab [23] and augmented it by adding a static object. The data consists of a human walking with 255 points tracked on the body. There is considerable articulation of the leg (including knees), but the arm does not significantly bend at the elbows. Also, no movement of head is present with respect to the torso during the sequence. We created a static background by adding a simple object (a sphere within a cube) to the point set. These 3D point tracks were converted to feature trajectories by projecting them using a moving orthographic camera translating and rotating around the scene. Since the arm is not identified as an articulated segment (due to lack of bending), it is reconstructed using the low-rank SFM algorithm. The background object was identified as the root, and a stationary sequence was identified when one of the legs was resting on the ground. We can observe that the 3D structure is accurately recovered and the synthesis is coherent (Figure 3). It can also be seen that for reconstruction of the arms, the method of metric reprojections [3] provides better reconstruction compared to hierarchical priors [2] in this case. Compared with the ground truth, average error in 3D locations of the reconstructed points is 1.2% using our method which is significantly better than 22.4% using the method of metric reprojections directly on the entire data. Tables providing detailed quantitative comparisons are included in supplementary material.

The motion segmentation results may not be accurate in all scenes. To study the effect of misclassification, we randomly changed the motion segmentation of a number of points and observed the accuracy of reconstruction. If a rigid point is incorrectly assigned as non-rigid, there was no noticeable loss in accuracy. However, if a point on the non-rigid or articulated segment was incorrectly labeled as rigid or articulated, there was some loss of accuracy. In Table 3 of Supplementary material, we present further results of our experiments. The segment assignment of a random number of selected non-rigid points were included in the nearest articulated segment for the first set of results. In the second case, they were assigned to rigid segments. Though the errors increased with the number of modified points, it always remained below the error from directly applying either [3] or [2].

## 6.2    Natural Videos

We demonstrate our method on three natural video sequences - Marple2, Tennis [24] and Mountain data sequence. Each of these is obtained using a moving camera capturing a scene with both rigid and non-rigid elements. The results shown in Figure 4 show that our algorithm successfully estimates the structure of the scene in each of these cases. The static background is correctly segmented in each case and the motion segments identified conform to the skeletal structure of the objects. Also, it can be seen that the synthesis step has accurately merged

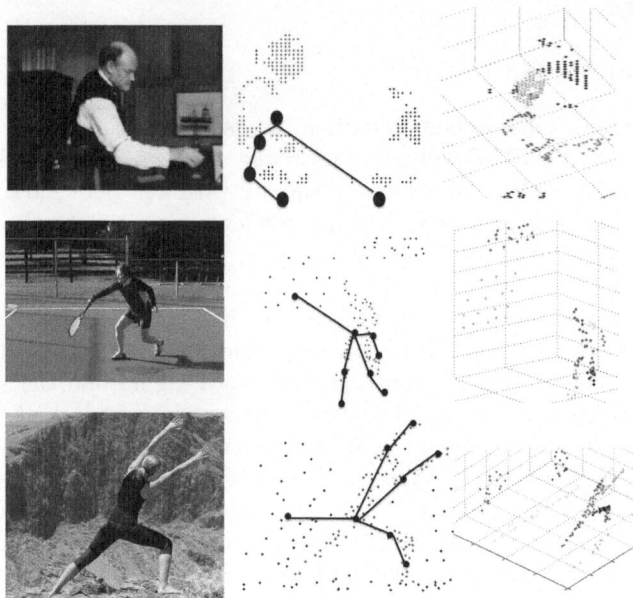

**Fig. 4.** Left Column: Frame from video, Central Column: Motion classification and subsequence tree (colors indicate motion classification: red indicates articulated segments, blue indicates non-rigid segments and black indicates rigid segments), Right column: Synthesized 3D reconstruction (colors indicate motion segments). The colors of central and right column are not related.

the individual reconstructions (the sizes and shapes of segments relative to each other are preserved).

## 7    Conclusion

Obtaining 3D structure from monocular videos of deforming objects is a challenging problem. Few existing algorithms can handle multiple types of motion in a scene. Our approach uses the notions of heterogeneity, articulation and stationarity and we present a scheme to perform motion classification and hence automatic selection of reconstruction algorithms for each scene object. Using sub-sequence stationarity graphs, these are stitched together to form a coherent structure. We tested our method on data from human motion capture for objective analysis and demonstrate on natural videos. We showed that our method performs significantly better than methods which try to apply a single model for the entire scene.

**Acknowledgement.** This work was made possible by National Science Foundation (NSF) Office of Polar Program grant ANT0636726.

# References

1. Bregler, C., Hertzmann, A., Biermann, H.: Recovering non-rigid 3d shape from image streams. In: CVPR, vol. 2, pp. 690–696 (2000)
2. Torresani, L., Hertzmann, A., Bregler, C.: Nonrigid structure-from-motion: Estimating shape and motion with hierarchical priors. PAMI 30, 878–892 (2008)
3. Paladini, M., Bue, A.D., Stosic, M., Dodig, M., Xavier, J., Agapito, L.: Factorization for non-rigid and articulated structure using metric projections. In: CVPR, pp. 2898–2905 (2009)
4. Taylor, J., Jepson, A., Kutulakos, K.: Non-rigid structure from locally-rigid motion. In: CVPR, pp. 2761–2768 (2010)
5. Ozden, K., Schindler, K., Van Gool, L.: Multibody structure-from-motion in practice. PAMI 32, 1134–1141 (2010)
6. Salzmann, M., Pilet, J., Ilic, S., Fua, P.: Surface deformation models for non-rigid 3d shape recovery. IEEE Transactions on Pattern Analysis and Machine Intelligence 29, 1481–1487 (2007)
7. Ross, D.A., Tarlow, D., Zemel, R.S.: Learning articulated structure and motion. Int. J. Comput. Vision 88, 214–237 (2010)
8. Vidal, R., Ma, Y., Piazzi, J.: A new GPCA algorithm for clustering subspaces by fitting, differentiating and dividing polynomials. In: CVPR, vol. 1, pp. 510–517 (2004)
9. Yan, J., Pollefeys, M.: Automatic kinematic chain building from feature trajectories of articulated objects. In: CVPR, pp. 712–719 (2006)
10. Del Bue, A., Llad, X., Agapito, L.: Non-rigid metric shape and motion recovery from uncalibrated images using priors. In: CVPR, vol. 1, pp. 1191–1198 (2006)
11. Fayad, J., Russell, C., Agapito, L.: Automated articulated structure and 3d shape recovery from point correspondences. In: ICCV (2011)
12. Rohith, M., Kambhamettu, C.: Estimation and utilization of articulations in recovering non-rigid structure from motion using motion subspaces. In: (J-HGBU 2011), ACM Multimedia 2011 (2011)
13. Roy-Chowdhury, A.: A measure of deformability of shapes, with applications to human motion analysis. In: CVPR, vol. 1, pp. 398–404 (2005)
14. Tresadern, P., Reid, I.: Articulated structure from motion by factorization. In: CVPR, vol. 2, pp. 1110–1115 (2005)
15. Akhter, I., Sheikh, Y., Khan, S., Kanade, T.: Trajectory space: A dual representation for nonrigid structure from motion. PAMI 33, 1442–1456 (2011)
16. Gotardo, P.F.U., Martinez, A.M.: Non-rigid structure from motion with complementary rank-3 spaces. In: CVPR, pp. 3065–3072 (2011)
17. Tresadern, P.A., Reid, I.D.: Video synchronization from human motion using rank constraints. CVIU 113, 891–906 (2009)
18. Shi, J., Malik, J.: Normalized cuts and image segmentation. In: CVPR (1997)
19. Tron, R., Vidal, R.: A benchmark for the comparison of 3d motion segmentation algorithms. In: CVPR (2007)
20. Oliensis, J., Hartley, R.: Iterative extensions of the Sturm/Triggs algorithm: Convergence and nonconvergence. PAMI 29, 2217–2233 (2007)
21. Rabaud, V.: Vincent's SFM Toolbox, http://vision.ucsd.edu/vrabaud/toolbox/
22. Hartley, R.I., Zisserman, A.: Multiple View Geometry in Computer Vision, 2nd edn. Cambridge University Press (2004) ISBN: 0521540518
23. CMU Graphics Lab Motion Capture Database, http://mocap.cs.cmu.edu//
24. Brox, T., Malik, J.: Large displacement optical flow: Descriptor matching in variational motion estimation. PAMI 33, 500–513 (2011)

# Locality-Constrained Active Appearance Model

Xiaowei Zhao[1,2], Shiguang Shan[1], Xiujuan Chai[1], and Xilin Chen[1]

[1] Key Lab. of Intelligent Information Processing of Chinese Academy of Sciences
(CAS), Institute of Computing Technology, CAS, Beijing 100190, China
[2] University of Chinese Academy of Sciences, Beijing 100049, China
mathzxw2002@gmail.com, {sgshan,chaixiujuan,xlchen}@ict.ac.cn

**Abstract.** Although the conventional Active Appearance Model (AAM) has achieved some success for face alignment, it still suffers from the generalization problem when be applied to unseen subjects and images. In this paper, a novel Locality-constraint AAM (LC-AAM) algorithm is proposed to tackle the generalization problem of AAM. Theoretically, the proposed LC-AAM is a fast approximation for a sparsity-regularized AAM problem, where sparse representation is exploited for non-linear face modeling. Specifically, for an input image, its $K$-nearest neighbors are selected as the shape and appearance bases, which are adaptively fitted to the input image by solving a constrained AAM-like fitting problem. Essentially, the effectiveness of our LC-AAM algorithm comes from learning a strong localized shape and appearance prior for the input facial image through exploiting its $K$-similar patterns. To validate the effectiveness of our algorithm, comprehensive experiments are conducted on two publicly available face databases. Experimental results demonstrate that our method greatly outperforms the original AAM method and its variants. In addition, our method is better than the state-of-the-art face alignment methods and generalizes well to unseen subjects and images.

## 1 Introduction

Face alignment is the process of moving and deforming a face model to match with the input facial image, which plays an important role in many computer vision problems, such as face recognition, facial expression analysis, face tracking in video, etc. Among sizable literatures on face alignment, the Active Shape Model (ASM) [1] and Active Appearance Model (AAM) [2] are the early popular approaches which attempt to fit the facial image with a statistical generative model.

As an extension of ASM, the power of AAM stems from statistically modeling the shape and appearance variations simultaneously through principal component analysis (PCA) on a set of labeled data. During the fitting procedure, the AAM is aligned by finding the model parameters that minimizing the distance between the observed and the synthesized facial appearance. As indicted by work [3], the AAM performs well if trained to work with a limited number of known subjects (e.g., person-specific Active Appearance Model). However, the alignment performance of AAM degrades quickly when it is trained on a large data

K.M. Lee et al. (Eds.): ACCV 2012, Part I, LNCS 7724, pp. 636–647, 2013.
© Springer-Verlag Berlin Heidelberg 2013

set and fitted to images that were not seen during the training procedure. We assert that this is mostly due to the fact that a single PCA model cannot well capture the non-linear appearance variation of a large training set, which contains larger variations (e.g., pose, expression, lighting, etc) than a small image set. Specifically, the learnt PCA model just preserves the statistically significant features of a training set, ignoring some subtle variations of images.

To tackle the generalization problem of AAM, two main kinds of approaches are proposed: discriminative and generative. The first approach learns a discriminative fitting function, which establishes a mapping between the facial appearance and the correct alignment. For example, Boosted Appearance Model (BAM) [4] exploits Haar-like features to model the appearance of faces, and learns a GentleBoost classifier to distinguish between correct and incorrect alignment. Then, the correct alignment can be obtained by maximizing the classification score. However, there is no guarantee that moving along the gradient of the learnt score function will always improve the alignment [5]. In order to overcome this limitation, Boosted Ranking Model (BRM) [5] proposes to learn a ranking function which is concave within the neighborhood of the correct alignment. Given a pair of images warped from different landmarks, the learnt GentleBoost-based ranking classifier can inform which alignment is better. Furthermore, a non-linear discriminative fitting approach is proposed by Saragih et al. [6], which learns a non-linear multivariate regressor through Boosting and directly predicts the update parameters in each iteration of AAM.

For generative approaches, there are many efforts to handle the multi-model distribution of shapes and appearances. Typically, Gaussian Mixture Model (GMM) is exploited to represent the non-linear shape and appearance variations [7,8]. Specifically, in literature [8], the multi-model appearance variations are captured by a mixture of probabilistic PCA (MPPCA) [9], noted as MPPCA-AAM. Then, the AAM alignment problem is formulated as a maximum likelihood problem, which can be easily solved by EM-algorithm. Besides the GMM methods, manifold learning technique can also be utilized to learn a non-linear prior for shapes and appearances [10]. However, the variations of facial shape and appearance are too complex to be characterized by a parametric distribution model.

In recent years, sparse representation is also utilized to model the complex non-linear distribution of facial shapes instead of PCA [11]. In their method, a novel Sparse Shape Composition model (SSC) is proposed to adaptively approximate the input shape by a sparse linear combination of training shapes. The effectiveness of SSC is validated on some real world medical applications. However, due to the high dimension (e.g., 40*50) of facial appearance, it is impractical to directly apply sparse representation to non-linear appearance modeling in AAM, which results in a computation-cost problem. Moreover, the multiple iteration times (at least 10 times) in the AAM fitting procedure also increases the computation cost. Fortunately, as empirically pointed by Yu et al., the results of sparse representation tend to be local: nonzero coefficients are often assigned to bases nearby to the encoded data [12]. So, the sparse representation-based method can be fast approximated by a $K$-nearest-neighbor ($K$-NN) search and then solving a constrained least square fitting problem [13].

In this paper, inspired by the empirical observations of Yu et al., we first reformulate the original Active Appearance Model as a sparse representation problem and then approximate it through introducing locality constraint, briefly called Locality-constrained Active Appearance Model (LC-AAM). Specifically, for an input image, we first find its $K$-nearest neighbors as the face bases and then adaptively fit to it by solving a constrained AAM-like fitting problem. The effect of locality constraint is twofold: (1) Learning the shape and appearance prior for the input facial image through exploring its $K$-nearest neighbors, which have similar patterns (e.g., pose, expression, subject, etc.). The person-specific AAM is just a special case of our LC-AAM, which requires that the images come from one specific person. (2) The global non-linear facial shape and appearance model is approximated by many localized linear models, which are specific to the input images and result in a faster convergence. To demonstrate the effectiveness of our method, comprehensive experiments are conducted by comparing our LC-AAM method with conventional AAM-based methods (e.g., the popular Inverse Compositional AAM (IC-AAM) [2], Simultaneously Inverse Compositional AAM (SIC-AAM) [3], and MPPCA-AAM [8]) and the state-of-the-art face alignment methods on two publicly available face databases, which contain multiple subjects and cover large variations in pose, expression and lighting, etc. Experimental results demonstrate that our proposed LC-AAM algorithm convincingly outperforms the conventional AAM-based methods. In addition, our method generalizes well to unseen subjects and images and is better than the state-of-the-art face alignment methods on the above-mentioned evaluation sets.

The remaining part of this paper is organized as follows. Section 2 gives a brief review of Active Appearance Model. Section 3 reformulates the original AAM problem as a sparsity-regularized AAM problem, which is future approximated by our Locality-constrained AAM algorithm. The formulation and implementation details are also presented in this section. Section 4 reports the experimental results and also the comparisons with the state-of-the-art methods. Section 5 concludes the paper.

## 2   Review of Active Appearance Model

In this section, we will first introduce the shape and appearance modeling of the conventional AAM, then describe the AAM based fitting algorithm. Some notations used in the following sections are also defined in this section.

### 2.1   Shape and Appearance Modeling

The AAM simultaneously characterizes the intrinsic variations of shape and appearance as linear combination of basis models of variation.

The shape $s$ of an AAM is represented by a set of 2D facial landmarks: $s = (x_1, y_1, x_2, y_2, \ldots, x_n, y_n)^{\mathrm{T}}$. The AAM allows a linear shape variation, which means that the shape instance $s$ can be expressed as follows:

$$s = s_0 + \sum_{i=1}^{M} \alpha_i s_i \tag{1}$$

where $s_0$ is the mean shape, $s_i$ is the $i$th shape basis, and the coefficients $\alpha = [\alpha_1, \alpha_2, \ldots, \alpha_M]^{\mathrm{T}}$ are the shape parameters to control the variation of $s$. The first four shape bases are designed to represent the global similar transformations, such as global translations in x and y direction, rotation, and scaling. The shape model of AAM is statistically learnt from a training set with annotated facial landmarks. Specifically, the training shapes are first geometrically aligned using the *Procrustes* analysis. Then eigenanalysis is applied to the aligned training shapes to obtain the mean shape and shape bases.

To learn the appearance model, each facial image $I$ should be warped into a "shape-normalized" frame, which is usually defined as the mean shape $s_0$. The warping function, noted as $W(\boldsymbol{u}; \alpha)$, is usually defined as a piecewise-affine warp from the mean shape $s_0$ to the shape of facial image. Here, $\alpha$ are the shape parameters of facial image $I$, and $\boldsymbol{u} = (x, y)^{\mathrm{T}}$ denote a set of pixels lie inside the mean shape $s_0$. So, the "shape-normalized" appearance of facial image $I$ is defined as $I(W(\boldsymbol{u}; \alpha))$. Then the AAM appearance model is computed by applying PCA to the collected "shape-normalized" appearances. Similarly to shape modeling, the appearance instance is generated using a linear combination of $L$ appearance bases:

$$A(\boldsymbol{u}) = A_0(\boldsymbol{u}) + \sum_{i=1}^{L} \beta_i A_i(\boldsymbol{u}) \tag{2}$$

where $A_0(\boldsymbol{u})$ is the mean appearance, $A_i(\boldsymbol{u})$ is the $i$th appearance basis, and the coefficients $\beta = [\beta_1, \beta_2, \ldots, \beta_L]^{\mathrm{T}}$ are the appearance parameters to control the variation of $A(\boldsymbol{u})$.

In the early literatures [14], the shape and appearance parameters are usually concatenated and a second level PCA is applied to these concatenated parameters to form a more compact representation. However, in this study, the shape and appearance model are taken into account separately.

## 2.2 Model Fitting

The fitting of AAM is to estimate the optimal shape and appearance parameters to minimize the discrepancy between the synthesized image $A(\boldsymbol{u}) = A_0(\boldsymbol{u}) + \sum_{i=1}^{L} \beta_i A_i(\boldsymbol{u})$ and the observed facial image $I(W(\boldsymbol{u}; \alpha))$. Here, $I$ is the test image, and $I(W(\boldsymbol{u}; \alpha))$ represents the warped "shape-normalized" facial image. Specifically, the AAM fitting algorithm is usually formulated as follows:

$$\min_{\alpha, \beta} \sum_{\boldsymbol{u} \in s_0} \left[ A_0(\boldsymbol{u}) + \sum_{i=1}^{L} \beta_i A_i(\boldsymbol{u}) - I(W(\boldsymbol{u}; \alpha)) \right]^2 \tag{3}$$

where the sum is performed over all of the pixels $\boldsymbol{u}$ in the base mesh $s_0$. The goal of AAM fitting is to minimize the expression in Eq.(3) simultaneously with respect to the shape parameters $\alpha$ and appearance parameters $\beta$.

Traditionally, Eq.(3) is solved by gradient decent method, which is computationally expensive. Recently, the computation cost of AAM fitting is greatly saved by the popular Inverse Compositional (IC) algorithm (i.e., IC-AAM) [2], in which the roles of the image and model are reversed and some time-consuming steps in AAM fitting are pre-computed and remain fixed in the iteration process. However, the IC-AAM only works well in the case that faces exhibit small amounts of variations.

### 2.3   Limitations of Active Appearance Model

Briefly, there are two main limitations for the conventional AAM, which are caused by the essentially non-linear variations of facial shape and appearance in a large data set.

Firstly, it is impossible to capture the complex non-linear shape and appearance variations of a large image set by just a single PCA model. Specifically, the learnt PCA model usually extracts the statistically significant features of the training set, ignoring some local details which are necessary for a more accurate alignment.

Secondly, in the AAM fitting procedure, the relationship between the appearance error (i.e., $\sum_{u \in s_0} [A_0(u) + \sum_{i=1}^{L} \beta_i A_i(u) - I(W(u; \alpha))])$ and the shape parameter update (i.e., $\alpha$) is assumed to be *close* to linear around the optimum, which is only right in the case that the face appearance variation is very small. However, it is hard to initialize the model parameters close enough to the correct alignment without any shape and appearance priors for the test image.

## 3   Locality-Constrained Active Appearance Model

In this section, to address the limitations of conventional AAM, it is reformulated as a sparsity-regularized AAM problem, where sparse representation is exploited to model the non-linear face representation of AAM. Subsequently, the sparsity-regularized AAM is further approximated by our proposed Locality-constrained AAM algorithm for a fast implementation.

### 3.1   Sparsity-Regularized Active Appearance Model

In this study, it is assumed that the shape and appearance of faces can be *sparsely* represented by faces of a large training set. Here, an explicit parametric model (e.g., PCA) is no longer needed. The aligned training shapes and the corresponding appearances are directly used as the shape and appearance bases. In this way, the original AAM is reformulated as the following sparsity-regularized AAM problem:

$$\min_{\alpha, \beta} \{ \sum_{u \in s_0} [\sum_{i=1}^{N} \beta_i A_i(u) - I(W(u; \alpha))]^2 + \lambda_1 \|\alpha\|_{l^1} + \lambda_2 \|\beta\|_{l^1} \} \qquad (4)$$

where $N$ is the number of faces in the training set, $s_0$ is the mean shape of all training faces, $A_i(u)$ is the "shape-normalized" appearance obtained by warped the facial image to the mean shape $s_0$, $\beta_i$ is the $i$th appearance model parameter, $\alpha$ are the shape parameters, $I(W(u;\alpha))$ is the observed "shape-normalized" appearance of the input facial image, and $\lambda_1, \lambda_2$ are the regularization coefficients, which add sparse constraints to the shape and appearance parameters $\alpha$ and $\beta$ respectively.

During the fitting procedure of sparsity-regularized AAM, the "analysis by synthesize" strategy is used to iteratively approximate the correct alignment. In each iteration, the "shape-normalized" facial appearance is first warped according to the current shape parameters $\alpha$. With the fixed $\alpha$ and the observed appearance $I(W(u;\alpha))$, the appearance parameters $\beta$ are calculated by solving a $l_1$ constrained optimization problem, Eq.(4). Then a new appearance is synthesized by the calculated appearance parameters $\beta$. To calculate the updated shape parameters, another $l_1$ constrained optimization problem (i.e., Eq.(4) with $\beta$ and $\sum_{i=1}^{N} \beta_i A_i(u)$ fixed), which aims to minimize the discrepancy between the observed appearance and the synthesized appearance. The correct alignment can be obtained until convergence or a maximum iteration number is reached.

However, as pointed out in section 1, the sparsity-regularized AAM is very time-consuming due to the high dimension $l_1$ optimization problem and multiple iterations in the fitting procedure.

## 3.2  Approximated Sparsity by Locality Constraint

Inspired by the theory analysis and empirical observations by Yu et al. [12], the sparse coefficients $\alpha$ and $\beta$ in Eq.(4) tend to be local and images with larger coefficients are more similar to the input image. So, to speed up the fitting procedure of sparsity-regularized AAM, locality constraint is introduced by us for a fast approximation.

Specifically, given an input image $I$ to be aligned, the sparsity constraint in Eq.(4) is replaced with our locality constraint, which is as follows:

$$\min_{\alpha,\beta}\{\sum_{u \in s_0}[\sum_{i=1}^{N} \beta_i A_i(u) - I(W(u;\alpha))]^2 + \lambda_1 \|\mathbf{d} \odot \alpha\|^2 + \lambda_2 \|\mathbf{d} \odot \beta\|^2\} \quad (5)$$

where $N$ is the number of faces in the training set, $A_i(u)$ is the appearance basis obtained by warping the train image to the mean shape $s_0$, $\beta_i$ is the $i$th appearance model parameter, $\alpha$ are the shape parameters, and $\lambda_1, \lambda_2$ are the regularization coefficients. Specifically, $\mathbf{d} = [d_1, d_2, \ldots, d_N]$ are the distances between the input image $I$ and the appearance bases $A(u) = [A_1(u), A_2(u), \ldots, A_N(u)]$, which add larger weights to the appearance bases nearer to $I$. Symbol $\odot$ denotes the element-wise multiplication.

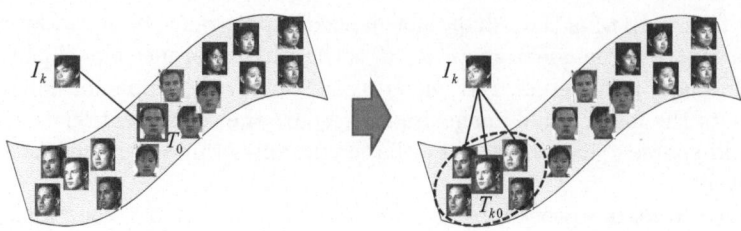

**Fig. 1.** Original AAM (*left*) vs. Locality-constrained AAM (*right*). $T_0$ is the mean template the whole training set, $T_{k0}$ is the mean template of the $K$-nearest neighbors of input image $I_k$.

In practice, Eq.(5) is fast implemented by directly setting the coefficients of the distant faces to be zero, i.e., selecting the $K$-nearest neighbors of $I$ as the shape and appearance bases, which is formulated as:

$$\min_{\alpha,\beta} \sum_{\boldsymbol{u}\in\overline{s}_0} [\sum_{i=1}^{K} \beta_i A_i(\boldsymbol{u}) - I(W(\boldsymbol{u};\alpha))]^2 \tag{6}$$

where $K$ is the number of selected nearest neighbors. It is important to note that $\overline{s}_0$ is the mean shape of the selected $K$-nearest neighbors.

Specifically, the optimization of Eq.(6) is similar to the conventional AAM-based fitting, which can be solved by gradient decent algorithm or the popular IC-AAM algorithm. Different from the conventional-AAM based methods, the appearance model used in our LC-AAM algorithm is localized linear, where the appearance variations are small and the relationship between the appearance error and the shape parameters is close to linear.

Figure 1 intuitively interprets why our LC-AAM algorithm works better than the original AAM. Specifically, in original AAM, the shape and appearance variations are characterized with a single Gaussian (PCA) model on the whole training set. However, the learnt PCA model cannot well characterize the non-linear feature of the whole training set. In comparison, our LC-AAM algorithm learns many localized linear models, which are specific for the input image, to approximate the global non-linear face model. Essentially, a stronger prior is learnt by exploring the $K$-nearest neighbors to constrain the shape and appearance subspace of input image. In addition, as illustrated in Figure 1, the input image $I_k$ is closer to the mean template $T_{k0}$ in LC-AAM, which is usually used to initialize the facial shape parameters, than the mean template $T_0$ in original AAM. So, it is much easier to converge to the correct alignment.

In our implementation, the neighbor samples are determined according to the measurement of the appearance similarity. Specifically, the face region is normalized by the automatically detected two eye centers [15,16] and the Euclidean distance is adopted to characterize the similarity of two faces. In addition, two kinds of feature descriptors are exploited to compute the similarity of faces, e.g., Histogram of Oriented Gradients (HOG) [17] feature and gray intensity value of image.

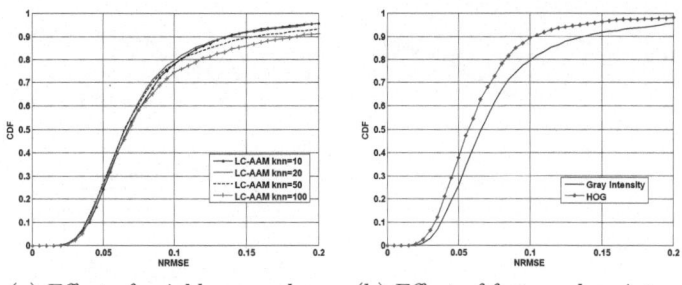

(a) Effect of neighbor number.    (b) Effect of feature descriptors.

**Fig. 2.** Performance variation of LC-AAM with different parameter configuration

## 4    Experiments

In this section, we evaluate the effectiveness of our LC-AAM algorithm[1] through comparing it with the conventional AAM-based methods and other state-of-the-art face alignment methods.

### 4.1    Databases and Evaluation Metric

Our evaluation experiments are conducted on two publicly available face data sets. Set 1 is randomly collected from CMU-PIE [18], FRGCv1[19], FERET [20], CAS-PEAL [21], and PubFig [22] face databases, which covers large variations in pose, expression, lighting and image conditions, etc. Totally, there are more than 7000 images in set 1 and 1500 images are randomly selected for testing, noted as T1. Set 2 is collected from Cohn-Kanade face database [23], which includes 486 image sequences (8796 static images) in nearly frontal view from 97 subjects. Each sequence begins with a neutral expression and proceeds to a peak expression. To demonstrate that the generalization capability of our method, 80 subjects are randomly collected for training, and the other remaining 17 subjects (consisting of 1519 images, noted as T2) for testing.

For evaluation metric, the normalized root-mean-squared error (NRMSE) relative to the ground truth is adopted as the error measure for the face alignment. The NRMSE is given as a percentage, computed by dividing the root mean squared error by the distance between the two eye centers. The cumulative distribution function (CDF) of NRMSE is used to evaluate the performance of face alignment algorithm.

### 4.2    Experimental Results

**Comparisons with Respect to Different Number of Neighbors.** To show how our method is affected by the number of nearest neighbors. We conduct

---

[1] The matlab code of our LC-AAM algorithm can be found at
http://vipl.ict.ac.cn/members/xwzhao

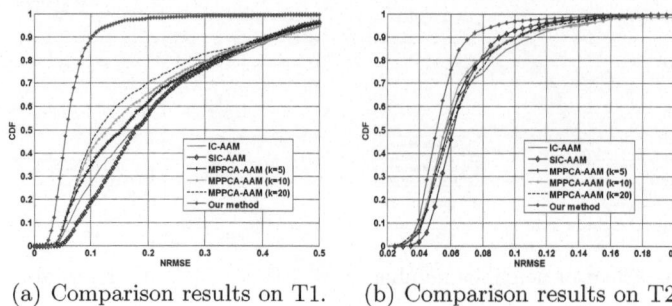

(a) Comparison results on T1.     (b) Comparison results on T2.

**Fig. 3.** Comparisons with original AAM and its variant methods

our experiments on T1 using $K$=10, 20, 50, 100 respectively. Moreover, the gray intensity is used to calculate the similarity of face images. From the experimental results, as shown in Figure 2(a), it is observed that $K$=20 is better than the other parameters. In addition, when a larger $K$ is selected, the alignment results become worse. So, in the following experiments, the number of nearest neighbors is set to 20.

**Comparisons with Different Feature Descriptors.** In this subsection, two kinds of feature descriptors are exploited to compute the similarity of image pairs: HOG feature and gray intensity. Specifically, for HOG feature, the block size, the number of orientation bins are set to $7 \times 7$ and 9 separately. The number of nearest neighbors is set to 20 in the comparison experiments.

The comparison experiments are conducted on T1. Experimental results, shown in Figure 2(b), demonstrate that the HOG feature is more suitable to calculate the similarity of faces than the gray intensity feature. The reason is that the HOG descriptor characterizes the boundary features of faces, eliminates some noise contained in gray pixel values.

**Comparisons with AAM and Its Variants.** In this subsection, we compare our algorithm with conventional AAM-based algorithms (e.g., IC-AAM, SIC-AAM, and MPPCA-AAM, etc.) on the above-mentioned two data sets. Specifically, the dimensionality of the shape and appearance models for IC-AAM and SIC-AAM is chosen by retaining 90% of the variance in the eigenvalues. For MPPCA-AAM, the number of Gaussian components is set to 5, 10, and 20 respectively. For our LC-AAM, the number of nearest neighbors is set to 20 and the HOG feature is exploited to calculate the similarity of image pairs. Moreover, the iteration number in the fitting procedure of all these methods is set to 25.

The comparison results are shown in Figures 3(a) and Figure 3(b), which demonstrate that our method greatly outperforms the conventional AAM-based methods. Specifically, in T1, which contains more pose variations than T2, our method achieves at least 40% higher than other methods when NRMSE is less than 0.1.

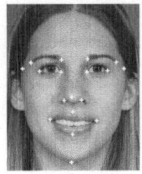

**Fig. 4.** Common facial landmarks of the evaluated methods

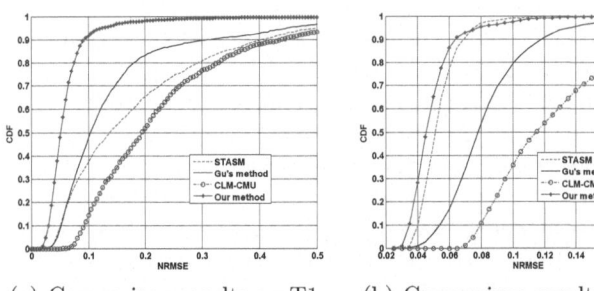

(a) Comparison results on T1.    (b) Comparison results on T2.

**Fig. 5.** Comparisons with state-of-the-art methods

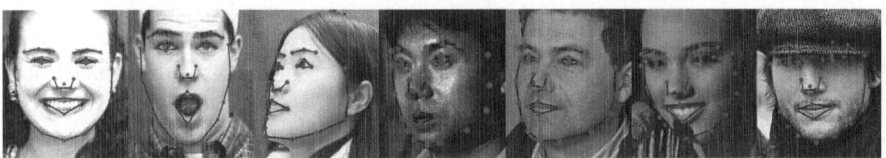

**Fig. 6.** Visualized example images of our method

**Comparisons with State-of-the-Art Methods.** In this subsection, we compare our algorithm with the state-of-the-art face alignment algorithms, such as MPPCA-ASM [24], STASM [25], and CLM-CMU [26]. Specifically, the MPPCA-ASM method is a kind of ASM-based approach, which exploits the mixture of probabilistic principal component analysis (MPPCA) to model the shape variations. In our previous study, the MPPCA-ASM algorithm performs well when the Gaussian component of MPPCA is set to 5, which corresponds to 5 different pose intervals in yaw direction. So, the number of Gaussian components is set to 5 in the following experiments. In our LC-AAM, the number of nearest neighbors is set to 20 and the HOG feature is adopted to calculate similarity of image pairs.

To perform a fair comparison, only the common 18 facial landmarks of these methods are used for performance evaluation, as shown in Figure 4. The comparison results are shown in Figures 5(a) and Figure 5(b) respectively. It is observed from the comparison results that our method greatly outperforms the other methods on T1. On T2, our method is comparable with STASM and is better than other methods. It is also interesting to note that the STASM algorithm performs well on near-frontal facial images (T2) but fails to work on images with large pose variation (T1). However, our method achieves consistently good alignment performance on these two test sets. Figure 6 shows some visualized example images of our method on challenging images.

## 5 Conclusion and Future Work

Instead of characterizing the facial shape and appearance distributions with a single PCA model, the original Active Appearance Model is reformulated as a sparsity-regularized problem. Then, based on the theory and empirical results of Yu et al., the sparse representation problem is further approximated by our Locality-constrained Active Appearance Model algorithm. For an input facial image, a strong shape and appearance prior is learnt by exploiting its $K$-similar patterns. Essentially, the effectiveness of our LC-AAM stems from learning many localized linear face model instead of a global non-linear face model. By comparison, the localized face model is more compact and much easier to converge to the correct alignment. The effectiveness of our method is validated through comprehensively comparisons with the original AAM method, the variant methods of AAM, and the state-of-the-art face alignment methods on two publicly available face databases. In addition, our proposed method generalizes well to unseen subjects and images than the original AAM and its variants.

**Acknowledgement.** This work is partially supported by Natural Science Foundation of China (NSFC) under contract Nos. 61025010, 61173065, and 61001193; and the FiDiPro program of Tekes.

## References

1. Cootes, T., Taylor, C., Cooper, D., et al.: Active shape models: Their training and application. CVIU 61, 38–59 (1995)
2. Matthews, I., Baker, S.: Active appearance models revisited. IJCV 60, 135–164 (2004)
3. Gross, R., Matthews, I., Baker, S.: Generic vs. person specific active appearance models. IVC 23, 1080–1093 (2005)
4. Liu, X.: Generic face alignment using boosted appearance model. In: CVPR, pp. 1–8 (2007)
5. Wu, H., Liu, X.: Face alignment via boosted ranking model. In: CVPR, pp. 1–8 (2008)
6. Saragih, J., Goecke, R.: A nonlinear discriminative approach to AAM fitting. In: ICCV, pp. 1–8 (2007)
7. Cootes, T.F., Taylor, C.J.: A mixture model for representing shape variation. IVC 17, 567–573 (1999)
8. van der Maaten, L., Hendriks, E.: Capturing appearance variation in active appearance models. In: CVPRWS, pp. 34–41 (2010)
9. Tipping, M.E., Bishop, C.M.: Mixtures of probabilistic principal component analyzers. Neural Computation 11, 443–482 (1999)

10. Etyngier, P., Sgonne, F., Keriven, R.: Shape priors using manifold learning techniques. In: ICCV (2007)
11. Zhang, S., Zhan, Y., Dewan, M., et al.: Towards robust and effective shape modeling: Sparse shape composition. Medical Image Analysis 16, 265–277 (2012)
12. Yu, K., Zhang, T., Gong, Y.: Nonlinear learning using local coordinate coding. In: NIPS, pp. 2223–2231 (2009)
13. Wang, J., Yang, J., Yu, K.: et al.: Locality-constrained linear coding for image classification. In: CVPR, pp. 3360–3367 (2010)
14. Edwards, G.J., Taylor, C.J., Cootes, T.: Interpreting face images using active appearance models. In: FG, pp. 300–305 (1998)
15. Zhao, X., Chai, X., Niu, Z., Heng, C., Shan, S.: Context constrained facial landmark localization based on discontinuous haar-like feature. In: FG, pp. 673–678 (2011)
16. Zhao, X., Chai, X., Niu, Z., Heng, C., Shan, S.: Context modeling for facial landmark detection based on non-adjacent rectangle (NAR) haar-like feature. Image and Vision Computing 30, 136–146 (2012)
17. Dalal, N., Triggs, B.: Histograms of oriented gradients for human detection. In: CVPR, pp. 886–893 (2005)
18. Sim, T., Baker, S., Bsat, M.: The cmu pose, illumination, and expression (PIE) database. In: FG (2002)
19. Phillips, P., Flynn, P., Scruggs, T.: et al.: Overview of the face recognition grand challenge. In: CVPR, pp. 947–954 (2005)
20. Phillips, P., Wechslerb, H., Huangb, J., et al.: The FERET database and evaluation procedure for face-recognition algorithms. IVC 16, 295–306 (1998)
21. Gao, W., Cao, B., Shan, S., et al.: The CAS-PEAL large-scale chinese face database and baseline evaluations. SMC, Part A: Systems and Humans 38, 149–161 (2008)
22. Kumar, N., Berg, A., Belhumeur, P.: et al.: Attribute and simile classifiers for face verification. In: ICCV, pp. 365–372 (2009)
23. Tian, Y.I., Kanade, T., Cohn, J.F.: Recognizing action units for facial expression analysis. IEEE T-PAMI 23, 97–115 (2001)
24. Gu, L., Kanade, T.: A Generative Shape Regularization Model for Robust Face Alignment. In: Forsyth, D., Torr, P., Zisserman, A. (eds.) ECCV 2008, Part I. LNCS, vol. 5302, pp. 413–426. Springer, Heidelberg (2008)
25. Milborrow, S., Nicolls, F.: Locating Facial Features with an Extended Active Shape Model. In: Forsyth, D., Torr, P., Zisserman, A. (eds.) ECCV 2008, Part IV. LNCS, vol. 5305, pp. 504–513. Springer, Heidelberg (2008)
26. Saragih, J., Lucey, S., Cohn, J.: Deformable model fitting by regularized landmark mean-shifts. IJCV 91, 200–215 (2011)

# Modeling Hidden Topics with Dual Local Consistency for Image Analysis

Peng Li, Jian Cheng, and Hanqing Lu

National Laboratory of Pattern Recognition, Institute of Automation,
Chinese Academy of Sciences, Beijing 100190, China
{pli,jcheng,luhq}@nlpr.ia.ac.cn

**Abstract.** Image representation is the crucial component in image analysis and understanding. However, the widely used low-level features cannot correctly represent the high-level semantic content of images in many situations due to the "semantic gap". In order to bridge the "semantic gap", in this brief, we present a novel topic model, which can learn an effective and robust mid-level representation in the latent semantic space for image analysis. In our model, the $\ell^1$-graph is constructed to model the local image neighborhood structure and the word co-occurrence is computed to capture the local word consistency. Then, the local information is incorporated into the model for topic discovering. Finally, the generalized EM algorithm is used to estimate the parameters. As our model considers both the local image structure and local word consistency simultaneously when estimating the probabilistic topic distributions, the image representations can have more powerful description ability in the learned latent semantic space. Extensive experiments on the publicly available databases demonstrate the effectiveness of our approach.

## 1 Introduction

Image representation is one of the most fundamental components for many image analysis and understanding tasks. A large variety of features have been proposed to characterize the content of images [1–3]. However, these low-level features cannot correctly represent the semantic content of images in many situations due to the so-called "semantic gap". Therefore, mid-level features are exploited by many researchers to bridge the gap. In recent years, the latent topic models, such as Probabilistic Latent Semantic Analysis (PLSA) [4], and Latent Dirichlet Allocation (LDA) [5], have been proposed to address this problem. The above-mentioned topic models can discover hidden topics in the latent semantic space based on a bag-of-words representation for the images, which can connect the low-level features and high-level semantic content. Due to the success of topic models, they have been widely adopted in many applications such as image classification, annotation, and retrieval [6–8].

However, most applications treat the topic model as a black box and each image or word is treated independently in topic modeling. There are still few efforts paid to explore how these hidden topics distribute and what correlations

K.M. Lee et al. (Eds.): ACCV 2012, Part I, LNCS 7724, pp. 648–659, 2013.
© Springer-Verlag Berlin Heidelberg 2013

exist among them. Therefore, the topic distributions estimated by the traditional models may not be accurate enough in some cases. According to recent research [9–11], data from images or texts are often found to lie on a low-rank non-linear manifold embedded in the high-dimensional space of the original data. Therefore, exploiting the intrinsic structure concealed in the data can help discover more accurate latent topics [12, 13]. Moreover, the words frequently co-occured in one image or text often have similar meanings and should be related to similar latent topics with a high probability. Thus, the word co-occurring information is also very essential to reveal the hidden semantics in the data.

To address the above issues, in this paper, we present a novel probabilistic topic model, named Dual Local Consistency Probabilistic Latent Semantic Analysis (DLC-PLSA), to model the latent topics with sparse neighborhood preserving embedding and local word consistency. Compared with the traditional models, our model has the following characteristics: (1) $\ell^1$-graph is constructed to model the sparse neighborhood structure of images and embedded into topic modeling. (2) the word co-occurring information is first incorporated into topic models to help discover more accurate latent topics. In this way, the topic model can estimate the probabilistic topic distributions and simultaneously consider the image neighborhood structure as well as the local word consistency in a uniform formulation. Therefore, our model is less sensitive to noise and has more discriminative power in the latent semantic space.

The rest of the paper is organized as follows: Section 2 gives a brief review of the related work. Section 3 presents the proposed topic model in detail. Extensive experimental results are reported in Section 4. Finally, we conclude our paper in Section 5.

## 2   Related Work

Image representation is very important for image analysis and understanding tasks. Due to the semantic gap between low-level features and the semantic content of images, mid-level representations have been widely exploited by many researchers. In recent years, the latent topic models, which can discover a latent semantic space, have attracted much attention. The latent topic models are originally proposed for document analysis. Latent Semantic Analysis (LSA) [14], which is the first latent topic model, uses a Singular Value Decomposition (SVD) of the term-document co-occurrence matrix to identify a latent semantic space. Despite its remarkable success in different domains, LSA has several deficits due to its unsatisfactory statistical formulation [4]. To address this issue, Hofmann proposed a generative probabilistic model named Probabilistic Latent Semantic Analysis (PLSA) [4]. PLSA models each word in a document as a sample from a mixture model, where the mixture components are multinomial random variables that can be viewed as representations of "topics". However, PLSA assumes that the probability distribution of each document on the hidden topics is independent and the number of parameters in the model grows linearly with the size of corpus. Latent Dirichlet Allocation (LDA) [5] is then proposed to overcome this problem by treating the probability distribution of each document over topics as a $K$-parameter hidden random variable rather than a large set of individual parameters, where $K$ is the number of hidden topics. When applying these models for image analysis, the images can be treated as documents and text words can be replaced by visual words, image regions and so on.

However, the traditional topic models treat each image or word individually in topic modeling without considering any local structure, the latent topic distributions learned by models may lack of discriminative power in many cases. In the past decade years, a variety of manifold-based approaches such as Isomap [15], Locally Linear Embedding (LLE) [9], Laplacian Eigenmaps [10] have been developed to explicitly discover the nonlinear manifold structure concealed in the data. Locality Preserving Projections (LPP) [16] and Neighborhood Preserving Embedding (NPE) [17] are the linear versions of Laplacian Eigenmaps and LLE, respectively. They are frequently added as regularization terms to many machine learning algorithms. Cai *et al.* propose a Laplacian Probabilistic Latent Semantic Indexing (LapPLSI) [12] model for document clustering, which models the hidden topics on document manifold by preserving the pairwise similarities of documents. Locally-consistent Topic Model (LTM) is proposed in [13], which uses KL-divergence instead of Euclidean distance to capture the document similarity. But the above methods just simply construct a $K$-NN graph to model the local document structure. However, as described in [18], there are some limitations of the $K$-NN graph. For example, it is very sensitive to data noises and one single global parameter may result in unreasonable neighborhood structure for certain data. More importantly, LapPLSI and LTM only take into account the local document structure while ignoring the word co-occurring consistency in topic modeling. The word co-occurring consistency represents how often two words co-occur in a document or an image. If two (visual) words frequently co-occur in a document (an image), they should also to be correlated to the same topic with a high probability. Therefore, incorporating the local word consistency is also very important for modeling more accurate hidden semntic topics.

## 3   The Proposed Approach

In this section, we present a novel topic model, named Dual Local Consistency Probabilistic Latent Semantic Analysis (DLC-PLSA). Different from the traditional topic models, our model considers the sparse image neighborhood structure and local word consistency simultaneously when estimating the latent topic distributions. Therefore, it can preserve more structure semantic information in the latent semantic space.

### 3.1   The PLSA Model

Our model is developed based on the Probabilistic Latent Semantic Analysis (PLSA) [4]. The PLSA model can be considered as a Bayesian network. The core of PLSA is a latent variable model for co-occurrence data which associates an unobserved topic variable $z_k \in \{z_1, \ldots, z_K\}$ with the occurrence of a word $w_j \in \{w_1, \ldots, w_M\}$ in a particular image $d_i \in \{d_1, \ldots, d_N\}$. As a generative model, PLSA is defined by the following scheme:

1. select an image $x_i$ with probability $P(x_i)$,
2. pick a latent topic $z_k$ with probability $P(z_k|x_i)$,
3. generate a word $w_j$ with probability $P(w_j|z_k)$.

As a result, one obtains an observation pair $(x_i, w_j)$, while the latent topic variable $z_k$ is discarded. Translating the data generation process into a joint probability model results in the expression

$$P(x_i, w_j) = P(x_i)P(w_j|x_i), \ \ P(w_j|x_i) = \sum_{k=1}^{K} P(w_j|z_k)P(z_k|x_i) \qquad (1)$$

The parameters can be estimated by maximizing the log-likelihood

$$l = \sum_{i=1}^{N} \sum_{j=1}^{M} n(x_i, w_j) \log P(x_i, w_j) \propto \sum_{i=1}^{N} \sum_{j=1}^{M} n(x_i, w_j) \log \sum_{k=1}^{K} P(w_j|z_k)P(z_k|x_i) \qquad (2)$$

where $n(x_i, w_j)$ is the number of occurrences of term $w_j$ in image $x_i$.

### 3.2 Embedding with Local Structure Consistency

With the PLSA model defined above, we will introduce how to embed the local structure of images and words into topic discovering in this subsection.

**Sparse Neighborhood Consistency.** In this part, we present a novel manifold learning approach based on traditional NPE method. Our method is motivated by the limitations of classical graph construction methods [9], [10] on robustness to data noise and data-adaptiveness, and recent advances in sparse coding [19], [20], [21]. With sparse representation, each sample can be reconstructed by the sparse linear superposition of the training data. The sparse reconstruction coefficients, used to deduce the weights of the $\ell^1$-graph, are derived by solving an $\ell^1$ optimization problem on sparse representation. Recent work in [18] has shown the $\ell^1$-graph is superior to the classical graphs in various machine learning tasks such as image clustering and subspace learning.

Suppose we have an underdetermined system of linear equations: $x = D\alpha$, where $x \in R^m$ is the vector to be approximated, $\alpha \in R^n$ is the vector for unknown reconstruction coefficients, and $D \in R^{m \times n}$ is the overcomplete dictionary with $n$ bases. Generally, a sparse solution is more robust and is able to facilitate the consequent identification of the test sample $x$. We seek the sparse solution to $x = D\alpha$ by solving the following optimization problem:

$$\min_{\alpha} \|\alpha\|_1, \quad s.t. \quad x = D\alpha \qquad (3)$$

This problem can be solved in polynomial time by standard linear programming method. In practice, there may exist noises on certain elements of $x$, and a natural way to recover these elements and provide a robust estimation of $\alpha$ is to formulate

$$x = D\alpha + \zeta = \begin{bmatrix} D & I \end{bmatrix} \begin{bmatrix} \alpha \\ \zeta \end{bmatrix} \tag{4}$$

where $\zeta \in R^m$ is the noise term. Then by setting $B = \begin{bmatrix} D & I \end{bmatrix} \in R^{m \times (m+n)}$ and $\alpha' = \begin{bmatrix} \alpha \\ \zeta \end{bmatrix}$, we can solve the following $\ell^1$-norm minimization problem with respect to both reconstruction coefficients and data noises:

$$\min_{\alpha'} \|\alpha'\|_1, \quad s.t. \quad x = B\alpha' \tag{5}$$

An $\ell^1$-graph summarizes the overall behavior of the whole dataset in sparse representation. The construction process is stated as follows.

1) **Inputs:** The image set denoted as the matrix $X = [x_1, x_2, \ldots, x_N]$, where $x_i \in R^M$
2) **Robust sparse representation:** For each image $x_i$ in the dataset, its robust sparse representation is achieved by solving the $\ell^1$-norm optimization problem

$$\min_{\alpha^i} \|\alpha^i\|_1, \quad s.t. \quad x_i = B^i \alpha^i \tag{6}$$

where $B^i = [x_1, \ldots x_{i-1}, x_{i+1} \ldots, x_N, I] \in R^{M \times (M+N-1)}$ and $\alpha^i \in R^{M+N-1}$
3) **Graph weight setting:** Denote the $G = \{X, W\}$ as the $\ell^1$-graph with the image set $X$ as graph vertices and $W$ as the graph weight matrix. We set $W_{ij} = \alpha_j^i$ if $i > j$, and $W_{ij} = \alpha_{j-1}^i$ if $i < j$.

After the $\ell^1$-graph is constructed, the neighborhood structure of the image dataset as well as the graph weights is derived simultaneously in a parameter-free manner. Then, similar to NPE, sparse neighborhood preserving embedding aims to preserve the neighborhood structure of the dataset in the latent topic space by minimizing

$$R_1 = \sum_{k=1}^{K} R_{1k} = \sum_{k=1}^{K} \sum_{i=1}^{N} (P(z_k|x_i) - \sum_{j=1}^{N} W_{ij} P(z_k|x_j))^2 \tag{7}$$

An intuitive explanation of minimizing $R_1$ is that if the image $x_i$ can be reconstructed by its neighbors in the feature space, the intrinsic structure should also be preserved in the latent topic space.

**Local Word Consistency.** Besides the image-level local structure, the word consistency is usually ignored and each word is treated individually in the existing topic models. However, the local word consistency is also very important for topic modeling. For example, it is a natural and intuitive assumption that frequently co-occurring words should share similar topics in the latent space. In this part, we will introduce how to maintain the local word consistency in our topic model.

We first compute the co-occurrence information $C_{ij}$ between word $w_i$ and word $w_j$ as follows:

$$C_{ij} = \frac{f_{ij}}{\sqrt{f_i} * \sqrt{f_j}} \tag{8}$$

where $f_{ij}$ is the number of images in which both word $w_i$ and word $w_j$ appeared and $f_i$ is the number of images in which word $w_i$ appeared.

After we get the co-occurrence matrix $C$, we maintain the local word consistency in the latent topic space by minimizing

$$R_2 = \sum_{k=1}^{K} R_{2k} = \sum_{k=1}^{K} \sum_{i,j=1}^{M} (P(w_i|z_k) - P(w_j|z_k))^2 C_{ij} \tag{9}$$

An intuitive explanation of minimizing $R_2$ is that if the word $w_i$ often co-occurred with $w_j$, their conditional distributions related to the latent topic $z_k$ should also be similar in the latent topic space.

**The Regularized Model.** In order to consider the local image and word structure simultaneously, we add $R_1$ and $R_2$ as regularized terms to the log-likelihood of PLSA model. Then we get our new latent topic model which aims to maximize the regularized log-likelihood as follows:

$$L = l - \lambda_1 R_1 - \lambda_2 R_2 = l - \lambda_1 \sum_{k=1}^{K} R_{1k} - \lambda_2 \sum_{k=1}^{K} R_{2k} \tag{10}$$

where $n(x_i, w_j)$ specifies the number of times the word $w_j$ occurred in image $x_i$, and $\lambda_{1,2}$ are the regularized parameters. When $\lambda_1 = \lambda_2 = 0$, our model degenerates to the traditional PLSA model. When $\lambda_1 = 0$, our model only considers the local word consistency. When $\lambda_2 = 0$, only the sparse neighborhood structure is preserved.

### 3.3   Model Fitting

When a probabilistic model involves unobserved latent variables, the EM algorithm [22] is generally used for the maximum likelihood estimation of the model. EM alternates two steps: (i) an expectation (E) step where posterior probabilities are computed for the latent variables, based on the current estimates of the parameters, (ii) a maximization (M) step, where parameters are updated based on maximizing the so-called expected complete data log-likelihood which depends on the posterior probabilities computed in the E-step.

As there are regularization terms in the log-likelihood of our model, the traditional EM algorithm cannot be applied directly. Here we use the generalized EM algorithm [23] for parameter estimation. The main difference between generalized EM and traditional EM is that generalized EM algorithm finds parameters that "improve" the expected value of the log-likelihood function rather than "maximizing" it.

Let $\phi = \{P(w_j|z_k)\}$ and $\theta = \{P(z_k|x_i)\}$ denote the parameters in our model.

**E-Step**

Our model adopts the same generative scheme as that of PLSA. Thus, we have the same E-step as that of PLSA. The posterior probabilities for latent variables are $P(z_k|x_i, w_j)$, which can be computed as follows:

$$P(z_k|x_i, w_j) = \frac{P(w_j|z_k)P(z_k|x_i)}{\sum_{l=1}^{K} P(w_j|z_l)P(z_l|x_i)} \tag{11}$$

**M-Step**

The relevant part of the expected complete log-likelihood for our model is

$$Q(\phi, \theta) = Q_1(\phi, \theta) - \lambda_1 R_1(\theta) - \lambda_2 R_2(\phi)$$

$$= \sum_{i=1}^{N} \sum_{j=1}^{M} n(x_i, w_j) \log \sum_{k=1}^{K} P(w_j|z_k)P(z_k|x_i)$$

$$- \lambda_1 \sum_{k=1}^{K} \sum_{i=1}^{N} (P(z_k|x_i) - \sum_{j=1}^{N} W_{ij} P(z_k|x_j))^2 \tag{12}$$

$$- \lambda_2 \sum_{k=1}^{K} \sum_{i,j=1}^{M} (P(w_i|z_k) - P(w_j|z_k))^2 C_{ij}$$

In the M-step, we improve the expected value of the log-likelihood function $Q(\phi, \theta)$. We have parameter values $\{\phi_r, \theta_r\}$ and try to find $\{\phi_{r+1}, \theta_{r+1}\}$ which satisfy $Q(\phi_{r+1}, \theta_{r+1}) \geq Q(\phi_r, \theta_r)$ in each step.

We first find $\{\phi_{r+1}^{(1)}, \theta_{r+1}^{(1)}\}$ which maximizes $Q_1(\phi, \theta)$ instead of the whole $Q(\phi, \theta)$. This can be done by the following equations which are the M-step re-estimation of PLSA:

$$P(w_j|z_k) = \frac{\sum_{i=1}^{N} n(x_i, w_j)P(z_k|x_i, w_j)}{\sum_{i=1}^{N} \sum_{m=1}^{M} n(x_i, w_m)P(z_k|x_i, w_m)} \tag{13}$$

$$P(z_k|x_i) = \frac{\sum_{j=1}^{M} n(x_i, w_j)P(z_k|x_i, w_j)}{\sum_{j=1}^{M} n(x_i, w_j)} \tag{14}$$

Clearly, $Q(\phi_{r+1}^{(1)}, \theta_{r+1}^{(1)}) \geq Q(\phi_r, \theta_r)$ does not necessarily hold. We then try to start from $\{\phi_{r+1}^{(1)}, \theta_{r+1}^{(1)}\}$ and decrease $R_1$ and $R_2$, which can be done through Newton-Raphson method [24]. Note that $R_1$ only involves parameters $P(z_k|x_i)$ while $R_2$ only involves parameters $P(w_j|z_k)$, we can update $\phi_{r+1}$ and $\theta_{r+1}$ respectively.

Given a function $f(x)$ and the initial value $x^{(t)}$, the Newton-Raphson updating formula to decrease (or increase) $f(x)$ is as follows:

$$x^{(t+1)} = x^{(t)} - \gamma \frac{f'(x^{(t)})}{f''(x^{(t)})} \tag{15}$$

where $0 \leq \gamma \leq 1$ is the step parameter. Since we have $R_{1k} \geq 0, R_{2k} \geq 0$, the Newton-Raphson method will decrease $R_{1k}$ and $R_{2k}$ in each updating step.

With $\phi_{r+1}^{(1)}$ and put $R_{1k}$ into the Newton-Raphson updating formula in Eqn. (17), we can get the closed form solution for $\phi_{r+1}^{(2)}, \phi_{r+1}^{(3)}, \ldots, \phi_{r+1}^{(m)}$, where

$$P(z_k|x_i)_{r+1}^{(t+1)} = (1 - \gamma_1)P(z_k|x_i)_{r+1}^{(t)} + \gamma_1 \sum_{j=1}^{N} W_{ij}P(z_k|x_j)_{r+1}^{(t)} \tag{16}$$

Similarly, we can also get the updating equation for $\theta_{r+1}$ as follows:

$$P(w_i|z_k)_{r+1}^{(t+1)} = (1 - \gamma_2)P(w_i|z_k)_{r+1}^{(t)} + \gamma_2 \frac{\sum_{j=1}^{M} C_{ij}P(w_j|z_k)_{r+1}^{(t)}}{\sum_{j=1}^{M} C_{ij}} \tag{17}$$

Every iteration of Eqn. (16) and (17) will make the topic distribution smoother. We continue the iteration of Eqn. (16) and (17) until $Q(\phi_{r+1}^{(t+1)}, \theta_{r+1}^{(t+1)}) \leq Q(\phi_{r+1}^{(t)}, \theta_{r+1}^{(t)})$. Then we test whether $Q(\phi_{r+1}^{(t)}, \theta_{r+1}^{(t)}) \geq Q(\phi_r, \theta_r)$. If not, we reject the values of $\{\phi_{r+1}^{(t)}, \theta_{r+1}^{(t)}\}$, and return the $\{\phi_r, \theta_r\}$ as the result of the M-step, and continue with the next E-step. The E-step and M-step are iteratively performed until the probability values are stable.

## 4    Experiments

In this section, we evaluate the performance of our model by comparing it with the state-of-the-art methods on image clustering task. Clustering is one of the most crucial techniques to organize the data samples. The latent topics discovered by the topic modeling approaches can be regarded as clusters. By representing the images in the latent space, topic models can assign each image to the most probable latent topic according to the estimated conditional probability distributions $P(z_k|x_i)$. Our experiments are conducted on three publicly available datasets: the Binary Alphadigits[1], the Scene-15 dataset [1], and the Caltech-101 dataset [25]. The weighting parameters $\lambda_1$ and $\lambda_2$ are tuned with cross validation from intervals [1,100] and [1000,1500] respectively. The values of the Newton step parameter $\gamma_1$ and $\gamma_2$ are both set to 0.1 in our experiment.

The Binary Alphadigits contains binary 20x16 digits of '0' through '9' and capital 'A' through 'Z' where there are 39 examples of each class. Thus we have 1404 images from 36 classes in total with each image represented by a 320-dimensional binary pixel vector. The topic models are applied to the images by representing each binary pixel as a word and each image as a document to generate K clusters. The Scene-15 dataset contains 4485 images from 15 categories, and the Caltech-101 dataset involves 9144 images from 101 object categories and a background category. A unique label has been assigned to each image in the datasets to indicate which category it belongs to, which serves as the ground truth for performance evaluation. SIFT [26] features are extracted and a 1000-D bag-of-words representation is generated for the Scene-15 and Caltech-101 dataset. Then all the models are performed on the bag-of-words to generate K clusters. The clustering accuracy (AC) is used to measure the clustering performance [27].

---

[1] http://www.cs.nyu.edu/~roweis/data.html

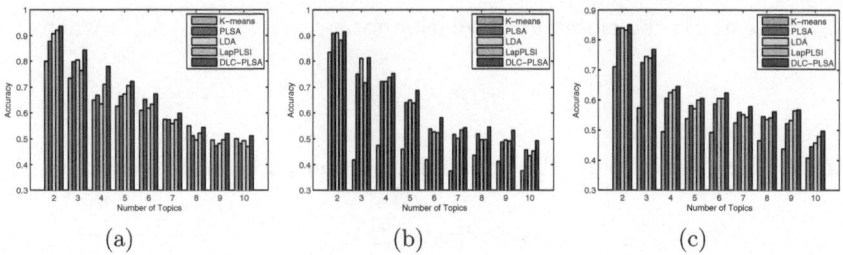

**Fig. 1.** Clustering results on (a) the Binary Alphadigits, (b) the Scene-15 dataset, and (c) the Caltech-101 dataset

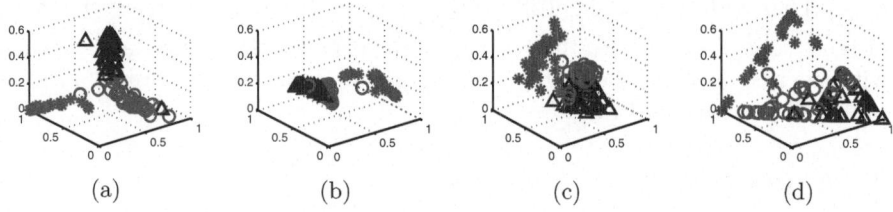

**Fig. 2.** Visualization view of image distribution in the latent topic space learned by different topic models. (a)The DLC-PLSA model. (b) The LapPLSI model. (c)The LDA model. (d)The PLSA model. (digit characters 'A' - 'C' in the Binary Alphadigits dataset, 'A': blue, 'B': green, 'C': red).

We evaluated the proposed DLC-PLSA model and compared it with the following algorithms: K-means clustering algorithm (K-means), Probabilistic Latent Semantic Analysis (PLSA) [4], Latent Dirichlet Allocation (LDA)[5], Laplacian Probabilistic Latent Semantic Indexing (LapPLSI) [12].

In order to make the experiments statistically meaningful, we conducted the evaluations with the cluster numbers ranging from two to ten. For each given cluster number k, k different categories were randomly selected from the datasets and provided to the clustering algorithms. Five test runs were conducted for each k, and the final performance scores were obtained by averaging the sores over the five test runs.

Figure 1 shows the clustering performance of all the algorithms on the Binary Alphadigits, the Scene-15 dataset and the Caltech-101 dataset, respectively. We can see that the topic models achieve better performance than the traditional K-means clustering method on the whole. But the PLSA and LDA model show lower performance than LapPLSI and DLC-PLSA because they do not consider any local discriminant structure when discovering the latent topics. Although the LapPLSI model considers the proximity between image pairs, it is not robust enough and sometimes even gets worse results than PLSA and LDA. The reason is that a $K$-NN graph is simply constructed to model the image structure, which is very sensitive to noise, and the local word consistency is also

**Table 1.** The influence of different regularized terms on the clustering accuracy of the Binary Alphadigits

| Topic number | 2 | 4 | 6 | 8 |
|---|---|---|---|---|
| $\lambda_1 \neq 0, \lambda_2 = 0$ | 0.926 | 0.722 | 0.648 | 0.528 |
| $\lambda_1 = 0, \lambda_2 \neq 0$ | 0.915 | 0.751 | 0.669 | 0.510 |
| $\lambda_1 \neq 0, \lambda_2 \neq 0$ | **0.935** | **0.780** | **0.673** | **0.544** |

**Table 2.** The influence of different regularized terms on the clustering accuracy of the Scene-15 dataset

| Topic number | 2 | 4 | 6 | 8 |
|---|---|---|---|---|
| $\lambda_1 \neq 0, \lambda_2 = 0$ | 0.906 | 0.733 | 0.522 | 0.518 |
| $\lambda_1 = 0, \lambda_2 \neq 0$ | 0.907 | 0.679 | 0.553 | 0.503 |
| $\lambda_1 \neq 0, \lambda_2 \neq 0$ | **0.914** | **0.752** | **0.581** | **0.545** |

ignored. Therefore, it cannot reach full discriminant power. Our DLC-PLSA model, which constructs the $\ell^1$-graph to model the neighborhood structure of images and incorporates the local word consistency into the model at the same time, can perform consistently better than other models.

In order to evaluate the performance of different regularized terms, we also compare the results of our model with different regularized terms by setting the regularization parameter $\lambda_1=0$ or $\lambda_2=0$ respectively on different topic numbers. The comparison results are shown in Table 1-3, from which we can see that the model with both the regularized terms always perform as well as or outperform the better one with only one regularized term. Moreover, the model with only the word regularized term also performs very consistently and sometimes get better results than the image regularized term, which proves that the local word consistency is also very important in topic modeling.

The visualization comparison of image distribution (digit characters 'A' - 'C' in the Binary Alphadigits dataset) in the latent topic space is shown in Figure 2. The comparison results show that the embedded representations of DLC-PLSA, which models the hidden topics with sparse neighborhood and local word consistency, have the best separability. Although LapPLSI considers the proximity of image pairs in topic modeling, it cannot separate characters 'A' and 'B' very well. We analyzed the reason and found that three 'noisy' images of character 'B' were very easily considered as neighbors by most images of character 'A' when constructing the $K$-NN graph, which affects the whole local structure significantly. In order to further show the impact of the noisy images on the performance of different models, we conduct an experiment by manually removing some noisy images in these three classes and the comparison clustering results are given in Table 4. We can see that the performance of LapPLSI is affected greatly by the noisy images, because it models the image structure on the K-NN graph. After removing the noisy images, its performance has a big improvement. In contrast, our model constructs $\ell^1$-graph to model the neighborhood structure of images and it can perform very consistently in both cases, which indicates that our model is more robust to noise and can discover more accurate latent topics.

**Table 3.** The influence of different regularized terms on the clustering accuracy of the Caltech-101 dataset

| Topic number | 2 | 4 | 6 | 8 |
|---|---|---|---|---|
| $\lambda_1 \neq 0, \lambda_2 = 0$ | **0.850** | 0.617 | 0.601 | 0.553 |
| $\lambda_1 = 0, \lambda_2 \neq 0$ | 0.844 | 0.626 | 0.613 | 0.559 |
| $\lambda_1 \neq 0, \lambda_2 \neq 0$ | **0.850** | **0.644** | **0.623** | **0.562** |

**Table 4.** The impact of noisy images on clustering accuracy (digit characters 'A', 'B', 'C') of different models

| | DLC-PLSA | LapPLSI | LDA | PLSA |
|---|---|---|---|---|
| Without removing the noisy images | 0.8718 | 0.6667 | 0.7949 | 0.7179 |
| Removing the noisy images | 0.8803 | 0.8034 | 0.8291 | 0.8205 |

## 5    Conclusion

In this paper, we have presented a novel topic model named DLC-PLSA. In our DLC-PLSA, the sparse neighborhood structure of the images and the local word consistency are preserved when modeling the latent topics. Therefore, our model can be less sensitive to noise and have more powerful description ability in the latent semantic space than the traditional topic modeling approaches. Experimental results on image clustering show that the DLC-PLSA model provides better representation and gets very consistent performance.

There are also some questions remained to be investigated in the future work. First, the idea of dual local consistency preserving can also be incorporated into other clustering methods or topic models. Second, the $\ell^1$-graph is unsupervised in our model. The label information can be used to construct a more discriminative graph. Finally, it is very interesting to explore new ways in order to capture the image or word correlations effectively.

**Acknowledgement.** This work was supported by National Natural Science Foundation of China (grant No. 61170127, 60975010, 61070104), Key project of Chinese Academy of Sciences (grant No. KGZD-EW-103-5).

## References

1. Lazebnik, S., Schmid, C., Ponce, J.: Beyond bags of features: Spatial pyramid matching for recognizing natural scene categories. In: CVPR, pp. 2169–2178 (2006)
2. Li, P., Wang, M., Cheng, J., Xu, C., Lu, H.: Spectral hashing with semantically consistent graph for image indexing. IEEE Transactions on Multimedia 14 (2012)
3. Li, Z., Yang, Y., Liu, J., Zhou, X., Lu, H.: Unsupervised feature selection using nonnegative spectral analysis. In: AAAI (2012)

4. Hofmann, T.: Unsupervised learning by probabilistic latent semantic analysis. Machine Learning 42, 177–196 (2001)
5. Blei, D., Ng, A., Jordan, M.: Latent dirichlet allocation. The Journal of Machine Learning Research 3, 993–1022 (2003)
6. Bosch, A., Zisserman, A., Muñoz, X.: Scene Classification Via pLSA. In: Leonardis, A., Bischof, H., Pinz, A. (eds.) ECCV 2006. LNCS, vol. 3954, pp. 517–530. Springer, Heidelberg (2006)
7. Monay, F., Gatica-Perez, D.: PLSA-based image auto-annotation: constraining the latent space. In: ACM Multimedia, pp. 348–351 (2004)
8. Cao, L., Li, F.: Spatially coherent latent topic model for concurrent segmentation and classification of objects and scenes. In: ICCV, pp. 1–8 (2007)
9. Roweis, S., Saul, L.: Nonlinear dimensionality reduction by locally linear embedding. Science 290, 2323–2326 (2000)
10. Belkin, M., Niyogi, P.: Laplacian eigenmaps for dimensionality reduction and data representation. Neural Computing 15, 1373–1396 (2002)
11. Tenenbaum, J., Silva, V., Langford, J.: A global geometric framework for nonlinear dimensionality reduction. Science 290, 2319–2323 (2000)
12. Cai, D., Mei, Q., Han, J., Zhai, C.: Modeling hidden topics on document manifold. In: CIKM, pp. 911–920 (2008)
13. Cai, D., Wang, X., He, X.: Probabilistic dyadic data analysis with local and global consistency. In: ICML (2009)
14. Deerwester, S., Dumais, S., Furnas, G., Landauer, T., Harshman, R.: Indexing by latent semantic analysis. Journal of the American Society for Information Science 41, 391–407 (1990)
15. Tenenbaum, J.: Mapping a manifold of perceptual observations. In: NIPS, pp. 682–688 (1997)
16. He, X., Niyogi, P.: Locality preserving projections. In: NIPS (2003)
17. He, X., Cai, D., Yan, S., Zhang, H.: Neighborhood preserving embedding. In: ICCV, pp. 1208–1213 (2005)
18. Cheng, B., Yang, J., Yan, S., Fu, Y., Huang, T.: Learning with $\ell^1$-graph for image analysis. IEEE Trans. on Image Processing 19, 858–866 (2010)
19. Donoho, D.: For most large underdetermined systems of linear equations the minimal $\ell^1$-norm solution is also the sparsest solution. Communications on Pure and Applied Mathematics 59, 797–829 (2004)
20. Meinshansen, N., Buhlmann, P.: High-dimensional graphs and variable selection with the lasso. The Annals of Statistics 34, 1436–1462 (2006)
21. Wright, J., Genesh, A., Yang, A., Ma, Y.: Robust face recognition via sparse representation. IEEE Trans. on Pattern Anal. Mach. Intell. 31, 210–227 (2009)
22. Dempster, A., Laird, N., Rubin, D.: Maximum likelihood from in complete data via the EM algorithm. Journal of the Royal Statistical Society 39, 1–38 (1977)
23. Neal, R., Hinton, G.: A view of the EM algorithm that justifies incremental, sparse, and other variants. In: Learning in Graphical Models (1998)
24. Press, W., Flannery, B., Teukolsky, S., Vetterling, W.: Numerical recipes in C: the art of scientific computing. Cambridge University Press (1992)
25. Li, F., Rob, F., Pietro, P.: Learning generative visual models from few training examples: an incremental bayesian approach tested on 101 object categories. In: CVPR Workshop on Generative Model Based Vision (2004)
26. Lowe, D.: Distinctive image features from scale-invariant keypoints. International Journal of Computer Vision 60, 91–110 (2004)
27. Xu, W., Liu, X., Gong, Y.: Document clustering based on non-negative matrix factorization. In: SIGIR, pp. 267–273 (2003)

# Design of Non-Linear Discriminative Dictionaries for Image Classification

Ashish Shrivastava, Hien V. Nguyen, Vishal M. Patel, and Rama Chellappa

UMIACS, University of Maryland, College Park, MD, USA

**Abstract.** In recent years there has been growing interest in designing dictionaries for image classification. These methods, however, neglect the fact that data of interest often has non-linear structure. Motivated by the fact that this non-linearity can be handled by the kernel trick, we propose learning of dictionaries in the high-dimensional feature space which are simultaneously reconstructive and discriminative. The proposed optimization approach consists of two main stages- coefficient update and dictionary update. We propose a kernel driven simultaneous orthogonal matching pursuit algorithm for the task of sparse coding in the feature space. The dictionary update step is performed using an approximate but efficient KSVD algorithm in feature space. Extensive experiments on image classification demonstrate that the proposed non-linear dictionary learning method is robust and can perform significantly better than many competitive discriminative dictionary learning algorithms.

## 1 Introduction

Sparse and redundant signal representations have recently drawn much interest in vision and image processing fields [1]. This is due in part to the fact that objects and images of interest can be sparse or compressible in some basis of a dictionary. We say a signal $\mathbf{x}$ is sparse in dictionary $\mathbf{D}$ when it can be well represented as $\mathbf{x} = \mathbf{D}\boldsymbol{\alpha}$, where $\boldsymbol{\alpha}$ is the sparse representation vector and $\mathbf{D}$ is a dictionary that contains atoms as its columns. The dictionary $\mathbf{D}$ can be analytic such as a redundant Gabor dictionary or it can be trained directly from data. It has been observed that learning a dictionary directly from training data rather than using a predetermined dictionary usually leads to better representation and hence can provide improved results in many practical image processing applications such as restoration and classification [1], [2], [3], [4]. Two well-known algorithms for learning a dictionary are the method of optimal directions (MOD) [5] and the KSVD algorithm [6]. While these approaches are purely generative, the design of discriminative dictionaries has also gained a lot of interest in recent years. Linear discriminant analysis (LDA) based basis selection and feature extraction algorithm for classification using wavelet packets was originally proposed in [7]. More recently, many other methods have shown significant improvements over purely reconstructive dictionaries, e.g. [8], [9], [10]. One of the major advantages of learning dictionaries which are simultaneously

K.M. Lee et al. (Eds.): ACCV 2012, Part I, LNCS 7724, pp. 660–674, 2013.
© Springer-Verlag Berlin Heidelberg 2013

reconstructive and discriminative is that they are known to be less sensitive to noise.

In many practical applications, data of interest lies on a non-linear structure. Linear dictionary learning methods such as MOD and KSVD are almost always inadequate for representing these nonlinear data. In [11], Nguyen *et al.* addressed this issue by learning dictionaries in the high dimensional feature space. Using kernel methods, they developed dictionary learning algorithms that take into account the nonlinear structure of data. They showed that their non-linear dictionary learning methods yield representations that are more compact than kernel PCA (Principal Component Analysis) and are able to handle the non-linearity better than their linear counterparts.

Several other methods have also been proposed for exploiting the non-linear structure of data by sparse coding in the feature space [12], [13]. In [14], Yuan and Yan propose a multi-task joint sparse representation for visual recognition. Their method is formulated as the solution to the problem of multi-task least squares regression problem with $\ell_{1,2}$ mixed-norm regularization. In [13], Zhang *et al.* propose a kernel version of the sparse representation-based classification algorithm which was originally proposed for robust face recognition [15].

The optimization approach presented in [11] is purely generative. It does not explicitly contain the discrimination term which is important for many

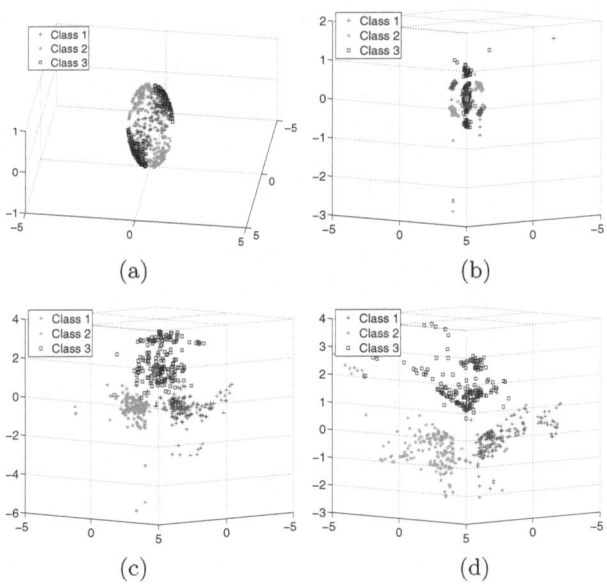

**Fig. 1.** A synthetic example showing the significance of the proposed method for classification. (a) Synthetic data which consists of linearly non separable 3D points on a sphere. Different classes are represented by different colors. (b) Sparse coefficients from KSVD projected onto learned SVM (Support Vector Machine) hyperplanes. (c) Sparse coefficients from a non-linear dictionary projected onto learned SVM hyperplanes. (d) Sparse coefficients from the proposed method projected onto learned SVM hyperplanes.

classification tasks. Using the kernel trick, when the data is transformed into a high dimensional feature space, the data from different classes may still overlap. Hence, by learning generative dictionaries for different classes in the feature space, one may not be able to capture the internal structure of the data in each class. This may lead to poor performance in classification. We propose a method for designing dictionaries in the feature space which are simultaneously reconstructive and discriminative.

Figure 1 presents an important comparison in terms of discriminative power of our approach with a few other methods. A scatter plot of the sparse coefficients obtained using different approaches show that our method is able to learn the underlying non-linear sparsity of data as well provide more discriminative representation.

This paper makes the following contributions:

- A non linear coefficient update which provides discriminative capability to the dictionary learning algorithm is proposed.
- A novel non-linear dictionary update algorithm based on approximate KSVD is presented.
- These two stages provide a framework for non-linear dictionary learning for classification in feature space.

## 2  Problem Formulation

We represent the data matrix as $\mathbf{X} = [\mathbf{X}_1, \ldots, \mathbf{X}_C] = [\mathbf{x}_1, \ldots, \mathbf{x}_N] \in \mathbb{R}^{d \times N}$ where $\mathbf{x}_i \in \mathbb{R}^d$ is a $d$ dimensional data sample, $\mathbf{X}_c \in \mathbb{R}^{d \times N_c}$ is the matrix of data samples in $c^{\text{th}}$ class, and $\mathbf{y} = [y_1, \ldots, y_N]$, where $y_i$ is the class label of data sample $\mathbf{x}_i$ and $C$ is the number of classes. We denote the number of samples in $c^{\text{th}}$ class by $N_c$ and total number of training samples by $N$, i.e. $N = N_1 + \cdots + N_C$. Linear dictionary $\mathbf{D}$ is denoted as the concatenation of $C$ sub-dictionaries $\mathbf{D} = [\mathbf{D}_1 \mathbf{D}_2 \ldots \mathbf{D}_C] \in \mathbb{R}^{d \times K}$ where $\mathbf{D}_c \in \mathbb{R}^{d \times K_c}$ is the dictionary for class $c$ and $K_c$ is the number of atoms in this dictionary. Here, $K(= K_1 + \cdots + K_C)$ is the total number of atoms in the dictionary $\mathbf{D}$. Similarly, the coefficient matrix is denoted by $\boldsymbol{\Gamma} = \begin{bmatrix} \boldsymbol{\Gamma}_1 \\ \vdots \\ \boldsymbol{\Gamma}_C \end{bmatrix} = [\boldsymbol{\gamma}_1, \ldots \boldsymbol{\gamma}_N] \in \mathbb{R}^{K \times N}$, where $\boldsymbol{\Gamma}_c \in \mathbb{R}^{K_c \times N}$ is the coefficient matrix corresponding to the $c^{\text{th}}$ class and $\boldsymbol{\gamma}_i$ is the coefficient vector for the $i^{\text{th}}$ data sample.

In the following sub-sections, we first present our formulation for designing a linear discriminative dictionary which, then, sets the ground for non-linear discriminative dictionary.

### 2.1  Linear Discriminative Dictionary Learning Model

In the linear case, we propose the following discriminative dictionary learning model

$$\hat{\mathbf{D}}, \hat{\boldsymbol{\Gamma}} = \min_{\mathbf{D}, \boldsymbol{\Gamma}} J(\mathbf{D}, \boldsymbol{\Gamma}; \mathbf{X}, \mathbf{y}) \text{ subject to } \|\boldsymbol{\gamma}_i\|_0 \leq T_0, \tag{1}$$

where the $\ell_0$ norm $\|\gamma\|_0$ counts the number of nonzero elements in the representation $\gamma$ and $T_0$ is a sparsity measure. The objective function $J$ is designed such that it captures discrimination as well as representation. It imposes Fisher type of discrimination on the sparse coefficients and enforces separability among dictionary atoms of different classes. It is defined as follows

$$J(\mathbf{D}, \mathbf{\Gamma}; \mathbf{X}, \mathbf{y}) = \sum_{c=1}^{C} \|\mathbf{X}_c - \mathbf{D}_c \mathbf{\Gamma}_c\|_F^2 - \lambda_1 F_1(\mathbf{D}, \mathbf{X}) + \lambda_2 F_2(\mathbf{D}), \qquad (2)$$

Here, $\|.\|_F$ denotes the Frobenius norm. The first term in Eq. (2) reduces the representation error. The second term essentially ensures that the sparse coding coefficients have small within-class scatter but large between-class scatter. Mathematically, it is defined as follows

$$F_1(\mathbf{D}, \mathbf{X}) = trace(\mathbf{D}^T \mathbf{S}_b \mathbf{D} - \mathbf{D}^T \mathbf{S}_w \mathbf{D}), \qquad (3)$$

where $\mathbf{S}_b = \frac{1}{N} \sum_1^C N_c (\mathbf{m}_c - \mathbf{m})(\mathbf{m}_c - \mathbf{m})^T$ and $\mathbf{S}_w = \frac{1}{N} \sum_{c=1}^{C} \sum_{\substack{i=1 \\ y_i=c}}^{N} (\mathbf{m}_c - \mathbf{m})(\mathbf{m}_c - \mathbf{m})^T$ are the between-class and within-class data scatter matrices, respectively. Here, $\mathbf{m}_c = \frac{1}{N_c} \sum_{\substack{i=1 \\ y_i=c}}^{N} \mathbf{x}_i$ is the mean of $c^{\text{th}}$ class data samples and $\mathbf{m} = \frac{1}{N} \sum_{i=1}^{N} \mathbf{x}_i$ is the mean of all the data samples. With this, $F_1$ can be rewritten as

$$F_1(\mathbf{D}, \mathbf{X}) = \sum_{k=1}^{K} \mathbf{d}_k^T \mathbf{S}_b \mathbf{d}_k - \sum_{k=1}^{K} \mathbf{d}_k^T \mathbf{S}_w \mathbf{d}_k. \qquad (4)$$

Where, $\mathbf{d}_k$ is the $k^{\text{th}}$ atom of dictionary $\mathbf{D}$. Finally, the third term in (2) is defined such that it enforces dissimilarity among atoms of different classes

$$F_2(\mathbf{D}) = \sum_{\substack{c=1 \\ j \neq c}}^{C} \|\mathbf{D}_c^T \mathbf{D}_j\|_F^2, \qquad (5)$$

where $\mathbf{D}_c$ refers to the set of those atoms which belong to class $c$. This enforces dissimilarity between the atoms of different classes.

## 2.2   Non-Linear Discriminative Dictionary (NLDD)

Let $\mathbf{\Phi} : \mathbb{R}^N \to G$ be a non-linear mapping from $\mathbb{R}^N$ into a higher dimensional feature space $G$. Since the feature space $G$ can be very high dimensional, in the kernel methods, Mercer kernels are usually employed to carry out the mapping implicitly. A Mercer kernel is a function $\tau(\mathbf{x}_1, \mathbf{x}_2)$ that for all data $\{\mathbf{x}_i\}$ gives rise to a positive semidefinite matrix $\mathcal{K}(i, j) = \tau(\mathbf{x}_i, \mathbf{x}_j)$. It can be shown that using $\tau$ instead of dot product in input space corresponds to mapping the data with some mapping $\mathbf{\Phi}$ into a feature space $G$. That is, $\tau(\mathbf{x}_i, \mathbf{x}_j) = \langle \mathbf{\Phi}(\mathbf{x}_i), \mathbf{\Phi}(\mathbf{x}_j) \rangle$. Some commonly used kernels include polynomial kernels $\tau(\mathbf{x}, \mathbf{y}) = \langle (\mathbf{x}, \mathbf{y}) + c \rangle^d$ and Gaussian kernels $\tau(\mathbf{x}, \mathbf{y}) = \exp(-\frac{\|\mathbf{x}-\mathbf{y}\|^2}{c})$, where $c$ and $d$ are the parameters.

We now show how the discriminative dictionary learning framework (1) can be kernelized.

We will use the following model for the dictionary in the feature space

$$\Phi(\mathbf{D}) = \Phi(\mathbf{X})\mathbf{A},$$

where $\mathbf{A} = [\mathbf{a}_1, \mathbf{a}_2, \dots, \mathbf{a}_K] \in \mathbb{R}^{N \times K}$ and $\Phi(\mathbf{X}) = [\Phi(\mathbf{x}_1)\Phi(\mathbf{x}_2)\dots\Phi(\mathbf{x}_N)]$. This model provides adaptivity via modification of the matrix $\mathbf{A}$ [16],[11]. First note that $\|\Phi(\mathbf{x}_i) - \Phi(\mathbf{X})\mathbf{A}_i\boldsymbol{\gamma}_i\|_2^2$ can be kernelized as follows,

$$\|\Phi(\mathbf{x}_i) - \Phi(\mathbf{X})\mathbf{A}_i\boldsymbol{\gamma}_i\|_2^2 = \mathcal{K}(\mathbf{x}_i, \mathbf{x}_i) + \boldsymbol{\gamma}_i^T \mathbf{A}_i^T \mathcal{K} \mathbf{A}_i \boldsymbol{\gamma}_i - 2\boldsymbol{\gamma}_i \mathbf{A}_i \mathcal{K}(\mathbf{X}, \mathbf{x}_i) \quad (6)$$

Next, the term $\mathbf{d}_k^T \mathbf{S}_b \mathbf{d}_k$ in (2) can be written in the feature space as

$$(\Phi(\mathbf{X})\mathbf{a}_k)^T \left( \frac{1}{N} \sum_{c=1}^{C} N_c (\mathbf{m}_c^{feat} - \mathbf{m}^{feat})(\mathbf{m}_c^{feat} - \mathbf{m}^{feat})^T \right) \Phi(\mathbf{X})\mathbf{a}_k, \quad (7)$$

where $\mathbf{m}_c^{feat} = \frac{1}{N_c} \sum_{\substack{i=1 \\ y_i=c}}^{N} \Phi(\mathbf{x}_i)$ and $\mathbf{m}^{feat} = \frac{1}{N} \sum_{i=1}^{N} \Phi(\mathbf{x}_i)$ are the mean vectors in the feature space. Equation (7) can be simplified as, $\mathbf{a}_k^T \mathbf{S}_b^{ker} \mathbf{a}_k$, where

$$\mathbf{S}_b^{ker} = \frac{1}{N} \sum_{c=1}^{C} N_c (\mathbf{m}_c^{ker} - \mathbf{m}^{ker})(\mathbf{m}_c^{ker} - \mathbf{m}^{ker})^T, \quad (8)$$

$\mathbf{m}_c^{ker} = \frac{1}{N_c} \sum_{\substack{i=1 \\ y_i=c}}^{N} \mathcal{K}(\mathbf{X}, \mathbf{x}_i)$ and $\mathbf{m}^{ker} = \frac{1}{N} \sum_{i=1}^{N} \mathcal{K}(\mathbf{X}, \mathbf{x}_i)$. Similarly, $\mathbf{d}_k^T \mathbf{S}_w \mathbf{d}_k$ (2) can be kernelized as $\mathbf{a}_k^T \mathbf{S}_w^{ker} \mathbf{a}_k$, where

$$\mathbf{S}_w^{ker} = \frac{1}{N} \sum_{c=1}^{C} \sum_{\substack{i=1 \\ y_i=c}}^{N} (\mathcal{K}(\mathbf{X}, \mathbf{x}_i) - \mathbf{m}_c^{ker})(\mathcal{K}(\mathbf{X}, \mathbf{x}_i) - \mathbf{m}_c^{ker})^T. \quad (9)$$

Finally, to kernelize the term in (5), we observe that the dot product of any two dictionary atoms in feature space can be written as

$$(\Phi(\mathbf{X})\mathbf{a}_i)^T (\Phi(\mathbf{X})\mathbf{a}_j) = \mathbf{a}_i^T \mathcal{K} \mathbf{a}_j. \quad (10)$$

Equipped with the above notations, the main problem can be formally stated as follows

$$\hat{\mathbf{A}}, \hat{\boldsymbol{\Gamma}} = \min_{\mathbf{A}, \boldsymbol{\Gamma}} J(\mathbf{A}, \boldsymbol{\Gamma}; \mathbf{X}, \mathbf{y}) \quad \text{subject to } \|\boldsymbol{\gamma}_i\|_0 \le T_0, \forall i \in \{1, \dots, N\}, \quad (11)$$

where

$$J(\mathbf{A}, \boldsymbol{\Gamma}; \mathbf{X}, \mathbf{y}) = \sum_{c=1}^{C} \|\Phi(\mathbf{X}_c) - \Phi(\mathbf{X})\mathbf{A}_c \boldsymbol{\Gamma}_c\|_F^2 - \lambda_1 F_1(\mathbf{A}, \mathbf{S}_b^{ker}, \mathbf{S}_w^{ker}) + \lambda_2 F_2(\mathbf{A}, \mathcal{K}),$$
$$(12)$$

$$F_1(\mathbf{A}, \mathbf{S}_b^{ker}, \mathbf{S}_w^{ker}) = \sum_{k=1}^{K} \mathbf{a}_k^T \mathbf{S}_b^{ker} \mathbf{a}_k - \sum_{k=1}^{K} \mathbf{a}_k^T \mathbf{S}_w^{ker} \mathbf{a}_k, \tag{13}$$

$$F_2(\mathbf{A}, \mathcal{K}) = \sum_{\substack{c=1 \\ j \neq c}}^{C} \|\mathbf{A}_c^T \mathcal{K} \mathbf{A}_j\|_F^2. \tag{14}$$

Here, $\mathbf{A}_c$ correspond to the atoms corresponding to class $c$. As the cost function (12) is jointly non-convex in $\mathbf{A}$ and $\mathbf{\Gamma}$, we adopt alternating optimization between coefficients $\mathbf{\Gamma}$ and $\mathbf{A}$. In what follows, we describe these steps in detail.

## 3   Computing Coefficients

To compute the coefficients, we fix $\mathbf{A}$ and find the best atoms indexed by $I$ on which we project the data. Hence, we solve the following optimization problem

$$\mathbf{\Gamma}^* = \arg\min_{\mathbf{\Gamma}} \|\mathbf{\Phi}(\mathbf{X}) - \mathbf{\Phi}(\mathbf{X})\mathbf{A}\mathbf{\Gamma}\|_F^2 - \lambda_1 F_1(\mathbf{A}, \mathbf{S}_b^{ker}, \mathbf{S}_w^{ker}) + \lambda_2 F_2(\mathbf{A})$$

$$\text{subject to} \quad \|\boldsymbol{\gamma}_i\|_0 \leq T_0, \quad \forall i \in \{1, \ldots, N\}. \tag{15}$$

In what follows, we describe how the well-known Simultaneous Orthogonal Matching Pursuit (SOMP) algorithm [17] can be extended to solve (15).

### 3.1   Supervised SOMP

Given a fixed dictionary $\mathbf{D}$ and examples $\mathbf{X}$, SOMP approximates all these samples at once using different linear combinations of the dictionary elements, while balancing the error in approximating the data against the total number of atoms that are used. It is a greedy algorithm that essentially solves the following optimization problem

$$\mathbf{\Gamma}^* = \arg\min_{\mathbf{\Gamma}} \|\mathbf{X} - \mathbf{D}\mathbf{\Gamma}\|_F^2 \quad \text{s. t.} \quad \|\mathbf{\Gamma}\|_{\text{row-0}} \leq T_0, \tag{16}$$

The SOMP algorithm can be extended to the supervised case where it includes the second and third terms of the cost function (2). The supervised SOMP can be obtained by changing the atom selection stage as follows

$$m = \arg\max_{p \in U} \sum_{\substack{i=1 \\ y_i = c}}^{N} |\langle \mathbf{r}_i^{(t-1)}, \mathbf{d}_p \rangle| + \lambda_1 (\mathbf{d}_p^T \mathbf{S}_b \mathbf{d}_p - \mathbf{d}_p^T \mathbf{S}_w \mathbf{d}_p) - \lambda_2 \sum_{\substack{j=1 \\ j \neq c}}^{C} \|\mathbf{D}_j^T \mathbf{d}_p\|_2^2. \tag{17}$$

where $m$ is the index of the selected atom at the current iteration and $\mathbf{r}_i^{(t-1)}$ is the residual for $i^{\text{th}}$ sample at $(t-1)^{\text{th}}$ iteration. In the next section, we show how this supervised SOMP algorithm can be kernelized to solve (15).

## 3.2  Supervised Kernel SOMP (KSOMP)

Note that residue for the $i^{\text{th}}$ sample in the feature space is

$$res_i = \mathbf{\Phi}(\mathbf{x}_i) - \mathbf{\Phi}(\mathbf{X})\mathbf{A}_I\boldsymbol{\gamma}_i^R, \tag{18}$$

where $\mathbf{A}_I$ is the set of selected elements indexed by $I$ and $\boldsymbol{\gamma}_i^R$ is the corresponding coefficient vector. Here, superscript $R$ denotes that the vector has been reduced to length of $I$ so that the remaining elements correspond to the atoms in $\mathbf{A}_I$. As will be evident later, this residue always appear as a dot product with $\mathbf{\Phi}(\mathbf{X})$. Hence we define,

$$\mathbf{r}_i = \mathbf{\Phi}(\mathbf{X})^T\left(\mathbf{\Phi}(\mathbf{x}_i) - \mathbf{\Phi}(\mathbf{X})\mathbf{A}_I\boldsymbol{\gamma}_i^R\right) \tag{19}$$

$$= \mathcal{K}(\mathbf{X}, \mathbf{x}_i) - \mathcal{K}(\mathbf{X}, \mathbf{X})\mathbf{A}_I\boldsymbol{\gamma}_i^R \tag{20}$$

The projection of the residue on the dictionary atom $\mathbf{a}_p$ can be computed as,

$$\langle\mathbf{\Phi}(\mathbf{X})\mathbf{a}_p, res_i\rangle = \mathbf{a}_p^T\left(\mathcal{K}(\mathbf{X}, \mathbf{x}_i) - \mathcal{K}(\mathbf{X}, \mathbf{X})\mathbf{A}_I\boldsymbol{\gamma}_i^R\right) = \langle\mathbf{r}_i, \mathbf{a}_p\rangle. \tag{21}$$

Equation 21 is the counter part of the dot product of candidate atom and residual in the feature space. Combining (21), with the definitions of scatter matrices in (8) and (9) we can write the atom selection stage of supervised kernel SOMP as

$$m = \arg\max_{p \in U} \sum_{\substack{i=1 \\ y_i=c}}^{N} |\langle\mathbf{r}_i^{(t-1)}, \mathbf{a}_p\rangle| + \lambda_1(\mathbf{a}_p^T\mathbf{S}_b^{ker}\mathbf{a}_p - \mathbf{a}_p^T\mathbf{S}_w^{ker}\mathbf{a}_p) + \lambda_2\sum_{\substack{j=1 \\ j\neq c}}^{C} \|\mathbf{A}_j^T\mathcal{K}\mathbf{a}_p\|_2^2.$$

$$\tag{22}$$

Finally, after selecting $I_c$ atoms of the $c^{\text{th}}$ class, the coefficients of the $i^{\text{th}}$ data sample can be computed as,

$$\boldsymbol{\gamma}_i^R = \left((\mathbf{\Phi}(\mathbf{X})\mathbf{A}_{I_c})^T(\mathbf{\Phi}(\mathbf{X})\mathbf{A}_{I_c})\right)^{-1}\left((\mathbf{\Phi}(\mathbf{X})\mathbf{A}_{I_c})^T\mathbf{\Phi}(x_i)\right)$$

$$= \left(\mathbf{A}_{I_c}^T\mathcal{K}\mathbf{A}_{I_c}\right)^{-1}\left(\mathbf{A}_{I_c}^T\mathcal{K}(\mathbf{X}, \mathbf{x}_i)\right). \tag{23}$$

The supervised kernel SOMP algorithm to compute coefficients $\mathbf{\Gamma}$ is summarized in Algorithm 1.

## 4    Dictionary Update

When $\mathbf{\Gamma}$ is fixed, we ignore $F_1$ and $F_2$ and solve the following optimization problem to update the dictionary

$$\mathbf{A}^* = \arg\min_{\mathbf{A}} \|\mathbf{\Phi}(\mathbf{X}) - \mathbf{\Phi}(\mathbf{X})\mathbf{A}\mathbf{\Gamma}\|_F^2. \tag{24}$$

This update can be computed efficiently by using the approximate kernel-KSVD algorithm [16] in the feature space.

---

**Algorithm 1:** supervised KSOMP

---

**Input:** $\mathbf{A}, \mathbf{h}, \mathcal{K}, \mathbf{y}, T_0$ .
**Output:** $\boldsymbol{\Gamma}$
*Initialization:* residual $(\forall i,)\mathbf{r}_i = \mathcal{K}(:,i)$, Set $(\forall c), I_c = [\ ]$, $\boldsymbol{\Gamma} = \mathbf{0}^{K \times N}$, $\mathbf{Q}_c = [\ ]$
**for** $t = 1, \ldots T_0$ **do**
    **for** $c = 1, \ldots C$ **do**
        $U = \{p = 1, \ldots, K\} \backslash I_c$
        compute $m$ using Eq. 22
        Set $I_c = I_c \cup m$
        Compute $\boldsymbol{\gamma}_i^R$ using Eq 23      $\forall i$, such that $y_i = c$.
        Set $\mathbf{r}_i = \mathcal{K}(:,i) - \mathcal{K}\mathbf{A}_{I_c}\boldsymbol{\gamma}_i^R$   $\forall i$, such that $y_i = c$
        $\boldsymbol{\Gamma}(I_c, i) \leftarrow \boldsymbol{\gamma}_i^R,$           $\forall i$, such that $y_i = c$
    **end**
**end**
**return** $\boldsymbol{\Gamma}$

---

## 4.1 Approximate Kernel KSVD

The following optimization problem is solved for each $\mathbf{a}_k$,

$$\mathbf{a}_k^* = \arg\min_{\mathbf{a}_k} \|\boldsymbol{\Phi}(\mathbf{X}) - \boldsymbol{\Phi}(\mathbf{X})\Big(\sum_{i \neq k} \mathbf{a}_i \boldsymbol{\gamma}_T^i + \mathbf{a}_k \boldsymbol{\gamma}_T^k\Big)\|_F^2 \tag{25}$$

$$= \arg\min_{\mathbf{a}_k} \|\boldsymbol{\Phi}(\mathbf{X})\mathbf{E}_k - \boldsymbol{\Phi}(\mathbf{X})\mathbf{a}_k \boldsymbol{\gamma}_T^k\|_F^2, \tag{26}$$

where $\mathbf{E}_k = \mathbf{I} - \sum_{i \neq k} \mathbf{a}_i \boldsymbol{\gamma}_T^i$. Furthermore, we need to consider only those samples which use $\mathbf{a}_k$. To do this we define the index set $I_k = \{j | 1 \leq j \leq K, \boldsymbol{\gamma}_T^k(j) \neq 0\}$ and a matrix $\boldsymbol{\Omega}_k \in \mathbb{R}^{N \times |I_k|}$ with 1's in the $(I_k(j), j)^{\text{th}}$ entry and 0's elsewhere.

---

**Algorithm 2:** Dictionary update stage using approximate kernel KSVD

---

**Input:** kernel matrix $\mathcal{K} \in \mathbb{R}^{N \times N}$, input labels $\mathbf{y} \in \mathbb{R}^{1 \times N}$ initial dictionary
       $\mathbf{A}_0 \in \mathbb{R}^{N \times K}$, coefficients matrix $\boldsymbol{\Gamma} \in \mathbb{R}^{K \times N}$.
**Output:** $\mathbf{A}$
*Initialization:* $\mathbf{A} \leftarrow \mathbf{A}_0,$
**for** $k = 1, \ldots K$ **do**
    $\mathbf{A}(:, k) = 0$
    $J = \{j \mid 1 \leq j \leq N, \boldsymbol{\Gamma}(k, j) \neq 0\}$
    $\mathbf{I}^R = \mathbf{I}(:, J)$
    $\boldsymbol{\gamma}_k^R = (\boldsymbol{\Gamma}(k, J))^T$
    $\mathbf{a}_k = \mathbf{I}^R \boldsymbol{\gamma}_k^R - \mathbf{A}\boldsymbol{\Gamma}_J \boldsymbol{\gamma}_k^R$
    $\mathbf{a}_k = \dfrac{\mathbf{a}_k}{\sqrt{\mathbf{a}_k^T \mathcal{K}\mathbf{a}_k}}$
    $\boldsymbol{\gamma}_k^R = (\mathbf{I}^R)^T \mathcal{K}\mathbf{a}_k - (\mathbf{A}\boldsymbol{\Gamma}_J)^T \mathcal{K}\mathbf{a}_k$
    $\boldsymbol{\Gamma}(k, J) = (\boldsymbol{\gamma}_k^R)^T$
    $\mathbf{A}(:, k) = \mathbf{a}_k$
**end**
**return** $\mathbf{A}$

Next, we define the reduced matrix $\mathbf{E}_k^R \triangleq \mathbf{E}_k \mathbf{\Omega}_k$, which consists of only those columns that use $\mathbf{a}_k$. Similarly, we reduce the length of the coefficient vector $\gamma_k$ and define a new column vector as $\gamma_k^R = (\gamma_T^k \mathbf{\Omega}_k)^T$. With this, the optimization problem can be rewritten as

$$\mathbf{a}_k^* = \arg\min_{\mathbf{a}_k} \|\mathbf{\Phi}(\mathbf{X})\mathbf{E}_k^R - \mathbf{\Phi}(\mathbf{X})\mathbf{a}_k(\gamma_k^R)^T\|_F^2 \quad \text{s.t.} \quad \|\mathbf{\Phi}(\mathbf{X})\mathbf{a}_k\|_2 = 1. \quad (27)$$

We use alternate optimization (fixing one variable and differentiating with respect to the other one) to compute $\mathbf{a}_k$ and $\gamma_k^R$,

$$\mathbf{a}_k = \frac{\mathbf{E}_k^R \gamma_k^R}{\sqrt{(\mathbf{E}_k^R \gamma_k^R)^T \mathcal{K} \mathbf{E}_k^R \gamma_k^R}}, \qquad \gamma_k^R = (\mathbf{E}_k^R)^T \mathcal{K} \mathbf{a}_k. \quad (28)$$

We summarize the procedure for approximate kernel KSVD in Algorithm 2.

---

**Algorithm 3:** Non-linear discriminative dictionary (NLDD) learning

**Input:**   Training Data $\mathbf{X} = [\mathbf{x}_1, \ldots, \mathbf{x}_N]$, class labels $\mathbf{y} = [y_1, \ldots, y_N]$, sparsity level $T_0$, parameters $\lambda_1, \lambda_2$.

**Output:** $\mathbf{A} = [\mathbf{A}_1, \ldots, \mathbf{A}_C]$

**Step 1:** (*Initialization*) Initialize each column of $\mathbf{A}$ with 1 at a random location. Compute kernel matrix $\mathcal{K}$, data scatter matrices $\mathbf{S}_b^{ker}$ and $\mathbf{S}_w^{ker}$.

**Step 2:** Compute sparse coefficients using Algorithm 1.

**Step 3:** Using sparse coefficients from step 2, update $\mathbf{A}$ using Algorithm 2 .

**Step 4:** Repeat steps 2 and 4 for pre-specified number of iterations.

**Step 5:** Remove those columns of $\mathbf{A}$ which were not used in last iteration.

**return A**

---

The complete NLDD algorithm of dictionary learning has been summarized in Algorithm 3

## 5   Classification

Once the dictionary has been learned, we use one of the following two methods of classification depending on the number of training samples per class.

**Case 1: (Large number of training samples per class).** When we have a large number of training samples per class (e.g digit recognition, gender recognition), we compute the per class reconstruction errors as follows

$$\epsilon_c(\mathbf{x}_t) = \|\mathbf{\Phi}(\mathbf{x}_t) - \mathbf{\Phi}(\mathbf{X})\mathbf{A}_c \gamma_t^*\|_2 \qquad \text{subject to} \quad \|\gamma_t\|_0 = T_0 \quad (29)$$

where $\mathbf{A}_c$ is the matrix corresponding to class $c$, $\mathbf{x}_t$ is the test sample, and $\gamma_t^*$ is the corresponding sparse coefficient computed using the kernel OMP algorithm [11] which solves the following problem

$$\gamma_t^* = \min_\gamma \|\mathbf{x}_t - \mathbf{\Phi}(\mathbf{X})\mathbf{A}_c \gamma\|_2 \qquad \text{subject to} \quad \|\gamma_t\|_0 = T_0. \quad (30)$$

Once the reconstruction errors are computed, the classification is done as follows

$$\text{class of } \mathbf{x}_t = \arg\min_c \epsilon_c(\mathbf{x}_t). \tag{31}$$

**Case 2: (Small number of training samples per class).** When the number of training samples per class is relatively small, one class is not expressive enough for a given test sample. Hence, while computing the sparse coefficients, we use the whole dictionary $\mathbf{D}$ and solve the following optimization problem,

$$\boldsymbol{\gamma}_t^* = \min_{\boldsymbol{\gamma}} \|\boldsymbol{\Phi}(\mathbf{x}_t) - \boldsymbol{\Phi}(\mathbf{X})\mathbf{A}\boldsymbol{\gamma}\|_2 \qquad \text{subject to} \quad \|\gamma_t\|_0 = T_0. \tag{32}$$

Now the reconstruction error for class $c$ is computed by using the elements of $\boldsymbol{\gamma}_t^*$ which correspond to the $c^{\text{th}}$ class. This can be written as,

$$\epsilon_c(\mathbf{x}_t) = \|\boldsymbol{\Phi}(\mathbf{x}_t) - \boldsymbol{\Phi}(\mathbf{X})\mathbf{A}_c\delta_c(\boldsymbol{\gamma}_t^*)\|_2 \tag{33}$$

where $\delta_c(.)$ is a characteristic function that selects the coefficients corresponding to class $c$. Classification based on only reconstruction error may be misleading in cases where two classes have very similar reconstruction errors. In such cases, we make the decision in favor of the class which gets the biggest contribution from the coefficient vector. To quantify this, we define a quantity $w_c(\boldsymbol{\gamma}_t^*) \triangleq \frac{\|\delta_c(\boldsymbol{\gamma}_t^*)\|_1}{\|\boldsymbol{\gamma}_t^*\|_1}$. The final classification is then done as

$$\text{class of } \mathbf{x}_t = \arg\min_c(\epsilon_c(\mathbf{x}_t) - \eta\, w_c(\boldsymbol{\gamma}_t^*)), \tag{34}$$

where $\eta$ is a constant that measures the importance of coefficient based classification.

## 6    Experiments and Results

In this section, we present several experimental results demonstrating the effectiveness of the proposed dictionary learning method for classification tasks. In particular, we present classification results on the AR face dataset [18], the extended Yale B face dataset [19][20], and the USPS digits [21] dataset. Comparison with other existing discriminative dictionary learning methods for image classification in [8] suggests that Fisher discrimination-based dictionary learning (FDDL) algorithm is among the best. Hence, we treat it as state-of-the-art and use it as a bench mark for comparisons. We also compare our method with that of kernel PCA (KPCA) [22] and kernel LDA (KLDA) [23]. In all of our experiments, we set the sparsity at test time to approximately 10% of the dictionary size. The dictionary size is chosen according to the size of available training data. When available data samples per class are relatively small (e.g. AR face recognition), we set the dictionary size same as the number of training samples. Conversely, when we have a large number of training samples per class, we limit the dictionary size to 100. The discriminative parameters $\lambda_1$ and $\lambda_2$ were experimentally selected so that they provide the best results. We set $\lambda_1$ and $\lambda_2$ equal to 0.7 and 0.4, respectively for all the experiments. For all the face recognition experiments we use the Gaussian kernel with $\sigma = 1.6$ and for digit recognition experiments we use the polynomial kernel of degree 4.

## 6.1 Digit Recognition

In the first set of experiments, we evaluate the performance of our method on the USPS digit dataset and compare it with some recent state-of-the-art methods namely, KSVD, FDDL [8], and kernel based methods KPCA, KLDA, kernel KSVD [11]. This dataset consists of 7291 training and 2007 test images. In this experiment, we randomly pick 200 training samples per class and 100 test samples per class. The results are shown in Table 1. It can be seen from the table that our method performs the best on this experiment with the USPS dataset.

**Table 1.** Recognition accuracy for the proposed method, compared to competing ones for digit recognition

| Algorithm | KSVD | FDDL | KPCA | KLDA | ker KSVD | NLDD |
|---|---|---|---|---|---|---|
| Accuracy (%) | 96.10 | 97.00 | 96.30 | 96.90 | 96.90 | **97.50** |

**Pre-images of Learned Atoms:** Recall that the $k^{\text{th}}$ kernel dictionary atom is represented by $\mathbf{\Phi}(\mathbf{X})\mathbf{a}_k$, where $\mathbf{a}_k \in \mathbb{R}^N$ is the representation of the kernel dictionary atom with respect to the base $\mathbf{\Phi}(\mathbf{X})$ in the feature space $G$. The pre-image of $\mathbf{\Phi}(\mathbf{X})\mathbf{a}_k$ is obtained by seeking a vector in the input space $\mathbf{d}_k \in mathbbR^N$ that minimizes the cost function $\|\mathbf{\Phi}(\mathbf{d}_k) - \mathbf{\Phi}(\mathbf{X})\mathbf{a}_k\|^2$. Due to various noise effects and the generally non-invertible mapping $\mathbf{\Phi}$, the exact pre-image does not always exist. However, the approximated pre-image can be reconstructed without venturing into the feature space using the techniques described in [23].

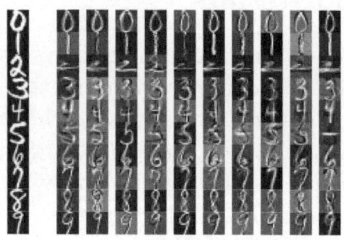

(a)                    (b)

**Fig. 2.** Pre-images of the learned dictionary atoms corresponding to the NLDD method. (a) class examples. (b) preimages of 10 dictionary atoms from each class.

Figure 2 shows the pre-images of the learned atoms corresponding the NLDD method. Note that our method is able to capture the internal common structure of data while maintaining the discriminative capability.

**Robustness of NLDD:** In this section, we evaluate the performance of the proposed method in the presence of various degradations such as missing pixels and noise. From each class, we randomly select 200 images for training and 100 images for testing. The first experiment presents the results for the situation where the test samples are corrupted by random Gaussian noise with different

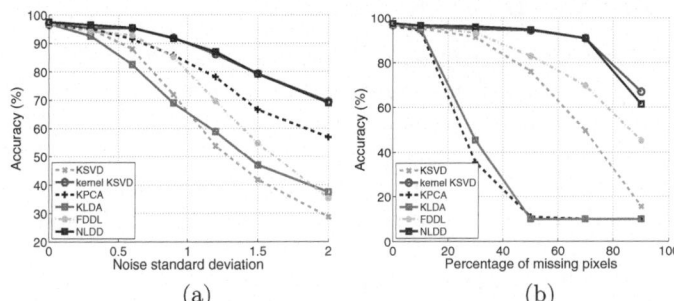

(a)                                         (b)

**Fig. 3.** Analysis of algorithms with noisy test data. (a) Accuracy with Gaussian noise. (b) Accuracy with missing pixels.

standard deviations as shown in Figure 3(a). The results obtained when pixels are randomly removed from the test images are shown in Figure 3(b).

In both experiments, Kernel-based dictionary learning methods such as kernel KSVD and NLDD perform much better than the other methods. As the distortion level increases the performance difference between kernel dictionaries and linear dictionaries become more dramatic. This demonstrates that non-linear dictionary learning can prove significantly better in some scenarios. Experiments described later show that having discriminative power along with non-linearity in dictinary learning can provide extra performance for classification.

## 6.2   AR Face Recognition

The AR dataset consists of 126 individuals with frontal faces captured in two sessions with different illuminations, expressions and occlusions. We follow the experimental setup of [8] and choose 50 male subjects and 50 female subjects with lighting and expression variations. The 7 images per subject from session 1 were used for training and 7 images with same lighting and expressions from session 2 were used for testing. The dimension of the images was reduced to 300 using PCA.

**Table 2.** Recognition accuracy for the proposed method, compared to competing ones for AR and Yale B face recognition

| Datset | SRC | SVM | DKSVD | FDDL | KPCA | KLDA | ker KSVD | NLDD |
|--------|------|------|-------|------|-------|-------|----------|--------|
| AR Face | 88.8 | 87.1 | 85.4 | 92.0 | 83.86 | 92.14 | 92.57 | **93.71** |
| Yale B | 90.0 | 88.8 | 75.3 | 91.9 | 88.09 | 92.02 | 91.84 | **94.62** |

The results are shown in Table 2 which shows around 2% improvement over FDDL and more than 1% improvement over kernel KSVD-based classification. Since the number of training images per class is only 7 we use the whole dictionary (case 2) for classification. Sparsity at test time was set to 23 and $\eta$ in (34) was set equal to 0.5. As can be seen from the table, our kernel-based discriminative dictionary learning method provides the best results. Here, SRC stands for sparse representation-based classifier and DKSVD for discriminative KSVD.

## 6.3   Extended Yale B Face Recognition

In this experiment we evaluate our algorithm on the extended Yale B dataset which has 38 subjects and about 64 images per subject with various illumination conditions. We follow the experimental set up as considered in [8]. We randomly select 20 images per subject for training and the rest for testing. Dimension of all the images have been reduced to 300 using PCA. Dictionary size of each class was set to 20 and at the test time, we use sparsity $T0 = 35$ and $\eta = 0.5$ for classification.

As shown in Table 2, NLDD performs the best and shows an improvement of about 3% over other competitive methods. This experiment shows that even in the presence of extreme illumination, our method is able to provide reasonable recognition performance.

## 6.4   Gender Recognition

In the final set of experiments, we evaluate the performance of our method on a two class problem of gender recognition. We choose 50 male subjects and 50 female subjects of the AR face database. We choose 14 faces per subject from both sessions. We train our algorithm, with first 25 males subjects and 25 female subjects and test our method with the remaining 25 male and 25 female subjects. The feature dimension was reduced to 300 using PCA. Results are presented in Table 3.

**Table 3.** Recognition accuracy for the proposed method, compared to competing ones for gender recognition recognition

| Algo. | SRC | SVM | DKSVD | FDDL | KPCA | KLDA | ker KSVD | NLDD |
|-------|-----|-----|-------|------|------|------|----------|------|
| Acc. (%) | 93.0 | 92.4 | 86.1 | 95.4 | 94.57 | 94.57 | 95.07 | **95.71** |

Since we have enough training samples per class, we classify based on the reconstruction error from each class (case 1). In this experiment, the sparsity was set equal to 30 for training as well as testing. As shown in the table, our method performance favorably over some of the competitive methods.

# 7   Discussions and Future Work

We have proposed an approach for learning discriminative and reconstructive dictionaries in a high dimensional features space. The proposed algorithm consists of two steps that iteratively update sparse coefficients and dictionary atoms. Sparse coefficients are updated using a variant of SOMP algorithm and the dictionary atoms are updated using an efficient kernel KSVD algorithm. Various experiments on popular face and digit recognition data sets have shown that our method is robust and can perform significantly better than many existing dictionary based recognition algorithms.

**Acknowledgement.** This work was partially supported by an ONR grant
N00014-12-1-0124.

# References

1. Rubinstein, R., Bruckstein, A., Elad, M.: Dictionaries for sparse representation
modeling. In: Proceedings of the IEEE, vol. 98 (2010)
2. Chen, Y.-C., Patel, V.M., Phillips, P.J., Chellappa, R.: Dictionary-Based Face
Recognition from Video. In: Fitzgibbon, A., Lazebnik, S., Perona, P., Sato, Y.,
Schmid, C. (eds.) ECCV 2012, Part VI. LNCS, vol. 7577, pp. 766–779. Springer,
Heidelberg (2012)
3. Patel, V.M., Wu, T., Biswas, S., Philips, P.J., Chellappa, R.: Dictionary-based face
recognition under variable lighting and pose. IEEE Transactions on Information
Forensics and Security 7, 954–965 (2012)
4. Shrivastava, A., Pillai, J.K., Patel, V.M., Chellappa, R.: Learning discriminative
dictionaries with partially labeled data. In: ICIP (2012)
5. Engan, K., Aase, S.O., Husoy, J.H.: Method of optimal directions for frame design.
In: ICASSP (1999)
6. Aharon, M., Elad, M., Bruckstein, A.M.: The K-SVD: an algorithm for designing of
overcomplete dictionaries for sparse representation. IEEE Trans. Signal Process. 54
(2006)
7. Etemand, K., Chellappa, R.: Separability-based multiscale basis selection and feature extraction for signal and image classification. TIP (1998)
8. Yang, M., Zhang, L., Feng, X., Zhang, D.: Fisher discrimination dictionary learning
for sparse representation. In: ICCV (2011)
9. Mairal, J., Bach, F., Ponce, J., Sapiro, G., Zisserman, A.: Supervised dictionary
learning. In: NIPS (2009)
10. Patel, V.M., Chellappa, R.: Sparse representations, compressive sensing and dictionaries for pattern recognition. In: ACPR (2011)
11. Nguyen, H.V., Patel, V.M., Nasrabadi, N.M., Chellappa, R.: Kernel dictionary
learning. In: ICASSP (2012)
12. Gao, S., Tsang, I.W.-H., Chia, L.-T.: Kernel Sparse Representation for Image Classification and Face Recognition. In: Daniilidis, K., Maragos, P., Paragios, N. (eds.)
ECCV 2010, Part IV. LNCS, vol. 6314, pp. 1–14. Springer, Heidelberg (2010)
13. Zhang, L., Zhou, W.D., Chang, P.C., Liu, J., Yan, Z., Wang, T., Li, F.-Z.: Kernel
sparse representation-based classifier. IEEE Trans. Signal Process. (2011)
14. Yuan, X.T., Yan, S.: Visual classification with multi-task joint sparse representation. In: CVPR (2010)
15. Wright, J., Yang, A.Y., Ganesh, A., Sastry, S.S., Ma, Y.: Robust face recognition
via sparse representation. PAMI 31 (February 2009)
16. Rubinstein, R., Zibulevsky, M., Elad, M.: Double sparsity: Learning sparse dictionaries for sparse signal approximation. IEEE Trans. Signal Process. 58 (2010)
17. Tropp, J.A., Gilbert, A.C., Strauss, M.J.: Algorithms for simultaneous sparse approximation. part i: Greedy pursuit. Signal Processing 86 (2006)
18. Martinez, A., Benavente, R.: The ar face database. CVC Technical Report No. 24
(1998)
19. Georghiades, A., Belhumeur, P., Kriegman, D.: From few to many: Illumination
cone models for face recognition under variable lighting and pose. PAMI (2001)

20. Lee, K., Ho, J., Kriegman, D.: Acquiring linear subspaces for face recognition under variable lighting. IEEE Trans. Pattern Anal. Mach. Intelligence 27 (2005)
21. Usps handwriten digit database,
    http://www-i6.informatik.rwth-aachen.de/~keysers/usps.html
22. Schölkopf, B., Smola, A., Müller, K.: Nonlinear component analysis as a kernel eigenvalue problem. Neural Comput. 10 (1998)
23. Scholkopf, B., Smola, A.J.: Learning With Kernels, Support Vector Machines, Optimization and Beyond. MIT Press (2001)

# Efficient Background Subtraction
# under Abrupt Illumination Variations

Junqiu Wang and Yasushi Yagi

The Institute of Scientific and Industrial Research, Osaka University
8-1 Mihogaoka, Ibaraki, Osaka, Japan
jerywangjq@gmail.com

**Abstract.** Background subtraction techniques require high segmentation quality and low computational cost. Achieving high accuracy is difficult under abrupt illumination changes. We develop a new background subtraction method in an expectation maximization (EM) framework. We describe foreground colors and illumination ratios using a few Gaussian mixture models. EM convergence is dependent on its initialization. We propose a novel initialization method that considers reflectance and illumination implicitly. Scene points occluded by a foreground object tend to have prominent illumination ratios since both the reflectance and illumination are different. We introduce a topological approach based on Morse theory to pre-classify pixels into foreground and background. Moreover, we only decompose the probability distributions in the initial step in our EM. Later iterations do not consider the probability distribution decomposition anymore. The experimental results demonstrate that our EM formulation provides high accuracy under abrupt variations in illumination. Additionally, in comparison with one of the state-of-the-art methods based on EM, our approach converges in fewer iterations, yielding computational savings.

## 1 Introduction

Real-time background subtraction is a key issue in a number of applications such as visual surveillance, tracking, detection, and augmented reality [1–3]. While previous investigations have demonstrated impressive results on many image sequences, few handle abrupt variations in illumination. In previous work, the background maintenance modules update background models to deal with gradual illumination changes. Unfortunately, this updating fails under abrupt changes in illumination.

Background subtraction aims to classify an image pixel into background or foreground. The classification relies on appearance differences between object and background. The color of scene points in an image is determined by its reflectance (or albedo) and illumination (or shading). Reflectance is a material-dependent property that does not change even if illumination conditions vary. A background scene point is only influenced by its illumination conditions. If a foreground object occludes a background scene point, both reflectance and

K.M. Lee et al. (Eds.): ACCV 2012, Part I, LNCS 7724, pp. 675–688, 2013.
© Springer-Verlag Berlin Heidelberg 2013

illumination will change. The corresponding ratio tends to be prominent compared with those in background. Therefore, pre-classification of image pixels into foreground and background is possible using image ratios. We introduce a topological method to fulfill this task. To be specific, we compute topological persistence in ratio images based on Morse theory [4]. Errors are unavoidable in the pre-classification step. We perform *Expectation Maximization* (EM) [5–7] to remove the errors.

We handle sudden illumination variations in an EM framework. An EM algorithm alternates between a responsibility assignment of a set of latent variables to input samples and parameter estimations of a few statistical models. EM has been widely used in background subtraction [1, 3, 8] because of its nice properties. We treat foreground and background labels as latent variables. We describe the pixels in the foreground using a *Gaussian Mixture Model* (GMM). The illumination ratios in the background are characterized by another GMM [3]. Based on the pre-classification result, we compute GMM component responsibility assignment and then parameter estimations for the GMMs.

Initialization plays an important role in the performance of EMs [5, 9]. Given a few labeled images, Pilet et al. [3] computed two types of texture distributions off-line. Next, the distributions were used to discriminate foreground and background in an input image. However, the off-line learning needs labeled images that are laborious to make. Additionally, whereas the distributions describe image pixels well in texture abundant regions, these are not reliable in smooth regions.

In this work, we compute the maximum channel in each pixel of the illumination ratio image. Then, we apply a topological method to pre-classify the ratio image. We only decompose the probability distribution in the first EM iteration. The pre-classification is used only in the first expectation step. Later expectation steps in the iterations do not involve in probability distribution decomposition anymore. Therefore, errors in the initialization do no affect the following EM iterations. Our experimental results verify that our formulation provides good performance.

The probability distribution in [3] is decomposed into a product of the illumination and the texture distributions. The decomposition is applied at each expectation step. We found this formulation deficient because errors at initialization might be propagated.

This paper is organized as follows: In Section 2, we briefly survey background subtraction techniques. After giving the computation of illumination ratios in Section 3, we introduce pre-classification using reflectance and illumination conditions implicitly in Section 4. Our formulation of EM inference is described in Section 5. Experiments are conducted in Section 6. We conclude our paper in Section 7.

## 2    Related Work

Background maintenance and foreground segmentation have been widely studied in recent decades [10–17]. Existing methods can be classified into three categories: pixel-based, texture-based, and pixel-texture-based methods – which each deal with illumination variations in their different ways.

Background modeling is fulfilled using single Gaussian distributions [18]. While single Gaussians are sufficient to model the pixel value with noises, they are unable to account for multi-modality. Friedman and Russell [8] described an incremental EM algorithm to handle illumination variations and background changes. Each pixel is classified according to the predefined labels corresponding to road, shadow, and vehicles. Staufer and Grimson [10] modeled each background pixel by a GMM. Such models are updated in a heuristic way. The number of the components in a GMM has an appropriate value according to its modality. Zivkovic and Heijden [19] automatically selected the number of GMM components and update the GMM parameters using an incremental EM. Their approach is one of the state-of-the-art background subtraction methods.

Besides these parametric representations, non-parametric density estimation has been applied in background subtraction. Elgammal et al. [14] built nonparametric representations for both background and foreground. Kernel density estimators were employed to characterize the pixels. However, all the above pixel-based methods provides poor segmentation results under abrupt illumination variations. Since image gradients are not sensitive to illumination variations, a local histogram of gradients are used to ameliorate the negative effects of illumination changes. Heikkila and Pietikainen [16] built a set of adaptive local

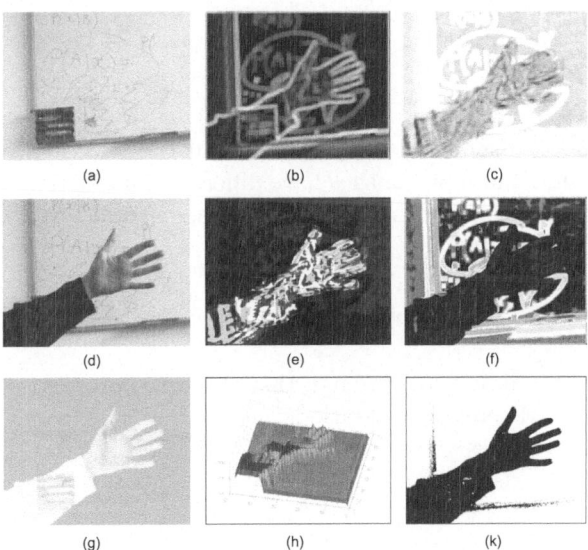

**Fig. 1.** (a) The background image. (b) The texture image. (c) The cross-correlation image. (d) The input image. (e) The foreground probability based on the texture distribution. (f) The background probability based on the cross-correlation distribution. (g) The illumination ratio image. (h) The maximum channel of the ratio image shown in 3D. (i) The pre-classification results.

binary pattern histograms (LBPs) for each pixel. Since the LBP representation includes regional contrast information that has certain invariances with respect to monotonic gray-scale changes, it is capable of dealing with certain illumination variations. Because texture-based methods consider contrast information in a certain neighborhood, ambiguities exist at object boundaries. This is a common drawback for most texture-based methods.

Li and Leung [17] integrate pixel and region information to detect changes in video sequences. They model texture based on the relationship between two gradient vectors, which is robust to gradual illumination variations.

Spatial continuity has been considered in a Markov Random Field (MRF) framework to improve the subtraction results. Sheikh and Shah [15] integrate foreground probabilities into a Maximum A Posteriori of MRF. An approach based on optimization by graph cut has been widely used in interactive [20] and automatic foreground segmentation [21]. A global optimization approach obviously is able to improve segmentation results at a price of increased computational complexity.

## 3   Illumination Ratios

Suppose $\{I_{i,m}\}_{i=\{1,2,...,n\}}$ and $\{I_{i,u}\}_{i=\{1,2,...,n\}}$ are pixel color vectors in a background image $m$ and an input image $u$, respectively. We have a set of latent variables $\{z_i\}_{i=\{1,2,...,n\}}$, where $z_i = 1$ (resp. $z_i = 0$) indicates pixel $i$ is in foreground (resp. background).

The color of scene points in an image is a product of its reflectance $R_i$ and illumination $L_i$ [22]:

$$I_i = L_i R_i, \tag{1}$$

where $L_i$ is a $3 \times 3$ diagonal matrix; $R_i \in \mathbb{R}^3$ and $I_i \in \mathbb{R}^3$.

The background and input images have different illumination conditions. We compute an illumination ratio between two pixels, one each form the background background and input images:

$$S_i = \frac{I_{i,u}}{I_{i,m}} = \frac{L_{i,u} R_{i,u}}{L_{i,m} R_{i,m}}. \tag{2}$$

If an image point is in the background, the reflectance properties should be the same $R_{i,m} = R_{i,u}$. Therefore, the ratio is

$$S_i = \frac{L_{i,u} \mathbf{1}^T}{L_{i,m} \mathbf{1}^T}, \tag{3}$$

where $\mathbf{1}^T$ is a unit $3 \times 1$ vector.

If an image point is in the foreground, the ratio (Eq. 2) is affected by both the difference of reflectance and illumination. It tends to be prominent in the ratio image compared with the background points. Although the scene points in the foreground might have similar reflectance with those in the background, this situation is difficult for all the background subtraction methods. We compute a ratio image for an image pair in Fig. 1. The hand and arm in the foreground stand out in Fig. 1(h). The probabilities obtained using the learned texture distributions are shown in Fig. 1(e) and (f).

## 4  Pre-classification for EM Initialization

We pre-classify image pixels as foreground and background using the ratio image. The foreground regions are usually conspicuous in the ratio image. The ratio image is composed of $3 \times 1$ vectors $S_i = (S_i^r, S_i^g, S_i^b)^T$, where $r$, $g$, $b$ indicate the RGB channels. We convert the ratio image into 1D by computing the maximum in the three channels:

$$S_i^{\max} = \max(S_i^r, S_i^g, S_i^b). \qquad (4)$$

We found that the maximum channel characterize foreground region prominence well. We pre-classify $S_i^{\max}$ using a topological approach.

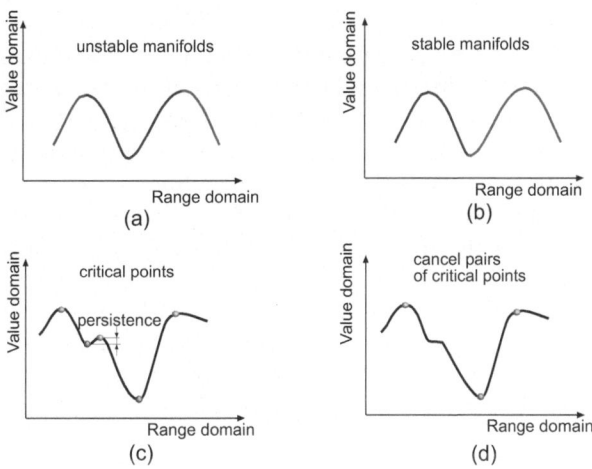

**Fig. 2.** Basics definitions of Morse theory

### 4.1  Basics of Morse Theory

Morse theory [23, 24] deals with differential topology of a manifold using differentiable functions of that manifold. A smooth map $f : \mathbb{M} \longrightarrow \mathbb{R}$ defined over a compact d-manifold $\mathbb{M}$ is a Morse function if all its critical points are non-degenerate. Here, the critical points of a function those points at which the differential of the function vanishes or does not exist. For a given local maximum and a local minimum, the set of points between them belong to a stable manifold. Stable and unstable manifolds are shown in Fig. 2. There are also unstable manifold if the set of points cross a local minimum. We can give labels according to the relationships between the critical points. The operations include label creation, copying and deletion as shown in Fig. 3.

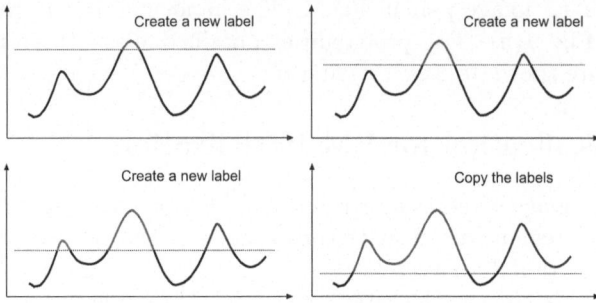

**Fig. 3.** Manifold analysis based on Morse theory

## 4.2 Pre-classification

We perform approximate density estimations using the improved Gauss transform [25? ], which is very efficient. The density estimation results are normalized and sorted into bins. We proceed from the maximum to the minimum densities. We keep computing the persistence between critical points. At the beginning of this process, a few stable topological structures emerges. After the emergence of the prominent components, the topology becomes stable until we meet the non-eminent components. We process from the minimum of the density estimations simultaneously. The stable topologies from the maximum and minimum find an agreement at a certain ratio value. We classify the eminent regions with stable topology as foreground objects. Many small regions obtained in the pre-classification result from noises, we discard these in the pre-classification.

The pre-classification results usually contain errors. This is predictable because the illumination ratios are not very discriminative in some cases. The errors can be removed in the EM iterations. The pre-classification results are described by $v(z|S_{i,u})$.

## 5 Our EM Formulation

We have two images as the input of our algorithm: a background image and an input image with illumination variations.

### 5.1 Color and Illumination Ratio Representation

We represent foreground appearance using a GMM with $C$ components:

$$p(I_{i,u}|z_i, \mu, \Sigma) = \sum_{c=1}^{C} \alpha_c \mathcal{N}(I_{i,u}|\mu_c, \Sigma_c),  \tag{5}$$

where $\mu_c$ and $\Sigma_c$ are the mean and the covariance matrix of the GMM, respectively; $\alpha_c$ is the $c^{th}$ mixture weight; $\mathcal{N}(I_{i,u}|\mu_c, \Sigma_c)$ is the 3-variate Gaussian pdf.

Similarly, we characterize the ratio image in the background using another GMM with $\overline{C}$ components:

$$p(S_i|z_i, \mu, \Sigma) = \sum_{c=C+1}^{C+\overline{C}} \alpha_c \mathcal{N}(S_i|\mu_c, \Sigma_c),\tag{6}$$

We have a uniform distribution accounting for the ambiguous pixels in the foreground because the foreground GMM cannot cover some of the pixels [3]. Ambiguous pixels occur with probability $\frac{1}{256^3}$. The uniform distribution is defined as

$$p(I_{i,u}|z_i, \mu, \Sigma) = \frac{\alpha_{C+\overline{C}+1}}{256^3}.\tag{7}$$

## 5.2   EM Inference

The purpose of our EM inference is to compute conditional probabilities of latent variables. The inference is formulated as a maximum likelihood estimation:

$$\theta^* = \arg\max_\theta \log \prod_i \sum_{z_i} p(I_{i,u}, S_i, z_i|\theta),\tag{8}$$

where $\theta = \{\mu, \Sigma, \alpha\}$.

**The Expectation Step.** The E step computes the responses from each component corresponding to point $i$ and improves the log likelihood of an auxiliary distribution $q^{(t+1)} = \mathrm{argmax}_q \mathcal{L}(q, \theta^{(t)})$, where $\mathcal{L}(q, \theta^{(t)})$ is the lower bound of the likelihood in the $t$-th iteration. $q$ is selected optimally as $q(z|S, I_u, \theta) = p(z|S, I_u, \theta^{(t)})$ [6].

The parameter set $\theta$ is unknown in the E step of the first iteration. We introduce the pre-classification results to initiate our EM. We compute the responsibilities of the GMM describing the foreground appearance based on the approximate foreground probabilities and a uniform initialization of the GMM:

$$r^{(t+1)}_{c=1...C} = \frac{1}{N_i}\alpha_c^{(t)}\mathcal{N}(I_{i,u}|\mu_c^{(t)}, \Sigma_c^{(t)})v(z = 1|S_{i,u}),\tag{9}$$

where $N_i$ is the normalization factor to be given later.

Then, we compute the responsibilities of the GMM characterizing the illumination ratio in the background by

$$r^{(t+1)}_{c=(C+1)...(C+\overline{C})} = \frac{1}{N_i}\alpha_c^{(t)}\frac{1}{\|J_c\|}\mathcal{N}(S_i|\mu_c^{(t)}, \Sigma_c^{(t)})v(z = 0|S_{i,u}),\tag{10}$$

where $J$ is the determinant of the Jacobian of function $S_i(I_{i,u})$ to complete the pdf [3].

We also compute the responsibilities of the ambiguous pixels based on the uniform distribution:

$$r^{(t+1)}_{i,c=(C+\overline{C}+1)} = \frac{1}{N_i}\alpha_{C+\overline{C}+1}^{(t)}\frac{1}{256^3}v(z = 1|S_{i,u}).\tag{11}$$

The normalization factor is computed by $N_i = \sum_{c=1}^{c=C+\overline{C}+1} r_{i,c}^{(t+1)}$.

After the first iteration of our EM, the parameter set $\theta$ is estimated in the M step. We will not include the pre-classification results $v(z|S_{i,u})$ in the E steps in the following iterations. The responsibilities are computed by

$$r_{c=1...C}^{(t+1)} = \frac{1}{N_i}\alpha_c^{(t)}\mathcal{N}(I_{i,u}|\mu_c^{(t)},\Sigma_c^{(t)}), \tag{12}$$

$$r_{c=C+1...C+\overline{C}}^{(t+1)} = \frac{1}{N_i}\alpha_c^{(t)}\frac{1}{\|J_c\|}\mathcal{N}(S_i|\mu_c^{(t)},\Sigma_c^{(t)}), \tag{13}$$

$$r_{i,c=(C+\overline{C}+1)}^{(t+1)} = \frac{1}{N_i}\alpha_{C+\overline{C}+1}^{(t)}\frac{1}{256^3}. \tag{14}$$

**The Maximization Step.** We compute the conditional expected values of the complete log likelihood based on the responsibilities computed in the E step. The component mixture weights are computed by

$$\alpha_c^{(t+1)} = \frac{\sum_{i=1}^n r_{i,c}^{(t+1)}}{n} \tag{15}$$

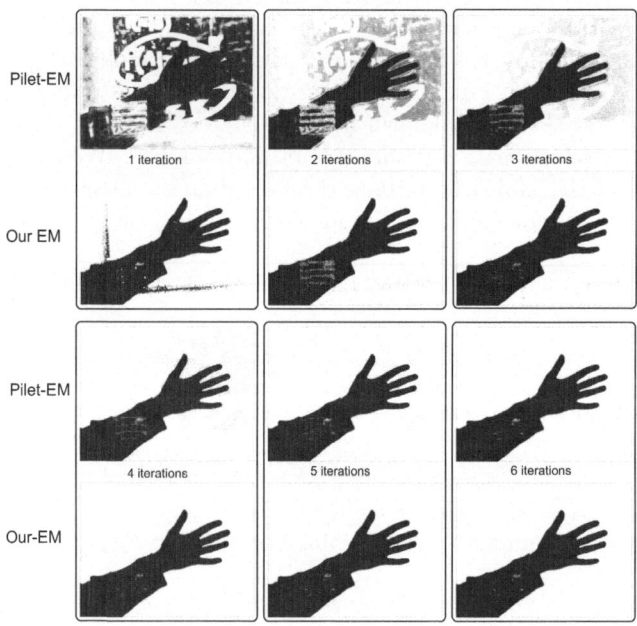

**Fig. 4.** The results of our EM and Pilet-EM after several iterations

We estimate the vector mean of the foreground GMM by

$$\mu_c^{(t+1)} = \frac{1}{N_c} \sum_{i=1}^{n} r_{i,c}^{(t+1)} I_{i,u}.$$ (16)

The covariance matrix of the foreground GMM is computed by

$$\Sigma_c^{(t+1)} = \frac{1}{N_c} \sum_{i=1}^{n} r_{i,c}^{(t+1)} (I_{i,u} - \mu_c)(I_{i,u} - \mu_c)^T.$$ (17)

Similarly, the mean and covariance matrix of the ratio GMM in the background are computed by

$$\mu_c^{t+1} = \frac{1}{N_c} \sum_{i=1}^{n} r_{i,c}^{(t+1)} S_i,$$ (18)

$$\Sigma_c^{(t+1)} = \frac{1}{N_c} \sum_{i=1}^{n} r_{i,c}^{(t+1)} (S_i - \mu_c)(S_i - \mu_c)^T.$$ (19)

The mixture component weights are computed by

$$N_c = \sum_{i=1}^{n} r_{i,c}^{(t+1)}$$ (20)

The probability of a pixel being described by the foreground GMM after $t + 1$ iterations is computed by

$$p^{(t+1)}(z = 1|\theta^*, I_{i,u}) = \sum_{c=1}^{C} r_{i,c}^{(t+1)}.$$ (21)

## 6   Experimental Results

In our experiments, we have pairs of images as input: one is the background model and the other is the input image. The illumination conditions in the two images have abrupt changes. We aim to estimate the probability of the foreground and background. This setting is more difficult than handling illumination variations in video sequences since less information is available here. To evaluate different background subtraction algorithms, we perform qualitative and quantitative comparisons. We have tested our algorithm on many image pairs. We show a few examples of our tested image pairs to demonstrate the performance of our algorithm.

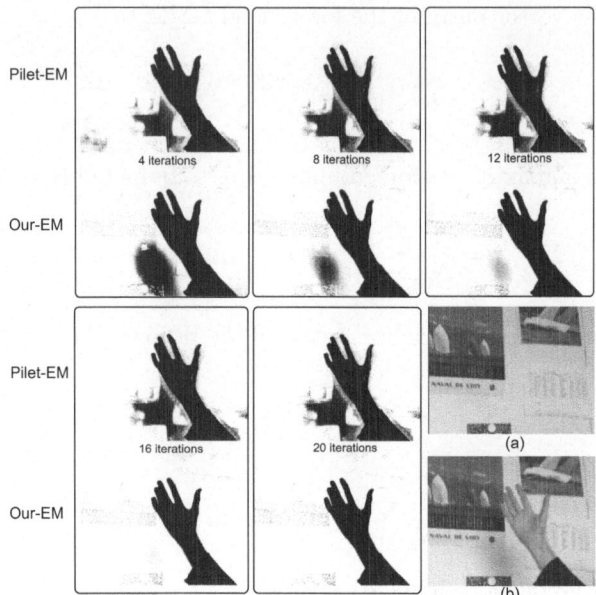

**Fig. 5.** The results of our EM and Pilet-EM after several iterations. (a) The background image. (b) The input image.

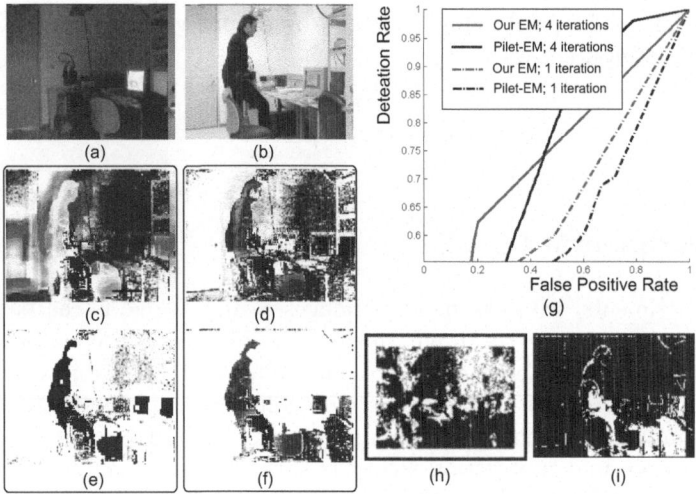

**Fig. 6.** The results of our EM, Pilet-EM [3], the LBP-based method [16], and the adaptive density estimation method [19]. (a) The background image. (b) The input image. (c) Pilet-EM result after 1 iteration. (d) Pilet-EM result after 4 iterations. (e) Our EM result after 1 iteration. (f) Our EM result after 4 iterations. (g) ROC curves of the results. (h) The result obtained using the texture-based method [16]. (i) The results from the adaptive density estimation method in [19].

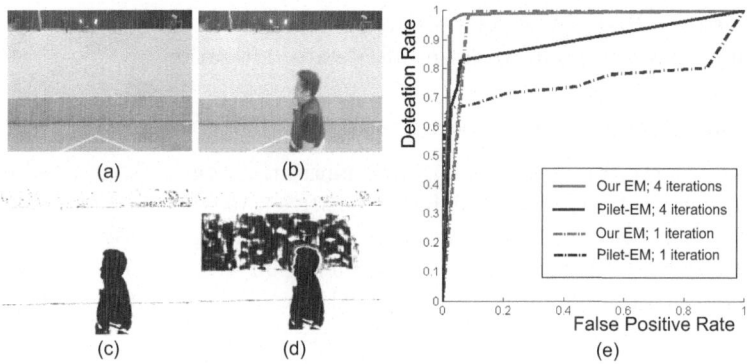

**Fig. 7.** The results of our EM and Pilet-EM. (a) The background image. (b) The input image. (c) Our EM result after 4 iterations. (d) Pilet-EM result after 4 iterations. (e) ROC curves of the results.

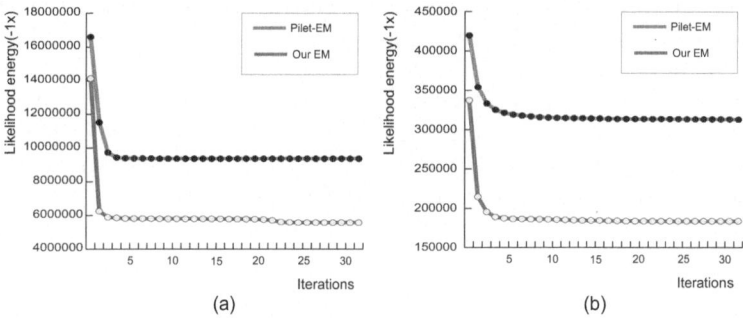

**Fig. 8.** Log likelihood value comparison between our EM and Pilet-EM. (a) The log likelihood of the image pair shown in Fig. 4. (b) The log likelihood of the image pair shown in Fig. 6.

## 6.1   Qualitative Comparison

Our EM usually takes fewer iterations to reach the same performance with the Pilet-EM. Therefore, our EM is more efficient than Pilet-EM. The first example is shown in Fig. 4. The background and input images are shown in Fig. 1. Our EM gives good accuracy after two iterations. Similar performance are not obtained in the first four iterations using Pilet-EM. The results of our EM are better than those of Pilet-EM in the first five iterations. Our results after three iterations do not change significantly. Although the Pilet-EM results after six iterations are similar to ours, the efficiency of our EM is clearly demonstrated.

The background and the input images with different illumination conditions in Fig. 5 are captured from Pilet et al.'s paper directly. The image pair might have misalignment due to processing error. In addition, noise is introduced as well. On this image pair, in the first few iterations, the results of our EM contain some errors in the region under the arm. However, the accuracy increases steadily.

In contrast, the Pilet-EM results retain the errors after many iterations, and in fact, exhibit almost no improvement after sixteen iterations.

## 6.2   Quantitative Comparison

We adopt two quality measures for our quantitative comparison: detection rate and false alarm rate. We prefer high true positive rates that indicate good detection with low probability of misclassifying a foreground point. We also track low false positive rates that signify good discrimination with low probability of classifying non-foreground points as foreground. Formally, we define detection rate $DR$ and false positive rate $FPR$ as $DR = \frac{TP}{TP+FN}$ and $FPR = \frac{FP}{TP+FP}$, where $TP$ denotes the number of true positives, $FN$ the number of false negatives, and $FP$ the number of false positives.

We have tested our method on a more difficult image pair from [11]. We show the results of our EM, Pilet-EM, the adaptive density estimation method [19], and the LBP-based method [16] in Fig. 6. The illumination conditions in the image pairs are very different. The adaptive density method [19] does not handle such abrupt illumination changes. It gives unsatisfying result. The LBP-based method [16] provides better result, thanks to its invariancy to illumination variations. However, its false positive rate is rather high. The Pilet-EM result is more reasonable than the adaptive density estimation and the LBP methods. We can figure out the shape of the person in the result. Unfortunately, it has much higher false positive rate than our EM result.

The results of another image pair are shown in Fig. 7. The background in this image pair is simple. However, the lighting conditions are complicated because of the inter-reflection. In addition, the green background board acts as a light source which violates white light assumption. While this problem is not well handled by Pilet-EM, our EM gives reasonable results.

## 6.3   Efficiency

We do not need the spatial likelihood model in [3]. Therefore, we do not have to label and train the texture histograms off-line. The online computation of the texture histograms is not necessary as well. However, we have to compute the topological analysis of the illumination ratios. This step turns out to have similar computational cost with the calculation of the cross-correlation histograms due to the use of fast density estimation method [? ].

According to the above performance analysis, our EM usually takes fewer iterations to reach a good accuracy. Thus, our algorithm runs more efficiently than Pilet-EM. Moreover, Pilet-EM has three more float multiplications in the expectation step after the first iteration because we only consider the pre-classification results in the first iteration.

## 6.4   Log Likelihood

The log likelihood is guaranteed to increase with EM iterations. In comparing the log likelihoods of Pilet-EM and our EM after several iterations, our EM clearly has higher log likelihood. In addition, the increase of our EM is faster than Pilet-EM. The log likelihood might indicate convergence of the EM. Thus,our EM converges in fewer iterations than Pilet-EM. Two comparisons are given in Fig. 8.

## 7    Conclusion and Future Work

We developed an EM-based background subtraction method. The EM is initialized based on pre-classification results using topology analysis. The probability decomposition is only performed in the first expectation step. Based on this strategy, initialization errors do not affect the following iterations. Our EM converged faster than the-state-of-the-art method. Moreover, we showed that our EM formulation can recover from errors more effectively.

We only deal with image pairs in this work. The performance of our method can be improved if we consider temporal and spatial continuities in image sequences. The textural information is helpful in the initialization, and integrating the merits of texture and the initialization in our method will be interesting. These issues reserve for future work.

**Acknowledgement.** This work was partly supported by the JST CREST "Behavior Understanding based on Intention-Gait Model" project.

## References

1. Stauffer, C., Grimson, W.E.L.: Learning patterns of activity using real-time tracking. IEEE Trans. Pattern Anal. Mach. Intell. 22, 747–757 (2000)
2. Wang, J., Yagi, Y.: Efficient kernel machines using the improved fast gauss transform. In: 2012 IEEE Int. Conf. on Systems, Man and Cybernetics (2012)
3. Pilet, J., Strecha, C., Fua, P.: Making Background Subtraction Robust to Sudden Illumination Changes. In: Forsyth, D., Torr, P., Zisserman, A. (eds.) ECCV 2008, Part IV. LNCS, vol. 5305, pp. 567–580. Springer, Heidelberg (2008)
4. Gyulassy, A., Bremer, P.T., Hamann, B., Pascucci, V.: A practical approach to morse-smale complex computation. IEEE Trans. Vis. Comput. Graph. 14, 1619–1626 (2008)
5. Dempster, A.P., Laird, N.M., Rubin, D.B.: Maximum likelihood from incomplete data via the em algorithm. Journal of the Royal Statistical Society. Series B (Methodological) 39, 1–38 (1998)
6. Neal, R., Hinton, G.: A view of the EM algorithm that justifies incremental, sparse, and other variants, Learning in Graphical Model. A Bradford Book (1998)
7. Verbeek, J.J., Vlassis, N.A., Krose, B.J.A.: Efficient greedy learning of gaussian mixture models. Neural Computation 15, 469–485 (2003)
8. Friedman, N., Russell, S.J.: Image segmentation in video sequences: A probabilistic approach. In: Proc. of UAI, pp. 175–181 (1997)
9. Melnykov, V., Melnykov, I.: Initialzing the em algorithm in guassian mixture models with an unknown number of components. Computational Statistics and Data Analysis 56, 1381–1395 (2012)

10. Stauffer, C., Grimson, W.E.L.: Adaptive background mixture models for real-time tracking. In: Proc. of CVPR, pp. 2246–2252 (1999)
11. Toyama, K., Krumm, J., Brumitt, B., Meyers, B.: Wallflower: Principles and practice of background maintenance. In: Proc. of ICCV, pp. 255–261 (1999)
12. Elgammal, A., Harwood, D., Davis, L.: Non-parametric Model for Background Subtraction. In: Vernon, D. (ed.) ECCV 2000, Part II. LNCS, vol. 1843, pp. 751–767. Springer, Heidelberg (2000)
13. Stenger, B., Ramesh, V., Paragios, N., Coetzee, F., Buhmann, J.M.: Topology free hidden markov models: Application to background modeling. In: Proc. of ICCV, pp. 294–301 (2001)
14. Elgammal, A.M., Duraiswami, R., Harwood, D., Davis, L.S.: Background and foreground modeling using nonparameteric kernel density for visual surveillance. In: Proceedings of the IEEE, vol. 90, pp. 1151–1163 (2002)
15. Sheikh, Y., Shah, M.: Bayesian modeling of dynamic scenes for object detection. IEEE Trans. Pattern Anal. Mach. Intell 27, 1778–1792 (2005)
16. Heikkila, M., Pietikainen, M.: A texture-based method for modeling the background and detecting moving objects. IEEE Trans. Pattern Anal. Mach. Intell. 28, 657–662 (2006)
17. Li, L., Leung, K.H.: Integrating intensity and texture differences for robust change detection. IEEE Trans. on Image Processing 11, 105–112 (2002)
18. Wren, C.R., Azarbayejani, A., Darrell, T., Pentland, A.: Pfinder: Real-time tracking of the human body. IEEE Trans. Pattern Anal. Mach. Intell. 19, 780–785 (1997)
19. Zivkovic, Z., van der Heijden, F.: Efficient adaptive density estimation per image pixel for the task of background subtraction. Pattern Recognition Letters 27, 773–780 (2006)
20. Rother, C., Kolmogorov, V., Blake, A.: "grabcut": interactive foreground extraction using iterated graph cuts. ACM Trans. Graph. 23, 309–314 (2004)
21. Criminisi, A., Cross, G., Blake, A., Kolmogorov, V.: Bilayer segmentation of live video. In: Proc. of CVPR, pp. 53–60 (2006)
22. Gehler, P.V., Rother, C., Kiefel, M., Zhang, L., Scholkopf, B.: Recovering intrinsic images with a global sparsity prior on reflectance. In: NIPS, pp. 765–773 (2011)
23. Milnor, J.: Morse theory. Princeton University Press (1963)
24. Matsumoto, Y.: An introduction to Morse theory. American Mathematical Society (2002)
25. Yang, C., Duraiswami, R., Davis, L.S.: Efficient kernel machines using the improved fast gauss transform. In: Proc. of NIPS, pp. 294–301 (2004)

# Naive Bayes Image Classification: Beyond Nearest Neighbors

Radu Timofte[1], Tinne Tuytelaars[1], and Luc Van Gool[1,2]

[1] ESAT-VISICS /IBBT, Catholic University of Leuven, Belgium
[2] D-ITET, ETH Zurich, Switzerland

**Abstract.** Naive Bayes Nearest Neighbor (NBNN) has been proposed as a powerful, learning-free, non-parametric approach for object classification. Its good performance is mainly due to the avoidance of a vector quantization step, and the use of image-to-class comparisons, yielding good generalization. In this paper we study the replacement of the nearest neighbor part with more elaborate and robust (sparse) representations, as well as trading performance for speed for practical purposes. The representations investigated are $k$-Nearest Neighbors ($kNN$), Iterative Nearest Neighbors ($INN$) solving a constrained least squares (LS) problem, Local Linear Embedding ($LLE$), a Sparse Representation obtained by $l_1$-regularized LS ($SR_{l_1}$), and a Collaborative Representation obtained as the solution of a $l_2$-regularized LS problem ($CR_{l_2}$). In particular, NIMBLE and K-DES descriptors proved viable alternatives to SIFT and, the NB$SR_{l_1}$ and NB$INN$ classifiers provide significant improvements over NBNN, obtaining competitive results on Scene-15, Caltech-101, and PASCAL VOC 2007 datasets, while remaining learning-free approaches (i.e., no parameters need to be learned).

## 1 Introduction

In [1], Boiman *et al.* introduced a novel, non-parametric approach for image classification, the Naive Bayes Nearest Neighbor classifier (NBNN). Given an image represented by a set of extracted features, and a priori sets/classes of such features with known label, NBNN is searching for the class to which the query features have the minimum cumulated distance. In spite of being a learning-free method and the lack of tuned parameters, this scheme achieves close to state-of-the-art results for image classification. This is due to: i) the lack of a vector quantization step, avoiding thus to introduce more discretization errors, and ii) the use of image-to-class comparisons instead of image-to-image, which allows to combine bits and pieces of information from multiple training images.

At the same time, NBNN also has its limitations. The most important one is the high computational cost during testing: computation time depends linearly on the number of extracted features from the query image and linearly to logarithmicly on the number of stored labeled features. Unfortunately, the performance heavily depends on the density of features: the more information, the better the results but the slower the evaluation. Some have also criticized

K.M. Lee et al. (Eds.): ACCV 2012, Part I, LNCS 7724, pp. 689–703, 2013.
© Springer-Verlag Berlin Heidelberg 2013

the Naive Bayes learning free approach, as it needs balanced data with similar density in feature space for all classes, which often is not the case, and also the feature independence assumption is questionable. Learning is the solution to these problems, as addressed by [2–4]. Here we do not follow this strand of work, but rather stick to the simplicity of the original, parameter-free NBNN based on Naive Bayes. Instead, we explore another, complementary direction for improving the results, by investigating alternative representations that can replace the Nearest Neighbor scheme. We believe it is easier to spot the relative power of different representations in a learning-free formulation. Adapting the learning-based extensions of NBNN of [2–4] to the Naive Bayes variants investigated here seems relatively straightforward.

NBNN starts from the basic Naive Bayes (NB) Classifier, and uses the distance to the Nearest Neighbor (NN) as an approximation of the log-probability for a single feature to belong to a certain class of features. This is a somewhat arbitrary choice, yet critical for the overall performance. Arguably, NN is not the best option. In sparse coding approaches for object classification [5], NN in the form of so-called 'hard assignment' was proven inferior to the 'soft-assignment' approaches such as $l_1$-regularized least squares. Moreover, the NN classifier has considerably lower performance than state-of-the-art classifiers such as Support Vector Machines or Sparse Representation-based Classifiers (SRC) for the recognition of faces [6], handwritten digits or traffic signs [7].

Replacing the NN with a different representation in the NB classifier formulation is not affecting the desirable properties of NBNN: i) discretization is still avoided, ii) the good generalization of 'image-to-class' is maintained, and iii) it is still a learning free method. The parameters of the representations are adjustable, but usually have known general values for which the performance is reasonably high on (largely) different features and settings.

The main contributions of this paper are as follows. We investigate more general variations of the Naive Bayes Classifier starting from sparse representations. We empirically evaluate $k$-Nearest Neighbors ($kNN$), Local Linear Embedding (LLE) [8], Iterative Nearest Neighbors ($INN$) [9], Sparse Representation with $l_1$-regularization ($SR_{l_1}$) [6], and the Collaborative Representation with $l_2$-regularization ($CR_{l_2}$) [10]. Except for the last one, all of these are sparse. Moreover, we use in the NB framework for the first time the recently proposed Kernel Descriptors [11] and compare them to the results obtained with NIMBLE features [12].

Another side contribution is the evaluation of speeding up strategies for Naive Bayes Classification. We show that with only a small overhead over the original NBNN introduced by computing the rich representations, we are able to improve the performance. Moreover, we evaluate schemes with asymmetric sampling density as in [4] and approximated nearest neighbors (ANN) [13], with respect to the impact on performance and the speedup achieved.

Section 2 of this paper reviews the NB classifier and the sparse representations based variants. Section 3 gives a time complexity analysis. Section 4 describes our experimental results. Section 5 discusses trade-offs between performance and speed for practical applications, and Section 6 concludes the paper.

## 2    Naive Bayes Classification

The NB classifier [1] is a probabilistic classifier working under strong independence assumptions. A query image is represented by a set $Q = \{q\}$ of features which are assumed to be independently sampled from a class-specific feature distribution $p(q|c)$. Assuming uniform priors $p(c)$, the classification then becomes

$$
\begin{aligned}
\hat{c} &= \arg\max_{c \in C} p(c|Q) &&= \arg\max_{c \in C}\{\textstyle\prod_{q \in Q} p(q|c)\} \\
&= \arg\min_{c \in C} -\log\{\textstyle\prod_{q \in Q} p(q|c)\} &&= \arg\max_{c \in C}\{\textstyle\sum_{q \in Q} \log p(q|c)\}
\end{aligned}
\tag{1}
$$

In the following we review some of the most popular techniques for defining a (sparse) representation for a query from a given set of samples and we show how the Naive Bayes Classifier can be adapted to use these representations.

### 2.1    $k$ Nearest Neighbors ($kNN$)

$kNN$ is a standard method for defining the locality of a sample. The parameters required are the similarity or distance measure necessary for ordering the neighbors and the number of nearest neighbors to be kept. Boiman $et$ $al.$ [1] have shown impressive results using NB and $1NN$ for image classification.

In the case of NB-$NN_k$, for a query image represented by its set of features $Q = \{q\}$, we compute the $k$-nearest neighbors from each class $c \in C$, notated $N_k^c(q)$, and the (squared) distance-to-class $d_q^c$ and the classification becomes

$$
\hat{c} = \arg\min_{c \in C} \sum_{q \in Q} d_q^c, \qquad d_q^c = \sum_{x \in N_k^c(q)} \|q - x\|^2
\tag{2}
$$

which corresponds to the class with the minimum cumulated distances to the query. It is assumed that $p(q|c) \sim \exp(-d_q^c)$. Here, we consider only neighborhood sizes: $k = 1$, $i.e.$ NB$NN_1$, which is the original NBNN [1], and $k = 5$, referred to as NB$NN_5$.

### 2.2    Local Linear Embedding ($LLE$)

LLE [8] was introduced as a non-linear dimensionality reduction method, and recently incorporated in the Locality-constrained Linear Coding (LLC) method [14].

For a given sample $q$ and the set $N_k(q)$ of $kNN$ from $all$ the labeled samples $X$, LLE solves:

$$
\min_w \|q - \textstyle\sum_{x \in N_k(q)} w_x x\|^2 , \qquad \text{subject to } \|w\|_1 = 1
\tag{3}
$$

where $w$ is a $k$-dimensional weights vector corresponding to the $kNN$, with its $l_1$-norm constrained to 1. In our experiments, we consider $5NN$ as in LLC [14].

The importance of each sample $x \in N_k(q)$ in the reconstruction of $q$ is given by the absolute value of the assigned weight, $\tilde{w}_x = |w_x|$, while the non-neighboring samples, $x \notin N_k(q)$, get $\tilde{w}_x = 0$. We further $l_1$-normalize the importance weights for a sample $q$ to sum to 1, yielding $\hat{w}^q = \tilde{w}/\|\tilde{w}\|_1$. Now the *likeliness* of $q$ to belong to class $c$ is given by:

$$d_q^c = \sum_{x \in X_c} \hat{w}_x^q \tag{4}$$

where $X_c$ is the subset of $X$ corresponding to the class $c$.

The decision for the NB$LLE$ classifier gives the class with the largest importance/likeliness in locally linear embedding the query image $Q$:

$$\hat{c} = \arg\max_{c \in C} \sum_{q \in Q} d_q^c \tag{5}$$

### 2.3    Sparse Representation with $l_1$-min ($SR_{l_1}$)

The power of $l_1$-regularized least squares or *lasso* is proven for problems such as face recognition [6] or dimensionality reduction [7]. Given the set of $M$ labeled samples $X = \{x\}$, a matrix is formed $\mathbf{X} = [x_1, x_2, \dots, x_M]$. Then, for a given sample $q$, we optimize over $w$ (we fix $\lambda = 0.3$):

$$\min_w \|q - \mathbf{X}w\|_2 + \lambda\|w\|_1 \tag{6}$$

For capturing the importance of the weights for the query $q$, we again take their absolute value $\tilde{w} = |w|$, as in [7], and further $l_1$ normalize them as in the case of $LLE$, yielding $\hat{w}^q = \tilde{w}/\|\tilde{w}\|_1$. Now the likeliness $d_q^c$ of $q$ to belong to class $c$ and the decision for the NB$SR_{l_1}$ classifier is taken similarly to NB$LLE$ (eqs. (4)(5)) and selects the class that scores the largest importance/likeliness in the sparse representations of the query image $Q$. In this form NB$SR_{l_1}$ has been used in [9].

### 2.4    Collaborative Representation ($CR_{l_2}$)

$CR_{l_2}$ [10] seen as $l_2$-regularized least squares can be as good as the $SR_{l_1}$ on face recognition under specific conditions, like high dimensional face representations and suitable features such as eigenfaces. A strong point of this approach is the existence of an algebraic solution for

$$\min_w \|q - \mathbf{X}w\|_2^2 + \lambda\|w\|_2^2 \tag{7}$$

(we fix $\lambda = 0.001$) such that the coding of $q$ over $X$ is given by

$$w = (\mathbf{X}^T\mathbf{X} + \lambda\mathbf{I})^{-1}\mathbf{X}^T q \tag{8}$$

For a specific class $c$ the regularized residuals are computed, as in [10]:

$$r_c^q = \|q - \mathbf{X}_c w_c\|_2 / \|w_c\|_2 \tag{9}$$

where $w_c$ is the (sub)vector of coefficients corresponding to the class $c$ samples from the whole representation $w$. Similarly $\mathbf{X}_c$ is the (sub)matrix of $\mathbf{X}$ containing only the samples corresponding to class $c$. The decision for $NBCR_{l_2}$ is then

$$\hat{c} = \arg\min_{c \in C} \sum_{q \in Q} r_q^c \tag{10}$$

corresponding to the class with minimum cumulated residuals to the query $Q$.

## 2.5   Iterative Nearest Neighbors ($INN$)

$INN$ [9] representation is an approximate solution to a LS decomposition with imposed coefficients/weights and optimized selected samples. $INN$ tries to fill the gap between fast $kNN$ approaches and powerful but slow sparse or collaborative representations ($SR_{l1}, CR_{l2}$). Given the set of labeled samples $X = \{x\}$, $k$ samples $s_i$ are picked iteratively optimizing

$$\arg\min_{\{s_i\}_{i=1}^K} \|q - \sum_{i=1}^K \frac{\lambda}{(1+\lambda)^i} s_i\|_2, \quad K = \lceil -\frac{\log(1-\beta)}{\log(1+\lambda)} \rceil \tag{11}$$

where $\lambda$ is set to 0.1 and $\beta$ is 0.95 as in [9], thus $K = 25$. Since the weights are nonnegative and sum up to 1, the likeliness of $q$ to belong to class $c$ is taken as:

$$d_q^c = \sum_{s_i \in X_c} w_{s_i}^q = \sum_{s_i \in X_c} \frac{\lambda}{(1+\lambda)^i} \tag{12}$$

where $X_c$ is the subset of $X$ corresponding to the class $c$ and $s_i$ is the $i$-th selected sample in the $INN$ representation.

The decision for the $NBINN$ classifier is taken similarly to $NBLLE$ (eq. (5))

# 3   Time Analysis

## 3.1   Time Complexity Analysis

$NBNN_k$ depends on the number of features from the query image, $N = |Q|$, the number of labeled features, $M = |X|$, the dimensionality of the features, $D$, and the number of nearest neighbors, $k$. The time complexity of a straightforward implementation is $O(NMD+NMk)$. Using the structure of the known data, and organizing it with standard data structures such as kd-trees or hashing tables, allows for a practical sub-linear search in $M$ for $k$ nearest neighbors, without loss of accuracy. However, the higher the dimensionality of the features, the lower the speedup achieved, to the point of no gain.

NB$LLE$ has a time complexity of $O(NMD + NMk + NMk^2D)$, where $O(NMk^2D)$ is the added time complexity introduced by solving the local linear embedding over $k$-nearest neighbors. In most practical cases $k \ll D$, thus NB$LLE$ is $k^2$ times slower than $NBNN_k$.

NB$INN$ is running iteratively $NN$, thus its time complexity is the number $K$ of iterations, equation (11), times the time complexity of NB$NN_1$, $O(NMDK)$.

NB$SR_{l_1}$ greatly depends on the $l_1$-minimization solver employed for solving equation (6). The feature sign algorithm solver used by us [15] has a time complexity, in the optimal case, of $O(MDs)$, where $s$ depends on the non-zero coefficients in the solution. The solutions tend to be very sparse, so $s$ is small. The time complexity of NB$SR_{l_1}$ is $O(NMDs)$ and, still, much slower than NB$NN_k$.

For NB$CR_{l_2}$, first computing the projection matrix of equation (8) greatly reduces the further computation time. The time complexity for this is $O(M^2D + M^3 + NMD)$, so depending heavily on the number of labeled features, $M$. If one uses the pseudoinverse [16] then we have $O(D^3 + D^2M + NMD)$.

With naive implementations all the NB variants presented are adding time complexity to that of the original NB$NN_1$ algorithm. Usually, in our settings, the running times are, from the fastest to the slowest, in the following order: NB$NN_1$ <NB$NN_k$ <NB$LLE$ ≈NB$INN$ ≪NB$SR_{l_1}$ <NB$CR_{l_2}$, where NB$SR_{l_1}$ and NB$CR_{l_2}$ can be orders of magnitude slower than the NB$NN_1$ classifier.

## 3.2 Approximations Analysis

At first glance, the presented NB variants are doomed to unfeasible computational burden. Luckily, all methods can be speeded up significantly using a number of approximations, as discussed next. First, as used in [14], $LLE$ can be seen as a local approximation of the richer LLC, which instead of $kNN$ is defined over the whole data. Also for $SR_{l_1}$ the performance is seen to degrade slowly when the labeled features used for the decomposition are reduced to a local neighborhood of sufficient size. In [5] only the top nearest neighbors are kept, reducing the computational burden and causing a drop in time complexity to $O(MD + Mk + kDs)$ for solving a single $l_1$-minimization. The same trick can be applied for $CR_{l_2}$, so the critical part remains the retrieval of the nearest neighbors.

**ANN.** The computational burden is now finding the $k$-nearest neighbors where $k$ is either 1 (NB$NN_1$ and NB$INN$), 5 (NB$NN_5$ and NB$LLE$), or 200 (NB$SR_{l_1}$ and NB$CR_{l_2}$). A lot of effort has been devoted to sub-linear searching by using the structure of the data, and accurate techniques such as kd-tree or hashing can be used especially when the feature dimensionality is low. In our case, the speedup over linear search is small with such approaches. Therefore, we employ approximated nearest neighbors. Here, we use the FLANN implementation [13]. At the price of lower accuracy (out of $k$-nearest neighbors, on average only 90% are accurately retrieved), we gain a substantial speedup. ANN was also used in [1, 4].

**Asymmetry.** A further improvement in running time of the NB variants can be obtained by sampling less densely. We experiment with an asymmetric scheme where we lower the sampling density on the training material (reducing $M$), or on the testing material (reducing $N$). Usually, the speedup obtained is equal to the subsampling ratios (except if combined with ANN, when it is significantly lower than the subsampling ratio in training material). [3] suggested reducing the sampling density and learning a metric in feature space to compensate for the loss in accuracy. [4] shows that reducing the sampling density in the query usually brings smaller than expected accuracy loss. We arguably show that it is better to keep as dense as possible the features on the query, exploiting all the information available in the query image. Reducing the sampling density for the known labeled features affects less the performance of the NB variants than sampling less densely on the query image. The reason behind this is: if the set of labeled features is sufficiently large, then it is likely to contain redundant data, and subsampling these features still keeps the overall distribution, while subsampling the query image results in loss of valuable data for classification.

## 4   Experimental Results

### 4.1   Feature Extraction

In our experiments we use both NIMBLE [12] and dense Gradient Kernel Descriptors (G-KDES) [11]. This choice is motivated by the reported performance of both features, consistently outperforming the more conventional SIFT [17] features. Moreover, the NIMBLE features are richer and achieve higher reported performance than SIFT while being an order of magnitude sparser. For NIMBLE we use the code of [12] and follow exactly the settings as in their paper (100 fixations per image and 500-dimensional feature descriptors). Due to its sparse extraction, the running time of the NB methods with NIMBLE is considerably lower than in the case of dense G-KDES or dense SIFT and it is therefore the first choice for most of the experiments we perform. For G-KDES we follow the settings from [11]: extracting dense G-KDES features over a regular grid with 8 pixels step and $16 \times 16$ pixels patches, after resizing the image to a maximum of $300 \times 300$ pixels. We further lower the dimensionality through PCA to 64.

We include the weighted relative image coordinates in our feature descriptors, as suggested in [1]. Without them there is a significant drop in performance for NBNN [4]. The image coordinates are normalized to $[0, 1]$ by dividing with the width and height of the image and added with an empirically fixed weight of $\sqrt{0.5}$ to the $l_2$-normalized feature descriptors. This is equivalent to the value 0.5 used in [12] to weight the square $l_2$ distances.

### 4.2   Implementation

In the case of $LLE$, we pick the $5NN$. This is motivated by [14], where the LLC framework performs best when the neighborhood size is 5. For solving (6) for the $SR_{l_1}$ representation, we use the feature sign search algorithm [15] run only on the top NNs to obtain approximated sparse coefficients. However, if the ratio of nearest neighbors $w.r.t.$ the total number of samples used for solving an approximated $SR_{l_1}$ representation is too small the loss in performance is significant [9]. Thus, we use 200-NN for the experiments up to 10000 training samples, 500-NN

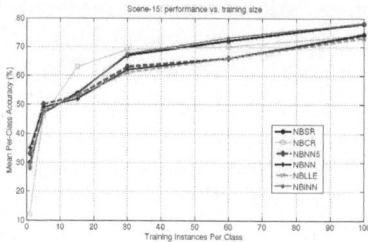

**Fig. 1.** Performance vs. training size on Scene-15

for up to 50000 and 2000-NN for up to 150000. Similarly to [5], for the feature sign algorithm, the parameter $\lambda$ is set to 0.3, which forces a very sparse representation. In case of $CR_{l_2}$, equation (7), we first compute the projection matrix, thus speeding up the subsequent computations. For the experiments with ANN we use [13] and build the data structure offline with a target of 90% correct neighbors in a $k$-NN query. Note that we are building one data structure for the whole pool of labeled features and we retrieve only once the 200-NN for each query feature. From these we pick the $k$-NN, for $NBNN_k$, for each class and, in absence of representatives, we take the largest distance to the retrieved samples. This approach was taken also in [9, 18]. In [18] the neighborhood size is tuned for best performance with FLANN, calling this method Local NBNN.

### 4.3   Scene-15

Scene-15 is a popular benchmark from [19]. We follow the common experimental settings, with a training partition of 100 images per class. We generate 20 random train/test splits and for each keep the performance as the average over per class accuracies. Finally we compute mean performance and standard deviation.

**Performance vs. Training Size.** First, we evaluate the impact of the number of training images per class on the performance using NIMBLE features (see Fig. 1). From Fig. 1 we see that considering more neighbors in the NB decision does not necessarily improve the performance. $NBNN_1$, $NBNN_5$ and NBLLE perform similarly. $NBCR_{l_2}$ is the best for 10 to 40 training images, while $NBSR_{l_1}$ takes the lead after 40 images. $NBINN$ is on par with $NBSR_{l_1}$.

**Performance vs. Feature Density** In Table 1 we report the accuracies for the NB variants under different uniform sampling densities of NIMBLE features in training and test images. Also the effect of using ANN is evaluated. We report mean classification rates and standard deviation for 20 trials for each setting. The best performance is achieved when sampling with the highest possible density in both training and testing images (78.2%-$NBINN$,77.8%-$NBSR_{l_1}$,74.3%-$NBNN_5$,74.2%-$NBNN$,73.7%-$NBCR_{l_2}$,73.1%-NBLLE). Reducing the density results in some performance loss, yet significantly speeds up all methods. Using only a single NIMBLE feature per image, the accuracy for $NBSR_{l_1}$ and $NBCR_{l_2}$ is still above 30% and 35%, respectively. This is mostly due to the

**Table 1.** Performance versus asymmetry in train/test and use of ANN on Scene-15

| #tr/#te features | With asymmetry | | | | | | | With ANN(target 90%) and asymmetry | | | | |
|---|---|---|---|---|---|---|---|---|---|---|---|---|
| | speedup | $NBNN_1$ | $NBNN_5$ | $NBCR_{l_2}$ | $NBSR_{l_1}$ | $NBINN$ | $NBLLE$ | speedup | $NBNN$ | $NBSR_{l_1}$ | $NBINN$ | $NBLLE$ |
| 1/1 | 10000x | 26.0±1 | 33.8±1 | 35.7±1 | 30.7±1 | 29.8±1 | 28.5±1 | 10000x | 25.92±1.3 | 30.63±0.9 | 29.13±1.7 | 28.49±0.8 |
| 5/5 | 400x | 52.2±1 | 59.8±1 | 63.2±1 | 58.8±1 | 58.2±1 | 53.1±1 | 500x | 52.19±1.0 | 58.83±1.2 | 56.95±1.9 | 53.05±0.6 |
| 10/10 | 100x | 62.3±1 | 65.6±1 | 68.3±1 | 68.7±1 | 68.4±1 | 62.5±1 | 200x | 61.26±1.1 | 66.29±1.1 | 65.86±1.0 | 61.37±1.2 |
| 20/20 | 25x | 67.0+1 | 70.6+1 | 70.0+1 | 71.1+1 | 71.6+1 | 66.4±1 | 75x | 66.86±1.0 | 71.44±0.8 | 70.61±1.5 | 66.45±0.7 |
| 50/50 | 4x | 72.1±1 | 74.1±1 | 72.2±1 | 75.5±1 | 76.2±1 | 70.5±1 | 12x | 71.30±0.7 | 74.33±0.7 | 74.18±1.4 | 69.00±1.8 |
| **100/100** | **(REF)** | **74.2±1** | **74.3±1** | **73.7±1** | **77.8±1** | **78.2±1** | **73.1±1** | 5x | 73.23±1.0 | 77.26±1.2 | 77.65±1.6 | 68.33±1.4 |
| 100/50 | 2x | 71.2±1 | 70.9±1 | 71.8±1 | 77.1±1 | 77.6±1 | 71.0±1 | 10x | 70.56±1.1 | 76.59±1.2 | 76.72±1.4 | 67.73±0.7 |
| 100/20 | 5x | 67.4±1 | 68.8±1 | 70.5±1 | 75.3±1 | 76.7±1 | 67.6±1 | 25x | 66.68±0.9 | 74.84±1.1 | 74.93±1.5 | 63.01±0.9 |
| 100/10 | 10x | 65.5±1 | 66.5±1 | 69.4±1 | 72.7±1 | 73.1±1 | 63.8±1 | 50x | 65.09±1.2 | 71.97±1.0 | 71.45±1.4 | 58.28±1.2 |
| 100/1 | 100x | 39.5±1 | 40.7±1 | 58.4±1 | 54.6±1 | 55.2±1 | 42.8±1 | 500x | 39.09±1.3 | 54.32±1.5 | 54.13±1.0 | 41.16±1.4 |
| 1/100 | 100x | 65.0±1 | 65.7±1 | 65.1±1 | 66.4±1 | 66.1±1 | 64.5±1 | 100x | 64.73±1.3 | 66.16±1.4 | 65.81±1.6 | 64.32±1.6 |
| 10/100 | 10x | 71.1±1 | 72.9±1 | 72.0±1 | 73.4±1 | 72.8±1 | 71.5±1 | 20x | 70.68±0.7 | 73.18±1.3 | 72.50±1.2 | 70.40±1.7 |
| 20/100 | 5x | 72.6±1 | 74.4±1 | 70.8±1 | 75.5±1 | 75.0±1 | 72.1±1 | 15x | 72.53±1.1 | 75.06±1.0 | 74.64±1.1 | 71.77±0.9 |
| 50/100 | 2x | 72.7±1 | 72.3±1 | 73.5±1 | 76.6±1 | 76.9±1 | 72.3±1 | 6x | 72.27±0.7 | 75.83±0.9 | 75.17±1.3 | 71.13±1.2 |

saliency guided NIMBLE feature extraction and the richness of the descriptor itself. The richer representations greatly improve over the standard $NN_1$ especially in the lower densities settings. Also note how for lower densities, $NBNN_5$ also does improve over the $NBNN_1$.

In an asymmetric setting, the performance decreases much faster when lowering the density in the query as compared to lowering the density for the training images, especially for $NBNN$. With only one feature per query image, $NBCR_{l_2}$ and $NBSR_{l_1}$ still give a reasonable performance (58% and 55%) vs. $NBNN_1$ (39%). In the reversed case, with one feature per training image, the drop in performance is much lower for all the methods, and $NBCR_{l_2}$ / $NBSR_{l_1}$ still reach 65%/ 66%. $NBINN$ is on par with $NBSR_{l_1}$ for all the settings.

**Performance vs. Running Time.** Note that subsampling can result in enormous speedups, with often acceptable drops in performance. For instance, with $NBSR_{l_1}$ a 100× speedup is achievable at the price of a 9.1% drop in performance (68.7% vs. 77.8%). $NBINN$ is 10× faster than and on par with $NBSR_{l_1}$. The ANN speedup increases with the size of the training, and decreases with feature dimensionality. Relaxing the target, by allowing more incorrect neighbors, lowers the performance but the gain in speed might pay off. One $NBNN$ experiment on Scene-15 using ANN and 100 NIMBLE features per image, takes less than 3 hours on a 2009 Core 2 Quad machine. $NBSR_{l_1}$ is slower, requiring about 4 hours, using a similar 200-NN retrieval per each feature. Nevertheless, the running time per query image per class is way below 1 second, which corresponds to the NBNN time reported in [1] (using dense SIFT).

**State-of-the-Art.** In Table 2 we compare the performance of the NB classifiers proposed here to state-of-the-art results reported in the literature. All these top methods are learning based, i.e. they require prior training and parameter estimation. The Naive Bayes methods, on the other hand, are learning-free and parameter-free to a large extent. One could tune $\lambda$ for $SR_{l_1}$ in equation (6), hoping in a better fit to the feature space used, but we did not try this. $NBSR_{l_1}$ and $NBINN$ methods improve over the standard $NBNN_1$ using either NIMBLE or G-KDES features. The gain in performance is more than 4% using $INN$ representations. The recently proposed, Kernelized NBNN with dense SIFT [4],

**Table 2.** Performance Comparison on Scene-15 and Caltech-101

| Scene-15 | | Caltech-101 | | |
|---|---|---|---|---|
| Method | 100 images | Method | 15 images | 30 images |
| ScSPM+SIFT [5] | $80.28 \pm 0.93$ | ScSPM+SIFT [5] | $67.0 \pm 0.5$ | $73.2 \pm 0.5$ |
| EMK+KDES [11] | 87.5 | EMK+KDES [11] | ? | 77.5 |
| LScSPM+SIFT [22] | **89.75±0.50** | GLP [21] | **70.34** | **82.6** |
| NBNN&BoF+SIFT [4] | $85 \pm 4$ | NBNN&phow+SIFT [4] | $69.2 \pm 0.9$ | $75.2 \pm 0.4$ |
| NBNN-$f_2$+SIFT [4] | $79 \pm 2$ | LLC+HOG [14] | 65.43 | 73.4 |
| NB-$NN$+NIMBLE | $74.2 \pm 1$ | NB-$NN$+NIMBLE | $70.1 \pm 1$ | $78.1 \pm 1$ |
| NB-$NN_5$+NIMBLE | $74.2 \pm 1$ | NB-$NN_5$+NIMBLE | $70.2 \pm 1$ | $78.2 \pm 1$ |
| NB-$SR_{l_1}$+NIMBLE | **77.8±1** | NB-$SR_{l_1}$+NIMBLE | **71.8±0.8** | **79.73±1.1** |
| NB-$INN$+NIMBLE | **78.2±1** | NB-$INN$+NIMBLE | **72.1±1.2** | **80.29±1.0** |
| NB-$CR_{l_2}$+NIMBLE | $73.7 \pm 1$ | NB-$CR_{l_2}$+NIMBLE | | |
| NB-$LLE$+NIMBLE | $74.0 \pm 1$ | NB-$LLE$+NIMBLE | $70.4 \pm 1$ | $78.2 \pm 1$ |
| NB-$NN$+G-KDES | $75.1 \pm 1$ | NBNN+SIFT [1]* | $65.0 \pm 1.1$ | 70.4 |
| NB-$NN_5$+G-KDES | $75.1 \pm 1$ | NBNN+NIMBLE [12]* | $70.8 \pm 0.7$ | $78.5 \pm 1.2$ |
| NB-$SR_{l_1}$+G-KDES | **78.7±1** | LocalNBNN+SIFT [18]* | $66.1 \pm 1.1$ | $71.9 \pm 0.6$ |
| NB-$INN$+G-KDES | **79.8±1** | | | |
| NB-$CR_{l_2}$+G-KDES | $74.5 \pm 1$ | | | |
| NB-$LLE$+G-KDES | $76.4 \pm 1$ | * indicates results without background class | | |

(a learning based method), has similar performance with the NB$SR_{l_1}$ and NB$INN$ methods. Our best performance is achieved by NB$SR_{l_1}$ with G-KDES features and is close in performance to the standard learned method Sparse Coding Spatial Pyramid Matching (78.7% vs. 80.3%). Note that kernelizing our methods and combining them with bag-of-features based methods as in [4] is likely to increase our results further (at the cost of switching to a learning-based scheme).

### 4.4 Caltech-101

On Caltech-101 [20] we report results both with NIMBLE and G-KDES features. In our evaluation (see Table 2), the performance of the NB$NN$ classifier with NIMBLE features compares to the one reported in the original paper [12] (note that their result is without considering the background class). All the NB variants achieve comparable or better results than the state-of-the-art. 70.3% at 15 images per class and 82.6% at 30 images is the best performance out of the state-of-the-art learning methods, achieved by the GLP method of [21]. NB$SR_{l_1}$ with NIMBLE features reaches 71.8%@15 and 79.73%@30, and NB$INN$ with NIMBLE features reaches 72.1%@15 and 80.29%@30. This is the best result using a single descriptor for Caltech-101 with 15 train images per class, to the best of our knowledge.

### 4.5 PASCAL VOC 2007

The PASCAL VOC 2007 [23] has a much higher variability in shape, pose, and position for the 20 annotated object classes than Caltech-101 or Scene-15. We are using NIMBLE features and report results with different sampling densities in training and test images respectively. We report for NB$INN$ the results from [9] and run only NB$NN$ and NB$SR_{l_1}$ since the other NB variants gave lower, less robust performance on the previous datasets.

For this challenge, we need to provide class confidences. The relative ranking among the classes for a specific image query is not sufficient, as some images contain instances of multiple classes. Using directly the score from equation (2) for NB$NN$ is not beneficial. The scores need to be brought to the same meaning, to be comparable across the image queries and not just for the class decision.

**Table 3.** Image classification results using PASCAL VOC 2007 dataset

| object class + #tr/#te | aero | bicyc | bird | boat | bottle | bus | car | cat | chair | cow | table | dog | horse | mbike | person | plant | sheep | sofa | train | tv | average |
|---|---|---|---|---|---|---|---|---|---|---|---|---|---|---|---|---|---|---|---|---|---|
| Best of VOC'07[23] | 77.5 | 63.6 | 56.1 | 71.9 | 33.1 | 60.6 | 78.0 | 58.8 | 53.5 | 42.6 | 54.9 | 45.8 | 77.5 | 64.0 | 85.9 | 36.3 | 44.7 | 50.9 | 79.2 | 53.2 | 59.4 |
| NB$INN$[9] | 69.8 | 63.8 | 48.5 | 61.9 | 26.6 | 58.9 | 74.8 | 52.9 | 51.6 | 36.0 | 42.5 | 40.8 | 75.7 | 62.2 | 82.8 | 22.1 | 28.9 | 41.3 | 74.1 | 46.0 | 53.1 |
| $INN$SPM[9] | 77.2 | 64.4 | 56.2 | 71.4 | 32.7 | 69.1 | 80.0 | 59.8 | 49.5 | 47.9 | 55.3 | 45.8 | 77.8 | 67.0 | 84.6 | 30.2 | 44.7 | 53.4 | 79.1 | 53.8 | **60.0** |
| NB$NN$+1/100 | 57.1 | 34.3 | 17.3 | 25.0 | 07.5 | 31.8 | 51.3 | 32.1 | 27.6 | 16.3 | 19.2 | 19.7 | 57.6 | 37.3 | 50.5 | 10.5 | 10.9 | 24.1 | 48.4 | 22.4 | 30.4 |
| NB$NN_S$+1/100 | 62.3 | 39.0 | 23.8 | 38.6 | 13.1 | 33.6 | 64.9 | 36.8 | 33.5 | 21.5 | 31.0 | 27.5 | 61.2 | 47.4 | 69.5 | 18.2 | 17.1 | 25.5 | 53.0 | 28.2 | 37.3 |
| NB$NN_S$+10/10 | 61.7 | 43.2 | 24.9 | 30.5 | 11.2 | 31.5 | 61.8 | 32.1 | 31.5 | 16.3 | 18.1 | 26.3 | 60.3 | 39.2 | 66.4 | 11.4 | 17.8 | 22.2 | 51.6 | 26.0 | 34.2 |
| NB$NN_S$+100/100 | 69.4 | 59.5 | 39.3 | 45.7 | 22.3 | 54.2 | 73.9 | 49.6 | 42.7 | 29.2 | 39.8 | 34.7 | 72.7 | 61.3 | 76.6 | 13.8 | 27.1 | 33.8 | 71.5 | 42.6 | 48.0 |
| NB$NN_S$+100/1000 | 70.7 | 59.3 | 40.3 | 47.4 | 23.0 | 57.4 | 74.3 | 50.7 | 42.2 | 32.9 | 43.7 | 35.7 | 72.9 | 61.8 | 78.1 | 14.5 | 29.1 | 34.8 | 73.1 | 44.9 | **49.3** |
| NB$SR_{l_1}$+1/1 | 36.9 | 17.1 | 09.2 | 13.7 | 04.8 | 14.4 | 32.0 | 11.2 | 21.0 | 04.4 | 14.2 | 16.0 | 18.2 | 16.5 | 52.7 | 06.3 | 02.9 | 09.2 | 17.6 | 08.4 | 16.3 |
| NB$SR_{l_1}$+10/10 | 62.0 | 47.2 | 28.4 | 41.7 | 12.4 | 35.7 | 66.1 | 36.7 | 37.9 | 18.8 | 20.3 | 28.8 | 62.8 | 45.0 | 72.6 | 09.7 | 17.7 | 24.4 | 57.7 | 32.8 | 37.9 |
| NB$SR_{l_1}$+100/100 | 67.9 | 63.2 | 46.1 | 50.7 | 21.6 | 56.6 | 75.2 | 54.5 | 46.4 | 34.2 | 40.9 | 41.4 | 73.5 | 62.1 | 81.4 | 21.1 | 26.9 | 41.9 | 72.7 | 44.9 | 51.2 |
| NB$SR_{l_1}$+100/1000 | 67.9 | 63.6 | 47.0 | 50.5 | 22.4 | 57.9 | 75.3 | 56.0 | 47.0 | 34.6 | 37.9 | 41.6 | 74.8 | 62.5 | 81.7 | 21.4 | 28.1 | 43.5 | 73.1 | 46.2 | **51.7** |

To this end, we consider the likelihood ratio between the probability of belonging to the class and the probability of not belonging to the class. This resembles the $f_2$ kernel from [4], and gives the following confidence function:

$$S = \sum_{q \in Q}(d_q^c - d_q^{\bar{c}}), \qquad d_q^{\bar{c}} = \sum_{x \in N_k^{\bar{c}}(q)} \|q - x\|^2 \qquad (13)$$

for a given query $Q$ and a class $c$, where $\bar{c}$ is the negative class. The NB$NN$ method with normalized scores is noted NB$NN_S$, where $k = 1$ as in NB$NN$.

In Table 3 we compare our different settings with the best results from the challenge. When using a strong asymmetry (just 1 feature per training image, 100 features per query image), we already achieve a mean average precision of 37.3% for NB$NN_S$. Using equal densities (100/100) we obtain a performance of 48.1%, which is 11% behind the best entry in the VOC2007 challenge. The sparse representations pay off and the NB$SR_{l_1}$ improves over NB$NN_S$ resulting in a mean average precision of 52% or only 7% below the top results. This is a good result, taking into account that the best entry in VOC2007 is a learning-based method, more complex than our learning-free approaches. Moreover, we used only the top 200$NN$ to compute the NB$SR_{l_1}$ decision, while NB$INN$ uses the whole training pool.

## 5    Discussion

**Computational Costs.** The main limitation of NB classifiers is the high computational cost. As shown in Section 3 the time complexity depends (usually) linearly on the number of training images, feature extraction density in training and testing, and feature dimensionality. All these made the deployment of NB$NN$ prohibitive in practice. It remained just a theoretical exercise. Even with exploiting the data structure and using ANN, NB$NN$ is quite slow in traditional settings, *i.e.* for $\sim 5,000$ SIFT features per image and 3,000 training images, it takes $\sim 1$ second per query image and class [1]. Here, we show how to temper the computational costs for NB schemes so they can be used in practice.

**Features.** The features are the building blocks in NB image classification. Ideally, features should be statistically significant for classification with a low dimensional representation and a low sampling density. The main stream literature

[1–4] heavily relies on the 128 dimensional SIFT features that for high classification performance require uniform sampling densities above 3,000 features per normalized $< 0.1$ mega pixels images. The recently proposed NIMBLE [12] features (500 dimensional, 100 sampling density) and G-KDES [11] features (200 dim., $< 1000$ density) proved to improve over SIFT based classification and come with (much) lower sampling densities. Using NIMBLE features gives two orders of magnitude speedup over the NBNN SIFT baseline. G-KDES features are also able to severely reduce (one order of magnitude) the running time of a NBNN SIFT baseline. The Matlab implementations as provided by [11, 12] are running in the range of seconds and can be optimized further.

**Training Size.** The number of training images per class heavily affects the performance. The larger their number the higher the classification rate but at the price of an increase in run time. From Fig. 1 we observe that for up to 5 training images per class, $NBCR_{l_2}$ is the worst performing method, while $NBNN_1$ and $NBNN_5$ are best. Collaborative Representation ($CR_{l_2}$) shows clearest benefit in performance in the middle range (10 up to 40 training images), while after 40 training images $NBCR_{l_2}$ performance scales less well *w.r.t.* the other NB variants. When more than 40 training images per class are available, $NBSR_{l_1}$ and $NBINN$ are clearly the best choices. To the limit, when infinite number of training images are available, it is expected that all NB variants with the exception of $NBCR_{l_2}$ converge in performance. A topic of further research is: how to filter the training features without loss in performance, *e.g.* by feature selection. Note that from Fig. 1 and Table 1 we see that the number of training images has a bigger impact than the sampling density of the extracted features: *e.g.* lowering from 100 to 50 the number of training images brings an 8% decrease in classification rates for $NBSR_{l_1}$, while reducing the feature density from 100 to 50 causes just a 2% drop. Each training image brings usually something new, while increased sampling over an image is likely to increase the redundancy of the features.

**Feature Density and Asymmetry.** What is better: higher sampling density in training or in query images? From Table 1 we see that for all the NB variants there is a higher drop in performance when we uniformly subsample in the query image than when we subsample in the training images. We achieve a 100 fold speedup by extracting a single NIMBLE feature either in each training image (causing a drop of 9% up to 12% in performance, depending on the method) or in the query (24% up to 35%). While in training the sampling density is less sensitive, for the query image the subsampling in fact removes important discriminant information for classification. For high feature densities $NBSR_{l_1}$ and $NBINN$ are our best choices. In very low sampling densities ($\leq 10$ per image), in either train or query or both, $NBCR_{l_2}$ gets on par or better than $NBSR_{l_1}$ and the other methods – promoting sparsity is less beneficial than using the whole data. It is worth mentioning that in lower densities $NBNN_5$ consistently outperforms $NBNN_1$ by stabilizing the assignments. While not tried, adjusting the neighborhood size to the pool size is expected to improve the results further.

**Approximations.** A consistent speed up can be obtained by using the structure of the data to drive the NN search. This is especially true when the feature dimensionality is low. Since NIMBLE features are 500 dimensional, we need to use approximated nearest neighbors. We control the chance of accurate neighbor retrieval to 90%, thus the drop in performance is marginal. Note that in our case, we achieve a maximal speedup of $5\times$. The larger the training pool, the bigger the speedup. Also, the representations can be computed approximatively using a local neighborhood as retrieved using ANN.

***State-of-the-Art.*** Using NIMBLE features instead of SIFT features in a standard setup brings up to two orders of magnitude speed up in a straightforward implementation. This allows us to provide results for large datasets such as PASCAL VOC 2007 (see Table 3) where $NBSR_{l_1}$ improves over $NBNN$ adapted for this task. For learning-free methods we show that representations such as $CR_{l_2}$, $SR_{l_1}$ or $INN$ are more suitable for high performance than the standard $NN$ under the standard Naive Bayes Image Classification formulation. The methods are validated on Scene-15, Caltech-101, and PASCAL VOC 2007. $NBINN$ shows improvements over $NBSR_{l_1}$ of 0.5% on Scene-15 and Caltech-101 (see Table 2) and of 1.4% on PASCAL VOC 2007 (see Table 3). Moreover, $INN$ while being on par with $SR_{l_2}$ it is much faster [9].

While we do not always outperform the state-of-the-art, it is surprising how close we get with our NB variants without any learning stage!

***Best Practice.*** For best performance, we suggest the use of NIMBLE features, high sampling densities in the query image (100 features per image), as many different training images as possible (not necessarily highly sampled), ANN for fast query feature neighborhood retrieval and more powerful sparse representation such as $SR_{l_1}$ or $INN$. When the labeled pool is small (tens of images per class) and feature dimensionality is large ($> 200$), $CR_{l_2}$ is a good option.

A good tradeoff between speed and performance is given by the following combination: NIMBLE features, low sampling densities (10 per image), ANN, and $NBNN_5/NBINN$ for very small training pool of samples, $NBCR_{l_2}$ for a small pool, or $NBSR_{l_1}/NBINN$ for large pools.

# 6   Conclusions

In this work we have studied the use of sparse representations in a learning-free, parameter-free setup given by the Naive Bayes Classifier formulation. In particular, the $NBSR_{l_1}$ and $NBINN$ give substantial improvements over the standard $NBNN$ approach which has the NN (hard assignment) as basis. Moreover, we have studied asymmetric schemes and the impact of the approximated nearest neighbors on the performance of the NB variants. Combined with recently introduced NIMBLE and G-KDES features, the $NBSR_{l_1}$ and $NBINN$ achieves state-of-the-art results for learning-free methods in all the considered benchmarks. Moreover, on Caltech-101, we establish a new state-of-the-art for single descriptor based methods. On PASCAL VOC 2007, we get close to the best entry of the challenge, a learned complex approach. Naive Bayes Classification is still promising. Further directions are to better subsample by feature selection and to explore kernelized versions of the NB variants, learning the priors, and, thus, further improving over our basic methods.

**Acknowledgement.** This work was partly funded by the Flemish IWT/SBO project ALAMIRE and the ERC research grant COGNIMUND.

# References

1. Boiman, O., Shechtman, E., Irani, M.: In defense of nearest-neighbor based image classification. In: CVPR. IEEE Computer Society (2008)
2. Behmo, R., Marcombes, P., Dalalyan, A., Prinet, V.: Towards Optimal Naive Bayes Nearest Neighbor. In: Daniilidis, K., Maragos, P., Paragios, N. (eds.) ECCV 2010, Part IV. LNCS, vol. 6314, pp. 171–184. Springer, Heidelberg (2010)
3. Wang, Z., Hu, Y., Chia, L.-T.: Image-to-Class Distance Metric Learning for Image Classification. In: Daniilidis, K., Maragos, P., Paragios, N. (eds.) ECCV 2010, Part I. LNCS, vol. 6311, pp. 706–719. Springer, Heidelberg (2010)
4. Tuytelaars, T., Fritz, M., Saenko, K., Darrell, T.: The NBNN kernel. In: ICCV (2011)
5. Yang, J., Yu, K., Gong, Y., Huang, T.S.: Linear spatial pyramid matching using sparse coding for image classification. In: CVPR, pp. 1794–1801. IEEE (2009)
6. Wright, J., Yang, A.Y., Ganesh, A., Sastry, S., Ma, Y.: Robust face recognition via sparse representation. PAMI 31 (2009)
7. Timofte, R., Van Gool, L.: Sparse representation based projections. In: BMVC (2011)
8. Roweis, S., Saul, L.: Nonlinear dimensionality reduction by locally linear embedding. In: IEEE ICCV, vol. 290, pp. 2323–2326 (2001)
9. Timofte, R., Van Gool, L.: Iterative nearest neighbors for classification and dimensionality reduction. In: CVPR (2012)
10. Zhang, L., Yang, M., Feng, X.: Sparse representation or collaborative representation: Which helps face recognition? In: ICCV (2011)
11. Bo, L., Ren, X., Fox, D.: Kernel descriptors for visual recognition. In: Advances in Neural Information Processing Systems (2010)
12. Kanan, C., Cottrell, G.W.: Robust classification of objects, faces, and flowers using natural image statistics. In: CVPR, pp. 2472–2479 (2010)
13. Muja, M., Lowe, D.G.: Fast approximate nearest neighbors with automatic algorithm configuration. In: VISAPP (1), pp. 331–340 (2009)
14. Wang, J., Yang, J., Yu, K., Lv, F., Huang, T., Gong, Y.: Locality-constrained linear coding for image classification. In: CVPR, pp. 3360–3367 (2010)
15. Lee, H., Battle, A., Raina, R., Ng, A.Y.: Efficient sparse coding algorithms. In: Schölkopf, B., Platt, J.C., Hoffman, T. (eds.) NIPS, pp. 801–808. MIT Press (2006)
16. Timofte, R., Van Gool, L.: Weighted collaborative representation and classification of images. In: ICPR (2012)
17. Lowe, D.G.: Distinctive image features from scale-invariant keypoints. International Journal of Computer Vision 60, 91–110 (2004)
18. McCann, S., Lowe, D.: Local naive bayes nearest neighbor for image classification. In: CVPR (2012)

19. Lazebnik, S., Schmid, C., Ponce, J.: Beyond bags of features: Spatial pyramid matching for recognizing natural scene categories. In: CVPR (2) (2006)
20. Fei-Fei, L., Fergus, R., Perona, P.: One-shot learning of object categories. IEEE Transactions on Pattern Analysis and Machine Intelligence 28(4), 594–611 (2006)
21. Feng, J., Ni, B., Tian, Q., Yan, S.: Geometric lp-norm feature pooling for image classification. In: CVPR, pp. 2697–2704. IEEE (2011)
22. Gao, S., Tsang, I.W.H., Chia, L.T., Zhao, P.: Local features are not lonely - laplacian sparse coding for image classification. In: CVPR, pp. 3555–3561 (2010)
23. Everingham, M., Van Gool, L., Williams, C.K.I., Winn, J., Zisserman, A.: The PASCAL Visual Object Classes Challenge 2007 (VOC 2007) Results (2007), http://www.pascal-network.org/challenges/VOC/voc2007/workshop/index.html

# Contextual Pooling in Image Classification

Zifeng Wu, Yongzhen Huang, Liang Wang, and Tieniu Tan

National Lab of Pattern Recognition Institute of Automation,
Chinese Academy of Sciences, Beijing 100190, China
{zfwu,yzhuang,wangliang,tnt}@nlpr.ia.ac.cn

**Abstract.** The original bag-of-words (BoW) model in terms of image classification treats each local feature independently, and thus ignores the spatial relationships between a feature and its neighboring features, namely, the feature's context. However, our intuition and empirical studies tell the importance of such spatial information. Although the global spatial information can be captured with the spatial pyramid matching scheme, the subject of capturing local spatial relationships between features is still open. In this paper, we propose a new method to embed such local spatial (context) information into the BoW model. A vector reflecting context information is firstly extracted along with each feature, context patterns are then code-specifically trained, and thus the context information is elegantly embedded into the BoW model by contextual pooling according to different context patterns. Extensive experiments on the PASCAL VOC 2007 dataset show that our method greatly enhances the BoW model, and achieves the state-of-the-art performance.

## 1   Introduction

Image classification has been one of the most active research areas in computer vision recently. In particular, the bag-of-words (BoW) model [1] has probably become the most widely-used approach to this purpose. A typical BoW model includes extracting local features, e.g., SIFT [2] descriptors, encoding the features by means of a pre-trained codebook, and finally performing classification with a classifier, e.g., SVM.

In previous work related to BoW, features with similar appearances are generally assigned to the same codeword and play the same role in generating the final representation. However, intuitively, they should play different roles if their contexts vary. For example, given two images in Fig. 1, each with wheel-like local features, marked by small red squares, traditional BoW will assign them to the same codeword, i.e., *wheel*, and similar representations will be generated. In this case, the wheel-like local features make little contributions in discriminating these two images. However, they can be easily differentiated if we consider their different contexts, i.e., the regions around the features marked by big blue squares in Fig. 1.

A feature's context can be considered as the relationships between the feature and other features in the same image. The original BoW model deals with each

K.M. Lee et al. (Eds.): ACCV 2012, Part I, LNCS 7724, pp. 704–715, 2013.
© Springer-Verlag Berlin Heidelberg 2013

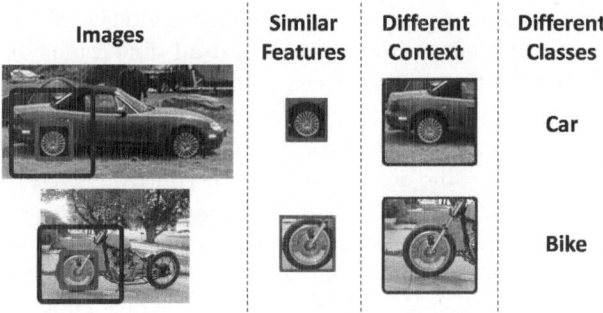

**Fig. 1.** Wheel-like features in different objects possess different contexts

feature independently, without considering the relationships between features at all. As a matter of fact, this model is limited in describing feature context information. To address this problem, we propose a contextual pooling strategy to capture the local spatial relationships between features. For each feature, we first extract its context vector, which reflects the distribution of other features within the feature's surrounding area. Afterwards, we learn context patterns using the context vectors collected from the training image set, code-specifically. Finally, we perform local pooling for multiple times, each of which corresponds to one context pattern. We name this process as the contextual pooling.

The main contribution of this paper is: to embed the local spatial information of local features, we map the features into a context space and perform multiple contextual pooling. Extensive experimental results obtained with different coding schemes on the PASCAL VOC 2007 dataset [3] demonstrate the effectiveness of our method.

The remainder of this paper is organized as follows: Section 2 reviews related work. Section 3 details our method, including context learning and contextual pooling. Section 4 presents experimental results prior to conclusion and future work in Section 5.

## 2 Related Work

### 2.1 Coding Schemes

Generally speaking, there are two key steps in the BoW model: coding and pooling. The coding phase focuses on independently describing each feature, in which we calculate the responses of features to different codewords. In the pooling phase, the responses are pooled together according to some strategies to derive an image-level representation.

In the past few years, various coding schemes have been proposed, such as histogram coding (VQ) [1], kernel codebook coding (KCB) [4], locality-constrained linear coding (LLC) [5] and saliency coding [6, 7]. The above listed schemes usually requires a large-scale codebook to perform well, which leads to higher computational cost in encoding. To our delight, there are other newly proposed high-dimensional schemes, which are both efficient and effective. Fisher coding (FK) [8] represents an image with a GMM, and all dimensions of the average first and second order differences between features and GMM centers are preserved. Super-vector coding (SV) [9] preserves all dimensions of the first order differences between features and codewords, and can thus better reconstruct an image than sparse coding and its extensions. In contrast to SV, FK encodes not only first order but also second order information so as to perform better. However, SV is much simpler in computation than FK. The selection of pooling scheme greatly depends on the adopted coding scheme. Widely-used pooling schemes include average pooling [1, 4, 8], weighted average pooling [9] and max pooling [5–7].

Above is still not an exhaustive list of existing coding schemes and their corresponding pooling schemes. We pick out two coding schemes for evaluation in this paper, i.e., SV [9], with weighted average pooling, and FK, with average pooling. SV and FK are both fast in calculation, and are the best two performers on many datasets. Thus, they are appropriate candidates for evaluation.

### 2.2   Context for Image Classification

While in the recent literature there has been great progress in the feature space i.e., different coding schemes, the topic of modeling the spatial information in the image space is still open. Toward this end, the spatial pyramid matching (SPM) scheme [10] is the most widely applied one, which can provide improvements co-operating with many coding schemes constantly. The success of SPM partly depends on the bias of photographers since it rigidly divides an image into blocks. Sometimes, however, the object in an image is appropriately aligned and rotated. And more often, the scenes where objects of the same category are located are similarly structured. When an image is shifted greatly, SPM tends to provide useless information.

One possible approach to addressing the problem of SPM is to capture local spatial information of features, which is the very approach that we adopt in this paper. The information in the image space can be interpreted as different kinds of context information, e.g., location and surroundings of a feature. The context of a feature refers to its spatially neighboring features in this paper. It should be emphasized that our work is different from those existing in the literature. In the first place, our work is quite different from the one in [11], though we use the same name, i.e., *feature context*. Wang et al. [11] present another way of dividing images according to 9 fixed reference points. However, we are exploring the context of each local feature by rearranging and pooling them within a context space.

Below are several other notable works about context. Rabinovich et al. [12, 13] adopt CRF (conditional random field) to capture the interaction between segmented local regions. Myeong et al. [14] explore object relationships with a graph-based context model. Morioka and Satoh [15] embed the relative spatial information of two features into a pair feature. Zhang et al. [16] embed context information into codewords. Features are extracted from images by detectors, and local feature groups (with members up to 3) are explored. Ito and Kubota [17] describe co-occurrence information of features and suggest that combining heterogeneous features, e.g., texture and shape information, is helpful for object classification. Su and Jurie [18] define 110 kinds of contexts by manual labeling for the purpose of providing abundant semantic information. Our work is different from theirs in at least one of the following aspects:

1. The context information in our method is heavily dense. We obtain each feature's context information by describing its surrounding area. In this process, the context information of all extracted features will be covered. Moreover, much more neighboring features are taken into account, compared with two in [15] and three in [16].
2. The context patterns in our method are automatically learned in a code-specific manner. This strategy does not depend on accurate segmentation or manual labeling. Moreover, we can adaptively learn richer context patterns and reduce the number of context patterns, compared with training a general context-book for all codes.
3. The utilization of context patterns is realized by means of multiple local pooling according to the pre-learned context-books, i.e., contextual pooling, which is very efficient and thus suitable for our heavily dense context information. The idea of contextual pooling is similar with the one of the scheme proposed by Boureau et al. [19], in spite that the ours is in the context space while the latter is in the feature space.

## 3 Method

The main idea of our method is to extract context vectors, learn context patterns and perform contextual local pooling. As illustrated in the middle part of Fig. 2, for each instance (marked by red small squares) of codeword *wheel* in an image, we extract its surrounding area as its corresponding context patch. These context patches are transformed into context vectors through a typical BoW process, so that the location of each feature in the context space is derived. Afterwards, as illustrated in the left part of Fig. 2, code-specific context patterns are obtained through unsupervised learning, to be detailed in Subsection 3.1. As illustrated in the right part of Fig. 2, features are pooled together according to different context patterns respectively, to be detailed in Subsection 3.2.

### 3.1 Context Learning

Suppose that we have densely extracted $M$ local features from an image, denoted by $\mathbf{a}_i$ $(i = 1, \cdots, M)$ respectively. These features can be extracted with any descriptors, e.g., SIFT [2]. In the original BoW model, only the appearance information is taken into account. Therefore, the $i$-th feature can be denoted as a tuple $f_i = (\mathbf{a}_i)$. In the case of the BoW model with spatial pyramid matching (SPM) [10], global spatial information, i.e., the absolute coordinates $\mathbf{l}_i$), is also considered. Therefore, a feature can be denoted as a tuple $f_i = (\mathbf{a}_i, \mathbf{l}_i)$.

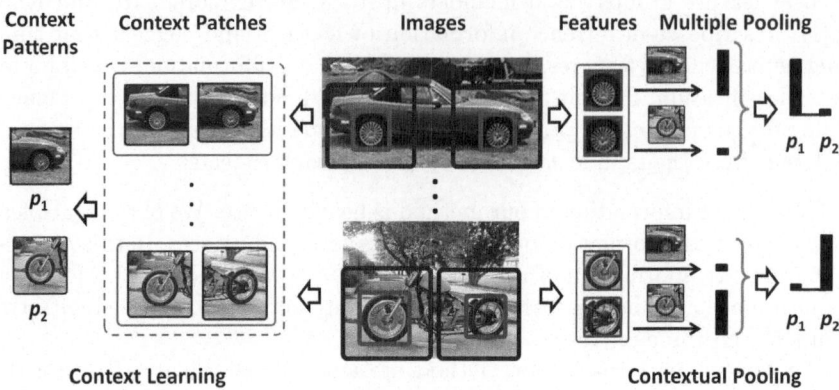

**Context Patterns** **Context Patches** **Images** **Features** **Multiple Pooling**

$p_1$

$p_2$

**Context Learning**

**Contextual Pooling**

**Fig. 2.** Pipeline of our method. $p_1$ and $p_2$ denote two different context patterns.

In our work, we put a context vector $\mathbf{c}_i$ into the description of features, i.e., $f_i = (\mathbf{a}_i, \mathbf{l}_i, \mathbf{c}_i)$. As illustrated in Fig. 2, for a feature $f_i$, we extract its surrounding area with a fixed size as the context patch and represent it with a context vector. There are various ways to generate such a vector. Particularly, in order to reflect the distribution of a feature's neighboring features, we propose to simply treat the context patch as a small image and perform a typical BoW process to calculate the context vector:

$$\mathbf{c}_i = \phi(\mathbf{l}_i, \mathbf{B}_c) \tag{1}$$

wherein $\mathbf{B}_c$ denotes a codebook for context description, and $\phi$ is the BoW representation of the context patch located at $\mathbf{l}_i$. Note that the codebook $\mathbf{B}_c$ is not required to be the same as the one for feature coding. The context vectors are hard voting based BoW representations of the context patches for efficiency. In our experiments, we try different settings, including different sizes of the context patches, sizes of $\mathbf{B}_c$, and SPM [10] configurations for context description.

With the context vectors collected from the training image set, we can train context patterns in a code-specific manner by $k$-means clustering. Supposing that we are using a codebook $\mathbf{B}$ (for feature coding) with $N$ codewords, denoted by $\mathbf{b}_j$ ($j = 1, \cdots, N$) respectively, we will obtain $N$ context-books, each with $T$ context patterns. For each codeword in $\mathbf{B}$, there will be a distinctive context-book $\mathbf{P}$, with each column $\mathbf{p}_t$ ($t = 1, \cdots, T$) denoting one context pattern.

## 3.2 Contextual Pooling

In this subsection, we embed the context information into BoW by contextual pooling according to the context patterns previously learned in Subsection 3.1. Suppose that we have extracted $M$ features $\mathbf{a}_i$ from an image, and that a codebook with $N$ codewords $\mathbf{b}_j$ is used. Let $\mathbf{v} \in \mathbb{R}^N$ denote the final representation of an image. For average pooling, we can calculate $\mathbf{v}$ in the original BoW model with [1]:

$$\mathbf{v} = [v_1, v_2, \cdots, v_N]^{\mathrm{T}} \tag{2}$$

$$v_j = \mathbf{z}_j^{\mathrm{T}} \cdot \mathbf{e} \tag{3}$$

$$\mathbf{e} = \mathbf{I} \in \mathrm{R}^M \tag{4}$$

wherein $v_j$ is the final representation with respect to codeword $\mathbf{b}_j$, and $\mathbf{z}_j \in \mathrm{R}^M$ is the coding responses of all the $M$ features to codeword $\mathbf{b}_j$.

The idea of local pooling is to pool multiple times and pool similar features together [19]. Local pooling can be redefined as:

$$\mathbf{v} = [\mathbf{v}_1^{\mathrm{T}}, \mathbf{v}_2^{\mathrm{T}}, \cdots, \mathbf{v}_N^{\mathrm{T}}]^{\mathrm{T}} \tag{5}$$

$$\mathbf{v}_j^{\mathrm{T}} = \mathbf{z}_j^{\mathrm{T}} \cdot [\mathbf{e}_1, \mathbf{e}_2, \cdots, \mathbf{e}_T] \tag{6}$$

$$\mathbf{e}_t(i) = \begin{cases} 1 \text{ if } f_i \in S_t \\ 0 \text{ else} \end{cases} \tag{7}$$

wherein $\mathbf{v}_j \in \mathrm{R}^T$ is the final representation with respect to codeword $\mathbf{b}_j$, $S_t$ is a set consisting of the features lying in the $t$-th pooling bin, and $\mathbf{e}_t \in \mathrm{R}^M$ is a mask vector depending on $S_t$. There are many instances of local pooling in the literature, e.g., the local pooling within the feature space [19] and the SPM scheme [10]. We can substantiate different local pooling schemes by replacing the definition of $S_t$ in Eq.(7). For example, if $S_t$ contains all the features lying in a spatial bin, the SPM scheme [10] is derived.

In contextual pooling, we perform local pooling according to a feature's context information. Accordingly, $S_t$ is made up of the features whose context vectors are assigned to the $t$-th context patterns. Within the framework of local pooling, we can rewrite Eq.(7) for contextual pooling as:

$$\mathbf{e}_t(i) = \begin{cases} 1 \text{ if } t = \underset{u=1,\cdots,T}{\arg\max} \|\mathbf{c}_i - \mathbf{p}_u\|_2 \\ 0 \text{ else} \end{cases} \tag{8}$$

wherein $\mathbf{c}_i$ is the context vector defined in Eq.(1), $\mathbf{p}_u$ is the $u$-th context pattern $\mathbf{p}_u$, i.e., the $u$-th column of a context-book $\mathbf{P}$. Note that $\mathbf{P}$ varies for different codewords. For example, the context-book with respect to codeword $\mathbf{b}_j$ will be adopted, when processing $\mathbf{z}_j$, i.e., the responses of features to codeword $\mathbf{b}_j$. The Euclidean distances between context vectors and context patterns are maximized in Eq.(8).

The above explanation of our method is presented supposing that each feature gives a scalar response to each codeword, and that average pooling is adopted. In the case of FK [8] and SV [9], the response of a feature to a codeword is a vector. And for sparse coding [5] and some other coding schemes, max pooling is adopted. However, we can derive the formulations for these situations by appropriately redefining Eq.(6). The details are omitted since the extension is straightforward.

# 4   Experiments

## 4.1   Experimental Settings

We test our method on the popular PASCAL VOC 2007 dataset. There are 9,963 images in the VOC 2007 dataset, belonging to 20 categories, e.g., bird, car and person. Images in VOC 2007 are of complicated backgrounds, carrying obvious variation in scale, illumination, viewpoint, occlusion, pose and so on. VOC 2007 is the latest one of the PASCAL VOC datasets with the labels on the test images fully released, and is thus convenient for offline validation. Moreover, the tendency of classification results on its succeeding datasets is basically the same. Therefore, VOC 2007 is an appropriate dataset for our evaluation. We follow the official experimental settings [3] and report mean average precision (AP).

In our experiments, gray-scale SIFT descriptors [2] are densely extracted every three pixels on four scales, with the width of SIFT spatial bins set to 4, 6, 8 and 10 pixels. GMMs for Fisher coding are trained with the Yael toolbox released by INRIA. Codebooks are trained by $k$-means clustering. SPM [10] is performed on three levels, i.e., $1 \times 1$, $2 \times 2$ and $3 \times 1$. LibSVMs [20] are trained as classifiers.

It should also be noted that we have re-implemented a framework of the BoW model for comprehensive comparison. As a result, there might be slight differences between the results in this paper and those reported by the original authors, due to re-implementation details, e.g., different sampling rates, and different strategies in normalization and reduction. Basically, our baseline is comparable with the results reported by Chatfield et al. in their extensive evaluation on coding schemes [21].

## 4.2   Parameter Evaluation

There is a parameter that should be fixed first in our method, i.e., the width of context patches $L$. For simplicity, we define the unit of $L$ as the SIFT step, i.e., 3 pixels. Intuitively, $L$ should not be too large, so as to keep context patches local, and not be too small, so as to make them discriminative enough. A preliminary experiment shows that classification results are not sensitive to $L$, if it varies within a certain range, i.e., $L \in [16, 32]$. In the next experiments, we let $L = 24$, which means that features located no more than 12 steps away from the center are considered as the context of the center feature, and that context patches are squares with a side length of 72 pixels.

There are two more parameters that should be tested, i.e., the size of the codebook for context description $N_c$, and the number of context patterns $T$. For the sake of efficiency, we always use SV with 128 codewords in this evaluation.

We first let $T = 4$ and test the influence of $N_c$. The results obtained with BoW and context pooling (CP) are depicted in Fig. 3. In the first column, the result obtained with our implementation of original BoW is given for reference. In the rest columns are results obtained with our method. It turns out that our method greatly improves the performance of BoW, and is also not sensitive to $N_c$ within the tested range. As $N_c$ increases, the performance grows slightly. $N_c$ is a key

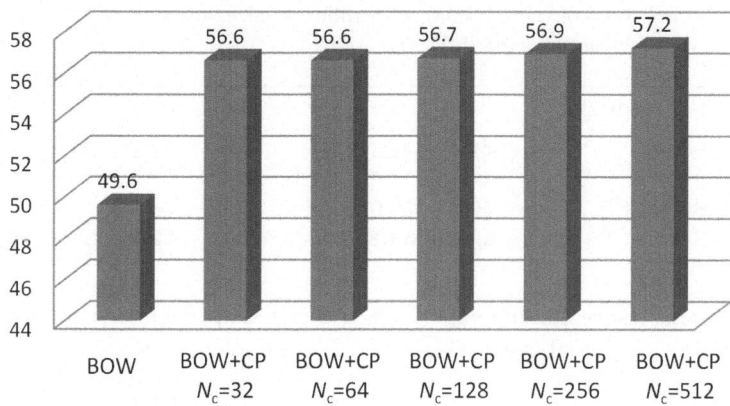

**Fig. 3.** Influence of the size of the codebook for context description

parameter which affects the computational cost in our method. Considering the tradeoff, we let $N_c = 128$ in our next experiments.

The following is the number of context patterns to be tested. The results are illustrated in Fig. 4. In the first column is the result obtained with our implementation of the original BoW model. In the second column, the result obtained with a globally trained context codebook is reported. An great improvement of 5.6% has been achieved. In other columns, the results obtained with code-specifically trained context codebooks are listed. The code-specific strategy (Column 5) further improves the performance by 2.2% compared with global strategy (Column 2), which indicates that two parts contribute to the overall improvement, i.e., the richness of context information and the learned code-specific context relationships. The performance of our method grows gradually as $T$ increases until $T > 8$. Considering the above results, we let $T = 8$ in our next experiments for the sake of effectiveness and efficiency.

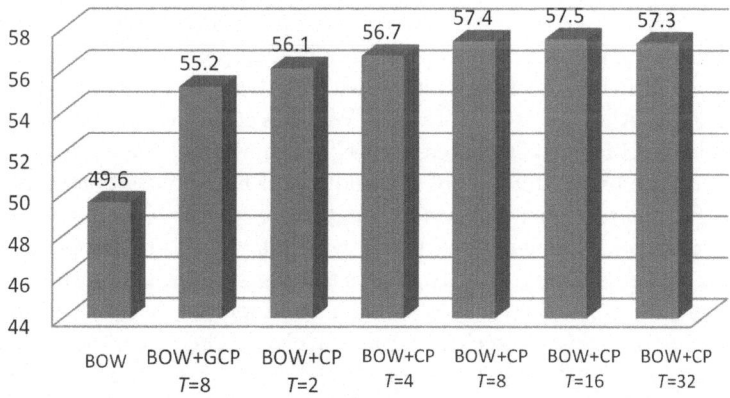

**Fig. 4.** Classification results obtained with different number of context patterns

**Table 1.** Performance of our method with different sizes of codebooks on PASCAL VOC 2007. Mean AP is reported in %.

| Codebook size | 16 | 32 | 64 | 128 | 256 | 512 |
|---|---|---|---|---|---|---|
| BOW | 41.4 | 44.5 | 47.1 | 49.6 | 52.2 | 53.5 |
| BOW+SPM | 49.0 | 51.7 | 54.1 | 56.0 | 57.7 | 59.0 |
| BOW+CP | 50.0 | 52.9 | 55.4 | 57.4 | 58.8 | 59.6 |
| BOW+CP+SPM | **52.4** | **54.8** | **57.0** | **58.5** | **59.8** | **60.7** |

Through out the remaining experiments, the three parameters in our method are fixed based on the above analysis, i.e., $L = 24$, $N_c = 128$, and $T = 8$.

## 4.3 Experimental Results and Analysis

We test our method on PASCAL VOC 2007 [3] and give analysis in this subsection.

In Table 1 is the performance of our method with different sizes of codebooks. It is demonstrated that contextual pooling greatly improves the performance of BoW, even better than the SPM scheme, namely, 1.5% better on average. Moreover, by combining contextual pooling with SPM, the performance improves further, which demonstrates that our method is complementary to SPM, i.e., our method captures the local spatial information, while SPM captures the global spatial information. The average overall improvement over BoW reaches 9.2%.

We then list in Table 2 the class-wise AP on PASCAL VOC 2007. It is demonstrated that obvious improvements are achieved for SV. Our method constantly outperforms the baselines for all the 20 categories. In the case of FK, our method wins on 17 categories. FK+SPM performs only slightly better than our method for two categories, i.e., boat and cat. Note that SPM captures the global spatial information, while contextual pooling captures the local spatial information. This is probably because that there happens to be less variation in background or spatial structure of those images belonging to these categories. There is a category, on which FK obtains the best performance, i.e., sheep. It is probably because that the spatial structure of the images labeled with sheep are so complicated that we can hardly capture any useful spatial information.

We compare the results of our method with the best results reported in the literature on PASCAL VOC 2007 in Table 3. We use a codebook with 512 codewords for SV, and a GMM with 256 centers for FK. As shown in Table 3, we achieve the best performance by combining our method with FK. Note that the source code of SV and FK has not been released by Chatfield et al. [21]. Therefore, the baseline of our method is implemented by us, which is close to their result, namely, 61.3%. Our implementation strictly follows the instructions in Chatfield's paper. Single feature descriptor, i.e., gray-scale SIFT, is adopted, no extra labels are used, and no flipping or any other techniques are involved. Therefore, the performance of our method is in fact better than our baseline by 0.7%. One of the best performers that we are aware of is the work of Zhou et al. [9]. They achieve a performance of 64.0% with a soft version of SV. However, according to the comments in

**Table 2.** Class-wise comparison of our method with our implemented baselines on PASCAL VOC 2007

| Category | SV | SV+SPM | SV+CP+SPM | FK | FK+SPM | FK+CP+SPM |
|---|---|---|---|---|---|---|
| aeroplane | 64.3 | 72.9 | **74.7** | 72.3 | 75.9 | **76.7** |
| bicycle | 64.5 | 65.7 | **66.4** | 65.2 | 66.8 | **67.8** |
| bird | 35.6 | 47.5 | **49.0** | 47.2 | 51.9 | **52.6** |
| boat | 67.0 | 69.2 | **70.3** | 70.8 | **72.4** | 72.2 |
| bottle | 24.5 | 27.8 | **30.1** | 32.1 | 30.8 | **32.9** |
| bus | 62.9 | 65.4 | **67.9** | 64.5 | 70.6 | **70.7** |
| car | 74.9 | 78.3 | **79.8** | 78.6 | 79.1 | **80.1** |
| cat | 52.2 | 58.8 | **59.1** | 57.7 | **61.9** | 61.6 |
| chair | 49.7 | 55.0 | **55.9** | 51.0 | 55.0 | **55.5** |
| cow | 39.2 | 46.6 | **47.2** | 50.0 | 51.1 | **51.6** |
| dinningtable | 42.2 | 54.3 | **58.6** | 48.8 | 57.7 | **60.3** |
| dog | 37.4 | 45.2 | **48.2** | 44.5 | 44.9 | **45.6** |
| horse | 75.1 | 76.8 | **77.3** | 77.7 | 78.3 | **78.5** |
| motorbike | 65.3 | 67.3 | **69.1** | 65.5 | **69.0** | 69.0 |
| person | 78.0 | 82.8 | **84.3** | 82.4 | 84.5 | **85.1** |
| pottedplant | 24.9 | 29.1 | **32.0** | 29.9 | 32.5 | **33.4** |
| sheep | 43.6 | 49.9 | **51.2** | **53.1** | 50.1 | 51.3 |
| sofa | 49.4 | 56.0 | **59.0** | 52.7 | 56.2 | **56.9** |
| train | 73.9 | 77.5 | **79.0** | 77.8 | 80.1 | **80.6** |
| tvmonitor | 44.6 | 54.5 | **55.5** | 55.8 | 57.0 | **57.8** |
| mean AP (%) | 53.5 | 59.0 | **60.7** | 58.9 | 61.3 | **62.0** |

Chatfield et al.'s paper, the result of 64% is achieved with nontrivial modifications such as using LDA to compute the SVM kernel and second order information as in the Fisher coding [21]. Another one of the best performers is the work of Su et al. [18]. To embed semantic context information into the BoW model, they introduce hundreds of context filters trained with extra manually labeled images. Based on the above fact, we skip both of them in the comparison, and 62.0% can thus be seen as the state-of-the-art obtained with single feature descriptor and linear classifier to the best of our knowledge.

### 4.4 Efficiency Analysis

The extra computational cost of our method is originated from extracting context patches and assigning features to context patterns. Directly calculating the context vectors leads to high computational complexity, i.e., $\mathcal{O}((L+1)^2 \cdot N_c \cdot M)$. However, the cost can be greatly reduced by caching incremental matrices in advance. For each codeword in $\mathbf{B}_c$, there will be a matrix, wherein the element in Row $i$ and Column $j$ denotes the number of the codeword's instances located in the element's upper-left direction. Afterwards, we can directly calculate the number of a codeword's instances within a rectangular region from the elements lying at the four corners of the region. Such a technique is applicable only if sum (average) pooling is adopted in describing the contexts of features.

**Table 3.** Comparison of our method with the state-of-the-art on PASCAL VOC 2007

| Method | Mean AP (in %) |
|---|---|
| Best of VOC07 [3] | 59.4 |
| LLC (CVPR10) [5] | 59.3 |
| Original SV (ECCV10) [9] | 59.8 |
| Original FK (ECCV10) [8] | 58.3 |
| SV by Chatfield et al. (BMVC11) [21] | 58.2 |
| FK by Chatfield et al. (BMVC11) [21] | 61.7 |
| Our method with SV | 60.7 |
| Our method with FK | **62.0** |

And this is part of the reason why we chose the VQ coding scheme for context description. In this way, the computational complexity for image representation will be $\mathcal{O}(N_c \cdot M + N \cdot M + T \cdot M)$. $T$ is very small, e.g., 4 or 8. Compared with the one of the original BoW model, i.e., $\mathcal{O}(N \cdot M)$, the main extra overhead is brought in by $N_c$, namely, the size of the codebook for context description. Note that our method is not sensitive to $N_c$, as illustrated in Fig. 3. For example, the performance obtain when $N_c = 32$ is only 0.1% lower than the one obtained when $N_c = 128$. In the case of VQ, KCB, LLC and some other coding schemes, $N$ is required to be much larger than 32 to achieve high performance, e.g., 25k [21]. Even for SV, $N$ should be up to 1,024 [21] or 2,048 [9]. Therefore, for these coding schemes, we can reduce $N_c$ so that $N_c \ll N$. In the case of FK, $N = 256$ [8, 21]. However, the computational cost of FK in coding is much higher than in pooling, which makes the $\mathcal{O}(N \cdot M)$ be the main time-consumer.

## 5    Conclusion and Future Work

In this paper, we have proposed a new scheme to capture the local spatial information between features, namely, contexts of features. The surrounding area of a feature is described with a context vector obtained through a typical BoW process, code-specific context patterns are learned with the obtained context vectors by clustering, and an image-level representation is generated by multiple pooling according to the learned context patterns. Extensive experiments on the PASCAL VOC 2007 datasets have shown the effectiveness of our method. The proposed method is complementary to the current dominant spatial pooling scheme, i.e., spatial pyramid matching, which captures the global spatial information. In addition, the extra computational cost can be effectively controlled by appropriately picking the parameters and speeding up the extraction of context patterns.

The follow-up work of this paper is to develop a better method for context learning. Currently, context patterns are trained in an unsupervised manner. In our future work, we will try supervised methods to enhance our system, which is supposed to be more discriminative.

**Acknowledgement.** This work is supported by National Natural Science Foundation of China (61135002, 61203252), Tsinghua National Laboratory for Information Science and Technology Cross-discipline Foundation (Y2U1011MC1).

# References

1. Csurka, G., Dance, C.R., Fan, L., Willamowski, J., Bray, C.: Visual categorization with bags of keypoints. In: ECCV (2004)
2. Lowe, D.G.: Distinctive image features from scale-invariant keypoints. International Journal of Computer Vision 2(60), 91–110 (2004)
3. Everingham, M., Van Gool, L., Williams, C.K.I., Winn, J., Zisserman, A.: The PASCAL Visual Object Classes Challenge 2007 (VOC 2007) Results (2007)
4. van Gemert, J.C., Veenman, C.J., Smeulders, A.W.M., Geusebroek, J.M.: Visual word ambiguity. IEEE Transactions on Pattern Analysis and Machine Intelligence 32, 1271–1283 (2010)
5. Wang, J., Yang, J., Yu, K., Lv, F., Huang, T.S., Gong, Y.: Locality-constrained linear coding for image classification. In: CVPR (2010)
6. Huang, Y., Huang, K., Yu, Y., Tan, T.: Salient coding for image classification. In: CVPR (2011)
7. Wu, Z., Huang, Y., Wang, L., Tan, T.: Group encoding of local features in image classification. In: ICPR (2012)
8. Perronnin, F., Sánchez, J., Mensink, T.: Improving the Fisher Kernel for Large-Scale Image Classification. In: Daniilidis, K., Maragos, P., Paragios, N. (eds.) ECCV 2010, Part IV. LNCS, vol. 6314, pp. 143–156. Springer, Heidelberg (2010)
9. Zhou, X., Yu, K., Zhang, T., Huang, T.S.: Image Classification Using Super-Vector Coding of Local Image Descriptors. In: Daniilidis, K., Maragos, P., Paragios, N. (eds.) ECCV 2010, Part V. LNCS, vol. 6315, pp. 141–154. Springer, Heidelberg (2010)
10. Lazebnik, S., Schmid, C., Ponce, J.: Beyond bags of features: spatial pyramid matching for recognizing natural scene categories. In: CVPR (2006)
11. Wang, X., Bai, X., Liu, W., Latecki, L.J.: Feature context for image classification and object detection. In: CVPR (2011)
12. Rabinovich, A., Vedaldi, A., Galleguillos, C., Wiewiora, E., Belongie, S.: Objects in context. In: ICCV (2007)
13. Galleguillos, C., Rabinovich, A., Belongie, S.: Object categorization using co-occurrence, location and appearance. In: CVPR (2008)
14. Myeong, H., Chang, J., Lee, K.: Learning object relationships via graph-based context model. In: CVPR (2012)
15. Morioka, N., Satoh, S.: Compact correlation coding for visual object categorization. In: ICCV (2011)
16. Zhang, S., Huang, Q., Hua, G., Jiang, S., Gao, W., Tian, Q.: Building contextual visual vocabulary for large-scale image applications. In: ACM Multimedia (2010)
17. Ito, S., Kubota, S.: Object Classification Using Heterogeneous Co-occurrence Features. In: Daniilidis, K., Maragos, P., Paragios, N. (eds.) ECCV 2010, Part II. LNCS, vol. 6312, pp. 209–222. Springer, Heidelberg (2010)
18. Su, Y., Jurie, F.: Visual word disambiguation by semantic contexts. In: ICCV (2011)
19. Boureau, Y., Roux, N.L., Bach, F., Ponce, J., Yann, L.: Ask the locals: multi-way local pooling for image recognition. In: ICCV (2011)
20. Chang, C., Lin, C.: Libsvm: a library for support vector machines. ACM Transactions on Intelligent Systems and Technology 2(27), 1–27 (2011)
21. Chatfield, K., Lempitsky, V., Vedaldi, A., Zisserman, A.: The devil is in the details: an evaluation of recent feature encoding methods. In: BMVC (2011)

# Spatial Graph for Image Classification

Zifeng Wu, Yongzhen Huang, Liang Wang, and Tieniu Tan

National Lab. of Pattern Recognition, Institute of Automation,
Chinese Academy of Sciences, Beijing 100190, China
{zfwu,yzhuang,wangliang,tnt}@nlpr.ia.ac.cn

**Abstract.** Spatial information in images is considered to be of great importance in the process of object recognition. Recent studies show that human's classification accuracy might drop dramatically if the spatial information of an image is removed. The original bag-of-words (BoW) model is actually a system simulating such a classification process with incomplete information. To handle the spatial information, spatial pyramid matching (SPM) was proposed, which has become the most widely used scheme in the purpose of spatial modeling. Given an image, SPM divides it into a series of spatial blocks on several levels and concatenates the representations obtained separately within all the blocks. SPM greatly improves the performance since it embeds spatial information into BoW. However, SPM ignores the relationships between the spatial blocks. To address this problems, we propose a new scheme based on a spatial graph, whose nodes correspond to the spatial blocks in SPM, and edges correspond to the relationships between the blocks. Thorough experiments on several popular datasets verify the advantages of the proposed scheme.

## 1 Introduction

Image classification has become one of the most active topics in the recent literature. In particular, the bag-of-words model (BoW) [1] has shown its effectiveness and applicability in terms of scene and object classification. In BoW, the occurrences of visual words are counted within the local feature set of each image respectively to generate a histogram, which is treated as a representation of the original image. Afterwards, we can just match the representations to figure out the similarity of two images, and furthermore to tell if they are of the same category.

In the original BoW model, the spatial information of visual words is not taken into account, which conflicts with our intuition and experience. We can better perceive the real world with the spatial information. A recent psychological study on recognizing jumbled images [2] demonstrates the importance of (global) spatial information and calls for research efforts in spatial modeling. In [2], an original image is divided into small blocks, which are then shuffled up randomly to obtain a jumbled image. For reference, this process is illustrated in Figure 1. The spatial information of visual words is missing in a jumbled image. As a result, subjects' classification accuracy might drop from 80% to 20% [2],

K.M. Lee et al. (Eds.): ACCV 2012, Part I, LNCS 7724, pp. 716–729, 2013.
© Springer-Verlag Berlin Heidelberg 2013

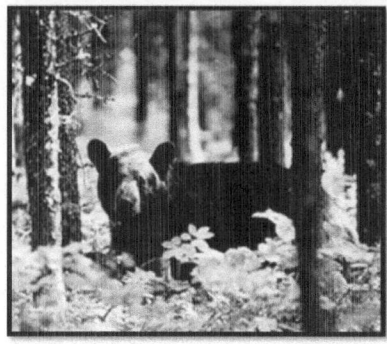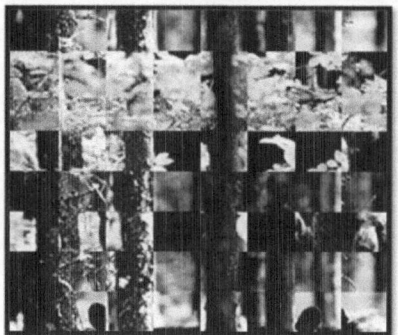

**Fig. 1.** An original image (left) and the corresponding jumbled image (right)

which shows the influence of spatial information in the classification process. The original BoW model, without any spatial information involved, simulates human's behavior in recognizing the jumbled image. In this way, we can hardly anticipate a good classification result.

Among all the efforts in spatial modeling, the spatial pyramid matching (SPM) scheme [3] is probably the most widely applied one. In SPM, an image is regularly divided into various blocks on several levels, as illustrated in Figure 2. The occurrences of visual words are then counted within these blocks respectively. Accordingly, we should match the representations from multiple corresponding blocks to find out if two images are of the same category. SPM can greatly improve the performance of BoW, and at the same time, it is easy to implement and of acceptable extra computational cost. As a result, SPM has already become an indispensable part in the BoW model.

In spite of the advantages, the blocks in SPM are treated independently. Two neighboring blocks are probably related considering that they are located close to each other, as illustrated in Figure 2. The spatial information of an image can be better reflected if the relation of spatial blocks are taken into account. However, the relation of blocks is completely ignored in SPM. To solve this problem, we propose a spatial modeling scheme based on a directed graph in this paper. In our scheme, blocks in SPM are represented by the nodes, and the relation of blocks which is missing in SPM is represented by the edges.

The main contribution of this paper is that we propose to embed the spatial information of an image into a spatial graph, by generating a series of histograms corresponding to nodes or edges of the graph. The proposed scheme is more flexible than SPM. Thorough experiments on 15 Scenes [3] and PASCAL VOC 2007 [4] show that this new scheme achieves better performance compared with SPM.

The remainder of this paper is organized as follows: Section 2 reviews the related work. Section 3 first introduces the original BoW model and its extension with SPM, and then proposes our scheme. Section 4 first explains the implementation details, and then reports and analyzes the experimental results. Finally, Section 5 concludes this paper.

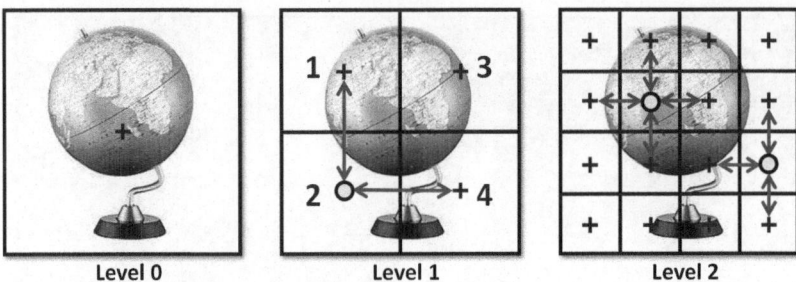

**Fig. 2.** SPM with 21 blocks on three levels: $1 \times 1$, $2 \times 2$ and $4 \times 4$. Middle: Bin 1 and Bin 2 are related to each other since they are neighbors, and so do Bin 2 and Bin 4. Right: More examples of relation between blocks.

## 2    Related Work

There is a great deal of work which takes the spatial information of visual words into account in the recent literature. They can be grouped into three major categories according to the adopted strategy for embedding spatial information.

The first is to embed spatial information into extended visual codes. Boureau et al. [5] embed local spatial information into macro-features which are extracted densely by concatenating small spatial neighboring local features. Morioka and Satoh [6] embed the relative spatial information of two visual words into a local pair-wise code. The pair-wise codes are obtained by clustering on pair-wise features extracted densely, each of which is a concatenation of two nearby local features. They further unify their work with the proximity distribution kernel [7] in [8], in order to combine the strengths of both, i.e., compactness and scale invariance. This kind of schemes focus on the local spatial information, but ignore the global spatial information.

The second is to express spatial information with an independent representation. The image-level representation of an image is the concatenation of a spatial section and an occurrence section obtained with the original bag-of-words (BoW) model [1]. Krapac et al. [9] propose to capture the spatial information of visual words with Fisher vectors. No matter how many dimensions a visual word owns (e.g., a visual word corresponds to a 129-dimensional vector in super-vector coding (SVC) [10]), the dimension of its spatial Fisher vector is the same. However, the performance is only comparable to the existing state-of-the-art schemes. The superiority of their scheme is thus about saving the memory and computational cost rather than improving the performance. Moreover, this superiority is true only if a high-dimensional coding scheme such as SVC is adopted.

The third is to pool spatially similar local features together to generate several representations and concatenate them, which is often referred to as spatial pooling. As a classic representative of the spatial pooling strategy, the spatial pyramid matching (SPM) scheme [3] is currently the most successful one, which is both effective and easy to implement. There are also some extensions of SPM. Harada et al. [11] train a discriminative spatial pyramid by optimizing the weights of blocks. Wang et al. [12] adopt a shape-context-like division strategy with respect to 9 fixed reference points. Yang et al. [13] propose a co-occurrence kernel for image matching instead of the original kernel adopted in SPM. Their model acts better than SPM on their land-use dataset, but on other popular datasets such as 15 Scenes [3], it only achieves a modest improvement. Our scheme proposed in this paper is also an instance of the spatial pooling strategy. However, different from the above three studies, we focus on embedding spatial information into a directed graph.

To build up an integrated BoW model, coding is an indispensable part. Recently, many researchers make great efforts in developing better coding schemes. Generally, the existing coding schemes can be grouped into three categories, namely, *probabilistic schemes*, e.g., hard voting (HV) [1], soft voting [14] and supervector coding (SVC) [10], *reconstruction-based schemes*, e.g., sparse coding [15] and locality-constrained linear coding (LLC) [16], and saliency-based schemes, e.g., saliency coding [17,18]. Probabilistic schemes, cooperating with average pooling (or weighted average pooling for SVC [10]), and reconstruction-based schemes, cooperating with max pooling, often show different characteristics in various aspects. Saliency-based schemes usually show similar characteristics with reconstruction-based schemes. Accordingly, we conduct experiments with SVC, as a representative of probabilistic schemes, and LLC, as a representative of reconstruction-based schemes in this paper.

## 3   Methods

Methods in this section mainly refer to the pooling stage in the BoW model. In other words, with the output of the coding stage, the question is what we should do to generate the final image-level representation. In the following, we first introduce the original BoW model, and then its extension with SPM. Afterwards, we will propose our scheme.

### 3.1   BoW

Suppose that the codebook consists of $K$ visual words, denoted by $c_j$ respectively. For an image, local features are extracted either with a feature detector or just by dense sampling. We assign each of these features to a visual word and record the occurrences of each visual word. Thus, a $K$-bin histogram is obtained for each image.

Let $X$ and $Y$ denote two images, and $\mathbf{x}$ and $\mathbf{y}$ denote their normalized histograms respectively. Supposing that we extract $M_X$ local features from $X$, denoted by $\mathbf{f}_i^X$ respectively, we can calculate $\mathbf{x}$ by:

$$\mathbf{x} = \mathbf{Z}_{k \times M_X}^X \cdot \mathbf{I}_{M_X}^X \tag{1}$$

wherein $\mathbf{Z}^X_{K \times M_X}$ is a matrix, each row of which (i.e., $\mathbf{z}^X_i$) corresponds to the coding output of the $i$-th feature, and $\mathbf{I}^X$ is a column vector whose entries are all one. In the case of HV, $\mathbf{z}_i$ is a vector with only one non-zero element, e.g., if $\mathbf{c}_j$ is the nearest code to $\mathbf{f}^X_i$, the $j$-th element of $\mathbf{z}_i$ will be one while the rest of its elements will be zero. Similarly, $\mathbf{y}$ is defined as:

$$\mathbf{y} = \mathbf{Z}^Y_{K \times M_Y} \cdot \mathbf{I}^Y_{M_Y}. \tag{2}$$

We can thus predict the similarity between the two images just by calculating the similarity between $\mathbf{x}$ and $\mathbf{y}$. Typically, it can be defined as the intersection kernel:

$$\kappa_{\mathrm{I}} = \min(\mathbf{x}, \mathbf{y})^{\mathrm{T}} \cdot \mathbf{I}_K. \tag{3}$$

Another common option is the linear kernel:

$$\kappa_{\mathrm{L}} = \mathbf{x}^{\mathrm{T}} \cdot \mathbf{y}. \tag{4}$$

### 3.2 BoW with SPM

No spatial information of visual words is considered in the original BoW model. To address this problem, SPM is proposed. The main idea of SPM is to match two images within a series of blocks on several levels. Those features matched on a high-resolution level will be excluded in matching on the following low-resolution levels.

The original definition of the SPM kernel is a little complicated [3], but it can be simply rewritten as the inner product of a weighting vector and the concatenation of every matching result within a separate block:

$$
\begin{aligned}
\kappa'_{\mathrm{I}} &= \min(\mathbf{x}, \mathbf{y})^{\mathrm{T}} \cdot \mathbf{w} \\
\mathbf{x} &= [\mathbf{x}^{\mathrm{T}}_{0,1}, \mathbf{x}^{\mathrm{T}}_{1,1}, \ldots, \mathbf{x}^{\mathrm{T}}_{1,B(1)}, \ldots, \mathbf{x}^{\mathrm{T}}_{L,1}, \ldots, \mathbf{x}^{\mathrm{T}}_{L,B(L)}]^{\mathrm{T}} \\
\mathbf{y} &= [\mathbf{y}^{\mathrm{T}}_{0,1}, \mathbf{y}^{\mathrm{T}}_{1,1}, \ldots, \mathbf{y}^{\mathrm{T}}_{1,B(1)}, \ldots, \mathbf{y}^{\mathrm{T}}_{L,1}, \ldots, \mathbf{y}^{\mathrm{T}}_{L,B(L)}]^{\mathrm{T}} \\
\mathbf{w} &= [w_0, w_1, \ldots, w_1, \ldots, w_L, \ldots, w_L]^{\mathrm{T}}
\end{aligned} \tag{5}
$$

wherein $\mathbf{x}_{l,b}$ and $\mathbf{y}_{l,b}$ denote the histograms of $X$ and $Y$ obtained within Bin $b$ on Level $l$, $L$ is the number of levels, $B(l)$ denotes a function returning the number of blocks on Level $l$, $\mathbf{w}$ denotes the weighting vector and $w_l$ denotes the weight on Level $l$. $\mathbf{x}_{l,b}$ and $\mathbf{y}_{l,b}$ are the product of a coding matrix and a mask vector like:

$$\mathbf{x}_{l,b} = \mathbf{Z}_{K \times M_X} \cdot \mathbf{v}_{l,b}. \tag{6}$$

Different from the original BoW model, spatial information of local features is required in SPM. Suppose that $M_{\mathbf{x}}$ local features are extracted from $X$ as $(\mathbf{f}^X_i, \mathbf{p}^X_i)$, wherein $\mathbf{p}^X_i$ denotes the location of $\mathbf{f}^X_i$ in the image. The $i$-th element of $\mathbf{v}_{l,b}$ can be defined as:

$$\mathbf{v}_{l,b}(i) = \begin{cases} 1 \text{ if } h(\mathbf{p}_i^X, l) = b \\ 0 \text{ else} \end{cases} \tag{7}$$

wherein $h(\mathbf{p}_i^X, l)$ is a function returning an index $\in \{1, 2, \ldots, B(l)\}$ denoting the block in which $\mathbf{p}_i^X$ lies on the specified Level $l$. Accordingly, the linear kernel with SPM is:

$$\kappa_L' = \mathbf{x}^T \cdot (\mathbf{y} \odot \mathbf{w}) \tag{8}$$

wherein $\odot$ denotes the element-wise multiplication.

## 3.3   Our Scheme

Our scheme is to match images with their spatial information embedded in a directed graph, so as to reflect the relation between neighboring blocks. The main idea is to represent an image with a series of histograms corresponding to the nodes and edges in a directed graph, as illustrated in Figure 3.

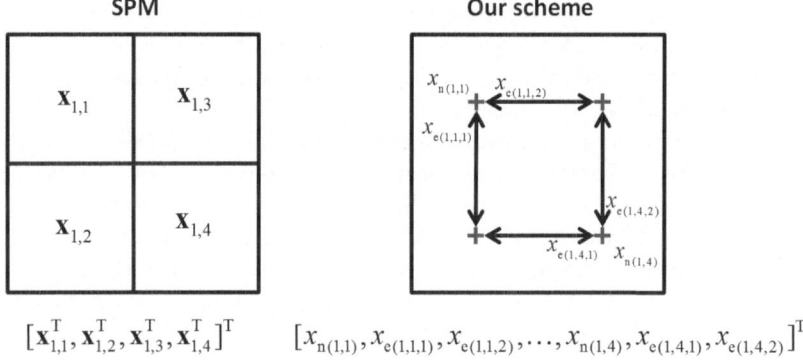

**Fig. 3.**   A comparison between SPM and our schemes on Level 1. $x_{n(l,n)}^j$: the $j$-th element of $\mathbf{x}_{\text{node}(l,n)}$. $x_{e(l,n,e)}^j$: the $j$-th element of $\mathbf{x}_{\text{edge}(l,n,e)}$. See the text for details.

In our scheme, the image-level representations are defined as:

$$\begin{aligned} \mathbf{x} &= [\mathbf{x}_{0,1}^T, \mathbf{x}_{1,1}^T, \ldots, \mathbf{x}_{1,N(1)}^T, \ldots, \mathbf{x}_{L,1}^T, \ldots, \mathbf{x}_{L,N(L)}^T]^T \\ \mathbf{x}_{l,n} &= [\mathbf{x}_{\text{node}(l,n)}^T, \mathbf{x}_{\text{edge}(l,n,1)}^T, \ldots, \mathbf{x}_{\text{edge}(l,n,E(l,n))}^T]^T \end{aligned} \tag{9}$$

wherein $\mathbf{x}_{\text{node}(l,n)}$ denotes the histogram of $X$ corresponding to Node $n$ on Level $l$, $\mathbf{x}_{\text{edge}(l,n,e)}$ denotes the histogram corresponding to the edge from Node $n$ on Level $l$ to its $e$-th neighbor, $N(l)$ denotes a function returning the number of nodes on Level $l$ and $E(l, n)$ denotes a function returning the outdegree of

Node $n$ on Level $l$. $\mathbf{x}_{\text{node}(l,n)}$ and $\mathbf{x}_{\text{edge}(l,n,e)}$ are each a product of the coding matrix and a mask vector:

$$\mathbf{x}_{\text{node}(l,n)} = \mathbf{Z}_{n \times m_X} \cdot \mathbf{u}_{l,n} \tag{10}$$

$$\mathbf{x}_{\text{edge}(l,n,e)} = \mathbf{Z}_{n \times m_X} \cdot \mathbf{u}_{l,n,e}. \tag{11}$$

The $i$-th element of $\mathbf{u}_{l,n}$ and $\mathbf{u}_{l,n,e}$ can be respectively defined as:

$$\mathbf{u}_{l,n}(i) = \begin{cases} 1 \text{ if } h_{\text{node}}(\mathbf{p}_i^X, l) = n \\ 0 \text{ else} \end{cases} \tag{12}$$

$$\mathbf{u}_{l,n,e}(i) = \begin{cases} 1 \text{ if } h_{\text{edge}}(\mathbf{p}_i^X, l, n) = e \\ 0 \text{ else} \end{cases} \tag{13}$$

wherein $h_{\text{node}}(\mathbf{p}_i^X, l)$ is an index $\in \{1, 2, \ldots, N(l)\}$ denoting the spatially nearest node to $\mathbf{p}_i^X$ on the specified Level $l$, and $h_{\text{edge}}(\mathbf{p}_i^X, l, n)$ is an index $\in \{1, 2, \ldots, E(l, n)\}$ denoting the nearest edge to $\mathbf{p}_i^X$ among all the edges originated from Node $n$ on Level $l$.

The above explanations are presented supposing that the sum (average) pooling scheme is adopted. However, there will be no difficulty in extending the formulations for weighted average pooling and max pooling. We omit the details since the extension is straightforward.

It is worthy noting that we introduce the representations of edges ($\mathbf{x}_{\text{edge}(l,n,e)}$) to reflect the relation between neighboring nodes. From this point of view, $\mathbf{u}_{l,n,e}$ defined in Equation (13) is not appropriate. What we want is to reflect the relation between Node $n$ and its neighbors, however, only the features belonging to Node $n$ are involved. To deal with this problem, we introduce the soft assignment mechanism into this process. In this way, $\mathbf{u}_{l,n}$ and $\mathbf{u}_{l,n,e}$ turn into weighting vectors. We will discuss the details in Section 4.1.

## 4    Experimental Results

### 4.1    Implementation Details

To implement our scheme, there are two main aspects that we must handle with. The first one is how to build up a directed graph, and the second one is how to assign local features to the nodes and edges in these graphs.

To build up the graph, we must first locate the nodes denoting different blocks. In this paper, we simply set the center of each block as a node $\mathbf{p}_{(l,n)}$, i.e., the location of Node $n$ on Level $l$. Afterwards, we assign an edge between two nodes on the same level if their corresponding blocks are neighbors, as illustrated in Figure 3.

Given a feature in an image, we should decide which node and edge it should be assigned to, as defined in Equations (12) and (13). As a common choice, we can conduct the node assignment with respect to the spatial Euclidean distances between features and nodes. Thus, $h_{\text{node}}$ in Equations (12) can be defined as:

$$h_{\text{node}}(\mathbf{p}_i^X, l) = \underset{n=1,\ldots,N(l)}{\arg\min} \; d_{\text{node}}(\mathbf{p}_i^X, l, n)$$

$$d_{\text{node}}(\mathbf{p}_i^X, l, n) = \left\| \mathbf{p}_i^X - \mathbf{P}_{(l,n)} \right\|_2. \tag{14}$$

We define $h_{\text{edge}}$ in Equation (13) as:

$$h_{\text{edge}}(\mathbf{p}_i^X, l, n) = \underset{e=1,\ldots,E(l,n)}{\arg\max} \; d_{\text{edge}}(\mathbf{p}_i^X, l, n, e)$$

$$d_{\text{edge}}(\mathbf{p}_i^X, l, n, e) = (\overrightarrow{P_{l,n} P_i^X} \cdot \overrightarrow{P_{l,n} P_{\text{neighbor}}^X})$$

$$\overrightarrow{P_{l,n} P_i^X} = \mathbf{p}_i^X - \mathbf{P}_{(l,n)} \tag{15}$$

$$\overrightarrow{P_{l,n} P_{\text{neighbor}}^X} = \mathbf{P}_{(l,neighbor(l,n,e))} - \mathbf{P}_{(l,n)}$$

wherein $neighbor(l,n,e)$ is a function returning the index $\in \{1,2,\ldots,N(l)\}$ of the $e$-th neighbor of Node $n$ on Level $l$. Here, we adopt the dot product as the distance between a feature and an edge. Compared with the spatial distance from a feature to a edge, the features which are close to a node will be smoothly assigned to the node's edges. As mentioned in Section 3.3, soft assignment is required for the motivation of our scheme. Fortunately, the treatment is in hand considering the distance, i.e., $d_{\text{node}}$ in Equation (14), and the similarity, i.e., $d_{\text{edge}}$ in Equation (15) have already been defined. We apply the Gaussian function for soft assignment:

$$d'_{\text{node}} = e^{-\lambda_n d_{\text{node}}^2} \tag{16}$$

$$d'_{\text{edge}} = \begin{cases} e^{-\lambda_e (d_{\text{edge}} - 0.5)^2} & \text{if } d_{\text{edge}} < 0.5 \\ 1 & \text{else} \end{cases} \tag{17}$$

wherein $\lambda_n$ and $\lambda_e$ are two parameters. And the elements of the weighting vectors in Equations (10) and (11) are obtained after normalization:

$$\mathbf{u}_{l,n}(i) = \frac{d'_{\text{node}}(\mathbf{p}_i^X, l, n)}{\displaystyle\sum_{n=1,\ldots,N(l)} d'_{\text{node}}(\mathbf{p}_i^X, l, n)} \tag{18}$$

$$\mathbf{u}_{l,n,e}(i) = \frac{d'_{\text{edge}}(\mathbf{p}_i^X, l, n, e)}{\displaystyle\sum_{e=1,\ldots,E(l,n)} d'_{\text{edge}}(\mathbf{p}_i^X, l, n, e)} \cdot \mathbf{u}_{l,n}(i). \tag{19}$$

Obviously,

$$\mathbf{u}_{l,n}(i) = \sum_{e=1,\ldots,E(l,n)} \mathbf{u}_{l,n,e}(i)$$

which means that

$$\mathbf{x}_{\text{node}(l,n)} = \sum_{e=1,\dots,E(l,n)} \mathbf{x}_{\text{edge}(l,n,e)}.$$

In other words, $\mathbf{x}_{\text{node}(l,n)}$ and $\mathbf{x}_{\text{edge}(l,n,e)}$ $(e = 1,\dots,E(l,n))$ are linearly correlated. Therefore, we can remove $\mathbf{x}_{\text{node}(l,n)}$ from the final representation without losing useful information. Notably, this is not always true as the strategy for generating the two weighting vectors varies.

## 4.2   Datasets and Experimental Settings

We evaluate our scheme on the 15 Scenes dataset [3] for scene classification, and the PASCAL VOC 2007 dataset [4] for object classification. In the 15 Scenes dataset, there are 4,485 images of natural scenes in total, belonging to 15 categories (e.g., bedroom, CALsuburb and industrial), each of which consists of 200 to 400 images. In the PASCAL VOC 2007 dataset, there are 9,963 images in total, belonging to 20 categories, e.g., bird, car and person. Images in VOC 2007 carry obvious variation in scale, illumination, viewpoint, pose, occlusion and so on. Generally speaking, the tendency of the resulting curves is similar on different VOC datasets, since they are of high overlap of the collected images (nearly 50% between VOC 2007 and VOC 2011). Most works in the recent literature report their results on VOC 2007 instead of the newer datasets because the labels on test images are fully released. For the sake of conveniences in evaluation and comparison with related work, we follow this policy.

For 15 Scenes, we follow the evaluation settings proposed in [3], i.e., randomly pick out 100 images from each category for training, and keep the remaining images for testing. We repeat the evaluation for 10 times and report the average classification accuracy and the standard deviation. For VOC 2007, we follow the official evaluation rules, i.e., train models on the *trainval* set, test on the *test* set, and report the mean average precision (mAP).

SIFT descriptors [19] are densely extracted every four pixels for all images on three scale, i.e., $16 \times 16$, $24 \times 24$ and $32 \times 32$ in pixels. The local features are L2-normalized as preprocessing. Codebooks are trained by the $k$-means clustering. Lib-linear SVMs [20] are trained as classifiers. For comparison, SPM [3] is performed on three levels, i.e., $1 \times 1$, $2 \times 2$ and $3 \times 1$. Accordingly, we build up graphs on three levels with the same setting. We do not follow the original SPM configuration in [3] for two reasons: first, the used configuration is of lower dimension and performs as well as or even better than the original one; second, there is no need to worry about the compatibility issues between the $3 \times 1$ level and the intersection kernel, since LLC and SVC are both designed for linear SVM. Cross-validation on training set shows that the optimal soft assignment parameters are relatively insensitive to the variation of code sizes and evaluation datasets. However, the optimal parameters tend to vary if the adopted coding scheme is different. Thus, we fix $\lambda_n$ and $\lambda_e$ for different kinds of coding schemes in our experiments. For SVC, $(\lambda_n, \lambda_e) = (32, 8)$, which are also appropriate for other probabilistic schemes. For LLC, $(\lambda_n, \lambda_e) = (16, 8)$, which are also appropriate for other reconstruction-based schemes.

It is worthy noting that we implement a general framework of the BoW model to ensure fair and comprehensive comparison. The results of BoW, SPM and our scheme reported in this paper are all obtained with this framework. As a result, there might be discrepancies between our results and those reported by the original authors.

## 4.3    Basic Results

To test the configurations of blocks and levels, we conduct a series of experiments with different combinations of levels. The detailed results are reported in Table 1. Only the results obtained with LLC on 15 Scenes are reported due to limited space, since the results for different coding schemes or datasets are basically the same. Results obtained with the representations on separate levels are also attached to show the contribution of different levels. Note that the last two rows are both on Level 2. Thus, the columns labeled by Pyramid in Row 3 denote the configuration: $1 \times 1$, $2 \times 2$ and $3 \times 1$, and those in Row 4 denote the configuration: $1 \times 1$, $2 \times 2$ and $4 \times 4$.

**Table 1.** Classification results obtained with LLC on 15 Scenes. The best results for different code sizes are shown in bold. Note that the last two rows are both on Level 2. See the text for details.

| Code size: | $n = 16$ | | $n = 512$ | | $n = 8192$ | |
|---|---|---|---|---|---|---|
| $L$ | Single level | Pyramid | Single level | Pyramid | Single level | Pyramid |
| $0\ (1 \times 1)$ | $35.0 \pm 0.6$ | | $64.5 \pm 0.6$ | | $77.1 \pm 0.7$ | |
| $1\ (2 \times 2)$ | $58.0 \pm 0.6$ | $58.7 \pm 0.5$ | $77.1 \pm 0.6$ | $77.4 \pm 0.6$ | $82.7 \pm 0.4$ | $83.0 \pm 0.4$ |
| $2\ (3 \times 1)$ | $55.2 \pm 0.5$ | $61.2 \pm 0.6$ | $76.1 \pm 0.5$ | $\mathbf{78.3 \pm 0.7}$ | $82.4 \pm 0.4$ | $\mathbf{83.3 \pm 0.3}$ |
| $2\ (4 \times 4)$ | $61.1 \pm 0.5$ | $\mathbf{61.7 \pm 0.3}$ | $76.7 \pm 0.3$ | $77.7 \pm 0.4$ | $80.4 \pm 0.2$ | $82.5 \pm 0.2$ |

The improvement in performance shown in Table 1 agrees with our anticipation. When $L = 0$, our scheme becomes an analogue of the original BoW model, where no spatial information is involved. When $L > 0$, the performance improves as $L$ increases, because finer spatial information is embedded. However, simply increasing the number of blocks does not always lead to better results. For example, the performance listed in Row 4 denoting the $4 \times 4$ level is inferior to the performance listed in Row 3 denoting the $3 \times 1$ level. The results demonstrate that our configuration is appropriate.

## 4.4    Comparison with SPM

We report the classification results of our scheme and SPM in Figure 4 for comparison on separate levels. The results of the original BoW model are also depicted for reference, and it again demonstrates the importance of spatial information. There are obvious gaps between SPM L1 and Graph L1, and between

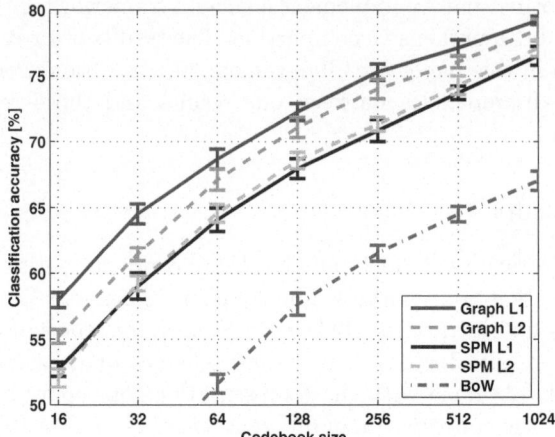

**Fig. 4.** Classification results obtained with representations on different levels separately on 15 Scenes. L1: $2 \times 2$. L2: $3 \times 1$.

**Table 2.** Classification results with LLC and different code sizes on VOC 2007

| Code size | BoW | SPM | Ours |
|:---------:|:----:|:----:|:----:|
| 16 | 16.0 | 24.0 | **27.0** |
| 128 | 24.5 | 35.4 | **38.2** |
| 1024 | 35.8 | 45.7 | **47.9** |
| 8192 | 48.4 | 55.5 | **56.3** |

SPM L2 and Graph L2. Some researchers would argue that the dimension of the representations in our scheme is higher. But note that higher-dimensional representations do not always lead to better results, as demonstrated in Section 4.3, and that Graph L2 is always better than Graph L1 though they both involve representations of the same dimension ($4n$). The results in Figure 4 can thus verify the effectiveness of our scheme on different levels.

To investigate the performance of our scheme with the representations on three levels all involved, we test our method on two datasets, i.e., 15 Scenes [3] and PASCAL VOC 2007 [4]. On the 15 Scenes dataset, our result is 83.3%, as listed in Table 1. The result in the original SPM paper [3] is 81.4%, and the one in [12] is 81.6%. The classification results on VOC 2007 are given in Table 2. The results of the original BoW model are also attached for reference. Table 2 demonstrates the great contribution of spatial modeling, since both SPM and our scheme outperform BoW greatly. In addition, our scheme consistently outperforms SPM with different code sizes on different datasets. Note that results in Table 2 are all obtained with the same $\lambda_n$ and $\lambda_e$. Therefore, it shows the insensitivity of the two parameters. We can draw a conclusion that our scheme cooperates fairly well with the representative of reconstruction-base schemes, i.e., LLC, considering

**Table 3.** Classification results with SVC and different code sizes on VOC 2007

| Code size: | $n = 16$ | | $n = 64$ | | $n = 256$ | |
|---|---|---|---|---|---|---|
| Category | SPM | Ours | SPM | Ours | SPM | Ours |
| aeroplane | 63.9 | **64.5** | 70.5 | **70.9** | 73.2 | **73.2** |
| bicycle | 52.4 | **53.7** | 58.2 | **60.3** | 62.4 | **63.3** |
| bird | 38.6 | **39.1** | 39.9 | **42.1** | 50.4 | **50.6** |
| boat | **64.7** | 64.4 | **69.3** | 68.4 | **70.8** | 70.2 |
| bottle | 19.9 | **20.1** | 21.4 | **22.8** | 24.7 | **26.0** |
| bus | 54.1 | **56.6** | 61.8 | **61.9** | **65.6** | 65.0 |
| car | 70.6 | **72.4** | 74.7 | **75.4** | 77.0 | **77.9** |
| cat | 48.4 | **49.5** | 55.9 | **57.9** | **59.9** | 59.8 |
| chair | 47.9 | **48.3** | 50.0 | **50.5** | **54.6** | 54.2 |
| cow | 35.0 | **36.6** | 41.5 | 41.5 | **44.4** | 44.2 |
| dinningtable | 47.9 | **50.4** | 50.3 | **51.8** | 53.2 | **53.2** |
| dog | **37.1** | 36.3 | 36.6 | **37.0** | 44.1 | **45.6** |
| horse | 72.6 | **73.7** | 74.5 | **76.2** | 76.9 | **78.1** |
| motorbike | 57.8 | **58.5** | 62.8 | **64.3** | 66.8 | **67.2** |
| person | 77.0 | **77.7** | 80.3 | **80.8** | 83.0 | **83.7** |
| pottedplant | 20.6 | **22.2** | 24.6 | **25.4** | 28.1 | **28.6** |
| sheep | **40.0** | 39.8 | 44.6 | **47.0** | 47.1 | **48.1** |
| sofa | 47.6 | **48.1** | 52.1 | **52.9** | 55.1 | **56.2** |
| train | 68.1 | **70.1** | 74.3 | **74.8** | 77.4 | **77.6** |
| tvmonitor | 39.9 | **43.2** | 48.7 | **50.4** | 53.4 | **55.1** |
| mean AP | 50.2 | **51.2** | 54.6 | **55.6** | 58.4 | **58.9** |

the reported results in Table 2. Notably, Wang et al. [16] reports higher results with LLC, i.e., 59.3%. However, this result is not reproducible even with their own released source code, and our results are more comparable with those reported by Chatfield et al. in their extensive survey paper on coding schemes [21]. To further investigate the performance of our scheme when cooperating with the representative of probabilistic coding schemes, i.e., SVC, we list the category-wise classification results on VOC 2007 in Table 3. The results again show that our scheme consistently performs better than SPM with different codes sizes.

### 4.5   Efficiency Analysis

The extra computational cost of our method is brought in by assigning features to nodes and edges of the spatial graph. The overall computational complexity for image representation is less than $\mathcal{O}(K \cdot M + N_{all} \cdot M)$, wherein $N_{all}$ denotes the total number of spatial regions. Usually, $N \ll K$. For example, in one of our experiments reported in Table 2, $K = 8192$, while $N_{all} = 13$. As a result, the additional cost of our method is ignorable.

## 4.6   Discussion

The original SPM scheme [3] grants different priority to different levels in order to balance their weights in the image-level representation. Harada et al. [11] even train the weights of different levels and blocks. Intuitively, such policy would boost the performance. However, we find empirically that re-weighting between levels gains limited improvements and brings in extra cost in practice. Using the same priority is a commonly-adopted policy in the recent literature, e.g., [21], a generally recognized survey on coding schemes.

Each node is a centroid of the local features extracted within a SPM block from the training image set, and each edge corresponds to a pair of neighboring blocks in SPM. The grid-like structure seems too rigid, and can be improved. We can make the nodes movable, the edges removable and the graph code-specific. Besides, supervised learning might generate discriminative spatial graphs and further boosts the performance.

A histogram on node reflects the occurrence of features in a block, and a histogram on edge reflects the occurrence of features which lie in one block and tend to shift into another. However, the histogram on a node is linearly correlated to those on its edges in our current implementation due to our assigning strategy. There might be a better strategy which preserves richer information. For example, the features definitely belonging to a block are assigned to the corresponding node, while the features tending to shift are assigned to histograms on edges.

## 5   Conclusion and Future Work

Among different strategies for spatial modeling, spatial pooling has been the most successful one. As a representative of spatial pooling schemes, SPM has become one standard part of an integrated BoW model due to its great simplicity and high performance. However, studies have shown that it is far from perfectly simulating human's behavior in perceiving spatial information. Two possible limitations of SPM include ignoring the relation of blocks. In this paper, we have proposed to capture the spatial information in images with a directed graph. Our scheme, which considers the relationship between spatial blocks, has shown its advantages in our experiments. In spite of the simplification in implementation, the proposed scheme has outperformed SPM with different kinds of coding schemes on several popular datasets.

After a period of achieving accomplishments in the feature space in terms of local feature detection, description and coding, it becomes more demanding for us to put more efforts in the work about the image space, i.e, capturing the spatial information contained in images. As one of the efforts towards this aim, the follow-up work of this paper is in two aspects: The first is to build up more flexible spatial graphs. The second is to find a better way to represent the relation of blocks so as to generate richer representation.

**Acknowledgement.** This work is supported by National Natural Science Foundation of China (61135003, 61203252), Tsinghua National Laboratory for Information Science and Technology Cross-discipline Foundation (Y2U1011MC1).

# References

1. Csurka, G., Dance, C.R., Fan, L., Willamowski, J., Bray, C.: Visual categorization with bags of keypoints. In: ECCV (2004)
2. Parikh, D.: Recognizing jumbled images: the role of local and global information in image classification. In: ICCV (2011)
3. Lazebnik, S., Schmid, C., Ponce, J.: Beyond bags of features: spatial pyramid matching for recognizing natural scene categories. In: CVPR (2006)
4. Everingham, M., Van Gool, L., Williams, C.K.I., Winn, J., Zisserman, A.: The PASCAL Visual Object Classes Challenge 2007 (VOC 2007) Results (2007)
5. Boureau, Y., Bach, F., LeCun, Y., Ponce, J.: Learning mid-level features for recognition. In: CVPR (2010)
6. Morioka, N., Satoh, S.: Building Compact Local Pairwise Codebook with Joint Feature Space Clustering. In: Daniilidis, K., Maragos, P., Paragios, N. (eds.) ECCV 2010, Part I. LNCS, vol. 6311, pp. 692–705. Springer, Heidelberg (2010)
7. Ling, H., Soatto, S.: Proximity distribution kernels for geometric context in category recognition. In: ICCV (2007)
8. Morioka, N., Satoh, S.: Compact correlation coding for visual object categorization. In: ICCV (2011)
9. Krapac, J., Verbeek, J., Jurie, F.: Modeling spatial layout with Fisher vectors for image categorization. In: ICCV (2011)
10. Zhou, X., Yu, K., Zhang, T., Huang, T.S.: Image Classification Using Super-Vector Coding of Local Image Descriptors. In: Daniilidis, K., Maragos, P., Paragios, N. (eds.) ECCV 2010, Part V. LNCS, vol. 6315, pp. 141–154. Springer, Heidelberg (2010)
11. Harada, T., Ushiku, Y., Yamashita, Y., Kuniyoshi, Y.: Discriminative spatial pyramid. In: CVPR (2011)
12. Wang, X., Bai, X., Liu, W., Latecki, L.J.: Feature context for image classification and object detection. In: CVPR (2011)
13. Yang, Y., Newsam, S.: Spatial pyramid co-occurrence for image classification. In: ICCV (2011)
14. van Gemert, J.C., Veenman, C.J., Smeulders, A.W.M., Geusebroek, J.M.: Visual word ambiguity. IEEE Transactions on Pattern Analysis and Machine Intelligence 32, 1271–1283 (2010)
15. Yang, J., Yu, K., Gong, Y., Huang, T.S.: Linear spatial pyramid matching using sparse coding for image classification. In: CVPR (2009)
16. Wang, J., Yang, J., Yu, K., Lv, F., Huang, T.S., Gong, Y.: Locality-constrained linear coding for image classification. In: CVPR (2010)
17. Huang, Y., Huang, K., Yu, Y., Tan, T.: Salient coding for image classification. In: CVPR (2011)
18. Wu, Z., Huang, Y., Wang, L., Tan, T.: Group encoding of local features in image classification. In: ICPR (2012)
19. Lowe, D.G.: Distinctive image features from scale-invariant keypoints. International Journal of Computer Vision 2(60), 91–110 (2004)
20. Fan, R., Chang, K., Hsieh, C., Wang, X., Lin, C.: Liblinear: a library for large linear classification. Journal of Machine Learning Research 9, 1871–1874 (2008)
21. Chatfield, K., Lempitsky, V., Vedaldi, A., Zisserman, A.: The devil is in the details: an evaluation of recent feature encoding methods. In: BMVC (2011)

# Knowledge Leverage from Contours to Bounding Boxes: A Concise Approach to Annotation

Jie-Zhi Cheng, Feng-Ju Chang, Kuang-Jui Hsu, and Yen-Yu Lin

Research Center for Information Technology Innovation, Academia Sinica, Taiwan
jzcheng@ntu.edu.tw, {fengju,kjhsu,yylin}@citi.sinica.edu.tw

**Abstract.** In the class based image segmentation problem, one of the major concerns is to provide large training data for learning complex graphical models. To alleviate the labeling effort, a concise annotation approach working on bounding boxes is introduced. The main idea is to leverage the knowledge learned from a few object contours for the inference of unknown contours in bounding boxes. To this end, we incorporate the bounding box prior into the concept of multiple image segmentations to generate a set of distinctive tight segments, with the condition that at least one tight segment approaching to the true object contour. A good tight segment is then selected via semi-supervised regression, which bears the augmented knowledge transferred from object contours to bounding boxes. The experimental results on the challenging Pascal VOC dataset corroborate that our new annotation method can potentially replace the manual annotations.

## 1 Introduction

Class based image segmentation [1–6] is the task of labeling pixels with several predefined object classes or background in an image. Distinct from the image driven segmentation task e.g., [7–11], class based image segmentation aims to not only identify the object classes of interest, but also determine the shapes or boundaries of these objects. Namely, it de facto involves in resolving two of the most fundamental problems in vision research: recognition and segmentation. Accordingly, it plays an essential role in many high-level computer vision applications, such as image and scene understanding.

Recently, significant progress for addressing the class based image segmentation has been made with the advances in many aspects, such as designing powerful visual features [1, 12], fusing information from various ways of image quantization [2, 4, 5], or exploring contextual relations between object classes [3, 6]. These approaches are implemented upon graphical models, especially *conditional random fields (CRFs)* [13], for the expressive power of modeling diverse cues and enforcing spatial consistency. However, learning graphical models in these approaches typically relies on a sufficient number of training data in the form of object *contours*. In general, the object contours are manually drawn or delineated by tools with intensive user interaction. Since learning complex graphical models typically requires large training data, the labeling cost of training data deems to be one of the major concerns for class based segmentation.

K.M. Lee et al. (Eds.): ACCV 2012, Part I, LNCS 7724, pp. 730–744, 2013.
© Springer-Verlag Berlin Heidelberg 2013

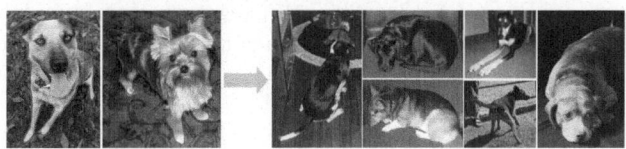

**Fig. 1.** Knowledge transfer from contours (*left*) to infer the unknown object contours enclosed by bounding boxes (*right*)

In this work, we introduce a concise annotation method to collect training data for class based image segmentation. Specifically, the annotation can be done with the drawing of bounding boxes. The bounding box annotation is pretty simple since we only have to click the four outer most boundary points of the object. Fig. 1 illustrates the problem setting of this study. Given a few contours as well as a set of bounding boxes of an object class, we would like to transfer the knowledge carried by the few contours to the bounding boxes. With the transferred knowledge, the object contour enclosed with the bounding box will be inferred as a training instance for the task of class based image segmentation. This work distinguishes itself with the following three main contributions.

First, we integrate the *bounding box prior* [14] into the concept of *multiple image segmentations* [2, 15, 16] as a new algorithm that automatically generates a set of *tight segments* [14] for each bounding box, and at least one of these tight segments would be close to the ground truth. An example of bounding box and its tight segments yielded by our approach are shown in Fig. 2. In this way, the task of figure-ground segmentation within this bounding box can be achieved by picking the best tight segment from the generated ones.

Second, we cast the tight segment selection for bounding boxes of an object class as a *semi-supervised regression* problem. Suppose that we are given a set of bounding boxes, and a few of them come with the object contours. In the regression problem, tight segments yielded from bounding boxes with ground truth serve as labeled training instances, while their target values for regression are set to reflect how well these segments approach the ground truth. As for tight segments without ground truth, we derive a difference upper bound of the target values of each segment pair in a bounding box. These bounds are formulated as additional constraints to regularize the learning process of the regressor. It alleviates the high risk of overfitting caused by the lack of labeled training instances. Once the regressor is obtained, the tight segment with the highest target value is selected for the bounding box.

The third contribution consists in the experiments conducted to demonstrate that our approach provides an effective alternate for manually labeled contours. We separately use the object contours obtained by manual drawings and the tight segments of bounding boxes picked by our approach as the training data for class based segmentation. Two state-of-the-art segmentation algorithms, i.e., [4, 5], are involved to compare the performances obtained by the two different sets of training data. The experimental results by each algorithm show that similar accuracy rates are achieved with either manual drawings or bounding box annotations on *PASCAL VOC* 2007 [17] segmentation task. It implies that the introduced annotation method can replace the tedious manual drawings.

## 2   Related Work

The literature of image segmentation is quite extensive, so our survey focuses on the key concepts relevant to the establishment of the proposed framework.

**Class Based Image Segmentation.** Approaches of this category, e.g., [1–6], aim to perform multi-class object recognition and segmentation simultaneously. Most of these segmentation approaches are established upon CRFs, since CRFs provide desirable abilities to concisely express the dependencies among random variables and observations, and enforce the consistency of labeling. For instance, Shotton et al. [1] propose a rich set of features to capture the texture, layout and contextual information of object classes in pixel level, and combine these features via solving an energy minimization problem over CRFs. Kohli et al. [3] and Gonfaus et al. [6] model the interaction between object classes by incorporating higher order potential functions into CRFs. Ladický et al. [4] integrate features extracted from different levels of image quantization by developing a hierarchical generalization of CRFs. Despite the effectiveness of these work, the annotation bottleneck for compiling sufficient training data remains unsolved.

**Figure-Ground Segmentation.** Some notable methods of this category, such as *graph-cut* [8], *GrabCut* [11], *constrained parametric min-cuts* [16], cast this task as an energy minimization problem over graph structures. A latter improvement of GrabCut is made by Lempitsky et al. [14] with the so-called *bounding box prior*. They show that the resulting foreground regions are sufficiently tight with respect to the given bounding boxes. Instead of working on individual images, the authors of [18–20] extend figure-ground segmentation for a set of images of an object class. This way, additional class-specific cues can be included to benefit figure-ground segmentation. Due to the inherent difficulty of unsupervised segmentation, the steps of segmenting objects and learning class models in [18–20] are carried out either alternately or sequentially. However, segmentation methods being aware of object classes may suffer from the problems caused by large intra-class variations or partial occlusions.

**Multiple Image Segmentations.** Classic image based segmentation methods, such as *normalized cuts* [7] or *mean-shift* [9], are developed with theoretic support. Nevertheless, the general conclusion [21] is still that the resulting segmentations typically are not good enough for discovering object contours. Since there is barely universal single-shot solution or parameter setting to segment out various objects with satisfactory results, the strategy of multiple image segmentations, e.g., [2, 15, 16, 22, 23], arises, in which many segmentations are computed with different segmentation algorithms, parameter settings, and/or seeds. In [15, 16], the authors assume that each object can be discovered by at least one segment. In [2], Pantofaru et al. propose to seek the most probable objects based on the intersections of multiple segments. Distinct from these approaches, we are motivated by the fact that the bounding box of an object can be acquired with low labeling cost (four clicks) but contains rich information for object inference. We couple the concepts of the bounding box prior and multiple image segmentations into a framework to estimate the object segments enclosed in the bounding boxes.

## 3  Inferring Multiple Tight Segments in a Bounding Box

In this section, we present an algorithm that automatically generates a set of *tight segments* for the bounding box of an object, and at least one of these tight segments would approach the object segment. Our goal in this step is to account for the information asymmetry between an object segment and its bounding box, since the latter can be determined once the former is given, but not vice versa. Specifically, we model the ambiguity in inferring the object segment from a bounding box by generating multiple segment hypotheses. If at least one of them is close to the object segment, the underlying task of inferring the object segment from a bounding box is reduced to a segment selection problem.

In the following, the approach by Lempitsky et al. [14] that yields one tight segment for a given bounding box is first reviewed. We then specify how to generalize their approach to obtain a few tight segments and make sure that at least one of them approaches the object contour.

### 3.1  Tight Segment via Bounding Box Prior

Let us consider a bounding box $\mathcal{I}$ of an object segment. We start by partitioning $\mathcal{I}$ into *superpixels* by mean-shift [9], which attains a fast and stable over-segmentation. In practice, the bandwidth parameters in mean-shift algorithm are adjusted by binary search, so that about 50 superpixels are obtained. Let $\mathcal{B}$ denote the set of the superpixels. A figure-ground segmentation or a segment can then be represented by a labeling vector $\ell = [l_p] \in \{0,1\}^{|\mathcal{B}|}$, where $l_p$ takes the value 1 if superpixel $p$ belongs to foreground, otherwise 0.

We are particularly interested in *tight segments* within bounding box $\mathcal{I}$. Here a segment is tight with respect to $\mathcal{I}$ if the smallest rectangle covering this segment is $\mathcal{I}$ itself. It is obvious that any non-tight segments won't be the object segment. In [14], Lempitsky et al. introduce the *crossing paths* of a bounding box, and prove that a segment is tight if and only if it intersects all the crossing paths. It turns out that a tight segment $\ell$ can be obtained by solving

$$\min_{\ell} \sum_{p \in \mathcal{B}} U_p \cdot l_p + \lambda \sum_{(p,q) \in \mathcal{E}} V_{p,q} \cdot |l_p - l_q| \tag{1}$$

$$\text{subject to} \quad \forall p \quad l_p \in \{0,1\}, \tag{2}$$

$$\forall C \in \Gamma \quad \sum_{p \in C} l_p \geq 1, \tag{3}$$

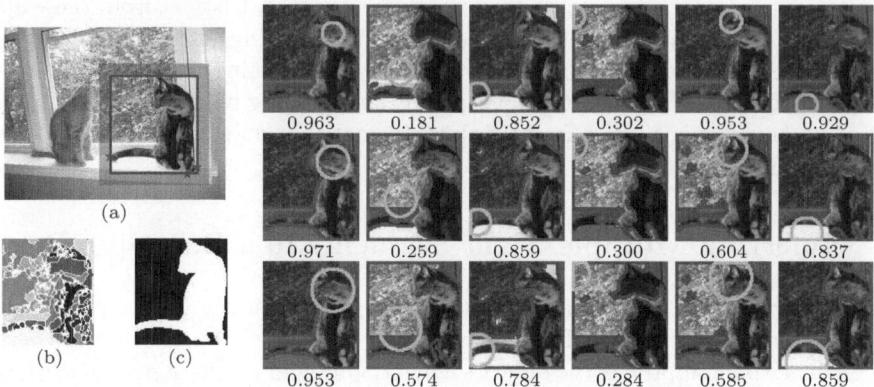

**Fig. 2.** (a) A bounding box defined by the four clicks (*purple stars*) for a kitty. Background seeds are placed in the blue highlighted region. (b) The superpixels of the bounding box. (c) The object segment (*ground truth*). (*Rest*) A few tight segments, marked by red contours, together with their accuracy by our approach. Each of them is generated with its respective seed region for foreground (cyan circle). These regions are sampled with different locations (*columns*) and radii (*rows*).

where $\mathcal{E}$ is the set of pairs of adjacent superpixels. The *unary potential* $U_p$ specifies the preference of assigning superpixel $p$ to either foreground or background. The *pairwise potential* $V_{p,q}$ ensures the smoothness between superpixel $p$ and $q$. The nonnegative coefficient $\lambda$ controls the importance tradeoff between the unary and pairwise terms. $\Gamma$ is the set of all the crossing paths of $\mathcal{I}$.

Note that the constraints (3) cause that the energy minimization problem (1) can no longer be solved by an efficient algorithm, like graph-cut [8]. Thus Lempitsky et al. instead solve a series of its linear relaxation, in which active constraints in (3) are added incrementally.

### 3.2   Multiple Tight Segments

The resulting segment by solving Eq.(1) is tightly enclosed by the given bounding box, and hence the aspect ratio of the object is maintained. Due to the unsupervised nature, a satisfactory figure-ground segmentation is not always guaranteed in our empirical test. When addressing bounding boxes of objects with multimodal color distributions and/or with clutter background, this shortcoming becomes even more evident. Alas, it is usually the case in nowadays benchmark databases of object segmentation, like MSRC-21 [1] or Pascal VOC [17].

We resolve this difficulty by implementing multi-segmentation relaxation. Namely, we generate a few tight segments with different *seeds* [16, 22], and relax the requirement to that at least one of them closely approaches the unknown object segment. It can be observed that apart from the property of tightness, the bounding box of an object also gives two additional hints for discovering the object segment: (1) Its outside borders provide strong cues for identifying the background in the bounding box; (2) It exists a few ROIs that are fully filled by the foreground. If we can retrieve one of them, it helps much in revealing the object segment. Specifically, we maintain the aspect ratio and expand the bounding box by 10%. The *background seeds* are the pixels outside the bounding box and inside the expanded one, i.e., those in the blue highlighted region in Fig. 2(a). We sample multiple sets of *foreground seeds* to account for the uncertainty on the locations and scales of those ROIs fully filled by the object. One circular seed region for foreground is constructed for the centroid of each superpixel and with each of predefined radii. The cyan circles in Fig. 2 show some of the seed regions for foreground.

We leverage the flexibility in developing potential functions $\{U_p\}$ and $\{V_{p,q}\}$ in Eq.(1), and derive one tight segment for each set of foreground seeds. A Gaussian mixture model $GMM_f$ with five components is learned with the foreground seeds in RGB color space. Similarly $GMM_b$ is acquired with the background seeds. For each superpixel $p$, the unary potential $U_p$ is defined as

$$U_p = \sum_{u \in p} \log P(c_u | GMM_b) - \log P(c_u | GMM_f), \qquad (4)$$

where $u$ is an image pixel and $c_u$ is its RGB color vector. On the other hand, the pairwise potential $V_{p,q}$ between superpixels $p$ and $q$ is given by

$$V_{p,q} = \sum_{u \in p, v \in q, (u,v) \in \mathcal{N}} \frac{1}{dist(u,v)} \cdot \exp\left(-\beta ||c_u - c_v||^2\right), \qquad (5)$$

where $\mathcal{N}$ is set of neighboring pixels. We use 8-connected neighbors, and $dist(u,v)$ is the Euclidean distance between pixels $u$ and $v$. $\beta$ is a positive constant. One tight segment is inferred by optimizing Eq.(1) with these redefined potentials in Eq.(4) and Eq.(5). The procedure is repeated for each combination of foreground seed regions and parameter settings ($\lambda$ in Eq.(1) and $\beta$ in Eq.(5)). Multiple tight segments of the bounding box are then produced.

An example is shown in Fig. 2. The left three figures give the bounding box, its representation in superpixels, and the ground truth (GT) respectively. The others are 18 of the yielded tight segments for the bounding box. We evaluate the goodness of a segment, say $\ell$, by $1 - \frac{XOR(R(\ell),GT)}{\#pixel}$, where $XOR$ is the function of *exclusive or*, and $R(\ell)$ is a binary vector that indicates each pixel in $\ell$ assigned to either foreground or background. Hereafter we will use the pixelwise XOR function to measure the goodness of a segment w.r.t. the ground truth, or the overlapping between two segments. From Fig. 2, it can be observed that seed regions for foreground located within the object and with proper radii often lead to satisfactory tight segments. Since the object must appears in some location of the bounding box with one particular scale, the seeding strategy with high chance will discover at least one tight segment close to the ground truth.

*Redundance Removal.* Each generated tight segment is parameterized by the location and scale of the seed region for foreground, and the values of $\lambda$ and $\beta$.

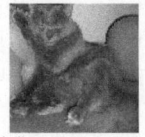
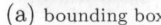
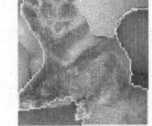
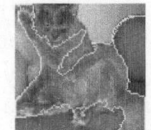
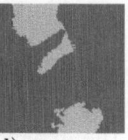

(a) bounding box    (b) tight segment A    (c) tight segment B    (d) XOR(A,B).

**Fig. 3.** For each pair of tight segments in a bounding box, an upper bound on the difference of their target values can be determined. See text for the details.

In our implementation, the number of the tight segments generated for a bounding box is in the order of $10^3$. Since many of them are redundant, we develop a $(1 - \epsilon)$-approximation procedure to compile the tight segmentations into a smaller set of representative ones. In initialization, all the tight segments are sorted in a queue according to their scores measured by *ratio cut* [24]. We *pop* the first tight segment, add it into the representative set, and remove all the tight segments of more than $1 - \epsilon$ overlapping with it from the queue. The process is done repeatedly until the queue is empty. It is obvious that the best tight segment remained in the representative set shares at least $1 - \epsilon$ overlapping with the original best one. We empirically set $\epsilon$ as 0.05 in all the experiments.

## 4   Semi-supervised Regression for Segment Selection

Given a few contours as well as a set of bounding boxes of an object class, we illustrate how to infer the object segments of these bounding boxes by solving a semi-supervised regression problem in this section.

### 4.1   Our Formulation

Consider a bounding box set $D$, which is collected from object segments of a class. A few bounding boxes in $D$ come with the object contours (ground truth), i.e., $D = L \cup U$, where $L = \{B_i, GT_i\}_{i=1}^{\ell}$, $U = \{B_i\}_{i=\ell+1}^{\ell+u}$, and $\ell << u$. We generate multiple tight segments for each bounding box $B_i$ by the procedure described above. That is, $B_i = \{\mathbf{x}_{ij}\}_{j=1}^{N_i}$, where $N_i$ is number of the yielded tight segments, and $\mathbf{x}_{ij}$ is the feature vector of the $j$th tight segment. Our goal is to infer the object segments of these bounding boxes. Since at least one tight segment with high probability is close to the object contour, this goal can be accomplished by picking the tight segment as close to object contour possible. We cast this task as a semi-supervised regression problem.

We start by creating the *labeled* training instances for the regression problem. Inspired by work [16, 22, 23] of ranking multiple segmentations or proposals, we treat each tight segment in a bounding box with the ground truth as one labeled instance, whose *target value* is set via computing the pixelwise XOR function w.r.t. the ground truth as mentioned before. A set of labeled training instances is then produced, i.e., $\{(\mathbf{x}_{ij}, y_{ij})\}_{(i,j) \in S_L}$, where $S_L = \{(i,j) | 1 \leq i \leq \ell, 1 \leq j \leq N_i\}$. Unlike [16, 22, 23] where sufficient training instances are available from other sources, we have too few labeled bounding boxes to stably derive the regressor. The unfavorable effect of *overfitting* hence may occur.

We resolve this problem by introducing the *unlabeled* tight segments. For each pair of tight segments in a bounding box, an upper bound on the difference of their target values can be derived without the ground truth. Let's illustrate it via Fig. 3. Given a pair of tight segments $A$ and $B$, the bounding box can be divided into two regions according to their labeling consistence, i.e., the magenta (consistent) and cyan (inconsistent) regions in Fig. 3(d). Suppose that the inconsistent part takes $\theta \times 100\%$ area of the bounding box. It can be verified that the difference between the target values of $A$ and $B$ is at most $\theta$, since the target value is defined as the percentage of *correct* pixels, and only the inconsistent region contributes to the difference of their target values. Thus a set of these bounds is yielded, i.e., $\{(\mathbf{x}_{ij}, \mathbf{x}_{ij'}, \theta_{ijj'})\}_{(i,j,j')\in S_U}$, where $S_U = \{(i,j,j')|\ell + 1 \leq i \leq \ell + u, 1 \leq j < j' \leq N_i\}$, and $\theta_{ijj'}$ is the bound between segments $\mathbf{x}_{ij}$ and $\mathbf{x}_{ij'}$ of bounding box $B_i$.

Integrating the labeled and unlabeled tight segments, the semi-supervised regression problem is formulated as the following constrained optimization problem

$$\min_{\mathbf{w},b,\{\xi_{ij}\},\{\rho_{ijj'}\}} \frac{1}{2}||\mathbf{w}||^2 + C_\ell \sum_{(i,j)\in S_L} \xi_{ij} + C_u \sum_{(i,j,j')\in S_U} \rho_{ijj'} \tag{6}$$

$$\text{subject to } \mathbf{w}^\top \mathbf{x}_{ij} + b - y_{ij} \leq \varepsilon + \xi_{ij}, \text{ for } (i,j) \in S_L, \tag{7}$$

$$y_{ij} - \mathbf{w}^\top \mathbf{x}_{ij} - b \leq \varepsilon + \xi_{ij}, \text{ for } (i,j) \in S_L, \tag{8}$$

$$\mathbf{w}^\top \mathbf{x}_{ij} - \mathbf{w}^\top \mathbf{x}_{ij'} \leq \theta_{ijj'} + \rho_{ijj'}, \text{ for } (i,j,j') \in S_U, \tag{9}$$

$$\mathbf{w}^\top \mathbf{x}_{ij'} - \mathbf{w}^\top \mathbf{x}_{ij} \leq \theta_{ijj'} + \rho_{ijj'}, \text{ for } (i,j,j') \in S_U, \tag{10}$$

where $\mathbf{w}$ and $b$ are parameters of the learned regressor, $f(\mathbf{x}) = \mathbf{w}^\top \mathbf{x} + b$. $\{\xi_{ij}\}$ and $\{\rho_{ijj'}\}$ are two sets of slack variables that are nonnegative, and are used to measure the degrees of violation in the corresponding constraints. $C_\ell$, $C_u$, and $\varepsilon$ are nonnegative constants whose values are determined via cross validation.

We now justify for the above optimization problem. The first two terms in Eq.(6) together with constraints in Eq.(7) and Eq.(8) jointly lead to the formulation of *support vector regression* [25]. The constraints in Eq.(9) and Eq.(10) result from pairs of unlabeled tight segments. In other words, the regressor is derived by not only fitting the labeled segments but also preserving the implicit structure of the unlabeled segments. Despite the complexity of Eq.(6), it is a *quadratic programming* (QP) problem, and there exist efficient solvers, e.g., *MOSEK* [26], for optimization.

The optimization problem still cannot be handled by a QP solver due to the large number of constraints in Eq.(9) and Eq.(10). However, this is not as hard a problem as it may seem at the first glance, since the *active* constraints in Eq.(9) and Eq.(10) are quite sparse. It implies that we can tackle this issue via the *cutting-plane method* [27] where a *working constraint set* is maintained by adding the most violated constraints incrementally. In our case, we start with a empty working set. At each iteration, we add the most violated constraint to the working set for each bounding box, if any. Iterations are repeated until no constraints can be added or a maximum number of iterations is reached.

Once the regressor, $f(\mathbf{x}) = \mathbf{w}^\top \mathbf{x} + b$, is obtained, we infer the object segment for each bounding box $B_i$ as the $j^*$th tight segment with $j^* = \arg\max_j f(\mathbf{x}_{ij})$.

### 4.2 The Adopted Features for Segment Description

We implement a set of *mid-level* features, suggested in [16, 23], for characterizing each tight segment, including 1) *Percentage of boundary pixels*: The ratio of the number of boundary pixels to the number of foreground pixels; 2) *Boundary edge strength*: The edge strengths along the object contour; 3) *Centroid*: The normalized coordinates of the mass center of the segment; 4) *Major and minor axis length*: The lengths of the major and minor axes of the ellipse that approximates the segment; 5) *Convexity and area*: The ratios of the number of foreground pixels to the area of the convex hull and to the whole bounding box; 6) *Foreground and background dissimilarity*: The dissimilarity is respectively measured by three visual features, i.e., color, *SIFT* [28], and *Texton* [1]. A pair of histograms, one for foreground and one for background, over the quantized clusters is yielded for each feature. The $\chi^2$ distance is employed for dissimilarity measure.

## 5    Experimental Results

To evaluate the performances of the proposed approach, three experiments are carried out on Pascal VOC 2007, a benchmark dataset for object segmentation. We investigate the validness of the assumption that there exists at least a good one in the pool of multiple tight segments in the first experiment. The efficacy of the semi-supervised regression model for segment selection is assessed in the second experiment. We demonstrate the effectiveness of using the bounding box annotations as training data for the class based image segmentation algorithms in the last experiment.

### 5.1    Dataset: Pascal VOC 2007

The Pascal VOC 2007 Segmentation Challenge contains 21 categories, including 20 object classes with the plus of background. Each object category contains about 30 to 100 annotated objects, except the class of person, which has more than 300 ones. Due to the large intra-class variations in this dataset, the annotation cost of segmentation is conceivably substantial. It hence serves as good test beds for corroborating our purpose of concise annotations, and for justifying the effectiveness of the proposed approach. In our work, the training and validation data in this dataset are used in the experiments I and II, and the selected tight segments by the semi-supervised regression models are treated as training data in the experiment III.

### 5.2    Experiment I: Multiple Tight Segments

The effectiveness of multiple segmentation strategy lives with the underlying assumption that there is at least one tight segment close to the object segment.

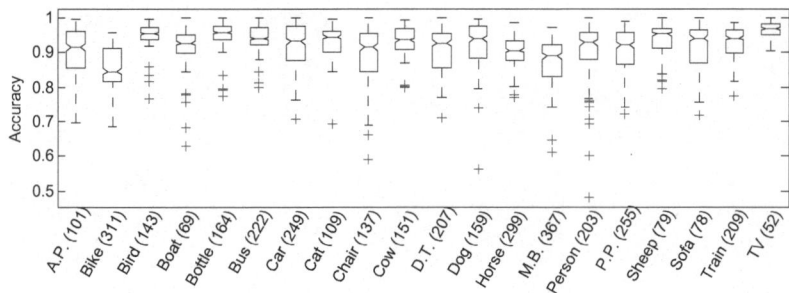

**Fig. 4.** Boxplot of the best accuracy rates of the best tight segments w.r.t. each of the 20 object classes. The edges of each box are the 25th and 75th percentiles. Outliers are marked as red-cross signs. The numbers of the generated tight segments are given.

To inspect if this assumption is held in our method, we crop the bounding box of each annotated object segment in the training and validation sets, and generate a set of tight segments for the bounding box. The resulting tight segments are compared to the annotated ground truths. Specifically, the input tight segments for the semi-supervised regression models of each class are first evaluated with the accuracy metrics. The tight segment with the highest accuracy of a bounding box is then regarded as the performance upper bound of the semi-supervised regression model. Figure. 4 depicts the MATLAB' boxplot of the best accuracy distributions of bounding boxes w.r.t. each of the 20 object classes. Meanwhile, the average numbers of the yielded tight segments are also reported in Fig. 4, with the variation from 52 to 367. The number of the yielded tight segments for each bounding box typically depends on the complexity of object appearance and the foreground/background discernibility. In general, it can be found that most bounding boxes hold *good* tight segments with accuracy rates higher than 0.9, except for those of class bike. However, the lowest Q1, i.e., the 25th percentile, of class bike is still higher than 0.8. This may set up a good foundation for the semi-supervised regression models to pick satisfying tight segment for the objects within the bounding boxes.

Figure. 5 lists several cases of the generated tight segments for visual assessment. The first three rows show the examples where the accuracy rates of the best tight segments are higher than 0.9. The last three rows give the cases where the proposed approach doesn't perform well, including objects constituted with fine details in the example of bike, objects sharing similarly color components with background in the latter example of dog, and objects co-presented with other objects in the example of motor bike.

## 5.3   Experiment II: Segment Selection for Object Contour Estimation

The experiment II is designed to assess the quality of the selected tight segments by the regressors derived via the proposed supervised (without constraints (9)

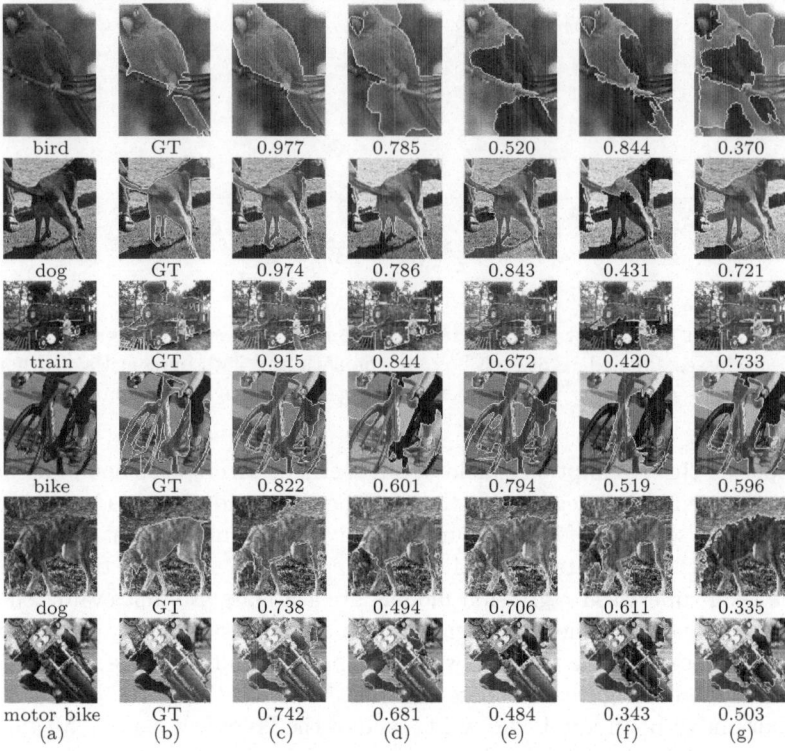

**Fig. 5.** Examples of the yielded multiple tight segments. (a) Bounding box. (b) Ground truth. (c) The best tight segment and its accuracy. (d) $\sim$ (g) Other tight segments.

and (10)) and semi-supervised regression models. Similar to the experiment I, the quality of the selected tight segment is evaluated with the accuracy metrics. To give comparative study, alternative segmentations from *GrabCut* [11] algorithm are involved in this experiment. The foreground model in GrabCut is initialized with the center 50% area of the bounding box, while the background model is fitted from the same background sample region of our method.

Both the supervised and semi-supervised models learn a regressor for each of the 20 object categories in Pascal VOC 2007. For each category, randomly selected 10% of bounding boxes come with the ground truths (object contours), while the rest are treated as unlabeled. In learning the regressors, all parameters ($C_\ell$ and $C_u$ in(6), $\varepsilon$ in (7)) are automatically determined via cross validation. The accuracy distributions of the tight segments selected by the semi-supervised regressor for each class are depicted with function `boxplot` in Fig. 6. Meanwhile, the average accuracy rates of each class w.r.t. the best tight segments in experiment I, the segments picked by supervised regressor, and the comparative segmentations from GrabCut are also plotted as the cyan triangles, magenta * signs, and green squares, respectively.

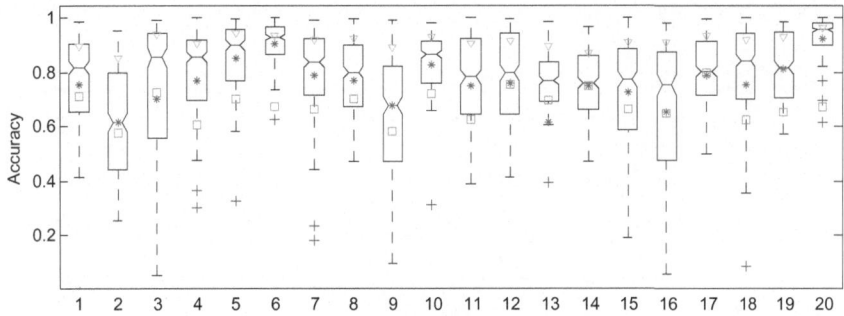

**Fig. 6.** The accuracy rates of the semi-supervised regressor (*plotted with* `boxplot`) are compared with those of the best tight segments (*cyan triangles*), of GrabCut (*green squares*), and of the supervised regressor (*magenta ∗ signs*)

It can be found in Fig. 6 that in most classes the tight segments selected by the semi-supervised regressor hold higher accuracy rates than the segments yielded by GrabCut or picked by the supervised regressor. It reveals that the additional constraints induced by unlabeled tight segments facilitate the training process, and lead to a regressor with low generalization error. The worst performance of our approach arrives at the 2nd class, i.e., `bike`. In this class, regressors learned by either supervised or semi-supervised models obtain similar accuracy rates around 0.6. The determined value of $C_u$ approaches zero in this class. It implies that satisfying the additional constraints is not helpful for reducing the validation error. We infer that it may result from the large intra-class variations.

To give visual assessment, Fig. 7 lists the tight segments selected from the supervised and semi-supervised regressors with the comparison to the ground truths, best tight segments, and the segmentation results by GrabCut.

### 5.4   Experiment III: Class Based Image Segmentation

The experiment III aims to verify the effectiveness of the concise annotations for the class based image segmentation methods. To this end, the tight segments selected by the supervised and semi-supervised regression models, GrabCut segments, and ground truths in the experiment II are treated as training annotations for two state-of-the-art class based segmentation methods [4, 5]. The yielded segments from the two variational regression models and GrabCut are pasted back to the original training and validation images for reasonable comparison to the ground truths. The two segmentation methods [4, 5] learnt from the distinctive four sets of annotations are further evaluated with the testing data of the PASCAL VOC 2007 Segmentation dataset.

Table 1 summarizes the averaged performances of the methods [4] and [5] w.r.t. the four sets of training data. In Table 1, the performances of the method [4] are first given, while the performances of the method [5] under the three settings, i.e., "CRF+N=0", "CRF+N=2", and "CRF+N=4", are then reported

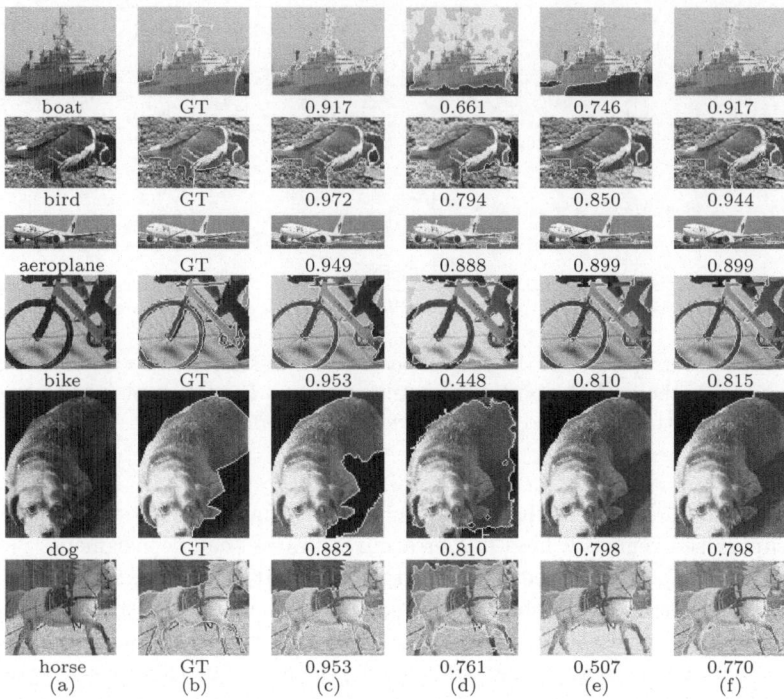

| | | | | | |
|---|---|---|---|---|---|
| boat | GT | 0.917 | 0.661 | 0.746 | 0.917 |
| bird | GT | 0.972 | 0.794 | 0.850 | 0.944 |
| aeroplane | GT | 0.949 | 0.888 | 0.899 | 0.899 |
| bike | GT | 0.953 | 0.448 | 0.810 | 0.815 |
| dog | GT | 0.882 | 0.810 | 0.798 | 0.798 |
| horse | GT | 0.953 | 0.761 | 0.507 | 0.770 |
| (a) | (b) | (c) | (d) | (e) | (f) |

**Fig. 7.** Inferred object segments by various approaches. (a) Bounding box. (b) Ground truth. (c) The best tight segment. (d) Segment yielded by GrabCut. (e) Segment selected via supervised regression. (f) Segment selected via semi-supervised regression.

**Table 1.** Quantitative results of methods [4, 5] on Pascal VOC Segmentation task w.r.t. annotations of the ground truth, GrabCut, supervised and semi-supervised regression models

| | Ground Truth | GrabCut | Supervised Reg. | Semi-Sup. Reg. |
|---|---|---|---|---|
| Hierarchical CRF [4] | **11.23** | 9.96 | 11.06 | 10.64 |
| CRF+$N = 0$ [5] | **14.10** | 12.47 | 13.29 | 13.33 |
| CRF+$N = 2$ [5] | 25.26 | 24.56 | **26.51** | **26.51** |
| CRF+$N = 4$ [5] | 23.92 | 21.31 | 24.81 | **24.85** |

respectively. Variable $N$ here indicates the neighborhood size in [5]. Referring to Table 1, the class based segmentations learnt from the two variations of our annotations achieve similar performances to the results of ground truth annotations. This promises our goal of using bounding boxes as concise annotations. The reason why the method [5] outperform to the method [4] may lie in that the hierarchical conditional random field model may highly rely on large training data to learn a powerful segmentation model.

Furthermore, it can be observed in the third and fourth rows of Table 1 that the accuracy rates with our annotations are slightly higher than the rates with ground truths. It may be because that the method [5] tends to overfit the difficult/noisy training data like the second dog case in Fig. 2, provided with precise annotations of manual drawings. Vague annotations resulted from our method may instead lower down the importance of this kinds of difficult training data, and lead to a surprisingly better performance.

## 6 Conclusions

A new concise annotation method for the task of class based image segmentation is introduced in this study. Guided by the bounding box prior, the proposed method first renders distinctive tight segments, and a good tight segment is further inferred by the supervised and semi-supervised regression models. The inferred tight segment from the given bounding box serves as a hidden object contour to train a complex graphical model for the class based image segmentation task. The results of three extensive experiments support the efficacy of our method. In the future, we will extend our inference model to account for the interaction between different classes, as the co-presentation of objects with different classes is the major limitation of our method. Moreover, performance evaluation on other challenging datasets is planned in our future work.

**Acknowledgement**. This study is conducted under the "III Innovative and Prospective Technologies Project" of the Institute for Information Industry which is subsidized by the Ministry of Economy Affairs of the Republic of China. It is also supported in part by grant NSC 101-2221-E-001-018.

## References

1. Shotton, J., Winn, J., Rother, C., Criminisi, A.: Textonboost for image understanding: Multi-class object recognition and segmentation by jointly modeling appearance, shape and context. IJCV (2009)
2. Pantofaru, C., Schmid, C., Hebert, M.: Object Recognition by Integrating Multiple Image Segmentations. In: Forsyth, D., Torr, P., Zisserman, A. (eds.) ECCV 2008, Part III. LNCS, vol. 5304, pp. 481–494. Springer, Heidelberg (2008)
3. Kohli, P., Ladický, L., Torr, P.: Robust higher order potentials for enforcing label consistency. IJCV (2009)
4. Ladický, L., Russell, C., Kohli, P., Torr, P.: Associative hierarchical CRFs for object class image segmentation. In: ICCV (2009)
5. Fulkerson, B., Vedaldi, A., Soatto, S.: Class segmentation and object localization with superpixel neighborhoods. In: ICCV (2009)
6. Gonfaus, J., Boix, X., van de Weijer, J., Bagdanov, A., Serrat, J., González, J.: Harmony potentials for joint classification and segmentation. In: CVPR (2010)
7. Shi, J., Malik, J.: Normalized cuts and image segmentation. TPAMI (2000)
8. Boykov, Y., Veksler, O., Zabih, R.: Fast approximate energy minimization via graph cuts. TPAMI (2001)
9. Comaniciu, D., Meer, P.: Mean shift: A robust approach toward feature space analysis. TPAMI (2002)
10. Felzenszwalb, P., Huttenlocher, D.: Efficient graph-based image segmentation. IJCV (2004)

11. Rother, C., Kolmogorov, V., Blake, A.: "GrabCut": Interactive foreground extraction using iterated graph cuts. In: SIGGRAPH (2004)
12. Shotton, J., Johnson, M., Cipolla, R.: Semantic texton forests for image categorization and segmentation. In: CVPR (2008)
13. Lafferty, J., McCallum, A., Pereira, F.: Conditional random fields: Probabilistic models for segmenting and labeling sequence data. In: ICML (2001)
14. Lempitsky, V., Kohli, P., Rother, C., Sharp, T.: Image segmentation with a bounding box prior. In: ICCV (2009)
15. Galleguillos, C., Babenko, B., Rabinovich, A., Belongie, S.: Weakly Supervised Object Localization with Stable Segmentations. In: Forsyth, D., Torr, P., Zisserman, A. (eds.) ECCV 2008, Part I. LNCS, vol. 5302, pp. 193–207. Springer, Heidelberg (2008)
16. Carreira, J., Sminchisescu, C.: Constrained parametric min-cuts for automatic object segmentation. In: CVPR (2010)
17. Everingham, M., Van Gool, L., Williams, C.K.I., Winn, J., Zisserman, A. (The PASCAL Visual Object Classes Challenge 2007 (VOC 2007) Results) (2007)
18. Winn, J., Jojic, N.: LOCUS: Learning object classes with unsupervised segmentation. In: ICCV (2005)
19. Cour, T., Shi, J.: Recognizing objects by piecing together the segmentation puzzle. In: CVPR (2007)
20. Alexe, B., Deselaers, T., Ferrari, V.: ClassCut for Unsupervised Class Segmentation. In: Daniilidis, K., Maragos, P., Paragios, N. (eds.) ECCV 2010, Part V. LNCS, vol. 6315, pp. 380–393. Springer, Heidelberg (2010)
21. Unnikrishnan, R., Pantofaru, C., Hebert, M.: Toward objective evaluation of image segmentation algorithms. TPAMI (2007)
22. Endres, I., Hoiem, D.: Category Independent Object Proposals. In: Daniilidis, K., Maragos, P., Paragios, N. (eds.) ECCV 2010, Part V. LNCS, vol. 6315, pp. 575–588. Springer, Heidelberg (2010)
23. Vicente, S., Rother, C., Kolmogorov, V.: Object cosegmentation. In: CVPR (2011)
24. Wang, S., Siskind, J.: Image segmentation with ratio cut. TPAMI (2003)
25. Vapnik, V.: Statistical Learning Theory. Wiley (1998)
26. The MOSEK Optimization Software, http://www.mosek.com/index.html
27. Joachims, T., Finley, T., Yu, C.N.: Cutting-plane training of structural SVMs. ML (2009)
28. Lowe, D.: Distinctive image features from scale-invariant keypoints. IJCV (2004)

# Efficient Pixel-Grouping Based on Dempster's Theory of Evidence for Image Segmentation

Björn Scheuermann[1], Markus Schlosser[2], and Bodo Rosenhahn[1]

[1] Leibniz Universität Hannover, Germany
{scheuermann,rosenhahn}@tnt.uni-hannover.de
[2] Technicolor Research & Innovation Hannover, Germany
markus.schlosser@technicolor.com

**Abstract.** In this paper we propose an algorithm for image segmentation using graph cuts which can be used to efficiently solve labeling problems on high resolution images or image sequences. The basic idea of our method is to group large homogeneous regions to one single variable. Therefore we combine the appearance and the task specific similarity with Dempster's theory of evidence to compute the basic belief that two pixels/groups will have the same label in the minimum energy state. Experiments on image and video segmentation show that our grouping leads to a significant speedup and memory reduction of the labeling problem. Thus large-scale labeling problems can be solved in an efficient manner with a low approximation loss.

## 1 Introduction

In the field of computer vision, discrete optimization using maximum flow algorithms has become very popular [1]. This has been driven by the fact that many problems such as image segmentation, stereo matching or shape matching are formulated using probabilistic models like Markov or conditional random fields (MRF or CRF respectively). The computation of the maximum a posteriori (MAP) solution for these models can be regarded as the discrete minimization of an energy function [2–4]. Many algorithms in literature are able to efficiently compute an approximate solution of the given optimization problem. Under some assumptions, e.g. such that the energy function is submodular, these methods are able to compute the exact minimum of the given energy function. We introduce an enhanced algorithm for grouping variables of the optimization problem which improves the general performance of maximum flow algorithms.

In parallel to the improvement of discrete energy minimization algorithms [3, 5, 6], the size of single images and image sequences increased significant. Compared to standard benchmark images, which have an approximate size of 120.000 pixels, nowadays commercial cameras capture images with many more pixels, e.g. up to 20 million. Since most energy functions for image segmentation or stereo matching contain one discrete variable per pixel, the minimization using maximum flow algorithms can be computationally extremely expensive. It has been shown that the given algorithms are not applicable if the data of

K.M. Lee et al. (Eds.): ACCV 2012, Part I, LNCS 7724, pp. 745–759, 2013.
© Springer-Verlag Berlin Heidelberg 2013

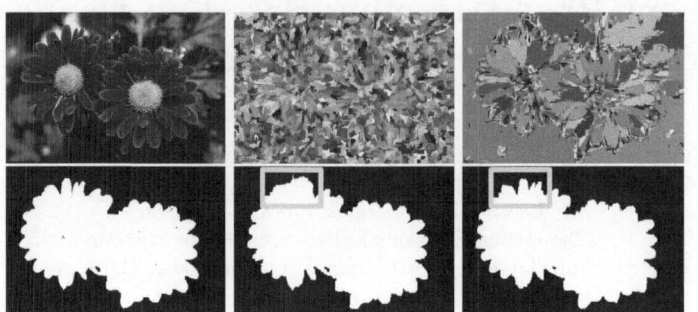

**Fig. 1.** Variable grouping for image segmentation. First row: original image; variable grouping of [9] with a budget of 1%; proposed variable grouping (COMPACTEDGE) with a budget of 1%; Second row: corresponding segmentation results. Using the same budget the proposed grouping is semantically more meaningful and leads to a smaller segmentation error.

the problem does not fit into the physical memory [7, 8]. This observation has inspired researchers to develop more efficient energy minimization methods [5, 10, 11].

**Related Work:** Research on solving discrete optimization problems using maximum flow / minimum cut algorithms for applications in computer vision can be divided into the following approaches:

**Augmenting Paths:** For computer vision problems, the most widely used algorithm is the Boykov and Kolmogorov augmenting paths algorithm [1, 12] (BK-algorithm). This algorithm efficiently solves moderately sized 2D and 3D problems with low connectivity.

**Push-Relabel:** Most parallelized maximum flow / minimum cut algorithms are based on the push-relabel scheme [8]. For huge and highly connected grid graphs these methods outperform the traditional BK-algorithm [1]. In contrast to these methods, the proposed algorithm does not use special hardware to approximate the optimal solution.

**Grouping of Variables / Graph Sparsification:** Besides the approaches to develop more efficient algorithms for the maximum flow / minimum cut problem, researchers are also trying to reduce the size of the labeling problem or the graph itself. One simple and widely used technique merges variables in the energy function into a smaller number of groups e.g. superpixels. Besides a number of well known image partitioning methods [13–16], Kim et al. presented a similar method [9] where the terms of the energy function and the algorithm proposed by Felzenszwalb and Huttenlocher [13] are used to decide if two variables should be merged. In [17] Scheuermann and Rosenhahn presented an algorithm for graph sparsification that does not change the optimal solution. The idea is to create a so called Slim Graph by merging nodes in the graph that do not change the maximum flow, meaning that these variables are guaranteed to have the same label in the minimum energy state. Lermé et al. proposed a similar approach for graph sparsification by maintaining the maximum flow [18].

**Multi-scale:** Our work is also related to multi-scale methods for image labeling. The idea is to first solve the problem at low resolution using standard techniques [19–21]. This can be interpreted as a grouping of pixels into regular non-overlapping groups. The result of the low-resolution labeling is refined at the high-resolution in a following optimization step, where most variables of the problem are fixed.

**Contribution:** We propose an algorithm that merges variables of the energy function to small sets of non overlapping groups, so that each group can be represented by one single variable. The merging follows the idea of [13] and [9] where the grouping is based on appearance or the terms of the energy function respectively. In contrast to [9], we combine the task-specific similarity and the appearance using Dempster's theory of evidence to compute the basic belief that two neighboring variables should be merged. Furthermore we do not directly penalize the size of a group by proposing new merging constraints (MAXEDGE and COMPACTEDGE), that follow our idea to allow large groups of variables in homogeneous regions. Instead of an accurate MAP our goal is to reduce to segmentation error. Therefore we use Dempster's theory of evidence that is complementary to the terms of the energy function. We evaluate our method on standard benchmark images to show that our grouping achieves a better performance than the methods of [13] and [9]. Furthermore we quantify our algorithm on video sequences and high-resolution images to show that the segmentation, performed on top of our grouping, results in a similar segmentation with a dramatic reduction in computational costs and memory requirements.

**Paper Organization:** In Section 2 we continue with a review of discrete energy minimization, which is the basis for our segmentation framework, and recall the idea of Dempster's theory of evidence. Section 3 introduces and explains the proposed grouping of variables. The details of our experiments and the analysis of the results are provided in Section 4. The paper finishes with a short conclusion.

## 2   Segmentation by Discrete Energy Minimization

The discrete energy $E : \mathcal{L}^n \to \mathbb{R}$ for the problem of binary image labeling addressed in this work can be written as the sum of unary $\varphi_i$ and pairwise functions $\varphi_{i,j}$

$$E(x) = \sum_{i \in \mathcal{V}} \varphi_i(x_i) + \sum_{(i,j) \in \mathcal{E}} \varphi_{i,j}(x_i, x_j), \tag{1}$$

where $x$ is the labeling, $\mathcal{V}$ corresponds to the set of all image pixels and $\mathcal{E}$ is the set of all edges between pixels in a defined neighborhood $\mathcal{N}$. For the problem of binary image segmentation, the label set $\mathcal{L}$ consists of a foreground $(fg)$ and a background ($bg$) labels. The unary function $\varphi_i$ is given as the negative log likelihood using a standard GMM model [6], defined as

$$\varphi_i(x_i) = -\log Pr(I_i \mid x_i = S), \tag{2}$$

where $S$ is either $fg$ or $bg$. The pairwise function $\varphi_{i,j}$ takes the form of a contrast sensitive Ising model, defined as

$$\varphi_{i,j}(x_i, x_j) = \gamma \cdot \text{dist}(i,j)^{-1} \cdot [x_i \neq x_j] \cdot \exp(-\beta\|I_i - I_j\|^2). \tag{3}$$

Here $I_i$ and $I_j$ describe the feature vectors of pixels $i$ and $j$, e.g. RGB-colors. The parameter $\gamma$ specifies the impact of the pairwise function. It has been shown that, using the defined unary and pairwise functions, the energy (1) is submodular and can hence be represented by a graph [12]. In this form, the global minimum of the energy can be computed with standard maximum flow algorithms [1].

To solve the labeling problem using maximum flow algorithms, the energy function needs to be represented by a graph. This can be done analogously to [12] by defining the graph $G = (\mathcal{V}_G, \mathcal{E}_G)$ as follows: the set of vertices is simply the set of pixels unified with two special vertices: $\mathcal{V}_G = \mathcal{V} \cup \{S, T\}$, where $S$ denotes the source and $T$ the sink. The set of edges consists of the set of all neighboring pixels plus edges between each pixel and the source and sink respectively: $\mathcal{E}_G = \mathcal{E} \cup \{(p, S), (p, T) \mid p \in \mathcal{V}\}$. The capacities $c(e)$ of each edge are defined analogously to Boykov et al. [12].

For the grouping of the variables, we follow the definitions given in [9] with our notation. A variable grouping of graph $G$ is a graph $G' = (\mathcal{V}'_G, \mathcal{E}'_G)$ with energy function $E'$ produced by a surjective map $m_G : \mathcal{V}_G \rightarrow \mathcal{V}'_G$ and the edge set $\mathcal{E}'_G = \{(s, t) \in \mathcal{V}'_G \times \mathcal{V}'_G \mid \exists (i, j) \in \mathcal{E}_G : m_G(i) = s \text{ and } m_G(j) = t\}$. Thus, the energy function for a variable grouping $G'$ reads:

$$E'(x) = \sum_{i \in \mathcal{V}} \varphi_i(\hat{x}_{m_G(i)}) + \sum_{(i,j) \in \mathcal{E}} \varphi_{i,j}(\hat{x}_{m_G(i)}, \hat{x}_{m_G(j)}), \tag{4}$$

where $\hat{x}$ is the labeling of the variable grouping. Solving this energy function on top of the grouping can be seen to correspond to the existing practice of using superpixels as a preprocessing step and defining the energy minimization problem on superpixels instead of pixels. Since most superpixels are directly derived from image properties, they perform poorly because the properties of the energy function, e.g. the unary term, are ignored. Figure 2 shows an example of a variable grouping and the corresponding graph based on the new energy function.

## 2.1   Dempster-Shafer Theory of Evidence

In this section we briefly review Dempster's theory of evidence, which is later used to define a similarity weight for two neighboring variables. The Dempster-Shafer theory of evidence, also called evidence theory, was introduced in the late 60s by A.P. Dempster [22], and more formally in 1976 by G. Shafer [23].

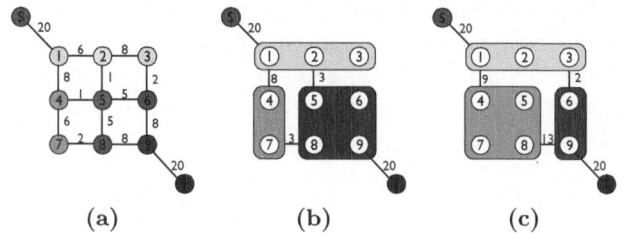

**Fig. 2.** Example variable grouping. The nodes from the original graph (a) are merged into three different groups of variables (b) and (c). The weights of the new graph are changed according to the new energy function. A good grouping (b) does not change the MAP solution of the original graph.

Later works [24, 25] applied it to image segmentation, and showed that it can be superior to Bayesian theory.

Evidence theory is a generalization of Bayesian theory which jointly represents inaccuracy and uncertainty information. The basic idea of the evidence theory is to define a so-called mass function on a hypotheses set $\Omega$. Let us note the hypotheses set $\Omega$ composed of $n$ single mutually exclusive subsets $\Omega_i$, symbolized by $\Omega = \{\Omega_1, \Omega_2, \ldots, \Omega_n\}$. In order to express a degree of confidence for each element $A$ of the power set $\wp(\Omega)$, an elementary mass function $m(A)$ is associated with it to indicate all confidences assigned to this proposition. The mass function $m$ is defined by: $m : \wp(\Omega) \to [0, 1]$ and must fulfill the following conditions:

$$(i) \quad m(\emptyset) = 0 \quad (ii) \quad \sum_{A_n \subseteq \Omega} m(A_n) = 1 \,. \tag{5}$$

The quantity $m(A)$ is interpreted as the belief strictly placed on hypothesis $A$. Compared to a Bayesian probability function, the mass function in evidence theory is the totality of belief. This belief is distributed on both simple and composed classes and models the impossibility to separate several hypotheses. Thereby the principal advantage of the evidence theory is characterized.

From the basic belief assignment $m$, a belief function $Bel : \wp(\Omega) \to [0, 1]$ can be defined as

$$Bel(A) = \sum_{A_n \subseteq A} m(A_n) \,, \tag{6}$$

with $A_n \in \wp(\Omega)$. The belief function is the mass of hypothesis $A$ plus the mass attached to all subsets of $A$.

This can be interpreted as the total belief committed to a hypothesis. $Bel(A)$ is then the total positive effect the body of evidence has on a value being in $A$. It quantifies the minimal degree of belief of the hypothesis $A$.

A particular characteristic of Dempster-Shafer evidence theory differs from Bayesian theory: If $Bel(A) < 1$, then the remaining evidence $1 - Bel(A)$ does not need necessarily refute $A$ (i.e. support its negation $\overline{A}$). That is, we do not have the so-called additivity rule $Bel(A) + Bel(\overline{A}) = 1$.

**Dempster's Rule of Combination.** To unify evidence from a variety of features we use *Dempster's rule of combination*. This rule combines two independent bodies of evidence, defined within the same frame of discernment, into one body of evidence. Let $m_1$ and $m_2$ be two mass functions associated to such independent bodies. Then the new body of evidence is defined by the mass function

$$m(A) = m_1(A) \otimes m_2(A) = \frac{\displaystyle\sum_{B \cap C = A} m_1(B)m_2(C)}{1 - \displaystyle\sum_{B \cap C = \emptyset} m_1(B)m_2(C)} . \tag{7}$$

Dempster's rule of combination computes a measure of agreement between two bodies of evidence and ignores the conflicting evidence through the normalization factor. Since Dempster's rule of combination is associative, we can combine information arising from more than two feature channels.

## 3   Dempster-Shafer Based Variable Grouping

In this section we describe the details of our approach and show the similarities and differences to existing approaches. Let us assume a score function $w$ measuring how similar two connected nodes are, such that small values indicate a strong similarity and large values dissimilarity. The idea of grouping nodes is as follows: (i) the first step is to sort all edges of the graph in ascending order so that edges with a small weight come first, (ii) for each edge in the list we merge nodes that fulfill a given constraint until we have sufficiently reduced the problem. The efficient graph-based segmentation method, proposed by Felzenszwalb and Huttenlocher [13], works exactly like this. To balance the size of a group and its internal coherence, a global criterion is used to decide if two groups can be merged. Algorithm 1 is identical to [13] and [9] using our notation. The merging constraint used in [13] and [9] is based on the so called internal difference

$$\text{Int}(C) = \max_{(i,j) \in \text{MST}(C, \mathcal{E})} w_{ij} ,$$

where $\text{MST}(C, \mathcal{E})$ is the minimum-weight spanning tree within the group $C$ with a set of edges $\mathcal{E}$. $\text{Int}(C)$ is small if the nodes in group $C$ are similar according to the defined edge weights. To decide whether two groups are merged, the algorithm compares the weight of the connecting edge between the two groups $C_1$ and $C_2$ and compares it with the internal difference $\text{Int}(C_i)$ of both groups. For our goal of grouping variables for energy minimization, this criterion makes sense since we want to build groups of variables that are similar and agree about their labeling. For the decision, [9, 13] use the function $\text{MInt}(C_1, C_2)$ defined as

$$\text{MInt}(C_1, C_2) = \min\{\text{Int}(C_1) + \tau(C_1), \text{Int}(C_2) + \tau(C_2)\} ,$$

where $\tau(C) = \frac{k}{|C|}$ penalizes the size of a group based on a free parameter $k$. According to Algorithm 1, when edge $w_{ij} \in \mathcal{E}_{\mathcal{G}}$ fulfills the equation

| **Algorithm 1.** Dempster-Shafer based Variable Grouping |
|---|

1: $(\mathcal{V}_\mathcal{G}', m) = \text{DempsterShaferGrouping}(G, \varphi, w)$
2: **Input:**
3:    $G = (\mathcal{V}_\mathcal{G}, \mathcal{E}_\mathcal{G})$ // an instance of the graph
4:    $\varphi_i, \varphi_{i,j}$ // node and edge energies
5:    $w : \mathcal{E}_\mathcal{G} \to \mathbb{R}$ // dissimilarity weights
6: **Output:**
7:    $\mathcal{V}_\mathcal{G}'$ // set of grouped variables
8:    $m$ // surjective map
9: **Algorithm:**
10:    $\mathcal{V}_\mathcal{G}' \leftarrow \mathcal{V}_\mathcal{G}, \mathcal{E}_\mathcal{G}' \leftarrow \mathcal{E}_\mathcal{G}$
11:    $m \leftarrow \{(i, i) \mid i \in \mathcal{V}_\mathcal{G}\}$
12:    $\pi \leftarrow \text{sort}(\mathcal{E}_\mathcal{G}, w)$ {sort weights in ascending order}
13:    **for** $e = 1, \ldots, |\pi|$ **do**
14:       $(i, j) \leftarrow \pi_e$
15:       **if** $m(i) = m(j)$ **then**
16:          **continue** {already merged}
17:       **end if**
18:       **if** $w_{ij}$ fulfills given constraint **then**
19:          merge $C_j$ and $C_j$ in $m, \mathcal{V}_\mathcal{G}'$
20:       **end if**
21:    **end for**

$$w_{ij} \leq \text{MInt}(C_i, C_j) \tag{8}$$

$C_i$ and $C_j$ are merged. As mentioned in [13], this graph based method is very efficient and easy to implement in $O(|\mathcal{E}_\mathcal{G}| \log |\mathcal{E}_\mathcal{G}|)$ time and memory.

## 3.1   Merging Function

The grouping resulting from the algorithms in [13] and [9] can be described as compact since the free parameter $k$ in $\tau(C)$ penalizes the size of a group. In [9] the goal was to produce compact groups of variables that will have the same label according to the minimum energy state. Therefore the weight functions are based on the unary or pairwise potentials of the energy function. In contrast, our goal is to group as many variables as possible that are likely to have the same label according to the minimum energy state and to the ground truth labeling.

To allow big groups of variables, e.g. in homogeneous regions, we propose new merging constraints based on the maximum weight among outgoing edges. Instead of using a global criterion, balancing the size and the internal coherence of a group we merge all nodes that are connected by a sufficiently small edge. E.g. one could use the function $w_{ij} \leq W$ to merge all nodes connected by an edge smaller than the parameter $W$. As we will show in the experiments this simple constraint does not produce groups that agree with either the minimum energy state or the ground truth. To produce groups of homogeneous variables, we propose two new merging constraints based on the local edge weights of two nodes. The first constraint takes into account the maximum value of any edge connected to one of the two nodes. Therefore two components connected by the edge $w_{ij}$ are grouped if

$$w_{max}(i,j) := \max\{w_{ik}, w_{lj} \mid (i,k),(l,j) \in \mathcal{E}_{\mathcal{G}}\} \leq W_1 \quad \text{(MAXEDGE)}. \quad (9)$$

This means that two nodes are merged if the weights of all edges adjacent to $(i,j)$, including the edge $w_{ij}$, are smaller than the parameter $W_1$, which indicates that these nodes are somewhat similar. In our experiments the threshold $W_1$ is computed according to the distribution of the edge weights (66% of the edge weights are smaller than $W_1$). The idea of the proposed constraint is to have large groups of variables in all images regions except the borders of the objects. If a node (pixel) is near the border of an object there should be one edge with a high weight. With (9) this edge guarantees that the node is not merged with any neighbor. As a second constraint we also include the global criterion based on the minimum-weight spanning tree and the size dependent function $\tau$, to balance the size of a group and its internal coherence, to allow somehow small compact groups of variables in regions that do not fulfill the MAXEDGE constrained, e.g. at the borders of an object. Thus, the decision is made according to

$$\text{MAXEDGE} \quad \text{or} \quad w_{ij} \leq \text{MInt}(C_i, C_j) \quad \text{(COMPACTEDGE)}, \quad (10)$$

The differences of the proposed merging functions are discussed in the experiment section.

## 3.2   Weight Functions

We consider three classes of weight functions $w_{ij}$. The first two are well known weight functions that shall serve as comparison with the proposed one.

**Felzenszwalb and Huttenlocher:** In [13] Felzenszwalb and Huttenlocher take the pixel difference as the grouping weight. If $I_i$ and $I_j$ are the feature vectors of pixels $i$ and $j$ in the image, the weight is set to the norm of the difference:

$$w_{ij}^{FH} = ||I_i - I_j||.$$

In our experiments on image segmentation, we will show that this method is not performing comparably, since the properties from the energy minimization problem are ignored.

**Kim et al.:** An approach very similar to [13] and ours, was proposed by Kim et al. in [9]. For comparison with the proposed method we use the defined UNARY-DIFF weight function. In our experiments on standard benchmark images this weight function outperformed the others for the problem of binary image segmentation. The weight is defined as

$$w_{ij}^{ud} = ||\varphi_i - \varphi_j||,$$

using the unary terms of the defined energy function. The weight describes the disagreement of the states between two variables and measure the task-specific similarity of two neighboring nodes.

**Dempster-Shafer Weighting Function:** Our proposed weight function includes the unary functions $\varphi_i$ and $\varphi_j$ and the pairwise terms $\varphi_{ij}$. Thereby we take into account the image information that are included in the pairwise function and the information included in the unary term, typically derived from a discriminative classifier. Hence the proposed weight function can be seen as a combination of the two earlier presented ones which combines the image features with the task specific unary functions. To combine both informations we use Dempster's theory of evidence. Therefore we define the weights based on the unary and pairwise functions

$$w_{ij}^{pairwise} = \varphi_{ij}(x_i, x_j) \quad \text{and} \quad w_{ij}^{unary} = ||\varphi_i - \varphi_j||. \tag{11}$$

Since the co-domain of the weights are different, we normalize them individually to $[0, 1]$. That means for two variables with a similar feature vector $w_{ij}^{pairwise} \approx 1$. For $w_{ij}^{unary}$ it means $w_{ij}^{unary} \approx 0$ if the negative log likelihood for two variables is similar for both states. Based on these weight functions, we define two mass functions over the hypothesis set $\Omega = \{\Omega_1, \Omega_2\}$, where $\Omega_1$ means that the two variables are similar and $\Omega_2$ that they are dissimilar:

$$
\begin{aligned}
m_1(\Omega_1) &= b_1 \cdot w_{ij}^{pairwise} \quad , m_1(\Omega_2) = b_1 \cdot (1 - w_{ij}^{pairwise}), \\
m_1(\emptyset) &= 0 \quad , m_1(\Omega) = b_1, \\
m_2(\Omega_1) &= b_2 \cdot (1 - w_{ij}^{unary}) \quad , m_2(\Omega_2) = b_2 \cdot w_{ij}^{unary}, \\
m_2(\emptyset) &= 0 \quad , m_2(\Omega) = b_2,
\end{aligned}
\tag{12}
$$

where $b_i$ describes the belief we put on the different information sources. In all our experiments we equally weight the believe with $b_1 = b_2 = 0.5$. Now we fuse the two mass functions with Dempster's rule of combination (7) and define the weights:

$$
\begin{aligned}
w_{ij}^{DS} &= 1 - Bel(\Omega_1) = 1 - m(\Omega_1) = 1 - m_1(\Omega_1) \otimes m_2(\Omega_1) \\
&= 1 - \left( \frac{m_1(\Omega_1) \cdot m_2(\Omega_1) + m_1(\Omega_1) \cdot m_2(\Omega) + m_1(\Omega) \cdot m_2(\Omega_1)}{1 - (m_1(\Omega_1) \cdot m_2(\Omega_2) + m_1(\Omega_2) \cdot m_2(\Omega_1))} \right)
\end{aligned}
\tag{13}
$$

In contrast to [9], the proposed weight function allows for the combination with other information sources, such as the user initialization, the optical flow in video sequences, depth images or appearance information of an object.

## 4   Experiments

Our proposed grouping allows us to compute an approximate segmentation. Since the resulting graph for the energy minimization is much smaller the segmentation result differs from the original MAP solution. Since the goal of our

**Table 1.** Comparison of the proposed algorithm and two similar methods proposed in [13] and [9]. All values are averaged over 50 benchmark images using stroke (lasso) initializations. As can be seen our proposed method COMPACTEDGE performed best in terms of quality with a smaller budget. The proposed MAXEDGE has the lowest minimum segmentation error with the drawback of a bigger budget. The graph visualizes $R_{se}(x)$ for one image and different budgets.

| Method | Avg. budget | Avg. $R_{mse}(x)$ | Avg. $R_{se}(x)$ |
|--------|-------------|-------------------|------------------|
| full MAP (reference) | 100 (100) | 0 (0) | 0.075 (0.058) |
| FH-alg [13] | 10.22 (10.22) | 209.74 (209.74) | 0.074 (0.063) |
| UNARYDIFF [9] | 10.72 (10.84) | 255.1 (219.08) | 0.073 (0.065) |
| **MAXEDGE** | 47.72 (15.21) | 58.42 (4.21) | 0.069 (0.058) |
| **COMPACTEDGE** | 6.25 (5.00) | 321.5 (63.52) | 0.061 (0.058) |

grouping is a low segmentation error, and not an accurate MAP, we quantify our algorithm using three performance measures: (i) the segmentation quality with respect to the ground truth solution, (ii) the minimum segmentation error of a grouping, and (iii) the ratio of runtimes solving the MAP-problems (including the time for the grouping). Following, we describe the three measures in detail:

**Segmentation Error:** The segmentation error is defined analogously to [2] as the ratio between the number of misclassified pixels and the number of pixels in unclassified regions:

$$R_{se}(x) = \frac{\sum_{i \in \mathcal{V}_\mathcal{G}} [x_i \neq x_i^{gt}]}{\text{no. pixels in unclassified regions}},$$

where $x^{gt}$ is the ground truth labeling.

**Minimum Segmentation Error:** Another measure to quantify the quality of a grouping is given by the minimum segmentation error, that counts the minimum number of misclassified pixels by an optimal segmentation.

$$R_{mse}(x) = \sum_{i \in \mathcal{V}'_\mathcal{G}} \min \left( \sum_{j \in m_{\mathcal{V}_\mathcal{G}}^{-1}(i)} [x_j^{gt} = fg], \sum_{j \in m_{\mathcal{V}_\mathcal{G}}^{-1}(i)} [x_j^{gt} = bg] \right).$$

**Ratio of Runtimes:** To compute the ratio of runtimes we compare the time to compute the grouping and solve the reduced problem with the time solving the original problem.

We present an evaluation of the proposed method on small scale images of the Microsoft segmentation benchmark, used by Blake et al. [2][1,2] as well as on

[1] http://research.microsoft.com/en-us/um/cambridge/projects/
visionimagevideoediting/segmentation/grabcut.htm
[2] http://www.eecs.berkeley.edu/Research/Projects/
CS/vision/grouping/segbench/

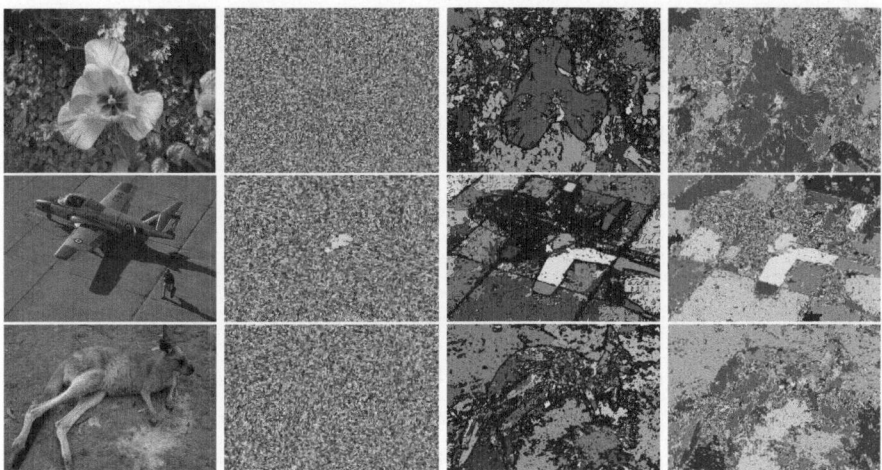

**Fig. 3.** Example for the different approaches for variable grouping. Columns: (i) original image; (ii) variable grouping using [9]; (ii) proposed method using MAXEDGE; (iv) proposed method using COMPACTEDGE; In contrast to [9] where the grouping produces superpixels that are comparable in size our proposed methods group large homogeneous regions to single variables.

large scale images with up to 26 million pixels found on the web. For the problem of binary video segmentation we used video sequences from the KTH action dataset [26][3] and videos provided by Sand and Teller[27][4]. In all experiments we use the same energy function proposed by Blake et al. [2] and the same set of parameters. The experiments were run on a MacBook Pro with 2.4 GHz Intel Core i5 processor and 4GB Ram. For all experiments we compare the proposed algorithm with the approaches of Felzenszwalb and Huttenlocher [13] and Kim et al. [9].

**Small-Scale Images:** Table 1 shows the evaluation of the proposed algorithm on the Microsoft segmentation benchmark in comparison to the works of Felzenszwalb and Huttenlocher and Kim et al.. Since independently the benefit of the proposed weight $w_{ij}^{DS}$ and the merging constraints is rather small, we only evaluate the combination that outperformed existing approaches.

We can observe that the combination of Dempster's theory of evidence and the proposed constraint has a smaller average segmentation error with an even smaller budget. The small minimum segmentation error using the MAXEDGE constraint highlights that our idea to group large homogeneous regions to one single variable makes sense and the proposed weights based on Dempster's theory of evidence reliably find those regions. In combination with small groups at the objects boundaries the proposed COMPACTEDGE constraint outperforms the existing approaches. See also Figure 3 for a visual comparison of the different approaches.

---

[3] http://www.nada.kth.se/cvap/actions/

[4] http://rvsn.csail.mit.edu/pv/

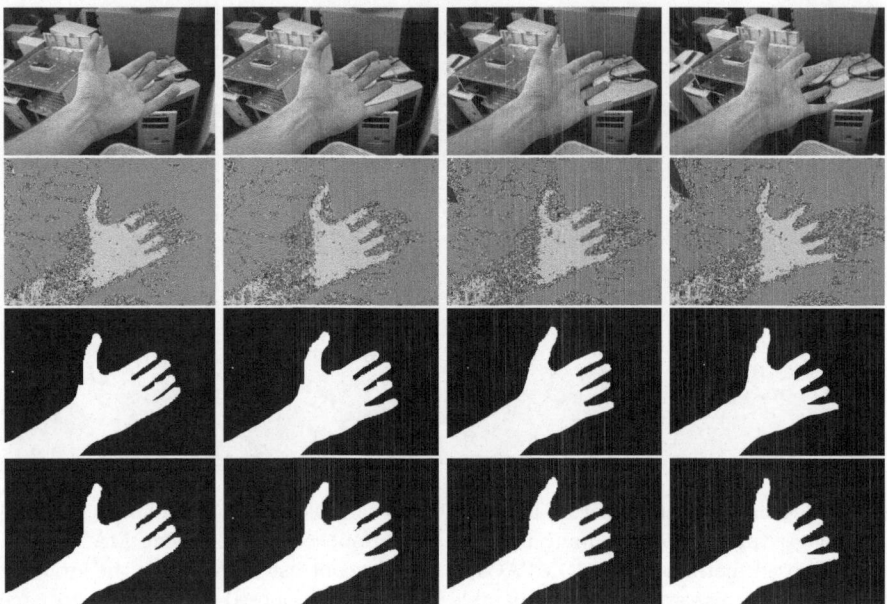

**Fig. 4.** Variable grouping for video segmentation. The columns correspond to the frames 5, 15, 25 and 38 of the hand sequence [27]. Rows: (i) original frame; (ii) variable grouping with the proposed algorithm; (iii) segmentation result solving the full MAP; (iv) segmentation result solving the approximated MAP. The segmentation results are almost identical even if the approximated solution used a Budget of 5%. The ratio of runtime for this example is $\approx 0.1$.

**High-Resolution Images:** To evaluate the segmentation quality and the possible speedup of the proposed method we used large-scale images with up to 20 MP and down sampled these images to several image-sizes. Similar to the experiments on small-scale images and video sequences the difference in segmentation quality is small and the reduction of runtime is dramatic for large images. As already shown by Delong and Boykov [8] the BK-algorithm is inefficient and unusable if the graph does not fit into the physical memory. For those large MAP inference problems the ratio of runtime was approximately 0.08 using a budget of 5%. Due to the limitations of the BK-algorithm the proposed method greatly extends its applications.

**Video-Sequences:** Our proposed algorithm can also be applied to group variables for the problem of video segmentation. To evaluate the performance of the proposed method we segmented different video-sequences. It can be seen from Figures 4 and 5 that the proposed algorithm achieves a similar segmentation like the full MAP solution with a much smaller budget and a dramatic reduction of runtime. E.g. for the hand video in Figure 4 (200 frames) we reduced the number of variables from 69.1 million to 3.5 million. For comparison of the results the full MAP solution was only computed for 40 frames since solving the full MAP problem for 200 frames was not possible due to memory reasons. The full MAP problem for the KTH-sequence shown in Figure 5 has 7 million variables and

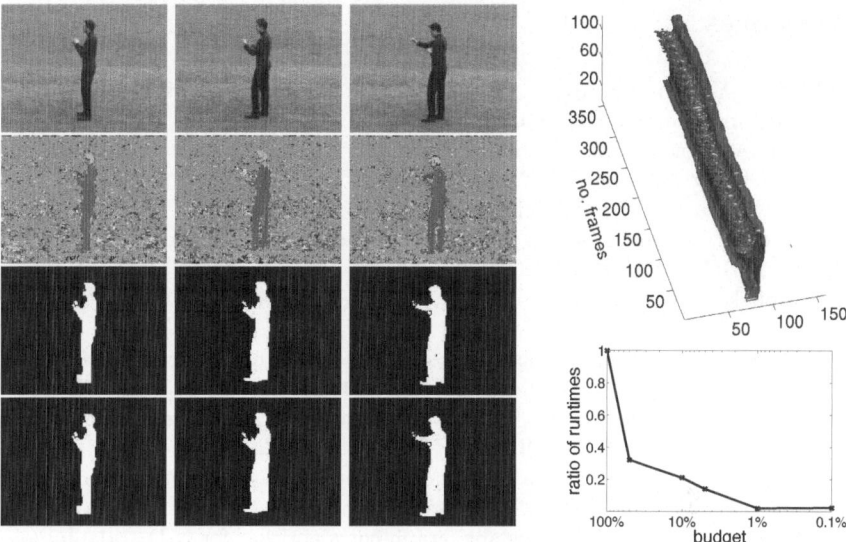

**Fig. 5.** Variable grouping for video segmentation. The columns correspond to the frames 20, 220 and 350 of the Boxing sequence from [26]. The last column visualizes the isosurface of our segmentation result and the ratio of runtime for a given budget. Rows: (i) original frame; (ii) variable grouping with the proposed algorithm; (iii) segmentation result solving the full MAP; (iv) segmentation result solving the approximated MAP. The segmentation results are almost identical even if the approximated solution used a Budget of 10%. The ratio of runtime for this example is $\approx 0.21$.

the results shown use an budget of approximately 10% resulting in 0.7 million variables with a comparable segmentation result. In all examples we initialized the segmentation with a few strokes in the first frame.

## 5  Conclusion

We presented an efficient algorithm for graph simplification of maximum a posteriori problems that is widely applicable to MAP inference problems in computer vision. It uses Dempster's theory of evidence and new constraints for the graph based grouping to group large homogeneous regions to one single variable of the problem. In our experiments on segmentation we demonstrated that the segmentation error using the proposed method is smaller or comparable to the full MAP solution. In several experiments on large-scale problems with millions of variables we demonstrate that the reduction in runtime is dramatic while the segmentation quality stays comparable.

# References

1. Boykov, Y., Kolmogorov, V.: An experimental comparison of min-cut/max-flow algorithms for energy minimization in vision. TPAMI 26, 1124–1137 (2004)
2. Blake, A., Rother, C., Brown, M., Perez, P., Torr, P.: Interactive Image Segmentation Using an Adaptive GMMRF Model. In: Pajdla, T., Matas, J(G.) (eds.) ECCV 2004. LNCS, vol. 3021, pp. 428–441. Springer, Heidelberg (2004)
3. Boykov, Y., Kolmogorov, V.: Computing geodesics and minimal surfaces via graph cuts. In: ICCV, pp. 26–33 (2003)
4. Lempitsky, V., Boykov, Y.: Global optimization for shape fitting. In: CVPR, pp. 1–8 (2007)
5. Kohli, P., Torr, P.H.S.: Efficiently solving dynamic markov random fields using graph cuts. In: ICCV, vol. 2, pp. 922–929 (2005)
6. Rother, C., Kolmogorov, V., Blake, A.: Grabcut: interactive foreground extraction using iterated graph cuts. SIGGRAPH 23, 309–314 (2004)
7. Boykov, Y., Veksler, O., Zabih, R.: Fast approximate energy minimization via graph cuts. TPAMI 23, 1222–1239 (2002)
8. Delong, A., Boykov, Y.: A scalable graph-cut algorithm for N-D grids. In: CVPR (2008)
9. Kim, T., Nowozin, S., Kohli, P., Yoo, C.D.: Variable grouping for energy minimization. In: CVPR, pp. 1913–1920 (2011)
10. Bhusnurmath, A., Taylor, C.: Graph cuts via $l_1$ norm minimization. TPAMI 30, 1866–1871 (2008)
11. Komodakis, N.: Towards More Efficient and Effective LP-Based Algorithms for MRF Optimization. In: Daniilidis, K., Maragos, P., Paragios, N. (eds.) ECCV 2010, Part II. LNCS, vol. 6312, pp. 520–534. Springer, Heidelberg (2010)
12. Boykov, Y., Jolly, M.: Interactive graph cuts for optimal boundary & region segmentation of objects in ND images. In: ICCV, vol. 1, pp. 105–112 (2001)
13. Felzenszwalb, P.F., Huttenlocher, D.P.: Efficient graph-based image segmentation. IJCV 59, 167–181 (2004)
14. Comaniciu, D., Meer, P., Member, S.: Mean shift: a robust approach toward feature space analysis. TPAMI 24, 603–619 (2002)
15. Levinshtein, A., Stere, A., Kutulakos, K.N., Fleet, D.J., Dickinson, S.J., Siddiqi, K.: TurboPixels: fast superpixels using geometric flows. TPAMI 31, 2290–2297 (2009)
16. Veksler, O., Boykov, Y., Mehrani, P.: Superpixels and Supervoxels in an Energy Optimization Framework. In: Daniilidis, K., Maragos, P., Paragios, N. (eds.) ECCV 2010, Part V. LNCS, vol. 6315, pp. 211–224. Springer, Heidelberg (2010)
17. Scheuermann, B., Rosenhahn, B.: SlimCuts: GraphCuts for High Resolution Images Using Graph Reduction. In: Boykov, Y., Kahl, F., Lempitsky, V., Schmidt, F.R. (eds.) EMMCVPR 2011. LNCS, vol. 6819, pp. 219–232. Springer, Heidelberg (2011)
18. Lermé, N., Létocart, L., Malgouyres, F.: Reduced graphs for min-cut/max-flow approaches in image segmentation. ENDM 37, 63–68 (2011)
19. Puzicha, J., Buhmann, J.: Multiscale annealing for grouping and unsupervised texture segmentation. IJCVIU 76, 213–230 (1999)
20. Kohli, P., Lempitsky, V., Rother, C.: Uncertainty Driven Multi-scale Optimization. In: Goesele, M., Roth, S., Kuijper, A., Schiele, B., Schindler, K. (eds.) Pattern Recognition. LNCS, vol. 6376, pp. 242–251. Springer, Heidelberg (2010)

21. Sinop, A.K., Grady, L.: Accurate Banded Graph Cut Segmentation of Thin Structures Using Laplacian Pyramids. In: Larsen, R., Nielsen, M., Sporring, J. (eds.) MICCAI 2006. LNCS, vol. 4191, pp. 896–903. Springer, Heidelberg (2006)
22. Dempster, A.P.: A generalization of Bayesian inference. Journal of the Royal Statistical Society 30, 205–247 (1968)
23. Shafer, G.: A mathematical theory of evidence. Princeton university press (1976)
24. Adamek, T., O'Connor, N.E.: Using Dempster-Shafer theory to fuse multiple information sources in region-based segmentation. In: ICIP, pp. 269–272 (2007)
25. Chaabane, S.B., Sayadi, M., Fnaiech, F., Brassart, E.: Dempster-Shafer evidence theory for image segmentation: application in cells images. IJSP (2009)
26. Schüldt, C., Laptev, I., Caputo, B.: Recognizing human actions: a local SVM approach. In: ICPR, pp. 32–36 (2004)
27. Sand, P., Teller, S.J.: Particle video: long-range motion estimation using point trajectories. In: CVPR, pp. 2195–2202 (2006)

# Video Segmentation with Superpixels

Fabio Galasso[1], Roberto Cipolla[2], and Bernt Schiele[1]

[1] Max Planck Institute for Informatics, Saarbrücken, Germany
[2] University of Cambridge, Cambridge, UK

**Abstract.** Due to its importance, video segmentation has regained interest recently. However, there is no common agreement about the necessary ingredients for best performance. This work contributes a thorough analysis of various within- and between-frame affinities suitable for video segmentation. Our results show that a frame-based superpixel segmentation combined with a few motion and appearance-based affinities are sufficient to obtain good video segmentation performance. A second contribution of the paper is the extension of [1] to include motion-cues, which makes the algorithm globally aware of motion, thus improving its performance for video sequences. Finally, we contribute an extension of an established image segmentation benchmark [1] to videos, allowing coarse-to-fine video segmentations and multiple human annotations. Our results are tested on BMDS [2], and compared to existing methods.

## 1 Introduction

Segmentation is a fundamental problem in computer vision with many applications such as action recognition, 3D reconstruction, or video indexing. Many powerful image segmentation (IS) methods exist (e.g. [3–9]) and there is common agreement to use multiple similarities based on brightness, color and texture over local image patches to achieve best image segmentation performance.

Video segmentation (VS) is far less researched due to its computational complexity and the inherent difficulties such as camera-motion, occlusions, changes in scale, perspective, illumination and contrast, or non-rigid deformations. Intuitively, besides *within-frame* similarities used for image segmentation, VS should also use *between-frame* similarities to connect and thus segment corresponding regions across multiple frames. While recent work on VS proposes a variety of such between-frame similarities [2, 10–13] there is no common agreement yet on which similarities are necessary for best performance.

The main contribution of the present work is thus a systematic analysis of different between- and within-frame similarities in a unified framework. Similarities are novel terms or derived from other VS methods. The major result of the analysis is to identify the most powerful similarities that in combination achieve best performance. We further contribute an extension to a hierarchical image segmentation (HIS) [1] including motion cues, which improves significantly its performance for video-segmentation. Finally, we extend an established IS benchmark [1] to evaluate coarse-to-fine VS results on multiple human annotations.

K.M. Lee et al. (Eds.): ACCV 2012, Part I, LNCS 7724, pp. 760–774, 2013.
© Springer-Verlag Berlin Heidelberg 2013

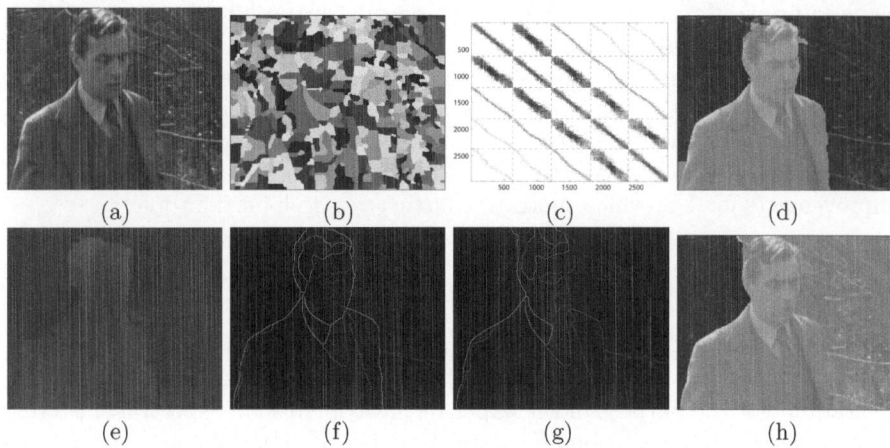

**Fig. 1.** (*Top row*) Proposed video segmentation model: we extract superpixels (b) with a novel motion-aware hierarchical image segmentation algorithm (MAHIS); we systematically analyze affinity matrices (c) based on novel and existing within- and between-frame superpixel similarities, and employ a spectral clustering framework to provide the final video segmentation (d). (*Second row*) The proposed MAHIS includes motion (e) and generates Ultrametric Contour Maps (f) which outperform the state-of-the-art (g) [1]. Note the ability of our video segmentation algorithm (d) to overcome the problems that standard image segmentation has for the right part of the image (h).

## 2    Related Work

A large body of literature on VS exists leveraging on appearance [11, 14–16], motion [2, 3, 12], or a combination of cues [10, 13, 17–23]. A variety of techniques is used, e.g. generative layered models [19, 20], graph-based models [15], mean-shift [17, 21], and techniques based on manifold-embedding and eigendecomposition, such as ISOMAP [12] and spectral clustering [2, 3]. Layered models [19, 20] have shown potential in learning general object motion and appearance, but are limited by their computational load. On the other hand graph-based [15] and meanshift techniques [21] may generalize to video sequences of arbitrary sizes, as they are based on local properties. We have chosen spectral clustering for our framework as it provides globally optimal solutions.

Recent works on VS have employed point trajectories [2], improving on the corresponding point track clustering literature [24, 25], and dense solutions are obtained with densification by non-linear diffusion [23] and graph-based methods [16]. Here we consider the dense video volume, arguing that sparse tracks do not capture the spatial cohesiveness of objects, as also maintained in [14].

Similarly to [11–13], we employ superpixels, which provide a desirable computational reduction and powerful within-frame representation. [11–13] extract region trajectories and provide video segmentations by respectively labelling them, in a CRF and ISOMAP framework. By contrast, we encompass an analysis of the between-frame affinities which they use. Our results are useful to improve the quality of their region trajectories.

Other work exists which extends the HIS of [1] to include motion cues. Most notably [26] evaluates frame differences and optical flow among multiple frames and applies twice the machinery of [1], outperforming [1] for occlusion boundary detection. Our extension to [1] is straightforward and provides significant improvements for VS, which motivates further research on the topic.

## 3    Framework

Many segmentation approaches exist that could serve as a general framework for our analysis of different within- and between-frame similarities for video segmentation. For the purpose of the paper we have opted to use spectral clustering [3, 27] given its long tradition and state-of-art performance in a number of areas including image [1] and video object segmentation [2, 12]. The mathematical theory is well understood, and the general framework is well established since the pioneering work on normalized cuts [3].

The algorithm is based on an affinity matrix $W$ formed of pair-wise similarity scores $w_{i,j}$ between data elements $i$ and $j$. For image segmentation these data elements are often the image pixels themselves [1, 3] or for video object segmentation these elements might be point trajectories [2, 12]. While $W$ is quadratic in the number of elements, it is typically sparse as only a local spatial(-temporal) neighborhood is considered, making the approach computationally viable.

The affinity matrix $W$ is employed to embed the data elements onto a manifold, by eigendecomposing the normalized graph Laplacian $L$:

$$L = D^{-\frac{1}{2}}(D - W)D^{-\frac{1}{2}} = V^T \Lambda V \tag{1}$$

where $D$ is a diagonal matrix with entries $d_{i,i} = \sum_j w_{i,j}$, matrix $V$ contains the eigenvectors, and the diagonal matrix $\Lambda$ contains the eigenvalues. The mapping into the manifold is given by taking the eigenvectors $\{v_0, v_1, \ldots, v_m\}$ corresponding to the $m + 1$ smallest eigenvalues $0 = \lambda_0 < \lambda_1 < \ldots, < \lambda_{m+1}$ (as $\lambda_0 = 0$, $v_0$ is constant and can be discarded). Partitioning or segmentation of the data elements can be obtained with standard clustering schemes.

This method is well suited to analyze the contribution of different within- and between-frame affinities by simply defining entries of the affinity matrix $W$ using single or a combination of affinities. Here we employ the above approach twice in a two-step framework. The first step results in a motion-aware hierarchical image segmentation (MAHIS) from which we obtain superpixels for the second step. This step uses pixel-based affinities that are calculated both from brightness, color, and texture [1], as well as from optical flow (see sec. 4).

The second step is superpixel-based and uses a variety of within- and between-frame affinities (see sec. 5) to obtain the video segmentation result. The motivation to use superpixels for video-segmentation is two-fold. First, a drastic reduction of the computational complexity is achieved since the number of data-elements to be considered is lowered by two orders of magnitude. And second,

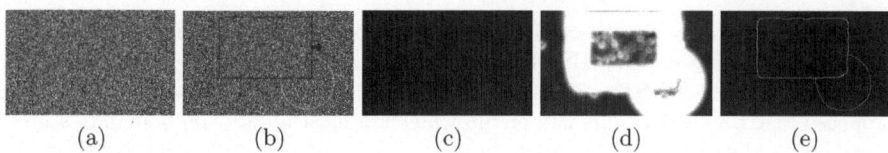

(a) (b) (c) (d) (e)

**Fig. 2.** (a,b) Two foreground objects move on a background with the same texture. None of the brightness, color and texture cues from the HIS algorithm of [1] detects the objects (c), which our motion cue (d) clearly identifies. Our proposed MAHIS provides the correct boundaries for the objects (e).

we can define richer and more powerful between-frame affinities than would be possible with pixel-based affinities alone.

Sec. 4 describes our motion-aware hierarchical image segmentation approach, sec. 5 the different between-frame affinities, and sec. 6 evaluated different combinations of those affinities in the context of video segmentation.

## 4 Motion-Aware Superpixels

Image segmentation is inherently ambiguous. In the frame shown in fig. 1(a), the jacket has a similar color as the background, clearly distinct from the skin and the shirt. Illumination and contrast help recover the true contours on the left contour of the body, but not the right contour. In fig. 1(g) the output of the image segmentation algorithm of [1] illustrates this expected result, also clear in the corresponding image segmentation in figure 1(h). On the other hand, the rich texture of the wood allows to accurately estimate optical flow, fig. 1(e), especially on the right side of the person, which perfectly complements appearance. By integrating our proposed motion cue into the algorithm of [1], we recover more respondent boundaries, fig. 1(f), and therefore superpixels.

Please note that not only the boundaries are better weighted, but the motion cue detects further boundaries in the image, as depicted in fig. 2 for a toy example. This further ensures that superpixels are conservatively representing the video without merging objects. On the other hand, the motion cue is zero for the static parts of the scene and the output is the same as from [1]. Here we describe our proposed MAHIS and validate it experimentally against [1].

### 4.1 Motion-Aware Hierarchical Image Segmentation

Optical flow has reached satisfactory maturity and suits the task of detecting motion. We use the dense optical flow algorithm of [28]. For each frame, horizontal $U(x,y)$ and vertical $V(x,y)$ optical flow components are composed by averaging the respective forward $U^+$ $V^+$ and backward $U^-$ $V^-$ estimates. The single-frame-averages smooth the flow and reduce the effect of outliers. A gradient is then computed for $U(x,y)$ and $V(x,y)$ with the histogram-based gradient operator, employed in [1] for the brightness BG, color CG and texture TG gradients. In particular, for both $U(x,y)$ and $V(x,y)$, we compute

**Table 1.** Our proposed image and video benchmark is used to compare our proposed VS and MAHIS against the HIS of [1] and the VS of [15] on BMDS [2]. All measures range $[0,1]$, higher is better; only VI ranges $[0,\infty)$, lower is better. (*First part*) Our proposed MAHIS outperforms HIS on most metrics, most notably on boundary scores. This clearly identifies MAHIS as the better candidate to extract superpixels for VS. (*Second part*) Our VS outperforms HIS and MAHIS. STT+LTT+STM+STA is identified as the minimal best set of affinities, in agreement with fig. 4. (*Third part*) Our proposed VS outperforms [15] on all fronts by large margins.

| | Boundary | | | Region | | | | | | |
| | | | | SC | | | PRI | | VI | |
| | ODS | OSS | AP | ODS | OSS | Best | ODS | OSS | ODS | OSS |
|---|---|---|---|---|---|---|---|---|---|---|
| HIS of [1] | 0.30 | 0.37 | 0.18 | **0.75** | 0.79 | 0.82 | **0.70** | 0.79 | **0.75** | 0.72 |
| Proposed MAHIS | **0.35** | **0.43** | **0.23** | 0.74 | **0.81** | **0.84** | 0.69 | **0.82** | 0.76 | **0.67** |
| VS: All | **0.35** | 0.41 | 0.22 | **0.80** | **0.85** | **0.87** | **0.78** | **0.86** | **0.71** | **0.56** |
| VS: ABA+LTT | 0.23 | 0.28 | 0.13 | 0.74 | 0.77 | 0.81 | 0.72 | 0.78 | 0.71 | 0.71 |
| VS: ABM+LTT | 0.21 | 0.25 | 0.11 | 0.74 | 0.76 | 0.80 | 0.72 | 0.77 | 0.71 | 0.71 |
| VS: STT | 0.16 | 0.20 | 0.08 | 0.74 | 0.75 | 0.78 | 0.72 | 0.75 | 0.71 | 0.70 |
| VS: STT+LTT | 0.20 | 0.24 | 0.12 | 0.74 | 0.76 | 0.79 | 0.72 | 0.77 | 0.71 | 0.71 |
| VS: STM | 0.32 | 0.33 | 0.22 | 0.74 | 0.76 | 0.78 | 0.72 | 0.78 | 0.71 | 0.69 |
| VS: STA | 0.19 | 0.25 | 0.11 | 0.74 | 0.75 | 0.76 | 0.72 | 0.75 | 0.71 | 0.71 |
| VS: STT+LTT+STM | 0.30 | 0.35 | 0.19 | 0.76 | 0.82 | 0.85 | 0.75 | 0.83 | 0.71 | 0.60 |
| VS: STT+LTT+STM+STA | **0.35** | 0.40 | 0.22 | **0.80** | **0.85** | **0.87** | **0.78** | **0.86** | **0.71** | **0.56** |
| VS: All-ABA | **0.35** | 0.41 | 0.22 | **0.80** | **0.85** | **0.87** | **0.78** | **0.86** | **0.71** | **0.56** |
| VS: All-ABM | **0.35** | 0.40 | 0.22 | **0.80** | **0.85** | **0.87** | 0.77 | **0.86** | **0.71** | 0.57 |
| VS: All-STT | 0.32 | 0.39 | 0.21 | 0.74 | 0.82 | 0.85 | 0.73 | 0.83 | 0.71 | 0.65 |
| VS: All-LTT | 0.30 | 0.33 | 0.19 | 0.74 | 0.78 | 0.79 | 0.72 | 0.80 | 0.71 | 0.67 |
| VS: All-STM | 0.24 | 0.29 | 0.13 | 0.74 | 0.76 | 0.80 | 0.72 | 0.77 | 0.71 | 0.70 |
| VS: All-STA | 0.31 | 0.36 | 0.19 | 0.76 | 0.82 | 0.86 | 0.75 | 0.83 | 0.71 | 0.60 |
| Our VS | **0.35** | 0.41 | 0.22 | **0.80** | **0.85** | **0.87** | **0.78** | **0.86** | **0.71** | **0.56** |
| VS of [15] | 0.20 | 0.23 | 0.10 | 0.74 | 0.76 | 0.78 | 0.72 | 0.76 | **0.71** | 0.71 |

the gradients $\Delta_\rho U(x,y,\theta)$ and $\Delta_\rho V(x,y,\theta)$ along 8 orientations $\theta \in (0,\pi]$ and 3 scale octaves $\rho$ (same parameters as [1]). Finally the flow gradient FG, for each orientation $\theta$ and scale $\rho$ sample, is given by the respective squared sums $\text{FG}_\rho(x,y,\theta) = \left[\Delta_\rho^2 U(x,y,\theta) + \Delta_\rho^2 V(x,y,\theta)\right]^{-\frac{1}{2}}$.

The new FG is then considered an additional channel, alongside BG, CG and TG, passed by the boundary detector to the spectral partitioning process, and finally to the OWT-UCM machinery which produces the hierarchical segmentation, following the pipeline and setup of [1]. The superpixels are conservatively extracted from the finest (over-)segmentation provided.

## 4.2   Experimental Evaluation

Our proposed MAHIS directly addresses the hierarchical image segmentation of video frames. For single images, or static frames, MAHIS provides identical result as the HIS of [1]. We thus test MAHIS on a video dataset including camera and object motion. Recently, [2] has provided the Berkeley motion segmentation dataset (BMDS), with 26 video sequences. The dataset includes persons, cars and other objects, and various degrees of motion. Our proposed MAHIS is evaluated against HIS of [1] at the provided ground truth frames.

We use the established evaluation metrics for HIS, for which benchmark code is publicly available [1]. The evaluation considers both boundaries and regions. The former are benchmarked using precision-recall. The latter are evaluated with three metrics: segmentation covering (SC) the degree of overlap between the ground truth and the machine segmentation; probabilistic rand index (PRI) the fraction of pairs of pixels consistently labelled; variation of information (VI) the distance between segmentations in term of mutual information and conditional entropy. For all metrics the optimal dataset scale (ODS) and optimal segmentation scale (OSS - namely OIS in [1]) are reported: best aggregated performance over the dataset for a fixed scale and for the best scale for each segmentation. Additionally the benchmark reports average precision (AP) for boundaries and Best for region SC, i.e. best selection of segments across scales.

Table 1(first part) illustrates the results: our proposed MAHIS outperforms [1] on most metrics. An improvement on the region metrics is desirable when extracting superpixels so as not to span multiple objects. An improvement in the boundary metric is also desirable so that superpixels on different objects are better separated. Most notably, the boundary ODS and OIS score outperform [1] by about 17%, our AP improves by 28%. These results clearly shows the potential of our proposed MAHIS for the extraction of superpixels for VS.

## 5    Superpixel Affinities for Video Segmentation

As discussed in sec. 3 the first step of our method extracts superpixels (sec. 4) and the second step uses within- and between-frame superpixel affinities to derive the final video segmentation result. This section motivates and introduces various affinities that are analyzed in sec. 6 alone and in combination.

There are two major dimensions that we explore in this paper to define affinities. The first dimension is the type of information used to calculate affinities. We use appearance (based e.g. on color, brightness, and texture) as well as motion and spatial overlap of superpixels in successive frames. The second dimension is time or the number of frames considered to calculate affinities. Besides within a single frame, one can also use affinities calculated across neighboring frames or even across a potentially large number of frames. Intuitively, affinities connecting superpixels across many frames may enable good video segmentation performance. However, in general, affinity matrices should be sparse to allow computationally viable eigendecompositions of the graph Laplacian.

Fig. 3 illustrates samples for four of the six affinity matrices introduced below. Superpixels are ordered with an increasing index, according to their top-down left-right position in the frame and to their frame. Dashed lines delineate the frame partitioning. Terms on the block diagonal correspond to within-frame

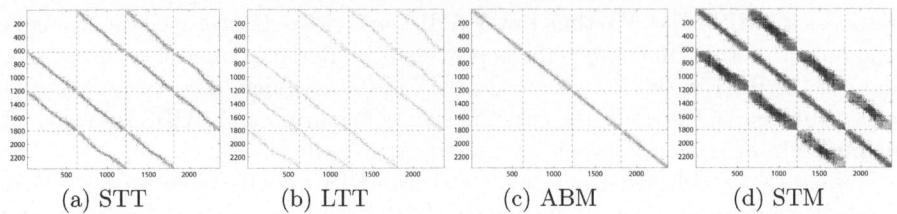

|   | (a) STT | (b) LTT | (c) ABM | (d) STM |

**Fig. 3.** Affinity matrices for 5 frames of sequence Marple1. Non-zero terms are colored blue to red. Note the different structure and sparsity of the affinity matrices. Affinity ABA has a similar structure as ABM and STA has a similar structure as STM.

affinities (e.g. ABM, fig. 3(c)) and terms off the block-diagonal correspond to between-frame affinities (e.g. STT and LTT, fig. 3(a,b)). In the following, affinity terms are grouped into three categories: between-frame, within-frame, and combined between- and within-frame affinities.

## 5.1   Between-Frame Affinities

The first two affinities measure the spatial overlap of superpixels in different frames. The first measure – STT – is taken from [12] that used it in the context of video-object segmentation. As STT is restricted to neighboring frames we define a new overlap term building on long-term point-trajectories [29].

**Short-Term-Temporal Affinity – STT.** [12] measures the similarity of superpixels by propagating the binary support mask of a superpixel with optical flow to neighboring frames and measuring their overlap by the Dice measure. Given superpixel $p^i_f$ at frame $f$ with binary mask $m_{p^i_f}$, and superpixel $p^j_{f'}$ at frame $f' = f \pm 1, 2$ with mask $m_{p^j_{f'}}$, the STT affinity score $w^{stt}_{p^i_f, p^j_{f'}}$ is given by:

$$w^{stt}_{p^i_f, p^j_{f'}} = \frac{2|m^{f'}_{p^i_f} \cap m_{p^j_{f'}}|}{|m^{f'}_{p^i_f}| + |m_{p^j_{f'}}|} \tag{2}$$

where $m^{f'}_{p^i_f}$ indicates the propagated mask of superpixel $p^i_f$ to frame $f'$.

**Long-Term-Temporal Affinity – LTT.** In order to calculate superpixel affinities across many frames that are potentially hundreds of frames apart we leverage on the recently introduced long-term point trajectories of [29]. Let $\Phi_{p^i_f} \subseteq \Upsilon = \{T^i\}_{i=1}^Q$ be a subset of all trajectories, containing those trajectories $T^i$ intersecting superpixel $p^i_f$. We define the LTT affinity score $w^{ltt}$ between superpixels $p^i_f$ and $p^j_{f'}$, $f' = f + N, N \neq 0$ to be the Dice coefficient between the intersection sets $\Phi_{p^i_f}$ and $\Phi_{p^j_{f'}}$ of the superpixels:

$$w^{ltt}_{p^i_f, p^j_{f'}} = \frac{2|\Phi_{p^i_f} \cap \Phi_{p^j_{f'}}|}{|\Phi_{p^i_f}| + |\Phi_{p^j_{f'}}|} \tag{3}$$

Figs. 3(a,b) illustrate the LTT and STT affinities. While both measure spatial overlap of superpixels there are two major differences. By design, LTT allows to calculate affinities between frames that can be hundreds of frames apart, due to the long-term nature of the point trajectories. However, since not all superpixels contain point trajectories, the LTT affinity matrix is much sparser than the STT matrix, although this only calculates affinities between superpixels in neighboring frames (in practice $\pm 2$ frames are used).

## 5.2   Within- and Between-Frame Affinities

One way to measure similarities between pixels across frames are spatiotemporal affinities based on appearance and/or motion [3, 17]. In order to overcome the computational complexity related to measuring pixel-affinities, [11] proposed to measure spatiotemporal affinities between superpixels instead. The first measure defined below – STA – is directly related to [11] and measures the appearance affinity. The second term – STM – focuses on the motion affinity of superpixels.

**Spatio-Temporal-Appearance Affinity – STA.** To score the appearance affinity we use the median brightness and color $\overline{Lab}_{p_f^i}$ of a superpixel $p_f^i$ using CIE Lab color space. The STA affinity between pairs of superpixels $p_f^i$ and $p_{f'}^j$ in a spatiotemporal neighborhood ($\pm 1$ frame, 2-layered neighborhood) is therefore:

$$w_{p_f^i, p_{f'}^j}^{sta} = \exp\left\{-\lambda_{sta} ||\overline{Lab}_{p_f^i} - \overline{Lab}_{p_{f'}^j}||\right\} \tag{4}$$

The affinity is inspired by [11]. More elaborate extensions use the $\chi^2$ distance between appearance histograms for video segmentation [15, 16].

**Spatio-Temporal-Motion Affinity – STM.** This term calculates affinities based on motion to allow grouping of superpixels of the same moving objects. Given the median optical flow $\overline{\mathbf{u}}_{p_f^i}$ of a superpixel $p_f^i$ the STM affinities $w^{stm}$ are calculated between superpixels $p_f^i$ and $p_{f'}^j$ in a spatio-temporal neighborhood ($\pm 1$ frames, 2-layered neighborhood) as:

$$w_{p_f^i, p_{f'}^j}^{stm} = \exp\left\{-\lambda_{stm} ||\overline{\mathbf{u}}_{p_f^i} - \overline{\mathbf{u}}_{p_{f'}^j}||^2\right\} \tag{5}$$

The STM affinity has been employed in numerous works for video segmentation [3], or in combination with an STA affinity [17]. These works use STM affinities between pixels, here we use it for superpixels.

## 5.3   Within-Frame Affinities

The terms defined here are complementary to STA and STM in the sense that they focus on the local similarities near the common boundary between superpixels rather than the median appearance and motion of the superpixels. The appearance based term – ABA – directly uses the contour maps of our MAHIS (sec. 4). The motion based term – ABM – is one of two terms used for occlusion boundary detection in [26].

**Across-Boundary-Appearance Affinity – ABA.** Motivated by the success of the HIS-algorithm [1] for hierarchical segmentation we propose to measure appearance affinity using our improved MAHIS algorithm. We define the affinity $w^{aba}$ between pairs of neighboring superpixels $p_f^i$ and $p_f^j$ as the average value $\bar{v}_f^{ij}$ of the ultrametric contour map (see fig. 1 for a ultrametric contour map) along the common boundary of the superpixels:

$$w_{p_f^i,p_f^j}^{aba} = \bar{v}_f^{ij} \tag{6}$$

**Across-Boundary-Motion Affinity – ABM.** While STM measures the similarity of the median motion of two superpixels, ABM measures the local similarity of motion along the common boundary of two superpixels. This measure allows to connect superpixels e.g. in the case of non-rigid motions where the median motion of the superpixels can be quite different but the motion on both sides of the common boundary between superpixels might be similar. We consider $\bar{\mathbf{u}}^f(\mathbf{x})$, a dense optical flow field [28], locally median filtered (first temporally ($\pm 2$ frames), then spatially (3 px radius within the superpixel)). Given $\Psi_f^{ij}$ the set of pixel pairs on opposite sides across the common boundary between $p_f^i$ and $p_f^j$, the ABM affinity $w^{abm}$ is defined as:

$$w_{p_f^i,p_f^j}^{abm} = \exp\left\{ -\lambda_{abm} \frac{\sum_{(\mathbf{x}_i^m,\mathbf{x}_j^m)\in\Psi_f^{ij}} ||\bar{\mathbf{u}}^f(\mathbf{x}_i^m) - \bar{\mathbf{u}}^f(\mathbf{x}_j^m)||^2}{|\Psi_f^{ij}|} \right\} \tag{7}$$

The ABM affinity has been proposed for occlusion boundary detection in [26], in combination with an affinity similar to ABA.

## 6   Experimental Validation

The VS literature does not yet provide a common benchmark or evaluation metric that is agreed upon and widely used such as the Berkeley image segmentation benchmark. Some work [15] only provide a qualitative evaluation, others introduce datasets and metrics [2, 11, 12], but few compare on a common dataset [2, 12, 23]. Here we use BMDS [2] (see also sec. 4.2), because it is a publicly available, of reasonable complexity and various papers show results for this dataset [2, 12, 23]. Following [11, 12], we perform dense clustering of the video sequences, and restrict the sequences to the first 100 frames. For each setting, we vary the number of clusters, in the range [1,600]. We assign each video segment to a ground truth label based on maximal region overlap, and score performance by global and average (over each ground truth frame) per-pixel labeling error, i.e. fraction of misclassified pixels. Note that the global per-pixel error is dominated by the large segments in the scene (often the background) and that the average error weights all ground-truth segments equally.

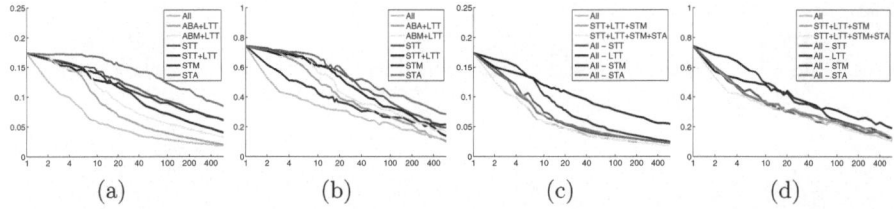

(a)                     (b)                     (c)                     (d)

**Fig. 4.** (a) Global and (b) average error curves comparing All combined affinities against the individual terms; (c) global and (d) average error curves comparing All against All minus one term. Please note the different scaling of the $y$-axis for (a,c). Curves are evaluated on BMDS [2]. We conclude from (c,d) that LTT and STM are most contributing to the VS performance and that the combination STT+LTT+STM+STA (green curve) equals the performance of All (cyan).

Fig. 4 presents the results: first we evaluate the performance of individual affinities to identify those contributing the most to VS, and then we aim to determine the minimal set providing best overall performance. The first two plots illustrate the performances of individual affinities and compare them to the overall best performance when using all affinities. Since ABA and ABM are within-frame affinities only we pair them with LTT to analyze their 'individual' performance, since LTT relates some superpixels only, it is paired with STT. Overall, the lowest error is obtained by all combined affinities (All, cyan, fig. 4(a,b)). As for the average error (fig. 4(b)), STM (blue) is the single best, followed by ABA+LTT (green) and ABM+LTT (yellow). STT+LTT (black) and STT (red) are slightly worse and the weakest affinity is STA (magenta). The ordering is nearly identical for the global error (fig. 4(a)) with the exception of ABA+LTT being best (green) and STM being one of the weaker overall (blue). While it can be concluded that STA does not perform well, none of the other affinities stands out to be better than any other.

The second two plots in fig. 4 reveal more insights into which of the affinities are essential to obtain the overall best performance when combined. For this we compare the performance of All (cyan) when taking out individual affinities, namely STM (All-STM, blue), LTT (All-LTT, black), STT (All-STT, red) and STA (All-STA, magenta). Note the significant drop in performance for the first two, All-STM(blue) and All-LTT(black), both for the global (fig. 4(c)) and the average error (fig. 4(d)). A less significant drop is observed for All-STT(red) and All-STA(magenta), while the performance is not altered when taking out the boundary affinities ABM and ABA (not reported due to space constraints). The performance of STT+LTT+STM+STA(yellow) nearly superposes All(cyan), therefore barely visible, while the performance drops slightly for STT+LTT+STM(green). Boundary terms surprisingly do not improve performance for VS, while they turned out useful to improve HIS [26].

These quantitative results are supported by qualitative results. Fig. 5 illustrates segmentation results when extracting 10 objects (i.e. clusters) from the video sequences Cars6 and People1. It shows (*column-wise*) All terms, the minimal best set STT+LTT+STM+STA, the temporal terms STT+LTT, the individual best

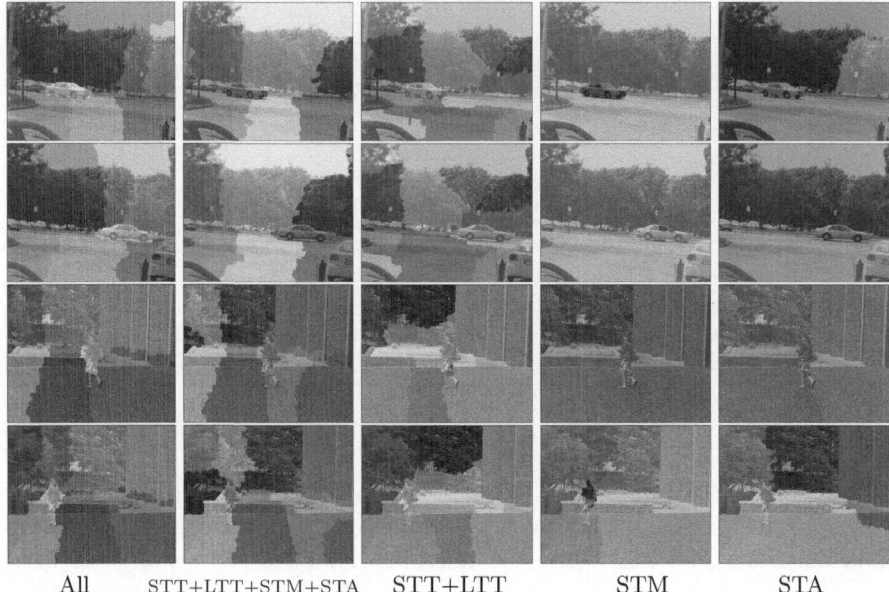

All     STT+LTT+STM+STA     STT+LTT     STM     STA

**Fig. 5.** 10-cluster video segmentations extracted from the video sequences Cars6 (*top two rows*) and People1 (*bottom two rows*). STT+LTT+STM+STA provides the same qualitative result as All affinities. STT+LTT: please note the "drag" effects generated by the imprecise optical flow at the contours of the moving objects. STM: the affinity gets more effective where the motion is larger, which makes STM the perfect complement to STT+LTT. STA: clusters are denoted by strong color differences. Although performing poorly, the term supplements the three motion affinities effectively.

performer STM, and the appearance term STA. As expected from the error metric All and STT+LTT+STM+STA provide the same qualitative results (while the random colors are different, the segmentation results are nearly identical). Temporal terms STT+LTT successfully track the image parts but suffer from "drag" effects in cases of large motion and imprecise optical flow. By contrast, STM addresses the moving objects, and employs the 10 object "allowance" to neatly segment them from the background. The appearance term STA segments the scene according to the strongest color differences. As from the numerical results, STT+LTT and STM are complementary motion terms, which are supplemented by STA, although the latter alone has a poor segmentation performance.

Finally, fig. 6 illustrates the use of our algorithm to extract a minimal number of clusters, as for obtaining object cut-outs. The figure also discusses some typical failure cases.

Next we discuss how we might obtain a commonly agreed upon evaluation metric. We believe that a cause for the lack of an established evaluation metric is mainly twofold: i) no standard format is given to write a segmentation output, i.e. the benchmark of [2] requires a conversion of the labelled video into point trajectories for evaluation; ii) the aspects of coarse-to-fine and over-segmentation

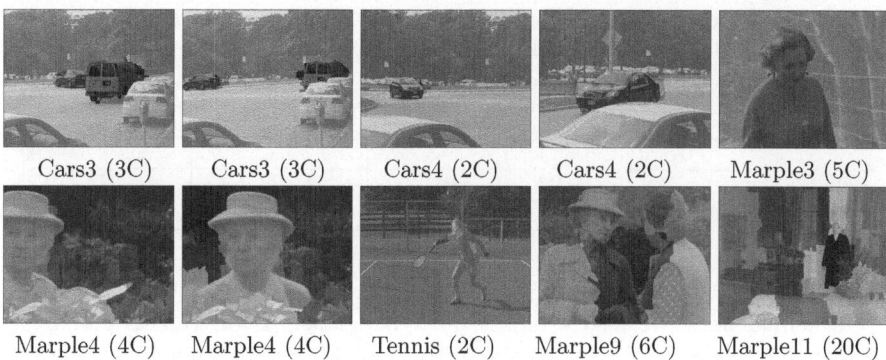

Cars3 (3C)     Cars3 (3C)     Cars4 (2C)     Cars4 (2C)     Marple3 (5C)

Marple4 (4C)   Marple4 (4C)   Tennis (2C)    Marple9 (6C)   Marple11 (20C)

**Fig. 6.** Video segmentations provided with a minimal number of clusters (C). The algorithm successfully segments objects in the first five examples. Marple9 and Marple11 are failure cases. Marple9: the right actress moves little, so it is wrongly segmented due to the misleading appearance differences; the left actress, also minimally moving, rotates the head but the motion is too small. Marple11: the person is not segmented even with 20 clusters, as he does not move and the scene boundaries are prevalent.

are not clearly addressed, i.e. the "right" video segmentation and number of clusters usually depends on the task, and may vary for the same video sequence.

These problems however have already been addressed for HIS [1], so that we propose to extend those established metrics to VS. We employ the same metrics as described in sec. 4.2, namely precision-recall for boundaries and SC, PRI and VI for regions, aggregating performance optimally for a fixed dataset scale (ODS) and for the best (video) segmentation scale (OSS). The extended benchmark uses video (spatio-temporal) segments, which it evaluates against all the ground truth frames altogether over the video sequence, thus addressing temporal consistency. The benchmark allows for evaluating coarse-to-fine VS on multiple ground truths, as for evaluating more general VS, without a specific defined task. We define the coarse-to-fine VS levels by varying the number of clusters in the range [1,600].

We evaluate the extended benchmark metrics on all BMDS videos, and report the results in table 1(second part) for the same setups of affinities as in fig. 4. These results confirm most findings of fig. 4: ABA+LTT and ABM+LTT are single best performers for the region evaluation, while the single best boundaries are provided by STM. On both boundary and region metrics, STT+LTT+STM+STA provides the same performance as All, while removing ABA and ABM from All does not alter performance. Interestingly, the best VS results (VS:All and VS:STT+LTT+STM+STA) are comparable to the best IS (MAHIS) on boundary metrics but neatly superior on region metrics, notwithstanding the additional temporal consistency constraint. This confirms the importance to consider segmentation as a spatio-temporal problem.

In table 1(third part), we also compare our VS with the algorithm of [15] (as implemented by [30]), which we outperform by ∼12% on regions and ∼80% on boundaries.

**Table 2.** Comparison with [2] on BMDS according to the benchmark of [2]. Both our 10-cluster (k=10) and 20-cluster (k=20) video segmentations are comparable in error to [2]. Notably we provide 100% density.

|  | Density | Overall error | Average error | Over-segmentation | Extracted objects |
|---|---|---|---|---|---|
| Our VS (k=10) | 100 | 9.92 | 16.52 | 6.77 | 17 |
| Our VS (k=20) | 100 | 5.84 | 15.20 | 16.27 | 18 |
| Method of [2] | 3.30 | 3.93 | 23.83 | 0.92 | 29 |

On a final note, we also evaluate our VS against [2] on BMDS employing their evaluation metric. Our average error is much lower although segmenting all pixels (density) rather than just a fraction; the number of extracted objects and overall errors are worse, although better for a larger number of clusters; the over-segmentation index is approximately fixed, given the number of clusters.

## 7    Conclusion and Future Work

We have proposed a model for unsupervised video segmentation based on clustering superpixels. We have analyzed a variety of affinities in isolation and in combination and have identified a minimal set that obtains best performance. While the use of superpixels necessarily results in an approximation we have shown that powerful affinity scores can be defined based on them and that good video segmentation performance can be obtained. A second contribution of the paper is the motion aware hierarchical image segmentation algorithm that is a direct extension of [1] to also include motion features improving their approach for image sequences. Finally, we have extended an established image segmentation benchmark to videos. We used it to evaluate our algorithm under different setups and to compare with a state-of-the-art algorithm [15]. The extended benchmark allows evaluating coarse-to-fine segmentations on multiple human ground truth annotations, although these are not yet provided by any video dataset.

## References

1. Arbelaez, P., Maire, M., Fowlkes, C., Malik, J.: From contours to regions: An empirical evaluation. In: CVPR (2009)
2. Brox, T., Malik, J.: Object Segmentation by Long Term Analysis of Point Trajectories. In: Daniilidis, K., Maragos, P., Paragios, N. (eds.) ECCV 2010, Part V. LNCS, vol. 6315, pp. 282–295. Springer, Heidelberg (2010)
3. Shi, J., Malik, J.: Normalized cuts and image segmentation. TPAMI (2000)
4. Comaniciu, D., Meer, P.: Mean shift: A robust approach toward feature space analysis. PAMI 24, 603–619 (2002)
5. Felzenszwalb, P.F., Huttenlocher, D.P.: Efficient graph-based image segmentation. IJCV 59 (2004)
6. Vese, L., Chan, T.: A multiphase level set framework for image segmentation using the mumford and shah model. IJCV 50, 271–293 (2002)

7. Pock, T., Cremers, D., Bischof, H., Chambolle, A.: An algorithm for minimizing the piecewise smooth mumford-shah functional. In: ICCV (2009)
8. Carreira, J., Sminchisescu, C.: Constrained parametric min-cuts for automatic object segmentation. In: CVPR (2010)
9. Endres, I., Hoiem, D.: Category Independent Object Proposals. In: Daniilidis, K., Maragos, P., Paragios, N. (eds.) ECCV 2010, Part V. LNCS, vol. 6315, pp. 575–588. Springer, Heidelberg (2010)
10. Levinshtein, A., Sminchisescu, C., Dickinson, S.: Spatiotemporal Closure. In: Kimmel, R., Klette, R., Sugimoto, A. (eds.) ACCV 2010, Part I. LNCS, vol. 6492, pp. 369–382. Springer, Heidelberg (2011)
11. Vazquez-Reina, A., Avidan, S., Pfister, H., Miller, E.: Multiple Hypothesis Video Segmentation from Superpixel Flows. In: Daniilidis, K., Maragos, P., Paragios, N. (eds.) ECCV 2010, Part V. LNCS, vol. 6315, pp. 268–281. Springer, Heidelberg (2010)
12. Galasso, F., Iwasaki, M., Nobori, K., Cipolla, R.: Spatio-temporal clustering of probabilistic region trajectories. In: ICCV (2011)
13. Cheng, H.T., Ahuja, N.: Exploiting nonlocal spatiotemporal structure for video segmentation. In: CVPR (2012)
14. Brendel, W., Todorovic, S.: Video object segmentation by tracking regions. In: ICCV (2009)
15. Grundmann, M., Kwatra, V., Han, M., Essa, I.: Efficient hierarchical graph-based video segmentation. In: CVPR (2010)
16. Lezama, J., Alahari, K., Sivic, J., Laptev, I.: Track to the future: Spatio-temporal video segmentation with long-range motion cues. In: CVPR (2011)
17. DeMenthon, D.: Spatio-temporal segmentation of video by hierarchical mean shift analysis. In: Statistical Methods in Video Processing Workshop (2002)
18. Greenspan, H., Goldberger, J., Mayer, A.: A Probabilistic Framework for Spatio-Temporal Video Representation amp Indexing. In: Heyden, A., Sparr, G., Nielsen, M., Johansen, P. (eds.) ECCV 2002, Part IV. LNCS, vol. 2353, pp. 461–475. Springer, Heidelberg (2002)
19. Kannan, A., Jojic, N., Frey, B.J.: Generative model for layers of appearance and deformation. In: AISTATS (2005)
20. Kumar, M.P., Torr, P., Zisserman, A.: Learning layered motion segmentations of video. IJCV 76, 301–319 (2008)
21. Paris, S.: Edge-Preserving Smoothing and Mean-Shift Segmentation of Video Streams. In: Forsyth, D., Torr, P., Zisserman, A. (eds.) ECCV 2008, Part II. LNCS, vol. 5303, pp. 460–473. Springer, Heidelberg (2008)
22. Lee, Y.J., Kim, J., Grauman, K.: Key-segments for video object segmentation. In: ICCV (2011)
23. Ochs, P., Brox, T.: Object segmentation in video: a hierarchical variational approach for turning point trajectories into dense regions. In: ICCV (2011)
24. Brostow, G.J., Cipolla, R.: Unsupervised bayesian detection of independent motion in crowds. In: CVPR (2006)
25. Sugimura, D., Kitani, K.M., Okabe, T., Sato, Y., Sugimoto, A.: Using individuality to track individuals: clustering individual trajectories in crowds using local appearance and frequency trait. In: ICCV (2009)
26. Sundberg, P., Brox, T., Maire, M., Arbelaez, P., Malik, J.: Occlusion boundary detection and figure/ground assignment from optical flow. In: CVPR (2011)
27. Ng, A.Y., Jordan, M.I., Weiss, Y.: On spectral clustering: Analysis and an algorithm. In: NIPS (2001)

28. Zach, C., Pock, T., Bischof, H.: A Duality Based Approach for Realtime TV-L$^1$ Optical Flow. In: Hamprecht, F.A., Schnörr, C., Jähne, B. (eds.) DAGM 2007. LNCS, vol. 4713, pp. 214–223. Springer, Heidelberg (2007)
29. Sundaram, N., Brox, T., Keutzer, K.: Dense Point Trajectories by GPU-Accelerated Large Displacement Optical Flow. In: Daniilidis, K., Maragos, P., Paragios, N. (eds.) ECCV 2010, Part I. LNCS, vol. 6311, pp. 438–451. Springer, Heidelberg (2010)
30. Xu, C., Corso, J.J.: Evaluation of super-voxel methods for early video processing. In: CVPR (2012)

# A Noise Tolerant Watershed Transformation with Viscous Force for Seeded Image Segmentation

Di Yang, Stephen Gould, and Marcus Hutter

Research School of Computer Science,
The Australian National University

**Abstract.** The watershed transform was proposed as a novel method for image segmentation over 30 years ago. Today it is still used as an elementary step in many powerful segmentation procedures. The watershed transform constitutes one of the main concepts of mathematical morphology as an important region-based image segmentation approach. However, the original watershed transform is highly sensitive to noise and is incapable of detecting objects with broken edges. Consequently its adoption in domains where imaging is subject to high noise is limited. By incorporating a high-order energy term into the original watershed transform, we proposed the viscous force watershed transform, which is more immune to noise and able to detect objects with broken edges.

## 1   Introduction

Image segmentation for identification of homogeneous regions in an image has been the subject of considerable research activities over the last three decades. Here, segmentation refers to the process of partitioning a digital image into multiple contiguous regions (sets of pixels, also known as super-pixels). Such representations, over regions rather than individual pixels, may be more meaningful and easier to analyse. For example, image segmentation can be used as a pre-processing step for locate objects in images. More formally, image segmentation can be thought of as the process of assigning a label to every pixel in an image such that pixels with the same label share certain visual characteristics and belong to the same region. Boundaries between regions are defined whenever neighbouring pixels differ in their assigned labels.

Most image segmentation approaches can be divided into two classes, namely region-based and edge-based. One of the earliest prototypes for region-based segmentation is the Mumford-Shah functional [1, 2], whose piecewise formulation is a spatially contiguous generalization of the Ising model [3]. Inspired by mean intensities employed in the Mumford-Shah functional, graph-based algorithms have been developed where globally optimal solutions (with respect to an energy function) can be obtained (e.g., graph-cuts [4] and watershed algorithms [5]). Other approaches, such as region-based level-sets (e.g., [1]), are similar but global optima cannot, in general, be guaranteed.

K.M. Lee et al. (Eds.): ACCV 2012, Part I, LNCS 7724, pp. 775–789, 2013.
© Springer-Verlag Berlin Heidelberg 2013

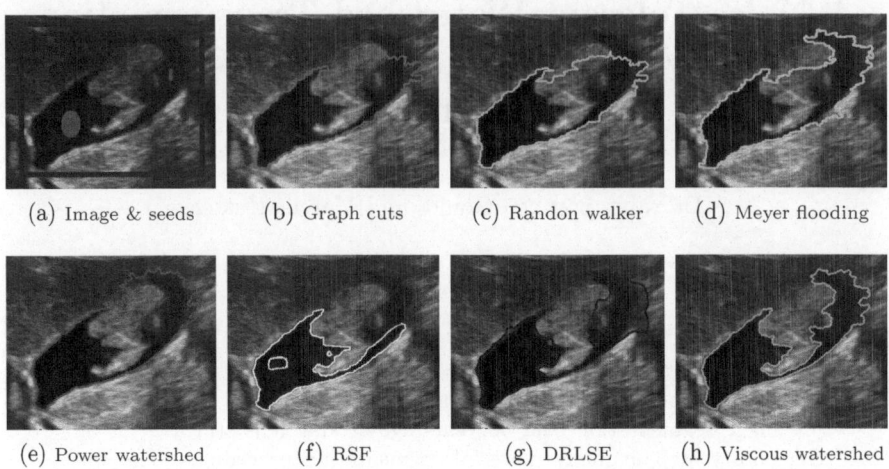

(a) Image & seeds          (b) Graph cuts          (c) Randon walker          (d) Meyer flooding

(e) Power watershed          (f) RSF          (g) DRLSE          (h) Viscous watershed

**Fig. 1.** Ultrasonic image segmentation: (a) Gallbladder sludge ultrasonic image with predefined seeds (from http://www.ultrasound-images.com). Results produced by various algorithms: (b) Graph cuts; (c) Random walker [10]; (d) Meyer flooding [11]; (e) Power watershed [12]; (f) Region scalable level-sets (RSF) [2]; (g) Distance regularized level-sets evolution (DRLSE) [13]; (h) Our viscous watershed.

Edge-based approaches often adopt line integrals along proposed boundaries to score segmentations. The Snakes active contour model [6] is an early example of this approach. Here, curvature and length constraints are encoded as regularity terms into the integration of squared image gradients. Some variational variants [7] successfully incorporate gradient vector flow energy into the integral to enhance robustness. Level-set methods [8] define a powerful curve propagation scheme which has been proposed as replacement to the arc-length function [9] in active contour models for curve evolution. Unfortunately the quality of solutions from these approaches rely on difficult to tune parameters which are image specific.

Watershed image segmentation was originally proposed by Digable and Lantuejoul [5], and later improved by Beucher and Lantuejoul [14]. The method has been demonstrated as a powerful, non-parametric and fast technique for region-based segmentation. In particular, watershed-based algorithms are widely used in image segmentation because of their efficiency and accuracy when applied to high-quality images. However, the watershed transformation suffers from poor robustness that results in significant fluctuations of the segmentation when contours are blurred or images are noisy. Moreover, the watershed transformation cannot find the outlines of objects with broken edges. Consequently, leaks and degeneracy may occur in results from watershed image segmentation (and indeed, other seeded image segmentation techniques). Figure 1, for example, highlights the failures of a number of segmentation algorithms on a low-quality image, whereas the performance of our algorithm is significantly better.

In this paper, we propose a new method that can significantly improve the robustness of the watershed transformation by incorporating a high-order energy term (that we designate *viscous force*). Our viscous force watershed transformation has two main advantages over the original watershed transformation:

1. Our high-order energy term can dramatically enhance the robustness of the watershed transformation thereby making it more tolerant to noise and other forms of image corruption.
2. Our viscous force watershed transformation can extract the contour of objects with broken edges, which is not possible using the conventional watershed transformation.

Importantly, our method retains the key strengths of the original watershed transform—it is simple and fast. This makes our method of particular relevance to application domains requiring segmentation of low-quality images (e.g. medical ultrasonic images as shown in Figure 1).

## 2    Background and Related Work

The essential idea behind the watershed transformation can be understood from a geographic analogy: We consider a grey-scale image as a topographic relief where the intensity of a pixel is represented by the height of the relief. When a drop of water falls on a topographic relief, it moves downhill coming to rest within a local basin. By filling the topographic relief with water up to the point where water from different local basins meet we can identify so-called watershed lines. As a result, the landscape (or image) is partitioned into regions separated by the watershed lines.

Despite its simplicity, the watershed transform suffers from several problems. Primary amongst these is its high sensitivity to variations in the image gradient resulting in significant over-segmentation of the image. To solve this problem, marker-based approaches have been proposed within the watershed framework (e.g., optimal spanning forest [15] or Meyer's flooding [11]). Here markers (or seeds) may be interactively placed by users or found automatically using prior information to constrain the segmentation of the image into desired regions.

The most recent marker-based watershed image segmentation method is the power watershed method [12], which casts the watershed algorithm as an energy minimisation problem. As a consequence the method unifies various marker-based image segmentation algorithms such as graph-cuts, random walker and shortest path optimisation algorithms. This is achieved by replacing the objective in the traditional watershed method with a pairwise energy terms, which, to some extent, can partially improve robustness. However, without introducing high-order energy terms, the power watershed method is still unable handle low quality images or images corrupted by noise.

To address the problem of image corruption, Meyer [16, 17] proposed the concept of viscous flooding. The idea of viscous flooding was inspired by morphological operations and geometrical constraints, and can be incorporated into the watershed segmentation algorithm in two different ways. The first, proposed by Meyer [16, 17], is to simulate a viscous fluid in the watershed line construction via the opening morphological operation. Here the magnitude of viscous force only depends on the radius of the morphological operation rather than neighbourhood intensity changes in the image.

The second method for incorporating viscous flooding into the watershed transformation is via the topological relief regularisation [18]. The essence of this approach is still based on morphological opening. However, the aim is to regularise topographic relief directly with a morphological operation rather than simulating the viscous fluid flooding as in the first approach [16]. Unlike these approaches, our method directly connects neighbouring intensity changes to the magnitude of the viscous force.

Edge-based image segmentation algorithms tackle the problem from a different perspective. Many of these algorithms are based on the level-sets method [8], which evolves a contour to segment regions from a rough initial boundary. The most recent level-sets method is the distance regularised level set evolution algorithm (DRLSE) [13]. However, level-sets are not limited to edge-based algorithms. The approach can also be extended to region-based segmentation (e.g., [1]). The most recent level-sets approach belonging to this category is the region scalable fitting level set (RSF) algorithm [2]. In both of these approaches, however, level-sets methods can not guarantee the globally optimal result.

All of the methods described above may be considered as addressing energies or external forces comprised of only unary and pairwise terms. Watershed segmentations (Power watershed or Viscous watershed) only consider the low order terms (e.g., opened sets). However, recent literature has found that the addition of external force defined with higher order terms can help improve performance in a variety of tasks [19, 20]. Although, level-set methods address image segmentation as energies and external forces comprised through pairwise terms, they failed to find the globally optimal result in most cases.

In this work, we propose a specific high-order term, which we call viscous force. By incorporating this term, we are able to address the drawbacks of previous approaches in dealing with noisy or corrupted images. Moreover, unlike the existing viscous watershed, our viscous force models neighbourhood intensity changes resulting in more precise and reliable segmentations.

## 3   Viscous Force into the Watershed Transformation

We begin our exposition by reviewing the fundamentals of the watershed transformation [11]. We then present our high-order viscous force term and show how it improves the segmentation accuracy and robustness without sacrificing the performance even under low-quality imaging scenarios. We examine special cases of this algorithm in the context of noisy images and images with missing boundaries.

We will consider a finite grid of pixels. We embed the set of pixels within an undirected graph, where the graph $D = (V, E)$ consists of a set $V = \{1, 2, \cdots, n\}$

of vertices (or nodes) denoting the pixels and a set $E \subseteq V \times V$ of pairs of vertices defining the connectivity structure, usually 4-connectivity or 8-connectivity. The set E consists of unordered pairs of nodes $(p, q)$ called an edge. In a weighted graph, a non-negative scalar (weight) is associated with each edge $(p, q) \in E$ in the graph. We can now define a digital greyscale image as a 3-tuple $D = (V, E, W(\cdot))$, where $(V, E)$ is a grid structured graph and $W(\cdot)$ is an edge weight function $W(p, q)$.

For many seeded image segmentation algorithms, the edge weights are determined by image intensity changes. One common format used by the graph-cuts and random walker segmentation algorithms is to set

$$W(p, q) = \exp(-\beta [I(p) - I(q)]^2), \tag{1}$$

where $I(p)$ is the image intensity at node (pixel) $p$. However, a special topographic relief function $W(\cdot) = T_f(\cdot)$ (mentioned later) will be employed in watershed segmentation.

Then, image segmentation proceeds to label each node (pixel) $p$ with a label from a fixed set $C = \{c_1, c_2, \cdots, c_n\}$ according to its corresponding edge weights. We first label some of the nodes (pixels) with these labels and treat them as seeds. Then the seeded image segmentation for producing a segmentation is to solve the problem [10, 12, 21]

$$\underset{x}{\arg\min} \quad \sum_{(p, q) \in E} W(p, q) [\![x_p - x_q]\!] \tag{2}$$
$$\text{subject to} \quad x(c_1) = 1, \ x(c_2) = 2, \cdots, \ x(c_n) = n$$

where $x_p$ denotes the unknown label of node (pixel) $p$. After establishing a function for the seeded image segmentation, there are some optimisation methods to search for the minima, for example region scalable level set (RSF) [2], graph cuts [4] and watershed algorithms [16].

As demonstrated in Figure 1, the above seeded image segmentation algorithms, associated with different optimisation methods, are unable to produce satisfactory segmentation results under low quality imaging. In other words, no mater what kind of optimisation method is employed by the seeded image segmentation, leaks and degeneracy frequently occur in the results under low quality imaging. That means the problem lies in the objective function rather than optimisation method. Thus, in this paper, we will incorporate a viscous force into the weight function, in order to produce a better weighted graph for segmentation.

## 3.1   Review of Watershed Transformation

We now describe how watershed segmentation simulates the fluid flooding and finds the watershed lines based on the established topographic relief.

Let the topographic relief $f(\cdot) \rightarrow [0, 255]$ have minima $\{m_k\}_{k \in K}$, shown in Figure 2 (a), for some index set $K \subseteq V$. The catchment basin $CB(m_i)$ of a

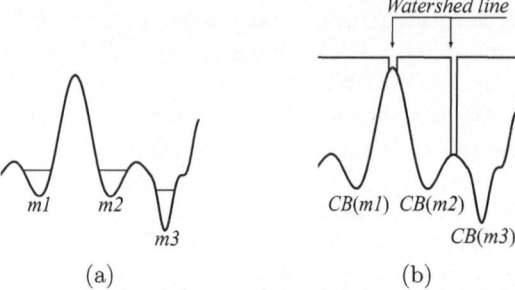

**Fig. 2.** Diagrams of minima, catchment basin and watershed line. From left to right: (a) Local minima of relief; (b) Yielded catchment basins and corresponding watershed lines.

minimum $m_i$ is defined as the set of nodes (pixels) $p \in V\backslash K$, which are topographically closer to $m_k$ with topographic distance $T_f(p, m_k)$ than to any other regional minimum $m_l$ with $T_f(p, m_l)$ (see Figure 2 (b)):

$$\mathrm{CB}(m_k) = \{p \in \mathrm{V}, k \in \mathrm{K} \mid \forall l \in \mathrm{K}\backslash\{k\} : f(m_k)+T_f(p, m_k) < f(m_l)+T_f(p, m_l)\}. \quad (3)$$

In an infinite graph, the watershed line of $f$ is the set of pixels that specify the boundaries between regions. Formally the watershed line is defined as the set of pixels that does not belong to any catchment basin (see Figure 2 (b)):

$$\mathrm{Wshed}(f) = \mathrm{V} \setminus \left[ \bigcup_{k \in \mathrm{K}} \mathrm{CB}(m_k) \right]. \quad (4)$$

Let Wshed denote the label for the watershed line — Wshed $\notin$ K. The watershed transform of $f$ is a mapping $\lambda : \mathrm{V} \to \mathrm{K} \cup \{\mathrm{Wshed}\}$, such that $\lambda(p) = k$ if $p \in \mathrm{CB}(m_k)$, and $\lambda(p) = \mathrm{W}$ if $p \in \mathrm{Wshed}(f)$. So the watershed transform of $f$ assigns labels to the points of V, such that different catchment basins are uniquely labelled, and a special label W is assigned to all points on the watershed line.

Initially, we assume that the image $I$ is lower complete; that means each pixel which is not in a minimum has a neighbour with a lower grey value. A plateau situation will be discussed later. The gradient magnitude $\|\nabla I(p)\|$ of $I$ at a pixel $p$ could be used to describe the topographic distance. But, in practice, the lower slope $LS(p)$ is actually calculated as the topographic distance due to computational efficiency. It is defined as the maximal slope linking $p$ to any of its neighbour of lower altitudes. Formally,

$$LS(p) = \max_{q \in N_G(p)} \left( \frac{I(p) - I(q)}{d(p, q)} \right), \quad (5)$$

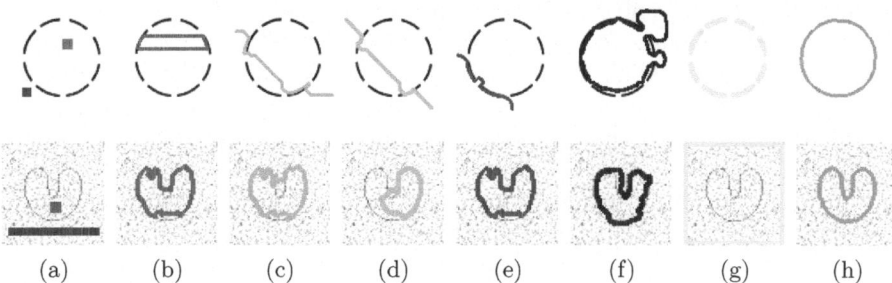

**Fig. 3.** Illustration of segmentations using predefined seeds in synthetic broken boundary and noise scenarios. (a) Image with seeds; (b - h) Segmentation results are yielded by Graph cuts, Random walker, Meyer flooding, Power watershed, DRLSE, RSF, and viscous force watershed, respectively. See text for details.

where $N_G(p)$ is the set of neighbours of the node (pixel) $p$ of the grid $D = (V, E)$, and $d(p, q)$ is the Manhattan distance between nodes (pixels) $p$ and $q$. Then, the topographic distance from $p$ to a neighbouring node $q$ is defined as

$$T_f(\nu_p, \nu_q) = \begin{cases} LS(p) \cdot d(p,q), & \text{if } I(p) > I(q) \\ LS(q) \cdot d(p,q), & \text{if } I(p) < I(q) \\ \frac{1}{2}(LS(p) + LS(q)) \cdot d(p,q), & \text{if } I(p) = I(q). \end{cases} \quad (6)$$

The topographical distance along a path $\pi = (p_0, \ldots, p_l)$ between $p_0 = p$ and $p_l = q$ in V is defined by:

$$T_f^\pi(p, q) = \sum_{i=0}^{l-1} T_f(p_i, p_{i+1}). \quad (7)$$

If an image is not lower complete the topographical distance between the interior pixels of a plateau will be identically zero. Thus, the Manhattan distance to the boundary of the plateau is usually computed instead of the topographic distance in this situation.

### 3.2 Watershed Transformation with Viscous Force

Let $D = (V, E, T_f)$ be a greyscale image. For any pair of vertices $p, q \in V$, consider all paths from $p_0 = p$ to $p_l = q$, whose vertices belong to the path $\pi = (p_0, p_2, \ldots, p_l)$ for which $\pi \subset V$.

Let $T_f^{\pi\star}(p, q)$ be the minimum-weight path among them. If $p_k$ is on the shortest path $T_f^{\pi\star}(p, q)$, then we can break this path into two sub-paths: one from $p$ to $p_k$ as $T_f^\pi(p, p_k)$, the other from $p_k$ to $q$ like $T_f^\pi(p_k, q)$. Then, each vertices $p_i$ on the shortest path $\pi^\star$ would satisfy the following properties:

$$T_f^{\pi\star}(p, q) = \begin{cases} T_f(p, q), & \text{if } (p, q) \in E \\ \arg\min_{p_k \in D, (p_k, q) \in E} \left[ T_f^{\pi\star}(p, p_k) + T_f^{\pi\star}(p_k, q) \right] & \text{otherwise.} \end{cases} \quad (8)$$

However, Equation 8 only considers vertices on the path and ignores other vertices in the neighbourhood. This property yields a weakness in the watershed transform, because "fluid" may leak out from broken edge or be interfered by noisy pixels (see Figure 3). Thus, we introduce a high-order term to the topographic distance calculation, in order to improve robustness of the watershed algorithm.

Intuitively, the idea of our high-order term can be motivated by the averaging the cost of all paths in the neighbourhood of a given path rather than the cost of the path itself. We expect the average path to be more robust to local topographic variations (e.g. broken edges and noise). This energy term presents as follows

$$\hat{T}_f^\pi(p,\, q) = \sum_{i=0}^{l-1} \left\{ T_f(p_i, p_{i+1}) + \frac{1}{2} \left[ \mathrm{VF}(p_i) + \mathrm{VF}(p_{i+1}) \right] \right\}. \tag{9}$$

where $\mathrm{VF}(p)$ is the energy function associated with $p$, which calculates the averaging topographic distance from point $p$ on the path to the other points in the neighbourhood. We define $\mathrm{VF}(p)$:

$$\mathrm{VF}(p) = \frac{1}{C} \ln \left\{ 1 + \sum_{q \in N_G(p)} \left[ 1 - e^{-C \cdot T_f(p,q)} \right] \right\}, \tag{10}$$

where $C$ is a positive constant, which controls the magnitude of the viscous force per pixel. Smaller values of $C$ produce a larger viscous force. In the other words, the viscous force effects vanish for large $C$. In our experiments, we found that setting $C = 0.005$ gives satisfactory results over a large range of images.

The size of the local neighbourhood $N_G(p)$ also affects the strength of the viscous force. When the neighbourhood is too large, the total viscous force may make fluid too thick to detect details of the topographic relief without a proper $C$, and our algorithm tends to over-smooth the image. Additionally, the computational cost of the viscous force depends on the size of this neighbouring set. We found that setting the neighborhood to $3 \times 3$ or $5 \times 5$ usually results in good performance. Then, equation 9 can be efficiently solved by the dynamic program, and Moore-Bellman-Ford algorithm is employed in this paper.

As shown in Figure 3(top row), the energy term assigns a high penalty value to the weighted path going through the window to make it expensive and stop the fluid from leaking out. Other seeded image segmentation approaches treat the broken edges as a plateau and give some unreasonable results.

In Figure 3(bottom row), the viscous force will result in a constant topographical path cost over local regions in noisy scenarios, which can neutralise the impact of noisy pixels. Other seeded image segmentation algorithms are affected by noisy pixels critically, so most of them cannot locate the boundaries of the structure or capture its shape.

After introducing the viscous force term into watershed transformation, we generate a new viscous force watershed transformation in equation 9 and 10. We

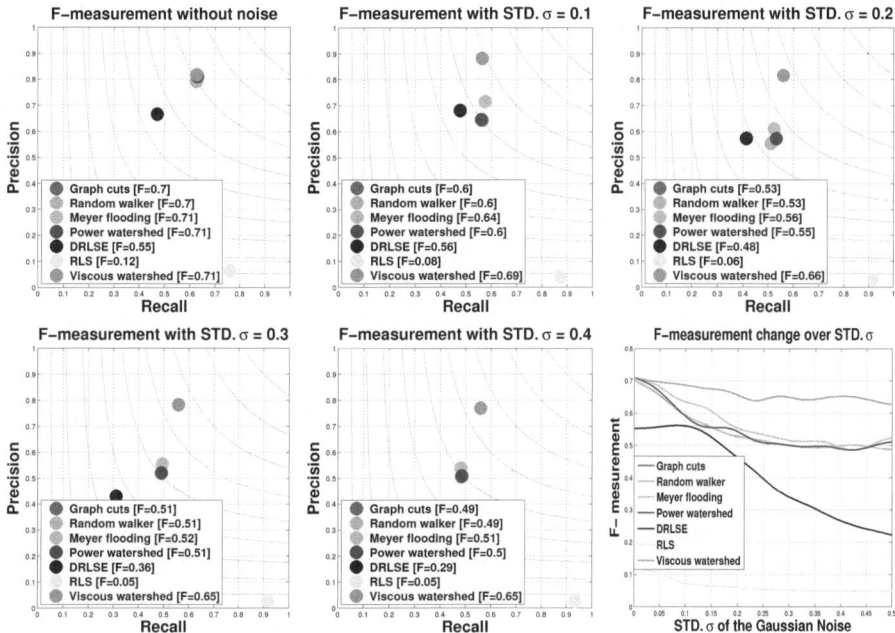

**Fig. 4.** Illustration of F-measurement drawing in $PR$-chart under the different magnitude of gaussian noise. Top row: F-measurement on original images, and F-measurement on images corrupted by gaussian noise with standard deviations, $\sigma = 0.1$, $\sigma = 0.2$. Bottom row: F-measurement on images corrupted by Gaussian noise with standard deviations, $\sigma = 0.3$, $\sigma = 0.4$, and changes of F-measurements over different levels of noise. Measurement software is provided by BSDS500 dataset.

can also incorporate our weight function, incorporating the viscous force, into other seeded image segmentation approaches via the generic framework described above (i.e. equation 2).

## 4    Experimental Results

We evaluate the performance of our proposed viscous force watershed transformation against other seeded watershed image segmentation algorithms and active contour models—specifically graph cuts, random walker, Meyer flooding, power watersheds, DRLSE, and RSF. Our experiments use the 50 image Grab-Cut dataset [22]. This dataset was first proposed for evaluating interactive image segmentation algorithms. It provides foreground segmentation masks which we use to generate the seeds by applying significant erosion.

Our viscous force watershed is targeted at low-quality image segmentation, (see in Figure 1). To evaluate performance in this regime we corrupt the images in the GrabCut dataset by adding zero-mean gaussian noise ($\sigma \in [0.1\ 0.4]$) to each pixel. Quantitative evaluation is then performed using the precision-recall chart

**Table 1.** F-measurement for boundary detection computed between the segmentations yielded by seven algorithms and ground truth images in GrabCut data set. †: $\Delta$ shows difference in F-measurement between our algorithm and the best algorithm among the remaining six.

| | $\sigma = 0$ | | $\sigma = 0.1$ | | $\sigma = 0.2$ | | $\sigma = 0.3$ | | $\sigma = 0.4$ | |
|---|---|---|---|---|---|---|---|---|---|---|
| | MedF | BestF | MedF | BestF | MedF | BestF | MedF | BestF | MedF | BestF |
| Graph cuts | 0.700 | 0.792 | 0.659 | 0.727 | 0.564 | 0.592 | 0.520 | 0.537 | 0.496 | 0.511 |
| Random walker | 0.701 | 0.793 | 0.660 | 0.728 | 0.564 | 0.592 | 0.520 | 0.537 | 0.496 | 0.512 |
| Meyer flooding | **0.711** | **0.819** | 0.684 | 0.781 | 0.616 | 0.679 | 0.539 | 0.580 | 0.512 | 0.549 |
| Power watershed | 0.709 | 0.810 | 0.671 | 0.743 | 0.556 | 0.586 | 0.515 | 0.534 | 0.496 | 0.510 |
| DRLSE | 0.552 | 0.666 | 0.557 | 0.673 | 0.537 | 0.647 | 0.422 | 0.503 | 0.322 | 0.383 |
| RSF | 0.119 | 0.165 | 0.104 | 0.179 | 0.066 | 0.112 | 0.056 | 0.091 | 0.051 | 0.093 |
| Viscous watershed | 0.710 | 0.817 | **0.697** | **0.801** | **0.676** | **0.845** | **0.639** | **0.754** | **0.641** | **0.757** |
| $\Delta^\dagger$ | **-0.001** | **-0.002** | **0.013** | **0.020** | **0.060** | **0.166** | **0.100** | **0.174** | **0.129** | **0.208** |

and F-measurement metrics developed by [23] for boundary quality evaluation. We also report ground truth covering and variation of information metric (VI) for region covering evaluation [23, 24].

## 4.1   Boundary Quality

The F-measurement is particularly meaningful in the context of boundary maps. It is reasonable to characterise higher level processing in terms of how true a signal is required for $R$ (recall) to be successful, and how much noise can be tolerated $P$ (precision). Then a balanced F-measurement can be calculated from these quantities.

Table 1 shows the quantitative results for the seven algorithms being tested under different Gaussian noise scenarios. We report two quantities. The first (MedF) reports the median F-measurement across the 50-image dataset, and the second (BestF) reports the best F-measurement over all images in the dataset. These metrics (BestF and MedF) range from 0 to 1 corresponding to bad and good matches, respectively.

Some qualitative results are shown in Figure 4. As these images and the quantitative results show, segmentations produced by our viscous watershed on original (noise free) images are as good as results produced by the other seeded image segmentation algorithms. The difference of quantitative measurements is marginal in the noise-free case, and the seeded image segmentation approaches all perform much better than DRLSE and RSF. However, when segmenting in the presence of Gaussian noise, our viscous force watershed method outperforms the other six algorithms.

Additionally, Figure 4 shows that the F-measurement metric of our viscous force watershed method drop much slower than the other algorithms as the magnitude of noise increases. In other words, viscous force is more robust to noise than the other seeded image segmentation algorithms.

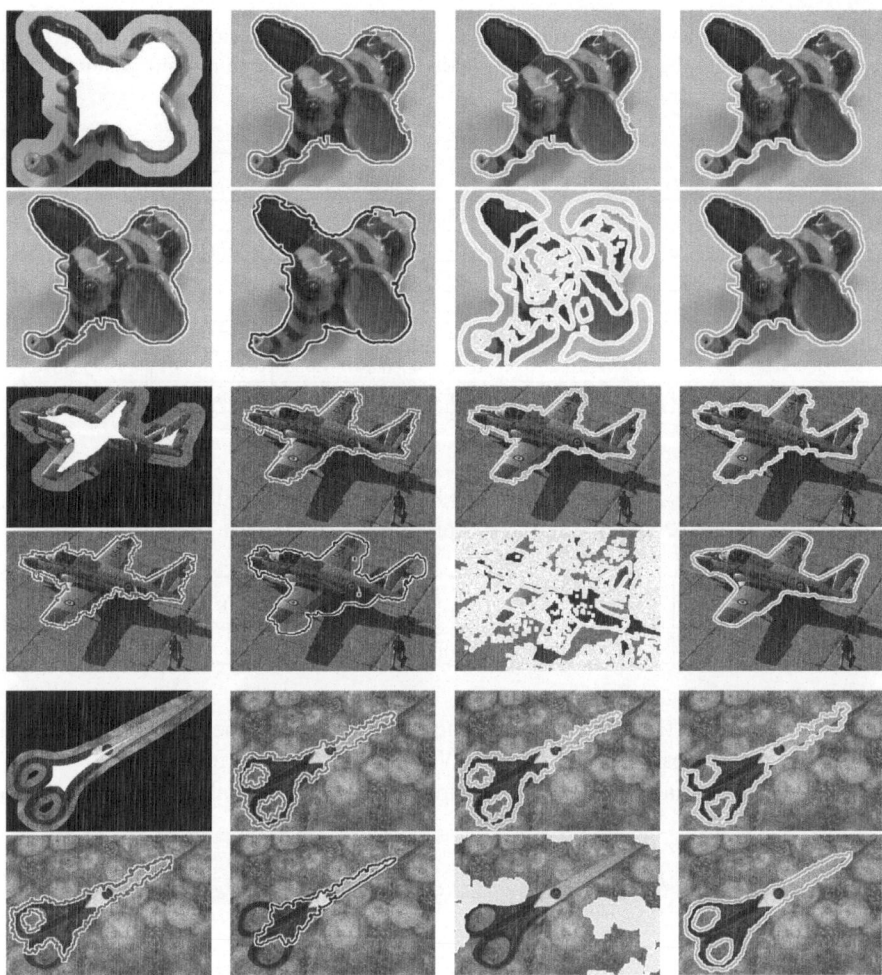

**Fig. 5.** Example segmentations on the GrabCut dataset images under different magnitudes of noise. For each image, **top row:** image with seeds, segmentations yielded by graph cuts, random walker, and Meyer flooding, **bottom row:** segmentations produced by power watershed, DRLSE, RSF and viscous watershed. From top to bottom, the ceramic elephant image is the original one without noise corruption, the fighter jet image is corrupted by a Gaussian noise with $\sigma = 0.1$, and the scissors image is corrupted by a Gaussian noise with $\sigma = 0.3$.

## 4.2 Region Quality

The Variation of Information metric (VI) was introduced for the purpose of label comparison [23, 24]. It measures the distance between two segmentations in terms of their average conditional entropies given by:

$$\mathrm{VI}(S, S') = H(S) + H(S') - 2I(S, S'),$$

**Table 2.** Region evaluation ground truth covering and Variation Information (VI), computed between the segmentations yielded by seven algorithms and ground truth images in GrabCut dataset.

| | $\sigma = 0$ | | $\sigma = 0.1$ | | $\sigma = 0.2$ | | $\sigma = 0.3$ | | $\sigma = 0.4$ | |
|---|---|---|---|---|---|---|---|---|---|---|
| | Cover | VI | Cover | VI | Cover | VI | Cover | VI | Cover | VI |
| Graph cuts | 0.971 | 0.200 | **0.954** | 0.295 | 0.939 | 0.373 | 0.937 | 0.386 | 0.937 | 0.384 |
| Random walker | 0.971 | 0.199 | 0.954 | 0.295 | 0.939 | 0.373 | 0.937 | 0.386 | 0.934 | 0.384 |
| Meyer flooding | **0.972** | 0.196 | 0.959 | 0.269 | 0.942 | 0.356 | 0.939 | 0.372 | 0.940 | 0.367 |
| Power watershed | **0.972** | **0.191** | 0.951 | 0.299 | 0.940 | 0.371 | 0.937 | 0.386 | 0.938 | 0.382 |
| DRLSE | 0.949 | 0.308 | 0.952 | 0.290 | 0.930 | 0.351 | 0.917 | 0.38 | 0.921 | 0.372 |
| RSF | 0.479 | 1.606 | 0.500 | 1.574 | 0.501 | 1.550 | 0.496 | 1.561 | 0.492 | 1.570 |
| Viscous watershed | **0.972** | 0.199 | **0.970** | **0.211** | **0.961** | **0.257** | **0.958** | **0.278** | **0.960** | **0.265** |

**Table 3.** Average executing time comparison among all these algorithms running on a 2.66GHz Intel Core2 Quad CPU Q9700 platform with Ubuntu 11.10

| Algorithm | Graph cuts | Random walker | Meyer flooding | Power watershed | DRLSE | RSF | Viscous watershed |
|---|---|---|---|---|---|---|---|
| exec. time | 247.4 ms | 2.6 ms | 6.8ms | 353.8 ms | 32.9s | 4.87s | 56.27ms |

where $H$ and $I$ are the entropies and mutual information between two segmentations $S$ and $S'$, respectively. Smaller VI means better segmentation.

Our second evaluation metric for region segmentation quality is ground truth covering defined as

$$\mathcal{O}(R, R') = \frac{|R \cap R'|}{|R \cup R'|}, \quad C(S' \rightarrow S) = \frac{1}{N} \sum_{R \in S} |R| \cdot \max_{R' \in S'} \mathcal{O}(R, R'),$$

where $R$ and $R'$ are the overlapped regions, the covering index $C$ of the ground truth $S$ by a segmentation $S'$ respect to $\mathcal{O}(\cdot)$, and, $N$ denotes the total number of pixels in the image.

The average over all 50 images of variation information and ground truth covering are shown in Table 2. According to these metrics the viscous force watershed performs better than all the other algorithms under noisy scenarios—its segmentation has the smallest value of Variation Information and the highest measurements in ground truth covering.

Last, we compare the running time of these different seeded image segmentation algorithms (see Table 3). Our method along with the other graph-based algorithms are much faster than the level sets approaches. Although, our method is slightly slower than the random walker and Meyer's flooding, it is still fast enough for many real-time applications.

**Table 4.** Performance evaluation on the pre-filtered images. Original images are corrupted by a Gaussian noise ($\sigma$=0.2), A Gaussian filter (size=15 $\times$ 15, $\sigma$=0.5).

| $\sigma$=0.2 | Graph C. | Random W. | Meyer F. | Power W. | DRLSE | RSF | Viscous W. |
|---|---|---|---|---|---|---|---|
| MedF | 0.600 | 0.600 | 0.628 | 0.587 | 0.569 | 0.067 | **0.676** |
| BestF | 0.604 | 0.604 | 0.630 | 0.598 | 0.665 | 0.1567 | **0.845** |
| cover. | 0.951 | 0.951 | 0.955 | 0.950 | 0.949 | 0.488 | **0.961** |
| VI | 0.309 | 0.309 | 0.286 | 0.313 | 0.296 | 1.587 | **0.257** |

### 4.3    Precision and Robustness

One may consider using a pre-filter to smooth the images before applying the segmentation algorithms as an alternative to our viscous force watershed method. However, as shown in Table 4, per-filtering may improve the segmenting performance slightly, but they are still not as good as our algorithm. We believe that this is because the pre-noise filter decreases noise magnitude at the cost of losing some high-frequency information. As such, precisely localizing boundaries and edges is compromised.

The affect of viscous force is different from pre-filtering. The viscous force watershed is designed to find an averaging weighted path over all paths around a certain minimum path in a neighbourhood. Thus, unlike the pre-filtering process, our method can not only enhance segmentation robustness, but can also preserve high-frequency information (precision) instead of filtering it along with the noise.

## 5    Discussion and Conclusion

In this paper we developed a high-order external energy term (viscous force) for image segmentation algorithms based on watershed. This energy term significantly improves the robustness of the watershed transformation. Specifically, our modification renders the watershed tolerant to noise and capable of segmenting object with broken edges.

Watershed-based algorithms have found many different applications in the computer vision field that go beyond image segmentation, such as stereo disparity map, video super-resolution and dynamic object detection [25–27]. By employing our viscous force formulation to improve robustness, the watershed transform may find even more applications within computer vision.

Our work, together with recent methods that unify the watershed transformation and graph-based segmentation techniques, suggest exciting future research directions. Most promising of these, perhaps, is the generalisation of our high-order viscous force approach to other seeded image segmentation algorithms including graph-cut and random walker via a unifying framework.

**Acknowledgement.** This work was kindly supported by ControlExpert GmbH, Langenfeld (Germany).

# References

1. Chan, T., Vese, L.: Active contours without edges. IEEE Trans. on Image Processing 10, 266–277 (2001)
2. Li, C., Kao, C.Y., Gore, J., Ding, Z.: Minimization of region-scalable fitting energy for image segmentation. IEEE Trans. on Image Processing 17, 1940–1949 (2008)
3. Binder, K.: Ising model. In: Hazewinkel, Michiel, Encyclopedia of Mathematics. Springer (2001)
4. Boykov, Y.Y., Jolly, M.P.: Interactive graph cuts for optimal boundary & region segmentation of objects in N-D images. In: ICCV, pp. 105–112 (2001)
5. Digabel, H., Lantuejoul, C.: Iterative algorithms. In: European Symposium on Quantitative Analysis of Microstructures in Materials Sciences, Biology and Medicinen, Caen, France, pp. 85–99 (1977)
6. Kass, M., Witkin, A., Terzopoulos, D.: Snakes: Active contour models. IJCV 1, 321–331 (1988)
7. Xu, C., Prince, J.L.: Snakes, shapes, and gradient vector flow. IEEE Trans. on Image Processing 7, 359–369 (1998)
8. Sethian, J.A.: Level Set Methods and Fast Marching Methods, 2nd edn. Cambridge University Press (1999)
9. Farouki, R.T.: Curves from motion, motion from curves. In: Curve and Surface Design: Saint- Malo. Vanderbilt Univ. Press (1999)
10. Grady, L.: Random walks for image segmentation. PAMI 28, 1768–1783 (2006)
11. Meyer, F., Beucher, S.: Morphological segmentation. Journal of Visual Communication and Image Representation 1, 21–46 (1990)
12. Couprie, C., Grady, L., Najman, L., Talbot, H.: Power watersheds: A new image segmentation framework extending graph cuts, random walker and optimal spanning forest. In: ICCV, pp. 731–738 (2009)
13. Li, C., Xu, C., Gui, C., Fox, M.: Distance regularized level set evolution and its application to image segmentation. IEEE Trans. on Image Processing 19, 3243–3254 (2010)
14. Beucher, S., Lantuejoul, C.: Use of watersheds in contour detection. In: International Workshop on Image Processing: Real-time Edge and Motion Detection/ Estimation, Rennes, France (1979)
15. Cousty, J., Bertrand, G., Najman, L., Couprie, M.: Watershed cuts: Thinnings, shortest path forests, and topological watersheds. PAMI 32, 925–939 (2010)
16. Meyer, F.: Topographic distance and watershed lines. Signal Processing 38, 113–125 (1994)
17. Meyer, F.: Inondation par des fluides visqueux. Technical report, Ecole des Mines de Pairs (1993)
18. Vachier, C., Meyer, F.: The viscous watershed transform. Journal of Mathematical Imaging and Vision 22, 251–267 (2005)
19. Alahari, K., Kohli, P., Torr, P.: Reduce, reuse and recycle: Efficiently solving multilabel MRFs. In: CVPR (2008)
20. Kohli, P., Kumar, M., Torr, P.: P3 beyond: Solving energies with higher order cliques. In: CVPR (2007)
21. Sinop, A.K., Grady, L.: A Seeded Image Segmentation Framework Unifying Graph Cuts And Random Walker Which Yields A New Algorithm. In: ICCV, pp. 1–8 (2007)
22. Rother, C., Kolmogorov, V., Blake, A.: Grabcut: interactive foreground extraction using iterated graph cuts. In: SIGGRAPH, pp. 309–314 (2004)

23. Martin, D.R., Fowlkes, C.C., Malik, J.: Learning to detect natural image boundaries using local brightness, color, and texture cues. PAMI 26, 530–549 (2004)
24. Arbelaez, P., Maire, M., Fowlkes, C., Malik, J.: Contour detection and hierarchical image segmentation. PAMI 33, 898–916 (2011)
25. Bertolini, G., Ramat, S.: Identification and recognition of objects in colour stereo images using a hierarchical som. In: Computer and Robot Vision, pp. 297–304 (2007)
26. Dailey, D., Cathey, F., Pumrin, S.: An algorithm to estimate mean traffic speed using uncalibrated cameras. IEEE Trans. on Intelligent Transportation Systems 1, 98–107 (2000)
27. Omer, O., Tanaka, T.: Region-based weighted-norm approach to video super-resolution with adaptive regularisation. In: ICASSP, pp. 833–836 (2009)

# Active Learning for Interactive Segmentation with Expected Confidence Change

Dan Wang, Canxiang Yan, Shiguang Shan, and Xilin Chen

Key Lab. of Intelligent Information Processing of Chinese Academy of Sciences
(CAS), Institute of Computing Technology, CAS, Beijing 100190, China
{dan.wang,canxiang.yan,shiguang.shan,xilin.chen}@vipl.ict.ac.cn

**Abstract.** Using human prior information to perform interactive segmentation plays a significant role in figure/ground segmentation. In this paper, we propose an active learning based approach to smartly guide the user to interact on crucial regions and can quickly achieve accurate segmentation results. To select the crucial regions from unlabeled candidates, we propose a new criterion, i.e. selecting the ones which maximize the expected confidence change ($ECC$) over all unlabeled regions. Given an image represented by oversegmented regions, our active learning based approach iterates following three steps: 1) selecting crucial unlabeled regions with maximal $ECC$; 2) refining the selected regions; 3) updating appearance models based on the refined regions and performing image segmentation. Specifically, a constrained random walks algorithm is employed for segmentation, since it can efficiently produce confidence for computing $ECC$ during active learning. Compared to the conventional interactive segmentation methods, the experimental results demonstrate our method can largely reduce the interaction efforts while maintaining high figure/ground segmentation accuracy.

## 1 Introduction

Interactive image segmentation is an active research area in recent decades [1–5]. From the perspective of computer vision, the task is to segment an interesting object from background with user's annotation [1-5]. A good interactive segmentation approach should fulfill three criteria: 1) user friendly interface; 2) accurate segmentation results; 3) smart guidance for the user.

For the first criterion, some previous methods often allow the user to iteratively specify some visual hints in different manners, such as drawing a box containing the object [4, 6], scribbling on the object and background regions [7, 8] and initializing contour points of the interesting object[1, 9]. Among all the methods, the interaction of scribbling [3] is very popular for it requires less accurate input from the user. The method allows a user coarsely mark some object regions rather than finely tracing near object contours. For the second criterion, lots of segmentation approaches, such as active contours [1], graph cut [3–5, 10], have been proposed to pursue high segmentation accuracy. Grady [10] presents a random walk segmentation algorithm, which takes user scribbles as input and can quickly produce segmentation results and the corresponding confidence.

K.M. Lee et al. (Eds.): ACCV 2012, Part I, LNCS 7724, pp. 790–802, 2013.
© Springer-Verlag Berlin Heidelberg 2013

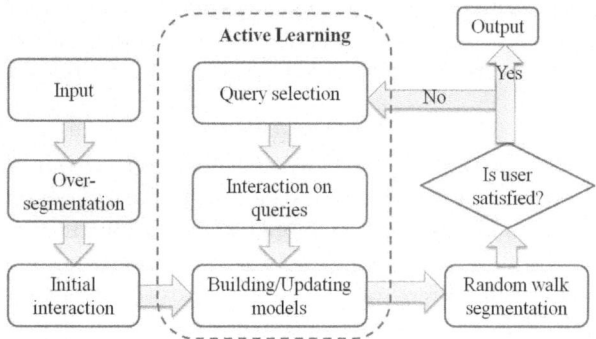

**Fig. 1.** Flowchart of active learning based interactive segmentation

Although many interactive segmentation systems have been built, the major efforts often focus on the first two criteria. It is still an open issue how to smartly guide the user interaction. The challenge is how to determine which unlabeled regions should be automatically recommended for interaction. For example, a user intends to segment an object with different color components. Experienced users may know it is crucial to supply scribbles on typical regions covering different color components, while the novices do not know that.

In order to effectively guide the user, we propose an active learning based approach for interactive segmentation. The approach actively selects crucial regions based on a new criterion, which targets to cause maximal expected confidence change $(ECC)$ after revealing the labels of selected regions. Figure 1 shows the flowchart of the proposed approach. Given an image, oversegmentation [11] is firstly performed and some initial interactions are provided by the user. Then we build appearance models (e.g. building Gaussian Mixture Models [4] of RGB values) for foreground and background and run a constrained random walks algorithm for segmentation. The active learning starts if current segmentation result is not perfect and the learning process consists of three steps: 1) selecting crucial regions with maximal $ECC$; 2) asking the user to answer the labels of queried regions; 3) updating appearance models by adding the queried regions to the labeled sets. After the active learning, the segmentation can re-execute based on the updated models. The procedure of active learning and segmentation will be iteratively performed, until a segmented result is satisfying.

## 2   Related Work

### 2.1   Interactive Segmentation

As an earlier study, active contour approaches [1] ask the user to outline an object contour and evolve the contour to true boundaries. However, the algorithm tends to get local optimum. The intelligent scissors [2] also explore boundary properties, which calculates the shortest path between the input points with Dijkstra's algorithm. Nevertheless, it needs too many user-labeled points along the boundaries. Recent studies mainly focus on region-based approaches [3–5, 10], among which the graph cut based methods are very popular [3–5]. They formulate the segmentation problem as a minimization of an energy function defined on a graph and the solution can be obtained by max-flow/min-cut algorithm [12]. As an extension, GrabCut [4] requires an input bounding box containing the object and can achieve perfect performance by iteratively adding other interaction hints. Moreover, the LazySnapping [5] utilizes both of region scribbles and boundary points. In spite of many advantages, the graph cut algorithm suffers from "short cut" problem and cannot estimate the confidence of segmentation.

In our method, a constrained random walks algorithm, which is an improved version of [10], is explored to perform segmentation. It is suited to our method, since it can fast produce segmentation results and provide the confidence of each node being foreground.

### 2.2   Active Learning

Active learning attracts growing interest in machine learning [13, 14] and Settles provides a comprehensive survey in [15]. There have been many proposed criteria for query selection such as uncertainty sampling and expected error reduction [13]. The uncertainty sampling generally considers only the local uncertainty of the label based on current information, while the expected error reduction criterion take into account the global impact on unlabeled instances.

There are relatively few works about active learning approaches in computer vision [16–20]. To the best of our knowledge, the most related work is the iCoSeg algorithm [18], which concentrates on reducing the user efforts when labeling a group of topically related images. However, the algorithm employs the uncertainty criterion to recommend informative regions, which is quite different from ours. The disadvantage of uncertainty based approaches is that the selected regions may have very little effects on other unlabeled regions. On the contrary, the maximal $ECC$ criterion always selects the regions which are expected to have the greatest influence on all unlabeled ones.

## 3   Proposed Approach

### 3.1   Overview

We briefly describe the proposed approach. Given an image in Figure 2(a) and the user inputs in Figure 2(b), the foreground/background appearance models are learned based on the labeled regions. Then a constrained random walks algorithm (Section 4) is employed to produce the initial segmentation in Figure 2(c). The active learning starts if the user is not satisfied with current result. It consists of three steps: 1) actively selecting crucial regions (shown red in Figure 2(d)) based on the proposed $ECC$ criterion; 2) asking the user for the labels of selected regions; 3) re-learning appearance models by adding the queried regions into the labeled sets. If the user is not satisfied, the active learning and segmentation will be iteratively performed.

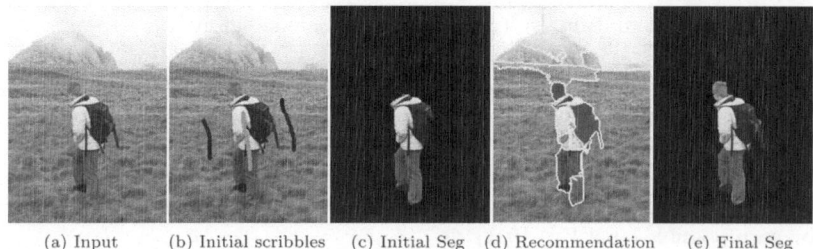

| (a) Input | (b) Initial scribbles | (c) Initial Seg | (d) Recommendation | (e) Final Seg |

**Fig. 2.** A real example using our active learning based approach. Green and Blue scribbles in (b) are initial inputs for foreground and background. (c) shows initial segmentation result. Red regions in (d) are selected for query and the yellow boundaries are produced by the oversegmentation algorithm in [11]. (e) is the final result.

Note that we employ a constrained random walks segmentation algorithm in [10]. Therefore, when the label of any region is revealed, it affects other unlabeled regions in two aspects: 1) the labeled region is added to seed sets and then propagate its information locally by a random walker; 2) it updates color models which are priors in random walks segmentation. Moreover, the image in Figure 2(d) are oversegmented by the mean shift algorithm [11], which is driven by the point density in feature space.

## 3.2 Formulation

We denote an image $X$ as $m$ non-overlapped regions. Formally, $X = \bigcup_{i=1}^{m} X_i$ and $X_i \cap X_j = \emptyset$ when $i \neq j$. Each region is denoted as $X_i = \{x_k^{(i)} | k = 1, \ldots, n_i\}$, where $n_i$ is the number of the pixels belonging to the $i^{th}$ region and $\sum_{i=1}^{m} n_i = n$ is the total number in the image $X$. The corresponding label for $i^{th}$ region is a binary variable, $Y_i \in \{0, 1\}$, where 0 corresponds to background and 1 corresponds to foreground.

Give the user scribbles, the image will be divided into a labeled region set $\mathcal{L}$ and an unlabeled set $\mathcal{U}$. We can learn GMM color models $\theta$ for foreground and background and perform random walks segmentation to produce initial labeling $\hat{Y}$ and confidence map $C$. Each unlabeled region $X_u$ will receive an estimated label $\hat{Y}_u$ and its confidence $C(\hat{Y}_u | X_u, \theta)$. Specifically, we define $C(\hat{Y}_u | X_u, \theta)$ as a signed confidence. Let $P_u$ be the probability of the region $X_u$ being foreground, which is obtained by averaging over all pixels in $X_u$, then the label confidence is

$$C(\hat{Y}_u | X_u, \theta) = \begin{cases} P_u, & \text{if } \hat{Y}_u = 1, \\ -P_u, & \text{if } \hat{Y}_u = 0. \end{cases}, (0 \leq P_u \leq 1) \tag{1}$$

**Expected Confidence Change (ECC).** If the user is not satisfied with the segmentation result, the active learning algorithm will start with query selection. Assume an region $X_q \in \mathcal{U}$ is selected for query, the GMM models $\theta$ will update to be $\theta_{+(X_q, Y_q)}$, which refers to the new model re-trained after adding the queried

---

**Algorithm 1.** Calculating $ECC$ for each unlabeled region $X_q$

---

**Input:**

    An image $X$, an unlabeled region $X_q$, the region set $\mathcal{L}$ and $\mathcal{U}$, current GMM models $\theta$, current segmentation $\hat{Y}$ and the confidence map $C$.

**Output:**

    Estimated $ECC$.

**Procedure:**

1: **for** each possible label $Y \in \{0,1\}$ **do**
2:     Retrain the GMM models based on $\mathcal{L} \cup \{(X_q, Y)\}$, denoted as $\theta_{+(X_q,Y)}$;
3:     Run random walks segmentation to obtain new labeling $\hat{Y}'$ and the corresponding confidence $C'$;
4: **end for**
5: Calculate the $ECC$ according to Equ. (4).

---

$(X_q, Y_q)$ to $\mathcal{L}$. The random walks algorithm will also re-execute based on the new GMM models and produce new labeling $Y'$ and new confidence map $C'$. For all unlabeled regions, the average Confidence Change ($CC$) by adding the pair of $(X_q, Y_q)$ will be

$$\Delta C_{+(X_q,Y_q)} = \frac{1}{|\mathcal{U}|} \sum_{X_u \in \mathcal{U}} \left| C'(\hat{Y}_u'|X_u, \theta_{+(X_q,Y_q)}) - C(\hat{Y}_u|X_u, \theta) \right|. \tag{2}$$

Since we do not know the real label of $X_q$, we can only estimate the expected confidence change through two possible labels $\{0,1\}$:

$$ECC(X_q) = \sum_{Y \in \{0,1\}} P(X_q|Y, \theta) \cdot \Delta C_{+(X_q,Y)}, \tag{3}$$

where $P(X_q|Y, \theta)$ refers to the likelihood of $X_q$ fitting to label $Y$, given the GMM models $\theta$. For clarity, we describe the computation of $ECC$ in Alg. 1.

**Weighted $ECC$.** In order to make the query selection more effective and efficient, we further explore a weighted variation of $ECC$. The weighted $ECC$ takes into account both of region size and the distance from each candidate unlabeled region to the seed ones. For each candidate region $X_q$,

$$ECC_w(X_q) = w_q \cdot ECC(X_q), \tag{4}$$

with
$$w_q = w_{size(q)} + \lambda \cdot w_{dist(q)}. \tag{5}$$

Here the first term $w_{size(q)} = n_q/n$ favors larger regions and the second term is related to the distance between the candidate region and the labeled regions. The factor $\lambda$ is empirically set to 1. Distance-based term is defined as

$$w_{dist(q)} \propto (-D_{q,\mathcal{F}} + D_{q,\mathcal{B}})/(D_{q,\mathcal{F}} + D_{q,\mathcal{B}}), \tag{6}$$

---

**Algorithm 2.** Procedure of active learning based interactive segmentation

---

**Input:**
　　An image $X$, the labeled regions $\mathcal{L}$ and the unlabeled $\mathcal{U}$, GMM models $\theta$, current
　　segmentation result $\hat{Y}$ and confidence map $C$ . Maximal iteration number $T$.
**Output:**
　　The estimated label vector $\hat{Y}'$.
**Procedure:**
　1: Initialize $t = 0$;
　2: **while** the user is not satisfied and $t < T$ **do**
　3: 　　**for** each query candidate $X_q \in \mathcal{U}$ **do**
　4: 　　　　Calculate weighted $ECC$ of $X_q$ according to Alg. 2;
　5: 　　**end for**
　6: 　　Select query regions according to Equ. (7);
　7: 　　Query the labels of regions $\{X_Q\}$ and receive answer $\{Y_Q\}$;
　8: 　　Update labeled set $\mathcal{L} = \mathcal{L} \cup \{(X_Q, Y_Q)\}$ and unlabeled set $\mathcal{U} = \mathcal{U} \backslash \{X_Q\}$;
　9: 　　Retrain GMM models $\theta' = \theta_{+\{(X_Q, Y_Q)\}}$ and predicet new labeling $\hat{Y}'$ with
　　　　random walks.
10: **end while**

---

where $D_{q,\mathcal{F}}$ and $D_{q,\mathcal{B}}$ is the normalized distance between 0 and 1. It measures
the average spatial distance between the centroid of $X_q$ and each user-labeled
region. The factor $w_q$ is scaled to $[0, 1]$ by Min-max normalization.

Note we are apt to select regions which are close to user-labeled foreground
and far from background regions. The intuition behind this setting is that regions near to the labeled foreground is also very possibly near to boundaries
which will provide crucial classification cues. On the other hand, regions far
away from the labeled background may contain color components, which are different from those of current background seeds. Therefore it can make the models
more accurate to add such regions to $\mathcal{L}$.

### 3.3  Query Selection

In brief, our basic idea for active learning is to greedily select queries from
unlabeled regions to maximize the expected confidence change ($ECC$) over all
unlabeled ones. Thus the region with largest $ECC$ will be recommended first:

$$X_Q = \underset{X_q \in \mathcal{U}}{\mathrm{argmax}}\, ECC(X_q). \tag{7}$$

The proposed active learning algorithm is described in Alg. 2.

**Batch-Mode Active Learning.** In the active learning based approach, if we
query the recommended regions in serial, i.e, one at a time, it will cost lots of
time to achieve satisfactory segmentation. Therefore, we employ the batch-mode,
which actively queries a group of regions at a time for learning, to accelerate
the process. Although there are several works on how to select the optimal set
for batch query [16, 21], we adopt a strategy with medium complexity, but is

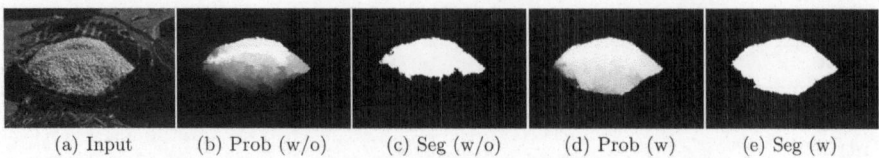

(a) Input    (b) Prob (w/o)    (c) Seg (w/o)    (d) Prob (w)    (e) Seg (w)

**Fig. 3.** The effect of the prior term on the probability map (Prob) and segmentation results (Seg). Green and blue scribbles are for foreground and background. 'w' denotes 'with prior' and 'w/o' denotes 'without prior'.

sufficiently effective for our approach. Specifically, we firstly choose a group of $k$ unlabeled regions with the largest $ECC$ to ensure the recommended ones are informative. Then we randomly sample $N_q$ from these $k$ candidates to ensure the recommended regions are diverse. In our implementation, $k = 8$ and $2 \leq N_q \leq 5$. For batch mode active learning, we denote the queried region sets as $\{X_Q\}$.

## 4   Constrained Random Walks for Segmentation

Random walks (RW) algorithm is employed for two reasons: 1) it can be efficiently computed; 2) it can provide the segmentation confidence, i.e. the probability of each pixel belonging to foreground. We briefly review the RW algorithm.

### 4.1   Preliminaries

Following the framework in [10], we formulate the segmentation problem on a graph $G = (V, E)$, with nodes $x \in V$ and edges $e \in E \subseteq V \times V$ with $n = |V|$. An edge, spanning two nodes $x_i$ and $x_j$, is denoted by $e_{ij}$. A weighted graph specifies a value $w_{ij}$ to each edge $e_{ij}$ called a weight. Given an image $\boldsymbol{X}$, each node represents a pixel and the nodes are locally connected via an 8-connected lattice. Given the user input, the nodes are partitioned into two sets, $\mathcal{L}$ and $\mathcal{U}$. The labeled set $\mathcal{L}$ consists of $\mathcal{L}^{\mathcal{F}}$ and $\mathcal{L}^{\mathcal{B}}$, which are foreground and background seeds. Let $p_i$ denote the probability of a walker starting from $x_i$ to reach a first foreground seed. Then producing a segmentation $\boldsymbol{Y}$ is to find a solution to

$$min \sum_{e_{ij} \in E} w_{ij}(p_i - p_j)^2, \tag{8}$$

$$\text{s.t.} \quad p_i = 1, \text{ if } x_i \in \mathcal{L}^{\mathcal{F}}; \ p_i = 0, \text{ if } x_i \in \mathcal{L}^{\mathcal{B}}.$$

One can analytically and quickly determine the solution [10]. Finally, each node $x_i$ is assigned a label $\hat{y}_i = 1$ if $p_i \geq 0.5$ or $\hat{y}_i = 0$ if $p_i < 0.5$. Denote the probability of each region $X_u$ belonging to foreground as $P_u$, which is the average probability of each pixel in $X_u$ belonging to the foreground. Then the region label $\hat{Y}_u$ will be $\hat{Y}_u = 1$ if $P_u \geq 0.5$ or $\hat{Y}_u = 0$ if $P_u < 0.5$.

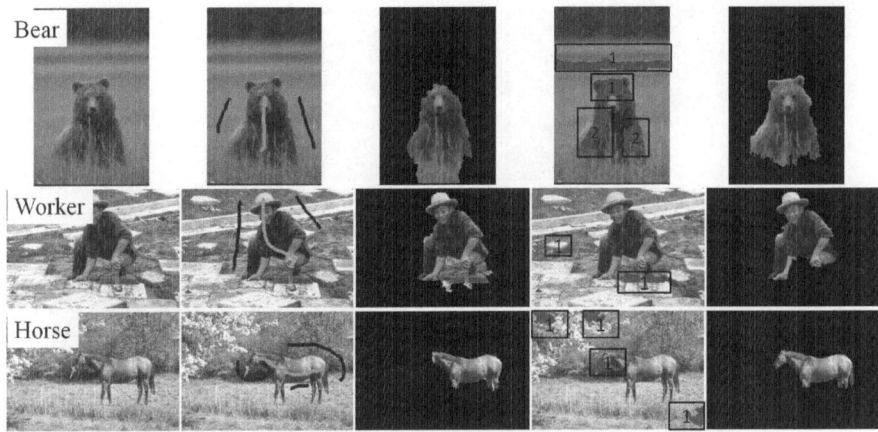

(a) Input     (b) Initial scribbles (c) Initial result (d) Recommendation (e) Final result

**Fig. 4.** Example results of the proposed approach. The number '1' and '2' labeled in (d) means the red regions are queried in the 1st and 2nd iteration of active learning.

## 4.2   Edge Weights

Generally, each edge weight is associated with the neighborhood distance [22]:

$$w_{ij} = exp\left(-(\beta\|\boldsymbol{I}_i - \boldsymbol{I}_j\|^2 + \|h_i - h_j\|^2)\right), \tag{9}$$

where $\boldsymbol{I}_i$ denotes the color vector and $h_i$ denotes the spatial position of pixel $i$. $\beta$ is a scaling factor. However, under such configurations, the probability of each node reaching foreground or background are quite sensitive to the seed positions. To deal with this problem, we integrate the prior models into the weight. Similar to [23], we define

$$w_{ij}^{new} = exp\left(-(\beta d_{ij}^2 + \|h_i - h_j\|^2)\right), \tag{10}$$

where

$$d_{ij}^2 = \|\boldsymbol{I}_i - \boldsymbol{I}_j\|^2 + \alpha\left(P_i^{\mathcal{F}} - P_j^{\mathcal{F}}\right)^2. \tag{11}$$

Here $P_i^{\mathcal{F}}$ is the normalized probability of the node $x_i$ belonging foreground:

$$P_i^{\mathcal{F}} = \left(-\log P(x_i|\mathcal{B})\right) / \left(-\log P(x_i|\mathcal{F}) - \log P(x_i|\mathcal{B})\right), \tag{12}$$

where $P(x_i|\mathcal{F})$ and $P(x_i|\mathcal{B})$ are the likelihoods of each node fitting to the foreground and background GMMs. The weight $\alpha \in [0,1]$ is defined as:

$$\alpha = \frac{1}{n}\sum_{i=1}^{n}\left|\frac{\log P(x_i|\mathcal{F}) - \log P(x_i|\mathcal{B})}{\log P(x_i|\mathcal{F}) + \log P(x_i|\mathcal{B})}\right|. \tag{13}$$

Note the second term in Equ. (11) plays a dominant role, when foreground and background colors are well separable. Figure 3 compares the probability maps and results calculated by random walks algorithms with and without priors.

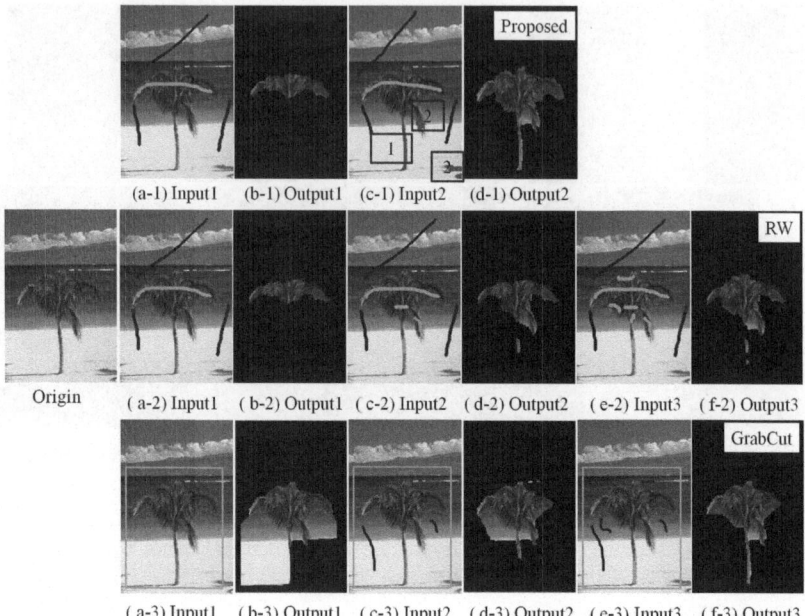

**Fig. 5.** Comparing user efforts of three algorithms. For our method, (c) in top row paints the recommended regions red, where the labeled number means the iteration number. For GrabCut, the green bounding box is the user input.

## 5    Experimental Results

We evaluate the proposed method in two aspects. Firstly, we evaluate how many efforts can be reduced by using our active learning based approach, compared with conventional segmentation algorithms. Secondly, we validate the superiority of $ECC$ for query selectioncompared with another typical criterion, i.e. uncertainty sampling [15]. For comparison, we select 20 representative challenging images from the GrabCut [4] and BSD database [24]. Among these images, foreground objects contain complex shapes or appearances in which color distributions of foreground and background are very similar. We manually label the ground truth and pixel-based accuracy is adopted to evaluate segmentation performance.

### 5.1    Interaction Effort Reduction Test

Figure 4 gives some qualitative results of the proposed approach. In Figure 4(d), the river regions in the 'bear' image, the regions near the left leg in the 'worker' image and some regions of horse head in the 'horse' image are selected for query. These selected regions are usually near the boundaries or have different appearance distribution from the scribbled ones. Therefore, querying such informative regions can largely reduce the user input to achieve perfect results.

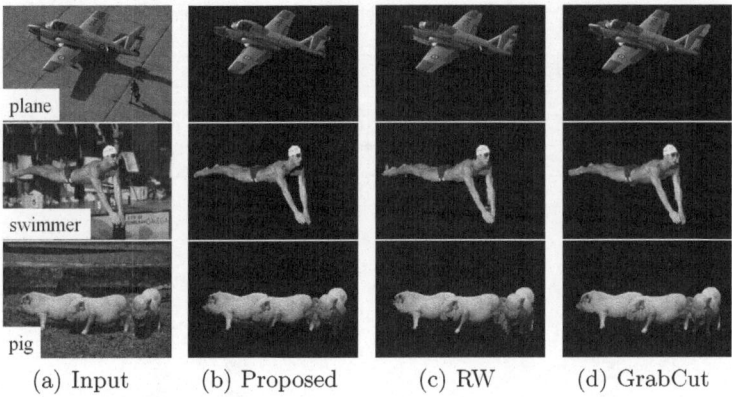

| (a) Input | (b) Proposed | (c) RW | (d) GrabCut |

**Fig. 6.** Final segmentation results of our method, random walks algorithm and Grab-Cut. The corresponding accuracies are reported in Table 1.

Figure 5 shows an example to qualitatively compare the user efforts of three methods: the proposed method, random walks (RW) [10] and GrabCut [4]. Note that the parameter $\beta$ in Equ. (10) is set to 300. The figure shows that random walks algorithm needs the user to successively add lots of scribbles to achieve perfect results and a few details are still missed (e.g. tree trunk regions). Likewise, GrabCut requires the user to draw a bounding box and finely give more inputs on foreground and background. Compared with these two algorithms, ours significantly reduces user efforts while preserving perfect segmentation result.

We further quantitatively compare the user efforts and segmentation accuracy of the three methods. We train 5 naive users with the interactive tools and compare the user efforts for the three images in Figure 6. Table 1 illustrates the average interaction times of the 5 users, when the segmentation accuracy of each image reaching to 97%. It can be seen that the proposed method can consistently achieve satisfactory results with least interactions. Moreover, we take one of the five users as an example and gives how the accuracy increases with this user's interaction times in Table 2. Figure 6 compares the final segmentations of different methods with this users' interactions. It is observed that the proposed method reduces the user interactions on these images while maintaining high accuracy, compared with other two methods. The main reason is that our method can actively recommend informative regions, while the user may aimlessly interact on regions which are no good for accuracy improvement.

**Table 1.** Average interaction times from 5 naive users

| Times | plane | swimmer | pig |
|---|---|---|---|
| GrabCut | 3.2 | 4.6 | 4.2 |
| RW | 4.0 | 3.6 | 4.6 |
| Proposed | 2.6 | 2.0 | 4.0 |

**Table 2.** The accuracy change with interaction times of one user (%)

| Times | plane | | | | | swimmer | | | | | pig | | | |
|---|---|---|---|---|---|---|---|---|---|---|---|---|---|---|
| | 1 | 2 | 3 | 4 | 5 | 1 | 2 | 3 | 4 | 5 | 1 | 2 | 3 | 4 |
| GrabCut | 92.8 | 97.7 | 98.9 | 99.2 | - | 79.4 | 95.6 | 97.0 | 98.8 | 98.9 | 94.4 | 95.2 | 97.7 | 97.9 |
| RW | 96.9 | 96.5 | 98.0 | 98.1 | 98.1 | 96.9 | 98.0 | 98.3 | 98.0 | 98.3 | 95.9 | 95.6 | 96.3 | 96.4 |
| Proposed | 96.9 | 98.0 | - | - | - | 96.9 | 98.2 | - | - | - | 95.9 | 95.4 | 97.0 | - |

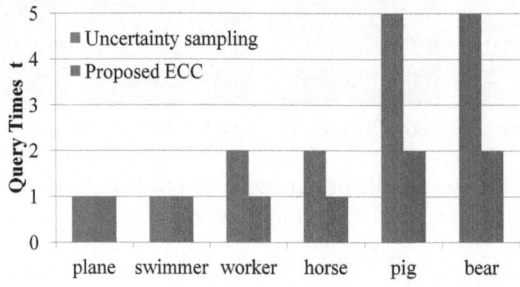

**Fig. 7.** Comparison of query times by using uncertainty sampling and the proposed *ECC* criterion. The smaller the value of $t$ is, the fewer user interactions are needed.

### 5.2 Maximal *ECC* Criterion Test

We compare the maximal *ECC* criterion with another competing criterion of query selection for active learning, called uncertainty sampling. Following the general setting, we use entropy to evaluate the uncertainty:

$$X_Q = \operatorname*{argmax}_{X_q \in \mathcal{U}} \sum_{Y \in \{0,1\}} \{-P(X_q|Y,\theta)\log P(X_q|Y,\theta)\}, \tag{14}$$

in which all notations are defined as in Section 3.

For fair comparison, we use the batch-mode for both of the *ECC* based and uncertainty based active learning. For the images in Figure 4 and Figure 6, each method iteratively queries informative regions and perform the Alg. 2 until the accuracy of 97% is reached. Figure 7 compares the query times for each method. It tells that we can achieve a fixed accuracy with fewer queries than uncertainty sampling does. This is due to the uncertainty sampling only considers local properties without predicting the global influence on other region labels.

## 6    Conclusion

We focus on how to actively recommend crucial regions to reduce user inputs. The main contribution lies in two aspects. Firstly, we propose an approach which can successively recommend informative regions based on random walks. Secondly, we propose a novel criterion, maximal *ECC*, which aims to select regions that will change most on the expected confidence over all unlabeled ones. Experiments on a challenging dataset demonstrate that compared with conventional interactive segmentation methods, our approach can significantly reduce user efforts and help more quickly achieve satisfactory results. Future work is to extend the proposed method to other application such as training set annotation.

**Acknowledgement.** This work is partially supported by National Basic Research Program of China (973 Program) under contract 2009CB320902; and Natural Science Foundation of China (NSFC) under contract Nos. 60833013 and 60832004.

# References

1. Kass, M., Witkin, A., Terzopoulos, D.: Snakes: Active contour models. IJCV 1, 321–331 (1988)
2. Mortensen, E.N., Barrett, W.A.: Interactive segmentation with intelligent scissors. In: Graphical Models and Image Processing, pp. 349–384 (1998)
3. Boykov, Y., Jolly, M.P.: Interactive graph cuts for optimal boundary amp; region segmentation of objects in n-d images. In: ICCV, pp. 105–112 (2001)
4. Rother, C., Kolmogorov, V., Blake, A.: "grabcut": interactive foreground extraction using iterated graph cuts. TOG 23, 309–314 (2004)
5. Li, Y., Sun, J., Tang, C.K., Shum, H.Y.: Lazy snapping. TOG 23, 303–308 (2004)
6. Lempitsky, V., Kohli, P., Rother, C., Sharp, T.: Image segmentation with a bounding box prior. In: ICCV, pp. 277–284 (2009)
7. Wang, J., Agrawala, M., Cohen, M.F.: Soft scissors: an interactive tool for realtime high quality matting. TOG (2007)
8. Vicente, S., Kolmogorov, V., Rother, C.: Graph cut based image segmentation with connectivity priors. In: CVPR, pp. 1–8 (2008)
9. Blake, A., Rother, C., Brown, M., Perez, P., Torr, P.: Interactive Image Segmentation Using an Adaptive GMMRF Model. In: Pajdla, T., Matas, J(G.) (eds.) ECCV 2004. LNCS, vol. 3021, pp. 428–441. Springer, Heidelberg (2004)
10. Grady, L.: Random walks for image segmentation. TPAMI 28, 1768–1783 (2006)
11. Comaniciu, D., Meer, P.: Mean shift: A robust approach toward feature space analysis. TPAMI 24, 603–619 (2002)
12. Boykov, Y., Kolmogorov, V.: An experimental comparison of min-cut/max- flow algorithms for energy minimization in vision. TPAMI 26, 1124–1137 (2004)
13. Roy, N., Mccallum, A.: Toward optimal active learning through sampling estimation of error reduction. In: ICML, pp. 441–448 (2001)
14. Zhu, X., Lafferty, J., Ghahramani, Z.: Combining active learning and semi-supervised learning using gaussian fields and harmonic functions. In: ICML Workshop on the Continuum from Labeled to Unlabeled Data in Machine Learning and Data Mining, pp. 58–65 (2003)
15. Settles, B.: Active learning literature survey. University of Wisconsin, Madison (2010)
16. Hoi, S.C.H., Jin, R., Zhu, J., Lyu, M.R.: Batch mode active learning and its application to medical image classification. In: ICML, pp. 417–424 (2006)
17. Joshi, A., Porikli, F., Papanikolopoulos, N.: Multi-class active learning for image classification. In: CVPR, pp. 2372–2379 (2009)

18. Batra, D., Kowdle, A., Parikh, D., Luo, J., Chen, T.: Interactively co-segmentating topically related images with intelligent scribble guidance. IJCV 93, 273–292 (2011)
19. Gosselin, P., Cord, M.: Active learning methods for interactive image retrieval. TIP 17, 1200–1211 (2008)
20. Vijayanarasimhan, S., Grauman, K.: What's it going to cost you?: Predicting effort vs. informativeness for multi-label image annotations. In: CVPR, pp. 2262–2269 (2009)
21. Guo, Y., Schuurmans, D.: Discriminative batch mode active learning. In: NIPS, pp. 593–600 (2007)
22. Grady, L., Schwartz, E.: Isoperimetric graph partitioning for image segmentation. TPAMI 28, 469–475 (2006)
23. Yang, W., Cai, J., Zheng, J., Luo, J.: User-friendly interactive image segmentation through unified combinatorial user inputs. TIP 19, 2470–2479 (2010)
24. Martin, D., Fowlkes, C., Tal, D., Malik, J.: A database of human segmented natural images and its application to evaluating segmentation algorithms and measuring ecological statistics. In: ICCV, pp. 416–423 (2001)

# Cross Anisotropic Cost Volume Filtering for Segmentation

Vladislav Kramarev, Oliver Demetz, Christopher Schroers, and
Joachim Weickert

Mathematical Image Analysis Group,
Faculty of Mathematics and Computer Science,
Campus E1.7, Saarland University, 66044 Saarbrücken, Germany
{kramarev,demetz,schroers,weickert}@mia.uni-saarland.de

**Abstract.** We study an advanced method for supervised multi-label
image segmentation. To this end, we adopt a classic framework which
recently has been revitalised by Rhemann et al. (2011). Instead of the
usual global energy minimisation step, it relies on a mere evaluation of
a cost function for every solution label, which is followed by a spatial
smoothing step of these costs. While Rhemann et al. concentrate on efficiency, the goal of this paper is to equip the general framework with
sophisticated subcomponents in order to develop a high-quality method
for multi-label image segmentation: First, we present a substantially improved cost computation scheme which incorporates texture descriptors,
as well as an automatic feature selection strategy. This leads to a high-
dimensional feature space, from which we extract the label costs using a
support vector machine. Second, we present a novel anisotropic diffusion
scheme for the filtering step. In this PDE-based process, the smoothing
of the cost volume is steered along the structures of the previously computed feature space. Experiments on widely used image databases show
that our scheme produces segmentations of clearly superior quality.

## 1   Introduction

Segmentation is one of the classical problems in image analysis. For the last four
decades, researchers have been developing a wide variety of different approaches
to this problem. In this paper, we consider a special instance of the segmentation
problem, so-called *supervised* segmentation. In this setting, we assume for every
class to be given an exemplary and reliable region in the image. In the field of
supervised segmentation, energy-based methods are most common today, where
the sought segmentation is the minimiser of a suitable cost function. Such a
function usually consists of at least two terms: A fidelity term, which relates the
unknown to the image, and a regularity term that implements prior knowledge
about the solution. The computation of a minimiser often renders itself very
difficult: First, in most cases the fidelity term cannot be solved directly for the
unknown which makes linearisation or relaxation steps necessary. Second, the
regularisation term usually couples the solution globally and by that makes a
pointwise minimisation impossible.

K.M. Lee et al. (Eds.): ACCV 2012, Part I, LNCS 7724, pp. 803–814, 2013.
© Springer-Verlag Berlin Heidelberg 2013

A framework which avoids the aforementioned difficulties was first introduced by Scharstein and Szeliski [1] and recently revisited by Rhemann et al. [2]. This so-called *Cost Volume Filtering* (CVF) framework describes a very versatile and general three-step procedure to find a good, spatially smooth configuration in a discrete solution space. In contrast to energy minimisation methods, the only requirement is an evaluable cost function. However, for certain other computer vision problems such as optic flow, the discreteness of the solution space constitutes a problem. Nevertheless, the framework is perfectly suited for the multi-class image segmentation problem. With this paper, we propose an advanced method for this task using the CVF framework.

**Our Contribution.** Although the general applicability of CVF to (binary) image segmentation has been shown in [2], this paper presents substantial improvements to this concept, yielding state-of-the-art results while sticking to the general framework. In detail, our contributions are twofold:

1. We improve the elementary cost computation in [2] by incorporating colour and texture information, leading to a high-dimensional feature space. In order to make the final cost calculation feasible and efficient, we propose an elaborate feature selection scheme which selects the most relevant features automatically. In this comparatively low-dimensional input space, we finally train a support vector machine with Gaussian kernels to compute the cost value.
2. Regarding the filtering stage, we propose the usage of a novel anisotropic diffusion filter which is steered by the feature space. Moreover, we embed the anisotropic smoothing into an interpolation scheme as known in the context of PDE-based image inpainting [3–5] and compression [6].

Right from the beginning, we want to stress that the main goal of our work is highest segmentation quality instead of lowest computation time, where [2] is focussed on. Nevertheless, also our method can be accelerated drastically by porting it to the GPU if necessary.

**Related Work.** The field of energy-based segmentation methods can be systematically split into discrete and continuous methods. Among the latter, the seminal model by Mumford and Shah [7] marked the starting point of many successful segmentation methods, e.g. [8, 9]. In [10], Brox et al. have shown in an unsupervised setting that incorporating motion information can improve the segmentation performance. Concerning discrete segmentation methods, graph cut methods [11–13] have become very popular in the last decade. In [14], Rother et al. demonstrate an interactive segmentation method and introduce a large image database with ground truth labelling data, which serves as a commonly used benchmark today. The work by Lellmann et al. [15] is situated in a similar setting as ours but focusses on a relaxation of the cost term, and is supplemented by a regularity term. Martin et al. also utilise color and texture descriptors [16] for boundary detection. Concerning the filtering step, Scharstein and Szeliski [1] propose so-called non-uniform diffusion to filter the costs. Yoon and Kweon [17] employ locally adaptive support weights which show close relationship to the bilateral filter [18]. In [2], Rhemann uses the guided image filter [19] as an approximation of the joint bilateral filter [20]. However, we advocate anisotropic PDE-based diffusion processes [21] to smooth the cost slices. Different strategies for PDE-based interpolation are studied in [3, 4, 6].

**Paper Organisation.** In the following section, we give an introductory explanation of the cost volume filtering framework. In Section 3 we give detailed explanations of our contributions: After discussing the cost computation scheme in Section 3.1, we subsequently introduce an anisotropic and supervised cost filtering strategy in Section 3.2. Our experiments in Section 4 show that the proposed segmentation method performs well in practice and competes with the state-of-the-art. We conclude the paper in Section 5.

## 2   Cost Volume Filtering

The *Cost Volume Filtering* (CVF) framework can be seen as a very general and versatile procedure comprising the following steps:

1. **Cost Computation.** First, the cost volume $f : \Omega \times \mathcal{L} \to [0, 1]$ is computed. In practice, a fidelity term is evaluated for every pixel of the image domain $\Omega$ and each possible label $\ell$ of the finite label space $\mathcal{L}$. The choice of this term depends on the application.
2. **Cost Smoothing.** In the second stage, the cost slices undergo a smoothing step. The most important property of this filtering step is that there is no direct coupling between the different label slices, i.e. a 2-D filter is applied to each cost slice separately. However, usually the smoothing is guided by the underlying image, which reflects the assumption that segment boundaries and image edges coincide.
3. **Minimisation.** The final step is to compute the pixelwise minimum of the cost volume and take this label as the result $r$:

$$r(x, y) = \operatorname{argmin}_{\ell \in \mathcal{L}} f_{\text{smoothed}}(x, y, \ell). \qquad (1)$$

This simple stepwise structure of CVF offers several advantages and disadvantages. In principle, any cost function can be used, because there are no requirements such as differentiability, convexity, linearity or even positivity. The filtering stage also offers many degrees of freedom; almost any scalar-valued smoothing method can be used, and the smoothing steps can be easily parallelised since there is no coupling between different labels. Finally, the minimisation is an efficient pointwise $\mathcal{O}(|\mathcal{L}|)$ operation.

On the other hand, unfortunately no energy function is known for CVF up to date, so almost no theoretical properties can be proven. Moreover, especially for continuous problems such as optic flow, the need for a finite solution space

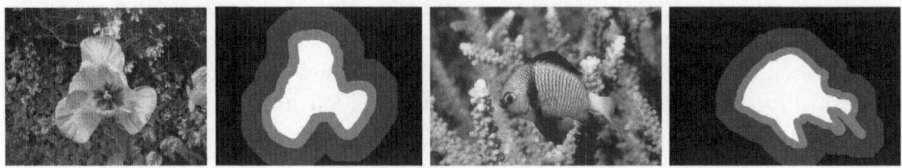

**Fig. 1.** Example images. While the flower can be well described by its colour statistics, obviously the fish exhibits very similar colours as the background. The second and last images show the associated given trimaps. Source: [14].

constitutes a severe restriction. However, the image segmentation problem is inherently finite and thus ideally suited for CVF.

## 3    Extensions for Supervised Segmentation

In the following sections, we consider the task of partitioning a colour image such that each component of the partition is assigned to one of $n \geq 2$ classes. Moreover, we are in a supervised segmentation setting, i.e. for each label $\ell \in \mathcal{L} = \{1, \ldots, n\}$ we are given an image region $\mathcal{T}_\ell \subset \Omega$ which definitely belongs to this class label. Figure 1 shows two exemplary images along with given user input. In these so-called trimaps, white and dark grey represent the user input for foreground and background, respectively. The black regions are not considered. Hence, the task is to classify each of the light grey pixels in the boundary region between fore- and background.

### 3.1    Cost Computation

The application of CVF to image segmentation is already addressed in [2], where the authors propose to compute the costs using colour statistics of the RGB channels. Apparently, this is the first solution which comes to mind. However, it exhibits several drawbacks in practice: The choice of the red, green and blue values as feature is redundant and not invariant against e.g. shadows or shading. In many cases, colour information is not a sufficiently relevant feature; see e.g. Figure 1. Moreover, the computation of the trivariate RGB histogram poses another problem: in order to cover all bins of the histogram fairly, a large number of samples from the training region is needed. In an interactive segmentation setting however, it can happen that size of the user input is very small. Hence, an overfit to the colour statistics in the training region can be the result.

Our method circumvents these problems in the following way: In a first step, we compute a large pool of features. Subsequently, we identify the most relevant ones using filter and wrapper methods [22]. Finally, the actual costs are determined by a support vector machine (SVM) with Gaussian kernels. The following paragraphs discuss these three steps in detail.

**Available Features.** We propose a pool of features which comprises a variety of colour and texture descriptors. Besides the red, green and blue channel, we also consider the hue, saturation, and value (HSV) representation. In the category of differential features, we compute the Gaussian smoothed gradient magnitude, first order derivatives in horizontal and vertical direction as well as the Laplacian magnitude averaged over 3 colour channels. Additionally, we incorporate the variance, skewness, kurtosis and entropy of the local histogram of disk shaped neighbourhoods of different radii. Such multi-scale descriptors have also shown their usefulness in [23, 24]. Additionally, we compute co-occurrence matrices for 16 different offset vectors in every pixel and include the quantities contrast and homogeneity [25] in our feature vector. In total, the mentioned concepts amount to a descriptor space of dimension 80.

**Feature Selection.** Although computationally very expensive, it would be possible to train an SVM directly in this high-dimensional feature space. However, usually only a few features are relevant for one particular image. Thus, also in terms of the classification performance it is a bad choice to always incorporate all features in the SVM. The goal of this paragraph is to discuss how we select the most relevant features in order to get a discriminative and at the same time low-dimensional feature space that our SVM will be trained in.

To be able to estimate the relevance of a certain set of features, we randomly divide the user input into a training and a validation set. This allows the application of the so-called wrapper method [22], which learns the SVM using the training set and assesses its classification performance on the validation set. This heuristic allows us estimate the relevance of a set of features just from the user input. Since the application of this strategy to all elements of the power set of the pool of features is computationally intractable, we consider colour and texture separately. The red, green and blue channels have the highest spatial resolution, hence we avoid to discard these in practice. The remaining colour features are selected by applying the wrapper method.

To find the most relevant texture features efficiently, we first compute the Fisher score [26] of every feature. Next, we filter the top 5 features and apply the wrapper method once more. A schematic overview of our strategy is depicted in Figure 2.

**Cost Evaluation.** After having selected the relevant features, we train a support vector machine (SVM) [27] with Gaussian kernels in a regression setting [28] in order to compute the costs. The final training can of course be performed incorporating all user input; a validation set is not necessary anymore. However, we can speed up the training phase by just randomly selecting 50% of the pixels without a significant impairment of accuracy. As for feature selection, we randomly split the input into training and validation sets to test different kernel and soft margin parameters in a grid search fashion [28].

A similar cost computation scheme also using colour and texture features can be found in [29]. However, the authors only considered local patch-based statistics as features and omitted the important intermediate feature selection step.

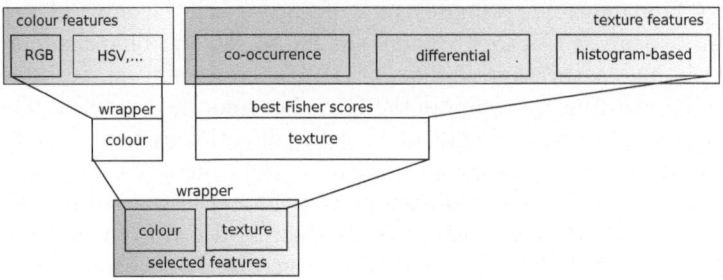

**Fig. 2.** Proposed feature selection strategy

In [29], the resulting segmentation was computed in a graph cut optimisation scheme with a spatial regularity prior.

The extension to the multilabel case $|\mathcal{L}| > 2$ is straightforward: For each label $\ell$, we perform the entire feature selection procedure and train the SVM in a one-vs-all strategy, i.e. during the computation for label $\ell$, the user input of all other labels is included to describe the negative class.

## 3.2   Anisotropic Diffusion Filtering

Once the cost volume has been computed, the properties and the behaviour of the filter are crucial for the final segmentation result. This filtering clearly stands in a close relationship to the regularisation term of energy-based methods: By choosing one particular regularisation term, the resulting smoothing process is determined automatically via the associated minimality conditions of the energy. Thus, for purely energy-based methods the choice of filtering processes is restricted. For CVF however, the cost smoothing filter can be chosen directly and without any restrictions.

In [2], the authors advertise the guided image filter [19] and rely on its efficiency and parallelisability. We instead propose to use *cross edge enhancing diffusion* (Cross-EED) as an extension of *edge enhancing diffusion* (EED) [21]. Both processes perform anisotropic diffusion and are described by the parabolic evolution equation

$$\partial_t u_\ell = \operatorname{div}\left(\boldsymbol{D}\,\boldsymbol{\nabla} u_\ell\right), \quad u_\ell(x,y,0) = f(x,y,\ell), \tag{2}$$

where $\boldsymbol{D} \in \mathbb{R}^{2\times 2}$ is the symmetric positive definite diffusion tensor, and $\boldsymbol{\nabla} = (\partial_x, \partial_y)^\top$ denotes the spatial gradient operator. Each slice of the computed cost volume $f(x,y,\ell)$ is embedded into a pseudo-temporal evolution $u_\ell(x,y,t)$ as its initial state at time $t = 0$. With progressing evolution time the amount of smoothing increases, and the resulting filtered cost slice is finally extracted at the stopping time $t_{\text{stop}}$:

$$f_{\text{smoothed}}(x,y,\ell) = u_\ell(x,y,t_{\text{stop}}). \tag{3}$$

**Alignment in Feature Space.** The difference between EED and Cross-EED is how the diffusion tensor is computed. For EED, the diffusion tensor is derived from the evolving signal itself. In case of cost volume filtering, this signal would coincide with the cost slices. More precisely, the eigenvalues of the tensor product of the pre-smoothed signal gradient are reweighed:

$$D(\nabla u) := g(\nabla u_\sigma \nabla u_\sigma^\top), \tag{4}$$

where $\nabla u_\sigma := K_\sigma * \nabla u$, and $K_\sigma$ denotes a two-dimensional Gaussian kernel with standard deviation $\sigma$. The anisotropic behaviour of this scheme is due to the positive, strictly monotonically decreasing function $g : \mathbb{R} \to \mathbb{R}^+$ that is applied to the eigenvalues of its argument. With EED, the signal is subject to a highly nonlinear evolution, which is known to smooth along edges in the cost volume but not across them [21].

The motivation for Cross-EED is that if a feature is considered to be relevant for the cost computation, then the spatial structures of this feature should also contain relevant information to steer the smoothing process. Thus, we propose to compute the diffusion tensor in the previously determined feature space. Assuming that the feature selection stage finally selected $k$ features, we align the diffusion along the spatial structures in this feature descriptor $h : \Omega \to \mathbb{R}^k$ as follows

$$D := g\left( K_\rho * \sum_{j=1}^{k} \nabla h_{j,\sigma} \nabla h_{j,\sigma}^\top \right). \tag{5}$$

Additionally, we introduce an outer integration scale $\rho$ in the latter equation, which leads to a coherence enhancing effect. This effect is known to tend to artistically and artificially-looking results for natural images. However, for cost filtering it has shown to be quite beneficial, due to its ability to fill holes and close small gaps in the cost slices [21].

Note that the resulting anisotropic evolution is linear, since the diffusion tensor is constant in time $t$ and does not depend on the evolving cost volume.

**Supervised Smoothing.** Up to now, the proposed cost smoothing takes as input the computed costs as well as the selected features, but disregards the information contained in the user input. Assuming that this auxiliary information is reliable, we alter the PDE from (2) into a scheme which interpolates the given data as follows [5]: Each slice of the cost volume undergoes an evolution where the user input serves as Dirichlet data and is kept fixed. In the other areas where no pre-segmentation is given, the computed costs serve as initialisation and are subject to the Cross-EED smoothing operator. This behaviour is realised by the PDE

$$\partial_t u_\ell = m \cdot (c_\ell - u_\ell) + (1 - m) \cdot \mathrm{div}\left(D \, \nabla u_\ell\right), \tag{6}$$
$$u_\ell(x, y, 0) = m \cdot c_\ell + (1 - m) \cdot f(x, y, \ell).$$

Let us explain the expressions $m$ and $c_\ell$. The mask function $m : \Omega \to [0, 1]$ switches between the diffusion process ($m=0$) and the given information ($m=1$). It is realised as the indicator function $\mathbb{1}$ of the union of all training regions

$$m = \mathbb{1}_{\mathcal{T}}, \qquad \mathcal{T} := \mathcal{T}_1 \cup \ldots \cup \mathcal{T}_n. \tag{7}$$

The costs we prescribe in these areas are denoted by $c_\ell : \Omega \to \{0,1\}$ and are minimal ($c_\ell = 0$) for pixels that belong to the training data and have the same label, and maximal ($c_\ell = 1$) for pixels belonging to a different label:

$$c_\ell = 1 - \mathbb{1}_{\mathcal{T}_\ell}. \tag{8}$$

This scheme is closely related to so-called inpainting schemes, which are known from the context of PDE-based image compression [6]. Note however, we are not computing the steady state of equation (6). Instead, our evolution is initialised with the computed costs and stopped at a certain time $t_{\text{stop}}$.

### 3.3    Iterative Application

Of course, it is possible to iterate the described framework. In particular, such an iterative minimisation constitutes an essential component of the GrabCut method [14]. In our setting, we update the user input regions $\mathcal{T}_\ell$ after each filtering stage. To this end, for every label $\ell$ we compute the 10% and 90% cost quantiles $q_\ell^{0.1}$ and $q_\ell^{0.9}$, respectively. Then each unclassified pixel is assigned to the user input of class $\ell$, if its filtered costs satisfy:

$$f_{\text{smoothed}}(x,y,\ell) < q_\ell^{0.1} \quad \text{and} \quad \forall_{\ell' \neq \ell}: \quad f_{\text{smoothed}}(x,y,\ell') > q_{\ell'}^{0.9}.$$

Thus, we consider a pixel reliable, if it has low costs for one label, and high costs for all other labels, and update $\mathcal{T}_\ell$ accordingly. Subsequently, we retrain the SVM using this new input and obtain refined costs. The following supervised smoothing step profits of the update in two aspects: Besides the new costs to be filtered, also the improved presegmentation is exploited for the mask $m$ as well as the prescribed costs $c_\ell$, cf. Equations (7) and (8).

## 4    Experiments

In order to show the performance of our method, we use the publicly available segmentation benchmark of Rother et al. [14]. Although the stages of our method introduce several free parameters, most of them can either be determined automatically or kept fixed for all images. Moreover, we apply an affine rescaling of the costs and features to the range $[0,1]$ before filtering, which also eases the parameter choice. For the cost filtering stage, we choose the Charbonnier diffusivity function $g(s^2) = 1/\sqrt{1 + s^2/\lambda^2}$ and the constant set of parameters $(\sigma, t_{\text{stop}}, \rho, \lambda) = (0.5, 5000, 0.5, 0.01)$ for all images.

Most of the running time of our sequential CPU implementation is spent in the multiple training phases of the SVM. Depending on the class overlap in

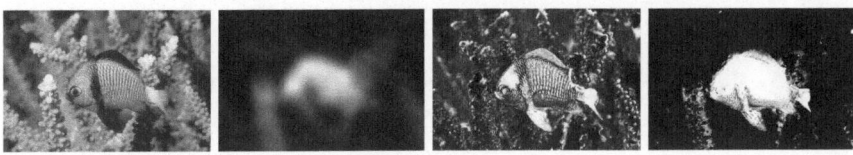

**Fig. 3.** Importance of texture features for cost computation. **From left to right:** (a) Input RGB image. (b) Gaussian smoothed Laplacian magnitude ($\sigma=12$). (c) Cost slice for background only using RGB features. Dark values indicate low costs. (d) Costs incorporating the feature from (b).

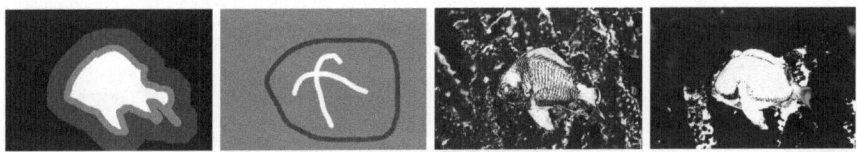

**Fig. 4.** Impact of reducing the user input. **From left to right:** (a) GrabCut input used to compute the costs in Fig. 3 (c) and (d). (b) Manually drawn smaller user input. (c) Cost slice using input (b) and only RGB features. (d) Costs computed from input (b) with texture feature.

feature space, the overall computation time varies between 10 seconds and a few minutes. On average, our method takes one minute per image of size $480 \times 320$ on a standard PC. Typically, a GPU implementation should be 40 times faster since all components are well parallelisable.

In our first experiment, we illustrate the usefulness of texture information. Figure 3 shows the image of a fish, which has almost the same colour distribution as its surrounding. In RGB space, the fish cannot be discriminated from the background (cf. Fig. 3(c)). On the contrary, by incorporating texture information, the fish can be distinguished: The raw number of misclassified pixels after cost computation drops from 19% to 6% just by incorporating texture features. In Figure 4, we examine the dependency of our method on the size of the user input. While the given user input of the GrabCut benchmark covers relatively large portions of the objects, we use a very sparse self-made trimap for comparison. The costs in Figure 4 (c) and (d) show that our method works almost as good with such more realistic user inputs and does not rely on a large number of feature points. In this special case of very small user input, the usage of texture information has shown to be extraordinarily beneficial.

The second experiment compares the proposed PDE-based smoothing against the filters in literature. The results in Figure 5 show that our anisotropic cost volume filtering clearly outperforms the guided image filter. Its anisotropic behaviour, especially in combination with the coherence enhancing effect, is perfectly suited to preserve small important details such as the feet, tail and wings, which cannot be preserved using the other filters.

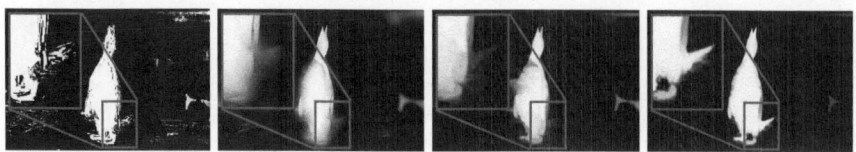

**Fig. 5.** Results of different smoothing filters. **From left to right: (a)** Input background cost slice for the penguin image. **(b)** Guided image filter. **(c)** Cross-EED without user input interpolation. **(d)** Cross-EED with interpolation.

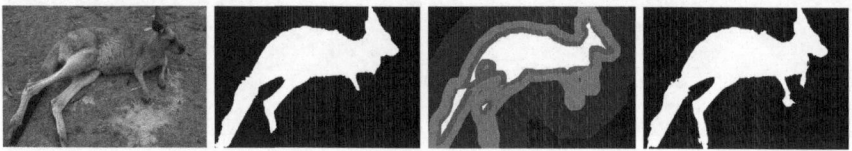

**Fig. 6.** Iterating the framework. **From left to right: (a)** Input kangaroo image. **(b)** Initial segmentation (error 7.2%). **(c)** User input. White depicts original user input, red visualises the updated input after the first iteration. **(d)** Final segmentation after second iteration (error 3.9%).

**Table 1.** Quantitative error comparison

|                  | CVF [2] | Grabcut [14] | Ours just RGB | Ours with texture | Ours iterated |
|------------------|---------|--------------|---------------|-------------------|---------------|
| Error unfiltered | -       | -            | 10.0 %        | 10.2 %            | 6.8 %         |
| Average Error    | 6.2 %   | 5.3 %        | 4.8 %         | 4.7 %             | 4.0 %         |

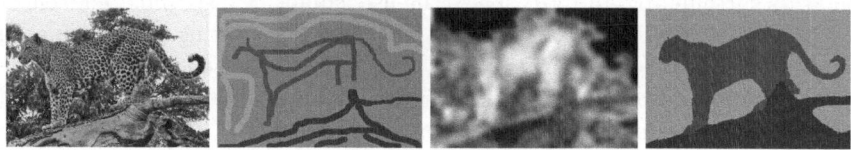

**Fig. 7.** Multi class segmentation example. **From left to right: (a)** Input image. **(b)** User input. **(c)** Automatically selected texture feature. **(d)** Final segmentation.

In Figure 6, we illustrate how iterating the framework improves the segmentation using the difficult kangaroo image. The given input regions expand towards the true object boundaries and the resulting segmentation includes previously undetectable parts of the kangaroo. Within 3 iterations, the average error on the whole GrabCut benchmark decreases from 4.7% to 4.0%.

In our fourth experiment, we segment an image into three classes (Fig. 7). In this example, the bright spots in the background make it impossible to discriminate the leopard without texture information. However, our feature selection strategy indentifies a suitable texture feature, and a highly accurate segmentation is possible.

Finally, Table 1 quantifies the performance of our segmentation method. To this end, we compute the average percentage of misclassified pixels in the unclassified region [13] over the whole set of 50 benchmark images from [14]. Note that we use a fixed set of parameters for all images. Compared to the method of Rhemann et al., our iterated approach reduces the error by 35%.

## 5   Conclusion

We improve the segmentation framework of Rhemann et al. [2] in several aspects. First, we incorporate texture information and present an elaborate cost computation and feature selection scheme. Additionally, we propose an anisotropic and supervised cost smoothing scheme that fully exploits the given user input. This smoothing process is steered by structures in the feature space and alignes the segmentation with them. By iterating the framework, we are able to outperform the state-of-the-art on the GrabCut benchmark.

In our ongoing research, we focus on improving the texture descriptors further. Besides Gabor or wavelet features, we are also interested in the potential of preprocessing these features with e.g. our anisotropic diffusion.

**Acknowledgements.** Funding by the Cluster of Excellence *Multimodal Computing and Interaction* is gratefully acknowledged.

## References

1. Scharstein, D., Szeliski, R.: Stereo matching with non-linear diffusion. In: Proc. Conf. on Computer Vision and Pattern Recognition, pp. 343–350. IEEE (1996)
2. Rhemann, C., Hosni, A., Bleyer, M., Rother, C., Gelautz, M.: Fast cost-volume filtering for visual correspondence and beyond. In: Proc. Conference on Computer Vision and Pattern Recognition, pp. 3017–3024. IEEE (2011)
3. Masnou, S., Morel, J.M.: Level lines based disocclusion. In: Proc. International Conference on Image Processing, vol. 3, pp. 259–263 (1998)
4. Bertalmío, M., Sapiro, G., Caselles, V., Ballester, C.: Image inpainting. In: Proc. SIGGRAPH, pp. 417–424. ACM (2000)
5. Weickert, J., Welk, M.: Tensor field interpolation with PDEs. In: Weickert, J., Hagen, H. (eds.) Visualization and Processing of Tensor Fields, pp. 315–325. Springer (2006)
6. Schmaltz, C., Weickert, J., Bruhn, A.: Beating the Quality of JPEG 2000 with Anisotropic Diffusion. In: Denzler, J., Notni, G., Süße, H. (eds.) Pattern Recognition. LNCS, vol. 5748, pp. 452–461. Springer, Heidelberg (2009)
7. Mumford, D., Shah, J.: Boundary detection by minimizing functionals, I. In: Proc. Conference Computer Vision and Pattern Recognition, pp. 22–26. IEEE (1985)
8. Koepfler, G., Lopez, C., Morel, J.M.: A multiscale algorithm for image segmentation by variational method. SIAM Journal Numerical Analysis 31, 282–299 (1994)
9. Chan, T.F., Vese, L.A.: Active contours without edges. Transactions on Image Processing 10, 266–277 (2001)

10. Brox, T., Rousson, M., Deriche, R., Weickert, J.: Colour, texture, and motion in level set based segmentation and tracking. Image Vision Computing 28, 376–390 (2010)
11. Boykov, Y., Veksler, O., Zabih, R.: Fast approximate energy minimization via graph cuts. Transactions on Pattern Analysis and Machine Intelligence 23, 1222–1239 (2001)
12. Boykov, Y., Jolly, M.P.: Interactive Graph Cuts for Optimal Boundary and Region Segmentation of Objects in $N$-D images. In: Proc. International Conference on Computer Vision, pp. 105–112. IEEE (2001)
13. Blake, A., Rother, C., Brown, M., Perez, P., Torr, P.: Interactive Image Segmentation Using an Adaptive GMMRF Model. In: Pajdla, T., Matas, J(G.) (eds.) ECCV 2004. LNCS, vol. 3021, pp. 428–441. Springer, Heidelberg (2004)
14. Rother, C., Kolmogorov, V., Blake, A.: "GrabCut": interactive foreground extraction using iterated graph cuts. In: Proc. SIGGRAPH, pp. 309–314. ACM (2004)
15. Lellmann, J., Becker, F., Schnörr, C.: Convex optimization for multi-class image labeling with a novel family of total variation based regularizers. In: Proc. Tenth International Conference on Computer Vision, pp. 646–653. IEEE (2009)
16. Martin, D., Fowlkes, C., Malik, J.: Learning to detect natural image boundaries using local brightness, color, and texture cues. Transactions on Pattern Analysis and Machine Intelligence 26, 530–549 (2004)
17. Yoon, K.J., Kweon, I.S.: Adaptive support-weight approach for correspondence search. Trans. on Pattern Analysis and Machine Intelligence 28, 650–656 (2006)
18. Tomasi, C., Manduchi, R.: Bilateral filtering for gray and color images. In: Proc. International Conference on Computer Vision, pp. 839–846 (1998)
19. He, K., Sun, J., Tang, X.: Guided Image Filtering. In: Daniilidis, K., Maragos, P., Paragios, N. (eds.) ECCV 2010, Part I. LNCS, vol. 6311, pp. 1–14. Springer, Heidelberg (2010)
20. Paris, S., Durand, F.: A Fast Approximation of the Bilateral Filter Using a Signal Processing Approach. In: Leonardis, A., Bischof, H., Pinz, A. (eds.) ECCV 2006. LNCS, vol. 3954, pp. 568–580. Springer, Heidelberg (2006)
21. Weickert, J.: Anisotropic Diffusion in Image Processing. Teubner, Stuttgart (1998)
22. Kohavi, R., John, G.H.: Wrappers for feature subset selection. Artificial Intelligence 97, 273–324 (1997)
23. Lowe, D.L.: Distinctive image features from scale-invariant keypoints. International Journal of Computer Vision 60, 91–110 (2004)
24. Dalal, N., Triggs, B.: Histograms of oriented gradients for human detection. In: Schmid, C., Soatto, S., Tomasi, C. (eds.) Proc. Conference on Computer Vision and Pattern Recognition, vol. 2, pp. 886–893 (2005)
25. Haralick, R.M., Shanmugam, K., Dinstein, I.: Textural features for image classification. Transactions of the Systems, Man and Cybernetics, 610–621 (1973)
26. Duda, R.O., Stork, D.G., Hart, P.E.: Pattern Classification, 2nd edn. Wiley (2000)
27. Vapnik, V.: The nature of statistical learning theory. In: Statistics for Engineering and Information Science. Springer (2000)
28. Schölkopf, B., Smola, A.: Learning with Kernels. MIT Press, Cambridge (2002)
29. Duchenne, O., Audibert, J.Y.: Fast interactive segmentation using color and textural information. Technical Report 06-26, CERTIS, ParisTech (2006)

# Author Index